THE PARALLEL BRAIN

THE PARALLEL BRAIN
The Cognitive Neuroscience of the Corpus Callosum

Eran Zaidel and Marco Iacoboni, *Editors*

A BRADFORD BOOK
THE MIT PRESS
CAMBRIDGE, MASSACHUSETTS
LONDON, ENGLAND

This book was set in Baskerville on 3B2 by Asco Type-
setters, Hong Kong, and was printed and bound in the
United States of America.

Library of Congress Cataloging-in-Publication Data

The parallel brain : the cognitive neuroscience of the
corpus callosum / edited by Eran Zaidel and Marco
Iacoboni.
     p. ; cm. — (Issues in clinical and cognitive
neuropsychology)
"A Bradford book."
Includes bibliographical references and index.
ISBN 0-262-24044-0 (hc : alk. paper)
   1. Corpus callosum. 2. Sensorimotor integration.
3. Cerebral hemispheres. 4. Alexia. I. Zaidel, Eran.
II. Iacoboni, Marco. III. Series.
   [DNLM: 1. Corpus Callosum—physiology. 2. Brain—
physiology. 3. Cognitive Science. 4. Dominance,
Cerebral. 5. Laterality. WL307 P222 2003]
QP382.2 .P37 2003
612.8'25—dc21   2001044328

Dedicated to the memory of Esther Zaidel

CONTENTS

PREFACE

This book originated in a NATO Advanced Science Institute held at Il Ciocco, Italy, on September 1–10, 1996. The Institute was entitled "The Role of the Corpus Callosum in Sensory-Motor Integration: Anatomy, Physiology and Behavior; Individual Differences and Clinical Applications." There were nearly 100 participants from 25 countries, including leading researchers on callosal structure and function. Most of the participants in the ASI contributed to this volume. Their original contributions were written in 1996, but all have been revised and updated in 1999–2000. A few additional contributors were invited to write new chapters on emerging relevant topics, notably neuroimaging.

This volume, however, is not a conference proceedings. Instead, it is meant to provide a unique perspective on the emerging field of Cognitive Neuroscience. It is designed to do so in two ways. First, it summarizes the state of the art of research on the human corpus callosum. Such treatment is sorely necessary because it has been at least a decade since the publication of the most recent overview. One can trace the development of human neuropsychology through the study of the corpus callosum, which, in turn, illuminates the study of hemispheric specialization. Hemispheric specialization remains a core problem in human neuropsychology because it recapitulates any aspect of the human condition, from perception and emotion to memory and language. Furthermore, hemispheric specialization and interhemispheric interaction serve as a model system for a fundamental problem of cognitive neuroscience: the problem of modularity and of intermodular communication. The study of the corpus callosum brings to this problem a neuroscientific arsenal, including neuroanatomy, neurophysiology, and behavior. The evolution of this study can be traced through a series of classical books, all based on conference proceedings, starting with Mountcastle's 1962 edited volume, *Interhemispheric Relations and Cerebral Dominance*, continuing with Russell, van Hof, and Berlucchi's 1979 edited volume, *Structure and Function of Cerebral Commissures*, and concluding with, Leporé, Ptito, and Jasper's edited 1986 volume, *Two Hemispheres—One Brain: Functions of the Corpus Callosum*. These volumes tend to be spaced a decade apart, and we are now overdue for the next installment. This book is meant to serve that role.

The second way this book is designed to provide a perspective on cognitive neuroscience is as an advanced didactic introduction to the field. Instead of providing a standard introduction by discussing the various systems of the mind/brain, such as perception, action, emotions, memory, language, and problem solving, this book uses the case study approach. It focuses on the simplest possible sequence of perception-decision-action as it occurs in the simple reaction time paradigm of Poffenberger (1912). The task could not be simpler: Press a button with one hand as soon as you detect a patch of light in the periphery of the visual field. But when the patch occurs in the visual field opposite to the responding hand, there must have occurred interhemispheric transfer prior to response. Transfer of what? A visual input code? A cognitive decision code? A motor response code? The book studies this task by considering, in turn, anatomical, physiological, and behavioral approaches, and by combining animal models, normal human studies, and evidence from clinical populations. In this way, the book introduces the basic methods of cognitive neuroscience, not in isolation but by focusing on the same central paradigm and problem. Learning best occurs in context, when attempting to answer a specific question. This book provides such a question-centered approach to cognitive neuroscience.

The format of the book is didactic and dynamic. Each of the five parts—anatomy, physiology, behavior, clinical studies, and a case study of pure alexia—includes several chapters that introduce the main findings, followed by commentaries that discuss and amplify those presentations. Each part concludes with an editorial commentary that summarizes the presentations and puts them in a larger context. These commentaries are also used to extend the coverage to more cognitive approaches.

The view that emerges from the book is that simple reaction time is not simple at all. The corpus callosum seems to consist of many parallel interhemispheric channels for communication and control. Even sensorimotor cross-callosal transfer is context-dependent and modulated by attention. This permits the two cerebral hemispheres to assume any of a variety of states or degrees of mutual independence. And that variety makes possible diverse cognitive processes.

This book owes its birth to NATO for generously making possible the original meeting in the true spirit of international cooperation. But our deepest debt is to the participants of the meeting, speakers and audience alike, who created a warm interactive atmosphere of a shared enthusiastic scientific exploration. Last but not least, that exploration was aided immensely by the scenery, food, and wine of Tuscany.

This work was supported in part by NIH grant NS 20187. Linda Capatillo-Cunliff was indispensable in organizing the meeting. Ian Gizer, Eric Mooshagian, and AnThu Vuong provided assistance in preparing the manuscript. Special thanks also to Dr. Joseph Janeti for advice and support throughout this project. Finally, we are indebted to Michael Rutter and Sara Meirowitz from MIT for their dedicated editorial assistance.

REFERENCES

LEPORÉ, F., M. PTITO, and H. H. JASPER, 1986. Two hemispheres—one brain: Functions of the corpus callosum. In *Neurology and Neurobiology*, vol. 17. New York: Alan R. Liss.

MOUNTCASTLE, V. B. (ed.), 1962. *Interhemispheric Relations and Cerebral Dominance*. Baltimore: Johns Hopkins University Press.

POFFENBERGER, A. T., 1912. Reaction time to retinal stimulation, with special reference to the time lost through nerve centers. *Arch. Psychol.* 23:1–73.

RUSSELL, I. S., M. W. VAN HOF, and G. BERLUCCHI (eds.), 1979. *Structure and Function of Cerebral Commissures*. Baltimore: University Park Press.

THE PARALLEL BRAIN

Introduction: Poffenberger's Simple Reaction Time Paradigm for Measuring Interhemispheric Transfer Time

ERAN ZAIDEL AND MARCO IACOBONI

The Poffenberger monograph

In 1912 the experimental psychologist A. T. Poffenberger, Jr., then an Assistant in the Psychology Department at Columbia University, published a 73-page monograph entitled "Reaction Time to Retinal Stimulation, with Special Reference to the Time Lost in Conduction Through Nerve Centers." The monograph was Volume 23 of the *Archives of Psychology*, edited by R. S. Woodworth, and it was also Volume XXI, Number 1 of the *Columbia Contributions to Philosophy and Psychology*. J. Mek and R. S. Woodworth supervised the study. This, then, was work in the mainstream of American experimental psychology. The study measured the time it takes a simple neural signal to cross from one hemisphere to the other as an example of "The time lost in the transmission of an impulse through a synapse within the human nervous system" (p. 2).

ANATOMIC RATIONALE Poffenberger's paradigm consisted of unimanual key presses to indicate detection of lateralized light flashes, namely, simple reaction time (SRT). When the right hand (Rh) responds to light in the right visual hemifield (RVF) or the left hand (Lh) responds to light in the left visual field (LVF), both sensory input and motor response are controlled by the same hemisphere ("uncrossed" or "direct" conditions), and there is no need for callosal relay. However, when the Rh responds to an LVF input or the Lh responds to an RVF input, callosal relay is necessary ("crossed" or "indirect" conditions). By subtracting reaction time (RT) in the uncrossed condition from RT in the crossed conditions and dividing by 2, we can obtain interhemispheric transfer time (IHTT).

Poffenberger considered both homotopic and heterotopic callosal channels, as well as noncallosal interhemispheric connections, that could mediate crossed responses but concluded, on empirical grounds, that the most likely callosal channel was an association tract connecting the motor areas in the two hemispheres through the central portion of the corpus callosum.

ASSUMPTIONS The overall rationale of Poffenberger's experiment presupposed that the measured RT could be fractionated into several serial additive information-processing stages with fixed processing latencies, to which Donder's subtraction method could then be applied. Specifically, these stages do not affect each other. Thus, according to this logic, the response hand did not affect hemispheric decision time. (However, modern work suggests that response hand blocking can prime the opposite hemisphere, so decision times are no longer symmetrical.) Poffenberger also assumed that contralateral motor control was faster than any possible ipsilateral motor control, so crossed responses must incorporate callosal relay.

ERAN ZAIDEL   Department of Psychology, University of California at Los Angeles, Los Angeles, California.
MARCO IACOBONI   Ahmanson Lovelace Brain Mapping Center, Neuropsychiatric Institute, Brain Research Institute, David Geffen School of Medicine, University of California at Los Angeles, Los Angeles, California.

METHODS Poffenberger used a light source mounted on the rim of a wheel driven by a motor and filtered and exposed for 4 ms through an aperture in the middle of a perimeter in front of the subject. Poffenberger noted that since it takes 165 ms to execute a saccade toward the peripheral stimulus, the lateralization of the stimulus was guaranteed. Peripheral retinal stimulation was accomplished by two methods. The first method required the subject to look straight ahead and then to move the eye gaze 45° sideways before each stimulus was presented at the center. The second involved rotating the subject's chair and requiring the subject to fixate straight ahead for the duration of a set of trials. Of course, these methods introduced differential possible spatial compatibility and hemispheric priming effects. Poffenberger tested four normal subjects, all graduate students in psychology at Columbia University.

Notable in its absence in the methodology was a hypothesis testing statistical analysis of the significance of the results.

DOMINANCE EFFECTS Poffenberger correctly noted that by averaging responses from both hands, possible effects of manual dominance were neutralize. A simple argument was applied to the possible differences in sensitivity between the nasal and temporal hemiretinae and to possible ocular dominance. Since ocular dominance was believed to be related to hemispheric dominance, this argument showed that relative hemispheric specialization for visual perception ("direct access") was neutralized by Poffenberger's average and subtraction method. Following (Liepmann and Maas, 1907), Poffenberger also considered the possibility that the left hemisphere (LH) was exclusively specialized for motor control. This would have invalidated the logic of the experiment. However, Poffenberger rejected the possibility that the LH controlled "coordinated movements," as were required in this experiment, on empirical grounds.

Poffenberger noted that his subject, T, a right-hander, responded faster by 0.6 ms with the right hand to RVF targets than with the left hand to LVF targets. His subject, P, a left-hander, responded faster by 5.5 ms with the left hand to left visual field targets than with the right hand to right visual field targets. Poffenberger speculated that this shows a right visual field advantage, that is, LH specialization, in T and a left visual field advantage, that is, right-hemisphere (RH) specialization, in P. However, this conclusion was curiously uncritical, since the observed pattern was equally consistent with a manual dominance effect, that is, an overall right-hand advantage in T and an overall left-hand advantage in

P. Poffenberger's conclusion may be explained by his failure to observe comparable hand differences in RT to foveal binocular stimulation.

MANIPULATION OF VISUAL PARAMETERS Poffenberger filtered the stimulus light source to create an input of pure white light, which could serve as a baseline for stimuli of different colors. But color was not manipulated in this experiment. Poffenberger did manipulate (1) stimulus retinal eccentricity, (2) left-eye versus right-eye viewing, (3) monocular versus binocular stimulation, and (4) body versus eye rotation for peripheral stimulation. Unfortunately, he found an effect of these parameters on overall RT but did not study their effect on the crossed-uncrossed difference (CUD).

Plotting the RT for the four response hand (rh) × stimulus visual field (VF) combinations for subject T from Poffenberger's Table I (1912, pp. 44–45), we see diverse patterns and CUDs varying from −9.8 to 14.8 ms. There was a tendency for the CUD to increase with decreasing eccentricities, but this may have been confounded with a practice effect, since the subject was tested in order with progressively smaller eccentricities. Inspection of Poffenberger's Table I suggests that negative CUDs occurred only for crossed eye-hand combinations, that is, right eye–left hand and left eye–right hand, especially for the 45° condition.

Exactly the same pattern emerges from a reanalysis of the data of Jeeves and Dixon (1990) using target eccentricities of 70°. This is true for right-handers using either unimanual or bimanual responses, and it is also true for left-handers using bimanual responses. The effect, then, is invariant for handedness and type of motor response. The most parsimonious explanation is that the visual pathways that cross the chiasm are stronger than the uncrossed pathways. This would work in concert with the anatomical ipsilateral h-VF advantage when the responding hand is ipsilateral to the viewing eye (i.e., Lh-LE and Rh-RE), but it would work against the anatomical ipsilateral h-VF advantage when the responding hand is contralateral to the viewing eye (i.e., Lh-RE or Rh-LE). This confound is eliminated in binocular viewing because the crossed pathways in the eye ipsilateral to the responding hand will likely dominate the response latency. Thus, crossed pathways are always used, and the algebraic model holds, provided that the crossed pathways are equally strong in both eyes.

Poffenberger showed that RT to foveal stimulation was faster with binocular than monocular presentations. He rejected on empirical grounds the interpretation of this as being due to intensity differences and suggested that it might have reflected a redundant target effect ("the dynamogenic effect"). Unfortunately, he did not analyze the effect of binocularity on lateralized targets and on the CUD.

MANIPULATION OF MOTOR PARAMETERS Poffenberger noted that manual dominance effects could be eliminated from the calculation of the CUD by averaging responses of both hands to both visual half fields. To estimate manual dominance, he measured left- and right-hand responses to foveal targets. He found greater hand differences with monocular than with binocular stimulation but could not explain this difference (Poffenberger, 1912, p. 60). Neither can we. But the discrepancy is unexpected and therefore important and potentially problematic to the anatomical model of the CUD as a measure of IHTT.

PRACTICE Poffenberger considered the effect of practice on RT in the SRT paradigm by noting changes in speeded responses to central presentations. He noted a systematic speeding up in subject T. but a slowing down in subject P. He interpreted the latter as a shift to a less conscious strategy. However, there was no attempt to study the effect of practice on the CUD.

SPATIAL COMPATIBILITY Poffenberger considered the possible confounding effect of spatial compatibility on the CUD, noting that "it is customary to react on the side from which the stimulus comes" (1912, p. 70). He rejected this objection on the grounds that spatial compatibility should decrease with decreasing eccentricity, whereas the CUD, if anything, tended to increase with decreasing eccentricity, at least for the two extreme positions of 45° versus 3°. This plausibility argument will not withstand the possibility that spatial compatibility has a separate effect on the CUD than the effect of anatomy.

HISTORICAL AWARENESS OF POFFENBERGER'S MONOGRAPH Poffenberger received his Ph.D. at Columbia in 1912. In the monograph he thanks Cattell and Woodworth for guiding the experiment. In time, Poffenberger came to succeed Woodworth as head of experimental psychology at Columbia (Boring, 1950). It is interesting that in Woodworth's classic *Experimental Psychology* (1938), Poffenberger's 1912 monograph was cited not for first demonstrating interhemispheric transmission time but for showing the facilitating effect of binocular over monocular presentations on simple reaction time.

Interest in measuring interhemispheric transmission time may be indicated by the number of citations of Poffenberger's monograph throughout the years. Figure 1 plots the number of citations, by half-decades, taken

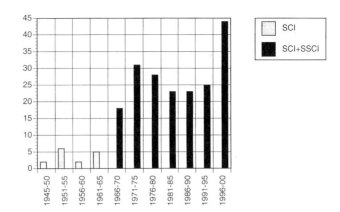

FIGURE 1. Number of citations for Poffenberger (1912) in five-year blocks from 1945 to 2000. SCI = Science Citation Index; SCI + SSCI = Science Citation Index and Social Science Citation Index.

from the Science Citation Index (1945–1965) and also from the Social Science Citation Index (after 1965). There is a steady increase in the number of citations in the 1970s, as research in behavioral laterality experiments in normal subjects accelerated, followed by a moderate decrease in the 1980s. The NATO conference that gave rise to this volume has reversed this trend. This can be seen in the dramatic increase in the number of citations for 1996–2000. The publication of this volume and renewed interest in interhemispheric transfer time for sensorimotor integration with the advent of new methodological tools (e.g., spatially localized ERP) and the availability of new clinical populations (e.g., partial callosotomy patients) promise to accelerate this trend.

The algebraic model

THE MODEL Consider an experiment in which the subject has to detect an unpatterned peripheral light flash and respond by pressing a button with one hand at a time. There are four stimulus visual hemifield × response hand conditions, and we can approximate the reaction time in each by partitioning it into schematized sequences of component mental operations, from visual registration V through stimulus detection D to motor programming MP and motor response M, including callosal relay CR. Let V_L denote speed of visual registration in the LH, D_L denote the speed of target detection in the LH, MP_R denote the speed of motor programming in the RH, M_R denote speed of motor output in the RH, CR_{LR} denote speed of callosal relay from the LH to the RH, and so on. When a target visual field is paired with response by the contralateral hand, then callosal relay is necessary at some stage of the

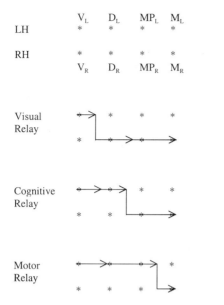

FIGURE 2. Alternative stages of interhemispheric relay in the SRT paradigm of Poffenberger. LH = left hemisphere, RH = right hemisphere, V_L = visual processing in the left hemisphere, V_R = visual processing in the right hemisphere, D_L = decision in the LH, D_R = decision in the RH, MP_L = motor programming in the LH, MP_R = motor programming in the RH, M_L = motor response in the LH, M_R = motor response in the RH.

information-processing sequence. Suppose relay occurs at an early visual stage, before stimulus detection, and that the decision, motor programming, and response all occur in the other hemisphere (visual relay; see Figure 2). Then the four stimulus visual field × response hand conditions yield the following:

1. LVF-Lh: $V_R +$ $D_R + MP_R + M_R$
uncrossed
2. LVF-Rh: $V_R + CR_{RL} + D_L + MP_L + M_L$
crossed
3. RVF-Rh: $V_L +$ $D_L + MP_L + M_L$
uncrossed
4. RVF-Lh: $V_L + CR_{LR} + D_R + MP_R + M_R$
crossed

We can incorporate D, MP, and M into one hemispheric processing component P and get the following:

1_v. LVF-Lh: $V_R +$ P_R uncrossed
2_v. LVF-Rh: $V_R + CR_{RL} + P_L$ crossed
3_v. RVF-Rh: $V_L +$ P_L uncrossed
4_v. RVF-Lh: $V_L + CR_{LR} + P_R$ crossed

We can now estimate callosal relay time or IHTT by the mean crossed-uncrossed difference (CUD):

5_v. CUD: $([2_v] + [4_v] - [1_v] - [3_v]) \div 2 =$
$(CR_{RL} + CR_{LR}) \div 2$

It is possible to compute a separate CUD for the Lh, for the Rh, for the LVF, and for the RVF, but as equations 6_v–9_v show, these estimates are confounded by hemispheric differences and may be negative. To get a pure estimate of IHTT, it is necessary to add the CUDs of the two VFs or of the two hands:

6_v. Lh CUD: $[4_v] - [1_v] = (V_L - V_R) + CR_{LR}$
7_v. Rh CUD: $[2_v] - [3_v] = (V_R - V_L) + CR_{RL}$
8_v. LVF CUD: $[2_v] - [1_v] = (P_L - P_R) + CR_{RL}$
9_v. RVF CUD: $[4_v] - [3_v] = (P_R - P_L) + CR_{LR}$

We can also compute a hand difference and a VF difference, as well as a difference between the two crossed conditions and a difference between the two uncrossed conditions:

10_v. Lh-Rh: $[1_v] + [4_v] - [2_v] - [3_v] =$
$2(P_R - P_L) + (CR_{LR} - CR_{RL})$
11_v. LVF-RVF: $[1_v] + [2_v] - [3_v] - [4_v] =$
$2(V_R - V_L) + (CR_{RL} - CR_{LR})$
12_v. [LVF-Rh] − [RVF-Lh]: $[2_v] - [4_v] =$
crossed difference $(V_R - V_L) +$
$(P_L - P_R) +$
$(CR_{RL} - CR_{LR})$
13_v. [LVF-Lh] − [RVF-Rh]: $[1_v] - [3_v] =$
uncrossed difference $(V_R - V_L) + (P_R - P_L)$

VISUAL, COGNITIVE, MOTOR, OR MIXED RELAY Consider a second scenario, in which the hemisphere that receives the initial light flash will detect the stimulus so that relay occurs after detection but before motor programming, that is, at a "cognitive" stage, perhaps through the posterior body of the corpus callosum that interconnects temporal cortices (Figure 2). Then, the four VF × rh conditions yield the following:

1. LVF-Lh: $V_R + D_R +$ $MP_R + M_R$
2. LVF-Rh: $V_R + D_R + CR_{RL} + MP_L + M_L$
3. RVF-Rh: $V_L + D_L +$ $MP_L + M_L$
4. RVF-Lh: $V_L + D_L + CR_{LR} + MP_R + M_R$

We can incorporate V + D into one input-processing component, IP, and similarly combine MP + M into one output-processing component, OP. Equations 1–13 now yield:

1c. LVF-Lh: $IP_R +$ OP_R
2c. LVF-Rh: $IP_R + CR_{RL} + OP_L$
3c. RVF-Rh: $IP_L +$ OP_L
4c. RVF-Lh: $IP_L + CR_{LR} + OP_R$
5c. CUD: $(CR_{RL} + CR_{LR}) \div 2$
6c. Lh CUD: $(IP_L - IP_R) + CR_{LR}$
7c. Rh CUD: $(IP_R - IP_L) + CR_{RL}$
8c. LVF CUD: $(OP_R - OP_L) + CR_{RL}$
9c. RVF CUD: $(OP_L - OP_R) + CR_{LR}$

10c. Lh−Rh: $2(\text{OP}_R - \text{OP}_L) + (\text{CR}_{LR} - \text{CR}_{RL})$
11c. LVF−RVF: $2(\text{IP}_R - \text{IP}_L) + (\text{CR}_{RL} - \text{CR}_{LR})$
12c. [LVF−Rh] − [RVF−Lh]: $(\text{IP}_R - \text{IP}_L) +$
$(\text{OP}_L - \text{OP}_R) +$
$(\text{CR}_{RL} - \text{CR}_{LR})$
13c. [LVF−Lh] − [RVF−Rh]: $(\text{IP}_R - \text{IP}_L) +$
$(\text{OP}_R - \text{OP}_L)$

A third possible scenario is that relay occurs after motor programming, that is, at a "motor" stage, presumably through the anterior body of the corpus callosum (Figure 2). Then the four VF × rh conditions yield the following:

1. LVF−Lh: $V_R + D_R + \text{MP}_R + \qquad M_R$
2. LVF−Rh: $V_R + D_R + \text{MP}_R + \text{CR}_{RL} + M_L$
3. RVF−Rh: $V_L + D_L + \text{MP}_L + \qquad M_L$
4. RVF−Lh: $V_L + D_L + \text{MP}_L + \text{CR}_{LR} + M_R$

We can incorporate V, D, and MP into one hemispheric component, P, and get the following:

1m. LVF−Lh: $P_R + \qquad M_R$
2m. LVF−Rh: $P_R + \text{CR}_{RL} + M_L$
3m. RVF−Rh: $P_L + \qquad M_L$
4m. RVF−Lh: $P_L + \text{CR}_{LR} + M_R$
5m. CUD: $(\text{CR}_{RL} + \text{CR}_{LR}) \div 2$
6m. Lh CUD: $(P_L - P_R) + \text{CR}_{LR}$
7m. Rh CUD: $(P_R - P_L) + \text{CR}_{RL}$
8m. LVF CUD: $(M_L - M_R) + \text{CR}_{RL}$
9m. RVF CUD: $(M_R - M_L) + \text{CR}_{LR}$
10m. Lh−Rh: $2(M_R - M_L) + (\text{CR}_{LR} - \text{CR}_{RL})$
11m. LVF−RVF: $2(P_R - P_L) + (\text{CR}_{RL} - \text{CR}_{LR})$
12m. [LVF−Rh] − [RVF−Lh]: $(P_R - P_L) +$
$(M_L - M_R) +$
$(\text{CR}_{RL} - \text{CR}_{LR})$
13m. [LVF−Lh] − [RVF−Rh]: $(P_R - P_L) +$
$(M_R - M_L)$

It is also possible that relay occurs through different channels in the two directions. Suppose CR_{LR} is motor but CR_{RL} is visual. Then the four VF × rh conditions yield the following:

1. LVF−Lh: $V_R + \qquad D_R + \qquad M_R$
2. LVF−Rh: $V_R + \text{CR}_{RL} + D_L + \text{MP}_L + M_L$
3. RVF−Rh: $V_L + \qquad D_L + \qquad M_L$
4. RVF−Lh: $V_L + \text{CR}_{LR} + D_L + \text{MP}_L + M_R$

Then we have the following:

5. CUD: $[(D_L - D_R) + 2\text{MP}_L +$
$(\text{CR}_{RL} + \text{CR}_{LR})] \div 2$
6. Lh CUD: $(V_L - V_R) + (D_L - D_R) + \text{CR}_{LR}$
7. Rh CUD: $(V_R - V_L) + \text{MP}_L + \text{CR}_{RL}$
8. LVF CUD: $(D_L - D_R) + (M_L - M_R) +$
$\text{MP}_L + \text{CR}_{RL}$

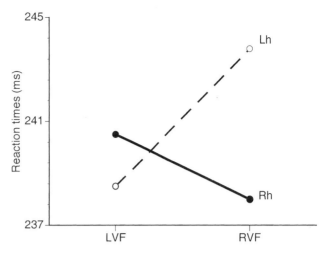

FIGURE 3. Overall visual field by response hand interaction of a meta-analysis on simple reaction time to lateralized flashes (Marzi et al., 1991). Lh = left hand, Rh = right hand, LVF = left visual field, RVF = right visual field.

9. RVF CUD: $(M_R - M_L) + \text{MP}_L + \text{CR}_{LR}$
10. Lh−Rh: $(D_R - D_L) + (\text{CR}_{LR} - \text{CR}_{RL})$
11. LVF−RVF: $2(V_R - V_L) + (D_R - D_L) +$
$(\text{CR}_{RL} - \text{CR}_{LR})$
12. crossed diff.: $(V_R - V_L) + (M_L - M_R) +$
$(\text{CR}_{RL} - \text{CR}_{LR})$
13. uncrossed diff.: $(V_R - V_L) + (D_R - D_L) +$
$(M_R - M_L)$

Of course, the CUD is no longer an estimate of IHTT! In particular, if D_R is large enough in relation to D_L, then the CUD is negative!

MARZI'S META-ANALYSIS   Marzi, Bisiacchi, and Nicoletti (1991) carried out a meta-analysis of SRT studies and obtained the pattern shown in Figure 3. In addition to the standard significant rh × VF interaction, they found an overall LVF advantage and an overall Rh advantage. There was also an asymmetry in the crossed conditions, with selectively long RVF-Lh responses and no difference between the two uncrossed conditions. These results mean that $[10_v] > 0$, $[11_v] < 0$, $[12_v] < 0$, and $[13_v] \approx 0$. It follows from equations $10_v–13_v$ that the meta-analysis is simultaneously consistent with all of the following three effects: (1) asymmetric transfer, (2) asymmetric hemispheric processing of the visual input, and (3) asymmetric hemispheric motor programming and response. In fact, assuming that $\text{CR}_{RL} < \text{CR}_{LR}$, the inequalities above yield $P_L < P_R$ and $V_R < V_L$. But the meta-analysis is also consistent with symmetric transfer and asymmetric processing: $\text{CR}_{LR} = \text{CR}_{RL}$, $V_R < V_L$ and $P_R > P_L$. Thus, the meta-analysis does not imply asymmetry in relay.

For the second scenario, cognitive relay, we get similar results. Given the same inequalities observed in the meta-analysis, we find that if $CR_{LR} > CR_{RL}$, then $OP_L < OP_R$ and $IP_R < IP_L$. Similarly, for motor relay, given the inequalities of the meta-analysis, we get that if $CR_{LR} > CR_{RL}$, then $M_L < M_R$ and $P_R < P_L$.

Modularity hypothesis

Poffenberger manipulated the strength of the input visual signal in the SRT paradigm by comparing monocular and binocular presentations. He noted that overall RT decreased with binocular input, but curiously, he did not analyze whether the CUD, that is, the IHTT, was affected as well. In 1971, Berlucchi and colleagues manipulated stimulus eccentricity, found that it did not affect the CUD, and concluded that interhemispheric transfer in the SRT paradigm is not visual. They reasoned that callosal fibers joining visual areas on the two sides are restricted to the neighborhood of the vertical meridian, so if transfer is visual, then more eccentric targets should take longer to transfer than less eccentric ones. Milner and Lines (1982) argued similarly (for acallosals, but the argument carries over to normals) that increased stimulus intensity increases the rate of neuronal recruitment in visual pathways, including interhemispheric ones.

More generally, one can articulate a modularity hypothesis according to which if interhemispheric transfer occurs through a particular callosal channel that interconnects specific cortical modules, then only the manipulation of a stimulus parameter that affects processing in those modules can affect the corresponding channel and thus interhemispheric transfer time in the same direction. Thus, only visual parameters can affect visual transfer, and visual parameters, such as intensity, eccentricity, or visual complexity, can affect only visual transfer. Similarly, cognitive parameters can affect cognitive transfer, and motor parameters can affect motor transfer. Thus, decision complexity should affect the transfer of cognitive/abstract information but not visual or motor transfer, whereas the complexity of the motor response pattern should affect motor transfer exclusively. Further, transfer along a particular visual pathway may be sensitive to one visual parameter (e.g., eccentricity) but not to another (e.g., intensity).

This view presupposes a decomposition of the information-processing sequence into several functionally independent components, including separate stages of visual analysis and motor programming. In this manner the visual and motor stages are modular (i.e., mutually impenetrable and encapsulated; Fodor, 1983). Thus, a change in visual parameters of the task may affect visual

analysis but no subsequent stages. If the CUD is invariant to the manipulation of a visual parameter, however, this does not necessarily imply nonvisual transfer. Transfer may be between visual areas that are far enough along not to be sensitive to the parameters used. Therefore, the CUD may be sensitive to other untried or as yet undiscovered visual parameters.

However, it is possible that the visual and motor stages are not modular. Transmission times for nonvisual pathways might therefore also be affected, cascade fashion, by changes in stimulus strength. The CUD in acallosal and commissurotomized patients could similarly result from nonvisual interhemispheric transfer or from the use of ipsilateral motor connections that are less effective than their contralateral counterpart (see Kinsbourne and Fisher, 1971; Zaidel, 1983; Jeeves and Milner, 1987; Trope et al., 1987). Nevertheless, it may still be possible to determine whether transfer occurs along visual or nonvisual pathways by manipulating two, rather than one, visual stimulus parameters.

If stimulus intensity and eccentricity manipulations have equivalent effects on the CUD, then the findings may still be equivocal, depending on whether or not modularity holds. However, if intensity and eccentricity

TABLE 1

Summary of the effects of motor, attentional, and visual manipulations on the CUD

	RT	CUD
Motor		
Di Stefano et al. '80, bimanual	+	+?
Iacoboni & Zaidel, '95, alt. fingers	−	+
Godbout et al., '95, three presses	+	
Godbout et al., '95, alt. hands		+
Attention		
Aglioti et al., '93, VF blocking	+	−
Iacoboni & Zaidel, spatial uncertainty	−	−
Iacoboni & Zaidel, RG within hems.	+	−
Iacoboni & Zaidel, RG between hems.	+	−
Braun et al., '95		
valid cues	+	−
invalid cues	+	−
Visual		
Berlucchi et al., '71, Eccentricity	+	−
Berlucchi et al., '77, Eccentricity	+	−
Milner & Lines, '82, Intensity	+	−
Lines et al., '84, Intensity	+	−
St. John et al., '87, Eccentricity	+	+

RG, redundancy gain

manipulations can be shown to have disparate effects on the CUD, while having comparable effects on overall reaction times, then transfer is probably occurring along visual pathways that are more sensitive to one of the two parameters (assuming that the same pathway mediates transfer in both manipulations).

Table 1 summarizes the effects of visual, motor, and attentional parameters on the CUD in normal subjects in studies extending up to 1995. The informative cases are those in which the manipulation affects overall RT. The standard visual parameters are intensity and eccentricity, and they usually affect overall RT but not the CUD. St. John and colleagues (1987) did find an effect of eccentricity on the CUD, but the difference was small (e.g., a 0.9 ms longer CUD at 2° than at 15°), and the majority of subjects did not show it.

Attentional parameters include blocking of target VF, spatial uncertainty of target location, redundancy gain, and precuing of target location. Again, there are effects on overall latency but not on the CUD. Motor manipulations include bimanual responses, alternating fingers or alternating hand responses, and number of response presses. In contrast to visual and attentional parameters, motor manipulations do affect the CUD. This is consistent with conclusion that interhemispheric transfer in the SRT paradigm of Poffenberger is at a late, motor, information-processing stage.

The algebraic model of the CUD assumes strong modularity and might not be valid. However, as a strong theoretical position, it serves to clarify opposing accounts of the CUD and to focus disconfirming evidence.

REFERENCES

AGLIOTI, S., B. BERLUCCHI, R. PALLINI, G. F. ROSSI, and G. TASSINARI, 1993. Hemispheric control of unilateral and bilateral responses to lateralized light stimuli after callosotomy and in callosal agenesis. *Exp. Brain Res.* 95:151–165.

BERLUCCHI, G., W. HERON, G. RIZZOLATTI, and C. UMILTÀ, 1971. Simple reaction times of ipsilateral and contralateral hand to lateralized visual stimuli. *Brain* 94:419–430.

BORING, E. G., 1950. *A History of Experimental Psychology*, 2nd ed. Englewood Cliffs, N.J.: Prentice-Hall.

BRAUN, C. M. J., S. DAIGNEAULT, S. MILJOURS, and A. DUFRESNE, 1995. Does hemispheric relay depend on attention? *Am. J. Psychol.* 108:527–546.

DISTEFANO, M., M. MORELLI, C. A. MARZI, and G. BERLUCCHI, 1980. Hemispheric control of unilateral and bilateral movements of proximal and distal parts of the arms as inferred from simple reaction time to lateralized light stimuli in man. *Exp. Brain Res.* 38:197–204.

FODOR, J. A., 1983. *The Modularity of Mind.* Cambridge, Mass.: The MIT Press.

GODBOUT, J. A., A. ACHIM, and C. M. J. BRAUN, 1995. Modulation motrice des dynamiques interhémisphériques dans le paradigme de Poffenberger [Abstract]. *Comptes Rendus du 18ième Congrès de la Société Québécoise de Recherche en Psychologie*, Ottawa, p. 72.

IACOBONI, M., and E. ZAIDEL, 1995. Channels of the corpus callosum: Evidence from simple reaction times to lateralized flashes in the normal and the split brain. *Brain* 118:779–788.

JEEVES, M. A., and N. F. DIXON, 1970. Hemisphere differences in response rates to visual stimuli. *Psychonomic Sci.* 20:249–251.

JEEVES, M. A., and A. D. MILNER, 1987. Specificity and plasticity in interhemispheric integration: Evidence from callosal agenesis. In *Duality and Unity of the Brain: Unified Functioning and Specialisation of the Hemispheres. Wenner-Gren International Symposium Series*, Volume 47, D. Ottoson, ed. Basingstoke: Macmillan, pp. 416–441.

KINSBOURNE, M., and M. FISHER, 1971. Latency of uncrossed and of crossed reaction in callosal agenesis. *Neuropsychologia* 9:471–473.

LIEPMAN, H., and O. MAAS, 1907. Fall von linksseitiger Agraphie und Apraxie bei rechtsseitiger Lähmung. *J. Psychol. Neurol.* 10:214–227.

LINES, C. R., M. D. RUGG, and A. D. MILNER, 1984. The effects of stimulus intensity on visual evoked potential estimates of interhemispheric transmission time. *Expl. Brain Res.* 57:89–984.

MARZI, C. A., P. BISIACCHI, and R. NICOLETTI, 1991. Is interhemispheric transfer of visuomotor information asymmetric? Evidence from a meta-analysis. *Neuropsychologia* 29:1163–1177.

MILNER, A. D., and C. R. LINES, 1982. Interhemispheric pathways in simple reaction time to lateralized light flash. *Neuropsychologia* 20:171–179.

POFFENBERGER, A. T., 1912. Reaction time to retinal stimulation, with special reference to the time lost in conduction through nerve centers. *Arch. Psychol.* 23:1–73.

ST. JOHN, R., C. SHIELDS, P. KRAHN, and B. TIMNEY, 1987. The reliability of estimates of interhemispheric transmission times derived from unimanual and verbal response latencies. *Hum. Neurobiol.* 6:195–202.

TROPE, I., B. FISHMAN, R. C. GUR, N. M. SUSSMAN, and R. E. GUR, 1987. Contralateral and ipsilateral control of fingers following callosotomy. *Neuropsychologia* 25:287–291.

WOODWORTH, R. S., 1938. *Experimental Psychology*. New York: Holt.

ZAIDEL, E., 1983. Disconnection syndrome as a model for laterality effects in the normal brain. In *Cerebral Hemisphere Asymmetry: Method, Theory and Application*, J. Hellige, ed. New York: Praeger, pp. 95–151.

I ANATOMY AND MORPHOMETRY OF THE CORPUS CALLOSUM

1 Callosal Axons and Their Development

GIORGIO M. INNOCENTI AND RAYMOND BRESSOUD

ABSTRACT Recently, the anterograde transport of biocytin, coupled with computerized three-dimensional reconstruction and analysis, has allowed a detailed description of the morphology of the terminal arbors of callosal axons interconnecting the visual areas of the cat. Callosal axons are specific in their topographical distribution both across areas and within each area. Furthermore, they distribute different numbers of boutons to their various target sites. On the basis of computer simulations the geometry of most callosal axons appears tailored to the task of activating their targets in precise synchrony. The latter aspect of the morphology of callosal axons may be important for generating assemblies of coactive neurons in the two hemispheres during visual perception. Callosal axons differentiate in stages, each characterized by a combination of target-aimed and exuberant growth. The latter is corrected by regressive events that eliminate large numbers of callosal axons, their branches, and synapses. Together, target-aimed and exuberant growth progressively restrict the arbors to their sites of termination. The role of vision in the development of callosal axons is documented by the finding that binocular deprivation of vision by suture of the eyelids decreases the number of juvenile callosal connections that are stabilized into adulthood and stunts the development of the individual arbors.

The corpus callosum interconnects mainly cortical neurons of the two cerebral hemispheres and is by far the largest fiber tract in the brain. It consists of about 23 million axons in the cat (Berbel and Innocenti, 1988) and about 56 million in the rhesus monkey (LaMantia and Rakic, 1990a).

Callosal connections are organized according to a number of specific rules, some of which have been known for several years.

First, in all species the majority of callosal axons originate from pyramidal neurons in layer III (Figure 1.1). The infragranular layers V and VI contribute axons to some callosal projections, particularly to feedback projections from higher to lower areas (reviewed in Innocenti, 1986; Kennedy, Meissirel, and Dehay, 1991).

GIORGIO M. INNOCENTI Division of Neuroanatomy and Brain Development, Department of Neuroscience, Karolinska Institutet, Stockholm, Sweden.
RAYMOND BRESSOUD Institut de Biologie Cellulaire et Morphologie, Lausanne, Switzerland.

The available electrophysiological and neurochemical evidence unequivocally establishes that the vast majority of these axons establish excitatory synapses. However, some axons probably terminate on inhibitory neurons and therefore have an inhibitory action on their targets (reviewed in Innocenti, 1986; Payne, 1994; Conti and Manzoni, 1994). The existence of a few directly inhibitory callosal axons seems probable in the cat (Hughes and Peters, 1992).

Second, each cortical area is connected with the corresponding area (homotopic callosal connections) and with noncorresponding areas in the contralateral hemisphere (heterotopic callosal connections; see Figure 1.2).

Third, each area is callosally connected to its own characteristic set of other areas. For example, the 17/18 region of the cat is connected to the contralateral 17/18 region as well as to peristriate areas such as 19 and 21a, the suprasylvian visual areas (Segraves and Rosenquist, 1982), and, in addition, to the insular cortex and to the claustrum (unpublished). The connections are usually reciprocal, and in general, areas that are callosally connected are also connected intrahemispherically (Figure 1.3). This suggests that areas in opposite hemispheres might communicate through a number of alternative intrahemispheric and interhemispheric routes, which might become differentially active in different functional conditions.

Fourth, callosal connections are unevenly distributed across the cortical areas (Figure 1.4; reviewed in Innocenti, 1986; Kennedy et al., 1991). In the visual system, callosal connections are restricted near the border between areas 17 and 18. This region represents the vertical meridian of the visual field and, in the cat, up to 20 degrees of visual field along it (Payne, 1994). A similarly restricted distribution of callosal connections is found in the primary somatosensory areas, along the representation of the body midlines, although part of the forepaw representation is also callosally connected. In addition to what was mentioned above, a different density of callosally projecting neurons was found in regions of the primary visual and somatosensory areas representing different sectors of the sensory peripheries

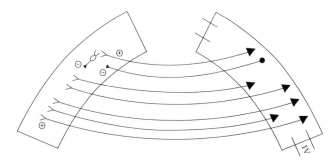

FIGURE 1.1. Schematic representation of layers of origin and type of callosal connections. In general, callosal axons originate from pyramidal neurons located above layer IV; fewer axons originate below layer IV. Most callosal axons are excitatory (+ and forked termination), although some of them probably terminate on inhibitory neurons (− and small triangles). A few nonpyramidal inhibitory neurons appear to establish callosal connections. For further explanations, see the text.

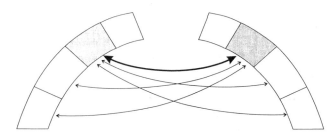

FIGURE 1.2. Schematic representation of the organization of callosal connections. An area (shaded) is strongly callosally connected (thick arrows) to its contralateral corresponding area (homotopic connections) as well as, more weakly (thin arrows), to noncorresponding areas (heterotopic connections). Connections are reciprocal and roughly symmetrical. However, the reciprocal connections between areas at different levels of cortical processing do not necessarily originate from the same layers (see the text). Nonsymmetrical connections can be generated experimentally, and they also must be expected to exist in anatomically or functionally asymmetric brains.

(Innocenti and Fiore, 1976; Caminiti, Innocenti, and Manzoni, 1979; Innocenti, 1980; Kennedy, Dehay, and Bullier, 1986). This suggested that the maps generated by thalamic afferents in the somatosensory areas are rescaled in the corpus callosum by virtue of the distribution of its neurons of origin (Innocenti, 1978) (see Figure 1.4). In addition, callosal connections might "filter out" other aspects of the cortical maps and distribute them to specific cortical sites. Indeed, both the neurons of origin of callosal projections and the callosal terminal axons were occasionally reported to be distributed in discrete "columnar" patches (reviewed and discussed in Innocenti, 1986; see also Olavarria and Abel, 1996).

The corpus callosum implements neuronal operations that lead to integrate or to lateralize the activity of the

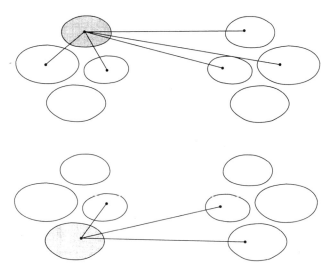

FIGURE 1.3. Schematized pattern of callosal connectivity among areas, four of which are represented for each hemisphere. As exemplified by the two shaded ones, each area forms callosal connections with a restricted set of contralateral areas; homotopic callosal connections are between corresponding areas, heterotopic connections between noncorresponding areas. The latter normally include areas that also receive intrahemispheric connections. For further explanations, see the text.

cerebral hemispheres. The structure of callosal connections provides precise indications of what some of the operations might be. In particular, the selective distribution of callosally projecting neurons and of their axons mentioned above suggested that callosal connections perform specific transformations of the cortical maps and therefore, in a broad sense, operations of a computational kind. This was stressed by the recent analysis of the morphology of individual callosal axons based on new anterograde axonal tracers and computer methods for the three-dimensional reconstruction and analysis (Houzel, Milleret, and Innocenti, 1994; Bressoud and Innocenti, 1999) (see Figure 1.5). At this new level of resolution, it became clear that by virtue of their geometry, individual callosal axons perform at least three types of operations; these are in the spatial (mapping), intensity (weighting), and temporal (synchronization or desynchronization) domains (Figure 1.6), as detailed below.

It should be stressed that the morphology of callosal axons is not unique in the cerebral cortex. On the contrary, there is consensus that except for their long trajectories, callosal axons are representative of corticocortical inter-areal and possibly intra-areal axons (Hubel and Wiesel, 1967; Innocenti, 1986; Kennedy et al., 1991). Thus, most or all the concepts that are coming into focus in structural or functional studies of the corpus callosum can probably be generalized to other cortical connections.

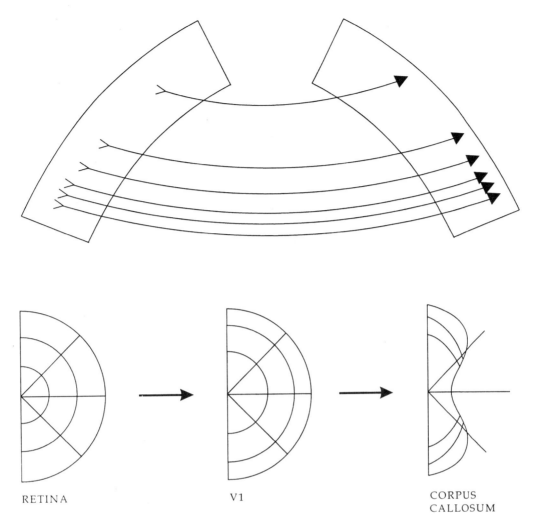

RETINA   V1   CORPUS CALLOSUM

FIGURE 1.4. Callosally projecting neurons (solid triangles) are usually unevenly distributed in a cortical area. As shown in the bottom panels, this results in the primary visual areas (17 and/or 18), in differential magnification, in the corpus callosum, of the various portions of the cortical retinotopic maps in which the central parts of the retina are already exaggerated.

Operations implemented by individual callosal axons

MAPPING Callosal axons implement connectional maps between the hemispheres. At the cellular level, this implies spatial transformations between the location of the cell body of origin and that of the terminal boutons of individual axons. The mapping applies at different levels of cortical organization.

Among-areas mapping As mentioned above, each cortical area establishes both homotopic and heterotopic connections with areas of the contralateral hemisphere. The question is whether the same cortical neuron can supply both homotopic and heterotopic callosal connections through bifurcating axons. In the visual system of the cat, which is apparently the only system that has been studied to this day, mature axons from areas 17 and 18 were found to establish diverging projections to either side of the contralateral 17/18 border but not (or very rarely), in addition, to other visual areas (Houzel et al., 1994; Bressoud and Innocenti, 1999). Similar results had been obtained with double retrograde labeling for callosal projections to 17/18 and suprasylvian areas (Segraves and Innocenti, 1985). Furthermore, callosal and intrahemispheric corticocortical projections from areas 17 and 18 originate from different neurons. This applies even in the case of projections to homologous areas of the two hemispheres such as those from areas 17 and 18 to the lateral suprasylvian areas (Segraves and Innocenti, 1985). Comparable results were obtained in the monkey (reviewed in Kennedy et al., 1991). Although callosally projecting neurons also have initial axon collaterals, these seem to remain confined relatively close to their cell body (Innocenti, 1980). Other callosal axons

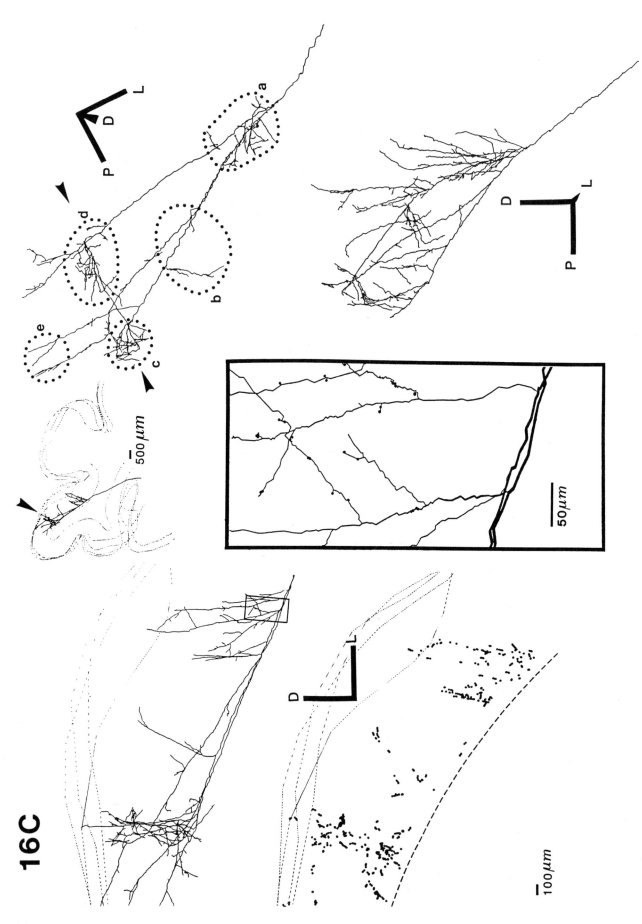

16C

14

FIGURE 1.5. Three-dimensional reconstruction of callosal axon 16C interconnecting the regions near the 17/18 borders of the cat. Middle-top panel: Arbor with outlines of some sections. Top-left panel: Front view of the arbor; the region in the box is shown enlarged in the middle-bottom panel, with the thickness of the branches proportional to their diameter (but not to the calibration bar). Bottom-left panel: Corresponding view of boutons with the bottom of layer VI marked by a thick dashed line. Top-right and bottom-right panels: Top and medial views of the arbor, respectively; terminal columns are encircled by dots and denoted by lowercase letters. Tapering of orientation bars point away from the viewer. The arrowheads point to the border between areas 17 and 18. Notice the disjunctive "columnar" termination of branches and boutons, with different numbers of boutons in different layers and columns. Notice also the complex branching pattern of the axon and the changes in axon diameter at some of the bifurcations. Reprinted from Houzel et al. (1994) with permission.

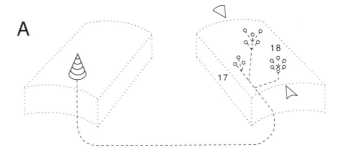

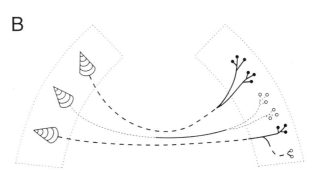

FIGURE 1.6. Operations performed, by virtue of their geometry, by callosal axons that interconnect areas 17 and 18 of the cat. Part A illustrates mapping and differential weighting. A point in one hemisphere, corresponding to the location of the cell body, is mapped into clusters of boutons (terminal columns) that are distributed in the contralateral cortex along the border between areas 17 and 18 (open triangles). Notice that the terminal columns contain different numbers of boutons, suggesting that the axon does not drive all the terminal columns with equal strength. Part B illustrates temporal transformations performed by axonal geometry. The top axon activates terminal columns simultaneously; the bottom axon with a delay due to axonal conduction within its terminal arbor; the activation of the intermediate axon is retarded in comparison to the others, owing to its smaller diameter. The active part of the axon is in solid black; the inactive part is interrupted.

originating in areas 17 and 18 target the border between areas 19 and areas 21a or 7. Still others reach the border between the posteromedial and posterolateral lateral suprasylvian areas (PMLS and PLLS). Nevertheless, only part of the heterotopic projections from areas 17 and 18 (Figure 1.7) is supplied by distinct axons for each areal border. Individual axons were also found that branch to PMLS/PLLS border *and* to the PMLS/21a border or else to the PMLS/PLLS *and* to the 19/21a border (Bressoud and Innocenti, 1999). A few neurons with axons bifurcating to both contralateral and ipsilateral areas 17 and 18 were also found in the deep layers of area PMLS using double retrogradely transported tracers (Segraves and Innocenti, 1985).

The findings mentioned above are potentially important, since they could mean that corticocortical outputs from one area use, in general, different "labeled lines," that is, neurons with different response properties. Alternatively, the lack of widely diverging axons might be the expression of limits in the total length of the axon that a cortical neuron can generate and/or maintain. This second interpretation appears less likely, since extremely long axons exist in the nervous system, including corticospinal axons and ascending axons from diffuse projection systems. Furthermore, a few callosal axons do branch to areas in the same hemisphere and in the opposite hemisphere or to different areas of the contralateral hemisphere (Segraves and Innocenti, 1985; Bressoud and Innocenti, 1999).

Thus, the existence of both individual and shared connections between areas seems to imply a high degree of flexibility in the generation of functionally linked neuronal assemblies in cortical areas of the two hemispheres.

Corticotopic mapping Callosal connections between areas of the two hemispheres have so far been considered to be orderly and point-to-point. This view, however, is no longer accurate. First, the tangential distribution of the terminal arbor of a single callosal axon often greatly exceeds the territory occupied by the cell body of the parent neuron, its dendrites included (Figures 1.5 and 1.7). Therefore, many individual callosal axons diverge to their site of termination. Furthermore, since the tangential extent of the callosal efferent zone (the volume containing callosally projecting neurons in one area) is wider than that of the callosal terminal territory (the volume containing the terminals of callosal axons), this implies convergence of callosal axons as well. Indeed,

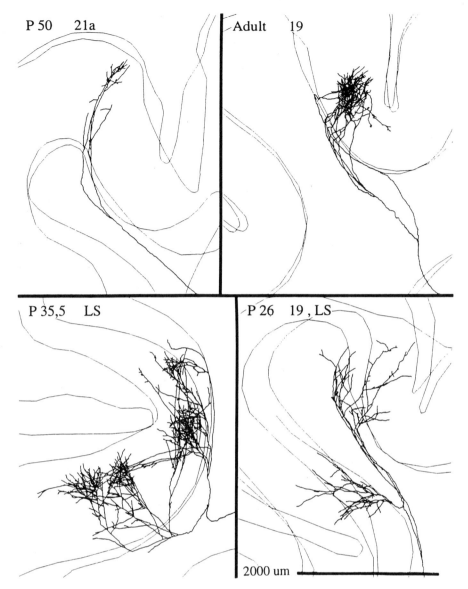

P 50   21a

Adult   19

P 35,5   LS

P 26   19 , LS

2000 um

FIGURE 1.7. Examples of three-dimensionally reconstructed callosal axons from primary visual areas 17 and 18 of the cat to the extrastriate areas 21a, 19, lateral suprasylvian (LS), as well as to 19 and LS. In each case, upper and lower boundaries of the gray matter in representative sections are also shown. The age of the animal is indicated in each case.

individual callosal axons have been seen to converge, at least partially onto the same target sites (Houzel et al., 1994; Bressoud and Innocenti, 1999). For the time being, only the values of divergence of callosal axons originating near the 17/18 border are known, to some extent. In the 17/18 region of the cat, individual axons can span tangentially between $100 \, \mu m^2$ and several thousand μm^2 (Houzel et al., 1994), with the greatest values of divergence in area 18. The degree of axonal divergence also varies among the callosal axons to the extrastriate visual areas. The highest divergence was found for axons to the lateral suprasylvian areas (probably equivalent to area MT in the monkey), and the smallest was found for those to area 21a (Bressoud and Innocenti, 1999) (see Figure 1.7). The degree of divergence of callosal axons might be related to the magnification factor of the retinotopic maps and to the size of individual receptive fields in the different areas. Given the large receptive fields found in area 18 and in the suprasylvian area, the divergence of callosal axons does not necessarily imply a mismatch between the retinal location of the receptive field of callosal axons and that of its target neurons.

The corticotopic mapping implemented by callosal axons in the primary visual areas might be the substrate for coarse stereopsis along the vertical meridian (discussed in Innocenti, 1986). In addition, it might correct for retinotopic mismatches in the callosal connections among visual areas (Olavarria, 1996).

Higher-order mapping Diverging callosal axons also implement mapping rules at levels of cortical organization beyond those considered above. Individual axons to the primary visual areas, to area 19, and to the visual areas in the suprasylvian sulcus of the cat often terminate with multiple clusters of boutons 300–600 μm across and separated by spaces 120–2770 μm wide (Houzel et al., 1994; Bressoud and Innocenti, 1999). The volumes containing the callosal boutons are called *terminal columns*. The visual areas, like most cortical areas, are organized in "columns" of neurons with similar functional properties. Callosal axons appear to respect, in their terminal distribution, this columnar organization. Indeed, it was demonstrated electrophysiologically that neurons in the primary visual areas have the same orientation specificity in the callosally as well as in the geniculocortically activated part of their receptive fields (Berlucchi and Rizzolatti, 1968). This suggests that, as intra-areal axons and axons from area 17 to area 18 of the same hemisphere (Gilbert and Wiesel, 1989), callosal axons interconnect cortical columns that recognize identical orientations of the visual stimulus. Further studies of the specific column-to-column connectivity in the different areas might clarify the previously discussed discrepancies among different studies, concerning the existence of segregated columns of callosally projecting neurons in cortical areas (Innocenti, 1986). Blurred columns of callosally projecting neurons were seen with retrograde transport in these areas (Boyd and Matsubara, 1994), while the identification of callosal terminal columns required the analysis of single axons.

Presumably, callosal axons implement still higher levels of topographical mapping. In several instances the diameter of the terminal clusters of callosal axons is inferior to what would be expected if the boutons were to occupy entirely one orientation column. Thus, only part of a column might receive callosal axons. Furthermore, callosal axons usually do not distribute to all layers in their site of termination, although in some cases they do. Most frequently, only the supragranular and infragranular layers receive boutons, not layer IV. This points to some complementarity between callosal axons and other afferents specific for layer IV, for example, thalamocortical axons or the recurrent projections from layer VI. It also points to levels of organization of cortical organization, which ought to be elucidated in the future.

Finally, it is not known whether the callosal axons synapse specifically on a given cell type. However, they might be selective for certain dendritic subdomains, since they appear to selectively contact dendritic spines rather than shafts (reviewed in Innocenti, 1986).

WEIGHTING   Individual callosal axons do not contribute the same number of boutons to different terminal columns. They also contribute different numbers of boutons to the different layers and can distribute to different layers in different columns. This applies to callosal axons to areas 17 and 18, as well as to those to extrastriate visual areas (Houzel et al., 1994; Bressoud and Innocenti, 1999). Usually, one or two of the columns receive many more boutons than the others. The maximal difference in the number of boutons found thus far across columns is about 1–50. Ratios of 1–10 or 1–20 are frequent (Houzel et al., 1994). The number of boutons per column is presumably determining the strength of the excitatory drive of the axon, the so-called synaptic weight of the axon in a given "terminal column." Therefore, the action potentials transmitted by a callosal axon might be differentially weighted at its sites of termination by the number of contacts. Unfortunately, nothing is known about the size of the callosal terminal boutons, their vesicular content, synaptic protein composition, quantal properties of transmitter release, and so on. All of these could also contribute to the synaptic weight of the axon at its different sites of termination.

TEMPORAL TRANSFORMATIONS   Several lines of evidence point to temporal parameters as a fundamental aspect of neural processing. Thus, neuronal subsystems characterized by the different conduction velocities of their axons exist in both the sensory and motor systems and implement different functions. In the visual system, faster-conducting axons appear to be involved in motion analysis, slower axons in form discrimination (Livingstone and Hubel, 1987). Furthermore, temporal transformations within the arbors of individual axons or between arbors belonging to different axons seem to be relevant for neural function. In the auditory system of birds, axons to the nucleus laminaris implement delay lines by distributing their action potentials to different targets with nonzero time lags (Carr and Konishi, 1990). Elsewhere, the different conduction length seems to be compensated by changes in axon diameter. This is true in systems as different as the motor neurons controlling the electric organ of fish (Bennett, 1968), the climbing fiber projection from the inferior olive to the cerebellar Purkinje cell (Sugihara, Lang and Llinas, 1993), and the intraretinal part of ganglion cell axons (Stanford, 1987). The degree of temporal precision necessary for neural operations has been a matter of debate, particularly for cerebral cortex. The issue is whether cortical neurons can use temporal resolutions in the millisecond range (Softky and Koch, 1993; Softky, 1994). In the auditory system of birds and in the neural structures that process or generate electrical signals in fish, temporal resolutions on the order of microseconds are used (reviewed in Carr, 1993).

Attention to the possibility that callosal axons might be involved in temporal transformation was raised by the observation that the geometry callosal axons seems occasionally uneconomical in terms of axoplasmic production and maintenance (Innocenti, Lehmann, and Houzel, 1994). In particular, callosal axons often possess branches that run in parallel to their targets for several millimeters or exchange branches between terminal columns several hundred microns apart (Houzel et al., 1994; Innocenti et al., 1994) (see Figure 1.5). In an attempt to clarify the possible functional consequences of the above-mentioned geometry, we ran simulations of action potential propagation along serially reconstructed visual callosal axons, based on the well-established relationship between conduction velocity and axon diameter (Innocenti et al., 1994). The simulation software (MAXSIM; Tettoni et al., 1996) allows generation of frequency histograms of the activation time of the individual boutons contributed by one axon to one or more sites of termination. The precision of the simulation is limited by a number of factors, including the accuracy of axon diameter measurements and the possibility that delays or accelerations of action potential propagation occur at the sites of axonal bifurcation, as is discussed elsewhere (Innocenti et al., 1994; Tettoni et al., 1996). Those intractable uncertainties aside, for visual callosal axons of the cat, the simulation returned interhemispheric conduction delays in the range of those measured electrophysiologically.

In the callosal axons analyzed to this date, we found a tendency for the geometry of the axon to maximize synchronous activation of spatially separate terminal columns with precision within 1 ms. The apparently wasteful geometry mentioned above is instrumental in generating such a synchronization. However, in terms of axoplasm production and maintenance, they do not represent the most parsimonious way of achieving synchronization. This suggests that other factors, in particular developmental constraints, influence the geometry of the axons (Innocenti, 1994). Callosal axons of the kind described above might participate in the synchronization of the activity of neuronal pools within and across the hemispheres demonstrated by single-unit analysis in animals (Engel et al., 1991; Nowak et al., 1995) and by EEG analysis in animals and the human (Kiper et al., 1999, Knyazeva et al., 1999). Accordingly, the interruption of callosal axons abolishes the synchronization.

Such a synchronization may be necessary for perceptual binding and figure/background segregation (Singer, 1995).

Although current research emphasizes the importance of synchronous activation of neuronal assemblies, the opposite—the desynchronization of neuronal assemblies—may play an equally important role in neural function. Indeed, a few axons with geometry appropriate for generating activation delays were also found. These axons run tangentially in the cortex contributing boutons serially to several terminal columns. An axon of this kind could activate separate cortical columns with a delay of up to 2 ms (Innocenti et al., 1994). Furthermore, callosal axons interconnecting the primary visual areas were found to vary in their diameter between about 0.5 and 2 μm. Axonal size might correlate with differences in the receptive field properties and connectivity of the parent cell bodies. McCourt, Thalluri and Henry (1990) found the fastest interhemispheric conducting axons for neurons of the S (simple) type. Axons with different diameter were found to converge on the same cortical sites. The simulations predicted that in a case of this kind, action potentials simultaneously initiated in the parent cell bodies would reach their target sites with important temporal delays (on the order of 2.5 ms) (Innocenti et al., 1994). The delays that are theoretically generated by conduction within the same axon or across axons are large in comparison to the average interhemispheric conduction delay in the cat (2.0–2.9 ms; Innocenti, 1995).

In conclusion, the analysis of individual callosal axons has focused attention on the morphological substrate of temporal transformations of interhemispheric interaction. The importance of these transformations for brain function can hardly be overemphasized. This is highlighted by the recent suggestion that increased interhemispheric delays caused by increased brain size may be a cause of hemispheric specialization in humans (Ringo et al., 1994). However, this provocative and stimulating hypothesis is not supported by the available electrophysiological data (reviewed in Innocenti, 1995). In fact, comparable mean interhemispheric conduction delays, on the order of 7–8 ms, were reported in the visual cortex of the rhesus monkey and the mouse in spite of the considerable difference in brain size. Cats and ferrets, whose brain size ranges between those of monkey and mouse, seem to be similar in their interhemispheric conduction delays, but these are definitely shorter than those in the other two species (about 2.9 ms). Curiously, the longest interhemispheric conduction delays were measured in rabbits (17 ms). Apparently, evolution managed to maintain comparable interhemispheric conduction delays, in spite of manifold increases in brain size. This was probably obtained by scaling the diameter of callosal axons to brain size, as preliminary evidence suggests (Innocenti, Aggoun-Zouaoui, and Lehmann, 1995). However certain species—in particular, the carnivores—might have faster interhemispheric conduction, possibly faster conduction in all the corticocortical pathways.

The formation of callosal connectional maps

Studies using retrogradely transported axonal tracers have demonstrated that callosal connections develop through a phase of exuberance in which more axons project into the corpus callosum than will be present in the adult (reviewed in Innocenti, 1986, 1991). The first unequivocally transient projections to be discovered were those originating from parts of the cortex that are no longer callosally connected in the adult such as most of area 17 and parts of the primary somatosensory areas. Transient callosal projections were also found in the cat between the primary auditory area and the visual area. Comparable results were reported in several other areas and species, including the rhesus monkey (Chalupa and Killackey, 1989).

The elimination of the transitory projections is due to selective elimination of axonal branches rather than neuronal death. The elimination is massive. For the whole corpus callosum it was estimated, on the basis of electron microscopic counts of callosal axons, to amount to at least 70% of the axons produced in both cats (Berbel and Innocenti, 1988) and monkeys (LaMantia and Rakic, 1990b). These findings were tentatively extrapolated to the developing human corpus callosum on the basis of measurements of corpus callosum sectional area (reviewed in Innocenti, 1991).

The production of transient projections, often topographically different from the adult ones, was found to be a very general phenomenon, not restricted to the callosal connections but applying also to intrahemispheric and corticosubcortical projections (reviewed in Innocenti, 1991). The overproduction of projections clearly provides the potential substrate for plastic changes in the developing brain. Indeed, neither the fate of normally maintained axons nor that of normally eliminated axons seemed rigidly predetermined. Instead, it was found to be modifiable by epigenetic events, including activity, integrity of the sensory periphery and of other brain regions, and hormonal and dietary influences (reviewed in Innocenti, 1991; Zufferey et al., 1999).

Studies with retrograde transport techniques, however, provided only limited and indirect information on the axons concerned. They failed to clarify the morphology of the developing axons and which relations they establish with the target regions. Both questions are important for understanding the functional role played by the transient connections in development and for clarifying the nature of the control that determines the fate of the juvenile axons.

Therefore, the methods for visualization, three-dimensional reconstruction and analysis of single axons, already used for the adult, were applied to developing callosal axons from the primary visual areas of the cat (Aggoun-Zouaoui and Innocenti, 1994; Aggoun-Zouaoui, Kiper, and Innocenti, 1996). The results clarified a number of factual and theoretical issues. The overall conclusion is that the formation of connectional maps includes a process of axonal differentiation involving both productive and regressive events. In this process, several growth stages can be identified. At each stage the axon exhibits exuberant growth, but the growth is progressively constrained within territories that gradually approach the adult distribution of the axon.

Stages in the differentiation of callosal axons

The stages of axonal differentiation described below (Figure 1.8) were originally determined from the analysis of callosal axons originating from, and terminating in, the primary visual areas of the cat, areas 17 and 18 (Aggoun-Zouaoui and Innocenti, 1994; Aggoun-Zouaoui et al., 1996). However they also apply to the projection from the primary visual areas to the peristriate areas (Bressoud and Innocenti, 1999) and perhaps to all callosal connections. The stages are schematized and purely descriptive. For individual axons there can be some temporal overlap between the events ascribed to two successive stages. Furthermore, at any age point, different axons can be at different stages of their development.

THE FIRST STAGE: AXONAL ELONGATION   This is essentially a prenatal event in the visual areas of the cat, although during the first postnatal week, axons from the primary visual areas continue to be added to the corpus callosum (see Aggoun-Zouaoui and Innocenti, 1994). The details of this important process are unknown. Apparently, a glial sling forms at the midline before the first callosal axons begin to cross and may be a prerequisite for the formation of the commissure (Silver et al., 1982; Silver, Edwards, and Levitt, 1993). The congenital or experimentally induced destruction of this bridge leads to callosal agenesis. The first callosal axons in the rat grow out of neurons in the cingulate cortex and might pioneer later growing axons (Koester and O'Leary, 1994). Radial glia seems to be involved in guiding callosal axons toward the cerebral cortex (Norris and Kalil,

AXONAL ELONGATION   CORTICAL BRANCHING & SYNAPTOGENESIS

SUBCORTICAL BRANCHING   PEAK OF SYNAPTOGENESIS

CORTICAL INGROWTH   ADULT

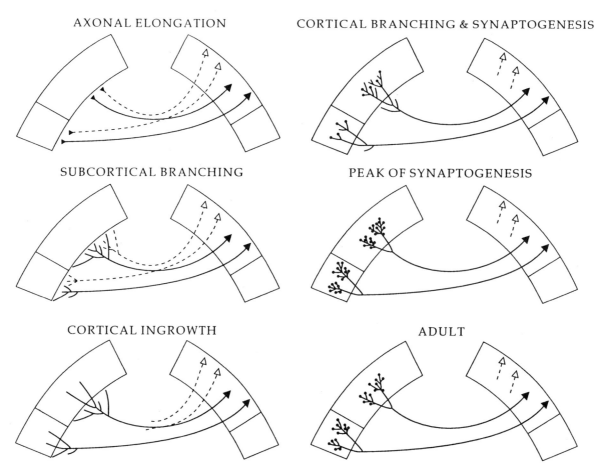

FIGURE 1.8. Schematic representation of stages in the differentiation of callosal terminal arbors in visual areas of the cat. The stages are axonal elongation, subcortical branching, cortical ingrowth, cortical branching, and synaptogenesis (the last two are here represented together). Notice that each stage is followed by partially regressive events, that is, elimination of long callosal axons (interrupted) between the second and third stage, of subcortical branches during synaptogenesis, and of synaptic boutons between the peak of synaptogenesis and adulthood. Neuronal cell bodies are represented by solid or open triangles, growth cones by small triangles at the end of the axonal branches, and synaptic boutons by dots. Some of the neurons (open triangles) eliminate their callosal axons without dying and presumably establish permanent connections in the ipsilateral hemisphere, presumably relatively close to their cell bodies (not shown).

1991). More information on this issue might arise from the study of axonal growth in acallosal strains of mice (Ozaki and Wahlsten, 1993).

Although at this stage the callosal axons are produced in excess, their growth is not unconstrained. Confirming previous results obtained with retrogradely transported axonal tracers (reviewed in Innocenti, 1986, 1991), most individual axons from areas 17 or 18 were found to grow either to the contralateral homologous areas, to area 19, to area 21a, or to the visual suprasylvian areas. Some axons, however, establish early branches to more than one area. As in the adult, these axons appear to be more numerous in the projections to extrastriate visual areas (Aggoun-Zouaoui and Innocenti, 1994; Innocenti and Bressoud, 1999). On the basis of previous work (reviewed in Innocenti, 1986, 1991), the callosally projecting neurons are also different from the intrahemispherically projecting ones. In the rat, callosally projecting neurons are also different, at this stage, from the subcortically projecting neurons in the same area (Koester and O'Leary, 1993). On the whole, it seems unavoidable to conclude that there might be subsets of intrinsically different cortical neurons and, in particular, of callosally projecting neurons. The growth of their axons appears to be differently regulated by substrate cues, resulting in specific projection patterns to the various areas of the contralateral hemisphere. This hypothesis is strengthened by the occasional observation of abrupt corrections in the trajectory of some of the axons after they had grown for some distance toward the "wrong" target (Bressoud and Innocenti, 1999). However, it must also be noticed that until the stage of subcortical branching (see below), callosal axons that are destined for elimination, such as those from area 17, and axons that are destined to be maintained, such as those from the 17/18 border, are indistinguishable.

THE SECOND STAGE: SUBCORTICAL BRANCHING   Time-lapse cinematography in the hamster (Halloran and Kalil, 1994) showed that callosal axons that have reached the subcortical white matter are in a dynamic state with continuous formation and retraction of new branches. This stage probably corresponds to the so-called waiting period described in the development of thalamocortical projections (see Aggoun-Zouaoui and Innocenti, 1994, for discussion and references).

Subcortical branching occurs in the visual areas of the cat during the first and second postnatal weeks. Therefore, it overlaps with the subsequent stage of growth into the gray matter, but it seems to end when branching in the gray matter begins. A substantial proportion of the branches remains confined to the white matter without aiming clearly to a specific cortical area. The others point to one or more target sites. Both the axons that are destined to be maintained and those that are destined for elimination branch. At this stage, however, differences emerge between the transient axons originating from area 17 and those originating from the 17/18 border. The former axons branch less abundantly, and their branches terminate more often in the white matter without aiming clearly at one cortical area.

It must be noticed that at this stage, the subcortical white matter contains a partially transient neuronal population, the cortical subplate, which is suspected to play a crucial role in guiding thalamic axons into the gray matter (reviewed by Allendoerfer and Shatz, 1994). The role of the subplate in the development of callosal connections is unknown. It might be relevant that differences in the branching patterns of the various populations of callosal axons emerge at this stage and that the branching is far more abundant close to the subplate of the various visual areas than elsewhere along the trajectory of the axon. Thus, at this stage, the subplate might provide cues for target-aimed growth of callosal axons.

THE THIRD STAGE: CORTICAL INGROWTH   The third stage begins around the end of the first postnatal week. Interestingly, only axons originating near the 17/18 border enter deeply into the gray matter. However, they avoid locations that are acallosal in the adult, such as most of area 17. Norris and Kalil (1992) observed a

comparable specific growth of callosal axons in the somatosensory cortex of the hamster. The majority of the transient axons from area 17 remain confined to the white matter or to the subplate. Only a few engage into the lower third of the gray matter in various areas, including area 17. Already at this stage, some axons enter the cortex with a disjunctive distribution of branches recalling the columnar pattern seen in the adult.

THE FOURTH STAGE: CORTICAL BRANCHING   This seems to begin almost as soon as the axons have entered the gray matter, that is, at the end of the first postnatal week in the most precocious axons found thus far. In the following weeks and up to around the beginning of the third postnatal month, the number of branches increases above that found in the adult. This growth blurs somewhat the previous disjunctive and quasi-columnar pattern of axonal ingrowth but remains confined to the regions where callosal axons are found in the adult.

THE FIFTH STAGE: SYNAPTOGENESIS   The fifth stage has been assessed, thus far, by examining axonal swellings at the light-microscopic level (for the morphological criteria that were used, see Aggoun-Zouaoui and Innocenti, 1994; Aggoun-Zouaoui et al., 1996). Although some boutons can be found at earlier ages in the region of the cortical subplate, boutons reminding those found in the adult appear in the gray matter only at the end of the second postnatal week. Over the following weeks, the number of boutons increases, and around the beginning of the third postnatal month, it reaches a peak well above the adult values. Boutons acquire from the beginning a layer-specific distribution and maintain it over the whole period of synaptogenesis. The first boutons appear in the infragranular layers, but then they become particularly numerous in the supragranular layers. As is mostly the case in the adult, they are sparse or absent in layer IV. Boutons also acquire, from the beginning, a disjunctive columnar distribution, which they maintain throughout synaptogenesis.

A precocious columnar distribution of terminating callosal axons was noticed in previous studies of the somatosensory areas of the rat, visual cortex of the cat, and the prefrontal cortex of the monkey (reviewed in Innocenti, 1986, 1991; see also Schwartz and Goldmann-Rakic, 1991; Norris and Kalil, 1992). In contrast, Elberger (see her 1994 review) has reported a massive and diffuse ingrowth of callosal axons in the visual areas of the cat and the rat. The reasons for these different findings are unclear. In Elberger's earlier studies, axons were labeled from the corpus callosum in conditions that do not allow an unequivocal identification of the nature of the labeled axons, as is discussed elsewhere (Aggoun-Zouaoui and Innocenti, 1994). More recent work from the same group using cortical application of biotinylated dextran amines (Ding and Elberger, 1994) reports a pattern of axonal growth into the cortex that is substantially different from that obtained in previous work and compatible, in our opinion, with what is described above.

Regressive events and selection in the differentiation of callosal axons

The growth stages described above lead to overproduction of callosal axons, branches in the white and in the gray matter, and synapses. They are followed by selection of axons, axonal branches, and synapses to be maintained and by elimination of the others. The elimination is massive. As was mentioned above, previous work has shown that at least 70% of the juvenile callosal axons are eliminated in both cat and monkey (Berbel and Innocenti, 1988; LaMantia and Rakic, 1990b). In addition, at the stage of subcortical branching, homotopic callosal axons from the 17/18 border have established, on average, about 10 branching points in the contralateral white matter. These are reduced to two in the adult. The number of branches in the gray matter near the 17/18 border was found to exceed 500 at the beginning of the third postnatal month, and it was down to 240 in the adult. The number of boutons reached about 2100 at the beginning of the third postnatal month, and it was down to the average adult value of about 300 by the end of the fifth month. It should be noticed that these values are only suggestive because the number of serially reconstructed axons is limited.

The overproduction of synapses is a well-documented phenomenon in the development of cerebral cortex (see Bourgeois and Rakic, 1993, for data and references). The concept was established on the basis of electron-microscopic estimates of synaptic density in sample volumes of cortical gray matter. However, the implications of the synaptic overproduction and elimination for connectivity remained unclear. In particular, the origin of the supernumerary synapses could not be defined, and it could have been expected that the synaptic elimination would cause important rearrangements in the topography of cortical connections. The results reported above reject this possibility by showing that the overproduction of synapses does not blur much, if at all, the topographical specificity of the connections. Therefore, rather than sharpening the topography of the projections, the synaptic elimination might adjust the strength of the connections between callosal axons and their postsynaptic targets.

Regulation of axonal differentiation and development of callosal connections

The stages of exuberant growth described above probably apply to other cortical axons (see Innocenti, 1991, 1995). Therefore, this mode of development raises several general questions about the mechanisms regulating the exuberant axonal growth as well as the selection for maintenance versus elimination of juvenile axonal branches and/or synapses.

The available information is mainly based on retrograde transport studies of the callosal axons and, to a lesser extent, of terminating callosal axons but using techniques that do not resolve the individual axons. Most of the relevant studies have been reviewed elsewhere (Innocenti, 1991). Only some essential findings will be summarized here, in particular some recent analysis of single callosal axons in visually deprived kittens (Zufferey et al., 1999).

VISUAL ACTIVITY Thus far, this is the most intensely explored factor regulating the development of callosal connections. In particular, deprivation of vision by bilateral suture of the eyelids appears to delete a large fraction of the callosal connections that are normally maintained, in addition to those that are normally eliminated (reviewed in Innocenti, 1991; see also Boire et al., 1995). Furthermore, the callosal axons that are not eliminated show severely stunted terminal arbors (Zufferey et al., 1999). Eye enucleation, thalamectomy, or lesion of thalamic radiation also plays a role (reviewed in Innocenti, 1991; see also Fish et al., 1991; Miller, Windrem, and Finlay, 1991).

On the whole, the maintenance or elimination of the juvenile callosal connections seems to require a signal conveyed via thalamic afferents. This signal might involve concurrent activation of thalamic and callosal afferents, as appears to be the case for intra-areal connections (Lowel and Singer, 1992; Schmidt et al., 1997). The importance of information from the retina in the development of callosal connections was stressed in a recent study in which redirecting retinal afferents to the auditory thalamus caused reorganization of the callosal connections in the auditory areas (Pallas, Littman, and Moore, 1999).

The mode of action of visual activity remains to be understood. Manipulation of visual activity thus far has failed to maintain the majority of the transient juvenile axons. Perhaps visual activity cannot override cellular specificities based on biochemical markers. However, the role of spontaneous activity generated along the visual pathways or by other cortical afferents has never been explored.

Interestingly, visual activity seems to modify the fate of juvenile callosal axons very early, as soon as they are establishing the very first synaptic boutons. Indeed, normal vision until the age of two weeks—that is, extending into the beginning of synaptogenesis—is sufficient to prevent the loss of callosal connections that normally follows binocular deprivation by eyelid suture (Innocenti, Frost, and Illes, 1985). At the end of the first postnatal week the arbors of callosal axons have not fully differentiated. Therefore, normal vision might play a constructive role in the differentiation of the arbor by validating or eliminating synapses soon after they have formed (discussed in Aggoun-Zouaoui et al., 1996). Consistent with this possibility, it was found that in kittens that were binocularly deprived of vision by eyelid suture, the differentiation of callosal axons interconnecting visual areas 17 and 18 of the two hemispheres is arrested at the early stages of intracortical branching and synaptogenesis (Zufferey et al., 1999). Nevertheless, surprisingly, if vision is allowed until these early stages, the process of axonal differentiation, including an almost normal branching and synaptogenesis, can proceed in the absence of vision (Zufferey et al., 1999).

ASYMMETRIC DEVELOPMENT OF THE HEMISPHERES Interestingly, when the two hemispheres develop differently from each other, the callosal connections can develop asymmetrically. This was first demonstrated by Cynader, Leporé, and Guillemot (1981) in kittens that were raised with chiasmatic transection and monocular occlusion. This resulted in the development of callosal connections from the seeing hemisphere to the hemisphere that receives from the occluded eye and decreased connections in the opposite direction. The consequences of unilateral thalamectomy or of unilateral lesion of the optic tract were studied in different systems and species (Cusick and Lund, 1982; Melzer, Rothblatt and Innocenti, 1987; Rhoades et al., 1987; Koralek and Killackey, 1990; Miller et al., 1991). The results are compatible with the hypothesis that the development of callosal connections is modified by information coming from the periphery through the thalamus. Unfortunately, the unavoidable transection of corticothalamic fibers and of other corticofugal and corticopetal axons weakens the interpretation. Interestingly, in all the above-mentioned studies, callosal connections developed asymmetrically. Asymmetrical callosal connections were also obtained after unilateral early lesions of the cortical gray matter of areas 17 and 18 produced with perinatal injections of ibotenic acid in the cat (Inno-

centi and Berbel, 1991). The injections deleted the infragranular layers as well as, partially, layer III, resulting in a cytoarchitectonic abnormality similar to congenital microgyria in humans. Callosal connections from the injured cortex to the normal cortex were also deleted. Instead, connections in the opposite direction were maintained. Transient callosal connections from the auditory to the injured visual cortex were also maintained.

The possibility that competition between callosal and other corticocortical axons might regulate the fate of the former was tested with early lesions of the somatosensory areas (Caminiti and Innocenti, 1981). It was found that a small number of transient callosal projections from SI to contralateral SII could be maintained when the target SII was deprived of association afferents from ipsilateral SI. This was not obtained with the deprivation of callosal afferents from contralateral SII. These results brought evidence compatible with the view that competition with other corticocortical afferents might regulate the selection of callosal connections. Nevertheless, a reorganization of the thalamocortical connections as a cause could not be excluded.

The formation of callosal connections after experimental manipulations that affect hemispheric symmetry might provide tools for understanding the development of interhemispheric interactions in lateralized brains such as the human (Rosen, Sherman, and Gallaburda, 1989).

Conclusions and perspectives

The studies summarized above stress the complexities and subtleties in the organization of adult callosal connections revealed by new anatomical methods and therefore widen our understanding of the morphological basis of interhemispheric interactions.

Several questions remain. First, the information about the individual callosal axons to "higher-order" visual areas is scanty, and nothing is known about those interconnecting higher association areas. Second, as this volume demonstrates, research on the corpus callosum has developed over several decades on a strong interdisciplinary basis. The challenge facing this particularly advanced field, but common to other areas of the neurosciences, is that of mapping structural, electrophysiological, and psychological data onto each other. Our analysis of adult material has tentatively identified basic operations that are performed by callosal axons. However, it is unclear how these operations are reflected at the levels of neuronal response properties and of visual perception. The role of callosal connections in "binding by synchrony" the activity of neurons in the two hemispheres in sensory processing (Engel et al., 1991) offers a promising direction for future investigations. One breakthrough in this area may come from the development of techniques for assaying the functionality of interhemispheric connections. The analysis of interhemispheric coherence of EEG signals during sensory stimulation may provide such a tool. Indeed, an increased interhemispheric coherence of EEG signals in the gamma band was observed in both animals and humans with stimuli that activate the callosal connections of the visual areas (Kiper et al., 1999; Knyazeva et al., 1999). With this technique the role of the corpus callosum in perceptual binding could be clarified by further investigations using chimeric figures (Levy, Trevarthen, and Sperry, 1972).

The studies of developing callosal connections stress their potential modifiability (plasticity) in early development. Callosal connections could be modified either by the altered growth of the axon, by the maintenance of axonal structures that are normally eliminated, or by the elimination of axonal structures that are normally maintained. Any of these modifications could occur at one or another stage of axonal differentiation detailed above. In addition, axonal morphology could be modified at myelination, not mentioned in the present review, in spite of its potential relevance for the temporal operations the axons perform. The stage of callosal synaptogenesis and the subsequent partial synaptic elimination are particularly important, since both events occur postnatally in humans and might be use-dependent. With the exception of myelination the other stages of axonal differentiation take place largely in utero and might be affected by prenatal events.

It is important to stress that the kind of plasticity exhibited by callosal axons in animal experiments is not necessarily of an adaptive kind. None of the animals with callosally modified connections have been tested in this respect. It should also be noticed that the information on the cellular mechanisms involved in the development of callosal connections is still extremely scanty. In particular, with the exception of preliminary studies on the maturation of some cytoskeletal proteins (reviewed in Innocenti, 1991), the biochemical events involved in the elimination or maintenance of callosal connections remain to be elucidated.

ACKNOWLEDGMENTS Supported by Swiss National Science Foundation grant 3100-039707.93 and Swedish Medical Research Council grant 12594. We wish to thank Mr. Philippe Gaudard, Mr. Eric Bernardi, and Mrs. Kristina Ingvarsson for their help at various stages in the preparation of this manuscript. This chapter was prepared in 1997 and partially updated in 1999.

REFERENCES

AGGOUN-ZOUAOUI, D., and G. M. INNOCENTI, 1994. Juvenile visual callosal axons in kittens display origin- and fate-related morphology and distribution of arbors. *Eur. J. Neurosci.* 6:1846–1863.

AGGOUN-ZOUAOUI, D., D. C. KIPER, and G. M. INNOCENTI, 1996. Growth of callosal terminal arbors in primary visual areas of the cat. *Eur. J. Neurosci.* 8:1132–1148.

ALLENDOERFER, K. L., and C. J. SHATZ, 1994. The subplate, a transient neocortical structure: Its role in the development of connections between thalamus and cortex. *Ann. Rev. Neurosci.* 17:185–218.

BENNETT, M. V. L., 1968. Neural control of electric organs. In *The Central Nervous System and Fish Behavior*, D. Ingle, ed. Chicago: The University of Chicago, pp. 147–169.

BERBEL, P., and G. M. INNOCENTI, 1988. The development of the corpus callosum in cats: A light and electron-microscopic study. *J. Comp. Neurol.* 276:132–156.

BERLUCCHI, G., and G. RIZZOLATTI, 1968. Binocularly driven neurons in visual cortex of split-chiasm cats. *Science* 159:308–310.

BOIRE, D., R. MORRIS, M. PTITO, F. LEPORE, and D. O. FROST, 1995. Effects of neonatal splitting of the optic chiasm on the development of feline visual callosal connections. *Exp. Brain Res.* 104:275–286.

BOURGEOIS, J.-P., and P. RAKIC, 1993. Changes of synaptic density in the primary visual cortex of the macaque monkey from fetal to adult stage. *J. Neurosci.* 13:2801–2820.

BOYD, J., and J. MATSUBARA, 1994. Tangential organization of callosal connectivity in the cat's visual cortex. *J. Comp. Neurol.* 347:197–210.

BRESSOUD, R., and G. M. INNOCENTI, 1999. Typology, early differentiation, and exuberant growth of a set of cortical axons. *J. Comp. Neurol.* 406:87–108.

CAMINITI, R., and G. M. INNOCENTI, 1981. The postnatal development of somatosensory callosal connections after partial lesions of somatosensory areas. *Exp. Brain Res.* 42:53–62.

CAMINITI, R., G. M. INNOCENTI, and T. MANZONI, 1979. The anatomical substrate of callosal messages from SI and SII in the cat. *Exp. Brain Res.* 35:295–314.

CARR, C. E., 1993. Processing of temporal information in the brain. *Ann. Rev. Neurosci.* 16:223–243.

CARR, C. E., and M. KONISHI, 1990. A circuit for detection of interaural time differences in the brain stem of the barn owl. *J. Neurosci.* 10:3227–3246.

CHALUPA, L. M., and H. P. KILLACKEY, 1989. Process elimination underlies ontogenetic change in the distribution of callosal projection neurons in the postcentral gyrus of the fetal rhesus monkey. *Proc. Natl. Acad. Sci. U.S.A.* 86:1076–1079.

CONTI, F., and T. MANZONI, 1994. The neurotransmitters and postsynaptic actions of callosally projecting neurons. *Behav. Brain Res.* 64:37–53.

CUSIK, C. G., and R. D. LUND, 1982. Modification of visual callosal projections in rats. *J. Comp. Neurol.* 212:385–398.

CYNADER, M., F. LEPORÉ, and J.-P. GUILLEMOT, 1981. Interhemispheric competition during postnatal development. *Nature* 290:139–140.

DING, S.-L., and A. J. ELBERGER, 1994. Confirmation of the existence of transitory corpus callosum axons in area 17 of neonatal cat: An anterograde tracing study using biotinylated dextran amine. *Neurosci. Lett.* 177:66–70.

ELBERGER, A. J., 1994. The corpus callosum provides a massive transitory input to the visual cortex of the cat and rat during early postnatal development. *Behav. Brain Res.* 64:15–23.

ENGEL, A. K., P. KÖNIG, A. K. KREITER, and W. SINGER, 1991. Interhemispheric synchronization of oscillatory neuronal responses in cat visual cortex. *Science* 252:1177–1179.

FISH, S. E., R. W. RHOADES, C. A. BENNETT-CLARKE, B. FIGLEY, and R. D. MOONEY, 1991. Organization, development and enucleation-induced alterations in the visual callosal projection of the hamster: single axon tracing with Phaseolus vulgaris leucoagglutinin and Di-I. *Eur. J. Neurosci.* 3:1255–1270.

GILBERT, C. D., and T. N. WIESEL, 1989. Columnar specificity of intrinsic horizontal and corticocortical connections in cat visual cortex. *J. Neurosci.* 9:2432–2442.

HALLORAN, M. C., and K. KALIL, 1994. Dynamic behaviors of growth cones extending in the corpus callosum of living cortical brain slices observed with video microscopy. *J. Neurosci.* 14:2161–2177.

HOUZEL, J.-C., C. MILLERET, and G. INNOCENTI, 1994. Morphology of callosal axons interconnecting areas 17 and 18 of the cat. *Eur. J. Neurosci.* 6:898–917.

HUBEL, D. H., and T. N. WIESEL, 1967. Cortical and callosal connections concerned with the vertical meridian of visual fields in the cat. *J. Neurophysiol.* 30:1561–1573.

HUGHES, C. M., and A. PETERS, 1992. Symmetric synapses formed by callosal afferents in rat visual cortex. *Brain Res.* 583:271–278.

INNOCENTI, G. M., 1978. Postnatal development of interhemispheric connections of the cat visual cortex. *Arch. Ital. Biol.* 116:463–470.

INNOCENTI, G. M., 1980. The primary visual pathway through the corpus callosum: Morphological and functional aspects in the cat. *Arch. Ital. Biol.* 118:124–188.

INNOCENTI, G. M., 1986. General organization of callosal connections in the cerebral cortex. In *Cerebral Cortex*, Vol. 5, E. G. Jones and A. Peters, eds. New York: Plenum Publishing Corporation, pp. 291–353.

INNOCENTI, G. M., 1991. The development of projections from cerebral cortex. In *Progress in Sensory Physiology*, Vol. 12. Berlin: Springer-Verlag, pp. 65–114.

INNOCENTI, G. M., 1994. Computational structure of central nervous system axons reflects developmental strategies. In *Structural and functional organization of the neocortex*, B. Albowitz, K. Albus, U. Kuhnt, H.-C. Nothdurf, and P. Wahle, eds. Berlin: Springer-Verlag, pp. 49–59.

INNOCENTI, G. M., 1995. Exuberant development of connections, and its possible permissive role in cortical evolution. *TINS* 18:397–402.

INNOCENTI, G. M., D. AGGOUN-ZOUAOUI, and P. LEHMANN, 1995. Cellular aspects of callosal connections and their development. *Neuropsychologia* 33:961–987.

INNOCENTI, G. M., and P. BERBEL, 1991. Analysis of an experimental cortical network: II. Connections of visual areas 17 and 18 after neonatal injections of ibotenic acid. *J. Neural Transplant. Plast.* 2:29–54.

INNOCENTI, G. M., and L. FIORE, 1976. Morphological correlates of visual field transformation in the corpus callosum. *Neurosci. Lett.* 4:245–252.

INNOCENTI, G. M., D. O. FROST, and J. ILLES, 1985. Maturation of visual callosal connections in visually deprived kittens: A challenging critical period. *J. Neurosci.* 5:255–267.

INNOCENTI, G. M., P. LEHMANN, and J.-C. HOUZEL, 1994. Computational structure of visual callosal axons. *Eur. J. Neurosci.* 6:918–935.

KENNEDY, H., C. DEHAY, and J. BULLIER, 1986. Organization of the callosal connections of visual areas VI and V2 in the macaque monkey. *J. Comp. Neurol.* 247:398–415.

KENNEDY, H., C. MEISSIREL, and C. DEHAY, 1991. Callosal pathways and their compliance to general rules governing the organization of corticocortical connectivity. In *Vision and visual dysfunction*, Vol. 3: *Neuroanatomy of the visual pathways and their development*, B. Dreher and S. Robinson, eds. London: Macmillan, pp. 324–359.

KIPER, D. C., M. G. KNYAZEVA, L. TETTONI, and G. M. INNOCENTI, 1999. Visual stimulus dependent changes in interhemispheric EEG coherence in ferrets. *J. Neurophysiol.* 82:3082–3084.

KNYAZEVA, M. G., D. C. KIPER, V. Y. VILDAVSKI, P. A. DESPLANDS, M. MAEDER-INGVAR, and G. M. INNOCENTI, 1999. Visual-stimulus-dependent changes in interhemispheric EEG coherence in humans. *J. Neurophysiol.* 82:3095–3107.

KOESTER, S. E., and D. D. M. O'LEARY, 1993. Connectional distinction between callosal and subcortical projecting cortical neurons is determined prior to axon extension. *Dev. Biol.* 160:1–14.

KOESTER, S. E., and D. D. M. O'LEARY, 1994. Axons of early generated neurons in cingulate cortex pioneer the corpus callosum. *J. Neurosci.* 14:6608–6620.

KORALEK, K.-A., and B. P. KILLACKEY, 1990. Callosal projections in rat somatosensory cortex are altered by early removal of afferents input. *Proc. Natl. Acad. Sci. U.S.A.* 87:1396–1400.

LaMANTIA, A.-S., and P. RAKIC, 1990a. Cytological and quantitative characteristics of four cerebral commissures in the rhesus monkey. *J. Comp. Neurol.* 291:520–537.

LaMANTIA, A.-S., and P. RAKIC, 1990b. Axon overproduction and elimination in the corpus callosum of the developing rhesus monkey. *J. Neurosci.* 10:2156–2175.

LEVY, J., C. TREVARTHEN, and R. W. SPERRY, 1972. Perception of bilateral chimeric figures following hemispheric deconnexion. *Brain* 95:61–78.

LIVINGSTONE, M. S., and D. H. HUBEL, 1987. Psychophysical evidence for separate channels for the perception of form, color, movement, and depth. *J. Neurosci.* 10:2156–2175.

LOWEL, S., and W. SINGER, 1992. Selection of intrinsic horizontal connections in the visual cortex by correlated neuronal activity. *Science* 255:209–212.

McCOURT, M. E., J. THALLURI, and G. H. HENRY, 1990. Properties of area 17/18 border neurons contributing to the visual transcallosal pathway in the cat. *Visual Neurosci.* 5:83–98.

MELZER, P., L. A. ROTHBLATT, and G. M. INNOCENTI, 1987. Lesions involving the optic radiation in kittens modify the postnatal development of corticocortical connections. *Neuroscience* 22:S223.

MILLER, B., M. S. WINDREM, and B. L. FINLAY, 1991. Thalamic ablations and neocortical development: Alterations in thalamic and callosal connectivity. *Cereb. Cortex* 1:241–261.

NORRIS, C. R., and K. KALIL, 1991. Guidance of callosal axons by radial glia in the developing cerebral cortex. *J. Neurosci.* 11:3481–3492.

NORRIS, C. R., and K. KALIL, 1992. Development of callosal

connections in the sensorimotor cortex of the hamster. *J. Comp. Neurol.* 326:121–132.

NOWAK, L. G., M. H. J. MUNK, J. I. NELSON, A. C. JAMES, and J. BULLIER, 1995. Structural basis of cortical synchronization. 1: Three types of interhemispheric coupling. *J. Neurophysiol.* 74:2379–2400.

OLAVARRIA, J. F., 1996. Non-mirror-symmetric patterns of callosal linkages in area 17 and 18 in cat visual cortex. *J. Comp. Neurol.* 366:643–655.

OLAVARRIA, J. F., and P. L. ABEL, 1996. The distribution of callosal connections correlates with the pattern of cytochrome oxidase stripes in visual area V2 of macaque monkeys. *Cereb. Cortex* 6:631–639.

OZAKI, H. S., and D. WAHLSTEN, 1993. Cortical axon trajectories and growth cone morphologies in fetuses of acallosal mouse strains. *J. Comp. Neurol.* 336:595–604.

PALLAS, S. L., T. LITTMAN, and D. MOORE, 1999. Cross-modal reorganization of callosal connectivity without altering thalamocortical projections. *Proc. Natl. Acad. Sci U.S.A.* 96:8751–8756.

PAYNE, B. R., 1994. Neuronal interactions in cat visual cortex mediated by the corpus callosum. *Behav. Brain Res.* 64:55–64.

RHOADES, R. W., S. E. FISH, R. D. MOONEY, and N. L. CHIAIA, 1987. Distribution of visual callosal projection neurons in hamsters subjected to transection of the optic radiations on the day of birth. *Dev. Brain Res.* 32:217–232.

RINGO, J. L., R. W. DOTY, S. DEMETER, and P. Y. SIMARD, 1994. Time is of the essence: A conjecture that hemispheric specialization arises from interhemispheric conduction delay. *Cereb. Cortex* 4:331–343.

ROSEN, G. D., G. F. SHERMAN, and A. M. GALABURDA, 1989. Interhemispheric connections differ between symmetrical and asymmetrical brain regions. *Neuroscience* 33:525–533.

SCHMIDT, K. E., D.-S. KIM, W. SINGER, T. BONHOEFFER, and S. LOWEL, 1997. Functional specificity of long-range intrinsic and interhemispheric connections in the visual cortex of strabismic cats. *J. Neurosci.* 17:5480–5492.

SCHWARTZ, M. L., and P. S. GOLDMANN-RAKIC, 1991. Prenatal specification of callosal connections in rhesus monkey. *J. Comp. Neurol.* 307:144–162.

SEGRAVES, M. A., and G. M. INNOCENTI, 1985. Comparison of the distributions of ipsilaterally and contralaterally projecting corticocortical neurons in cat visual cortex using two fluorescent tracers. *J. Neurosci.* 5:2107–2118.

SEGRAVES, N. M., and A. C. ROSENQUIST, 1982. The afferent and efferent callosal connections of retinotopically defined areas in cat cortex. *J. Neurosci.* 2:1090–1107.

SILVER, J., M. A. EDWARDS, and P. LEVITT, 1993. Imnmunocytochemical demonstration of early appearing astroglial structures that form boundaries and pathways along axon tracts in the fetal brain. *J. Comp. Neurol.* 328:415–436.

SILVER, J., S. E. LORENZ, D. WAHLSTEN, and J. COUGHLIN, 1982. Axonal guidance during development of the great cerebral commissures: Descriptive and experimental studies, in vivo, on the role of preformed glial pathways. *J. Comp. Neurol.* 210:10–29.

SINGER, W., 1995. Time as coding space in neocortical processing: a hypothesis. In *The cognitive neurosciences*, M. S. Gazzaniga, ed. Cambridge, MA/London, GB: MIT Press, pp. 91–104.

SOFTKY, W., 1994. Sub-millisecond coincidence detection in active dendritic trees. *Neuroscience* 58:13–41.

SOFTKY, W., and C. KOCH, 1993. The highly irregular firing of cortical cells is inconsistent with temporal integration of random EPSPS. *J. Neurosci.* 13:334–350.

STANFORD, L. R., 1987. Conduction velocity variations minimize conduction time differences among retinal ganglion cell axons. *Science* 238:358–360.

SUGIHARA, I., E. J. LANG, and R. LLINAS, 1993. Uniform olivocerebellar conduction time underlies Purkinje cell complex spike synchronicity in the rat cerebellum. *J. Physiol.* 470:243–271.

TETTONI, L., P. LEHMANN, J.-C. HOUZEL, and G. M. INNOCENTI, 1996. Maxsim, software for the analysis of multiple axonal arbors and their simulated activation. *J. Neurosci. Methods* 67:1–9.

ZUFFEREY, P. D., F. JIN, K. NAKAMURA, L. TETTONI, and G. M. INNOCENTI, 1999. The role of pattern vision in the development of cortico-cortical connections. *Eur. J. Neurosci.* 11:2669–2688.

COMMENTARY 1.1

The Effects of Early Injury to the Cortical Plate on Callosal Connectivity

GLENN D. ROSEN

In their paper, Innocenti and Bressoud elegantly describe the development and final disposition of individual callosal axons. They emphasize that these axons rarely subsume point-to-point interactions between homologous regions of the cerebral cortex but probably activate distinct neuronal populations (Houzel, Milleret, and Innocenti, 1994; Innocenti, Aggoun-Zouaoui, and Lehmann, 1995). Using simulations, Innocenti and colleagues further point out that as far as optimal spatiotemporal resolution is concerned, these elaborate patterns of axonal arborization are not the "most economical" possible and are therefore most likely the result of sequential processes of exuberance and retraction during development (Innocenti, Lehmann, and Houzel, 1994). Toward that end, four stages of callosal development are outlined, each of which is characterized by these periods of exuberance and specification. Further, at each of these stages, there are a number of intrinsic and extrinsic factors that can affect the eventual disposition of axonal arbors (Innocenti, 1995). In this commentary I will concentrate on one of these factors: the effects of early damage to the cerebral cortex on the formation of callosal connectivity.

It has long been known that damage to the brain during development affects typical patterns of neuronal connectivity. In hamsters, unilateral neonatal lesions of the superior colliculus result in restructuring of afferent connections (Schneider, 1981). Specifically, these lesions cause optic fibers to cross the midline, where they compete successfully for available terminal space in the intact superior colliculus. In monkeys, prenatal unilateral

removal of portions of the frontal cortex results in significant displacement of connections (Goldman and Galkin, 1978). There is additional evidence that neuropathological events occurring during the period of neuronal migration to the cortex might have profound effects both on the eventual laminar disposition of neurons and on the patterns of intrinsic connectivity. For example, injection of ibotenic acid into the visual cortex of cats on postnatal days 2 and 3 causes death primarily of infragranular neurons and the subsequent formation of microgyric-like cortex (Innocenti and Berbel, 1991a). Furthermore, this microgyric cortex receives projections from auditory areas AI and AII—projections that are normally eliminated during development (Innocenti and Berbel, 1991b). Cerebral hypoxia, induced by neonatal carotid ligation in cats, results in a marked increase in efferent projections from visual cortex to the opposite hemisphere (Miller et al., 1993). Finally, disturbed interhemispheric connectivity has been associated with a spontaneously occurring microgyrus in the rat (Rosen et al., 1989a). Specifically, four-layered cortex was seen surrounding a microsulcus consisting of infolded, fused molecular layers and containing ectopic neurons. The pattern of callosal termination within this microgyrus did not show the normal pattern of lamination; in its place was a band of dense axonal termination with projection-rich bridges to deeper cortical layers (Rosen et al., 1989a).

Because spontaneously occurring microgyria are rare in experimental animal species, a method for inducing a microgyrus would be a useful tool to further evaluate the connectional consequences of focal cortical lesions during neuronal migration. Regions of focal cerebrocortical microgyria are reliably induced in neonatal rat neocortex by placement of a freezing probe on the skulls of newborn rats (Dvorák and Feit, 1977; Humphreys et al., 1991). We have explored the effect of these induced microgyria on patterns of interhemispheric connectivity in

GLENN D. ROSEN Dyslexia Research Laboratory and Charles A. Dana Research Institute, Beth Israel Deaconess Medical Center; Division of Behavioral Neurology, Beth Israel Deaconess Medical Center, Boston, Massachusetts; Harvard Medical School, Boston, Massachusetts.

two series of experiments. In the first experiment, we cut the corpora callosa of microgyric rats and stained for degenerating axon terminals; in the second experiment, we injected tracers (biotinylated dextran amine: BDA) directly into microgyria and into homologous regions of the opposite hemisphere.

The first of the series of experiments showed that the most obvious changes in the patterns of callosal axonal terminations occurred in and around the areas of the neocortical microgyria. There was an increase in the density of callosal terminations in the microgyrus when it was located in an area that normally received callosal terminations. In general, however, this increase was not as striking as that seen in the previously reported spontaneous microgyrus (Rosen et al., 1989a). Exuberant patches of callosal termination were found immediately medial or lateral to the region of microdysgenesis that either were not seen in homologous regions of control brains or were gross distortions of patches that were normally present. There was a decrease in the pattern of axonal terminations in the entire contralateral hemisphere when compared either to controls or to the patterns of termination within the ipsilateral hemisphere. Areas lateral to the homologous regions also showed a relative decrease in axonal degeneration, although there was relative preservation of callosal terminations in areas medial to the homologous area (Rosen et al., 1989b).

To confirm and extend these findings, we injected an in vivo tracer (BDA) into the microgyric and control cortices of adult animals. In these animals the microgyria were placed into the primary somatosensory cortex (Par1, HL, and FL; after Zilles, 1985). In general, we found patterns of interhemispheric connectivity that were consistent with the results reported above. In comparison to controls, there was an overall decrease in efferent projections from the microgyric cortex to the opposite hemisphere. A finding of perhaps greater interest involved the specific locations of the callosal patterns of termination in the microgyric animals. In control (sham lesioned) cases we found the expected results, namely, that homotopic callosal projections were the rule. In the microgyric cases, on the other hand, we found appropriately directed connections to homotopic areas in some but not all rats. Thus, there was often a significant diminution or complete absence of homotopic callosal fibers in the opposite hemisphere. In addition, heterotopic projections to frontal and secondary sensorimotor cortices were noted. These heterotopic projections were particularly notable for their density and for the fact that they were rarely seen in control subjects. Finally, projections from homotopic regions in the hemisphere opposite to the malformation terminated

densely most often in the medial portions of the microgyrus or avoided it entirely (Rosen et al., 2000).

These results may best be considered in the light of knowledge of the ontogeny of callosal connectivity. During early development, callosal cells of origin are represented diffusely in the neocortex (Innocenti and Clarke, 1984), and as the brain matures, they become restricted to discrete columnar and laminar locations. Axons of these cells cross the midline of the corpus callosum between P0 and P3 in the rat. They are diffusely distributed beneath the cortical plate until they begin to penetrate it widely (but not homogeneously) between P3 and P6 and reach their mature pattern by P12. This progressive restriction of both callosal cells of origin and their terminations is thought to result from axonal pruning rather than from the death of neurons. It is therefore possible that the increase in afferent connectivity to these injured areas could be the result of the preservation of processes that would normally be eliminated. Nerve growth factor and other trophic factors are released during injury to nervous tissue, and the presence of such trophic factors in the area of a lesion may diminish ontogenetic axonal pruning. The increased number of callosally projecting neurons that are seen in the cats with carotid ligation would presumably also reflect increased survival of developmentally transient projections, a phenomenon that is directly demonstrated by Innocenti and Berbel (1991b) in ibotenic-injected cats.

Alternatively, it could be that the increase in heterotopic connections is the result of increased sprouting of axodendritic processes. If increased sprouting were the primary cause of the increase, then one would not expect differences in the number of neurons projecting to the lesioned area from the opposite hemisphere when compared to the projections seen in undamaged brains. Although we have not addressed this issue in these experiments, Miller and colleagues have seen an increase in such callosally projecting neurons to hypoxic-ischemic visual cortex (Miller et al., 1993). On the other hand, in the current paper, Innocenti shows that the presence of heterotopic callosal projections in visual cortices can result from axonal sprouting. Although we can't yet make definitive statements, it appears unlikely that axonal sprouting alone is a major factor in the increase of afferent connections to the damaged hemisphere.

Finally, these abnormal connections might reflect transient projections that are normally eliminated during development or perhaps the introduction of novel projections by the release of some trophic factor associated with the cortical injury. As was mentioned above, Innocenti and Berbel (1991b) have demonstrated the maintenance of otherwise transient projections following induction of microgyria in the visual cortex of cats. We have not conducted the experiments to determine whether there is maintenance of transient projections in this system or whether novel projections are induced by the induction of microgyria.

Areas of focal microdysgenesis and microgyria are seen in individuals with developmental dyslexia (Galaburda et al., 1985). It had been hypothesized that these focal developmental abnormalities are related to the cognitive deficits of dyslexia, either because they directly provoke cerebral reorganization even at a distance or because their presence serves as an indicator of such reorganization stemming from an (as yet) unidentified common etiologic factor. The results outlined here lend some support to the first of these two possibilities.

ACKNOWLEDGMENTS The work reported in this commentary was supported, in part, by Grant HD20806 from the Public Health Service of the United States. Thanks also go to my collaborators, Albert M. Galaburda, Gordon F. Sherman, Peter Humphreys, and Deborah Burstein.

REFERENCES

DVORÁK, K., and J. FEIT, 1977. Migration of neuroblasts through partial necrosis of the cerebral cortex in newborn rats: Contribution to the problems of morphological development and developmental period of cerebral microgyria. *Acta Neuropathol. (Berl.)* 38:203–212.

GALABURDA, A. M., G. F. SHERMAN, G. D. ROSEN, F. ABOITIZ, and N. GESCHWIND, 1985. Developmental dyslexia: Four consecutive cases with cortical anomalies. *Ann. Neurol.* 18:222–233.

GOLDMAN, P. S., and T. W. GALKIN, 1978. Prenatal removal of frontal association cortex in the fetal rhesus monkey: Anatomical and functional consequences in postnatal life. *Brain Res.* 152:451–485.

HOUZEL, J.-C., C. MILLERET, and G. INNOCENTI, 1994. Morphology of callosal axons interconnecting areas 17 and 18 of the cat. *Eur. J. Neurosci.* 6:898–917.

HUMPHREYS, P., G. D. ROSEN, D. M. PRESS, G. F. SHERMAN, and A. M. GALABURDA, 1991. Freezing lesions of the newborn rat brain: A model for cerebrocortical microgyria. *J. Neuropathol. Exp. Neurol.* 50:145–160.

INNOCENTI, G. M., 1995. Exuberant development of connections, and its possible permissive role in cortical evolution. *Trends Neurosci.* 18:397–402.

INNOCENTI, G. M., D. AGGOUN-ZOUAOUI, and P. LEHMANN, 1995. Cellular aspects of callosal connections and their development. *Neuropsychologia* 33:961.

INNOCENTI, G. M., and P. BERBEL, 1991a. Analysis of an experimental cortical network: I. Architectonics of visual areas 17 and 18 after neonatal injections of ibotenic acid; similarities with human microgyria. *J. Neur. Transplant.* 2:1–28.

INNOCENTI, G. M., and P. BERBEL, 1991b. Analysis of an experimental cortical network: II. Connections of visual areas 17 and 18 after neonatal injections of ibotenic acid. *J. Neur. Transplant.* 2:29–54.

INNOCENTI, G. M., and S. CLARKE, 1984. The organization of immature callosal connections. *J. Comp. Neurol.* 230:287–309.

INNOCENTI, G. M., P. LEHMANN, and J.-C. HOUZEL, 1994. Computational structure of visual callosal axons. *Eur. J. Neurosci.* 6:918–935.

MILLER, B., D. NAGY, B. L. FINLAY, B. CHANCE, A. KOBAYASHI, and S. NIOKA, 1993. Consequences of reduced cerebral blood flow in brain development: I. Gross morphology, histology, and callosal connectivity. *Exp. Neurol.* 124:326–342.

ROSEN, G. D., D. BURSTEIN, and A. M. GALABURDA, 2000. Changes in efferent and afferent connectivity in rats with cerebrocortical microgyria. *J. Comp. Neurol.* 418:423–440.

ROSEN, G. D., A. M. GALABURDA, and G. F. SHERMAN, 1989a. Cerebrocortical microdysgenesis with anomalous callosal connections: A case study in the rat. *Int. J. Neurosci.* 47:237–247.

ROSEN, G. D., P. HUMPHREYS, G. F. SHERMAN, and A. M. GALABURDA, 1989b. Connectional anomalies associated with freezing lesions to the neocortex of the newborn rat. *Soc. Neurosci. Abstr.* 15:1120.

SCHNEIDER, G. E., 1981. Early lesions and abnormal neuronal connections. *Trends Neurosci.* 4:187–192.

ZILLES, K., 1985. *The Cortex of the Rat: A Stereotaxic Atlas.* Berlin: Springer-Verlag.

COMMENTARY 1.2

Binocular Input Elimination and the Reshaping of Callosal Connection

MAURICE PTITO AND DENIS BOIRE

Innocenti and Broussoud have has presented a fascinating series of experiments showing how callosal axons grow and form adult connections. They further stress that these connections perform specific transformations of the callosal cortical maps that are, in a broad sense, of a computational nature. The callosal connections develop through a period of exuberance in which many more axons project in the corpus callosum of the growing organism than in adulthood. It is well known that the manipulation of the visual environment affects the development of visual callosal connections. Various experimental conditions performed on neonates, such as dark rearing (with bilateral eyelid suture or bilateral enucleation or with alternating monocular occlusion), produce a subnormal number of callosally projecting neurons in areas 17 and 18 of the cerebral cortex. In addition, an abnormally wide distribution of callosal neurons in the primary visual cortex has been observed following enucleation, whereas rearing in the dark and lid suture result in a somewhat narrower than normal distribution (see Boire et al., 1995, for a review). This widespread distribution of callosally projecting neurons in areas 17 and 18 has also been observed in surgically induced strabismus, monocular enucleation, and monocular eyelid suture in kittens. It thus seems that visual experience does influence the distribution of callosal neurons by modulating the developmental elimination of some immature callosal axons, which normally leads to a characteristically restricted tangential distribution of callosal neurons (see reviews by Innocenti, 1986, 1994). Boire et al. (1995) have previously studied the

role in callosal development of binocular input to the visual cortex, and we will report here some of the anatomical data obtained in split-chiasm kittens as to the number and distribution of callosally projecting neurons in areas 17 and 18.

The section of the optic chiasm at the midline in the adult cat eliminates a large amount of retinal projections to the contralateral lateral geniculate nucleus (LGN) and hence to the visual cortex. The visual information entering one eye is, in this condition, restricted to the ipsilateral hemisphere. However, that information, stemming from the temporal hemiretina, can be relayed to the contralateral hemisphere via the corpus callosum (see Chapter 6 in this book for a review). Binocularity is still maintained in the callosal recipient zone, although the number of binocularly driven cells is dramatically reduced (Berlucchi and Rizzolatti, 1968). In kittens, splitting the chiasmatic decussation results in less severe physiological and behavioral deficits (see Boire et al., 1995, for a review) and might be suggestive of a rearrangement of callosal connections.

Methods

The anatomical methods used in this experiment have been previously described (Boire et al., 1995) and will be only briefly presented here. Four kittens at 12 days old, under deep general anesthesia, underwent the splitting of the optic chiasm (OC) using a transbuccal approach (Boire et al., 1995). They were then raised in the animal colony for about 759 days. They received large unilateral injections of horseradish peroxydase (40% HRP, 10–12 0.5-μl injections) in the visual cortex so as to retrogradely label the callosally projecting neurons in the opposite hemisphere (Innocenti and Frost, 1980). Following a two-day survival period, the animals were deeply anesthetized and transcardially perfused. The brains were then dissected, stored overnight in 30% su-

MAURICE PTITO   Ecole d'Optometrie, Université de Montréal, Montreal, Quebec, Canada; Department of Neurology and Neurosurgery, Montreal Neurological Institute, McGill University, Montreal, Quebec, Canada.

DENIS BOIRE   Ecole d'Optometrie, Université de Montréal, Montreal, Quebec, Canada.

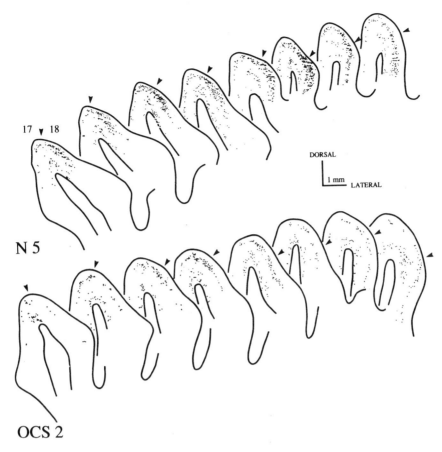

FIGURE 1.9. Distribution of HRP-labeled callosal neurons in coronal sections through areas 17 and 18 of one normal (N5) and one split chiasm cat (OCS 2). Note the abundance of callosal cells in the supragranular layers compared to the infragranular ones.

crose, and sectioned while frozen in the coronal plane at 80 μm. A one in two series of sections was then reacted for HRP histochemistry using the tetramethyl benzidine technique (Mesulam, 1978) to visualize the retrogradely filled callosal cells while the other series was stained with cresyl violet to confirm the completeness of the optic chiasm split.

In all brains, HRP-labeled callosal neurons in a series of sections spaced 320 μm apart and encompassing the caudal 13–15 mm of the cortex were charted at 250× using a computer-controlled microscope. We also measured for each brain the mediolateral width of the cortical volume containing callosal neurons (the callosal efferent zone or CZ) at the three levels that divide the rostrocaudal extent of area 17 into four equal parts.

Results

The distribution of labeled callosal cells in normal adult cats was compared with that obtained in the split-chiasm ones. In normal cats, callosal neurons form a band run-ning rostrocaudally along the border between areas 17 and 18 and extending 1–3 mm either side of the border. In areas 17 and 18, callosal neurons are distributed in two radially separated, superposed laminae in layers III and IV (supragranular layers or subzone a) and layer VI (infragranular layer or subzone c). Neurons in the two subzones were easily distinguished, and the two subdivisions are illustrated in Figure 1.9. There are many more callosal neurons in subzone a than in subzone c, the average number of neurons per section in subzones a and c being 263.5 and 39.1, respectively.

In the split-chiasm cats the radial distribution of callosal cells in areas 17 and 18, as illustrated in Figure 1.9 (OCS 2), is not altered by the surgery. As in normal cats, callosal cells are distributed in two distinct, radially separated, superposed laminae in layers III/IV and layer VI. The callosal efferent zone in areas 17 and 18 contains 29.2% of the normal number of labeled callosal neurons in subzone a and 94.3% of the normal number in subzone c. The average number of retrogradely labeled cells per section in subzones a and c of the split-chiasm cats was 77.04 and 36.86, respectively. It thus

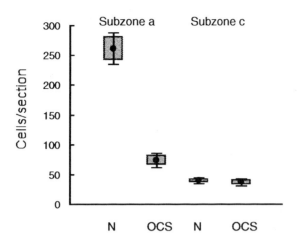

FIGURE 1.10. Box-and-whisker plot showing the mean number of HRP-labeled callosal neurons per section in areas 17 and 18 of normal and OCS cats. Note the drastic reduction of callosal cells in subzone a of the split-chiasm cats. Box: 95% confidence interval; whiskers: 99% confidence interval.

in the supragranular layers of areas 17–18 and leaves intact the number of callosal cells in the infragranular layers. This reduction in the number of callosal neurons in the visual cortex is similar to what has been found in visual deprivation experiments such as binocular eyelid suture (Innocenti and Frost, 1980) and seems to be related to the natural postnatal reshaping of callosal connections, that is, the elimination of axons that cortical neurons transiently send through the corpus callosum (Berbel and Innocenti, 1988). The neonatal section of the optic chiasm may exaggerate this normal elimination of callosal axons. Our results support such an assumption based on the observations that (1) the most significant effect of early chiasmatomy happens when the optic chiasm is split before the stabilization/elimination process is complete and (2) that subzone a is postnatally the principal source of transient callosal projections and undergoes much more severe natural reduction that does subzone c (Innocenti and Caminiti, 1980).

seems that subzone a is much more affected than subzone c (Figure 1.10).

Concerning the tangential distribution of callosally projecting neurons, we demonstrated that for both normal and split-chiasm cats, the density of cells peaked near the 17/18 border and diminished progressively with increasing distance from the border (see Figure 1.9). The callosal zone, for both groups of animals, is relatively wide in the caudal 3 mm of the cortex and progressively narrows further rostrally. However, in the split-chiasm cats, the mediolateral width of subzone a appears to be somewhat less than in normal animals, particularly in the rostral portion. The mean width of the callosal zone for the operated animals was 4.51 mm, and that for the normals was 5.96 mm. Although it seemed that the callosal zone for the split-chiasm cats was narrower than that for normal animals, the difference was not statistically significant.

Discussion

Neonatal section of the optic chiasm produces a loss of about 70% of the normal population of callosal neurons

REFERENCES

BERBEL, P., and G. M. INNOCENTI, 1988. The development of the corpus callosum in cats: A light- and electron-microscopic study. *J. Comp. Neurol.* 276:132–156.

BERLUCCHI, G., and G. RIZZOLATTI, 1968. Binocularly driven neurons in visual cortex of split-chiasm cats. *Science* 159:308–310.

BOIRE, D., R. MORRIS, M. PTITO, F. LEPORE, and D. FROST, 1995. Effects of neonatal splitting of the optic chiasm on the development of feline visual callosal connections. *Exp. Brain Res.* 104:275–286.

INNOCENTI, G., 1986. General organization of callosal connections in the cerebral cortex. In *Cerebral Cortex*, Vol. 5, E. G. Jones and A. Peters, eds. New York: Plenum, pp. 291–353.

INNOCENTI, G., 1994. Some new trends in the study of the corpus callosum. *Behav. Brain Res.* 64:1–8.

INNOCENTI, G. M., and R. CAMINITI, 1980. Postnatal shaping of callosal connections from sensory areas. *Exp. Brain Res.* 38:381–394.

INNOCENTI, G. M., and D. O. FROST, 1980. The postnatal development of visual callosal connections in the absence of visual experience or of the eyes. *Exp. Brain Res.* 39:365–375.

MESULAM, M. M., 1978. Tetramethyl benzidine for horseradish peroxydase neurohistochemistry: A non-carcinogenic blue reaction product with superior sensitivity for visualizing neural afferents and efferents. *J. Histochem. Cytochem.* 26:106–117.

2 Corpus Callosum Morphology in Relation to Cerebral Asymmetries in the Postmortem Human

FRANCISCO ABOITIZ, ANDRÉS IDE, AND RICARDO OLIVARES

ABSTRACT In this chapter we present data of fine callosal structure in postmortem humans revealing regional differences in fiber composition that indicate differences in interhemispheric transfer between primary/secondary sensorimotor areas, on the one hand, and higher-order cortical regions, on the other. In addition, we review evidence from studies concerning a negative relation between interhemispheric communication and brain lateralization in the human as indexed by anatomical asymmetry in the Sylvian fissure and on individual differences in this relation. Since the topic of anatomical asymmetry in perisylvian regions is now a debated issue, it is necessary to delve into some details about the morphology of the Sylvian fissure. Therefore, the chapter begins with a review of callosal anatomy in the postmortem human at both the macroscopic and microscopic levels, continues with a critical review of the current status of anatomical asymmetry in the posterior language region and its relationship to callosal structure, and ends with an evolutionary discussion of the original role of the corpus callosum in placental mammals and its possible participation in the generation of lateralization in the human brain.

Among other things, the brain of placental mammals is unique in that it bears a main fiber tract connecting the two cerebral hemispheres: the corpus callosum. In the human this tract consists of possibly more than 200,000,000 fibers (Aboitiz et al., 1992a). Comparing this number with the approximately 1,000,000 fibers in the optic nerve gives an idea of the potential complexity of interactions that may occur during interhemispheric interaction. However, fundamental questions, such as the adaptive value of the corpus callosum or what role may callosal function play in the development and the

evolutionary origin of brain lateralization, are still matters of debate.

In this context we will address two related problems regarding the role of the corpus callosum in brain function. The first is the question of what the advantage of having a corpus callosum is to placental mammals. The obvious answer is interhemispheric communication. But why is interhemispheric communication so important to them? There are many large-brained species among reptiles, birds, monotremes (the platypus and the echidna), and marsupials that seem to do well with a much more limited extent of interhemispheric connectivity through the anterior and pallial commissures. From a comparative viewpoint the increased levels of interhemispheric interaction that we observe in placental mammals cannot be considered simply a consequence of having a large and complex brain. Rather, there must be specific adaptive reasons for the origin and maintenance of the corpus callosum in this group.

The second problem is that although the corpus callosum participates in lateralized function in the human brain, there has been some controversy as to whether (both in development and phylogeny) the callosum plays a role in the generation of lateralization or whether hemispheric specialization may itself affect callosal function. It has been repeatedly proposed that the corpus callosum is important for the appearance of functional lateralization in the mammalian brain, although hemispheric differences in function are well documented for nonmammalian brains without a corpus callosum, perhaps indicating distinct mechanisms involved in the generation of brain asymmetry in different vertebrates (Bradshaw and Rogers, 1993; Bisazza, Rogers, and Vallortigara, 1998). Two kinds of ideas regarding the role of the callosum in the generation of mammalian lateralization have been proposed: that it contributes to lat-

FRANCISCO ABOITIZ Departamento de Psiquiatría, Pontificia Universidad Católica de Chile, Santiago, Chile.
ANDRÉS IDE Departamento de Morfología Experimental, Facultad de Medicina, Universidad de Chile, Santiago, Chile.
RICARDO OLIVARES Facultad de Ciencias, Veterinarias, Universidad de Chile, Santiago, Chile.

eralization through asymmetric inhibitory interactions between the hemispheres (Cook and Beech, 1990; Bradshaw and Rogers, 1993) and that an intact corpus callosum is required for the maintenance of brain symmetry; when callosal function is impaired for some reason, asymmetry develops as a consequence of hemispheric isolation (Ringo et al., 1994; Witelson, 1995). The first concept implies that brain asymmetry might further develop with increasing inhibitory interhemispheric connectivity; the second suggests an inverse relationship between callosal connectivity and brain asymmetry. In addition to these two possibilities, hemispheric specialization may induce alterations in interhemispheric communication, and consequently, the corpus callosum should have more restricted functions in a lateralized brain. Some clues to the first question on the adaptive value of the corpus callosum may be found through the study of regional variation in fiber composition in the postmortem human, while we expect to shed light on the second problem of the callosal role in brain lateralization by analyzing individual variability of the corpus callosum.

More specifically, in this chapter we will discuss evidence for regional variability in fiber composition in the human corpus callosum, with a functional interpretation concerning the special role in midline fusion of callosal fibers connecting sensory (especially visual) areas. Then recent findings regarding structural asymmetry in the human brain (especially the Sylvian fissure and planum temporale) and its relationship to lateralized linguistic function will be reviewed. Since this is a controversial topic, it will be discussed in some detail. After this, the relationship between callosal fiber connectivity and the degree of anatomical asymmetry will be analyzed, and a developmental mechanism relating hemispheric asymmetry and callosal connectivity will be proposed. The chapter ends with a phylogenetic discussion of callosal function in mammals and its possible role in the origin of brain lateralization.

The corpus callosum: Its anatomy and variability

As has been mentioned, the corpus callosum consists of nerve fibers connecting the cerebral cortices of the two cerebral hemispheres. During embryonic development and also in phylogeny, it originates as a component of the hippocampal (pallial) commissure, an ancient fiber tract that connects the medial cortices (hippocampi) of the two hemispheres (Rakic and Yakovlev, 1968). Eventually, the corpus callosum separates from the hippocampal commissure and locates in the dorsal part of the hippocampal formation, becoming the main fiber tract connecting the two hemispheres. There is a topographic

organization of callosal fibers in relation to the cortical regions that they connect; that is, fibers connecting frontal regions travel through the front of the corpus callosum, while fibers connecting occipital cortices tend to travel in the posterior part of this structure. In this way, a map of the different cortical regions can be established along the callosum (Pandya and Seltzer, 1986). However, in smaller-brained animals such as the cat and the rat, the segregation of callosal fibers belonging to distinct cortical areas is less clear-cut (Nakamura and Kanaseki, 1989; Clarke et al., 1995; Kim, Ellman, and Juraska, 1996). A commonly used and straightforward method to subdivide the corpus callosum is the partition proposed by Witelson (1995), in which the corpus callosum has been arbitrarily divided into three regions according to maximal straight length (see the top part of Figure 2.1). The anterior third (denominated by the genu) is a rather bulbous region that contains fibers connecting prefrontal cortices. The middle third is the midbody of the corpus callosum, a slender region that contains projections from motor, somatosensory, and auditory cortices. The posterior third is divided into the posterior fifth (the splenium), which in anteroposterior sequence contains temporoparietal and occipital (visual) fibers, and the isthmus, a region between the midbody (middle third) and the splenium (posterior fifth), which is believed to contain fibers connecting superior temporal and parietal regions, including perisylvian areas, related to language processes (Witelson, 1995).

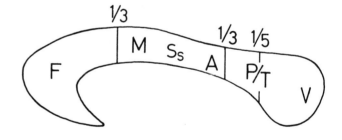

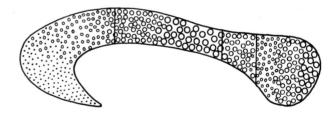

FIGURE 2.1. Top: Diagram of the corpus callosum, indicating the regions through which fibers connecting different cortical areas pass. F, frontal; M, motor; S$_S$, somatosensory; A, auditory; P/T, parieto-temporal; V, visual. Bottom: Distribution of fiber diameters in different callosal regions.

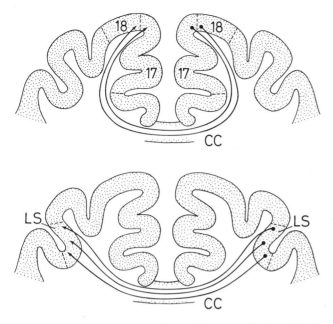

FIGURE 2.2. Top: Callosal cells and their terminations in the contralateral cortex in the primary and secondary visual cortices of the cat are concentrated in the midline of the visual field. Bottom: Callosal cells in higher-order visual cortices are dispersed throughout the respective area. (Modified from Berlucchi, 1972.)

Many callosal fibers are homotopical, that is, they connect equivalent regions on the two sides of the brain. Callosal cells and nerve terminals that connect early-processing sensory areas (somatosensory, auditory and especially visual) and motor regions tend to be restricted to the borders between left and right areas rather than being dispersed along the surface (Berlucchi, 1972; Innocenti, 1986; Clarke and Miklossy, 1990). In these regions there is a sophisticated topographic map of the sensory surface, and callosal cells and terminals are located in the region representing the sensory or motor midline (Figure 2.2). Since each hemisphere contains a representation of the contralateral sensory or motor field, it has been postulated that callosal cells participate in fusing the two hemirepresentations in each hemisphere. In the case of the visual system, midline fusion is important to maintain a continuity of the visual scene, and in some animals, such as humans, it is also useful for depth vision at and around the midline. Interestingly, the auditory areas are slightly different from visual and somatosensory areas in that the representation of the sensory surface (the cochlea) is tonotopic, that is, organized in stripes that represent auditory tones rather than spatial locations. Callosal cells here are also located in a band transverse to these isofrequency contours in the borders of the areas (Innocenti, 1986).

In so-called higher-order or association areas in the temporoparietal and frontal lobes, increasingly abstract and complex aspects of sensory and motor processing take place, and the topography of the sensory/motor surface becomes blurred. In many of these regions, cells respond much better to stimuli characteristics than to the location of the stimulus in the sensory field. Callosal cells and terminals connecting these regions are dispersed along the respective cortical areas instead of being restricted to the borders that represent the midline (Berlucchi, 1972; Innocenti, 1986).

Fiber composition of the corpus callosum: Regional differences, interhemispheric delays, and dependence on age

There is a direct relationship between the velocity of electrical conduction and the diameter of nerve fibers, such that thick fibers conduct their impulses faster than thin ones. Another factor that increases conduction velocity is myelin wrapping. Myelinated fibers are much faster conductors than unmyelinated ones. As seen in the light microscope, human callosal fiber diameters range from 0.4 to 15 µm in diameter, but the most commonly observed fiber diameters are between 0.6 and 1 µm. Unmyelinated fibers seem to be scarce (about 5% of the total, except in the genu, where they may make up about 16%; see Aboitiz et al., 1992a), although, in general, postmortem human tissue is of suboptimal quality for determining the numbers of very thin unmyelinated fibers. The fiber composition of the corpus callosum shows regional differences that match the topographic arrangement of cortical areas (Aboitiz et al., 1992a) (see Figure 2.3). Fast-conducting, large-diameter fibers (larger than 3 µm in diameter) are especially abundant in the posterior body and the posterior splenium, which correspond in rostrocaudal sequence to the representation of motor, somatosensory, and auditory areas (posterior body) and visual cortex (posterior splenium). On the other hand, callosal regions representing higher-order areas are mainly composed of small-diameter, slower-conducting fibers. The callosal region with a highest density of thin, lightly myelinated and non-myelinated fibers is the genu, which, as has been mentioned, connects frontal areas. This is of interest because, as we said above, callosal cells connecting primary and secondary sensorimotor areas are relatively few, restricted to a narrow strip in the border of the area that represents the sensory or motor midline; in higher-order areas, callosal cells can be found all along the respective regions (see Innocenti, 1986). In primary and secondary visual and somatosensory cortices, fast-conducting, gigantic callosal fibers may be involved in fusing the two

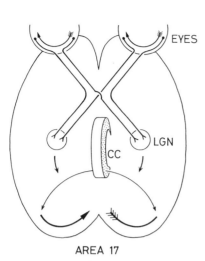

FIGURE 2.3. Diagram indicating the task of midline fusion for callosal cells in the primary visual cortex. In each hemisphere the visual cortex has a representation of the contralateral visual hemifield that is connected to the contralateral hemisphere through callosal fibers, thus establishing a continuity between the two hemirepresentations.

sensory or motor hemirepresentations in both hemispheres, while in auditory areas they may represent an additional stage of fast bilateral interaction in the auditory pathway that serves to localize sounds in space (Aboitiz et al., 1992a). Early stages of sensory processing probably require fast interhemispheric interaction, especially in regions representing the visual midline, where depth perception is achieved. In higher-order cortical areas, where intrinsic processing may take long enough to render the interhemispheric delay less critical, conduction velocity may not be such a stringent requirement. Note that fibers connecting prefrontal areas, which participate in long-term organization of behavior, are the thinnest and bear the highest proportion of unmyelinated fibers of the whole corpus callosum.

The interhemispheric distance between sensory areas is around 100–130 mm in the human. Interhemispheric transmission delay can be estimated to be of about 19–25 ms for the most abundant fibers between 0.4 and 1 μm in observed diameter. This fits the reported interhemispheric transmission times reported by evoked potentials (see Aboitiz et al., 1992a). Behavioral experiments in humans indicate that the shortest interhemispheric delays for simple motor reaction time tasks take around 3 ms, a time that fits the population of large-diameter fibers (larger than 3 μm) that tend to connect sensorimotor areas, while delays for more complex tasks take on average around 45 ms, fitting the population of

thinnest myelinated and unmyelinated fibers that correspond to association or higher-order areas. However, delays of around 45 ms may be an overestimate, since, especially for complex tasks, it is sometimes difficult to distinguish interhemispheric transmission times from inherent hemispheric differences in computational speed (Aboitiz et al., 1992a). In this context, it is of interest to mention that Grafstein (1963) found that unmyelinated callosal fibers produce an evoked potential of longer latency and of opposite sign than myelinated fibers. Keeping in mind the difficulties of interpreting these results, one role of unmyelinated fibers may perhaps be thought of as an aftereffect of the excitation or inhibition (via excitation of inhibitory interneurons) produced by faster, myelinated fibers, thereby modulating the temporal dimension of the interhemispheric stimulus.

We (Aboitiz et al., 1996) have recently observed an increase in the numbers of relatively large (larger than 1 μm) and very large-diameter (larger than 3 μm) callosal fibers with age (at least until 68 years old). At least some interhemispheric functions may increase transmission velocity with age, perhaps related to the automatization of certain neural strategies after continued use. It is known that the course of myelination depends on the functional state of the nerve fibers in the optic nerve (Fernández et al., 1993). Therefore, it is possible that, in general, large-diameter callosal fibers correspond to relatively automatic neural circuits that become established early in ontogeny, such as those involved in midline fusion in primary sensory areas. Some other automatic circuits may become established later and even during adult life, thus increasing the proportions of large-diameter fibers with age.

After separating by sex and considering the different segments of the corpus callosum, it was found that in females fibers larger than 1 μm in diameter increased in numbers in the anterior and posterior thirds only. In the midbody (but not in the splenium), fibers larger than 3 μm in diameter also increased their numbers with age. In males, however, the relationship between very large-diameter fibers and age disappeared after the callosum was divided into distinct segments. This indicates that in females there is an age-related increase of relatively fast interhemispheric transfer (fibers larger than 1 μm) in regions connecting higher-order areas of the frontal and temporoparietal lobes (corresponding to fibers larger than 1 μm of the anterior and posterior thirds), while the largest fibers involved in very fast transfer increase in the callosal midbody that connects motor, somatosensory, and auditory areas. However, there is no significant age dependency in the very large visual fibers of the posterior splenium that represent visual areas. On the other hand, although in males gigantic fibers (larger than 3 μm) increased with age in the whole callosum, we could not detect any callosal region in which this relationship was concentrated. Perhaps in males the age relationship with these very large fibers is dispersed along the corpus callosum, not relating to a particular, localized kind of function. The possibility that females and males differ in the fiber types that increase with age is reminiscent of other findings in the rat (Juraska and Kopcic, 1988) in which different fiber types respond to different specific environmental conditions in the two sexes (see below).

Individual differences in the human corpus callosum

A controversial line of research has suggested the existence of individual differences in callosal gross anatomy, mainly in regard to handedness and sex. Differences in the cross-sagittal size of the corpus callosum may have functional significance, as a larger total or partial callosal size reflects an increased number of small-diameter fibers as seen in light microscopy (Aboitiz et al., 1992a). The sparse large-caliber fibers of more than 3 μm are so variable in density that they fail to show a relationship with callosal size. An additional factor contributing to callosal size is myelin deposition, which also has functional correlates, since, as we discussed, increased myelination is associated with higher conduction velocity and hence shorter interhemispheric transmission time.

Some studies indicate a more bulbous splenium in females than in males, while other studies report a sex difference in the size of the isthmus in favor of females. Other findings suggest no sex differences in callosal morphology or fiber composition (for a review, see Aboitiz and Ide, 1998; see also Bishop and Wahlsten, 1997; Oka et al., 1999). Taking into account all the conflicting reports on callosal sex differences, probably the safest conclusion at this point is that if they exist, they are not robust (but see Bishop and Wahlsten, 1997). This perhaps contrasts with the striking difference in brain size between the sexes (Aboitiz, Scheibel, and Zaidel, 1992c). Peters (1988) has argued that sex differences in brain weight relate to cortical areas connected with sensorimotor surfaces but not to higher-order areas involved in cognition, which make the bulk of callosal fibers (see above). However, as yet there is no strong evidence in his support. A diferent explanation may come from the work of Haug (1987) and Witelson, Glezer, and Kigar (1995), who reported that cortical cell density is higher in females than in males, which may result in similar numbers of cortical cells in the two sexes (Haug, 1987). If this is the case, and if the proportion of cells projecting to the corpus callosum does not differ across the sexes, similar callosal sizes and fiber numbers might be expected in males and females. However, the above

findings must be taken with caution. Pakkenberg and Gundersen (1995) estimate that males have a larger total number of cortical neurons than females (the difference being of the same magnitude as the brain size difference), which does not agree with the above hypothesis.

Anatomical asymmetries in perisylvian regions

Another variable that has been found to correlate with callosal structure is brain lateralization. This makes sense, since the two lateralized hemispheres must interact with each other through the corpus callosum to generate coherent behavior. Some callosal functions that are of direct relevance for a lateralized brain are interhemispheric transfer, in which information presented to the noncompetent hemisphere may be transferred through the corpus callosum to the contralateral hemisphere to be adequately processed; interhemispheric inhibition, in which one hemisphere inhibits certain processes on the contralateral side, thus either enhancing or masking hemispheric asymmetry; and hemispheric monitoring, in which the two hemispheres solve the same task in parallel and the results of both processing chains are compared through the corpus callosum at different stages of the neural sequence (Zaidel et al., 1995).

Brain lateralization may be indexed in a variety of ways, two of the most common being dichotic listening, in which different syllables are presented simultaneously to each ear and the subject usually reports the syllable presented directly to the hemisphere that is dominant for language, and handedness, in which the most useful classification has consisted of separating subjects into consistent right-handers and nonconsistent right-handers rather than into dextrals and sinistrals (Witelson, 1995). There is an important relationship between functional lateralization (hereafter referred to as *lateralization*) and anatomical asymmetry (hereafter referred to as *asymmetry*) in the human brain, which will be reviewed in the next section. Next, we will analyze in some detail the relationship between brain asymmetry/lateralization and interhemispheric connectivity.

Only after Geschwind and Levitsky's (1968) classic paper did the concept that the human brain is structurally asymmetrical become widely accepted. In an analysis of 100 human brains, Geschwind and Levitsky found that the planum temporale, a planar cortical field located in the posterior floor of the Sylvian fissure (the Sylvian fossa), was larger on the left in 65% of the cases and larger on the right in 11%. Symmetric plana were found in 24% of the specimens. In the left hemisphere the planum temporale is located in a region that overlaps with Wernicke's area, the posterior language re-

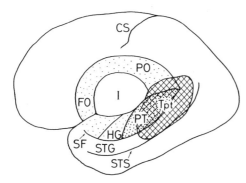

FIGURE 2.4. Lateral view of a left hemisphere, with the Sylvian fissure (SF) opened to expose the insula (I) and the floor of the Sylvian fissure. In the latter, the planum temporale (PT, densely dotted) is located behind Heschl's gyrus (HG). Cytoarchitectonic area Tpt is indicated with crosshatching. CS, central sulcus; FO, frontal operculum; PO, parietal operculum; STG, superior temporal gyrus; STS, superior temporal sulcus. As in all figures, anterior is to the left side.

gion. This asymmetry is associated with a longer Sylvian fissure on the left side (Galaburda, 1995; Witelson, 1995). The planum temporale corresponds roughly to a cytoarchitectonic area called Tpt, which is strongly asymmetric toward the left side, having a volume up to seven times larger in the left than in the right (Galaburda et al., 1978) (see Figure 2.4). Asymmetries in the Sylvian fissure can be observed in 31-week-old fetuses or even earlier, and in the newborn they already have the distribution observed in adults (Chi, Dooling, and Gilles, 1977; see also Witelson, 1995).

In vivo studies relating anatomical asymmetry and functional laterality

In vivo imaging techniques such as carotid angiography and computerized tomography were initially critical for establishing a relationship between behavioral lateralization and anatomical asymmetry. More recently, magnetic resonance imaging (MRI) studies of cerebral asymmetries in the language areas of living subjects have been performed, confirming the concept of a relationship between anatomical asymmetry and functional laterality in Wernicke's area (Aboitiz and Ide, 1998). In general, the strongest behavioral indicator of anatomical asymmetry in language regions is linguistic lateralization to the left and its reduction in left-handers (as determined, for example, by dichotic listening, hemifield tachistoscopy or the sodium amytal test). Indeed, there is a good correlation between right-handedness and left-language dominance (Witelson, 1995). Perhaps language lateralization evolved from a brain already lateralized for manual functions in the left hemisphere and for

certain visuospatial functions in the right (Bradshaw and Rogers, 1993). An interesting finding is that, among left-handers, those who have an inverted writing posture tend to show leftward asymmetry of the planum temporale, while those with noninverted writing have a rightward asymmetry (Foundas, Leonard, and Heilman, 1995). Using MRI, Habib and colleagues (1995) found two leftward asymmetric parameters: the size of the planum temporale and the distance between the central sulcus and the end of the Sylvian fissure. These two asymmetries were not correlated; that is, in a given individual, presence of asymmetry in one region does not predict that the other region will be asymmetric. Although each of these asymmetry measures correlates with handedness, the two combined showed a much stronger correlation with manual preference. This is consistent with a recent report (Ide et al., in press) showing several anatomical asymmetries in different surface regions of the human brain even though there is no correlation between them. This indicates that the overall morphological pattern rather than that of a specific measure may yield better estimates of lateralization of function.

Sex differences

Recent reports on autopsy material (Aboitiz et al., 1992c; Witelson and Kigar, 1992; Ide et al., 1996) indicate that sex differences in Sylvian asymmetries are not significant. In a postmortem study, Witelson and Kigar (1992) determined that the horizontal segment of the Sylvian fissure (see below) tends to be larger bilaterally in right-handed than in nonconsistent right-handed men. In females there were no differences. In general, many studies have determined that when an anatomical relationship exists between functional laterality and structural asymmetry, it is more significant in males than in females (Aboitiz and Ide, 1998). However, this difference may be marginally significant or simply not robust, resulting in discrepant findings across studies when sample sizes are at the limit of statistical power.

Morphology of the Sylvian fissure and of the planum temporale and their variability

Since the advent of neuroimaging techniques it is of the greatest interest to establish the precise arrangements of cortical areas in different sulci and gyri, especially for regions such as the planum temporale and cytoarchitectonic area Tpt. This is of importance also because there is an immense individual variability in the morphology of the Sylvian fissure. A qualitative and quantitative analysis of the variability of this region has been re-

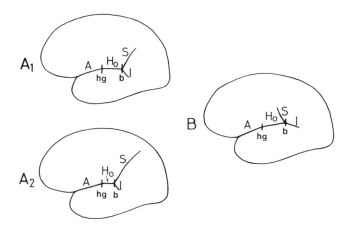

FIGURE 2.5. Three common types of Sylvian fissure: In A₁ and A₂ the superior or ascending branch (S) is longer than the inferior branch. In A₁ the horizontal ramus (Ho) is relatively long (27.5% of the cases); in A₂ the horizontal ramus (Ho) is rather short, but the ascending branch (S) is very long and deep (33.75% of cases). In B the superior ramus (S) is distorted and directed forward (21.25% of cases). The remaining 17.5% of the cases belong to different types.

TABLE 2.1
Distribution of major Sylvian fissure types according to hemispheres. Values in each cell indicate number of cases. (Data from Ide et al., 1996. N = 40, @0 males, 20 females; χ² = 8.22, p < 0.05). No significant sex differences were found.

Fissure Type	Number of Cases in Left Hemisphere	Number of Cases in Right Hemisphere	Total
A1	10	12	22
A2	09	18	27
B	13	04	17
Other types	08	06	14
Total	40	40	80

cently performed (Ide et al., 1996). Anatomically, the Sylvian fissure divides into an anterior segment that ends posteriorly in the gyrus of Heschl (containing the primary auditory area). Behind the gyrus of Heschl there is a horizontal segment containing the lateral extension of the planum temporale and the Sylvian fossa. More posteriorly, the Sylvian fissure bifurcates into two, usually more superficial ascending and descending rami (see Figure 2.5). There are two main types of Sylvian fissure. In the standard type, the ascending ramus is longer and deeper than the descending one. Two subtypes can be distinguished within the standard type, according to the relative length of the horizontal segment (compare types A₁ and A₂ in Figure 2.5), type A₂ being more common in the right hemisphere (Table 2.1). Ide and colleagues

(1996) have also described a type of fissure (Figure 2.5B) that is characterized by a long horizontal segment and a sometimes small, but at other times relatively long, fissure that is directed upward and forward (instead of upward and backward). This type of fissure is more common in the left hemisphere (Table 2.1), and corresponds in many cases to what other authors have described as the absence of an ascending ramus. The interpretation is that the upward/forward-directed ramus described by Ide and colleagues (1996) is a distorted and sometimes vestigial superior branch.

Distinct fissurization patterns may result from differences in the relative growth of specific cortical regions, which in turn may be directly associated with divergent modes of cortical processing. In particular, the position of the planum temporale and area Tpt may differ in the distinct fissure types reported here, an issue of relevance for studies that incorporate imaging analyses. Witelson and Kigar (1992) and later Ide and colleagues (1996) have suggested that in some cases (particularly in the case of the fissure type A₂ in Figure 2.5, which may correspond to Witelson and Kigar's "V-type"), the planum temporale perhaps runs into the ascending branch of the Sylvian fissure. In the other cases (especially type B) it appears that the planum temporale is restricted to the horizontal segment of the Sylvian fissure. Since type A₂ is more common on the right, this position of the planum may reflect the development of cortical areas related to right hemisphere skills or the reduction in the size of areas related to left hemisphere skills, while the type B fissure, which is more common on the left, may be related to the development of cortical areas involved in linguistic skills. In this context, although many studies highlight the size difference between the left and right plana (Beaton, 1997; Shapleske et al., 1999), the above and other recent findings (e.g., Loftus et al., 1993; Jäncke et al., 1994) emphasize a difference in the position of the planum temporale (or the Sylvian fossa) in the two sides rather than an asymmetry in overall planum size. Additional studies are urgently needed to settle the question of a correspondence between variability at the level of gross anatomy and variability at the level of cortical cytoarchitectonics.

Brain asymmetry and interhemispheric communication: Anatomical aspects and possible sex differences

In the human, MRI and postmortem studies have detected an inverse relationship between total callosal size and functional brain lateralization as determined by several behavioral parameters, including handedness (Witelson, 1995). When the sexes are separated, it has been observed that the callosal isthmus (the region between the posterior third and the posterior fifth) correlates negatively with visual behavioral laterality measures in males but not in females (Witelson and Goldsmith, 1991; Clarke and Zaidel, 1994). Supporting these findings, Habib and colleagues (1991) determined that the total size and the size of the anterior half of the corpus callosum were larger in nonconsistent than in consistent right-hander males. However, they also found that the posterior midbody was larger in consistent than in nonconsistent right-handed females, a result that was not found by Clarke and Zaidel (1994).

Aboitiz and colleagues (1992b, 1992c) analyzed the relationships between callosal connectivity and hemispheric specialization, as indexed by the degree of perisylvian asymmetry. The Sylvian fissure was measured from Heschl's gyrus to the end of the ascending branch, and the magnitude of the asymmetry (regardless of direction) was plotted against callosal measures. An inverse relationship was found between asymmetry and the size and fiber numbers in the isthmus that was specific for males, supporting the above findings. At the level of fiber composition, in males the significant correlation was observed for the numbers of small, medium-sized, and moderately large fibers of the isthmus (between 0.4 and 3 μm in diameter) but not for the fibers larger than 3 μm. However, in a small segment immediately posterior to the isthmus (the anterior third of the splenium), small and medium-sized fibers (between 0.4 and 1 μm) showed a significant, negative correlation with asymmetries, this time only in females. This may indicate either a differential mapping of asymmetric regions of males and females or that distinct cortical regions are asymmetric in the two sexes. However, we cannot reject the possibility that in both males and females the isthmus and the anterior splenium contain fibers connecting asymmetric areas, the observed sex differences resulting from the high interindividual variability and the relatively small sample used in the study (10 subjects of each sex). Another intriguing finding is that only in males, fibers with diameters between 1 and 3 μm correlated with asymmetry, perhaps indicating that in males but not females, relatively fast interhemispheric transfer is affected by the asymmetry of language-related areas. When the correlation between the asymmetry levels of the different components of the Sylvian fissure and callosal connectivity was tested, no significant relationship was found, presumably because these components involve smaller cortical regions whose contribution to the total fibers in the isthmus becomes less important.

The above indicates that in the human, increasing anatomical asymmetry and increasing functional lateralization tend to be associated with a decreased inter-

hemispheric communication, especially in males. Thus, the interplay between callosal connectivity and hemispheric asymmetry may be of great importance during the development of language lateralization. Some findings in rats tend to support this conclusion, as the density of somatomotor callosal terminals decreases as volumetric cortical asymmetries increase (Rosen, Sherman, and Galaburda, 1989). However, later the same group (Rosen et al., 1990) found no relationship between anatomical asymmetry measures and callosal size in different mice strains. Other results in rodents indicate a complex, if not confusing, relationship between asymmetry and callosal connectivity (Bradshaw and Rogers, 1993). Some findings are compatible with models of inhibitory callosal interactions that mask an underlying hemispheric asymmetry (Denenberg, 1981). The controversial nature of some of these findings aside, it is possible that during human development, the relationship between corpus callosum and brain lateralization is different than in other species. Below, we will discuss a possible model for the interaction between anatomical asymmetry and callosal connectivity in the human, followed by a discussion of the role of the corpus callosum in the phylogeny of placental mammals, including its possible role in the origin of brain lateralization.

Developmental aspects of the relationship between callosal connectivity and hemispheric asymmetry

As was mentioned above, many callosal connections tend to be homotopical, that is, they connect equivalent regions in both hemispheres (Innocenti, 1986, 1995a, 1995b). However, in the newborn, callosal connections are overdeveloped, many of them connecting areas that are devoid of callosal projections in the adult. In the perinatal period there is a massive decrease in the number of callosal fibers (LaMantia and Rakic, 1990), producing the adult pattern of restricted callosal connections (Innocenti, 1986, 1995a, 1995b). It has been postulated that if two homotopic cortical areas are asymmetric, there will be a higher than normal process of callosal fiber retraction during this period owing to topographic and functional incongruities between the two regions (Aboitiz et al., 1992b, 1992c). Alternatively, an increased retraction of callosal terminals may induce the generation of hemispheric asymmetry and lateralization, especially in males (Witelson and Nowakowski, 1991; Witelson, 1995), presumably owing to the emphasis on intrahemispheric processing and progressive isolation of the two hemispheres. Witelson and Nowakowski found that very premature infants show a high proportion of left-handedness, which they interpret as showing that the normal course of callosal axon loss has been interfered with, resulting in loss of laterality. Supporting this view, Lassonde, Bryden, and Demers (1990) report that subjects with callosal agenesis tend to be more lateralized than control subjects, as seen in dichotic listening tests (note that this diverges from the findings in acallosal mice mentioned above). However, in this proposed mechanism there is no explanation of why language should be localized to the left instead of the right. Furthermore, evidence indicates that anatomical asymmetry (see above) seems to appear earlier in development than the period of callosal axon retraction, which apparently takes place between the thirty-fifth gestational week and the first postnatal month (Clarke et al., 1989). A likely possibility is that the two factors reinforce each other; that is, after early-generated anatomical asymmetries have induced an increased retraction of terminals in the corpus callosum, the reduced callosum itself plays a role enhancing the incipient functional lateralization by constraining the communication between the two hemispheres. In this way, the development of language dominance would depend on the interplay between anatomically asymmetric structures and their respective degree of interhemispheric communication.

One interesting and recurrent finding is that the relationship between callosal connectivity and hemispheric asymmetry tends to be stronger in males. This might imply that in females the process of perinatal reaccommodation of connectivity is not as intense as in males. For example, if asymmetry determines an increased retraction of callosal terminals in males, for some reason in females there might be less competition between axons, resulting in a less intense regression of projections than in males, which in turn would imply that, at least for some processes, females might be able to tolerate a higher level of interhemispheric interaction with increasing hemispheric specialization than males. Perhaps sex hormones have an effect on the process of terminal retraction in late neural development, thus causing the proposed developmental differences between sexes. Sex hormones have been reported to modulate callosal morphology (Moffat et al., 1997; Fitch and Denenberg, 1998). Furthermore, different fiber types can have different sensitivities to sex hormones, yielding the observed finding of a negative correlation of the number of relatively thick fibers with asymmetry only in males. It has been reported (Juraska and Kopcic, 1988) that male rats that are raised in an enriched environment tend to develop larger myelinated callosal axons than those raised in an isolated environment. Female rats that are raised in an enriched environment tend to show increased numbers of callosal fibers rather than increased fiber size. Recall that among humans, relatively large fi-

bers (between 1 and 3 μm in diameter) showed a negative correlation with asymmetries only in males, which might suggest that males but not females tend to respond to different developmental conditions (be they increasing hemispheric asymmetry or an enriched environment) by changing the proportions of relatively large-diameter fibers (Aboitiz et al., 1992b). Nevertheless, our more recent findings indicate that age-related increases in the numbers of large-diameter callosal fibers tend to be female-specific (Aboitiz et al., 1996; see above), indicating that sex differences in the process of myelination and fiber growth may follow rather complex rules.

Evolutionary speculations based on postmortem anatomy in the human

The results presented in this chapter support the concepts of regional variation and of individual diversity in callosal fiber composition in the human. The first class of findings unveiled a difference between commissural connections of primary and secondary sensorimotor versus higher-order cortical areas in terms of the requirements of interhemispheric transfer time. On the basis of these results, we will propose a phylogenetic scenario for the origin of callosal function that is based on the emphasis in midline fusion tasks. This process is not well developed in the telencephalon of other vertebrates, as they lack a major telencephalic commissure, but also because most topographical sensory information is processed at lower brain levels, that is, in the midbrain. Next, a tentative scenario for the evolution of callosal connectivity both in placental mammals and in the lateralized human brain will be proposed.

The origin of the corpus callosum in the brain of placental mammals

The evolutionary origin of mammals is marked among other things by the elaboration of a six-layered neocortex and a general expansion of the brain. In addition, visual projections that in reptiles project mainly to the midbrain shift in mammals to the cerebral cortex (cerebral hemispheres) via the lateral geniculate nucleus of the thalamus (Aboitiz, 1992, 1995). In reptiles and birds, sophisticated topographic maps of the visual field, somatosensory surface, and the auditory space tend to be located in the optic tectum of the midbrain (equivalent to the superior colliculus in mammals; see Stein and Meredith, 1993), while in the cerebral hemispheres the regions equivalent to the mammalian sensory cortices have poorly defined maps of the respective sensory surfaces (Ulinski, 1990; Aboitiz, 1992, 1995). In the optic tectum there is a commissure (the tectal commissure) that plays the role of fusing the two visual hemifields in reptiles. We suggest that, as a consequence of the relative reduction of the optic tectum and the associated displacement of the topographic sensory information to the cerebral cortex, selective pressure developed in early mammals for an efficient commissural system in the cerebral hemispheres that could perform midline fusion particularly in the visual system. Monotremes and marsupials bear a six-layered neocortex with topographic sensory maps but have no corpus callosum. Instead, they have a well-developed anterior commissure (and sometimes an associated fasciculus aberrans) containing fibers that connect frontal, somatosensory, auditory, and visual cortices (Granger, Masterton, and Glendenning, 1985; Bradshaw and Rogers, 1993). However, this is not a "smart" route to follow, since visual areas located in the occipital lobe have to send fibers traveling all the way forward to the anterior commissure and then return to the contralateral occipital lobe to perform midline fusion. (There are also fibers crossing through the hippocampal commissure, but they seem to be relatively few.) A more efficient design is to send the axons via a shortcut. As we mentioned above, embryological evidence indicates that this was the solution attained by placental mammals: Commissural fibers from visual cortex may have started crossing through the hippocampal commissure, which turned out to be of advantage in terms of visual processing. Eventually, a fiber tract differentiated from the hippocampal commissure and developed as the corpus callosum. Why did monotremes and marsupials not find this simple solution? Perhaps they did not need it. The superior colliculus (optic tectum) is relatively well developed in primitive mammals, and thus midline fusion may still be performed in the midbrain to a large extent, even though the cerebral cortex is already processing topographic relations. In other words, the shift of topographic sensory information from the midbrain to the mammalian cerebral cortex may have been a gradual process in which midline fusion was among the latest functions to be fully transferred to the cerebral hemispheres. Marsupials and monotremes thus represent intermediate stages in this process.

Midline fusion is still an important callosal function in modern mammals. Preliminary findings in our laboratory (Olivares, Michalland, and Aboitiz, 1995) indicate that frontally looking species such as carnivores and primates tend to have a relatively larger posterior third of the corpus callosum than do laterally looking species such as ungulates and rodents. Although it is not certain to what extent these fibers connect homologous areas, the findings are consistent with a higher proportion of posterior (i.e., visually related) callosal fibers in frontally looking species than in laterally looking ones, since the former tend to develop depth vision and therefore the task of midline fusion may be of more importance than in other species. Additionally, it is of interest that among placental mammals there is a good correlation between brain size and total callosal area (with an exponent approximating 0.75; see Olivares et al., 1995), although cetaceans have a smaller callosum than many other mammals (Glezer et al., 1988). The visual system of cetaceans is not as developed as that of other large-brained mammals, and perhaps tasks such as midline fusion are not of high relevance. Furthermore, the inferior and superior colliculi are relatively large in these species, and it is possible that many commisural interactions associated with echolocation are achieved in the mesencephalon.

The above scenario proposes that the main adaptive value of the corpus callosum relates to the process of midline fusion in sensorimotor regions of the neocortex. However, we have seen that callosal fibers connecting these areas are relatively few, most callosal projections belonging to higher-order or association cortices. Together with developing midline tasks, the corpus callosum probably became involved in coordination of more subtle processing between the two hemispheres. It may have worked as a monitoring system to check for different stages of parallel processing in the two hemispheres and as a way to transfer sensory and motor information to the other hemisphere, especially in relation to learning and plasticity. More generally, there has been a tendency in mammals to develop corticocortical connections between different regions as the number of cortical areas increases, and since a straightforward path between the hemispheres was available through the corpus callosum, interhemispheric connections became no exception to this trend. Thus, we claim that the main evolutionary advantage of having a corpus callosum relies, at least initially, more on cortical midline fusion than on interhemispheric communication between higher-order areas, although the latter benefited from the origin of the corpus callosum. In later stages of eutherian (placental mammal) evolution, the callosum may have permitted appropriate synchrony of processes in the two hemispheres and, at the same time, the transfer of information from one side to the other (which might not occur to the same degree in animals whose hemispheres are disconnected), and this may have enhanced the processing capacity of the brain.

The corpus callosum and the evolution of brain lateralization

It is practically impossible that the two hemispheres will work in exactly the same manner; furthermore, in ontogeny they might tend to deviate from each other in their processing strategies. With the increase in cortical areas in mammalian evolution, the two hemispheres perhaps tended to diverge in their processing sequences if not interacting properly. The corpus callosum may have compensated for intrinsic differences in neural processing between the hemispheres by monitoring parallel processing in the two sides (Zaidel et al., 1995) or through inhibitory interactions. Inhibitory connections may sometimes mask inherent asymmetries in the two hemispheres that are to the disadvantage of the animal (Denenberg, 1981). However, in some species, including hominids, lateralized functions appeared that were of high adaptive value, such as visuospatial processing in the right hemisphere and particularly linguistic processing in the left hemisphere. In this case, instead of compensating for the asymmetry generated in the two hemispheres, the corpus callosum worked as a pathway for transfer of relevant information to the specialized hemisphere. Inhibitory callosal interactions may have begun to block incompatible strategies in the two hemispheres. Other asymmetric functions remained processed in parallel in the left and the right sides, each hemisphere using a different strategy and being reciprocally monitored with the contralateral side at different computational stages through the corpus callosum (Zaidel et al., 1995).

The above scenario implies that although the corpus callosum has a role in the origin of lateralization, it is not the cause of it. Brain asymmetry might initially develop as a specialization of neural processing that is intrinsic to each hemisphere, in a manner analogous to the developmental model suggested above. A different, but not alternative, model (Ringo et al., 1994) suggests a direct role for the callosum in the evolutionary origin of lateralization. These authors proposed that in phylogeny, a longer interhemispheric delay due to increased brain size might produce an emphasis on local processing within each hemisphere, resulting in hemispheric isolation, which in turn would facilitate hemispheric asymmetry and lateralization. Thus, according to Ringo and colleagues (1994), hemispheric lateralization for language might be partially a byproduct of having a larger brain. In this context, Jerison (1991) and later Schütz and Preissl (1996) reported no differences in average callosal fiber diameter between the mouse and the macaque, suggesting that conduction velocity remains constant despite an increased interhemispheric distance, thereby effectively increasing interhemispheric delay in larger brains. Preliminary findings by two of us (F. A. and R. O.) tend to support this conclusion, though also indicating that the largest callosal fibers tend to be thicker (and hence faster-conducting) in large-brained species compared to small-brained ones (Figure 2.6). This sug-

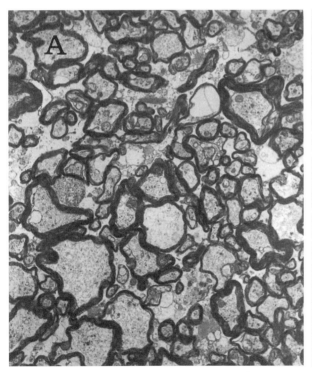
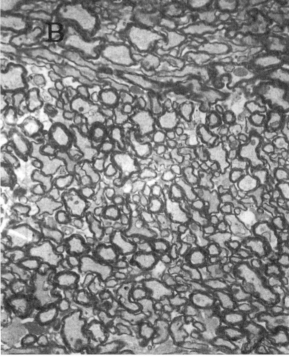

FIGURE 2.6. Electron micrograph of the midsplenium of the corpus callosum of (left) a horse and (right) a rat, indicating the appearance of large-diameter fibers in the callosums of large-brained species. 15,400× E.M.

gests that a subpopulation of large, fast-conducting fibers tends to compensate for the increasing interhemispheric distance by increasing their axon diameter and conduction velocity.

Since the timing requirements are most stringent for sensorimotor areas, perhaps the population of large, fast-conducting fibers increases in size and numbers especially in callosal regions connecting these areas (Aboitiz et al., 1992a). Comparing the sizes of axons connecting visual areas 17/18 in the mouse and cat, Innocenti (1995a; see also Innocenti et al., 1995) reports an increase in fiber diameters in the cat. However, brain volume might not be the only factor, as behavioral specializations can also influence callosal fiber composition. Across species, no relationship was found between interhemispheric conduction delay in the 17/18 border and brain size when comparing studies performed by different authors (four species were compared: mouse, rabbit, cat, and monkey; see Innocenti, 1995a). Interestingly, the shortest interhemispheric delay (antidromic stimulation) is found in the cat (between 2 and 3 ms), and the monkey has a delay comparable to that of the mouse (7 to 8 ms) despite the approximately tenfold difference in interhemispheric distance. The rabbit has an unusually long interhemispheric delay (about 17 ms average), which perhaps relates to the poorly developed area of binocular vision and the strong emphasis on lateral vision in this species. The relatively short interhemispheric delays in cat and monkey may relate to the fact that both are frontally eyed species with a high degree of binocularity and depth perception, for which fast interhemispheric conduction may be especially useful. These results point to the possibility that besides brain size, callosal fiber composition may depend on behavioral and perceptual specializations such as the degree of stereopsis, again supporting the concept of an important role of the corpus callosum in midline fusion, especially in the visual system.

To what extent an increased interhemispheric distance plays a role in the evolutionary origin of brain lateralization needs to be determined by comparative studies analyzing interhemispheric transmission times in both sensory and higher-order areas and in species with different brain sizes and with different degrees of brain lateralization. In any case, Ringo and colleagues (1994) leave the question open of why the left hemisphere specializes in linguistic-type task and the right in visuospatial tasks instead of vice versa. A right hemisphere superiority in visuospatial tasks has been observed in small mammals (Bradshaw and Rogers, 1993), indicating that at least there are other factors involved in the generation of brain asymmetry. Nevertheless, just as in the developmental model proposed above, in phylogeny a decreased callosal function (be it a consequence of less interhemispheric fibers or an increased transmission delay) may perhaps have served to enhance functional lateralization between the two hemispheres, particularly in the case of males (Witelson and Nowakowski, 1991; Aboitiz et al., 1992b, 1992c).

Final comment

We have reviewed some of our findings on regional fiber composition and of individual variability in callosal structure in the postmortem human and other species, together with anatomical analyses of the human Sylvian fissure, its asymmetry, and its relationship to brain lateralization and to callosal connectivity. In our view, these results shed light on two main questions: the original adaptiveness of the corpus callosum in placental mammals, which we propose has to do with the generation of tasks related to midline fusion in the telencephalon, and the relationship between callosal connectivity and hemispheric laterality in the human, in both ontogenetic and phylogenetic terms. An inverse relationship between callosal connectivity and brain lateralization holds in the human, which is apparently the result of early-generated anatomical asymmetry producing a decreased interhemispheric connectivity, especially in males. Eventually, perhaps a reduced interhemispheric communication serves to increase functional laterality. In phylogeny the relationship between callosal connectivity and hemispheric asymmetry is less clear, although comparative studies providing interesting findings are forthcoming.

ACKNOWLEDGMENTS This work has been supported by FONDECYT grant 1940450 (Chile) and DTI grant M3604 9633 (Chile).

REFERENCES

Aboitiz, F., 1992. The evolutionary origin of the mammalian cerebral cortex. *Biol. Res.* 25:41–49.

Aboitiz, F., 1995. Homology in the evolution of the cerebral hemispheres: The case of reptilian dorsal ventricular ridge and its possible correspondence with mammalian neocortex. *J. Brain Res.* 4:461–472.

Aboitiz, F., and A. Ide, 1998. Anatomical asymmetries in language-related cortex and their relation to callosal function. In *Handbook of Neurolinguistics*, B. Stemmer and H. Whitaker, eds. San Diego: Academic Press, pp. 393–404.

Aboitiz, F., E. Rodríguez, R. Olivares, and E. Zaidel, 1996. Age-related changes in fibre composition of the human corpus callosum: Sex differences. *Neuroreport* 7:1761–1764.

Aboitiz, F., A. B. Scheibel, R. S. Fisher, and E. Zaidel, 1992a. Fiber composition of the human corpus callosum. *Brain Res.* 598:143–153.

Aboitiz, F., A. B. Scheibel, R. S. Fisher, and E. Zaidel, 1992b. Individual differences in brain asymmetries and fiber composition in the human corpus callosum. *Brain Res.* 598:154–161.

ABOITIZ, F., A. B. SCHEIBEL, and E. ZAIDEL, 1992c. Morphometry of the human corpus callosum, with emphasis on sex differences. *Brain* 115:1521–1541.

BEATON, A. A., 1997. The relation of planum temporale asymmetry and morphology of the corpus callosum to handedness, gender and dyslexia: A review of the evidence. *Brain Lang.* 60:255–322.

BERLUCCHI, G., 1972. Anatomical and physiological aspects of visual function of the corpus callosum. *Brain Res.* 214:239–259.

BISAZZA, A., L. J. ROGERS, and G. VALLORTIGARA, 1998. The origins of cerebral asymmetry: A review of evidence of behavioural and brain lateralization in fishes, reptiles and amphibians. *Neurosci. Biobehav. Rev.* 22:411–416.

BISHOP, K. M., and D. WAHLSTEN, 1997. Sex differences in the human corpus callosum: Myth or reality? *Neurosci. Biobehav. Rev.* 21:581–601.

BRADSHAW, J., and L. ROGERS, 1993. *The Evolution of Lateral Asymmetries, Language, Tool Use, and Intellect.* New York: Academic Press.

CHI, J. G., E. C. DOOLING, and F. H. GILLES, 1977. Left-right asymmetries of the temporal speech areas in the human fetus. *Arch. Neurol.* 34:346–348.

CLARKE, J. M., and E. ZAIDEL, 1994. Anatomical-behavioral relationships: Corpus callosum morphometry and hemispheric specialization. *Behav. Brain Res.* 64:185–202.

CLARKE, S., F. DERIBAUPIERRE, V. M. BAJO, E. M. ROUILLIER, and R. KRAFTSIK, 1995. The auditory pathway in cat corpus callosum. *Exp. Brain Res.* 104:534–540.

CLARKE, S., R. KRAFTSIK, H. VAN DER LOOS, and G. M. INNOCENTI, 1989. Forms and measures in adult and developing human corpus callosum: Is there sexual dimorphism? *J. Comp. Neurol.* 280:213–230.

CLARKE, S., and J. MIKLOSSY, 1990. Occipital cortex in man: organization of callosal connections, related myelo- and cytoarchitecture, and putative boundaries of functional visual areas. *J. Comp. Neurol.* 298:188–214.

COOK, N. D., and A. R. BEECH, 1990. The cerebral hemispheres and bilateral neural nets. *Intern. J. Neurosci.* 52:201–210.

DENENBERG, V. H., 1981. Hemispheric laterality in animals and the effects of early experience. *Behav. Brain Sci.* 4:1–49.

FERNÁNDEZ, E., N. CUENCA, J. R. CEREZO, and J. DEJUAN, 1993. Visual experience during postnatal development determines the size of optic nerve axons. *Neuroreport* 5:365–367.

FITCH, R. H., and V. H. DENENBERG, 1998. A role of ovarian hormones in sexual differentiation of the brain. *Behav. Brain Sci.* 21:311–352.

FOUNDAS, A. L., C. M. LEONARD, and K. M. HEILMAN, 1995. Morphologic cerebral asymmetries and handedness: The pars triangularis and planum temporale. *Arch. Neurol.* 52:501–508.

GALABURDA, A. M., 1995. Anatomic basis of cerebral dominance. In *Brain Asymmetry*, R. J. Davidson and K. Hugdahl, eds. Cambridge, MA: MIT Press, pp. 51–73.

GALABURDA, A. M., M. LE MAY, T. KEMPER, and N. GESCHWIND, 1978. Left-right asymmetries in the brain. *Science* 199:852–856.

GESCHWIND, N., and W. LEVITSKY, 1968. Human brain: Left-right asymmetries in temporal speech region. *Science* 161:186–187.

GLEZER, I. I., M. S. JACOBS, and P. J. MORGANE, 1988. Implications of the 'initial brain' concept for brain evolution in cetacea. *Behav. Brain Sci.* 11:75–116.

GRAFSTEIN, B., 1963. Postnatal development of the transcallosal evoked response in the cerebral cortex of the cat. *J. Neurophysiol.* 26:79–99.

GRANGER, E. M., R. B. MASTERTON, and K. K. GLENDENNING, 1985. Origin of interhemispheric fibers in acallosal opposum (with a comparison to callosal origins in rat). *J. Comp. Neurol.* 241:82–98.

HABIB, M., D. GAYRAUD, A. OLIVA, J. REGIS, G. SALAMON, and R. KHALIL, 1991. Effects of handedness and sex on the morphology of the corpus callosum: A study with magnetic resonance imaging. *Brain Cogn.* 16:41–61.

HABIB, M., F. ROBICHON, O. LÉVRIER, R. KHALIL, and G. SALAMON, 1995. Diverging asymmetries of temporo-parietal cortical areas: A reappraisal of Geschwind/Galaburda theory. *Brain Lang.* 48:238–258.

HAUG, H., 1987. Brain sizes, surfaces, and neuronal sizes of the cortex cerebri: A stereological investigation of man and his variability and a comparison with some mammals. *Am. J. Anet.* 180:126–142.

IDE, A., C. DOLEZAL, M. FERNÁNDEZ, E. LABBÉ, R. MANDUJANO, S. MONTES, P. SEGURA, G. VERSCHAE, P. YARMUCH, and F. ABOITIZ, 1999. Hemispheric differences in variability of fissural patterns in parasylvian and cingulate regions of human brains. *J. Comp. Neurol.* 410:235–242.

IDE, A., E. RODRÍGUEZ, E. ZAIDEL, and F. ABOITIZ, 1996. Bifurcation patterns in the human Sylvian fissure: Hemispheric and sex differences. *Cereb. Cortex* 6:717–725.

INNOCENTI, G. M., 1986. General organization of callosal connections in the cerebral cortex. In *Cerebral Cortex*, Vol. 5, E. G. Jones and A. Peters, eds. New York: Plenum, pp. 291–354.

INNOCENTI, G. M., 1995a. Cellular aspects of callosal connections and their development. *Neuropsychologia* 33:961–988.

INNOCENTI, G. M., 1995b. Exhuberant development of connections, and its possible permissive role in cortical evolution. *Trends Neurosci.* 18:397–402.

INNOCENTI, G. M., D. AGGOUN-ZOUAOUI, and P. LEHMANNN, 1995. Cellular aspects of callosal connections and their development. *Neuropsychologia* 33:961–988.

JÄNCKE, L., G. SCHLAUG, Y. HUANG, and H. STEINMETZ, 1994. Asymmetry of the planum parietale. *Neuroreport* 5:1161–1163.

JERISON, H. J. 1991. *Brain size and the evolution of mind.* Fifty-ninth James Arthur Lecture on the Evolution of the Human Brain, American Museum of Natural History, New York.

JURASKA, J. M., and J. R. KOPCIC, 1988. Sex and environmental influences on the size and ultrastructure of the rat corpus callosum. *Brain Res.* 450:1–8.

KIM, J. H. Y., A. ELLMAN, and J. M. JURASKA, 1996. A reexamination of sex differences in axon density and number in the splenium of the rat corpus callosum. *Brain Res.* 740:47–57.

LaMANTIA, A. S., and P. RAKIC, 1990. Axon overproduction and elimination in the corpus callosum of the developing rhesus monkey. *J. Neurosci.* 10:2156–2175.

LASSONDE, M., M. P. BRYDEN, and P. DEMERS, 1990. The corpus callosum and cerebral speech lateralization. *Brain Lang.* 38:195–206.

Loftus, W. C., M. J. Tramo, C. E. Thomas, R. L. Green, N. A. Nordgren, and M. S. Gazzaniga, 1993. Three-dimensional quantitative analysis of hemispheric asymmetry in the human superior temporal region. *Cerebral Cortex* 3:348–355.

Moffat, S. D., E. Hampson, J. C. Wickett, P. A. Vernon, and D. H. Lee, 1997. Testosterone is correlated with regional morphology of the corpus callosum. *Brain Res.* 767:297–304.

Nakamura, H., and T. Kanaseki, 1989. Topography of the corpus callosum in the cat. *Brain Res.* 485:171–175.

Oka, S., O. Miyamoto, N. A. Janjua, N. Hongo-Fujiwara, S. Nagao, H. Kondo, T. Minami, T. Toyoshima, and T. Itano, 1999. Re-evaluation of sexual dimorphism in the human corpus callosum. *Neuroreport* 10:937–940.

Olivares, R., S. Michalland, and F. Aboitiz, 1995. Interspecies morphometric analysis of the corpus callosum. *Notic. Biol.* 3:141.

Pakkenberg, B., and H. J. Gundersen, 1995. Solutions to old problems in quantitation of the central nervous system. *J. Neurol. Sci.* 16 (Suppl.), 65–67.

Pandya, D. N., and B. Seltzer, 1986. The topography of commissural fibers. In *Two Hemispheres One Brain: Functions of the Corpus Callosum*, D. Ottrosson, ed. New York: Alan Liss, pp. 47–73.

Peters, M., 1988. The size of the corpus callosum in males and females: Implications of a lack of allometry. *Can. J. Psychol.* 42:313–324.

Rakic, P., and P. I. Yakovlev, 1968. Development of the corpus callosum and cavum septi in man. *J. Comp. Neurol.* 132:45–72.

Ringo, J. L., R. W. Doty, S. Demeter, and P. Y. Simard, 1994. Time is of the essence: A conjecture that hemispheric specialization arises from interhemispheric conduction delay. *Cereb. Cortex* 4:331–343.

Rosen, G. D., G. F. Sherman, K. Emsbo, C. Mehler, and A. M. Galaburda, 1990. The midsagittal area of the corpus callosum and total neocortical volume differ in three inbred strains of mice. *Exp. Neurol.* 107:271–276.

Rosen, G. D., G. F. Sherman, and A. M. Galaburda, 1989. Interhemispheric connections differ between symmetrical and asymmetrical brain regions. *Neuroscience* 33:525–533.

Schütz, A., and H. Preissl, 1996. Basic connectivity of the cerebral cortex and some considerations on the corpus callosum. *Neurosci. Biobehav. Rev.* 20:567–570.

Shapleske, J., S. L. Rossell, P. W. R. Woodruff, A. S. David, 1999. The planum temporale: A systematic, quantitative review of its structural, functional and clinical significance. *Brain Res. Rev.* 29:26–49.

Stein, B. E., and M. A. Meredith, 1993. *The Merging of the Senses.* Cambridge, MA: MIT Press.

Ulinski, P. S., 1990. The cerebral cortex of reptiles. In *Cerebral Cortex*, Vol. 8A: *Comparative Structure and Evolution of the Cerebral Cortex*, E. G. Jones and A. Peters, eds. New York: Plenum Press, pp. 139–215.

Witelson, S. F., 1995. Neuroanatomical bases of hemispheric functional specialization in the human brain: Possible developmental factors. In *Hemispheric Communication: Mechanisms and Models*, F. L. Kitterle, ed. Hillsdale, NJ: Lawrence Erlbaum Associates, pp. 61–84.

Witelson, S. F., I. I. Glezer, and D. L. Kigar, 1995. Women have greater density of neurons in posterior temporal cortex. *J. Neurosci.* 15:3418–3428.

Witelson, S. F., and C. H. Goldsmith, 1991. The relationship of hand preference to anatomy of the corpus callosum in men. *Brain Res.* 545:175–182.

Witelson, S. F., and D. L. Kigar, 1992. Sylvian fissure morphology and asymmetry in men and women: Bilateral differences in relation to handedness in men. *J. Comp. Neurol.* 323:326–340.

Witelson, S. F., and R. S. Nowakowski, 1991. Left out axons make men right: A hypothesis for the origin of handedness and functional asymmetry. *Neuropsychologia* 29:327–333.

Zaidel, E., F. Aboitiz, J. Clarke, D. Kaiser, and R. Matteson, 1995. Sex differences in interhemispheric relations for language. In *Hemispheric Communication: Mechanisms and Models*, F. L. Kitterle, ed. Hillsdale, NJ: Lawrence Erlbaum Associates, pp. 85–176.

COMMENTARY 2.1

Complexity of Human Interhemispheric Connections

STEPHANIE CLARKE

Francisco Aboitiz, Andres Ide, and Ricardo Olivares review very interesting evidence concerning regional differences in axonal diameters within the corpus callosum, an inverse relation between the degree of hemispheric asymmetry and callosal size, and models of the development of this relationship in ontogeny and in phylogeny. They argue that diameters of callosal axons reflect their cortical origin, large axons originating in sensory and motor cortices and small axons in association cortices. On the basis of reports that the changes in callosal size associated with different degrees of hemispheric asymmetry affect some parts of the corpus callosum but not others, the authors argue that the variable regions within the corpus callosum are those that convey fibers from asymmetric regions. Finally, they propose that in both ontogeny and phylogeny the density of callosal connections arising from a cortical region may be influenced by the degree of asymmetry between this region and the homotopic one in the opposite hemisphere. All three arguments rely on the assumptions that there is a rather precise topographic arrangement of axons within the corpus callosum according to their origin and that callosal connections are essentially homotopical. One of my criticisms is that these fundamental assumptions may be false, since human tracing studies indicate that both aspects of interhemispheric connectivity may be more complex than presumed.

Interhemispheric pathways in the human brain

Relatively little is known about interhemispheric pathways in the human brain. This is partly owing to methodological difficulties. Techniques that can be applied to the human brain either have low sensitivity (retrograde

STEPHANIE CLARKE Division de Neuropsychologie, Centre Hospitalier Universitaire Vaudois, Lausanne, Switzerland.

degeneration, demyelination techniques, detection of macrophage or glia reaction) or are very time consuming (Nauta method for anterogradely degenerating axons). Our current beliefs on human interhemispheric connectivity are mostly extrapolations from work on nonhuman primates. However, there may be particular requirements of human cognitive functions that are met by the human but not by other primate brains.

Topography within the corpus callosum

It is generally assumed that there is a topographical arrangement of axons within the corpus callosum according to their origin. However, actual anatomical evidence from human studies is very limited and sometimes contradictory. Callosal axons from the occipital cortex cross in the splenium, mostly in its lower part; the degeneration of this pathway has been shown after small lesions with the Weigert-Pal stain (Dejerine and Dejerine-Klumpke, 1895; Van Valkenburg, 1908) and with the Nauta method (Clarke and Miklossy, 1990). Callosal axons from the anterior parts of the frontal lobe cross within the genu as demonstrated with the Glees method in a case of frontal leucotomy (Beck, Meyer, and Le Beau, 1951). Several attempts have been made to trace callosal pathways from the temporal lobe using myelin stains after localized lesions (Zingerle, 1912; Van Buren and Yakovlev, 1959); the callosal bundles could not be traced to the midsagittal plane, probably owing to their "dilution" with other, nonaffected fiber bundles (for discussion, see Clarke et al., 1995). Axons from the posterior parietal and posterior temporal cortex have been reported to cross in the splenium and possibly also in the posterior part of the body of the corpus callosum, those from the lower frontal and anterior parietal convexity in the genu and those from the upper frontal and anterior parietal convexity in the anterior two thirds of the body; relatively discrete signs of Wallerian degeneration (myelin pallor, loss of fibers, presence of phagocytes) were observed there after lesions in the corresponding parts of the hemispheres (De Lacoste, Kirkpatrick, and Ross, 1985). Thus, the genu and the splenium, but not the body, are likely to contain relatively tight bundles of axons originating in restricted cortical regions and arranged topographically according to their origin. However, none of the published observations can affirm that a given bundle in the splenium or genu contains all callosal fibers from a given cortical region.

Corpus callosum versus anterior commissure

The distribution of interhemispheric fibers between the corpus callosum and the anterior commissure is even less clear than the topographical order within the corpus callosum. Fiber dissection studies have shown that the human anterior commissure conveys fibers from parts of the orbitofrontal and polar temporal structures, including the amygdala (Klinger and Gloor, 1960). In the macaque monkey, tracing studies have demonstrated that the anterior commissure receives fibers from all the above structures but also from virtually the entire temporal cortex (Demeter, Rosene, and Van Hoesen, 1990).

We have studied the contribution of different cortical regions to the anterior commissure in the human by using the Nauta method for anterogradely degenerating axons in cases with circumscribed hemispheric lesions (Di Virgilio et al., 1999). A large number of degenerating axons were found in the anterior commissure in a case with a lesion spreading over the middle third of the inferior temporal, the fusiform, and the parahippocampal gyri as well as the hippocampal formation but sparing the amygdala, the anterior perforated substance, the olfactory tubercle, the diagonal band of Broca, and the prepiriform cortex. Degenerating axons were present in the anterior commissure, although in smaller numbers, in four other cases with lesions in the inferior part of the occipitotemporal cortex and in the middle frontal gyrus (two cases), the superolateral occipital convexity (one case), and the fundus of central fissure (one case). In cases with lesions involving the inferior occipital cortex, the splenium was also analyzed, and degenerating axons were found in its inferior part (Clarke and Miklossy, 1990). No degenerating axons were found in two cases without lesions and in a case with a lacuna inferomedial to the left pallidum (not encroaching on the posterior limb of the anterior commissure). Thus, the human anterior commissure conveys axons from a much larger territory than previously assumed. In particular, there is a heavy contribution from the inferoposterior part of temporal cortex. The suggestion that cortical regions on the frontoparietooccipital convexity also contribute to

the anterior commissure, even if weakly, is puzzling and worth further investigation. Furthermore, the inferior part of the occipitotemporal cortex appears to project through both the corpus callosum and the anterior commissure.

Homotopic and heterotopic callosal connectivity

It is often assumed that human callosal connections exist predominantly between homotopic regions of the cortex. At the same time what is considered a homotopic connection is rarely specified. Homotopy could be considered at the level of lobes, areas (Brodmann's areas, functional areas such as V1 and V2), or topographic representations within a given area (e.g., the same parts of the visual field). Recent evidence from human tracing studies, using the Nauta method for anterogradely degenerating axons in cases with circumscribed lesions, suggests that heterotopic interhemispheric connections are numerous and widespread.

Heterotopic connections between lobes were demonstrated in two instances. The right calcarine region was shown to send interhemispheric connections not only to the whole occipital cortex, but also to the posterior part of the temporal and parietal cortices, including regions proposed to be involved in specifically human functions such as the angular gyrus (Clarke et al., 1995, and unpublished results). The middle portion of the inferior temporal, the fusiform, and the parahippocampal gyri and of the hippocampal formation on the right side was shown to send relatively dense heterotopic connections to the posterior part of the superior temporal gyrus, the planum temporale, and the supramarginal and the angular gyri (corresponding to Wernicke's area) as well as weak connections to the posterior part of the inferior frontal gyrus (corresponding to Broca's area; see Di Virgilio and Clarke, 1997).

Heterotopic connections were demonstrated within the occipital lobe (Clarke and Miklossy, 1990). Heterotopic connections were observed from the medial to the lateral part and from the superolateral to the superomedial part of the occipital cortex.

Heterotopic connections between visual areas were demonstrated in a case with a small lesion in the upper part of Brodmann's area 19. As derived from the pattern of interhemispheric and intrahemispheric connections (Clarke and Miklossy, 1990; Clarke, 1994), the lesion was most likely in the putative human equivalent of macaque area PO/V6. Most of the interhemispheric connections originating in the damaged cortex terminated in the symmetrical region of the opposite hemisphere but some also in other parts. Among the latter were the boundaries between visual areas V1 and V2 and between areas V3 and V3A, as well as areas V4 and V5.

What does corpus callosum morphology tell us about callosal connections?

The rather unsatisfactory reply is that callosal morphology is most likely a poor correlate of specific callosal connections for several reasons:

1. Interindividual comparison of callosal morphologies is reputably difficult even if obvious pitfalls are avoided (for discussion, see, e.g., Clarke et al., 1989). Identification of corresponding regions in different corpora callosal remains often hazardous.

2. A roughly ordered arrangement of axons within the corpus callosum according to their origin appears to be present in the genu and the splenium but not in the body.

3. The pathway taken by heterotopic callosal axons has not been investigated. The possibility that they travel in very different parts of the corpus callosum than the homotopic axons originating or terminating within the same region cannot be excluded.

4. Cortical regions that are known to be asymmetrical in the human might well receive (described here for the planum temporale) and give rise to widely heterotopic callosal connections.

REFERENCES

BECK, E., A. MEYER, and J. LE BEAU, 1951. Efferent connexions of the human prefrontal region with reference to fronto-hypothalamic pathways. *J. Neurol. Neurosurg. Psychiatr.* 14:295–302.

CLARKE, S. 1994. Association and intrinsic connections of human extrastriate visual cortex. *Proc. R. Soc. Lond. B* 257:87–89.

CLARKE, S., F. DE RIBAUPIERRE, V. M. BAJO, E. M. ROUILLER, and R. KRAFTSIK, 1995. The auditory pathway in cat corpus callosum. *Exp. Brain Res.* 104:534–540.

CLARKE, S., R. KRAFTSIK, H. VAN DER LOOS, and G. M. INNOCENTI, 1989. Forms and measures of adult and developing human corpus callosum: Is there sexual dimorphism? *J. Comp. Neurol.* 280:231–253.

CLARKE, S., and J. MIKLOSSY, 1990. Occipital cortex in man: Organization of callosal connections, related myelo- and cytoarchitecture, and putative boundaries of functional visual areas. *J. Comp. Neurol.* 298:188–214.

DE LACOSTE, M. C., J. B. KIRKPATRICK, and E. D. ROSS, 1985. Topography of the human corpus callosum. *J. Neuropathol. Exp. Neurol.* 44:578–591.

DEJERINE, J., and A. DEJERINE-KLUMPKE, 1895. *Anatomie des centres nerveux.* Paris: Rueff et Cie.

DEMETER, S., D. L. ROSENE, and G. W. VAN HOESEN, 1990. Fields of origin and pathways of the interhemispheric commissures in the temporal lobe of macaques. *J. Comp. Neurol.* 302:29–53.

DI VIRGILIO, G., and S. CLARKE, 1997. Direct interhemispheric visual input to human speech areas. *Hum. Brain Mapp.* 5:347–354.

DI VIRGILIO, G., S. CLARKE, G. PIZZOLATO, and T. SCHAFFNER, 1999. Cortical regions contributing to the anterior commissure in man. *Exp. Brain Res.* 124:1–7.

KLINGER, J., and P. GLOOR, 1960. The connections of the amygdala and of the anterior temporal cortex in the human brain. *J. Comp. Neurol.* 115:333–369.

VAN BUREN, J. M., and P. I. YAKOVLEV, 1959. Connections of the temporal lobe in man. *Acta Anat.* 39:1–50.

VAN VALKENBURG, C. T. 1908. Zur anatomie der projektions- und balkenstrahlung des hinterhauptlappens sowie des cingulum. *Monatsschr. Psychiatrie Neurologie* 24:320–339.

ZINGERLE, H. 1912. Ueber einseitigen schläfenlappendefekt beim menschen. *Z. Psychologie Neurologie* 18:205–238.

3 Brain Size: A Possible Source of Interindividual Variability in Corpus Callosum Morphology

LUTZ JÄNCKE AND HELMUTH STEINMETZ

ABSTRACT   Applying in vivo magnetic resonance morphometry in healthy adults and reviewing published work on postmortem brains, we uncovered that the relationship between forebrain volume and the midsagittal size of the corpus callosum (CC) follows a geometrical rule according to which larger brains have a relatively smaller midsagittal CC. This allometric relationship is taken as support for the hypotheses of Ringo and coworkers suggesting that brain size may be an important factor influencing interhemispheric connectivity and lateralization. According to this theory, larger brains would be more lateralized than smaller brains. Because female and male brains on average differ in terms of brain size, this sexual dimorphism might explain the well-known gender differences with respect to functional lateralization.

The corpus callosum (CC) is the main fiber tract connecting the cerebral hemispheres, and it has been estimated that about 200–350 million fibers run through this structure in the human brain (Aboitiz et al., 1992a, 1992b). The CC seems to be important in the transfer and facilitation of sensorimotor and associative information between the hemispheres. It is thought that the cross-sectional size of the CC may indicate the number of small-diameter fibers crossing through (Aboitiz et al., 1992a), implying that a larger callosal area may indicate a higher capacity for interhemispheric transfer of associative information. Because the midsagittal CC size is so easy to measure either in postmortem material or on magnetic resonance images (MRI), it is one of the human brain structures to receive particular attention. There is some evidence suggesting that the morphology of the CC may be related to language dominance (Clarke

et al., 1993a; Clarke and Zaidel, 1994), gender (De Lacoste-Utamsing and Holloway, 1982; Oka et al., 1999), handedness (Witelson, 1985, 1989; Witelson and Goldsmith, 1991; Witelson and Nowakowski, 1991), Down syndrome (Wang et al., 1992), dysphasia (Njiokiktjien and Sonneville, 1991), schizophrenia (Woodruff, McManus, and David, 1995), depression (Wu et al., 1993), epilepsy (Atkinson et al., 1996), Tourette syndrome (Baumgardner et al., 1996; Moriarty et al., 1997), posttraumatic stress disorder (De Bellis et al., 1999), Alzheimer's disease (Hampel et al., 1998; Lakmache et al., 1998), alcohol abuse (Estruch et al., 1997; Oishi, Mochizuki, and Shikata, 1999), and dyslexia (Hynd et al., 1995). The sometimes conflicting results in CC morphology were interpreted in two ways. The common interpretation has been that a larger CC midsagittal area (total CC or CC subarea) reflects increased interhemispheric connectivity resulting in (or due to) increased ambilaterality (Witelson, 1989). This interpretation is at variance with the interpretation by Clarke and coworkers (1993a) that the CC size indicates the number of fibers that subserve inhibiting or interfering processes located in the dominant hemisphere. In the light of these controversies and considering the enormous variability in CC size across the subgroups tested, we employed whole-brain in vivo magnetic resonance morphometry to investigate the anatomical relationship between CC midsagittal size and forebrain volume. This approach may also provide an empirical evaluation of the recently suggested relationship between brain size and lateralization (Ringo, 1991; Ringo et al., 1994), and it might help to explain the large interindividual variability in callosal size. In particular, we were interested in answering the following questions:

1. Is there an allometric relationship between callosal size and brain size?

LUTZ JÄNCKE   Department of Psychology, Division of Neuropsychology, University of Zurich, Zurich, Switzerland.

HELMUTH STEINMETZ Department of Neurology, Johann Wolfgang Goethe University, Frankfurt, Germany.

2. If there is a relationship between callosal size and brain size, does this relationship follow a geometrical rule?

3. Is there a true influence of gender in this relationship?

4. Is handedness or brain lateralization related to callosal size?

The relationship between corpus callosum size and forebrain volume

Several attempts have been made to relate brain and CC size measures in humans. In general, most postmortem studies found small but significant linear correlations between both measures (Zilles, 1972; Witelson, 1985, 1989; Highley et al., 1999). However, recent large studies using MRI to estimate brain size by one or a few cross-sectional brain area measures revealed no significant CC/brain size relationship (Mall, 1909; Kertesz et al., 1987; Clarke et al., 1989). These results were taken as evidence for a lack of an allometric CC/brain size relationship. In our own study (Jäncke et al., 1997) we measured forebrain volume and the size of the midsagittal CC area in 120 young, healthy adults (49 women, 71 men, mean age $\pm$ S.D. $= 25.7 \pm 4.7$ years) using in vivo magnetic resonance morphometry of the brain (128 contiguous sagittal 1.17-mm-thick sections). In that study we found a mean $\pm$ S.D. total brain volume of 1.120 ± 0.110 liter for women and 1.240 ± 0.110 liter for men. Taking into account a specific gravity of fresh postmortem brain tissue of 1.04–1.09 kg/liter (Blinkov and Glezer, 1968) and the up to 9% increase in brain volume during the first hours after death (presumably owing to the absorption of cerebrospinal fluid) (Appel and Appel, 1942), our brain volume measurements obtained in living subjects correspond exactly to what one would expect from these postmortem data. With these in vivo measurements of brain volume we evaluated the CC/brain volume relationship. Because total brain volume is mostly determined by forebrain volume (brain volume—hindbrain volume), the following analysis is focused on forebrain volume (FBV).

When relating midsagittal CC size to FBV, one has to consider that CC size is measured as an area (mm^2) and FBV as a volume (mm^3). In addition, CC area is part of the FBV and thus contributes to FBV. As a first approach in relating CC size to FBV, one might argue that brains of different size are geometrically similar. In Euclidean geometry, two triangles are geometrically similar if corresponding sides are in a constant ratio and corresponding angles are equal. In addition, if two triangles are equiangular, then their corresponding sides are

proportional. Such geometric similar bodies are often called isometric. The same considerations pertain to any other geometrically similar figures and can be extended to three-dimensional figures as well. Now consider two cubes of different sizes. Because all corresponding linear measurements of the two cubes are in the same proportion and all corresponding angles are equal, the two cubes are geometrically similar or isometric. However, the surface areas of the two cubes do not change in the same ratio as their linear dimensions, but rather with the square of the linear ratio. Similarly, the volumes of the cubes change in proportion to the third power of their linear dimensions. Say that the larger cube has a side twice as long as a side of the smaller cube. The surface area of the larger cube will then be 2^2, or four, times as large as the smaller cube, and its volume will be 2^3, or eight, times as great. The same rules apply to any other geometrically similar or isometric three-dimensional bodies, whatever the shapes. According to this rule, the size of a cross-sectional area of a three-dimensional object does not increase proportionally to the volume of this object, but only to the two-thirds power of the volume. With respect to our problem of relating CC cross-sectional area to FBV, we can write:

$$CC = constant \times FBV^{2/3} \qquad (3.1)$$

This equation states that as FBV increases, the cross-sectional CC area does not increase in the same proportion, but only in proportion to the two-thirds power of FBV. Another fact that is related to that rule is that smaller bodies have, relative to their volumes, larger surface areas than larger bodies of the same shape. With respect to our problem, this can be expressed by dividing Equation (3.1) by FBV:

$$CC/FBV = constant \times FBV^{2/3}/FBV$$
$$CC/FBV = constant \times FBV^{-1/3} \qquad (3.2)$$

These equations can be transformed logarithmically, revealing the following equations, which are much easier to handle with conventional statistical software:

$$\log CC = \log constant + \tfrac{2}{3} \times \log FBV \qquad (3.3)$$
$$\log(CC/FBV) = \log constant + (-\tfrac{1}{3}) \times \log FBV \qquad (3.4)$$

To test whether the CC/FBV relationship followed the geometrical rule, we calculated Equations (3.3) and (3.4) and compared the slopes of interest with the hypothetical slopes derived from the geometrical rule ($\tfrac{2}{3} = 0.67$ or $-\tfrac{1}{3} = -0.33$). If a cross-sectional area/volume relationship follows the geometrical rule, the slopes are 0.67 in Equation (3.3) and -0.33 in Equation (3.4). In this case smaller brains have, relative to their volumes, larger

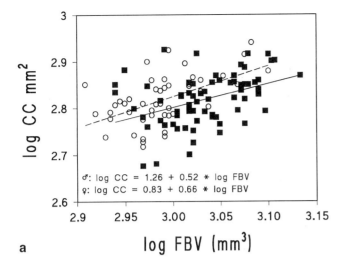

a

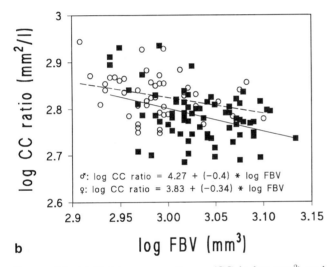

b

FIGURE 3.1. (a) Total corpus callosum (CC in log mm²) and forebrain volume (FBV in log l). (b) Total corpus callosum ratio (CC/FBV in log mm²/l) and forebrain volume (FBV in log l). Data are taken from Jäncke et al., 1977. Open circles indicate women, and solid squares indicate men. Regression slopes for women are dashed.

cross-sectional CC areas than larger brains of the same shape.

In Figure 3.1a the cross-sectional CC area is plotted against the FBV on logarithmic coordinates. For this scattergram we obtained significant regressions (females: $r^2 = 0.30$; males: $r^2 = 0.17$) with slopes of 0.66 (females) and 0.52 (males). Both slopes significantly differed from 1, indicating that log CC area increases less than proportional to log FBV. More important, both slopes do not differ significantly from 0.67, indicating that these relationships followed the geometrical rule. If, instead, CC area per unit FBV (CC ratio) is plotted (Figure

3.1b), the regression line shows that the relative surface area decreases with increasing FBV. The slopes of these regression lines are −0.34 (females) and −0.48 (males). When total CC is divided into subareas (anterior third, middle third, isthmus, and splenium, according to Witelson, 1989), the relationship between CC area measurements and FBV remains fairly stable. A further result of these analyses is that there are no substantial gender differences with respect to the CC/FBV relationships. Thus, the geometrical rule is appropriate for describing the CC/FBV relationship for both genders not only for the total CC but also for CC subareas (for details, see Jäncke et al., 1997).

To cross-validate our results, we reviewed the literature for studies giving total CC size and precise brain size measures. We found only studies relying on post-mortem analyzed brains (Bean, 1906; Mall, 1909; Zilles, 1972; De Lacoste-Utamsing and Holloway, 1982; Holloway and De Lacoste, 1986; Weber and Weis, 1986; Demeter, Ringo, and Doty, 1988; Witelson, 1989; De Lacoste, Adesanya, and Woodward, 1990; Aboitiz, Scheibel, and Zaidel, 1992c). From these studies, mean CC area size as well as mean brain weight were derived and plotted on logarithmic coordinates.[1] For this scattergram (Figure 3.2a) we obtained significant regressions (female: $r^2 = 0.16$; male: $r^2 = 0.42$) with slopes of 0.56 (females) and 0.71 (males). When CC ratios (CC/brain weight) are plotted as function of brain weight (Figure 3.2b), the regression line shows that the relative surface area decreases with increasing FBV. The slopes of these regression lines are −0.48 (females) and −0.28 (males). Thus, these analyses confirm our data. Taken together, the data demonstrate that the CC/brain size relationship follows the geometrical rule implying that the cross-sectional CC area increases less than proportional to brain size. It follows from this relationship that larger brains have relatively smaller cross-sectional callosal areas.

Because cross-sectional CC area and small diameter callosal axon number are positively related in humans (Aboitiz et al., 1992b), our result suggests that the degree of interhemispheric connectedness may indeed decrease with an enlarging brain. This provides first empirical support of the aforementioned conjecture by Ringo and coworkers that brain size may be an important factor

---

[1] Because Weber and Weis (1986) presented only cerebrum weight, we estimated total brain weight by adding hindbrain weight derived according to Blinkov and Glezer (1968). De Lacoste and coworkers (1990) presented only brain weights of brains, excluding the rhombencephalon. Therefore, brain weight was adjusted according to Blinkov and Glezer (1968).

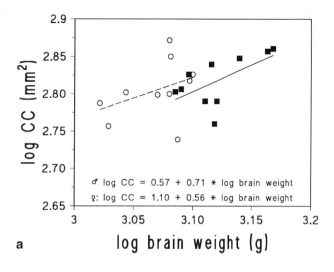

a

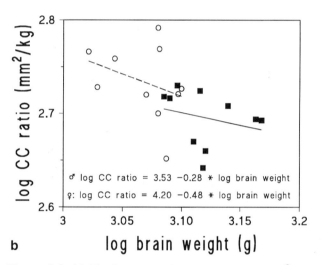

b

FIGURE 3.2. (a) Total corpus callosum (CC in log mm²) and brain weight (BW in g). (b) Total corpus callosum ratio (CC/BW in log mm²/kg) and brain weight (BW in log g). Data are taken from published postmortem studies (see text for further details). Open circles indicate women, and solid squares indicate men. Regression slopes for women are dashed.

influencing interhemispheric communication (Ringo, 1991; Ringo et al., 1994).

Is there a true gender difference in the cross-sectional size of the corpus callosum?

Whether there are gender differences in the size or the shape of the CC is a long-standing question. The first author who evaluated gender differences in callosal area size was Bean (1906), who found a larger genu in males. Shortly thereafter, Mall (1909), using a modern approach including a blind procedure (not used by Bean), failed to

find differences in the CC that could be attributed to gender. This debate was reestablished by a postmortem study by De Lacoste-Utamsing and Holloway (1982), who reported that women might have a wider and more bulbous splenium than men and that even the overall size of the CC might be absolutely larger in women (Holloway and De Lacoste, 1986). The majority of follow-up studies failed to replicate these results (Weber and Weis, 1986; Kertesz et al., 1987; Oppenheim et al., 1987; Byne, Bleier, and Huston, 1988; Demeter et al., 1988; Clarke et al., 1989, 1993b; Hayakawa et al., 1989; Weis et al., 1989; Elster, Di Persio, and Moody, 1990; Going and Dixson, 1990; Allen et al., 1991; Emory et al., 1991; Habib et al., 1991; Aboitiz et al., 1992c; Steinmetz et al., 1992, 1995; Holloway et al., 1993; Pujol et al., 1993; Johnson et al., 1994; Pozzilli et al., 1994; Rauch and Jinkins, 1994). For a thorough discussion of this issue, see also Bishop and Wahlsten (1997). Nevertheless, most authors found a larger relative CC in women (i.e., CC relative to brain or skull size) or larger relative posterior portions of the CC in women (i.e., splenium or isthmus relative to total CC) (Kertesz et al., 1987; Reinarz et al., 1988; Clarke et al., 1989; Witelson, 1989; De Lacoste et al., 1990; Elster et al., 1990; Allen et al., 1991; Habib et al., 1991; Steinmetz et al., 1992, 1995; Holloway et al., 1993; Johnson et al., 1994; Clarke and Zaidel, 1994). A typical result based on our previously described sample of 120 young and healthy subjects is shown on Figure 3.3a. This figure illustrates that there is no gender difference in callosal size, either for the total CC or for the CC subareas (which are defined according to criteria suggested by Witelson (1989) and Jäncke and coworkers (1997). However, callosal size related to FBV revealed a stronger gender difference, with women showing the largest CC ratios (Figure 3.3b). The common interpretation of this sexual dimorphism would be that it reflects increased interhemispheric connectivity due to increased female ambilaterality especially for temporoparietal cognitive functions (McGlone, 1980).

In light of the data presented in the preceding paragraph, one might ask whether there is a true gender effect on relative CC area size or whether the relative CC size might be affected by a more general brain volume effect. To examine whether there was a true gender difference in the CC ratios (CC/FBV), we divided our sample into FBV quintiles, with 24 brains per quintile (Figure 3.4). For each FBV quintile, *t*-tests were calculated to compare FBV and CC measurements between the genders. They revealed no significant gender differences, except for the third quintile, made up of brains with FBV values of approximately 1.0 liter. For this group we found a larger total CC and CC ratio in women. Subsequent analyses revealed that this gender

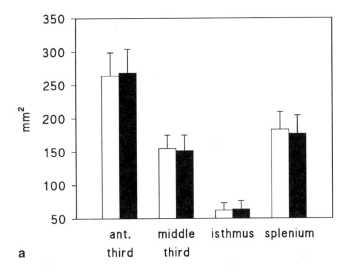

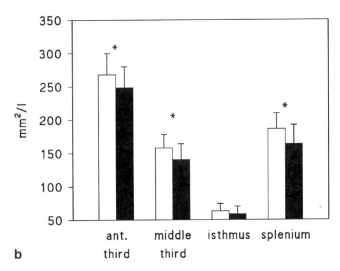

FIGURE 3.3. (a) Mean CC subarea measures for women (white bars) and men (black bars). (b) Mean CC ratios (CC subarea divided by FBV) for women (white bars) and men (black bars). Vertical lines indicate standard deviations.

difference was restricted to the middle third and the splenium. However, because this quintile comprised 5 female and 19 male brains, a sampling error is possible.

In our opinion these data suggest that brain volume is the main factor affecting relative callosal size. Because the CC/brain size relationship follows a geometric rule, larger brains will be associated with smaller CC ratios than smaller brains. Since on average women have smaller brains, they will have larger CC ratios. More important, women with large brains do show small CC ratios, while men with small brains show large CC ratios. Thus, the size of the CC and the CC ratio depend mainly on brain size and not on gender per se.

Corpus callosum and brain lateralization

Witelson was the first to suggest that hand preference, interacting with gender, might also affect CC morphology (Witelson, 1985, 1989; Witelson and Goldsmith, 1991; Witelson and Nowakowski, 1991). In her postmortem studies, nonconsistently right-handed men showed larger total CC areas than consistently right-handed men or women. This suggested a relationship between laterality and callosal size, at least in men. Subsequent in vivo imaging studies, however, revealed equivocal results. Whereas some investigators replicated the findings of Witelson and coworkers for absolute and relative CC subarea measurements (Elster et al., 1990; Habib et al., 1991; Cowell, Kertesz, and Denenber, 1993; Clarke and Zaidel, 1994; Moffat, Hampson, and Lee, 1998), others could not confirm significant influences of handedness (Nasrallah et al., 1986; Kertesz et al., 1987; O'Kusky, Strauss, and Kosaka, 1988; Reinarz et al., 1988; Steinmetz et al., 1992, 1995; Jäncke et al., 1997).

Further support that the CC is involved in the processing of lateralized functions comes from dichotic listening studies. Dichotic listening is a frequently used index of cerebral lateralization (Bryden, 1988; Hugdahl, 1992). The expected finding with verbal stimuli is a right ear advantage that is believed to result from left hemisphere lateralization of language function and greater efficiency of the contralateral auditory pathways in the simultaneous stimulation condition (Kimura, 1967). It is thought that the CC may serve a critical function in transmitting verbal information from the left ear via the right hemisphere to the language areas on the left (Kimura, 1967). This callosal transfer model has received support from studies on split-brain patients in whom complete left ear extinction has been observed (e.g., Zaidel, 1976). Sectioning of the anterior third of the CC, as well as sectioning of the splenium, maintains an intact left ear performance (Eslinger and Damasio, 1988; Risse et al., 1989). The remaining critical sector is consistent with anatomical knowledge about the interhemispheric connections of the auditory cortices (Sidtis, 1988). In fact, it is most likely that auditory interhemispheric transfer occurs through the isthmus (Alexander et al., 1988).

It has been speculated that the anatomical variation in CC size or shape is of functional significance for cerebral lateralization (Witelson, 1989). If behavioral measures of interhemispheric functions are related to morphometric measures of callosal connectivity, then left ear performance should correlate with CC size (because left ear stimuli are transmitted via the CC to the language areas in the left hemisphere). Laterality measures (e.g., right minus left ear performance) should

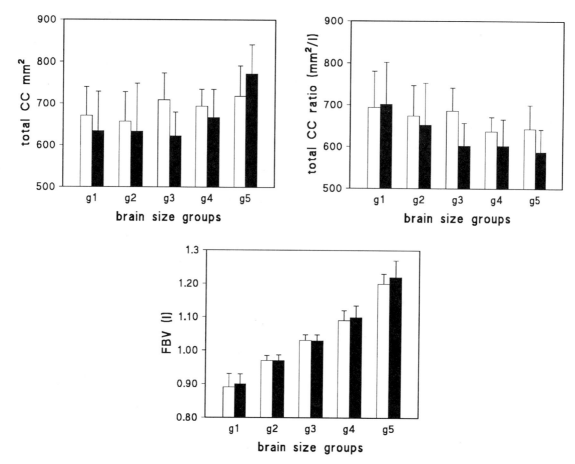

FIGURE 3.4. Mean total CC and CC ratios as a function of brain size groups (g1 to g5). Brain size in terms of FBV of the five brain size groups is depicted in the lower panel.

correlate negatively with the size of the posterior body of the callosum (isthmus and splenium), where interhemispheric auditory fibers are presumed to be located in humans. This predicted structure-function relationship is based on the assumption that a larger callosal area is associated with more fibers and/or larger-diameter fibers, which, in turn, permit more efficient callosal transfer in this difficult task.

Witelson (1987) was the first to test this hypothesis. She applied the dichotic listening test to 13 terminally ill male cancer patients whose brains were later analyzed in for callosal morphology. She found that the size of the isthmus was negatively correlated with the difference between right and left ear accuracy of the dichotic listening task ($r = -0.55$). Five studies examining callosum measures obtained from MRI and dichotic listening scores in normal subjects have produced equivocal findings. O'Kusky and coworkers (1988) found significant negative correlations of a dichotic listening laterality index with total callosum area, as well as with two anterior callosum measures. Hines and coworkers (1992)

discovered a trend of a negative relationship between the size of the splenium and a laterality index in dichotic listening. Clarke and coworkers (1993b) found no correlations between left ear performance and size of the CC, but they did find a negative correlation between right ear score and size of the CC. They interpret their results as indicating an interhemispheric inhibitory-facilitatory function of callosal connections. Two further studies found no relationship between midsagittal callosal measures and dichotic listening test results (Kertesz et al., 1987; Jäncke and Steinmetz, 1994).

Because there have been only a few studies of the relationship between behavioral laterality effects and callosum morphology, there is a need for further investigation of this topic. We therefore examined the relationship between handedness and midsagittal corpus callosum area in our sample of 120 young and healthy subjects. We applied Annett's handedness questionnaire (Annett, 1970) because this handedness classification has been validated with hand skill measures (Jäncke, 1996). As is shown in Figure 3.5, we discovered no substantial

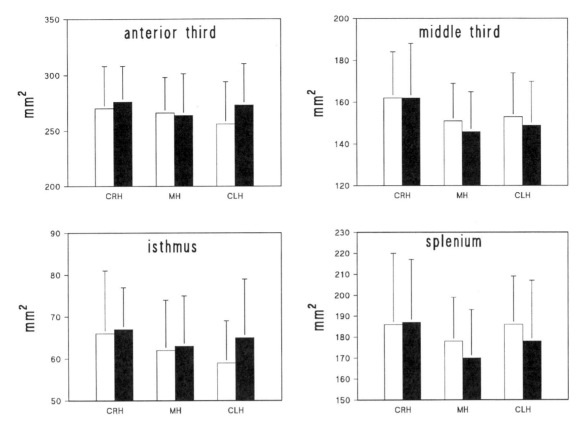

FIGURE 3.5. Mean CC subarea measures for consistent right-handers (CRH), consistent left-handers (CLH), and mixed-handers (MH) as a function of gender (women: white bars; men: black bars). Vertical lines indicate standard deviations.

influence of handedness on CC size for either males or females. The same negative finding was found for callosal ratios (Figure 3.6). Thus, we could not confirm larger CC measurements in nonconsistent right-handers, mixed-handers, or consistent left-handers when compared to consistent right-handers. This is in agreement with the majority of studies investigating possible relationships between CC size and handedness (Nasrallah et al., 1986; Kertesz et al., 1987; O'Kusky et al., 1988; Reinarz et al., 1988; Steinmetz et al., 1992). In our sample, consistent right-handers even showed a larger midbody than other handedness groups, which is in contrast to previous reports of opposite handedness effects (Witelson, 1989; Denenberg, Kertesz, and Cowell, 1991; Habib et al., 1991; Cowell et al., 1993; Clarke and Zaidel, 1994). However, it should be mentioned that two of the latter studies (Denenberg et al., 1991; Cowell et al., 1993) were reanalyses of data for which a prior report (Kertesz et al., 1987) had failed to identify a gender or handedness difference, that the postmortem sample of Witelson (Witelson, 1989) was relatively heterogeneous, and that the effect reported by Clarke and Zaidel (1994) remained small. While our data may add further confusion to this part of the ongoing discussion, it appears fair

to say that an influence of handedness on CC size or shape must remain questionable.

Since handedness is only moderately related to brain asymmetry, it is necessary to examine further behavioral laterality measures and their relationship to callosum size. We therefore applied a consonant-vowel dichotic listening recall test (Jäncke, Steinmetz, and Volkmann, 1992) to young, healthy subjects (26 males and 24 females) in whom the CC was measured using MRI. This sample was divided according to median-split into subjects with larger (17 men and 18 women) and smaller brains (16 women and 19 men). For each brain size group, Pearson product-moment correlations were determined between the midsagittal CC subareas and (1) the dichotic listening recall scores for superior ear accuracy, (2) those for inferior ear accuracy, and (3) the dichotic listening ear difference scores. It should be reiterated here that if behavioral measures of interhemispheric transfer functions are related to morphometric correlates of callosal connectivity, then inferior ear performance (left ear performance in right-handers and right ear performance in some left-handers) should correlate positively, and laterality measures (e.g., superior minus inferior ear performance) should correlate nega-

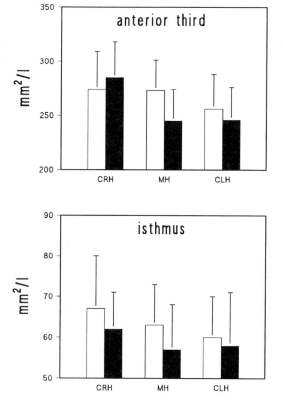

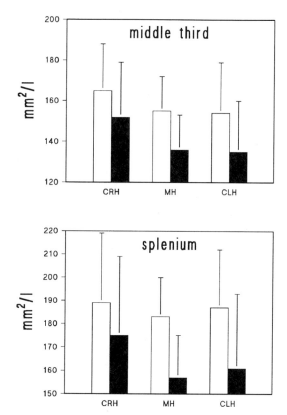

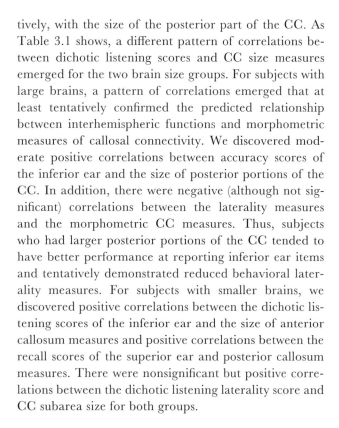

FIGURE 3.6. Mean CC ratios for consistent right-handers (CRH), consistent left-handers (CLH), and mixed-handers (MH) as a function of gender (women: white bars, men: black bars). Vertical lines indicate standard deviations.

tively, with the size of the posterior part of the CC. As Table 3.1 shows, a different pattern of correlations between dichotic listening scores and CC size measures emerged for the two brain size groups. For subjects with large brains, a pattern of correlations emerged that at least tentatively confirmed the predicted relationship between interhemispheric functions and morphometric measures of callosal connectivity. We discovered moderate positive correlations between accuracy scores of the inferior ear and the size of posterior portions of the CC. In addition, there were negative (although not significant) correlations between the laterality measures and the morphometric CC measures. Thus, subjects who had larger posterior portions of the CC tended to have better performance at reporting inferior ear items and tentatively demonstrated reduced behavioral laterality measures. For subjects with smaller brains, we discovered positive correlations between the dichotic listening scores of the inferior ear and the size of anterior callosum measures and positive correlations between the recall scores of the superior ear and posterior callosum measures. There were nonsignificant but positive correlations between the dichotic listening laterality score and CC subarea size for both groups.

These findings may be important in two ways:

1. They do not confirm the results of Clarke and co-workers (Clarke et al., 1993a; Clarke and Zaidel, 1994), and therefore, they mitigate the functional interpretation given by these authors that callosal size reflects an interhemispheric inhibitory-facilitatory function of callosal connections.

2. Different patterns of anatomical-behavioral correlations emerged for the two brain size groups. While the pattern observed for subjects with large brains was in line with the predicted anatomical-behavioral relationship, the correlations obtained for subjects with smaller brains did not follow this prediction. It is possible that the fibers crossing the midline are involved in different interhemispheric functions depending on brain size.

However, one has to keep in mind that dichotic listening tests might not be a particularly reliable measure of lateralization or interhemispheric transfer. Ear asymmetry may also be influenced by factors unrelated to laterality, such as competitive attentional biases between the ears, individual differences in the capacity of ipsilateral auditory pathways, and variations in processing strategies (Hugdahl and Andersson, 1986; Bryden, 1988; Jäncke,

TABLE 3.1

Correlation coefficients for 50 subjects divided according to brain volume into two groups (large and small brain groups) between anatomical area measures of the corpus callosum and behavioral measures from a dichotic listening task.

	Superior Ear Report	Inferior Ear Report	Laterality Index
Large brains (n = 25)			
Anterior third	+0.30	+0.30	−0.12
Middle third	+0.29	+0.45*	−0.14
Isthmus	+0.04	+0.38*	−0.24
Splenium	+0.19	+0.37*	−0.07
Small brains (n = 25)			
Anterior third	+0.38	+0.45*	+0.10
Middle third	+0.55*	+0.40*	+0.26
Isthmus	+0.54*	+0.33	+0.32
Splenium	+0.48*	+0.22	+0.35

*$p < 0.05$.

1994; Asbjornsen and Bryden, 1996). Therefore, we cannot rule out that these factors might have attenuated relationships between dichotic listening scores and CC measurements in our study. Similarly, owing to the relative complexity of the tasks employed here, the dichotic listening test results may reflect not only interhemispheric transfer but intrahemispheric processing as well.

Our working hypothesis was based on the so-called *callosal transfer model.* According to this model, only the dominant hemisphere processes auditory-verbal stimuli, so laterality effects are expected to reflect callosal transfer from the nondominant to the dominant half of the brain. In contrast, the *direct access model* has suggested that the nondominant hemisphere is also capable of processing auditory-verbal information but less efficiently than the contralateral one (Zaidel, Clarke, and Suyenobu, 1990). According to this model, dichotic listening results would reflect efficiency of information processing within each hemisphere. Zaidel (1983) argues from data with split brain patients that dichotic listening to nonsense consonant-vowel syllables is callosal relay. But the task used here may have different properties.

In addition, one has to question whether midsagittal CC size is indeed a valid index of the conduction velocity of callosal axons. The study by Aboitiz and coworkers (1992b) demonstrated that CC subarea sizes are positively related only to the number of small-diameter (slow-conducting) callosal fibers but not to the number of large-diameter (fast-conducting) axons crossing through. Unfortunately, we do not know which class of fibers is involved in the callosal transfer of auditory information as investigated here.

Nevertheless, the positive finding of our study was that the size of almost all CC subareas correlated with the dichotic listening accuracy scores (for either the superior or the inferior ear). In general, subjects with larger CC areas demonstrated better accuracy scores. Stimulus detection tasks have shown that recall and discrimination rates are very strongly associated with stimulus complexity and cognitive capacity (intelligence) (Jensen, 1982). Interestingly, a previous study found evidence for a link between CC area size and verbal fluency, a further variable that is closely associated with cognitive capacity (Hines et al., 1992; Strauss, Wada, and Hunter, 1994). Thus, it appears possible that precision and speed of cognition, essentials of intelligence, are somehow related to callosal size.

Conclusion

A major aim of this presentation is to demonstrate that at least a part of the large interindividual variability in callosal size might be explained by brain size differences. Our analysis revealed that the CC/brain size relationship follows a geometrical rule implying that the cross-sectional CC area increases less than proportional to brain size (FBV or weight). It follows from this relationship that larger brains have relatively smaller cross-sectional CC areas. Nevertheless, this allometric relationship with FBV explained not more than 30% of the total variability in CC size observed in our sample, demonstrating that the thickness of the CC is still influenced mainly by other factors. The majority of callosal fibers are thought to originate from association cortices and subserve higher-order functions (Innocenti, 1986;

Pandya and Seltzer, 1986; LaMantia and Rakic, 1990; Aboitiz et al., 1992a). Thus, as was previously hypothesized by Peters (Peters, 1988), a possible lack of an allometric relationship between the size of the brain and the association cortices could account for at least some of the variation in CC size that remains unexplained by the CC/FBV relationship.

Additional variance of CC morphology may be added by environmental factors. In animal studies of postnatal development of the CC, the number of callosal axons in neonates exceeds that of young adults, suggesting that normal development involves the remodeling of axonal projections between the two hemispheres with a subsequent elimination of callosal axons (Innocenti and Frost, 1979; Clarke et al., 1989; LaMantia and Rakic, 1990; Innocenti, this volume; Rosen, this volume). However, this reduction in the number of callosal axons, reflecting the selective elimination of axon collaterals or callosal neurons during the early postnatal period, can be manipulated experimentally by altering sensory or motor experience during early development (Innocenti, Fiore, and Caminiti, 1977; Berrebi et al., 1988). Studies of humans have suggested a considerable degree of callosal plasticity during brain development until adulthood, possibly induced by environmental stimulation (Allen et al., 1991; Pujol et al., 1993; Schlaug et al., 1995).

The lack of a principal gender difference in the CC/FBV relationship implies that small brains exhibit larger CC ratios, irrespective of gender. Thus, FBV was the main factor explaining the gender difference in our sample of 120 young, healthy subjects. However, it remains to be determined in future experiments whether gender might exert additional impact on CC morphology.

On the basis of present anatomical knowledge, a functional interpretation of this inverse relationship between forebrain size and relative callosal size must remain speculative. Let us assume that the packing densities and branching patterns of callosal neurons and axons do not depend on brain size. In that case our data would indicate that the degree of interhemispheric connectedness decreases with increasing human brain size. This would concur with theoretical predictions made by Ringo and coworkers (Ringo, 1991; Ringo et al., 1994). They argued that as brain size is scaled up, there must be a decrease in interhemispheric connectivity, owing to the increasing time constraints of transcallosal conduction delay. Consequently, functionally related neuronal elements would cluster in one hemisphere, so increasing brain size would be the driving force in the phylogeny of hemispheric specialization. With regard to callosal connectivity, our morphometric data provide the first empirical support of this conjecture.

Our finding that CC size is related to FBV should motivate future studies to normalize CC measures to brain size measures, similar to what it was originally proposed by De Lacoste et al. (1990). Brain size turns out to be an important variable in aging, in psychopathology, and perhaps in cognitive capacity. Thus, it is necessary to rule out that subgroup differences in callosal morphology are not solely a function of brain size. Let us consider a study designed to compare CC size between mixed- and right-handers. The mean brain size of the mixed-handers might be slightly larger by sampling errors. Then it is most likely that the CC size measures of the mixed-handers are slightly larger than those of the right-handers. Therefore, it would be more appropriate to use brain size-normalized CC size measures or to compare handedness subgroups with similar brain size measures. In general, this problem can be extended to any study comparing CC size between subgroups, whether they are normal, dysphasic, autistic, schizophrenic, or whatever.

Previous in vivo MRI studies have tried to address this challenge by measuring total midsagittal cross-sectional area of both cerebral hemispheres to predict brain size (Clarke and Zaidel, 1994; Kertesz et al., 1986; Rauch and Jenkins, 1994). However, the postmortem study of De Lacoste and coworkers (De Lacoste-Utamsing and Holloway, 1982) demonstrated that such measures cannot be used to predict brain weight because the correlation between midsagittal surface area and brain weight is rather low ($r = 0.40$, $r^2 = 0.20$). Therefore, it is necessary to measure brain volume more directly.

Our results supporting the conjecture that brain asymmetry might be linked to brain size may stimulate future research in a number of ways. An important question will be whether brains of different sizes differ in neuronal packing density and branching patterns of callosal axons. It will also be worth examining the relationship between brain size, established behavioral (language lateralization) asymmetries, and structural asymmetries (e.g., planum temporale and planum parietale asymmetry) (Steinmetz et al., 1991; Aboitiz et al., 1992c; Jäncke et al., 1994). If there is indeed a relationship between brain size and asymmetry, larger brains should demonstrate stronger anatomical and functional asymmetries. This then may provide clues for the phylogeny of hemispheric dominance in the higher primates (Ringo, 1991; Ringo et al., 1994).

REFERENCES

ABOITIZ, F., A. B. SCHEIBEL, R. S. FISHER, and E. ZAIDEL, 1992a. Fiber composition of the human corpus callosum. *Brain Res.* 598:143–153.

ABOITIZ, F., A. B. SCHEIBEL, R. S. FISHER, and E. ZAIDEL,

1992b. Individual differences in brain asymmetries and fiber composition in the human corpus callosum. *Brain Res.* 598:154–161.

ABOITIZ, F., A. B. SCHEIBEL, and E. ZAIDEL, 1992c. Morphometry of the Sylvian fissure and the corpus callosum, with emphasis on sex differences. *Brain* 115:1521–1541.

ALEXANDER, M. P. and R. L. WARREN, 1988. Localization of callosal auditory pathways: a CT case study. *Neurology* 38:802–804.

ALLEN, L. S., M. RICHEY, Y. CHAI, and R. GORSKI, 1991. Sex differences in the cerebral cortex and the corpus callosum of the living human being. *J. Neurosci.* 11:933–942.

ANNETT, M., 1970. A classification of hand preference by association analysis. *Br. J. Psychol.* 61:303–321.

APPEL, F. W., and E. M. APPEL, 1942. Intracranial variation in the weight of the human brain. *Human Biol.* 14:235–250.

ASBJORNSEN, A. E., and M. P. BRYDEN, 1996. Biased attention and the fused dichotic words test [published erratum appears in *Neuropsychologia* 34 (11):1141]. *Neuropsychologia* 34:407–411.

ATKINSON, D. S. J., B. ABOU-KHALIL, P. D. CHARLES, and L. WELCH, 1996. Midsagittal corpus callosum area, intelligence, and language dominance in epilepsy. *J. Neuroimaging* 6:235–239.

BAUMGARDNER, T. L., H. S. SINGER, M. B. DENCKLA, M. A. RUBIN, M. T. ABRAMS, M. J. COLLI, and A. L. REISS, 1996. Corpus callosum morphology in children with Tourette syndrome and attention deficit hyperactivity disorder. *Neurology* 47:477–482.

BEAN, R. B., 1906. Some racial pecularities of the negro brain. *Am. J. An.* 5:353–432.

BERREBI, A. S., R. FITCH, D. RALPHE, J. DENENBERG, V. FRIEDRICH, and V. H. DENENBERG, 1988. Corpus callosum: Region-specific effects of sex, early experience and age. *Brain Res.* 438:216–224.

BISHOP, K. M., and D. WAHLSTEN, 1997. Sex differences in the human corpus callosum: Myth or reality? *Neurosci. Biobehav. Rev.* 21:581–601.

BLINKOV, S. M., and I. I. GLEZER, 1968. *Das Zentralnervensystem in Zahlen und Tabellen.* Jena: VEB Gustav Fischer Verlag.

BRYDEN, M. P., 1988. Correlates of the dichotic right-ear effect. *Cortex* 24:313–319.

BYNE, W., R. BLEIER, and L. HUSTON, 1988. Variations in human corpus callosum do not predict gender: A study using magnetic resonance imaging. *Behav. Neurosci.* 102:222–227.

CLARKE, J. M., R. B. LUFKIN, and E. ZAIDEL, 1993a. Corpus callosum morphometry and dichotic listening performance: Individual differences in functional interhemispheric inhibition? *Neuropsychologia* 31:547–557.

CLARKE, J. M., R. B. LUFKIN, and E. ZAIDEL, 1993b. Corpus callosum morphometry and dichotic listening performance: Individual differences in functional interhemispheric inhibition? *Neuropsychologia* 31:547–557.

CLARKE, J. M., and E. ZAIDEL, 1994. Anatomical-behavioral relationships: Corpus callosum morphometry and hemispheric specialization. *Behav. Brain Res.* 64:185–202.

CLARKE, S., R. KRAFTSIK, H. VAN DER LOOS, and G. M. INNOCENTI, 1989. Forms and measures of adult and developing human corpus callosum: Is there sexual dimorphism? *J. Comp. Neurol.* 280:213–230.

COWELL, P. E., A. KERTESZ, and V. H. DENENBERG, 1993. Multiple dimensions of handedness and the human corpus callosum. *Neurology* 43:2353–2357.

DE BELLIS, M. D., M. S. KESHAVAN, D. B. CLARK, B. J. CASEY, J. N. GIEDD, A. M. BORING, K. FRUSTACI, and N. D. RYAN, 1999. AE Bennett Research Award. Developmental traumatology. Part II: Brain development [see comments]. *Biol. Psychiatry* 45:1271–1284.

DE LACOSTE, M. C., T. ADESANYA, and D. J. WOODWARD, 1990. Measures of gender differences in human brain and their relationship to brain weight. *Biol. Psychiatry* 28:931–942.

DE LACOSTE-UTAMSING, M. C., and R. L. HOLLOWAY, 1982. Sexual dimorphism in the human corpus callosum. *Science* 216:1431–1432.

DEMETER, S., J. L. RINGO, and R. W. DOTY, 1988. Morphometric analysis of the human corpus callosum and anterior commisure. *Human Neurobiol.* 6:219–226.

DENENBERG, V. H., A. KERTESZ, and P. E. COWELL, 1991. A factor analysis of the human's corpus callosum. *Brain Res.* 548:126–132.

ELSTER, A. D., D. A. DI PERSIO, and D. M. MOODY, 1990. Sexual dimorphism of the human corpus callosum studied by magnetic resonance imaging: Fact, fallacy and statistical confidence. *Brain Dev.* 12:21–325.

EMORY, L. E., D. H. WILLIAMS, C. M. COLE, E. G. AMPARO, and W. J. MEYER, 1991. Anatomic variation of the corpus callosum in persons with gender dysphoria. *Arch. Sex. Behav.* 20:409–417.

ESLINGER, P. J., and H. DAMASIO, 1988. Anatomical correlates of paradoxic ear extinction. In *Handbook of Dichotic Listening*, K. Hugdahl, ed. New York: Wiley, pp. 139–160.

ESTRUCH, R., J. M. NICOLAS, M. SALAMERO, C. ARAGON, E. SACANELLA, J. FERNANDEZ-SOLA, and A. URBANO-MARQUEZ, 1997. Atrophy of the corpus callosum in chronic alcoholism. *J. Neurol. Sci.* 146:145–151.

GOING, J. J., and A. DIXSON, 1990. Morphometry of the adult human corpus callosum: Lack of sexual dimorphism. *J. Anat.* 171:163–167.

HABIB, M., D. GAYRAUD, A. OLIVA, J. REGIS, G. SALAMON, and R. KHALIL, 1991. Effects of handedness and sex on the morphology of the corpus callosum: A study with brain magnetic resonance imaging. *Brain Cogn.* 16:41–61.

HAMPEL, H., S. J. TEIPEL, G. E. ALEXANDER, B. HORWITZ, D. TEICHBERG, M. B. SCHAPIRO, and S. I. RAPOPORT, 1998. Corpus callosum atrophy is a possible indicator of region- and cell type-specific neuronal degeneration in Alzheimer disease: A magnetic resonance imaging analysis. *Arch. Neurol.* 55:193–198.

HAYAKAWA, K., Y. KONISHI, T. MATSUDA, M. KURIYAMA, K. KONISHI, K. YAMASHITA, and R. OKUMURA, 1989. Development and aging of brain midline structures: Assessment with MR imaging. *Neuroradiology* 172:171–177.

HIGHLEY, J. R., M. M. ESIRI, B. MCDONALD, M. CORTINA-BORJA, B. M. HERRON, and T. J. CROW, 1999. The size and fibre composition of the corpus callosum with respect to gender and schizophrenia: A post-mortem study. *Brain* 122:99–110.

HINES, M., L. CHIU, L. A. MCADAMS, P. M. BENTLER, and J. LIPCAMON, 1992. Cognition and the corpus callosum: Verbal fluency, visuspatial ability, and language lateralization related to midsaggital surface areas of callosal subregions. *Behav. Neurosci.* 106:3–14.

HOLLOWAY, R. L., P. J. ANDERSON, R. DEFENDINI, and C. HARPER, 1993. Sexual dimorphism of the human corpus callosum from three independent samples: Relative size of the corpus callosum. *Am. J. Phys. Anthropol.* 92:481–498.

HOLLOWAY, R. L., and M. C. DE LACOSTE, 1986. Sexual dimorphism in the human corpus callosum: An extension and replication study. *Human Neurobiol.* 5:87–91.

HUGDAHL, K., 1992. Brain lateralization: Dichotic listening studies. In *Encyclopedia of Neuroscience: Neuroscience Year 2*, B. Smith and G. Adelman, eds. Cambridge, Mass.: Birkhauser, pp. 23–26.

HUGDAHL, K., and L. ANDERSSON, 1986. The "forced-attention paradigm" in dichotic listening to CV-syllables: A comparison between adults and children. *Cortex* 22:417–432.

HYND, G. W., J. HALL, E. S. NOVEY, D. ELIOPULOS, K. BLACK, J. J. GONZALEZ, J. E. EDMONDS, C. RICCIO, and M. COHEN, 1995. Dyslexia and corpus callosum morphology. *Arch. Neurol.* 52:32–38.

INNOCENTI, G. M., 1986. What is so special about callosal connections. In *Two Hemispheres—One Brain: Functions of the Corpus Callosum*, F. Lepore, M. Ptito, and H. H. Jasper, eds. New York: Alan R. Liss, pp. 75–82.

INNOCENTI, G. M., L. FIORE, and R. CAMINITI, 1977. Exuberant projections into the corpus callosum from the visual cortex of newborn rat. *Neurosci. Lett.* 4:237–242.

INNOCENTI, G. M., and D. O. FROST, 1979. Abnormal visual experience stabilizes juvenile patterns of interhemispheric connections. *Nature* 280:231–234.

JÄNCKE, L., 1994. Hemispheric priming affects right-ear advantage in dichotic listening. *Int. J. Neurosci.* 74:71–77.

JÄNCKE, L., 1996. The hand performance test with a modified time limit instruction enables the examination of hand performance asymmetries in adults. *Percept. Mot. Skills* 82 (3, Pt. 1):735–738.

JÄNCKE, L., G. SCHLAUG, Y. HUANG, and H. STEINMETZ, 1994. Asymmetry of the planum parietale. *NeuroReport* 5:1161–1163.

JÄNCKE, L., J. F. STAIGER, G. SCHLAUG, Y. HUANG, and H. STEINMETZ, 1997. The relationship between corpus callosum size and forebrain volume. *Cereb. Cortex* 7:48–56.

JÄNCKE, L., and H. STEINMETZ, 1994. Interhemispheric transfer time and corpus callosum size. *NeuroReport* 5:2385–2388.

JÄNCKE, L., H. STEINMETZ, and J. VOLKMANN, 1992. Dichotic listening: What does it measure? *Neuropsychologia* 30:941–950.

JENSEN, A. R., 1982. Reaction time and psychometric g. In *A Model for Intelligence*, H. J. Eysenck, ed. New York: Springer, pp. 93–132.

JOHNSON, S. C., T. FARNWORTH, J. B. PINKSTON, E. D. BIGLER, and D. D. BLATTER, 1994. Corpus callosum surface area across the human adult life span: Effect of age and gender. *Brain Res. Bull.* 35:373–377.

KERTESZ, A., S. E. BLACK, M. POLK, and J. HOWELL, 1986. Cerebral asymmetrics on magnetic resonance imaging. *Cortex* 22:117–127.

KERTESZ, A., M. POLK, J. HOWELL, and S. E. BLACK, 1987. Cerebral dominance, sex, and callosal size in MRI. *Neurology* 37:1385–1388.

KIMURA, D., 1967. Functional asymmetry of the brain in dichotic listening. *Cortex* 3:163–168.

LAKMACHE, Y., M. LASSONDE, S. GAUTHIER, J. Y. FRIGON, and F. LEPORE, 1998. Interhemispheric disconnection syndrome in Alzheimer's disease. *Proc. Natl. Acad. Sci. U.S.A.* 95:9042–9046.

LAMANTIA, A., and P. RAKIC, 1990. Axon overproduction and elimination in the corpus callosum of the developing rhesus monkey. *J. Neurosci.* 10:2156–2175.

MALL, F. P., 1909. On several anatomical characters of the human brain, said to vary according to race and sex, with especial reference to the weight of the frontal lobe. *Am. J. Anat.* 9:1–32.

McGLONE, J., 1980. Sex differences in human brain asymmetry: A critical survey. *Behav. Brain Sci.* 3:215–263.

MOFFAT, S. D., E. HAMPSON, and D. H. LEE, 1998. Morphology of the planum temporale and corpus callosum in left handers with evidence of left and right hemisphere speech representation. *Brain* 121:2369–2379.

MORIARTY, J., A. R. VARMA, J. STEVENS, M. FISH, M. R. TRIMBLE, and M. M. ROBERTSON, 1997. A volumetric MRI study of Gilles de la Tourette's syndrome. *Neurology* 49:410–415.

NASRALLAH, H. A., N. C. ANDREASEN, J. A. COFFMAN, S. C. OLSON, V. D. DUNN, J. C. EHRHARDT, and S. M. CHAPMAN, 1986. A controlled magnetic resonance imaging study of corpus callosum thickness in schizophrenia. *Biol. Psychiatry* 21:274–282.

NJIOKIKTJIEN, C., and L. SONNEVILLE, 1991. Abnormal morphogenesis of the corpus callosum. II: Morphometry. In *The Child's Corpus Callosum*, G. Ramaekers and C. Njiokiktjien, eds. Amsterdam: Suyi Publications, pp. 310–318.

OISHI, M., Y. MOCHIZUKI, and E. SHIKATA, 1999. Corpus callosum atrophy and cerebral blood flow in chronic alcoholics. *J. Neurol. Sci.* 162:51–55.

OKA, S., O. MIYAMOTO, N. A. JANJUA, N. HONJO-FUJIWARA, M. OHKAWA, S. NAGAO, H. KONDO, T. MINAMI, T. TOYOSHIMA, and T. ITANO, 1999. Re-evaluation of sexual dimorphism in human corpus callosum. *NeuroReport* 10:937–940.

O'KUSKY, J., E. STRAUSS, and B. KOSAKA, 1988. The corpus callosum is larger with right hemisphere cerebral speech dominance. *Ann. Neurol.* 24:379–383.

OPPENHEIM, J. S., B. C. P. LEE, R. NASS, and M. S. GAZZANIGA, 1987. No sex-related differences in human corpus callosum based on magnetic resonance imagery. *Ann. Neurol.* 21:604–606.

PANDYA, D. N., and B. SELTZER, 1986. The topography of commisural fibers. In *Two Hemispheres—One Brain. Functions of the Corpus Callosum*, F. Lepore, M. Ptito, and H. H. Jasper, eds. New York: Alan R. Liss, pp. 47–73.

PETERS, M., 1988. The size of corpus callosum in males and females: Implications of a lack of allometry. *Can. J. Psychol.* 42:313–324.

POZZILLI, C., S. BASTIANELLO, A. BOZZAO, A. PIERALLINI, F. GIUBILEI, C. ARGENTINO, and L. BOZZAO, 1994. No differences in corpus callosum size by sex and aging. *J. Neuroimaging* 4:218–221.

PUJOL, J., P. VENDRELL, C. JUNQUE, J. L. MARTI VILATA, and A. CAPDEVILA, 1993. When does human brain development end? Evidence of corpus callosum growth up to adulthood. *Ann. Neurol.* 34:71–75.

RAUCH, R. A., and J. R. JINKINS, 1994. Analysis of cross-sectional area measurements of the corpus callosum adjusted for brain size in male and female subjects from childhood to adulthood. *Behav. Brain Res.* 64:65–78.

REINARZ, S. J., C. E. COFFMAN, W. R. SMOKER, and J. C. GODERSKY, 1988. MR imaging of the corpus callosum: Normal and pathologic findings and correlation with CT. *Am. J. Roentgenol.* 151:791–798.

RINGO, J. L., 1991. Neuronal interconnection as a function of brain size. *Brain Behav. Evol.* 38:1–6.

RINGO, J. L., R. W. DOTY, S. DEMETER, and P. Y. SIMARD, 1994. Time is of the essence: A conjecture that hemispheric specialization arises from interhemispheric conduction delay. *Cereb. Cortex* 4:331–343.

Risse, G. L., J. Gates, G. Lund, R. Maxwell, and A. Rubens, 1989. Interhemispheric transfer in patients with incomplete section of the corpus callosum. *Arch. Neurol.* 46:437–443.

Schlaug, G., L. Jäncke, Y. Huang, J. F. Staiger, and H. Steinmetz, 1995. Increased corpus callosum size in musicians. *Neuropsychologia* 33:1047–1055.

Sidtis, J. J., 1988. Dichotic listening after commisurotomy. In *Handbook of Dichotic Listening*, K. Hugdahl, ed. pp. 161–162.

Steinmetz, H., L. Jäncke, A. Kleinschmidt, G. Schlaug, J. Volkmann, and Y. Huang, 1992. Sex but no hand difference in the isthmus of the corpus callosum [see comments]. *Neurology* 42:749–752.

Steinmetz, H., J. F. Staiger, G. Schlaug, Y. Huang, and L. Jäncke, 1995. Corpus callosum and brain volume in women and men. *NeuroReport* 6:1002–1004.

Steinmetz, H., J. Volkmann, L. Jäncke, and H. J. Freund, 1991. Anatomical left-right asymmetry of language-related temporal cortex is different in left- and right-handers. *Ann. Neurol.* 29:315–319.

Strauss, E., J. Wada, and M. Hunter, 1994. Callosal morphology and performance on intelligence tests. *J. Clin. Exp. Neuropsychol.* 16:79–83.

Wang, P. P., S. Doherty, J. R. Hesselink, and U. Bellugi, 1992. Callosal morphology concurs with neurobehavioral and neuropathological findings in two neurodevelopmental disorders. *Arch. Neurol.* 49 (4):407–411.

Weber, G., and S. Weis, 1986. Morphometric analysis of the human corpus callosum fails to reveal sex-related differences. *J. Hirnforsch.* 27:237–240.

Weis, S., G. Weber, E. Wenger, and M. Kimbacher, 1989. The controversy about a sexual dimorphism of the human corpus callosum. *Int. J. Neurosci.* 47:169–173.

Witelson, S. F., 1985. The brain connection: The corpus callosum is larger in left-handers. *Science* 229:665–668.

Witelson, S. F., 1987. Hand preference and sex differences in the isthmus of the corpus callosum. *Soc. Neurosci. Abstr.* 13:48–48.

Witelson, S. F., 1989. Hand and sex differences in the isthmus and genu of the human corpus callosum: A postmortem morphological study. *Brain* 112 (Pt. 3):799–835.

Witelson, S. F., and C. H. Goldsmith, 1991. The relationship of hand preference to anatomy of the corpus callosum in men. *Brain Res.* 545:175–182.

Witelson, S. F., and R. S. Nowakowski, 1991. Left out axons make men right: A hypothesis for the origin of handedness and functional asymmetry. *Neuropsychologia* 29:327–333.

Woodruff, P. W., I. C. McManus, and A. S. David, 1995. Meta-analysis of corpus callosum size in schizophrenia. *J. Neurol. Neurosurg. Psychiat.* 58 (4):457–461.

Wu, J. C., M. S. Buchsbaum, J. C. Johnson, T. G. Hershey, E. A. Wagner, C. Teng, and S. Lottenberg, 1993. Magnetic resonance and positron emission tomography imaging of the corpus callosum: Size, shape and metabolic rate in unipolar depression. *J. Affect. Disord.* 28:15–25.

Zaidel, E., 1976. Language, dichotic listening, and the disconnected hemispheres. In *Conference on Human Brain Function*, D. O. Walter, L. Rogers, and J. M. Finzi-Fried, eds. Los Angeles: Brain Information Service/BRI Publications Office, UCLA, pp. 103–110.

Zaidel, E., J. M. Clarke, and B. Suyenobu, 1990. Hemispheric independence: A paradigm case for cognitive neuroscience. In *Neurobiology of Higher Cognitive Functions*, A. B. Scheibel and A. F. Wechsler, eds. New York: Guilford, pp. 297–355.

Zilles, K., 1972. Biometrische analyse der frischvolumina verschiedener prosencephaler hirnregionen von 78 menschlichen, adulten gehirnen. *Gegenbaurs morphologisches Jahrbuch Leipzig* 118:234–273.

COMMENTARY 3.1

Size Differences in the Callosum: Analysis Beyond the Main Effects

PATRICIA E. COWELL

The investigation of regional neuroanatomy along dimensions of interest such as male-female differences is a complex task. It might seem at first glance a simple job to compare the size of a brain region in one group of research subjects to the size of the same region in another group. However, even the most straightforward comparisons of neurobiological measures can be contaminated or influenced by variability in the data that is related to factors outside the purview of the particular research in question. For example, a comparison of temporal lobe size in men and women to examine anatomical sex differences in this part of the brain may be affected by other aspects of the subjects' biographies (e.g., age, medical history) or neurobehavioral profiles (e.g., brain size, hand preference) even though these were not the original or primary foci of the study. When the relationships between such other factors and the research measures of interest are not well understood themselves, the task of accounting or correcting for their influence is a difficult one. Moreover, if these contaminating effects of outside factors are strong enough, even the most straightforward interpretation of a basic research comparison may be called into question.

The corpus callosum (CC), shown in Figure 3.7, is one brain structure that has been the source of both considerable interest and debate in the area of individual differences in human and animal research. Yet investigation of this structure's anatomy has been clouded by multiple methodological weaknesses, including small sample sizes, disagreement on which units of measurement to use, and analytic approaches that failed to account for the influence of factors such as age when examining sex differences (for further discussion, see Denenberg et al., 1989, 1991; Cowell et al., 1992, 1993, 1994a; Bishop and Wahlsten, 1997). Also, researchers

PATRICIA E. COWELL Department of Human Communication Sciences, University of Sheffield, Sheffield, United Kingdom.

have studied the CC to great extent without having a complete understanding of its relationship to the whole brain. Clearly, the overall size of an organism's head or brain has some influence on the size of the structures contained within, but brain size, in its many possible forms of measurement, has a complex and not well-understood relationship with regional anatomical measures such as the callosum. In research in which the effects of brain size are not considered, it is possible that group differences simply reflect variation in the size of the whole brain. Alternatively, when the effects of brain size are removed from analyses of the CC in an inappropriate fashion, the result may be data that are over-corrected or undercorrected.

Jäncke and Steinmetz's model of CC/brain size relationships

In light of the confusion and controversy surrounding the study of regional CC anatomy in humans, Jäncke and Steinmetz set out to systematically investigate the relationship between the CC and brain size with the aid of a mathematical model. These authors used a geometric model to explore the neuroanatomical relationships between the callosum and the rest of the brain as defined by the midsagittal CC area and the volume of the forebrain (FBV).

In the geometric model, two neuroanatomical relationships were expressed as the following rules:

$$CC = \text{constant} \times FBV^{2/3} \quad (3.1)$$

$$CC/FBV = \text{constant} \times FBV^{-1/3} \quad (3.2)$$

These formulas were then logarithmically transformed for ease of statistical manipulation and display to:

$$\log CC = \log \text{constant} + (2/3) \times \log FBV \quad (3.3)$$

$$\log CC/FBV = \log \text{constant} + (-1/3) \times \log FBV \quad (3.4)$$

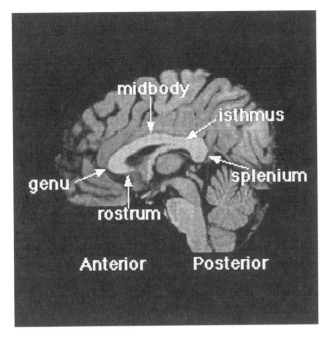

FIGURE 3.7. Midline view of the human brain from a magnetic resonance image. The corpus callosum has been labeled to show the names that are often used to refer to the various anatomical regions of this structure.

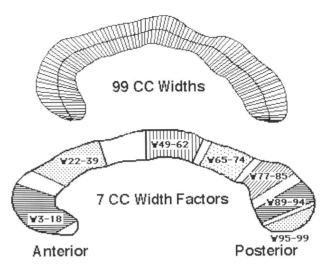

FIGURE 3.8. The method used by Denenberg, Cowell, and colleagues to measure the human corpus callosum involved three steps: (1) drawing an outline of each midsagittal corpus callosum from a magnetic resonance image; (2) digitizing the CC and measuring 99 widths along the longitudinal axis such that the sum of the widths was a minimum (upper picture); and (3) entering the 99 widths with other CC and brain measures into a factor analysis to derive clusters of widths (lower picture) to subdivide the CC into regions. (This figure has been adapted from Cowell et al., 1993, with permission from Lippincott-Raven Publishers.)

Equations (3.3) and (3.4) were then applied to actual CC and FBV measures obtained from magnetic resonance images (MRIs) of 49 women and 71 men. Fitting the data to the model revealed that (1) CC area increased less than proportionately to brain size and (2) CC area taken as a proportion of brain size actually *decreased* as brain size increased.

Significant regressions between CC area and FBV using logarithmic coordinates provided further supporting evidence of the CC-to-brain-size relationship.

As will be discussed in sections below, Jäncke and Steinmetz's research (Jäncke et al., 1997) represents a novel approach to one of the most vexing and neglected areas in the field of regional neuroanatomical research: specifying the nature of relationships between the whole brain and its parts.

Comparison to Denenberg and colleagues' factor analysis model

Denenberg and colleagues (1991) are one of the few other research groups who have systematically studied the anatomy of the CC in rodents and humans with a mathematical model (Denenberg et al., 1989, 1991; Cowell et al., 1994a). In these studies, the midsagittal CC was subdivided into 99 widths along its longitudinal axis. CC area, perimeter, length, and noncallosal measure of brain size (brain weight for rats, midline brain

area for humans) were also collected (see Figure 3.8). The CC data for 104 human subjects and 155 rats were then modeled with a multivariate correlational technique called a factor analysis. Separate analyses were performed for each species. The pattern of results that emerged characterized the intercorrelational relationships among the multiple CC and brain measures.

In both the human and rat analyses, a total of eight factors resulted, of which seven comprised intercorrelated clusters of CC widths. CC area did not correlate uniquely with any cluster, and brain size was associated with an eighth factor. Among the many implications of this factor analytic model to CC and brain anatomy, the one most relevant to Jäncke and Steinmetz's model is that CC area and the seven width clusters were not strongly related to measures of brain size in humans or rats.

Midsagittal brain area, forebrain volume, total cerebral volume, and brain weight are among the various indicators of brain size used by scientists. Pearson correlations, factor analysis, and now Jäncke and Steinmetz's model are among the various methods used to relate CC size to brain size. In light of Denenberg and colleagues' (Denenberg et al., 1989, 1991; Cowell et al., 1994a) factor analyses in rats and humans, Jäncke and Steinmetz's work indicates that results and interpretations of explorations into the nature of the CC's relationship with the rest of the brain are affected by the particular measures and methods chosen to represent the CC and brain size (see Bishop and Wahlsten (1997) for a review). As Jäncke and Steinmetz have shown, the manner in which any particular relationship between CC size and brain size is expressed also depends on the relative weights or mathematical operations applied to the CC and brain size measures before modeling or analysis. Attempts to use correlational methods with untransformed measures of CC and brain size have met with varying degrees of success in trying to define the link between CC and brain size. Numerous approaches, including Denenberg and colleagues' factor analyses of callosal widths, have found that regional CC size was not highly related to brain size. Such "null findings" may indicate more about the measures and methods used in a particular study than about an absence of any systematic relationships between the callosum and the brain. As shown by Jäncke and Steinmetz's work, relationships between the CC and brain size have far-reaching implications for many aspects of neurobehavioral research.

Application of Jäncke and Steinmetz's model to the study of group differences in CC anatomy: Brain size as a correction factor in the study of group differences in regional CC size

On the basis of evidence derived from their modeling of the relationships between CC area and FBV, Jäncke and Steinmetz conclude that brain volume is one of the main factors affecting CC size and, in turn, interhemispheric communication. They observed that women with larger brains had smaller CC/FBV ratios and that men with smaller brains had larger CC/FBV ratios. This finding supports their assertion that CC size is determined largely by brain size rather than sex. Similarly, the authors propose that sex differences in brain size may be primarily responsible for carrying sex differences in callosal size. As FBV has been shown to relate in a systematic fashion to CC size, the authors examined sex differences in CC area and CC subareas using raw data and also CC/FBV ratios. For a sample of 120 subjects, only the CC/FBV ratio comparisons revealed any trace of sex differences, females having slightly larger CC/FBV ratios than men.

There are two aspects of this comparison that deserve comment. The first is the question of how, having established a connection between CC size and some measure of brain size, one goes about correcting the CC data to remove those brain size effects. The second point concerns the multidimensional nature of the CC, its plasticity across the life span, and how factors other than

FBV (e.g., age) also contribute to sex differences in CC anatomy. The fact that the relationship between CC and FBV described by Jäncke and Steinmetz accounts for not more than 30% of variation in the CC is relevant to both of these points.

Once the relationship between a measure of global brain size and a particular neuroanatomical region has been established, the issue of how to remove the effects of brain size so that the region of interest—in this case, the CC—can be studied in isolation is not entirely clear. Several methods have been published in the literature (see Bishop and Wahlsten, 1997), and each has its own advantages and disadvantages. One of the most widely used methods is removal of the contaminating factor (here, brain size) through analysis of covariance, that is, regression of brain size from the region of interest (here, the CC). This method is optimal for data in which the relationship between brain size and the CC is constant for the comparison groups. However, it is not clear how one should proceed when the very relationship between the whole brain and the CC differs between comparison groups. This latter concern is particularly relevant to the study of the CC in patients with neuropsychiatric, neurobehavioral, or neurodevelopmental disorders and in studies of development or aging in which brain size also changes over time.

Another method that has been used to correct regional measures for brain size is to calculate region/whole-brain ratios or percentages. In my own experience, neuroanatomical regions that correlate moderately or highly with head or brain size (roughly, a correlation coefficient equal to or greater than 0.600 for a sample of 30–100 subjects) typically reveal the same results in group comparisons, regardless of which corrections are performed. However, if the correlations are low, the risk of further contaminating the data by an overcorrection factor arises if one opts for the ratio rather than one of the more selective covariance methods. After satisfying oneself that comparisons of ratio and covariance/regression methods of correction are equivalent, then certainly the ratio data offer a greater degree of ease in interpretation over the covariance/regression methods. Bishop and Wahlsten (1997) also agree that percentages can be simpler to conceptualize than residuals.

If there is no correlation between the callosum and brain size, then there is no statistical basis for correcting the regional CC data before analysis. However, researchers who have not corrected for brain size owing to weak or inconsistent relationships between their particular CC and brain size measures may still find themselves in the position of having to defend their research against criticisms that variation in brain size is responsible for their results. The following logical argument provides support for the uniqueness of results in the CC on the basis of regional specificity of effects, whether or not the data require corrections for brain size. Theoretically, the whole brain subsumes all the complexities of its component parts, but as a single volumetric measure, it cannot simultaneously account, statistically or otherwise, for the fact that the interactive effects of variables such as sex, age, or hand preference may be restricted to one CC region. The CC is a fiber tract composed of axons from many cortical zones, and hence, region-specific effects are unlikely to be the result of variation in brain size alone.

Application of Jäncke and Steinmetz's model to the study of group differences in CC anatomy: Stability or sex differences in the CC/brain size relationship?

An important aspect of Jäncke and Steinmetz's model is that the slopes derived for their mathematical functions were equivalent for men and women. The authors cite this as evidence to support a relatively constant relationship between the CC and FBV for both sexes. The work of Mack and colleagues (1993) on the rat CC suggests that if brain size is measured by brain weight and the relationship between the regional CC measures and brain weight is expressed with a simple correlation of nontransformed data, there appear to be some differences in the relationships between brain size and regional CC size as a function of sex and hormonal status. For example, in rats, correlations among regional CC widths and brain weight were low to moderate, but their patterns were inconsistently so for males compared to females, ovariectomized females, and ovariectomized females with estrogen replacement (Mack et al., 1993).

When comparing results across studies, it is critical to understand that stability of CC/brain size relationships between the sexes is subject to the same intricacies and complexities as are the basic CC/brain size relationships described above. Whether application of Jäncke and Steinmetz's modeling techniques using an FBV measure would lead to a result in rats paralleling that seen in humans is a matter to be tested empirically. Nevertheless, it is noteworthy that application of Jäncke and Steinmetz's model to CC area and brain weight reported in 10 postmortem studies in humans did appear to follow similar patterns as their own data analysis with CC area and FBV using MRI.

Beyond the removal of sex effects related to brain size

Is there significant sex-related variance in CC size after FBV has been removed? According to Jäncke and Steinmetz, probably not. However, the removal or correction of main sex effects through FBV does not necessarily rule out the possibility that complex interactive effects of sex with other factors still contribute to a substantial portion of the remaining 70% of variation in CC size that is unrelated to FBV. Some of my own work has shown that subregions of the CC are particularly sensitive to sex differences but that the nature of these differences is largely a function of age (Cowell et al., 1992). We found that in men the anterior CC widths increased with age up to the third decade of life, after which the width of anterior CC declined. In contrast, the same anterior CC regions in women continued to increase in width through the fifth decade of life and declined with advancing age thereafter. Hence, the anterior CC widths appear slightly larger in men in the third decade of life but larger in women by the fifth decade of life. Only the anteriormost and posteriormost CC regions showed significant interactive effects of sex and age, a finding that offers further argument against the notion that all sex differences are related to overall brain size alone. A similar pattern of regional sensitivity to the interactive effects of sex and age was found in a study of outlying cortical volumes, where the frontal lobe was more affected by the differential effects of age on men and women than the temporal lobe or other brain regions (Cowell et al., 1994b). These interactive effects of sex and age in outlying cortex were robust to corrections for head size. Indeed, they were significant for uncorrected regional volumes, ratios of regional volumes to head size (cranial volume), and regional volumes from which head size had been regressed.

The work on regional interactive effects of sex and age, viewed in consideration with Jäncke and Steinmetz's CC/FBV relationships, suggests that most main effects of sex in the CC may be attributable to brain size but that more complex dimorphisms may still be revealed when one uses a developmental trend analysis and takes into account differential patterns of cortical plasticity in men and women as a function of age and neuroanatomical region. In general, sex differences expressed as complex interactions with other neurobehavioral variables of interest may remain even after removal of overall male-female differences related to brain size. The conceptual parallel in an analysis of variance framework would be a callosal measurement examined in two age groups of men and women (i.e., younger men and women plus older men and women) that yielded a statistically significant main effect of sex and a sex by age interaction. Such an outcome could result from a situation in which, for example, (1) callosal size was larger in both male age groups than in both female age groups and (2) callosal size decreased in men but increased in women as a function of age. If these same data were subjected to an analysis of covariance to correct for whole brain size, the result might be a statistically significant sex by age interaction, a significant effect of the covariate, and a reduction or elimination of the main effect of sex. (This example assumes a moderate to high correlation between callosal and whole brain size that is relatively constant within each of the four sex by age groups.) The point here is that it is possible to remove sex differences in callosal size that are linked to differences in brain size, but this will not necessarily factor out the unique interactive relationships between sex and other factors such as age.

Finally, before one discounts the existence of the effects of sex on the human CC, it is necessary to consider that when factors contributing to individual differences in humans (e.g., prenatal environment, rearing conditions, age) were carefully controlled in animal studies, the effects of both naturally occurring and experimentally manipulated hormones were both statistically significant and reproducible (Fitch et al., 1990, 1991a, 1991b). Moreover, the effects of hormones on CC development in the rat were also regionally distinct and not found to be wholly attributable to changes in brain weight or body size alone (Fitch et al., 1990, 1991a, 1991b; Mack et al., 1993).

Neurobehavioral implications of Jäncke and Steinmetz's model

Jäncke and Steinmetz further demonstrate the salience of the relationship between FBV and CC size when they divided subjects on the basis of FBV and then correlated measures of dichotic listening performance within the large- and the small-brained groups. Their results showed a different pattern of correlations for the two groups in a fashion similar to what other researchers have demonstrated when subdividing groups by sex and hand preference (Zaidel, Clarke, and Suyenobu, 1990). The results serve not only as further functional validation of the importance of FBV in CC size and function, but also emphasize the importance of the within-group comparison (Cowell et al., 1995).

In view of their proposal that FBV plays a major role in the determination of CC size, Jäncke and Steinmetz explore the relationship between hand preference and regional CC anatomy. Their study measured hand preference using the Annett handedness questionnaire, and subjects were classified as either right-handers, mixed-handers, or left-handers. On the basis of this classification, there were no significant group differences. However, Cowell and colleagues (1993) showed that both direction and degree were salient dimensions of hand preference with respect to regional CC size (see

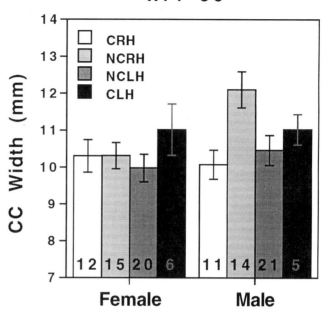

FIGURE 3.9. Data from Cowell and colleagues (1993) showing width of the callosal isthmus as measured by CC factor width 77–85 in 104 human subjects as a function of sex and hand preference. (Group sample sizes are at the base of each bar.) Nonconsistent right-handed (NCRH) men had larger regional widths than consistent right-handed (CRH) men. In both men and women left-handers, consistency had the opposite effect as in right-handers; consistent left-handers (CLH) had larger widths than nonconsistent left-handers (NCLH). When the four handedness groups were pooled across sex, a significant hand by consistency effect was the result, with the NCRH and CLH groups having larger isthmal width than CRH and NCLH groups. (These data have been adapted from Cowell et al., 1993, with permission from Lippincott-Raven Publishers.)

Figure 3.9). Furthermore, direction and degree of hand preference interacted with sex, and these effects were regionally specific to the callosal isthmus. Our study showed that nonconsistent right-handers had larger CC isthmuses than consistent right-handers, but only in men. A different effect was found for left-handers whereby consistent left-handers of both sexes had larger CC isthmuses than nonconsistent left-handers. By collapsing nonconsistent right-handers and nonconsistent left-handers into one group of mixed-handers, Jäncke and Steinmetz may have inadvertently obscured size differences in the CC by ignoring the independent dimensions of direction and degree of manual laterality.

Conclusions: The multidimensional nature of the CC

Whether one considers the effects of brain size, sex, age, hand preference, or any other combination of factors on the CC, its multidimensional nature becomes readily apparent. The complexity of interrelations between the CC, brain size, and the influences of individual difference were highlighted in a study of the CC in language- and learning-impaired (LLI) children (Cowell et al., 1995). We found that there was a significant correlation between prenatal risk and CC size in LLI children but not in their age- and IQ-matched controls. A similar phenomenon was found in overall cerebral volume. In both the CC and cerebral volume, higher risk was associated with smaller neuroanatomical size. Despite the fact that risk is correlated with both cerebral volume and CC area in LLI children, the two anatomical measures themselves were not correlated. This seemingly non-intuitive pattern of results was interpreted as evidence for the multidimensional nature of the measures involved. It was hypothesized that the cerebral volume was affected by one dimension of risk, whereas the CC area was affected by another, independent dimension of the risk measure.

The case described above lends credence to the possibility that even after accounting for a significant proportion of the CC's variation with an overall measure of brain size, there are still multiple dimensions of CC anatomy to explore with respect to the interactive effects of sex, age, hand preference, and so forth. One might venture so far as to speculate that even after the same numeric proportion of variance is accounted for by removing brain volume effects from CC size in men and women, one still does not necessarily know, on the basis of one set of anatomical measurements, that whole brain and callosal anatomy were developmentally linked via identical mechanisms. Indeed, figuring out whether such statistical effects represent unitary or "separate developmental pathways" is one of the challenges faced by researchers in this area (Bishop and Wahlsten, 1997, p. 591).

In conclusion, Jäncke and Steinmetz make a very strong case for the importance of FBV and its allometric relationships with midsagittal CC area. Accounting statistically for the main effects of brain size and related sex differences in overall CC size represents a key component of future efforts to investigate the gross anatomy of this structure. Only through a firm understanding of region/whole brain relationships can researchers move forward in their exploration of the complex interactions between the CC, demographic, clinical, and neurocognitive factors of interest.

REFERENCES

BISHOP, K. M., and D. WAHLSTEN, 1997. Sex differences in the corpus callosum: Myth or reality? *Neurosci. Biobehav. Rev.* 21:581–601.

COWELL, P. E., L. S. ALLEN, A. KERTESZ, N. S. ZALATIMO, and V. H. DENENBERG, 1994a. Human corpus callosum: A stable mathematical model of regional neuroanatomy. *Brain Cogn.* 25:52–66.

COWELL, P. E., L. S. ALLEN, N. S. ZALATIMO, and V. H. DENENBERG, 1992. A developmental study of sex and age interactions in the human corpus callosum. *Dev. Brain Res.* 66:187–192.

COWELL, P. E., T. L. JERNIGAN, V. H. DENENBERG, and P. TALLAL, 1995. Language and learning impairment and prenatal risk: An MRI study of the corpus callosum and cerebral volume. *J. Med. Speech Lang. Pathol.* 3:1–13.

COWELL, P. E., A. KERTESZ, and V. H. DENENBERG, 1993. Multiple dimensions of handedness and the human corpus callosum. *Neurology* 43:2353–2357.

COWELL, P. E., B. I. TURETSKY, R. C. GUR, D. L. SHTASEL, R. I. GROSSMAN, and R. E. GUR, 1994b. Sex differences in aging of the human frontal and temporal lobes. *J. Neurosci.* 14:4748–4755.

DENENBERG, V. H., A. S. BERREBI, and R. H. FITCH, 1989. A factor analysis of the rat's corpus callosum. *Brain Res.* 97:271–279.

DENENBERG, V. H., A. KERTESZ, and P. E. COWELL, 1991. A factor analysis of the human's corpus callosum. *Brain Res.* 548:126–132.

FITCH, R. H., A. S. BERREBI, P. E. COWELL, L. M. SCHROTT, and V. H. DENENBERG, 1990. Corpus callosum: Effects of neonatal hormones on sexual dimorphism in the rat. *Brain Res.* 515:111–116.

FITCH, R. H., P. E. COWELL, L. M. SCHROTT, and V. H. DENENBERG, 1991a. Corpus callosum: Demasculinization via perinatal anti-androgen. *Int. J. Dev. Neurosci.* 9:35–38.

FITCH, R. H., P. E. COWELL, L. M. SCHROTT, and V. H. DENENBERG, 1991b. Corpus callosum: Ovarian hormones and feminization. *Brain Res.* 542:313–317.

JÄNCKE, L., J. F. STAIGER, G. SCHLAUG, Y. HUANG, and H. STEINMETZ, 1997. The relationship between corpus callosum size and forebrain volume. *Cereb. Cortex* 7:48–56.

MACK, C. M., R. H. FITCH, P. E. COWELL, L. M. SCHROTT, and V. H. DENENBERG, 1993. Ovarian estrogen acts to feminize the female rat's corpus callosum. *Dev. Brain Res.* 71:115–119.

ZAIDEL, E., J. CLARKE, and B. SUYENOBU, 1990. Hemispheric independence: A paradigm case for cognitive neuroscience. In *Neurobiological Foundations of Higher Cognitive Function*, A. Scheibel and A. Wechsler, eds. New York: Guilford Press, pp. 297–355.

COMMENTARY 3.2

Individual Differences in Corpus Callosum Morphometry: To Normalize or Not to Normalize for Brain Size

JEFFREY M. CLARKE

The advent of magnetic resonance imaging (MRI) has provided a relatively simple and straightforward means of obtaining anatomical measures of interhemispheric connectivity in individual subjects via measures of midsagittal corpus callosum area. Despite the dozens of studies that have investigated individual differences in corpus callosum morphometry, a basic question still remains: whether or not corpus callosum measures should be normalized for individual differences in brain size. This has an important bearing on, for example, studies of sex differences in callosum size, since male brains are, on average, about 10% heavier and larger than female brains. In a continuation of their thorough investigations of corpus callosum morphometry issues, the chapter by Jäncke and Steinmetz has undertaken an important study of the normalization issue. They provide convincing evidence that midsagittal corpus callosum area and forebrain volume are related by geometric principles, whereby individual differences in corpus callosum area are accompanied by even greater relative differences in brain volume. That is, brain volume increases at a faster rate than corpus callosum area. This finding may at last resolve the seemingly paradoxical finding of highly reliable sex differences in brain size despite weak or no sex differences in total corpus callosum area (i.e., a lack of allometry between brain size and corpus callosum area; see Peters, 1988). Although most studies do not find a statistically significant sex difference in nonnormalized total callosum area, the pattern across studies is for larger means in males than for females. A meta-analysis has indeed shown that total

callosum area is slightly, but significantly, larger in males than in females (Driesen and Raz, 1995). Since brain volume increases at a faster rate than corpus callosum area, Jäncke and Steinmetz's observation would explain why there is greater statistical power in detecting sex differences in brain size (a statistically reliable effect) than in corpus callosum area (a less reliable effect). Importantly, Jäncke and Steinmetz demonstrate that the same geometric relationship between callosum area and brain size holds for both males and females, indicating that brain size, rather than sex per se, is a determinant of callosum size.

Given the evidence for a geometric relationship, Jäncke and Steinmetz argue that larger brains have proportionally smaller corpus callosum areas than smaller brains, and hence larger brains have proportionally less interhemispheric connectivity than smaller brains. This interpretation assumes that both corpus callosum area and brain volume are related to the number of neurons and/or neuronal connections within these structures. As Jäncke and Steinmetz point out, the human evidence indicates that corpus callosum area is proportional to the number of interhemispheric fibers that pass through it (Aboitiz et al., 1992a). Large corpora callosa have more interhemispheric fibers than do small corpora callosa. The relationship between brain size and total number of cerebral neurons is less clear. Pakkenberg and Gundersen (1995) report that female brains have, on average, significantly fewer neocortical neurons than males, a finding that parallels the smaller brain volume in females than in males. This finding suggests that neuronal densities are the same in males and females and that total number of cerebral neurons is indeed related to brain size. However, both Haug (1987) and Witelson, Glezer, and Kigar (1995) found opposite results, where-

JEFFREY M. CLARKE University of North Texas, Denton, Texas.

by neuronal densities were markedly higher in female brains than in male brains. These latter findings suggest that males and females tend to have an equal number of cerebral neurons despite having different brain sizes. If the total number of cerebral neurons is fixed for different brain sizes, while the number of interhemispheric neurons increases with increasing brain size (i.e., total callosum neurons is related to callosum size, and callosum size is, in turn, related to brain size by the geometric principle), then larger brains should have greater, not less, interhemispheric connectivity. In this case, normalizing callosum area for brain size would be inappropriate, as this would result in a measure of interhemispheric connectivity that is precisely the opposite of what it should be. Clearly, further research is required to unambiguously determine the true relationship between brain size and total neuronal counts before one can confidently conclude that corpus callosum area should or should not be normalized for individual differences in brain size.

An alternative normalization approach that has been frequently implemented is to use regional subdivisions of the corpus callosum normalized for total corpus callosum area (i.e., proportional area). This approach determines whether regionally specific, and presumably functionally specific, callosum areas have a greater representation in some individuals or groups than others. Despite the presence and importance of heterotopic callosum fibers, the majority of callosum fibers are homotopic and are arranged in a topographic arrangement with functionally distinct cerebral regions (e.g., Pandya and Seltzer, 1986). Topographically localized functions in the corpus callosum have been demonstrated in patients with lesions of discrete callosum regions, which results in systematic disconnection syndromes for a specific sensory or motor modality (see Clarke and Zaidel, 1994). Using proportional normalization procedures, Steinmetz and colleagues (1992), Witelson (1989), and Clarke and Zaidel (1994) have found the isthmus of the corpus callosum to be proportionally larger in females than in males. Most other studies that have failed to find a sex difference in the isthmus have used isthmus measures that are different from those used in these three studies. The isthmus interconnects visuoperceptual and posterior language areas that may be related to sex differences in these respective functions. Below, I will discuss how this sex difference in isthmus size is influenced by handedness factors. Note that this proportional normalizing procedure emphasizes the relative representation of different callosum subregions rather than the absolute number of interhemispheric fibers within a subdivision. Again, only with further investigation can we be certain which of these measures is a more appropriate index of the extent of functional interhemispheric connectivity.

If there is a relationship between corpus callosum size and hemispheric asymmetries (functional and/or anatomical), then one would expect to find corpus callosum measures to vary with handedness, since there are reliable handedness differences in laterality measures. As Jäncke and Steinmetz note, the majority of studies have not been able to find reliable main effects of handedness in corpus callosum measures. This may be a statistical power issue, since a meta-analysis of seven studies found a small but significant handedness effect whereby the corpus callosum tends to be larger in left-handers than in right-handers (Driesen and Raz, 1995). More reliable effects, at least for the isthmus, are apparent when both handedness and sex are considered. Although Jäncke and Steinmetz did not find interactions of sex and handedness in callosum measures, four other studies did find a significant interaction for the isthmus (Witelson, 1989; Denenberg et al., 1991; Habib et al., 1991; Clarke and Zaidel, 1994). The common finding from these four studies was larger isthmus sizes in mixed-handed males than in consistently right-handed males and no handedness difference for females (see Clarke and Zaidel, 1994). Thus, a handedness effect for the isthmus is apparent for males but not for females. This effect appears to depend on classifying participants by consistency of hand preferences rather than by writing hand or direction of hand preference (Clarke and Zaidel, 1994; however, see Steinmetz et al., 1992).

Just as sex differences have been found in callosum measures when handedness is considered, similar sex differences in callosum morphometry have also been demonstrated when anatomical and behavioral hemispheric asymmetries are taken into account. Aboitiz, Scheibel, and Zaidel (1992b) found a relationship, again only in males, between isthmus size and anatomical measures of hemispheric asymmetries. Isthmus size was negatively related to hemispheric asymmetries in both Sylvian fissure length and planum temporale area. Note that this finding is consistent with the handedness findings above: Males with more lateralized brains tend to have smaller isthmus sizes, whereas for females, laterality measures are unrelated to isthmus size. This pattern appears again when a behavioral laterality measure is considered from a lexical decision task with semantic priming (Clarke and Zaidel, 1994). For males a negative relationship was found between isthmus size and hemispheric asymmetries in semantic priming, while in females there was no significant relationship. Taken together, these findings point to a relationship between hemispheric asymmetries and isthmus size in males but not in females. It is encouraging that such consistent findings are emerging from such a variety of approaches. This sex difference may be due in part to a sex difference in the fiber composition of the isthmus. For both males and females, isthmus size correlates with the number of small-diameter isthmus fibers; however, only for females does isthmus size correlate with the number of large-diameter fibers as well (Aboitiz, 1991, Table 4.4). This sex difference may be important if large- and small-diameter fibers subserve different interhemispheric functions, as has been previously suggested (Aboitiz et al., 1992a). Importantly, other callosum regions, such as the anterior splenium, may be related to hemispheric asymmetries for females but not for males (Zaidel, Aboitiz, and Clarke, 1995).

As Jäncke and Steinmetz note, several studies have examined correlations between callosum morphometry measures and behavioral laterality measures from dichotic listening tasks. Across all of these studies, there is a tendency for total corpus callosum size to be larger in individuals with smaller behavioral laterality measures, although this effect is often small and nonsignificant. Importantly, only two of these studies (Jäncke and Steinmetz, 2003; Clarke, Lufkin, and Zaidel, 1993) examined correlations between corpus callosum measures and separate *weak ear* (i.e., the ear associated with poorer accuracy, typically the left ear) and *strong ear* (typically the right) scores. Both groups of researchers point out the importance of comparing separate weak ear and strong ear correlations, since in the majority of individuals, verbal stimuli that are presented to the weak ear require interhemispheric transfer via the corpus callosum to be fully processed, while strong ear stimuli do not. Despite using a similar task (consonant-vowel recall), these two studies obtained opposite results. Jäncke and Steinmetz found partial support for a sensory-interhemispheric transfer model associated with callosum size (weak ear scores tended to be higher in individuals with larger corpora callosa; however, positive correlations were also found for strong ear scores, which is inconsistent with a pure sensory-transfer explanation). Clarke and colleagues' (1993) findings, on the other hand, are consistent with a nonsensory, functional interhemispheric inhibition relationship with callosum measures (weak ears scores were not significantly correlated with callosum size, while strong ear scores were worse in individuals with larger callosum measures). The inconsistencies between the results of these two studies are disturbing, especially given the similarities in the methodologies. Differences in the behavioral laterality findings may partly explain the divergent results. In an earlier study, Jäncke, Steinmetz, and Volkmann (1992) reported that their consonant-vowel recall task resulted in small mean laterality indices that were identical for right- and left-handers (i.e., laterality index $e = 0.04$). When the same laterality indices are calculated from our results (Clarke et al., 1993) and are compared to those obtained by Jäncke and colleagues (1992), we find a laterality index that is five times larger for our right-handers ($e = 0.20$) and twice as large for our left-handers ($e = 0.08$), and this represents a significant handedness difference. Apparently, there are significant sampling, cultural, and/or procedural differences between the two studies that account for these different outcomes. However, this is still an inadequate explanation as to why opposite anatomical-behavioral correlation findings were obtained, and this deserves further investigation.

In sum, inconsistencies among studies of individual differences in corpus callosum size may in part be attributed to different measurement approaches, and Jäncke and Steinmetz have taken important steps toward determining the most appropriate approach. Future endeavors will want to shift from relatively arbitrary subdivisions of the corpus callosum (e.g., into halves, thirds, and fifths) to more sophisticated procedures that take into account neurocellular differentiation for different callosum regions, systematic morphometric features of the callosum (e.g., Denenberg et al., 1991), and evidence from patients with discrete callosum lesions that produce selective disconnection syndromes.

REFERENCES

Aboitiz, F., 1991. *Quantitative morphology and histology of the human corpus callosum and its relation to brain lateralization.* Doctoral dissertation, University of California at Los Angeles.

Aboitiz, F., A. B. Scheibel, R. S. Fisher, and E. Zaidel, 1992a. Fiber composition of the human corpus callosum. *Brain Res.* 598:143–153.

Aboitiz, F., A. B. Scheibel, and E. Zaidel, 1992b. Morphometry of the Sylvian fissure and the corpus callosum, with emphasis on sex differences, *Brain* 115:1521–1541.

Clarke, J. M., R. B. Lufkin, and E. Zaidel, 1993. Corpus callosum morphometry and dichotic listening performance: Individual differences in functional interhemispheric inhibition? *Neuropsychologia* 31:547–557.

Clarke, J. M., and E. Zaidel, 1994. Anatomical-behavioral relationships: Corpus callosum morphometry and hemispheric specialization. *Behav. Brain Res.* 64:185–202.

Denenberg, V. H., A. Kertesz, and P. E. Cowell, 1991. A factor analysis of the human's corpus callosum. *Brain Res.* 548:126–132.

Driesen, N. R., and N. Raz, 1995. The influence of sex, age, and handedness on corpus callosum morphology: A meta-analysis. *Psychobiology* 23:240–247.

Habib, M., D. Gayraud, A. Oliva, J. Regis, G. Salamon, R. Khalil, 1991. Effects of handedness and sex on the morphology of the corpus callosum: A study with brain magnetic resonance imaging. *Brain Cogn.* 16:41–61.

Haug, H., 1987. Brain sizes, surfaces, and neuronal sizes of the cortex cerebri: A stereological investigation of man and his variability and a comparison with some mammals. *Am. J. Anat.* 180:126–142.

JÄNCKE, L., and H. STEINMETZ, 2003. Brain size: A possible source of interindividual variability in corpus callosum morphology. In *The Parallel Brain: The Cognitive Neuroscience of the Corpus Callosum*, M. Iacoboni and E. Zaidel, eds. Cambridge, MA: MIT Press.

JÄNCKE, L., H. STEINMETZ, and J. VOLKMANN, 1992. Dichotic listening: What does it measure? *Neuropsychologia* 30:941–950.

PAKKENBERG, B., and H. J. GUNDERSEN, 1995. Solutions to old problems in the quantitation of the central nervous system. *J. Neurol. Sci.* 16 (Suppl.):65–67.

PANDYA, D. N., and B. SELTZER, 1986. The topography of commissural fibers. In *Two Hemispheres—One Brain: Functions of the Corpus Callosum*, F. Leopore, M. Ptito, and H. H. Jasper, eds. New York: Alan R. Liss, pp 47–73.

PETERS, M., 1988. The size of the corpus callosum in males and females: Implications of a lack of allometry. *Can. J. Psychol.* 42:313–324.

STEINMETZ, H., L. JÄNCKE, A. KLEINSCHMIDT, G. SCHLAUG, J. VOLKMANN, and Y. HUANG, 1992. Sex but no hand difference in the isthmus of the corpus callosum. *Neurology* 42:749–752.

WITELSON, S. F., 1989. Hand and sex differences in the isthmus and genu of the human corpus callosum. *Brain* 112:799–835.

WITELSON, S. F., I. I. GLEZER, and D. L. KIGAR, 1995. Women have greater density of neurons in posterior temporal cortex. *J. Neurosci.* 15:3418–3428.

ZAIDEL, E., F. ABOITIZ, and J. M. CLARKE, 1995. Sexual dimorphism in interhemispheric relations: Anatomical-behavioral convergence. *Biol. Res.* 28:27–43.

4 Morphometrics for Callosal Shape Studies

FRED L. BOOKSTEIN

ABSTRACT Procrustes analysis and the thin-plate spline, two new methods for biometrical analysis of curving form, together greatly enhance the power of quantitative studies of callosal shape. This chapter introduces these methods informally and explains why they are more powerful than their predecessors. In a comparison of the brains of chronic schizophrenics with normal brains, a highly localized remodeling of the ventricular boundary of the isthmus in the midsagittal plane distinguishes the groups much more effectively than does the general run of quantitative neuroanatomical differentia for this disease. In another study, the shape of the callosum of healthy elderly males is found to be considerably and reliably different from that of elderly females in the region of the splenium. In a third study, callosal shape is found to be strikingly associated with callosal function in a study of 30 adult males diagnosed with prenatal alcohol damage. In all these studies, statistical significance can be demonstrated rigorously, and shape effects can be localized accurately, even though there are considerably more variables than cases. The combination of Procrustes analysis and thin-plate spline visualization may prove useful in a wide range of epigenetic or syndromal studies of the geometry of this important structure.

Recently, there have been important theoretical and practical advances in morphometrics, the statistics of biological shape and shape change. These developments did not come primarily at the hands of biomedical researchers. Rather, they have arisen since the late 1980s out of advances in probability theory, pattern analysis, and interpolation theory during the preceding decade. Although they have proved quite useful in a variety of prototype biological and biomedical applications, the new methods are not yet well known outside a small expert circle. Most discussions and examples appear in technical journals or conference volumes that are scrutinized far more often by those of us who build tools than by neuroscientists in search of quantitative tools to use. Most accessible, perhaps, are two recent review articles by Bookstein (1998, 1999) and, for the more

mathematically oriented, a new graduate text (Dryden and Mardia, 1998).

The purpose of this note is to motivate the reader's deeper study of these new methods by pointing to otherwise subtle callosal shape findings that are produced quite straightforwardly with their aid. For an argument introducing and defending a method as unfamiliar as this, the conventional outline of biomedical papers—methods, then results, then discussion—is not particularly helpful. One needs, rather, to explain the methods by the results they produce: to introduce the methods and results at the same time. Hence, my presentation here is in the nature of an informal lecture emphasizing the surprising precision and power of analyses of what is, after all, a rather familiar data resource: outlines of the corpus callosum near the midsagittal plane. I hope thereby to call the new methodology to the attention of a sophisticated professional community who are likely in need of just such a toolkit at this time.

The corpus callosum in schizophrenia

The data for the first example comprise outlines of the corpus callosum in nearly midsagittal parasagittal sections extracted from ordinary clinical-quality magnetic resonance (MR) images of 13 schizophrenic patients and 12 normal adults (the patients' psychiatrists, actually). Original data collection was not at all elegant; it entailed manually outlining the callosum on these MR images one at a time. In this first example, slices were thick (5 mm), and so the rostrum was illegible. The group to which the image pertained (house staff or schizophrenic patient) was not known to the person carrying out the tracing. The full data set of 25 outlines is shown in Figure 4.1; solid lines are from doctors, dashed lines are from patients. There are 26 points in each outline. The groups are group-matched for age and sex; cases and most nearly midsagittal slices were selected by my colleague John DeQuardo, M.D.

FRED L. BOOKSTEIN Institute of Anthropology, University of Vienna, Austria; Institute of Gerontology, University of Michigan, Ann Arbor, Michigan.

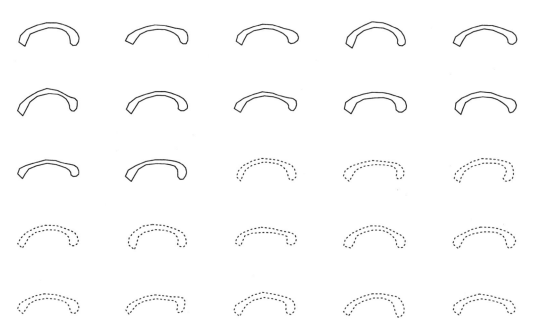

FIGURE 4.1. A typical data set for studies of callosal shape: tracings of 25 callosal outlines from thick midsagittal MR images. Solid lines: normals; dotted lines: schizophrenics. The outlines are 26-point polygons of semilandmarks as explained in the text.

In the jargon of morphometrics (see Slice et al., 1995), these data points are not landmark points having Latinate names and clearly punctate anatomical-histological definitions specimen by specimen. Instead, as is typically the case for studies of higher brain structures, they are semilandmarks that represent curving structures (in two dimensions, outlines like these) rather than discrete locations. The particular 26 points here were produced by a method of "sliding" that took into account the presence of some ancillary landmark points as explained and diagrammed by Bookstein (1997a, 1997c). Each of the 26 points is located along the callosal boundary in a manner that is optimal (in a sense to be explained below) given the locations of the other 25 points for its case and the sample Procrustes average of all the forms from both groups.

Analysis of biological shape by the Procrustes method

In ordinary language the shape of a geometric or pictorial object is described by measurements (for instance, angles or ratios of distances or areas) that do not change when the object is moved, rotated, or enlarged or reduced on the page or in your hands. The translations, rotations, and changes of scale that we are ignoring constitute the similarity group of transformations of the plane. When the "objects" are point sets like that in Figure 4.1, it turns out to be useful to say that their shape simply is the set of all point sets that "have the same shape."

We need a distance measure for shapes defined in this way. If we were talking just about sets of labeled points, a reasonable formula for squared distance would be the usual Pythagorean sum of squared distances between corresponding points over the list. It is reasonable to define shape distance as the minimum of these sums of squares over the classes that are involved in the definition of "shape"—over the classes of point sets generated by the similarity group that the notion of shape explicitly disregards. The squared shape distance between one point set A and another point set B might then be taken as the minimum summed squared Euclidean distances between the points of A and the corresponding points in point sets C as C ranges over the whole set of shapes having the same shape as B.

For this definition to make sense, we have to fix the scale of A. The mathematics of all this is most elegant if the sum of squares of the points of A around their center of gravity is constrained to be exactly 1. (The square root of this sum of squares is usually called centroid size.) The resulting squared Procrustes distance is proportional to the sum of the areas of the circles in Figure 4.2. A small adjustment of the definition is required to make it symmetric in A and B, a property that one would reasonably expect anything called a distance to have. Notation is easiest if one uses complex numbers. Write the two sets of landmarks, each one centered at $(0,0)$ and of centroid size unity, as vectors of complex numbers z_i with $\Sigma z_i = 0$ and $\Sigma z_i \bar{z}_i = 1$. (The overbar is the operation of complex conjugation, reflection in the x-

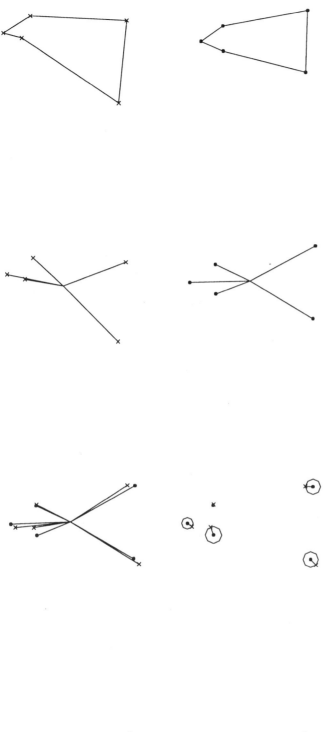

axis.) Then the Procrustes distance between z and z' is $\arccos |\Sigma z_i \bar{z}_i'|$, where $|w|$ is the complex modulus $\sqrt{w\bar{w}}$. The arccosine is taken in radians; Procrustes distance is a dimensionless number between 0 and $\pi/2$. For an extended and rigorous development of this non-Euclidean geometry, see Dryden and Mardia (1998).

To average ordinary numbers, you add them up and then divide by their count. Because we can't add up shapes or divide, we borrow instead a different characterization of the ordinary average: It is also the least-squares fit to those numbers, the quantity about which they have the least sum of squared distances. Since we already have a distance between shapes, we inherit a notion of average in this way as soon as we have an algorithm for minimizing that sum of squares. That turns out not to be too difficult. One picks a tentative average, fits every form of the sample to it, substitutes the average of the fits for the previous guess at the average, and iterates. For biologically realistic data sets, this algorithm is guaranteed to converge to a shape that has the minimum summed squared distances to the original forms—just how you'd want the average shape to behave. Formally, in the complex notation introduced a few lines above, this average shape is the first principal component of the sample summed Hermitian outer product $\Sigma z\bar{z}^t$, where $z\bar{z}^t$ is the $k \times k$ matrix whose ijth entry is $z_i \bar{z}_j$ (k is the number of landmarks). For the data set here, with $k = 26$ landmarks, the result—the sample Procrustes average—is displayed at the left in Figure 4.3.

When any or all of the points subject to this sort of analysis are semilandmarks (the "sliding" points introduced above), an additional step is inserted in this algorithm, whereby these points are simultaneously slid along their several estimated tangent directions at the same time the forms are fitted to the emerging average one by one. (In effect, we are free to continue minimizing sums of squared distances over all the other outline

lines shown. Third row left: The centroids are superposed, and then one form is rotated over the other so that the sum of squared distances between corresponding landmarks is a minimum. Third row right: With the construction lines erased, the squared Procrustes distance between the pair of forms is that sum of squared distances. It is proportional to the total area of the circles. Bottom row: The Procrustes computation of average shape. Left: Emergence of an average form (solid circles) from the alternation of two-form superpositions, as above, with averages of the resulting superposed locations (big black dots). Right: Resulting sample scatter of linearized shapes, made up of five separate scatters of shape coordinates. The information in this scatter is the domain of all multivariate manipulations of landmark data, such as the group mean comparisons in this chapter.

FIGURE 4.2. Procrustes superposition. Upper row: Two forms of five homologous landmarks. Second row: Each form is rescaled so that the sum of squares of the distances to the centroid of its landmarks is 1. This is the sum of squares of the five

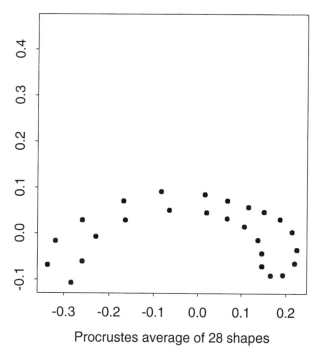

Procrustes average of 28 shapes

sample Procrustes scatter

FIGURE 4.3. Procrustes analysis of the data set in Figure 4.1. Left: Procrustes average shape, full sample. Right: Scatter of Procrustes fits of each specimen to the average shape. In this and all subsequent Procrustes plots, axes are in units of Pro-crustes distance, which is dimensionless. There is an apparently outlying arc at the lower left here, corresponding to the form in the third row, fifth column of Figure 4.1; its presence does not affect the multivariate findings reported.

points that these "might have been" while continuing adequately to represent the same outlines.) All the semi-landmarks slide at once so as to minimize their joint bending energy (see below) with respect to their tentative average, just as the rest of the Procrustes algebra ends up minimizing the joint Procrustes distance of all specimens from the average. The slipping step is a straightforward linear matrix operation in the coordinates of each configuration. For formulas and details, see Bookstein (1997c).

After we have computed the average, we can put each individual shape down over the average using the similarity transformation that made the sum of squares from the average a minimum in its particular case. Continuing the notation above, this superposition is (approximately) $z \to z(\Sigma z \bar{A})/|\Sigma z \bar{A}|$, where A is the Procrustes average just computed. For the data set here, there results the diagram at the right Figure 4.3. These points, the Procrustes shape coordinates of our sample, describe the variation of the whole set of shapes around the average in terms of variations "at" the component points separately. Any analyses that follow this construction of coordinates are of shape only. The information about scale that was sequestered when centroid size was standardized remains available for group comparisons (here, the groups differ by about 3% in average centroid size, which is not significant) or for studies of allometry (cor-

relation of size with shape), group differences, and the like. We will not need these additional analyses in either of the examples here, but they have not been precluded.

Group shape differences and their significance tests

Shape coordinates help us to carry out many familiar operations of ordinary scientific statistics. Figure 4.4, for example, shows two averages of points from the preceding scatter corresponding to the means for the subgroups of this data set in which we are the most interested: the average for the normal brains (the doctors') versus the average for the patients'.

The comparison in the figure began with 52 coordinates (x and y for each of 26 points) but lost four of these degrees of freedom when the forms were translated, rotated, and scaled to all fit the same sample average. The 48 dimensions of variability remaining are quite a bit more than the pooled sample size here, $12 + 13 = 25$, so it is not at all obvious how to proceed with a conventional significance test for the improbability of the difference shown in the figure on a null hypothesis of no group difference.

Most good morphometric data sets are of this form—more coordinates than cases—and hence much of the time spent developing this new morphometrics was devoted to the specific problem of rigorous statistical test-

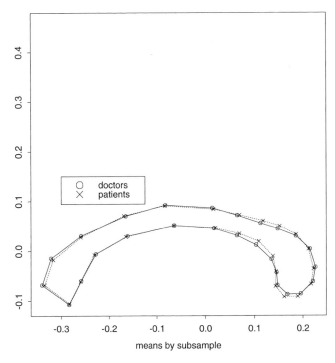

means by subsample

FIGURE 4.4. Procrustes mean shapes for the two subgroups of Figure 4.1.

ing under these conditions (cf. Bookstein, 1996). It turns out that these problems of dimensionality are much less severe than they seemed. The 48 variables remaining are not just any set of 48 measurements; they are coordinates of corresponding points that, after the Procrustes maneuver, do not vary much in location in two-dimensional Euclidean space. Their statistical analysis is thereby susceptible to a clever maneuver that was originally laid out by Colin Goodall (1991). If, for purposes of testing, we are willing to treat all the points as equivalent and, likewise, all the ways in which the shape of their configurations can vary, then we can mount a powerful test of the presence of any group difference by paying no attention to any aspect of the sample variation except net Procrustes distances of each form from the others and from the mean.

The argument begins with a suspiciously symmetric "null model," according to which each point of the data set arises from the same grand mean by pure uncorrelated Gaussian noise of the same small variance in every direction at every landmark separately. Under this model, if one has no prior knowledge about just how the shapes are likely to differ, the best statistic for testing group differences in mean shape is exactly the Procrustes distance we have just introduced, and its distribution on the null is borne in an F-ratio that can be evaluated and tested no matter how many points there are or how few specimens per group. The F in question looks just like

any other F-ratio from your introductory biostatistics course: a between-group sum of squares divided by a within-group sum of squares, multiplied by an integer fraction and looked up in an F-table. In this application the integer fraction and the degrees of freedom are functions of the number of landmarks as well as the sample sizes. The formula, which is appropriate on the assumptions opening this paragraph, regardless of the number of landmarks or cases, reads as follows: The quantity

$$\frac{\mathcal{N}_1 + \mathcal{N}_2 - 2}{\mathcal{N}_1^{-1} + \mathcal{N}_2^{-1}} \frac{\|\bar{F}_1 - \bar{F}_2\|^2}{\Sigma_{\text{cases}}\|F - \bar{F}_i\|^2}$$

is distributed as the statistician's $F_{2k-4,\,(2k-4)(\mathcal{N}_1+\mathcal{N}_2-2)}$. Here $\mathcal{N}_1$ and $\mathcal{N}_2$ are the two group sample sizes, $\bar{F}_1$ and $\bar{F}_2$ are the group average shapes in the common (pooled) Procrustes registration, and $\|\cdot\|^2$ is squared Procrustes distance. The numerator of the ratio at the right is the squared distance between mean shapes—the sum of the squared separations between the paired points in Figure 4.4. The denominator is the sum of all squared Procrustes residuals (which have been assumed sufficiently small) from the group means over landmarks and cases.

Although this formula is interesting, the assumptions underlying the claimed F-distribution are quite unrealistic in many settings. They are violated, for instance, whenever variation in points close together is correlated (which is certainly the case for adjacent points along smooth curves), whenever deviations at a distance are correlated (which is certainly the case for symmetrical or nearly symmetrical forms), and whenever some landmarks are noisier than others or more variable in certain directions than others, no matter how small the underlying shape variation. Nevertheless, the statistic itself, that squared Procrustes distance $\|\bar{F}_1 - \bar{F}_2\|^2$ in the numerator, is a very useful summary of all the difference between the mean shapes. It can be exploited whenever one has decided that all the measurable a priori causes of these correlations have been adjusted out. The denominator is a fine summary of all the within-group shape variation under a similar caveat.

Regardless of Goodall's assumptions, then, one can use the Procrustes statistic $\|\bar{F}_1 - \bar{F}_2\|^2$ as a very useful summary measure of shape effect size as long as one computes its distribution realistically rather than by recourse to tables. For this purpose it is most useful to construct the reference distribution by permutation test (Good, 2000). In this approach, the actual Procrustes distance between group mean shapes, such as the two in Figure 4.4, is referred not to a table of F-ratios but to the actual distribution of such distances computed after the assignment of groups to specimens is randomly per-

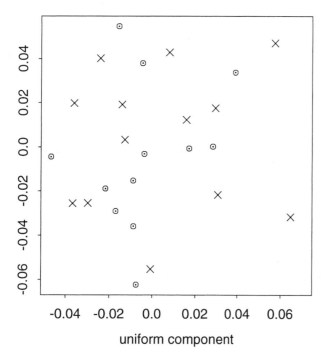

uniform component

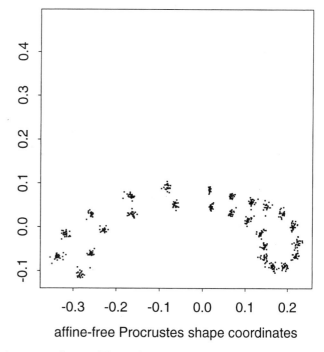

affine-free Procrustes shape coordinates

FIGURE 4.5. Aspects of the uniform adjustment. Left: Procrustes optimal uniform component; there are no differences in central tendency by group. Right: Uniform-free Procrustes shape coordinates. The variance here is less than half of that of the analogous unadjusted plot in Figure 4.3.

muted. For instance, in the present data set, the first 12 specimens are normals (doctors), and the last 13 are patients; one permutation might declare the doctors to be cases 3, 5, 7, 9, 10, 11, 15, 18, 19, 20, 23, and 25 and the patients to be the other cases. The exact significance level of a Procrustes distance between group means like these is the fraction of permutations that produce a difference at least as large while wholly ignoring the actual information about grouping. In practice, one need not take all the combinations—there are more than five million for this sample of 13 cases versus 12—but a suitably extensive random sampling. In this paper, every permutation test involved 1000 permutations. (It sounds as if we are ignoring the denominator of the equation above. Actually, as explained by Bookstein (1997b), the numerator and denominator here sum to a constant— the total variation of the full data set—and so the permutation test ends up a function of the numerator, the pseudogroup mean Procrustes distance, alone.)

To apply this test to a data set such as this one, it is important to partial out all factors that are known in advance to contribute large-scale variability that is unrelated to the hypothesis at hand. In modern morphometrics there are a good many rigorous ways of partialing out such factors in advance. One method, which is useful in the present context, is removal of the so-called uniform term, the extent to which specimens differ by deformations that take square graph paper into a uniform grid of identical parallelograms. Changes like these, while they can be quite interesting, account for correlated displacements of all the landmarks at once, which can easily overwhelm the signal from any local shape difference encoded in a small arc of callosal boundary.

In the Procrustes toolkit, this uniform term is computed by a fixed formula (see Bookstein, 1996, 1997b) that is determined once and for all by the Procrustes geometry around the mean form. Here this term accounts for more than half of all the shape variation in the data. Figure 4.5 shows the estimate of this component (think of it as height of the arch; notice that it does not discriminate the groups) and also, at the right, the variation remaining after this adjustment. It is clear by comparison with Figure 4.3 that this Procrustes-optimal adjustment for uniform variation greatly sharpened the precision with which other comparisons can be assessed.

A permutation test applied to the unadjusted data in Figure 4.3 results in a significance level of about 25% for the group mean shape difference in Figure 4.4. Applied to the residuals in Figure 4.5, the same test finds that out of 1000 permutations, only 12 produced a Procrustes distance between pseudogroup means as large as the difference shown in Figure 4.4. That is, the two mean shapes in question, the doctors' and the patients', differ significantly in the nonuniform component of shape at about the 1.2% significance level. This degree of im-

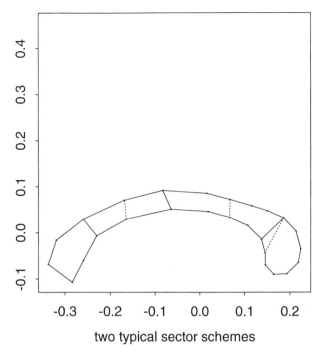

two typical sector schemes

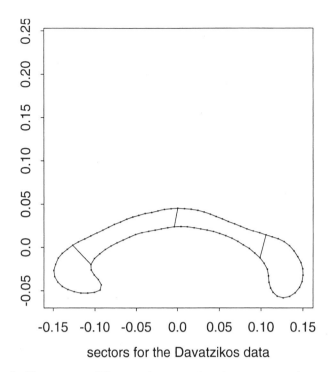

sectors for the Davatzikos data

FIGURE 4.6. Simulation of the approach by sector areas. Left: For the mean shape in Figure 4.3. Right: For the mean shape from Figure 4.10. No schemes of this type show statistically significant group differences in area ratios after an appropriate correction for the multiple comparisons involved.

plausibility on the null hypothesis (no difference) is sufficient to justify a search for further substantive features.

It is instructive to compare this overall approach to significance testing with the conventional counterpart, which would typically reduce the comparison of groups to a matter of areas of various sectors of the callosum (see, e.g., Semrud-Clikeman et al., 1994; Riley et al., 1995). Diverse sets of sectors, such as the two sketched at the left in Figure 4.6, never manage to recover a set of sectors for which the difference of relative areas, doctors versus patients, is significant even at the 5% level when tested by the corresponding omnibus T^2 test (or, if you like, when tested by ordinary t-ratio but then corrected Bonferroni-style for the number of sectors). In the Procrustes method, by contrast, there is only one statistic to be tested—the summary statistic was always summed all the way around the outline, even though our findings will be limited to much smaller regions when we discuss them—and hence there was no associated "correction." The true p-value of the group difference here is arithmetically the same 1.2% that is reported by the permutation test.

Thin-plate splines for the relation of two shapes

Thus, we have a significant shape difference in the non-uniform subspace between the averages of these two samples of callosal outlines. From the representation in Figure 4.4, however, it is difficult to say in exactly what feature(s) this difference might be expressed. To render shape differences legible, we turn to an idea as old as the invention of artistic perspective in the Renaissance. We can show the changes of all the points in Figure 4.3 as one coherent graphical display by imagining one of the averages—say, the normals (the dots)—to have been put down on ordinary square graph paper. Call it the starting shape. We deform the paper so that the dots now fall directly over the other set of points, the set constituting the target shape. At the left, Figure 4.7 shows what happens to the grid.

Naturally, it matters what deformation one uses. Part of the modern efflorescence of modern morphometric methodology depends on the mathematical properties of one particular choice, the thin-plate spline, that minimizes yet another sum of squares. In this context, we are minimizing the summed squared second derivatives (integrated over the whole plane) of the map in the figure—something like the summed squared deviations of the shapes of the little squares from the shapes of their neighbors and thus a measure of local information in the mapping. It is quite remarkable that the function we want can be written out in full in elementary notation. Let the landmarks of the form on which the grid is squared be denoted P_i; $i = 1, \ldots, k$, in one single image,

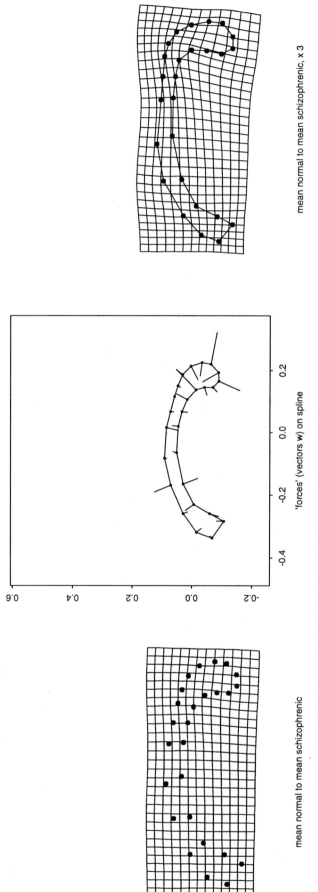

mean normal to mean schizophrenic

'forces' (vectors w) on spline

mean normal to mean schizophrenic, x 3

FIGURE 4.7. Thin-plate spline visualizations for the comparison of group mean shapes in Figure 4.4. Left: The actual mean difference as a deformation. Center: Coefficients (w_{ix}, w_{iy}) of the nonlinear part of the spline, indicating, by their perpendicularity to the mean outline, that the points have been "slipped" along the outline everywhere except at the corners, that is, that these points are not landmarks but semilandmarks. Right: The same spline extrapolated threefold. Its summary by a pair of discrete features, the shrinkage at genu and the directional displacement of the isthmus-splenium boundary, is now quite clear.

and write $U_{ij} = U(P_i - P_j)$, where U is the function $U(r) = r^2 \log r$. Then build up matrices

$$K = \begin{pmatrix} 0 & U_{12} & \dots & U_{1k} \\ U_{21} & 0 & \cdots & U_{2k} \\ \vdots & \vdots & \ddots & \vdots \\ U_{k1} & U_{k2} & \dots & 0 \end{pmatrix}, \quad Q = \begin{pmatrix} 1 & x_1 & y_1 \\ 1 & x_2 & y_2 \\ \vdots & \vdots & \vdots \\ 1 & x_k & y_k \end{pmatrix},$$

and

$$L = \begin{pmatrix} K & Q \\ Q^t & O \end{pmatrix}, \quad (k+3) \times (k+3),$$

where O is a 3×3 matrix of zeros. The thin-plate spline $f(P)$ having heights (values) h_i at points $P_i = (x_i, y_i)$, $i = 1, \dots, k$, is the function

$$f(P) = \sum_{i=1}^{k} w_i U(P - P_i) + a_0 + a_x x + a_y y$$

where

$$W = (w_1 \dots w_k\, a_0\, a_x\, a_y)^t = L^{-1} H$$

with

$$H = (h_1\, h_2 \dots h_k\, 0\, 0\, 0)^t.$$

In the application to two-dimensional landmark data, we compute two of these splined surfaces, one in which the vector H is loaded with the x-coordinates of the landmarks in a second form and one for the y-coordinates. The resulting map $(f_x(P), f_y(P))$ is now a deformation of one picture plane onto the other that maps landmarks onto their homologues and has the minimum integrated sum of squared second derivatives of any such interpolant. The reader who enjoys playing with graphic software can build this useful mapping tool direct from these equations and explore its properties on any convenient computer or might instead download our Edgewarp program package, which centers on a graphics engine producing these maps for any sets of landmarks (see the section below entitled "Software"). The bending energy of such a spline, analogue of the physical energy of the metaphorical underlying plate, is the scalar quantity $H_{kx}^t L_k^{-1} H_{kx} + H_{ky}^t L_k^{-1} H_{ky}$, where H_{kx} and H_{ky} are the vectors of the k nonzero elements of H for the Cartesian coordinates of the "target" landmarks separately and L_k^{-1} is the upper left $k \times k$ submatrix of L^{-1}. This is also the quantity that is minimized to slide the sliding landmarks. For additional identities and an intuitive introduction to all these concepts, see Bookstein (1991).

To return to the main argument: At left in Figure 4.7 is the map given by the data of Figure 4.4 when the grid squared on the normal mean is deformed to match the syndromal mean. In the center panel of the figure is a nonstandard auxiliary illustration showing the forces on the spline, the vectors (w_{ix}, w_{iy}) of the preceding nota-

tion. Most of these vectors are perpendicular to the outline at the point from which they spring. (Where they are not perpendicular, it is owing to the effect of landmark points distinct from the callosal outline itself, points that are not shown in the graphics here.) That perpendicularity is the evidence that these points were slipped along their contours in the course of the digitizing, as I claimed without explanation when this data set was introduced in Figure 4.1. The spacing on one form was arbitrary (but reasonable); the spacing on all the others is determined mainly by this criterion of perpendicularity.

The left panel of Figure 4.7 is correctly drawn but remains hard to decipher nevertheless. It is not yet straightforward to state exactly what the shape change is, just what kind of process is being displayed here. For the purpose of interpreting figures like these, it is often very useful, after statistical testing is complete, to improve the visualization by an extrapolation of the shape change under consideration. (One of the advantages of the thin-plate spline interpolant is that this operation is linear in the data.) From a threefold extrapolation of the same grid, at right in the figure, it is now apparent how this group difference ought to be summarized. There are two spatially disparate features of the syndromal effect

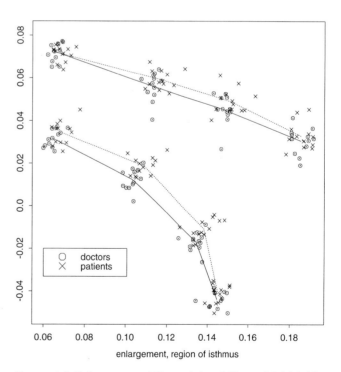

FIGURE 4.8. Enlargement of Figure 4.4 and Figure 4.5 (right) in the region of the isthmus. The reshaping of the lower arc here is responsible for most of the statistical significance of the overall group difference. A Procrustes fit of just these eight points results in an even clearer localization of the shape difference between these two groups.

on callosal shape. One is in genu: a generalized shrinking of the feature. (In the data set at hand, this effect should not be given too much credence, as the original slices from which these outlines were extracted were so thick that the region of rostrum was not reliably discernible.) More interesting is the change toward the posterior, in the splenium and the arc of isthmus just above. The underside of the isthmus appears to be substantially displaced in an upward-posterior direction. The difference is rather more one of location than one of area.

With this hint in hand, we know where to look. Drawing from the original scatter, Figure 4.8 enlarges this interesting region where the isthmus springs from the splenium. At this scale, it is possible to indicate the group origin of each outline point: The doctors' data points are shown by circles, the patients' by crosses. At the semilandmark that has shifted most in Figure 4.8—second from the left in the lower segment—the groups are separated in the direction normal to the curve by a very substantial amount. Discarding the rest of the information in the outline, Bookstein (1997c) repeats the Procrustes analysis using only this subset of eight points and shows that in the resulting projection the doctors and the patients are separated at this locus with only two classification errors. The separation is by 1.75 times the standard deviation of the normative subsample, the largest effect I have ever seen reported in any neuroanatomical study of schizophrenia. The statistical significance of the overall comparison of mean outline shapes owes wholly to this sharp shape difference in one short arc of the ventricular boundary of the isthmus. Recall that was an overall significance test, a test for the presence of any

substantial difference of location along any subarc or set of subarcs. The significance of any difference is tested first, globally. It is the overall level, not any Bonferroni correction of local findings, that applies to the study as a whole.

A second data set: Sexual dimorphism of the aged human callosum

The data for the second example, courtesy of Christos Davatzikos of Johns Hopkins University, began their geometric life quite differently. As explained by Davatzikos and colleagues (1996), these callosal outlines were produced completely automatically by a so-called active contour method on each of 16 images (eight from elderly males, eight from elderly females). On one form, they were evenly spaced. The sets of 100 semilandmarks for each of the other 15 forms were selected on the polygonal outlines by an elastic method of "slipping" with respect to the evenly spaced points on the first form. This elastic slipping method is very close in spirit to the thin-plate spline slip used in the preceding example. The full data set, 100 points for 16 cases, is shown in Figure 4.9. It is then put into the Procrustes superposition over its own Procrustes average; the result is the well-behaved scatter at the left in Figure 4.10.

The group mean outlines (solid line for females, dotted line for males) are shown at right in the same figure. They look considerably more divergent in shape than the group averages of the preceding example; on the other hand, these samples are smaller and the points more numerous. A straightforward application of the methods demonstrated so far results in a significance

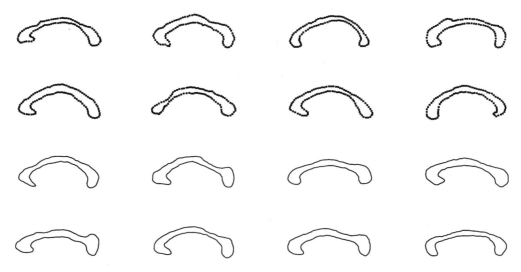

FIGURE 4.9. A second data set: 16 callosal outlines of healthy elderly. Upper two rows: males. Lower two rows: females. (From Davatzikos et al., 1996.)

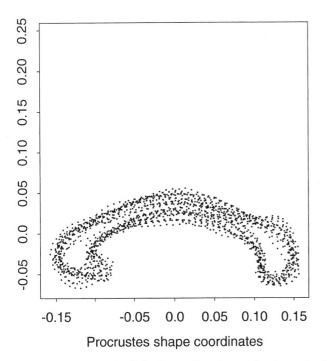

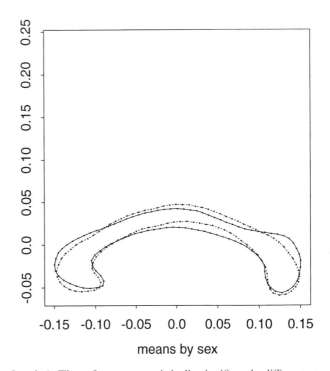

Procrustes shape coordinates

means by sex

FIGURE 4.10. Analysis of the Davatzikos data set by the tools of this toolkit. Left: Procrustes shape coordinates for 16 cases of 100 semilandmarks each. Right: Mean shapes by sex (solid line: females). These forms are statistically significantly different at the 0.5% level by the direction-restricted permutation test described in the text.

level of about 8% for the difference. Partialing out the uniform term, as we did before (Figure 4.5), does not strengthen this finding. (There is also a difference of 7% in centroid size, just significant at the 0.05 level. The areas of these callosa likewise differ by about 7% in mean, but there is much more scatter, as befits a quantity with dimensions of square centimeters, so the area difference is not significant, even though the size difference is significant.)

We need, rather, to turn to another device from our modern morphometric toolkit. In the Procrustes formulation, distances between matched points are computed by using all the information available: two coordinates per point. In the originally acquired data and in the Procrustes scatter, these are stored as x- and y-coordinates. But they are more profitably considered in another coordinate system, one varying in orientation from point to point: the system of tangent and normal to the mean outline curve. The real import of data sets like these characterizes outlines mainly in the direction perpendicular to the (typical) curve. The usual Procrustes formula, by attending to shifts in both directions, is incorporating too great a degree of noise into the computation for the signal here to emerge clearly. We can correct this problem by reducing the "distance" squared and summed in the Procrustes formula to only one of its coordinates, the one that has the information we seek: the distance nor-

mal to the average curve. (The sampled points in the first example are too widely separated for this statistic to apply there.) Following this modification, the permutation test goes forward exactly as before: The true summed squared normal difference between the group averages is calibrated against the distribution of that same sum of squares, all the way around the outline, when group is randomized over the 16 cases. There are 12,869 other groupings of this data set into eight versus eight; we take 1000 of these at random. Out of the thousand, only five permutations generated pseudogroups having a larger summed squared distance taken in this locally directional sense. In other words, the two group mean shapes in Figure 4.10 are statistically significantly different at about the 0.5% level. Compare the report of this same data set by Davatzikos and colleagues (1996), in which this same contrast could not be shown to be statistically significant by analysis of areas.

As in the first example, it remains to extract the features of this difference—to put the contrast into words—and again, the thin-plate spline is the best available tool. At the left in Figure 4.11 is the spline, extrapolated twofold, from the average of the male forms to the average for the females. There is clearly a reshaping of the region of the splenium involving some directional size change and some adjustment of its connection with the isthmus. In a somewhat focused-down version of the

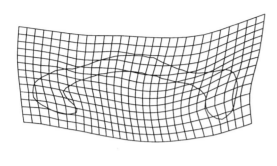

deformation, male --> female, x 2

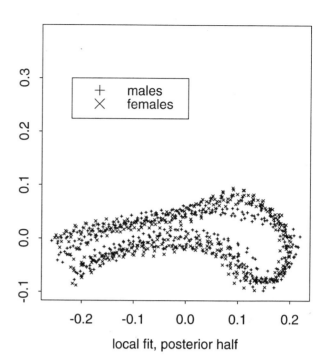

local fit, posterior half

FIGURE 4.11. Localizing the difference in Figure 4.10. Left: Thin-plate spline for two times the difference of means by sex. Notice the substantial reshaping of the splenium. Right: Recomputation of Procrustes scatter restricted to the posterior half of the form. The separation at the upper margin of the splenium is now almost perfect; it accounts for the significance of the contrast as a whole.

entire Procrustes analysis, for the posterior half of the form, we can see some of this difference in the nearly perfect separation of the outlines by sex in the vicinity of the "bump" at the top of the splenium in the right panel.

In an earlier draft, the decision to focus the previous paragraph on the vicinity of the splenium was defended as merely an interesting place to look; but recently, it has become possible to bring it to the analyst's attention by a wholly automatic procedure that is much more in keeping with the spirit of other chapters of this volume, such as Thompson's. Figure 4.12 demonstrates a technique that has just been introduced for group comparisons of landmark or semilandmark data in two or three dimensions: summary of these extended splined grids by a hierarchy of discrete localized features that look like creases, organized patterns surrounding maxima or minima of ratios of homologous distance elements. At the left is the analytic computation corresponding to our informal report of Figure 4.11, the precise location and orientation of the global maximum of strain from the male to the female mean form. The maximum strain, computed analytically from the spline's explicit formula, is 1.413. If we were to replace the female mean form, then, by the form that deviated from the male form by a multiple of $0.413^{-1} = -2.42$ of the actual transformation here—the form for which landmarks shifted 2.42-fold as far in the opposite direction—then this optimal

derivative would be precisely zero, giving the appearance of a crease in the grid, as shown at right in Figure 4.12. Algebraically, if the grid in Figure 4.11 corresponds to the spline $M \rightarrow F$, where M and F are the male and female mean forms in the Procrustes geometry, respectively, then the new figure is the result of applying the standard splining technique to the map $M \rightarrow (M - 2.42(F - M))$. (Also, the original Cartesian system has been rotated so that the direction in which strain was artificially sent to zero is now the y-axis of the original coordinate system.)

There results a remarkable diagram indeed. However distorted the form of the "callosum" here, its message about the geometry of the original dimorphism, male mean versus female mean, is startlingly clear. We knew that this strain had to be aligned with the boundaries of the callosal outline in its vicinity, as there is no possibility of shear along that boundary in the algorithm that Davatzikos used to assign homology; but we did not know that it would prove as spatially focal as it is here seen to be. The crease organization that ordinarily looks like a 90° rotation of a pair of abutting parentheses,) (, here takes on an appearance like an hourglass instead: a highly local squeezing inward (in the real data, extension outward) at the posterior end of an arch that otherwise manifests a more or less constant strain in this direction. The width of this "waist" is roughly the same as that

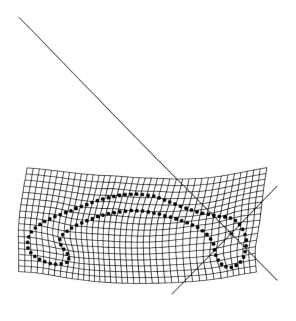 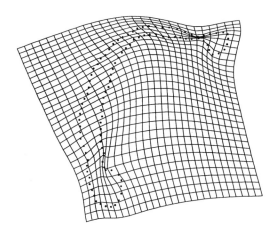

extremum of deformation tensor, M-F   the same extrapolated -2.42fold to a crease

FIGURE 4.12. The same, now localized automatically by the method of creases (Bookstein, 2000). Left: Global extremum of the larger principal strain of the derivative of the thin-plate spline mapping at left in Figure 4.11. This maximum strain is 1.413 along the approximately northeast-southwest direction drawn. Right: Negative fractional extrapolation of the trans- formation from male mean to female mean by a factor of $(1 - 1.413)^{-1} = -2.42$. While the callosal form itself is hugely distorted, the extreme directional derivative is thereby con- verted to an isolated zero, around which the grid takes a characteristic and very helpful appearance.

of the "bump" in the right-hand panel of Figure 4.11. There is an additional center of compression in the crease picture, at the crook of genu, showing a simi- larly localized aspect of relative female hypertrophy at a slightly lower value of maximum strain. (It was presaged at the far left in the grid of Figure 4.11, just as the crease here was already visualized at the far right.) In between these two foci of compression, the extrapolation in Figure 4.12 is quite smoothly graded; we might have anticipated this in the smooth rectilinearity of the grid cells within the arch in Figure 4.11.

In a comparison of a mere eight forms of each gender, it would be unwise to speculate further on this localiza- tion. But the technique of creases is likely to be a great aid to hypothesis generation in larger samples, for which the underlying uncertainty of these foci is often less. For the underlying calculus (which, though novel, is an ele- mentary application of some classic twentieth century results in differential geometry), significance tests, pa- rameterizations, and additional possibilities, see Book- stein (2000).

Covariance between callosal shape and function

A third data set augments the formalization of callosal shape with direct measurements of neuropsychological function on a simple test battery. The following discus- sion is a small part of a far more extensive investigation reported in detail by Bookstein and colleagues (2002).

For this application, callosal "outlines" were actually digitized as chains of three-dimensional points that lay on the local axis of symmetry of appropriate anatomical cross sections. These points were then slipped to mini- mize net bending energy, as discussed earlier, and finally projected onto a common synthetic "midsagittal plane" for analysis. The resulting curves incorporate one true landmark (rostrum, a good three-dimensional point) along with 39 semilandmarks; after Procrustes fitting, there are $40 \times 2 = 80$ shape coordinates. This geometry was recorded for 30 adult males from the Seattle area who had been diagnosed with either fetal alcohol syn- drome or fetal alcohol effects (Institute of Medicine, 1996). The neuropsychological battery here, extracted from a much larger protocol of 260 tests over 6 hours, included five measures of reaction time in each of three experimental conditions (simple, choice, and interhemi- spheric transfer) combining laterality of visual stimulus with laterality or contralaterality of motor response. (This does not constitute a proper battery for testing callosal function per se, as the total allocated time was only 4 minutes, corresponding to only 48 separate ex- perimental stimuli.)

Analysis here is by the method of partial least squares (PLS), which is a singular-value decomposition of the covariance matrix between the callosal shape coordinates and the ranks of the 15 neuropsychological measures, followed by interpretation of the singular vectors as coefficients of linear combinations of the two blocks. PLS can be thought of as a combination of regression analysis and factor analysis; it extracts profiles of behavior that optimally covary with dimensions of shape and also produces scores (latent variables) characterizing the study's subjects on these paired dimensions. For a didactic explanation of the matrix algebra underlying this method, along with an explanation of its differences from canonical correlations analysis and structural equations modeling, see Bookstein and colleagues (1996).

The cross-modality signal relating callosal shape to these functional measures was dominated by the uniform term introduced above, which accounts for almost 60% of the cross-block covariance signal in this data set. (This is unlike the situation in the first example, in which the uniform term contributed no useful information to the descriptive task, the group discrimination.) A single uniform shear correlated 0.40 (Figure 4.13, left panel; $p \sim 0.03$) with a profile of behavior emphasizing left-side reaction time, and RT standard deviation, in the simple experimental condition (press a button with the hand on the side that the visual stimulus is on). The more complex conditions contribute essentially nothing to this structure-behavior covariance: Squared direction cosines of the first singular vector total 0.88 for the five measures in the first experimental condition versus 0.09 for the second and only 0.03 for the third. This is the case even though the first principal component of the three sets of five reaction time measures weights the three almost equally (0.32, 0.34, 0.34).

The callosal shape correlated with greater reaction times (poor performance) is somewhat thinned in the splenium, as shown at upper center in Figure 4.13, and a bit attenuated. The size of these arches, set down point by point in the left panel, is not correlated either with this feature of shape or with the corresponding profile of performance deficit. (The unit of this size measure is millimeters, and the nearest simply phrased measure is callosal length.) A suitable test for the scientific content of this analysis might examine the distribution of the extent to which covariation with callosal shape is concentrated in the first (simple) subtest only; the corresponding tail probability is $p \sim 0.008$. There is no significant signal in the relation of callosal shape to either of the other subtests.

The deficit in reaction time speed in this simple condition does not correlate with full-scale IQ (right panel)

in this sample, nor does the relation differ between subjects with ($\times$) and without ($+$) the facial stigmata that differentiate fetal alcohol syndrome from fetal alcohol effects. This independence of the teratogenesis from both the facial features and the IQ deficits according to which patients qualify for social services bears directly on public policies regarding treatment of people who are diagnosed with prenatal alcohol damage (Bookstein et al., 2002).

Discussion

I am not competent to discuss the psychiatric, gerontological, or neurological meaning of any of these findings. (Indeed, I look forward very much to receiving my copy of this volume just so that I can learn some of the neurobiology of the callosum as it may relate to these sturdy statistical contrasts.) It may be useful, nevertheless, if I pursue some of the morphometric issues here. Why is it that the new methods are so much more powerful than the traditional approach to cause-and-effect analysis via sectioning the area of the arch? There are three general reasons, I would argue, that this new toolkit of methods ought to replace the old in studies of the callosum: the richness of this parametric treatment of shape, the reliance on omnibus statistical tests rather than ad hoc Bonferroni corrections of localized analyses, and the power of the associated visualizations.

STUDYING SHAPE DIFFERENCES PER SE The standard sectoral approach studies only the area inside the callosal form. Such approaches incorporate no representation of shapes of individual callosa by any parameter vector that can be diagrammed, regionalized, or tested by formal statistical procedure. They are thus ineffective at detecting changes that alter shape without much altering area. In the second example here, just such an effect was found: Group difference in the region of the isthmus is mainly of position, much less of relative area. In the first example, the change at isthmus incorporates some areal shrinkage but also some displacement. The areal approach is clearly much less likely to find such changes than, say, the relative enlargement of splenium. The splenium sector, shown at the right in Figure 4.6, occupies a fraction of the total callosal area that differs in a ratio of 17% between the sexes. This difference is significant at $p \sim 0.03$ by conventional t-test (before the Bonferroni correction). By contrast, the difference of position of the border at the upper right in the right panel of Figure 4.7, a different descriptor of the same shape difference, is significant at about $p \sim 0.003$ by t-test in the normal direction. Put most tersely, there is

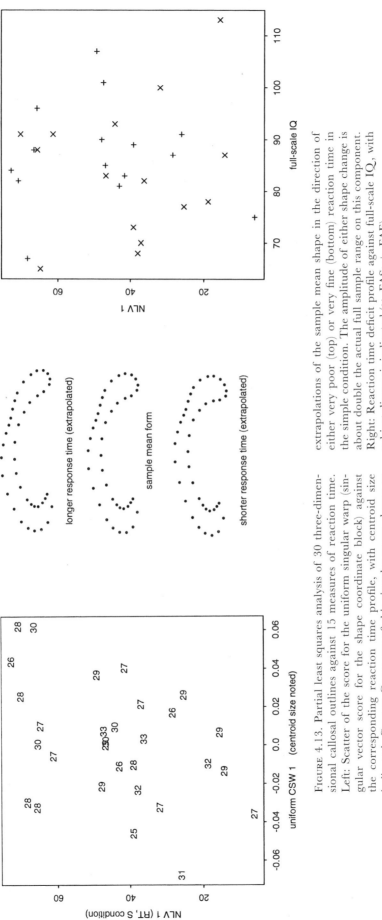

FIGURE 4.13. Partial least squares analysis of 30 three-dimensional callosal outlines against 15 measures of reaction time. Left: Scatter of the score for the uniform singular warp (singular vector score for the shape coordinate block) against the corresponding reaction time profile, with centroid size indicated. Center: Geometry of this singular warp, drawn as extrapolations of the sample mean shape in the direction of either very poor (top) or very fine (bottom) reaction time in the simple condition. The amplitude of either shape change is about double the actual full sample range on this component. Right: Reaction time deficit profile against full-scale IQ, with subject diagnosis indicated (×, FAS; +, FAE).

89

considerably more information in shape than in area and therefore many more ways of reporting effects on shape than effects on area. In general, description by the areal-ratio scalar, like any other scalar description, uses one parameter (the determinant) from the three that together describe the tensor field of afine derivatives (Bookstein, 1999), and so discards about two-thirds of the information available for discussions of variability.

STATISTICAL TESTS   In the context of a size standardization there is no overall area distance between forms. The areal methods, whether the standard comparisons sector by sector or Davatzikos's little area elements, are forced to report significance tests for multiple comparisons: multiple sectors, multiple grid squares. Claims of overall significance level must be tempered thereafter by the need for Bonferroni correction; indeed, in Davatzikos's data set, no areas were left significant after this procedure, and so no inference about the difference between the genders was reported at all, even though we saw above that their average outline shapes are actually different at about the 0.5% level by an appropriate test. By contrast, the combination of Procrustes and permutation procedures here takes the correlation of adjacent sectors, adjacent grid cells, and so forth into account quite automatically in a way that the Bonferroni-corrected methods simply cannot. Whereas the conventional methods are all ad hoc, providing varying mean differences and varying significance levels depending on the number and placement of sectors, the toolkit here incorporates one unitary multivariate test for the significance of an overall shape difference of outlines in the full shape space or in any feature-specific subspace. For instance, in the third example the statistical test took the built-in subspace of uniform shears (largest-scale shape changes) for granted and exploited it to test instead the apparent concentration of the structure/function finding in one particular behavioral channel.

The failure of the standard methods to produce an explicit representation of shape per se is particularly unfortunate because the statistical properties of size-normalized shape (as, for instance, series of ratios) are strongly dependent on the choice of a size measure to use for normalizing. The properties of the choice here, centroid size, are the subject of theorems (cf. Bookstein, 1998a) that justify its use in this application. Other measures, such as overall length, lead to correlations among derived scores that can interfere quite badly with the detection of group differences.

VISUALIZATIONS   In the conventional approach, no average shapes are produced, only averaged areas, and findings and visualizations are in all the same coin of bar graphs with error bars. In Davatzikos's method, findings were presented as areal ratios but could not be tested, and there was no representation of sample variation around the averaged outlines. By contrast, our analysis of semilandmarks all around the boundary uses the entire picture plane to communicate the nature of whatever findings are significant. In the first example the findings include the shrinkage of one callosal component (genu) and the displacement of another; in the second example the findings are of a quite different flavor, emphasizing a complex shape difference in the mean shape of the splenium without any corresponding large-scale shift. One does not need to have adumbrated the right flavor of finding from this list in advance of the analysis because the multivariate statistical workup deals with any shape difference whatever, regardless of geometry, location, or scale. The scientist is thereby free to report whatever differences can be seen in the deformation figures; it is not those features that are tested, but instead the simple, unitary claim that the groups have different shapes (examples 1 and 2) or that different shapes correspond to different profiles of neuropsychological function (example 3).

Software

Software that carries out most of these computations is publicly available. Those of you with a modern workstation might FTP to my web site, brainmap.med. umich.edu, go to the directory pub/edgewarp or pub/edgewarp3.1, and there grab a program and a manual to browse through. The Edgewarp software family, constructed by my colleague William D. K. Green, includes a variety of programs for digitizing two-dimensional and three-dimensional medical images, averaging the shape information they bear, and averaging the images after unwarping to those average shapes. There are versions for many modern Unix workstations and also for Linux, the Unixlike operating system for PCs. I would also gladly share the source files in Splus (a commercial statistical package) that produced all the statistical analyses and diagrammatic figures here.

ACKNOWLEDGMENTS   Preparation of this contribution was supported by NIH grants DA09009 and GM37251 to Fred L. Bookstein. I thank John DeQuardo, the University of Michigan, for the subjects and the selection of image planes underlying the schizophrenia data set here (example 1), Christos Davatzikos of Johns Hopkins University for the gerontological data set (example 2), and Ann Streissguth, grant AA10836, and the Fetal Alcohol and Drug Unit at the University of Washington for the fetal alcohol structural and behavioral data (example 3).

REFERENCES

BOOKSTEIN, F. L., 1991. *Morphometric Tools for Landmark Data.* New York: Cambridge University Press.

BOOKSTEIN, F. L., 1996. Biometrics, biomathematics, and the morphometric synthesis. *Bull. Math. Biol.* 58:313–365.

BOOKSTEIN, F. L., 1997a. Biometrics and brain maps: The promise of the morphometric synthesis. In *Neuroinformatics: An Overview of the Human Brain Project, Progress in Neuroinformatics*, Vol. 1, S. Koslow and M. Huerta, eds. Hillsdale, N.J.: Lawrence Erlbaum, pp. 203–254.

BOOKSTEIN, F. L., 1997b. Shape and the information in medical images: A decade of the morphometric synthesis. *Computer Vision and Image Understanding* 66:97–118.

BOOKSTEIN, F. L., 1997c. Landmark methods for forms without landmarks: Localizing group differences in outline shape. *Med. Image Analysis* 1:225–243.

BOOKSTEIN, F. L., 1998. A hundred years of morphometrics. *Acta Zool.* 44:7–59.

BOOKSTEIN, F. L., 1999. Linear methods for nonlinear maps: Procrustes fits, thin-plate splines, and the biometric analysis of shape variability. In *Brain Warping*, A. Toga, ed. New York: Academic Press, pp. 157–181.

BOOKSTEIN, F. L., 2000. Creases as local features of deformation grids. *Med. Image Analysis*, 4:93–110.

BOOKSTEIN, F. L., A. STREISSGUTH, P. SAMPSON, and H. BARR, 2002. Corpus callosum shape and neuropsychological deficits in adult males with heavy fetal alcohol exposure. *NeuroImage* 15:233–251.

BOOKSTEIN, F. L., A. STREISSGUTH, P. SAMPSON, P. CONNOR, and H. BARR, 1999. Corpus callosum shape hypervariation covaries with neuropsychological deficits in adult males with heavy fetal alcohol exposure. *Arch. Gen. Psychiatry*, under re-review.

DAVATZIKOS, C., M. VAILLANT, S. M. RESNICK, J. L. PRINCE, S. LETOVSKY, and R. N. BRYAN, 1996. A computerized approach for morphological analysis of the corpus callosum. *J. Comput. Assis. Tomogr.* 20:88–97.

DRYDEN, I., and K. V. MARDIA, 1998. *Statistical Shape Analysis.* New York: Wiley.

GOOD, P., 2000. *Permutation Tests*, 2nd ed. New York: Springer-Verlag.

GOODALL, C. R., 1991. Procrustes methods in the statistical analysis of shape. *J. Roy. Statist. Soc.* B53:285–339.

INSTITUTE OF MEDICINE, 1996. *Fetal Alcohol Syndrome: Diagnosis, Epidemiology, Prevention, and Treatment.* Washington, D.C., National Academy Press.

RILEY, E. P., S. MATTSON, E. SOWELL, T. JERNIGAN, D. SOBEL, and K. JONES, 1995. Abnormalities of the corpus callosum in children prenatally exposed to alcohol. *Alcohol. Clin. Exp. Res.* 19:1198–1202.

SEMRUD-CLIKEMAN, M., P. FILIPEK, J. BIDERMAN, R. STEINGARD, D. KENNEDY, P. RENSHAW, and K. BEKKEN, 1994. Attention deficit hyperactivity disorder: Magnetic resonance imaging morphometric analysis of the corpus callosum. *J. Am. Acad. Child Adolesc. Psychiatry* 33:875–881.

SLICE, D., F. L. BOOKSTEIN, L. MARCUS, and F. J. ROHLF, 1995. *A Glossary for Geometric Morphometrics.* Electronic publication: http://life.bio.sunysb.edu/morph/gloss1.html.

5 Mapping Structural Alterations of the Corpus Callosum During Brain Development and Degeneration

PAUL M. THOMPSON, KATHERINE L. NARR, REBECCA E. BLANTON, AND ARTHUR W. TOGA

ABSTRACT In this chapter we review current neuroimaging research on the structure of the corpus callosum. The corpus callosum is the main fiber tract connecting the two brain hemispheres, consisting of approximately 200–350 million fibers in humans. Given the corpus callosum's importance in communicating perceptual, cognitive, mnemonic, learned, and volitional information between the hemispheres, it has not surprisingly been a focus of many studies examining structural and functional neuropathology. We and other groups have investigated callosal abnormalities in Alzheimer's disease, multi-infarct dementia, schizophrenia, attention deficit hyperactivity disorder, and multiple sclerosis and during normal and aberrant development. Nonetheless, extreme variations in brain structure make it difficult to design computerized strategies that detect and classify abnormal structural patterns. Intense controversy exists on the question of whether different callosal regions undergo selective changes in each of these disease processes. Additional controversy surrounds studies that have identified specific differences in callosal structure related to sex, handedness, IQ, and musical ability and in studies comparing monozygotic and dizygotic twins. Anatomically specific relationships between callosal structure, cortical asymmetry, and a range of cognitive measures have generated great interest, in view of the light they shed on the organization of brain function and the nature of interhemispheric communication. In our review, we emphasize the many recent mathematical and methodological advances in the field. Imaging and computational methods are discussed for analyzing dynamic patterns of growth and degeneration. We also review progress in constructing a probabilistic reference system for the human brain, which can be used to analyze callosal anatomy. In particular, computerized strategies are described that (1) detect abnormal callosal structure in disease, (2) relate callosal anomalies to changes in cortical asymmetry and variability, and (3) relate callosal changes found in development and normal aging to changes found in Alzheimer's Disease and schizophrenia.

CHALLENGES IN MAPPING THE CORPUS CALLOSUM The rapid growth in brain-imaging technologies has been matched by an extraordinary increase in the number of investigations focusing on the structural and functional organization of the brain. An extensive amount of research has been directed toward analyzing the structure and function of the corpus callosum, the main fiber tract connecting the two brain hemispheres, which consists of approximately 200–350 million fibers in humans (Aboitiz et al., 1992a, 1992b). Surgical transection of this structure in humans provides evidence that the corpus callosum functions to communicate perceptual, cognitive, mnemonic, learned, and volitional information between the two brain hemispheres (Bogen et al., 1965). Given the importance of sensory, motor, and cognitive callosal relay between hemispheres, it is not surprising that this anatomical region has been a focus of studies examining structural and functional neuropathology.

Because of the corpus callosum's key role as the primary cortical projection system, any focal or diffuse abnormalities of bilaterally connected cortical regions may be expected to have secondary effects on homotopically distributed fibers in the callosum. These effects are observable at both cellular and gross anatomic scales (Innocenti, 1994). Effects on regional callosal structure have been reported in schizophrenia (Woodruff, McManus, and David, 1995; DeQuardo et al., 1996), attention deficit hyperactivity disorder (Giedd et al., 1994; Baumgardner et al., 1996), relapsing-remitting multiple sclerosis (Pozzilli et al., 1991; Rao et al., 1989a, 1989b), Alzheimer's disease (Hofmann et al., 1995; Vermersch et al., 1996; Janowsky, Kaye, and Carper, 1996), multi-infarct dementia (Yoshii, Shinohara, and Duara, 1990),

PAUL M. THOMPSON, KATHERINE L. NARR, REBECCA E. BLANTON, AND ARTHUR W. TOGA   Laboratory of Neuro Imaging, Department of Neurology, Division of Brain Mapping, UCLA School of Medicine, Los Angeles, California.

and a range of neurodevelopmental disorders and dysplasias (Sobire et al., 1995).

STRUCTURAL CHANGES Analysis of regional neuroanatomy and callosal structure are key factors in the radiological assessment of a wide range of neurological disorders. Nonetheless, extreme variations in brain structure make it difficult to design computerized strategies that detect and classify abnormal structural patterns. Intense controversy exists on the question of whether different callosal regions undergo selective changes in each of these disease processes. To distinguish abnormalities from normal variants, a realistically complex mathematical framework is required to encode information on anatomical variability in homogeneous populations (Grenander and Miller, 1994; Mazziotta et al., 1995). Additional controversy surrounds studies that have identified specific differences in callosal structure related to gender (DeLacoste-Utamsing and Holloway, 1982), handedness (Witelson, 1985), IQ (Strauss, Wada, and Hunter, 1994), and musical ability (Schlaug et al., 1995) and studies comparing monozygotic and dizygotic twins (Oppenheim et al., 1989). Anatomically specific relationships between callosal structure, cortical asymmetry, and a range of cognitive measures have generated great interest, in view of the light they shed on the organization of brain function and the nature of interhemispheric communication.

In this chapter we review current neuroimaging research on callosal structure. We emphasize the many recent mathematical and methodological advances in the field. A range of imaging and computational methods are discussed for analyzing and understanding the extremely complex dynamic processes that affect callosal anatomy in the healthy and diseased brain. We also review progress in constructing a probabilistic reference system for the human brain, which can be used to analyze callosal anatomy (Mazziotta et al., 1995; Thompson et al., 1997, 1998a). Magnetic resonance imaging (MRI)–based image archives from large human populations are stratified into subpopulations according to age, disease state, gender, and other demographic criteria to produce population-specific representations of anatomy. The resulting brain atlases encode information on population variability, with the goal of identifying group-specific patterns of brain structure. Computerized strategies are developed to (1) detect abnormal structure in disease, with a particular focus on the corpus callosum, (2) relate detected callosal anomalies to changes in the three-dimensional patterns of cortical asymmetry and structural variability, and (3) relate callosal changes found in development and aging to changes found in Alzheimer's disease and schizophrenia.

GROWTH PATTERNS Later in the chapter, we discuss methods for mapping dynamic patterns of growth at the corpus callosum. The callosum undergoes profound changes in morphology, fiber composition, and myelination during brain development, and these patterns are dramatically altered in disease. In many ways, static representations of callosal structure are ill suited to determining the dynamic effects of development and disease. Several algorithms are used to create four-dimensional quantitative maps of complex growth patterns across the corpus callosum, based on time series of pediatric MRI scans (Thompson et al., 1998a; Thompson and Toga, 1998). Mathematical techniques are designed to analyze local growth rates, revealing the local magnitude and principal directions of dilation or contraction. Serial scanning of human subjects, coupled with computational methods for analyzing the changing callosal geometry, show promise in enabling disease and growth processes to be tracked in their full spatial and temporal complexity.

Maps of the corpus callosum

Neuroimaging studies of the corpus callosum are easier to understand if its elaborate internal organization is considered. The corpus callosum connects the cortical surfaces of the two brain hemispheres, and there is a topographically specific organization of callosal fibers in relation to the cortical regions they connect. Tract-tracing studies using anterograde or retrograde labels such as biocytin or rhodamine-labeled latex microspheres (Innocenti, 1994) have established the topographic distribution of callosal connections at the cortex in several species. A massive perinatal loss of callosal axons, lasting from the thirty-fifth gestational week to the end of the first postnatal month (Clarke et al., 1989; LaMantia and Rakic, 1990), is thought to lead to a restricted pattern of adult callosal connections (Innocenti, 1994). In the adult callosum the genu (or anterior third) connects prefrontal cortices; the midbody (middle third) connects motor, somatosensory, and auditory cortices; and the splenium (posterior fifth) carries temporal, parietal, and occipital (visual) fibers. Perisylvian fibers from superior temporal and parietal cortex relay information from critical language and association areas and cross mainly in the isthmus (just anterior to the splenium; see Figure 5.1). To a certain degree, callosal fiber types are also organized topographically. Fast-conducting, large-diameter (>3 μm) sensorimotor fibers are concentrated in the posterior midbody and splenium, while thinner, more lightly myelinated fibers are found at the genu. These fibers at the genu offer a lower conduction velocity, connecting prefrontal regions implicated in longer-term planning and organization of behavior (Aboitiz et al., 1992a). Nonetheless, the idea of a sharply defined cortical map at the callosum has been mitigated by recent anterograde tracer studies in humans (Di Virgilio and Clarke, 1997). These suggest that heterotopic connections (i.e., between nonequivalent cortical areas in each brain hemisphere) are numerous and widespread, even in the genu and splenium where callosal axons are most highly segregated.

PARTITIONING APPROACHES   Because there are no gross anatomical landmarks that clearly delimit anatomically or functionally distinct callosal regions, several geometric partitioning schemes have been designed to subdivide the callosum into subregions whose fiber topography is expected to be different (Figure 5.1). These partitions define subregions that might be affected differently in development or disease and whose structural parameters (such as size, shape, or MRI signal intensity) might correlate more or less strongly with cognitive test data that evaluate different channels of interhemispheric communication (Clarke and Zaidel, 1994).

Vertical partitions   Most studies of gender and handedness effects on callosal structure have been based on the Witelson (1989) partition (see Figure 5.1c). This scheme defines callosal subdivisions based on fractions of its maximum anterior-posterior length. Nonetheless, the curvature and shape variability of the midsagittal callosum can bias the proportions of callosal area represented in each of the resulting segments. This difficulty has led several investigators (e.g., Clarke et al., 1989) to base their partitions on a curvilinear reference line (Figure 5.1d), which takes the global curvature of the callosum into account.

RADIAL PARTITIONS   On the basis of the centroid, or center of mass, of the corpus callosum, angular rays can be defined (Figure 5.1e) that intersect the callosal boundary above and below. These rays can be used to produce an equiangular partition with 100 separate elements (Figure 5.1e) (see Rajapakse et al., 1996). Clarke and colleagues (1989) partition this medial reference line into nodes of equal separation, before defining 30 sectors based on the shortest line through each node connecting outer and inner boundaries (Figure 5.1d). Stievenart and colleagues (1997) partition the callosum by defining rays normal to a series of equidistant nodes on the ventral callosal boundary (Figure 5.1g), which provide the basis for thickness and curvature measurements. Allen and colleagues (1991) noted that the tip of the rostrum is occasionally difficult to identify, which may add error in defining the curvilinear partitions

while affecting only the rostral sector in the straight-line-based approaches (Figures 5.1a and 5.1c).

To avoid making arbitrary definitions, Denenberg, Kertesz, and Powell (1991) performed a factor analysis to determine a "natural" partition of the callosum. Thickness measurements were obtained from a population of 104 normal adults (by connecting 100 equally spaced points on the inner and outer callosal boundaries; see Figure 5.1f), and these measures were used to determine seven regions with consistent variations (seven factors). While the partitioning scheme chosen ultimately depends on the application objectives and the scale of the expected structural effects (Bookstein, 1996), many apparent conflicts among different callosal studies derive from hidden or overt methodological differences, as will be seen in the following sections.

Sex differences in the corpus callosum

Intense controversy surrounds reports of regional sex differences in the anatomy of the corpus callosum (DeLacoste-Utamsing and Holloway, 1982; Clarke et al., 1989; Beaton, 1997; Bishop and Wahlsten, 1997; cf. Allen and Gorski, 1990; Allen et al., 1989). In 1982, DeLacoste-Utamsing and Holloway found that the area of the splenium (defined as the posterior fifth of the callosum) was larger in five female brains than in nine male brains examined postmortem ($p < 0.0895$, without correction for multiple comparisons or for brain weight), despite the fact that male brains were heavier overall and total callosal area did not differ. In 1986 the same group reported total callosal area and maximal splenial width (SW; see Figure 5.1d) to be greater postmortem in eight females (age: 53–87 years) than in eight males (35–81 years). The result for maximal splenial width was also found postmortem in fetuses ($N = 32$, 19 males, 11–40 weeks gestation; see Holloway and DeLacoste-Utamsing, 1986).

Three subsequent studies, however (Bleier, 1985; Demeter, Rongo, and Doty, 1985; Nasrallah, 1985), reported a failure to confirm the original findings of a sex difference in adult postmortem specimens. The fetal result was also not replicated by Clarke and colleagues, (1989) ($N = 32$, 16 males, 20–42 weeks gestation); the same study, however, reported a larger fraction of callosal area in the posterior fifth in adult females (using a curvilinear reference line; see Figure 5.1d; $N = 58$, 32 males), although this effect was not detectable in a smaller subsample of MRI scans ($N = 12$, 5 males). Clarke and colleagues also reported a larger bulbosity index in postmortem adult females ($p < 0.003$, $N = 46$, 27 males, one outlier excluded). The bulbosity measure was designed to provide a nondimensional index of splenial shape, by comparing splenial and presplenial thicknesses. Defined as $(T_{max} - T_{min})/T_{min}$, this measure is based on the maximal (T_{max}) and minimal (T_{min}) presplenial thicknesses found among the posterior 10 thickness measurements. In this scheme, thickness values were measured in a 30-segment radial partition (Figure 5.1d) using the shortest line connecting outer and inner boundaries which also passed through equally spaced nodes on the curvilinear reference line.

AGE × SEX INTERACTION EFFECTS   Witelson (1989, 1991) detected an age-related decrease in total callosal size (without correction for overall brain size) in male but not female postmortem specimens ($N = 62$; 23 males aged 26–69 years, mean age 54; 39 females aged 35–65 years, mean age 52). Similarly, Burke and Yeo (1994) found a greater age-related decline in callosal area in males ($N = 97$ MRI scans; all subjects right-handed; 38 males). If gender-related changes in callosal size with age are confirmed (i.e., if an age × sex interaction occurs; cf. Byne, Bleier, and Houston, 1988), comparisons between the sexes at even slightly different ages could be prone to misinterpretation. Some callosal studies have been criticized for comparing subject groups with large age variations (Beaton, 1997). Age-related effects may be exacerbated in developmental and embryonic studies, where gestational or chronological age might not be a reliable index of developmental state. In pediatric studies, significant age-related changes may occur over periods of weeks or months (Allen et al., 1991; Thompson et al., 1998a).

In view of possible age-related effects, Allen and colleagues (1991) performed a large-scale age-matched MRI study ($N = 122$; 61 males aged 16–78, mean 42.1 years; 61 females aged 16–79, mean 42.9 years). In this study, the maximum width of the splenium (SW; see Figure 5.1d) was found to be significantly greater in adult females (without adjustment for head size), as was a different measure of bulbosity, namely, the percentage by which the average width of the splenium (defined, again, as the posterior fifth in a curvilinear partition) exceeded the average width of the adjacent sectors. A 23.2% greater value was found in females when the bulbosity coefficient measured how much splenial widths exceeded the average width of the rest of the posterior half. No individual sector area was sexually dimorphic ($p > 0.05$ after Bonferroni correction), irrespective of whether areas were expressed as a proportion of total callosal area and whether or not areas were defined by using a straight-line or curvilinear partition (Figure 5.1).

BRAIN SIZE EFFECTS   Additional controversy surrounds the practice of expressing measures of specific brain

structures as a proportion of overall brain size, which is known to be significantly different between the sexes. The mean volume of the forebrain, where all callosal fibers originate, is about 9% higher in adult young men than in age-matched women (men: 1.08 ± 0.11 l ($N = 71$, age: 25.3 ± 4.6), women: 0.99 ± 0.10 l ($N = 49$, age: 26.3 ± 4.9); see Jäncke et al., 1997). A similar 10% sex difference in mean postmortem brain weight has also been reported by Pakkenberg and Voigt (1964).

In considering size differences for specific brain structures, it is important to know whether a group difference can be explained by a mere difference in overall brain volume or whether it reflects the influence of additional factors (sex, handedness, disease conditions) independent of brain volume effects. In an attempt to factor out the effects of gross variations in brain size, early studies of the callosum used the ratio of total callosal area to a measure of whole brain (or forebrain) size. Weight measures were typically used in postmortem studies, while volume or midsagittal cerebral area were used as correction factors in neuroimaging studies. Although these corrections are performed because total callosal area is correlated with brain weight ($r = 0.29$; see Bishop and Wahlsten, 1997), it was found that, despite this correction, the callosal area/brain weight ratio is still highly correlated with brain weight even though brain weight has supposedly been divided out ($r = -0.314$; $N = 95$; see Bishop and Wahlsten, 1997). This indicates that ratio measures do not fully adjust for brain size. To assess the effects of various factors on regional callosal measures, brain size measures should instead be added as a covariate in ANCOVA or multiple correlation type analyses. Unfortunately, even these linear statistical models expect callosal measures to vary linearly with extraneous parameters such as brain size. Ultimately, a power law might be more appropriate, as will be seen in the next sections.

Jäncke and colleagues (1997) suggested that a log-linear relation exists in adults between total callosal area (CC) and forebrain volume (FBV), with CC = constant × (FBV)^p. Estimates of the power p (0.66 in females, 0.52 in males) were based on significant regressions in an MRI cohort of 120 subjects. Since callosal area increases less than linearly with forebrain volume (i.e., $p < 1$) and since women have smaller brains on average, the ratio of total callosal size to brain volume will automatically be larger in women in the absence of other factors. This indicates a general brain size effect, which takes place independent of gender, so the altered proportion is not a specialized feature of the structure being analyzed (Clarke et al., 1989; Jäncke et al., 1997).

As a brain size correction, the pth power of FBV, estimated empirically from the sample, is likely to provide

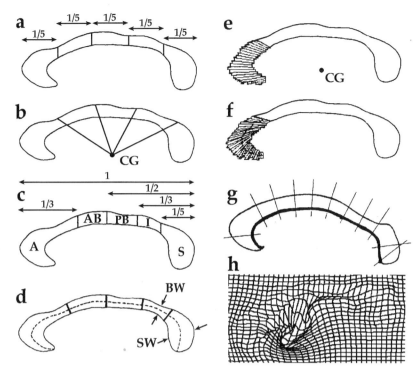

FIGURE 5.1. Common partitioning schemes for regional analysis of the corpus callosum. In view of the topographically specific relation between callosal regions and the cortical regions they connect, several partitioning approaches have been devised to allow separate analysis of different callosal sectors. Vertical partitions subdivide the callosum based on fractions of its maximal anterior-posterior length. Vertical fifths (a) (e.g., Duara et al., 1991; Larsen et al., 1992) or equal angular sectors, relative to the callosal centroid, labeled CG (b), are commonly used. Variants of the radial partition have used rays emanating from the midpoint of the line joining the inferior rostrum and inferior splenium (Weis et al., 1993). (c) A variant of the widely used Witelson partition (Witelson, 1989) further subdivides the anterior third (A) into rostrum, genu, and rostral midbody, using an additional vertical line (Rajapakse et al., 1996). Angular rays from the callosal centroid (CG) can be used to produce a partition with 100 equiangular elements (e) (Rajapakse et al., 1996). The center of these elements can also be used to derive a curvilinear reference line (d) (Clarke et al., 1989). By using a set of nodes to partition this line into 5, as in (d), or 30 (Clarke et al., 1989) equal segments, a slightly different set of sectors can be defined on the basis of the shortest line through each node connecting inner and outer callosal boundaries. These shortest lines form the basis for maximal splenial width (SW) and minimal body width (BW) measurements (Clarke and Zaidel, 1994), and derived bulbosity measures (Clarke et al., 1989). Alternatively, sets of 100 nodes equally spaced along inner and outer boundaries (f) can be joined directly (Denenberg et al., 1991) before a factor analysis to determine a natural partition. Stievenart and colleagues (1997) partition the callosum by defining rays (g) normal to a series of equidistant nodes on the ventral callosal boundary. Finally, approaches based on deformable templates (h) measure the deformation required to match a digital template of the callosum with callosal outlines from individual subjects. A rectilinear grid, ruled over the template callosum, can be passively carried along in the deformation to reveal patterns of shape difference or shape change over time. A simulated deformation is shown in part (h). Statistics of these deformation maps can be used to localize and test the significance of patterns of shape differences (Davatzikos et al., 1996; Bookstein, 1997; Thompson and Toga, 1998). (Schematics shown here are adapted from diagrams created by Witelson, 1989; Clarke et al., 1989; Clarke and Zaidel, 1994; Rajapakse et al., 1996; and Stievenart et al., 1997.)

a useful covariate for multivariate statistical tests, if removal of brain size effects is required. However, an even more general model might be required if the value of the exponent p were also found to depend on gender. In addition, the ratio of callosal area to an area-based measure of brain size, namely, the sum of cerebral areas in an axial and a sagittal cut (Rauch and Jinkins, 1994), has been found to rise rapidly with age from birth to age 20 years. This ratio rose from 1% to 4% across this 20-year span (although no gender differences were detected in the overall rate of increase; see Rauch and Jinkins, 1994). As a result, sex differences in any proportion measures (such as splenial area as a proportion of total callosal area) must be interpreted with caution, since any association between sex or age and the ratio's denominator can create a substantial effect. As a result, significant sex differences in ratio measures have often been found to disappear when analysis of covariance is used on the same data (Bishop and Wahlsten, 1997).

MEASUREMENT USING DEFORMABLE BRAIN ATLASES
Engineering approaches based on deformable templates (Figure 5.1h) have also been applied to detect differences in callosal shape due to sex, disease, or growth processes (Davatzikos et al., 1996; Bookstein, 1997; Thompson et al., 1997, 1998a). The basic idea of these approaches is outlined in the next few sections.

Digital brain atlases are templates that represent labeled anatomical structures from a typical subject or specimen in a three-dimensional coordinate system. Design of a brain atlas to represent human populations is complicated by drastic cross-subject variations in anatomy, and a fixed atlas based on a single subject may fail to represent the anatomy of new subjects. Typical solutions to this problem involve deformable, probabilistic, or hybrid atlases, which expand the atlas concept to represent large human populations (Mazziotta et al., 1995; Thompson et al., 1997; Thompson and Toga, 1998; for a review, see Toga and Thompson, 1998).

Deformable atlases are brain atlases that can be adapted to reflect the anatomy of new subjects (Evans et al., 1991; Christensen, Rabbitt, and Miller, 1993; Gee, Reivich, and Bajcsy, 1993; Sandor and Leahy, 1995; Rizzo et al., 1995; Haller et al., 1997). Image warping algorithms, specially designed to handle three-dimensional neuroanatomical data, apply complex profiles of dilation and contraction to a digital brain atlas, reconfiguring it into the shape of the patient's anatomy (see Figure 5.2). Any successful warping transform for individualizing a brain atlas must be high-dimensional, that is, it must allow any segment of the atlas anatomy to dilate, contract, twist, and even rotate to bring the atlas into structural correspondence with the target scan at a very local level (Christensen, Rabbitt, and Miller, 1996). Interestingly, the complex profiles of dilation and contraction that are required to warp an atlas onto the new subject's brain provide an exquisitely detailed map of the anatomical shape differences between that subject's brain and the atlas. Differences in regional shape can be assessed by applying vector and tensor field operators to the transformation field required to locally deform one brain volume into another (Figure 5.3) (see Thompson et al., 1998a; Thirion, Prima, and Subsol, 1998). This type of approach has been used to detect sex differences in callosal shape and has recently been extended to produce a probabilistic atlas for pathology detection.

SEX DIFFERENCES To examine sex differences at the callosum, Davatzikos and colleagues (1996) derived a digital template of the callosum from the Talairach brain atlas (Talairach and Tournoux, 1988). This template was then deformed, using image warping, to match individual callosal outlines from eight male and eight female subjects' MRI scans. Analysis of the required deformation fields showed that in some areas the average dilation for the female group was greater than the average dilation for the male group. Dilation values were defined mathematically as the local Jacobian determinant, or local expansion factor, of the deformation field (see Figure 5.1h), and these values were normalized with respect to total callosal area. The sex difference was most prominent in a vertical strip that crossed the splenial region. Evidence for a local sex difference was expressed as an effect size, indicating that the sex difference in mean dilation values exceeded the overall standard deviation of the dilation values in parts of the splenium (Davatzikos et al., 1996).

Shape-theoretic approaches

The data acquired by Davatzikos and colleagues (1996) was subsequently reanalyzed by Bookstein (1997) using shape-theoretic methods. In the Procrustes methods, developed for the statistical analysis of biological shape (Bookstein, 1989, 1997), a series of points are spread out along the callosal boundary and used to derive a warping field that matches one boundary with another. Affine components of neuroanatomical difference are first factored out by rotating and scaling configurations of point landmarks in each subject into least-squares correspondence with a Procrustes mean shape. Residual deformations that reflect individual anatomical differences are then expressed in terms of an orthogonal system of principal deformations derived from the bending energy matrix of the differential operator which governs the deformation (Bookstein, 1997). The deformations

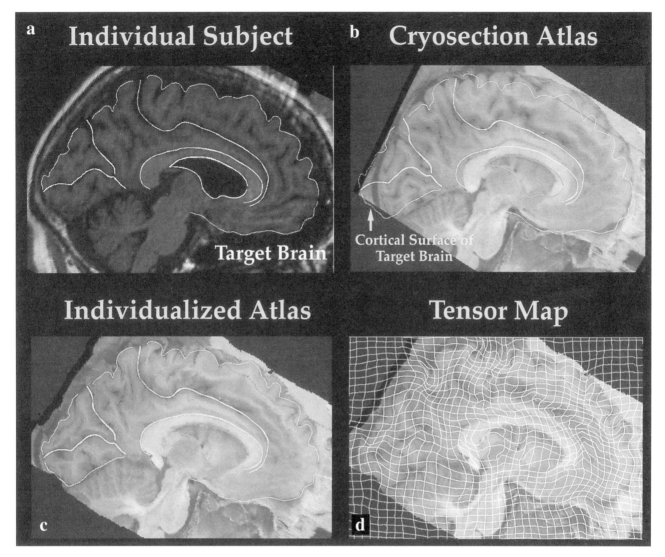

a Individual Subject

b Cryosection Atlas

Target Brain

Cortical Surface of
Target Brain

Individualized Atlas

Tensor Map

c

d

FIGURE 5.2. A deformable brain atlas mapping a three-dimensional digital cryosection volume onto three-dimensional MRI volumes. The result of warping a three-dimensional cryosection brain atlas (a) into the shape of a target MRI anatomy of (b) is shown (c), with callosal and cortical landmarks of the target anatomy superimposed. Note the reconfiguration of the callosum, as well as major occipital lobe sulci, into the shape of the target anatomy. This type of registration of callosal, sulcal, and cytoarchitectural boundaries can be used to measure neuroanatomic differences in individual subjects or groups (see Figures 5.5–5.10). Three-dimensional mapping of very local differences in structure (d) is possible only with a high-dimensional warping technique (Christensen et al., 1996; Davatzikos et al., 1996; Thompson and Toga, 1996). (See Color Plate 1.)

produced by image warping algorithms that match biological shapes are often governed by a differential operator that controls the way in which one anatomy is deformed into the other (for a technical review, see Thompson and Toga, 1998). Examples include the Cauchy-Navier operator of linear elasticity $(\lambda + \mu) \cdot \nabla(\nabla \bullet) + \mu \nabla^2$, used by Davatzikos and colleagues (1996) and by Thompson and Toga (1998), and the biharmonic, or thin-plate spline operator, ∇^4, used by Bookstein (1989, 1997). The properties of the governing operator can be used to make the deformation reflect the mechanical properties of deformable elastic or fluid media.

In Bookstein's approach (1989), a number of modes of variation, based on the eigenvectors of the covariance matrix of landmark positions, can be determined to describe the main factors by which the instance shapes tend to deform from the generic shape. Of particular relevance are methods used to define a mean shape, and distances between shapes (Procrustes distances), in such a way that conventional statistical procedures can be applied to characterize shape differences between two groups. In his reanalysis of the callosal data acquired by Davatzikos and colleagues (1996), Bookstein (1997) used a permutation test to determine whether the Procrustes

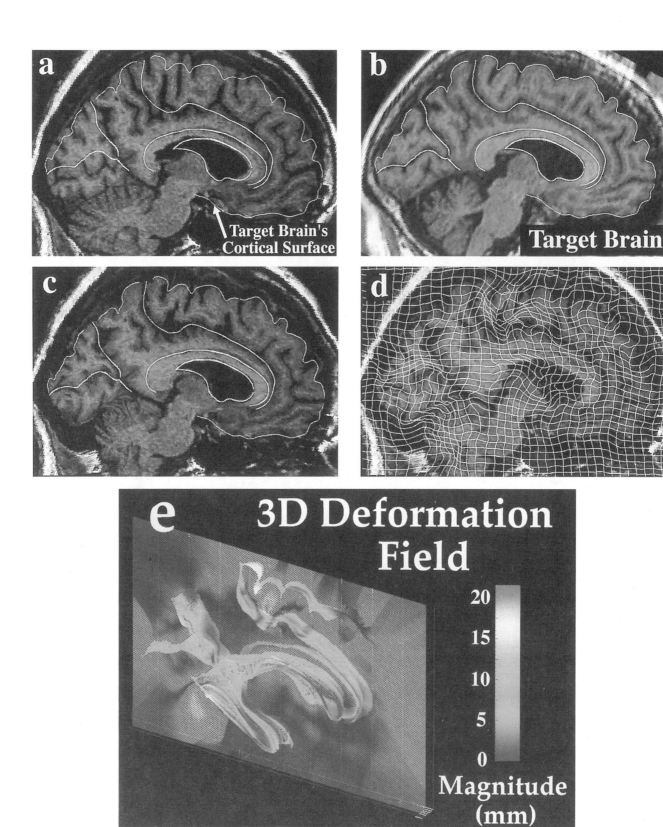

FIGURE 5.3. Three-dimensional image-warping measures patterns of anatomic differences. T_1-weighted MR sagittal brain slice images from (a) a normal elderly subject's scan; (b) a "target" anatomy, from a patient with clinically determined Alzheimer's disease; and (c) the result of warping the reference anatomy into structural correspondence with the target. Note the precise nonlinear registration of the callosal and cortical boundaries, the desired reconfiguration of the major sulci, and the contraction of the ventricular space and cerebellum. The complexity of the recovered deformation field is shown by ap-

ANATOMY AND MORPHOMETRY OF THE CORPUS CALLOSUM

shape distance between the mean callosal shapes was significantly greater when the outlines were split into male and female groups than when groupings were randomly assigned. As indicated by the effect size analysis of Davatzikos and colleagues (1996), this shape-theoretic analysis identified a shape difference between the sexes in the posterior half of the callosal boundary ($p \sim 0.03$). These approaches are also being applied to detect callosal shape anomalies in schizophrenia (DeQuardo et al., 1996; Bookstein, 1997).

ORTHOGONAL FUNCTIONS AND FOURIER SERIES APPROACHES Shape-theoretic approaches, described above, express shape differences between anatomical boundaries in terms of statistically orthogonal functions, namely, principal components of covariations of position (Bookstein, 1997). Geometrically orthogonal functions, such as elliptical Fourier series (Staib and Duncan, 1992), Oboukhoff expansions (Joshi, Miller, and Grenander, 1998), and spherical harmonics (Thompson and Toga, 1996; Joshi et al., 1998) have also been used to represent anatomical shapes. These representations provide a spatial frequency-based decomposition of an object and describe its overall shape efficiently using a few parameters, which can be analyzed statistically. Owing to their representation efficiency and ability to represent a large class of shapes, elliptical Fourier series have also been used in automated methods to find the callosal boundary in MRI images (Staib and Duncan, 1992). This contour detection method operates by tuning the Fourier coefficients of an estimated callosal shape, until a goodness-of-fit measure is optimized. Elliptical Fourier series also provide a means to generate average callosal shapes for specific subject groups, and they have been used to quantify large-scale changes in callosal anatomy during brain development (Ferrario et al., 1996).

---

plying the two in-slice components of the three-dimensional volumetric transformation to a regular grid in the reference coordinate system. This visualization technique (d) highlights the complexity of the warping field in the posterior frontal and cingulate areas, corresponding to subtle local variations in anatomy between the two subjects. To monitor the smooth transition to the surrounding anatomy of the deformation fields initially defined on the surface systems, the magnitude of the warping field is visualized (e) on models of the surface anatomy of the target brain, as well as on an orthogonal plane slicing through many of these surfaces at the same level as the anatomical sections. Note the smooth continuation of the warping field from the complex anatomic surfaces into the surrounding brain architecture and the highlighting of the severe deformations in the premarginal cortex, ventricular, and cerebellar areas. (See Color Plate 2.)

Local shape operators In view of the large number of harmonics required to represent complex shapes, descriptors based on orthogonal functions are less suitable for detecting local structural differences. Small-scale shape differences, such as callosal differences that may exist due to sex or handedness, are likely to be detected optimally by using local shape operators such as the delta filter (Bookstein, 1997) and other tensorial operators that act on deformation fields to quantify local shape differences (Thompson and Toga, 1998; see also Thirion and Calmon, 1997; Thirion et al., 1998). These operators are used to detect growth patterns at the callosum and to detect multiple sclerosis lesion growth (Thirion and Calmon, 1997). The statistical significance of these local deformation maps can be assessed by modeling the dilation maps as a log-normal distributed random scalar field (cf. Ashburner et al., 1997; Thirion et al., 1998) or by estimating the parameters of a Gaussian random vector field as a means to assess shape differences between groups (see later in the chapter; see also Thompson and Toga, 1997, 1998; Cao and Worsley, 1998). Nonetheless, it seems that any method, however powerful, must be combined with large sample sizes and be carefully controlled for extraneous demographic factors such as age, head size, and handedness. Only then is the controversy over sex differences in callosal anatomy likely to be resolved.

Development of the corpus callosum

EMBRYONIC PERIOD Growth of the normal human brain occurs in a highly regular and well-defined manner. Anatomical neuronal development progresses in a posterior-to-anterior fashion as well as a ventral-to-dorsal fashion. Growth of the corpus callosum also occurs in an orderly manner. The development of the corpus callosum is initiated between 8 and 17 weeks of gestation (Rakic and Yakovlev, 1968). A thickening of the telencephalon, along the rostral wall, forms the lamina reuniens, which is the precursor to the white matter bundles of the anterior commissure and corpus callosum. As cells from the lamina reuniens migrate superiorly, they form the massa, which will form the bed for the extension of the crossing fibers of the corpus callosum (Barkovich and Norman, 1988). The corpus callosum does not develop homogeneously, and axons of the genu develop first, followed by the body and splenium. One exception to this anterior to posterior growth pattern is the rostrum. This is the last component of the callosum to project crossing fibers, at approximately 18–20 weeks gestation (Rakic and Yakovlev, 1968).

The major components of the corpus callosum are established prenatally, yet development is far from complete at birth. Although neuronal differentiation has concluded at birth, myelination of cortical axons has just begun. Myelination is the process whereby axons become encased by myelin sheaths. This process insulates axons and enhances the speed of neuronal conduction (Yakovlev and Lecours, 1967). Myelination of the central nervous system generally occurs in a caudal-to-rostral fashion. Spinal cord and brain stem pathways myelinate first, during prenatal stages, and frontal and association areas of the cerebrum myelinate postnatally (Barkovich and Kjos, 1988). Continued myelination has been reported as late as the third decade of life, and this may reflect increased efficiency in the synthesis of information (Yakovlev and Lecours, 1967).

Paralleling the growth processes in the cerebrum, myelination of callosal axons also proceeds in a posterior to anterior fashion and may be the primary component of the growth observed at the callosum (Georgy, Hesselink, and Jernigan, 1993). Rakic and Yakovlev (1968) report that the corpus callosum more than doubles in size between birth and 2 years of age. Barkovich and Kjos (1988) also observed that the newborn corpus callosum appears thin and flat, with substantial thickening occurring around 3 months of age. Substantial area increases are seen in the splenium, followed by more gradual increases in the body and rostrum (Kier and Truwit, 1996). As was noted earlier, the genu of the corpus callosum consists mainly of fibers that traverse inferior frontal and anterior/inferior parietal regions, while the splenium carries fibers from homologous visual and visual association areas (DeLacoste, Kirkpatrick, and Ross, 1985). The observed pattern of callosal development is therefore not surprising; sensorimotor and visual areas may be most important as the neonate develops binocular vision and becomes coordinated in various body movements such as grasping objects (Von Hoftsten, 1984; Barkovich and Kjos, 1988). Prefrontal and posterior association areas may initially be less important to the infant, as these regions integrate sensory experiences and subserve higher cognitive processes such as planning (Diamond, 1990). Increases in corpus callosum size may reflect increases in the complexity of interactions between an infant and its environment.

CHILDHOOD AND ADOLESCENCE   The most dramatic developmental changes of the corpus callosum occur during the first years of life, yet continued maturational changes have been reported until late childhood and adolescence (Pujol et al., 1992; Giedd et al., 1996). Pujol and colleagues (1992) measured total callosal area in a cohort of 90 subjects and found area increases until the third decade of life. In addition, cross-sectional studies of total callosal area have corroborated increases in

callosal volume until adulthood (Schaefer et al., 1990; Allen et al., 1991; Rauch and Jinkins, 1994). More regional assessments of callosal development have been obtained in a group of children ranging in age from 4 to 18 (Rajapakse et al., 1996; Giedd et al., 1996). Developmental increases were found primarily in the area of the splenium and isthmus regions. No corresponding age effects were detected in the genu, rostrum, and body. Morphological changes of the corpus callosum have also been observed with increasing age (Ferrario et al., 1996). Dramatic maturational changes were seen as the callosum transformed from thin and flat in infants, with no bulbous enlargements, to a thicker, rounder genu and splenium in teens. As in the adult studies, measurements of sexual dimorphism in the corpus callosum of children and adolescents have produced conflicting results. No significant sex differences were found in splenial area or shape in a postmortem sample of children ranging in age from birth to 14 years (Bell and Variend, 1985). In contrast, gender differences in callosal shape as well as total callosal area have been reported in infants as young as newborn to 14 months of age (Clarke et al., 1989).

Several authors have postulated reasons for such patterns of growth in the brain from birth to late adolescence. Neuronal cell division and migration has been reported as complete before birth (Carlson, Earls, and Todd, 1988). Postnatal anatomical reorganization may arise primarily from processes such as naturally occurring cell death, synaptic pruning, and myelination. Huttenlocher (1990) proposed that brain reorganization occurs into late childhood and adolescence owing to synaptic refinement of functional pathways. At birth, diffuse projections have been observed in callosal connections across visual, auditory, and somatosensory cortex in young primates, kittens, and rodents (Ivy and Killackey, 1981; Feng and Brugge, 1983; Innocenti, 1994). Transient callosal projections between areas have also been reported and may suggest excess cortical connectivity during early childhood (Carlson et al., 1988).

With age, diffuse and transient axonal projections are selectively retracted, a process that is termed *synaptic refinement*. Selective elimination of axons originating from cortical locations has been observed in both cats and monkeys, in which more than half of the axons produced are eliminated from the callosum during development. Furthermore, synaptic refinement has been observed in human frontal and visual cortex (Huttenlocher, 1990). Functional consequences of such refinements have been studied by using PET (Chugani, Phelps, and Mazziotta, 1987). Cerebral blood flow measurements decreased and became less diffuse with age, suggesting that less neural activity is required with increasing maturation of cognitive skills. While significant reductions in axonal projections have been reported in the corpus callosum, increases in total area have been reported. Callosal connections that are not eliminated may be strengthened by increases in axonal diameter and myelin deposition (Carlson et al., 1988). As a consequence, the speed and efficiency of the interhemispheric transfer of information may be enhanced. Brown and Jaffe (1975) suggest that the two hemispheres might not be completely specialized at birth. Refinement of axonal connections and increases in axonal size may reflect continued development in functional specialization of the cerebral hemispheres. Thus, growth of the callosum into late adolescence and early adulthood may reflect a balance between synaptic refinement and increases in myelination and diameter of axonal projections. These processes may ultimately serve to increase functional specialization of the hemispheres, allowing acquisition of more agile and finely coordinated skills.

CHILDHOOD DISORDERS

Attention deficit hyperactivity disorder Attention deficit hyperactivity disorder (ADHD) has been characterized as a disorder in attentional and motor systems and is thought to arise from deficits in frontal lobe circuitry. The corpus callosum has been studied in ADHD to assess possible abnormalities in commissural circuits. Decreases in the area of the splenium (Semrud-Clikeman et al., 1994; Lyoo et al., 1996), the genu (Hynd et al., 1991), and the rostrum and rostral body have all been reported (Giedd et al., 1994; Baumgardner et al., 1996). Findings of reductions in anterior callosal regions (genu, rostrum, and rostral body) suggest abnormalities of information transfer in prefrontal, premotor, and anterior cingulate regions (Witelson, 1989). These callosal deficits coincide well with data suggesting that anterior cingulate and prefrontal regions are involved in attentional regulation (Steere and Arnsten, 1995). However, posterior association areas have been suggested to play a role in sustained attention, and deficits here may explain abnormalities found in posterior regions of the callosum (Semrud-Clikeman et al., 1994).

Autism Social and cognitive abnormalities suggest that autism might be a disorder of information processing (Saitoh et al., 1995). Autistic children fail to make eye contact and rarely use language to communicate (Cole and Cole, 1993). Structural abnormalities have included regional brain enlargement in posterior, temporal, and occipital but not frontal cortices (Piven et al., 1997). The corpus callosum has been examined to assess a possible excess cortical connectivity resulting from such enlargements. The splenium of the corpus callosum

was reported as smaller in autistic patients compared to controls, with a trend for reductions in isthmus/posterior body regions (Saitoh et al., 1995; Piven et al., 1997). Yet a lack of differences in corpus callosum volume between autistic patients and normal controls has also been cited (Gaffney et al., 1987). The discrepancy between regional enlargement of brain hemispheres and decreases in posterior regions of the corpus callosum might suggest increases in ipsilateral connections, with concomitant decreases in contralateral callosal connections. This suggests that autism may be a disorder arising from detrimental increases in ipsilateral connections.

Down syndrome Down syndrome is the most frequent genetic cause of mental retardation and is a chromosomal disorder, with patients having one more chromosome than normal (Cole and Cole, 1993). Corpus callosum abnormalities have been reported, with associated decrements in anterior regions (Wang et al., 1992). These results are not surprising, because Down syndrome patients also have reductions in frontal lobe volume (Jernigan et al., 1993). Furthermore, it has been reported that subjects with Down syndrome display poor verbal fluency and impaired performance in problem-solving strategies (Wang et al., 1992). Thus, in the case of Down syndrome, interhemispheric transfer of semantic information may be compromised by deficits in frontal lobe and anterior callosal regions.

Dyslexia Dyslexia has been characterized as a disability in reading performance observed in conjunction with average or above average intelligence (Hynd et al., 1995). More specifically, it has been suggested that some dyslexics have deficits in the phonological processing of information (Rumsey et al., 1992). Studies of callosal morphology in dyslexia have reported a smaller callosal genu (Hynd et al., 1995), as well as larger splenium and total callosal area (Duara et al., 1991; Njiokiktjien, de Sonneville, and Vaal, 1994). Furthermore, Hynd and colleagues (1995) found correlations between reading achievement and the relative size of the splenium and genu in dyslexic patients. Abnormalities of the corpus callosum in dyslexic patients may imply a role for the corpus callosum in the interhemispheric transfer of phonological information. Evidence for this comes from findings that callosal agenesis patients are impaired in phonological as compared to lexical reading (Temple et al., 1990).

Fetal alcohol syndrome Fetal exposure to alcohol can have several morphological effects, such as central nervous system and facial abnormalities, depending on the timing of maternal exposure to alcohol and the quantity consumed (Johnson et al., 1996). Several abnormalities of the corpus callosum have been reported in this disorder (Riley et al., 1995; Johnson et al., 1996; Swayze et al., 1997). Abnormalities include complete or partial agenesis, thinning of the posterior body, and area decreases in rostral regions. Deficits of the corpus callosum may arise from excessive or premature cell death, as well as an inhibition of axons that cross the midline (Swayze et al., 1997). Johnson and colleagues (1996) hypothesize that the teratogenic effects of alcohol may suppress neuronal activity and thus impair activity-dependent neuronal development. Results such as these suggest that callosal development may be an activity-dependent process, which is particularly susceptible to the harmful effects of alcohol.

Tourette's syndrome Tourette's syndrome is characterized by vocal and motor tics and has commonly been referred to as a disorder involving the basal ganglia (Hyde et al., 1995). Total corpus callosum volume has been examined in adult patients and was found to be significantly reduced (Peterson, Leckman, and Duncan, 1994). On the other hand, increases in the size of the rostrum have been reported in child and adolescent populations, even after correcting for intracranial volume (Baumgardner et al., 1996). It was suggested that a larger corpus callosum in childhood may cause an overcompensation in synaptic refinement and result in a smaller corpus callosum in adulthood. Baumgardner and colleagues (1996) further propose that a callosal enlargement in childhood may amplify interhemispheric transfer of information, thus decreasing control of a behavior specialized to a particular hemisphere.

Mapping dynamic growth patterns during development

TEMPORAL MAPS OF BRAIN STRUCTURE Current structural brain imaging investigations focus on the analysis of three-dimensional models of brain structure, derived from volumetric images acquired at a single time point from each subject in the study. In many ways, static representations of structure are ill suited to determining the dynamic effects of brain development or disease. However, serial scanning of human subjects, when combined with a powerful set of warping and analysis algorithms, can enable disease and growth processes to be tracked in their full spatial and temporal complexity.

Three-dimensional image warping algorithms, specially designed to handle neuroanatomical data, provide a means to compute extremely complex maps of anatomical differences between different subjects (Figures 5.2 and 5.3) (Thompson and Toga, 1996). Maps of anatomical change can also be generated by warping scans acquired from the same subject over time (Thirion et al., 1998; Thompson et al., 1998a). In a changing morphology, warping algorithms enable one to model structural changes that occur over prolonged periods, such as developmental, aging, or disease processes, as well as structural changes that occur more rapidly, as in recovery following trauma or tumor growth. A four-dimensional approach, which uses serial scanning and specialized image-warping algorithms, can provide critical information on local patterns and rates of tissue growth, atrophy, shearing, and dilation that occur in the dynamically changing architecture of the brain (Toga, Thompson, and Payne, 1996; Thompson et al., 1998a).

WARPING ALGORITHMS Any comprehensive framework for modeling temporal change in three-dimensional brain structure must draw on methods for quantitating its material transformation between pairs of images acquired at successive time points. Warping algorithms are central to all of these approaches. The warp is a four-dimensional model. It specifies the displacement of every anatomical point in the brain across the disease or developmental stage spanned by the two images. As such, it permits complete morphometric quantitation of the dynamic effects of the underlying biological processes on the geometry of the brain and its substructures. It allows points, surfaces, and curved anatomical interfaces to be matched up in a pair of image sets. As a result, changes in volumes, surface areas, orientations, and distances and in metrical relationships between substructures—as well as measures of dilation rates, contraction rates, and rates of shearing and divergence of the cellular architecture—may be computed locally, for all structures, directly from the warping field. The warping field assigns a displacement for every anatomical point across a time step so that curves, surfaces, and volumes in an early image may be reidentified in a later one. This enables relative areas, lengths, and volumes to be compared over time. Derivatives of these quantities with respect to time allow growth rates to be quantified locally for any structure; spatial derivatives of the warping field allow shearing and dilation to be measured locally and compared for different substructures.

MAPPING GROWTH PATTERNS IN FOUR DIMENSIONS In our initial human studies (Thompson et al., 1998a; Thompson and Toga, 1998), we developed several algorithms to create four-dimensional quantitative maps of growth patterns in the developing human brain, based on time series of high-resolution pediatric MRI scans. Deformation processes recovered by the warping algorithm were analyzed by using vector field operators to produce a variety of tensor maps. These maps were

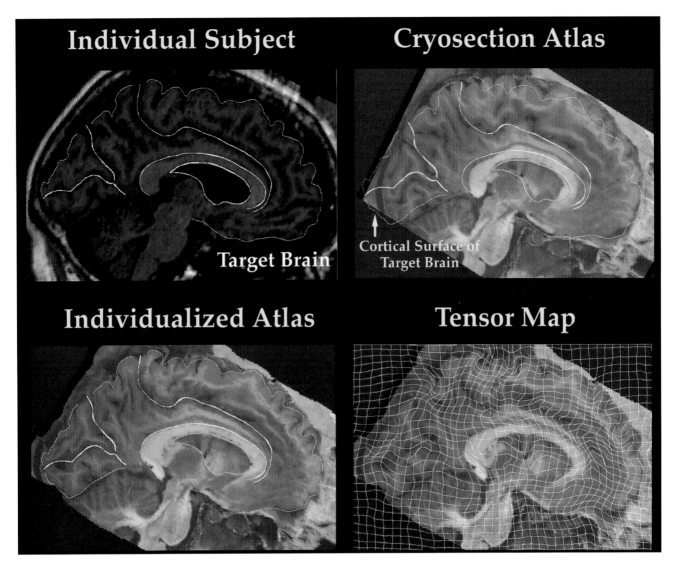

Individual Subject — Target Brain

Cryosection Atlas — Cortical Surface of Target Brain

Individualized Atlas

Tensor Map

Plate 1. A deformable brain atlas mapping a three-dimensional digital cryosection volume onto three-dimensional MRI volumes. The result of warping a three-dimensional cryosection brain atlas (a) into the shape of a target MRI anatomy of (b) is shown (c), with callosal and cortical landmarks of the target anatomy superimposed. Note the reconfiguration of the callosum, as well as major occipital lobe sulci, into the shape of the target anatomy. This type of registration of callosal, sulcal, and cytoarchitectural boundaries can be used to measure neuroanatomic differences in individual subjects or groups (see Figures 5.5–5.10). Three-dimensional mapping of very local differences in structure (d) is possible only with a high-dimensional warping technique (Christensen et al., 1996; Davatzikos et al., 1996; Thompson and Toga, 1996). (See Figure 5.2.)

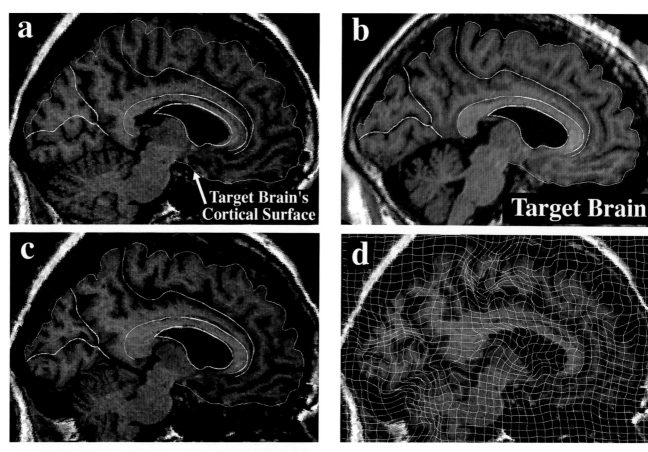

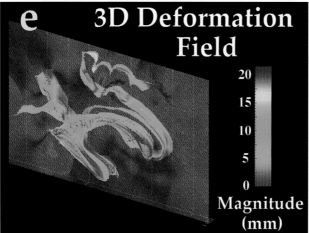

Plate 2. Three-dimensional image-warping measures patterns of anatomic differences. T_1-weighted MR sagittal brain slice images from (a) a normal elderly subject's scan; (b) a "target" anatomy, from a patient with clinically determined Alzheimer's disease; and (c) the result of warping the reference anatomy into structural correspondence with the target. Note the precise nonlinear registration of the callosal and cortical boundaries, the desired reconfiguration of the major sulci, and the contraction of the ventricular space and cerebellum. The complexity of the recovered deformation field is shown by applying the two in-slice components of the three-dimensional volumetric transformation to a regular grid in the reference coordinate system. This visualization technique (d) highlights the complexity of the warping field in the posterior frontal and cingulate areas, corresponding to subtle local variations in anatomy between the two subjects. To monitor the smooth transition to the surrounding anatomy of the deformation fields initially defined on the surface systems, the magnitude of the warping field is visualized (e) on models of the surface anatomy of the target brain, as well as on an orthogonal plane slicing through many of these surfaces at the same level as the anatomical sections. Note the smooth continuation of the warping field from the complex anatomic surfaces into the surrounding brain architecture and the highlighting of the severe deformations in the pre-marginal cortex, ventricular, and cerebellar areas. (See Figure 5.3.)

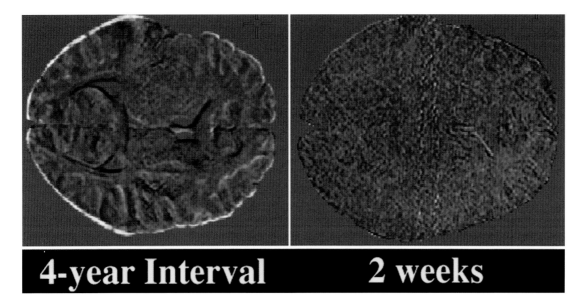

4-year Interval   **2 weeks**

Plate 3. Growth patterns in the developing human brain. A young normal subject was scanned at the age of 7 and again four years later, at the age of 11, with the same protocol (data from Thompson et al., 1998a). Scan histograms were matched and rigidly registered, and a voxel-by-voxel map of intensity differences (left) reveals global growth. In a control experiment, identical procedures were applied to two scans from a 7-year-old subject acquired just 2 weeks apart, to detect possible artifactual change due to mechanical effects and due to tissue hydration or CSF pressure differences in the young subject between the scans. These artifacts were minimal, as shown by the difference image, which, as expected, is largely noise. Rigid registration of the scans does not localize anatomical change but is a precursor to more complex tensor models of structural change (see the main text and Figures 5.5 and 5.6), which not only map local patterns of differences or change in three dimensions, but also allow calculations of rates of dilation, contraction, shearing, and torsion (Toga et al., 1996; Thompson et al., 1998a). (See Figure 5.4.)

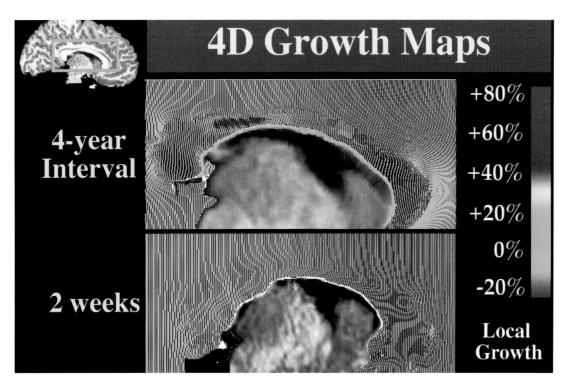

4D Growth Maps

4-year Interval

2 weeks

+80%
+60%
+40%
+20%
0%
-20%

Local Growth

Plate 4. Local analysis of callosal growth patterns using vector field operators. Vector field operators help to emphasize patterns of contractions and dilations, emphasizing their regional character. Here, the color code shows values of the local Jacobian of the warping field, which indicates local volume loss or gain. Pronounced neuroanatomical growth is observed during the 4-year interval (upper panel). This contrasts sharply with the negligible change detected over a 2-week time span (lower panel). (See Figure 5.6.)

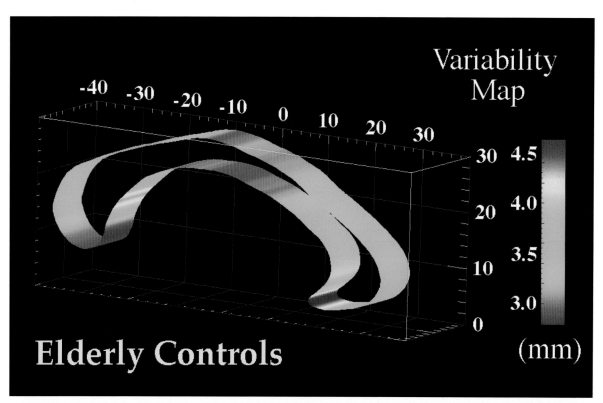

Variability Map

Elderly Controls (mm)

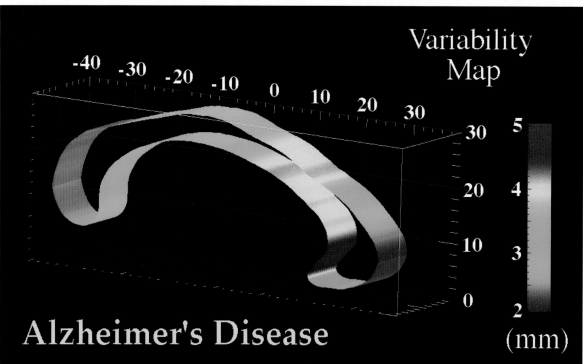

Variability Map

Alzheimer's Disease (mm)

Plate 5. Maps of stereotaxic variability at the corpus callosum in patients with Alzheimer's disease and in elderly normal subjects. Separate maps of local variability were constructed for (a) Alzheimer's patients and (b) control subjects, expressing (in color) the r.m.s. variation of callosal points in each subject group around an average boundary representation of the callosum, at the midsagittal plane of Talairach stereotaxic space. Unlike the asymmetry and variability maps in Figure 5.9, these are strictly two-dimensional maps, since the midsagittal analysis of callosal morphology is conducted in a single vertical plane. Average boundary representations have therefore been thickened for visualization purposes only. Two trends are apparent. Although the variability measure peaks at the rostrum, this may be an artifact due to the difficulties of defining an unambiguous anatomical limit for the inferior aspect of the rostrum. Nevertheless, the pronounced rise in variability at the rostral midbody in AD (b) may reflect disease-related enlargement of the third ventricle, which forms its inferior boundary. (See Figure 5.8.)

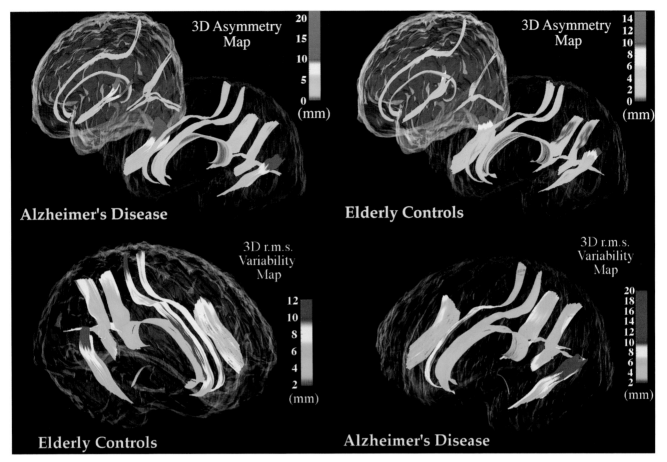

Plate 6. Population-based maps of three-dimensional structural variation and asymmetry. Statistics of three-dimensional deformation maps can be computed to determine confidence limits on normal anatomic variation. Three-dimensional maps of anatomical variability and asymmetry are shown for 10 subjects with Alzheimer's disease (age: 71.9 ± 10.9 years) and 10 normal elderly subjects matched for age (72.9 ± 5.6 years), gender, handedness, and educational level (Thompson et al., 1998). Normal Sylvian fissure asymmetries (right higher than left, $p < 0.0005$), mapped for the first time in three dimensions, were significantly greater in AD than in controls ($p < 0.0002$; top panels). In the three-dimensional variability maps derived for each group (lower panels), the color encodes the root mean square magnitude of the displacement vectors required to map the surfaces from each of the 10 patients' brains onto the average. Confidence limits on three-dimensional cortical variation (lower right panel), exhibited severe increases in AD from 2–4 mm at the corpus callosum to a peak standard deviation of 19.6 mm at the posterior left Sylvian fissure. (See Figure 5.9.)

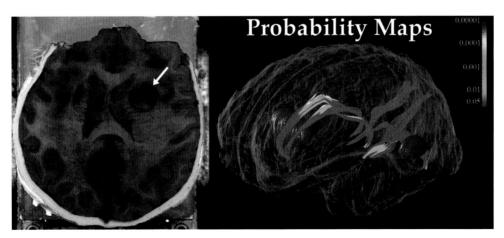

Plate 7. Distortions in brain architecture induced by tumor tissue: probability maps for ventral callosum and major sulci in both hemispheres. Color-coded probability maps (b) quantify the impact of two focal metastatic tumors (illustrated in red; see also cryosection blockface) (a) on the ventral callosal boundary, as well as the parieto-occipital and anterior and posterior calcarine sulci in both brain hemispheres. (See Figure 5.10.)

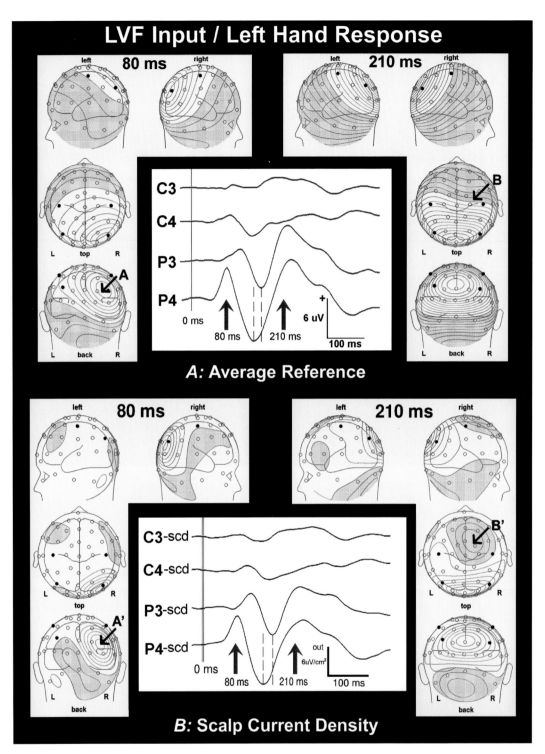

Plate 8. (a) Average-referenced scalp isopotential contour maps with left and right central and parietal voltage waveforms (indicated as solid circles among the electrode locations drawn on the maps) from a 63-channel study using the Poffenberger task with LVF input and left-hand responses (grand mean of five subjects). The arrows indicate the times at which the map views are drawn. Stippled (blue) areas correspond to negative voltage (0.6 μV/line). Displayed ERP epoch is −25 ms to 425 ms poststimulus. Note the widespread positivity of the visual P1 shown at 80 ms, and the ill-defined motor response over right central regions. (b) SCD maps and Laplacian waveforms from the identical data as shown in part (a) plotted at equivalent sensitivity (0.6 μV/cm²). The activation at 80 ms is now restricted to the posterior regions of the right hemisphere, as expected, given LVF input. The 210-ms maps also now reveal a right central focus, in keeping with the execution of left-hand responses. The Laplacian waveforms show greater peak latency delays between left and right parietal regions and less early activity at C4 than seen in part (a). Stippled (blue) areas correspond to inward current, red areas correspond to outward current, both derived from scalp voltage. (See Figure 8.3.)

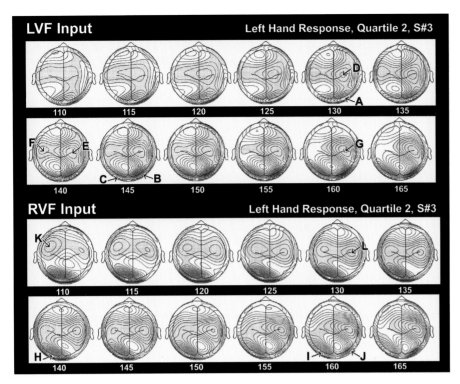

Plate 9. Top-view SCD maps at 5-ms intervals from 110 to 165 ms poststimulus, separately for LVF and RVF data from the second quartile of the left-hand RT distribution for subject 3. Stippled (blue) regions correspond to inward scalp current derived from scalp potential. Red isocontours correspond to outward scalp current. Plotted sensitivity is 0.5 μV/cm². Responses to LVF input reveal posteriorly the expected initial lateralization followed by callosally mediated bilateral activa-tion. Central regions show an initial bilateral activation pat-tern that resolves into the unilateral right-hemisphere focus associated with the left-hand response. Posterior responses to RVF input are of opposite lateralization compared to those of LVF input, as expected. The central response pattern sug-gests a visuomotor routing of left-hemisphere visual-to-motor activation, followed by motor-related left-to-right interhemi-spheric transfer. See the text for details. (See Figure 8.7)

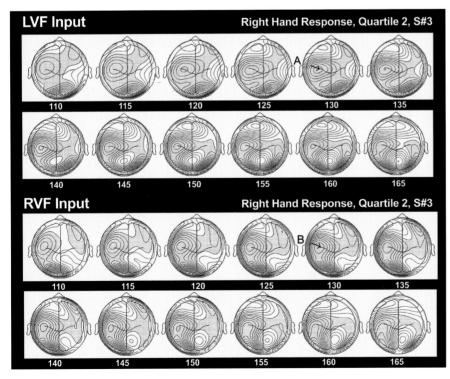

Plate 10. Top-view SCD maps at 5-ms intervals from 110 to 165 ms poststimulus, separately for LVF and RVF data from the second quartile of the right-hand RT distribution for sub-ject 3. Stippled (blue) regions correspond to inward scalp current. The plotted sensitivity is 0.5 μV/cm². While the pos-terior activation pattern is nearly identical to that seen in Figure 8.7, the change of responding hand is clearly visible in the shift to left central activation independent of input visual field (A and B). (See Figure 8.8.)

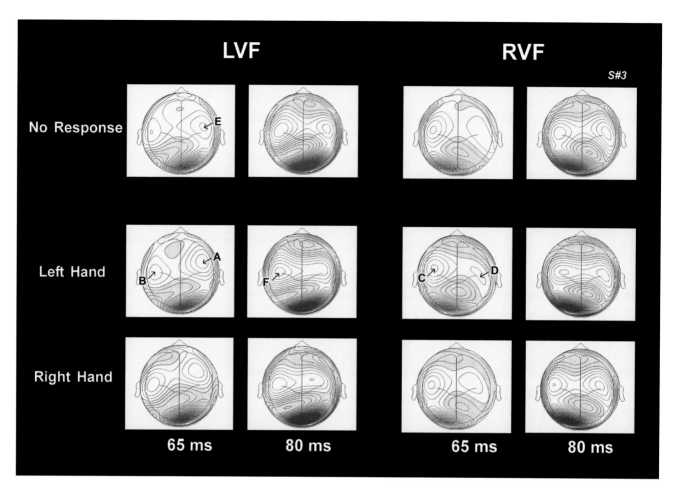

Plate 11. Top-view SCD maps for all stimulus and response conditions from the retest of subject 3 are plotted at high sensitivity (0.1 μV/cm², λ = 1 x 10⁻⁵) at 65 and 80 ms poststimulus. These across-RT data (120–600 ms) have $n \approx 1350$. $N \approx$ 735 for the passive view control conditions. Both LVF and RVF stimuli show a larger focus of activity over central regions ipsilateral to the hemisphere receiving visual input. The LVF data suggest that there may be an effect of response condition, with larger initial ipsilateral central activations seen in the reaction time conditions. At 80 ms, central regions contralateral to the hemisphere receiving visual input show equal or greater activity than seen ipsilateral to the stimulated hemisphere at 65 ms. This may reflect a very early visually generated central interhemispheric transfer. Stippled (blue) areas represent inward current flow. Red areas correspond to outward current. See the text for more details. (See Figure 8.12.)

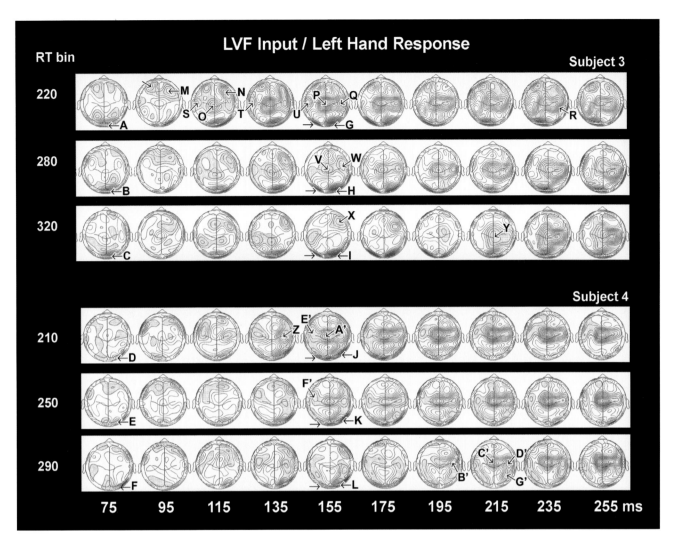

Plate 12. Top-view SCD map time series ($\lambda = 1 \times 10^{-7}$) from 75 to 255 ms poststimulus for the intrahemispheric LVF/LH condition for the retest of subjects 3 and 4. The data are displayed by RT bin, with each value the midpoint of a 10-ms range (*n*'s for subject 3 were 86, 105, and 55 for RT bins 220, 280, and 320, respectively; *n*'s for subject 4 were 49, 76, and 37 for RT bins 210, 250, and 290, respectively). The stability of the posterior visual response across RT is evident. The patterns of central activation for both subjects markedly differ, the faster two RT bins sharing similar overall activation patterns that are lower in magnitude for the middle RT bin. For both subjects, the slowest RTs show a delayed activation pattern. These data illustrate the multiplicity of motor regions of both hemispheres active during performance of intrahemispheric task conditions and highlight individual differences in spatiotemporal activation patterns during performance of simple RT. Stippled (blue) regions correspond to inward scalp current, red to outward current. Plotted sensitivity is 0.5 $\mu V/cm^2$ for subject 3 and 0.6 $\mu V/cm^2$ for subject 4. See the text for a detailed explanation of activation patterns. (See Figure 8.13.)

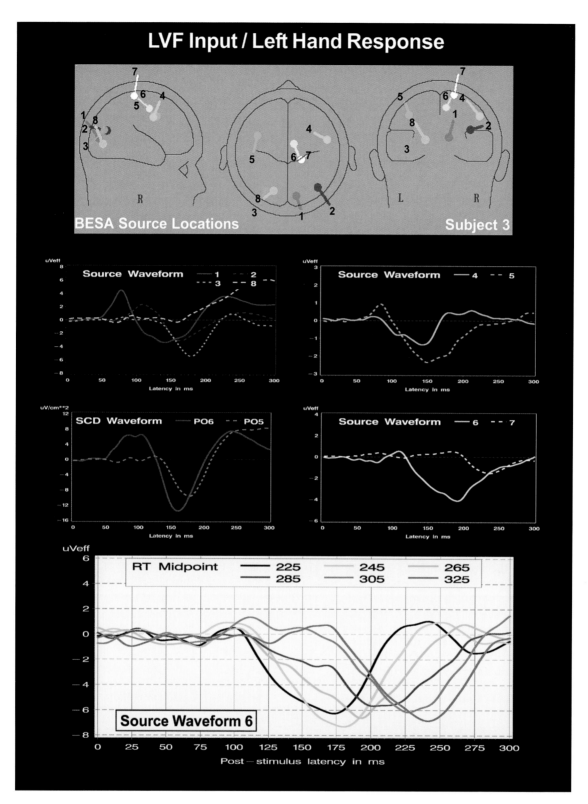

Plate 13. (a) BESA dipole locations and orientations for the LVF input/left-hand response condition for subject 3. See the text for caveats and functional interpretations of each dipole. (b) Source waveform overlays based on the BESA solution depicted in part (a) and comparison with SCD waveforms from parieto-occipital sites. Across-RT data. (c) Waveforms from each of six 20-ms RT bins for source 6 are overplotted. Peak latencies reliably track RT for all bins; however, the response onset times do not. Note that responses from bins 225–285 begin within the same 15-ms period. This suggests that the slope/rate of motor-related cortical activation is reflected in RT. The slowest responses (bins 305 and 325) do not follow this pattern. There is a ~70-ms delay relative to the first four bins before a response is initiated, with a slope comparable to the faster responses. This suggests different routes of response-related activations for these reaction times compared with reaction times in the 215- to 295-ms range. See the text for further details. (See Figure 8.15.)

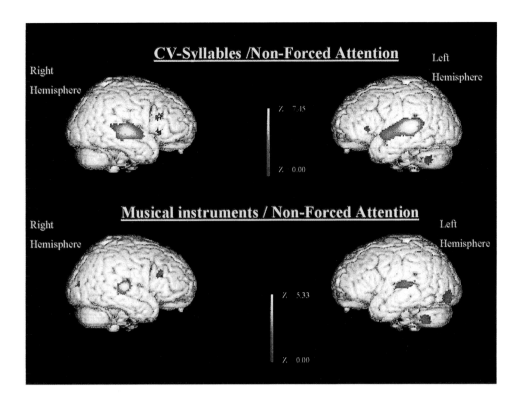

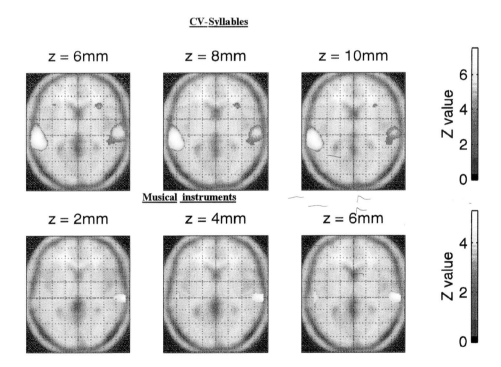

Plate 14. ¹⁵O-PET activation images after presentation of CV syllables (upper row in both panels), and musical instruments (lower row in both panels). The upper panel shows significant clusters of activation plotted onto lateral views of a brain template. The lower panel shows the same data plotted on axial slices. (Data from Hugdahl et al., 1999a.) (See Figure 12.2.)

**NF Attention:
"Attend both ears"**

**FR Attention:
"Attend right ear"**

**FL Attention:
"Attend left ears"**

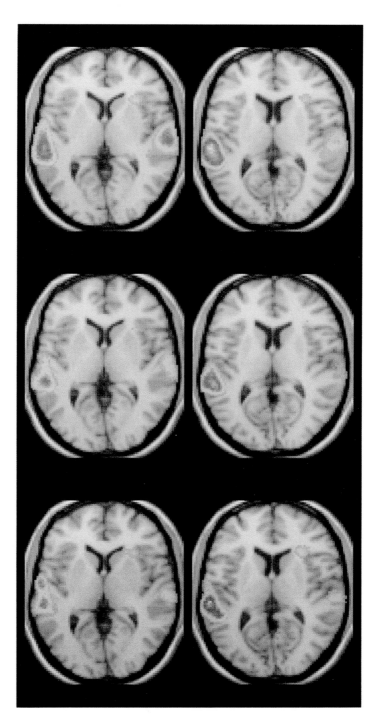

Plate 15. 15O-PET activation images during the NF, FR, and FL attention conditions plotted onto axial slice brain templates across the superior temporal gyrus and planum temporale. The left column is 2 mm above the AC-PC midline; the right column is 8 mm above the AC-PC midline. Note the relative attenuation of activation during the FR and FL conditions compared to the NF attention condition. (Data from Hugdahl et al., 2000.) (See Figure 12.5.)

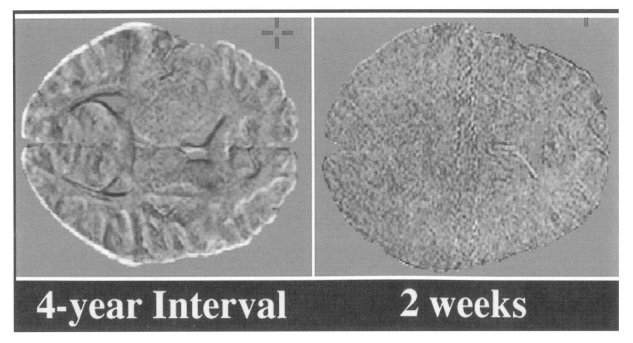

FIGURE 5.4. Growth patterns in the developing human brain. A young normal subject was scanned at the age of 7 and again four years later, at the age of 11, with the same protocol (data from Thompson et al., 1998a). Scan histograms were matched and rigidly registered, and a voxel-by-voxel map of intensity differences (left) reveals global growth. In a control experiment, identical procedures were applied to two scans from a 7-year-old subject acquired just 2 weeks apart, to detect possible artifactual change due to mechanical effects and due to tissue hydration or CSF pressure differences in the young subject between the scans. These artifacts were minimal, as shown by the difference image, which, as expected, is largely noise. Rigid registration of the scans does not localize anatomical change but is a precursor to more complex tensor models of structural change (see the main text and Figures 5.5 and 5.6), which not only map local patterns of differences or change in three dimensions, but also allow calculations of rates of dilation, contraction, shearing, and torsion (Toga et al., 1996; Thompson et al., 1998a). (See Color Plate 3.)

designed to reflect the magnitude and principal directions of dilation or contraction; the rate of strain; and the local curl, divergence, and gradient of flow fields representing the growth processes recovered by the transformation.

Three-dimensional $(256^2 \times 124$ resolution$)$ T_1-weighted fast SPGR (spoiled GRASS) MRI volumes were acquired from young normal subjects (mean age: 8.6 ± 3.1 years) at intervals ranging from 2 weeks to 4 years. Pairs of scans were selected to determine patterns of structural change across the interval between the two scans. These scan pairs were preprocessed, with a radio frequency bias field correction algorithm, and rigidly registered using automated image registration software (Woods, Mazziotta, and Cherry, 1993). Registered scans were then histogram-matched, and a preliminary map of differences in MR signal intensities between the two scans was constructed (Figure 5.4). While difference maps help to determine whether structural change has occurred in such diseases as dementia (Freeborough, Woods, and Fox, 1996), these maps do not localize change, nor do they provide three-dimensional measures of dilation, contraction, or shearing of anatomical

regions. To address this, parametric mesh models (Thompson et al., 1996a, 1996b, 1997, 1998a) were created to represent a comprehensive set of deep sulcal, callosal, caudate, and ventricular surfaces at each time point. Surface models based on manually digitized data were averaged across multiple trials ($\mathcal{N} = 6$) to minimize error. The deformation field that is required to match the surface anatomy of one scan with the other was extended to the full volume using a continuum-mechanical model based on the Cauchy-Navier operator of linear elasticity (Thompson and Toga, 1998). Deformation processes recovered by the warping algorithm were then analyzed using vector field operators to produce a variety of tensor maps (Figures 5.5 and 5.6). These maps were designed to reflect the magnitude and principal directions of dilation or contraction, the rate of strain, and the local curl, divergence, and gradient of flow fields representing the growth processes recovered by the transformation.

TENSOR MAPS OF GROWTH   In contrast to the near-zero maps of change recovered at short time intervals (2 weeks), tensor maps of growth spanning large time in-

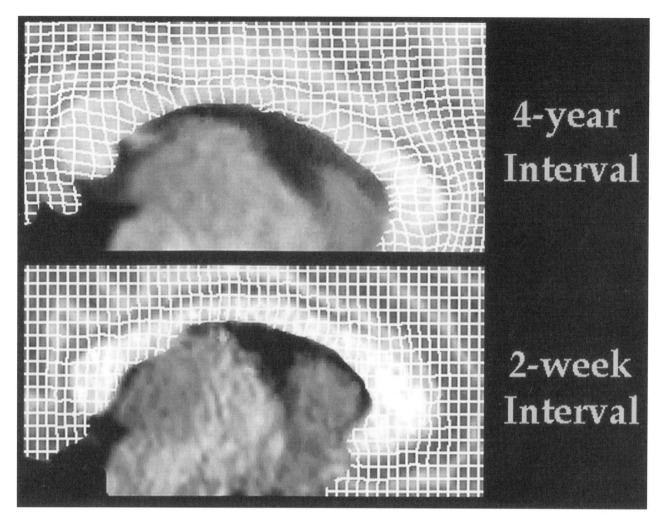

4-year
Interval

2-week
Interval

FIGURE 5.5. Tensor maps of callosal growth. A complex pattern of growth is detected in the corpus callosum of a young normal subject (upper panel). This map illustrates structural change occurring in the 4-year period from 7 to 11 years of age. The effects of the transformation are shown on a regular grid ruled over the reference anatomy and passively carried along in the transformation that matches it with the target. Despite minimal changes in overall cerebral volume, callosal growth is dramatic, with peak values occurring at the isthmus. The pattern of growth contrasts with the near-zero maps of change observed between scans acquired over a 2-week interval (lower panel).

tervals (4 years) showed complex and heterogeneous patterns of change. In one subject who was scanned at ages 7, 9, and 11, comparative stability of lobar and thalamic anatomy and negligible changes at the cortex were accompanied by pronounced focal growth of the callosal isthmus (Figure 5.5), ventricular enlargement, and loss of caudate tissue.

GROWTH IN CALLOSAL ANATOMY To further characterize the growth process at the callosum (Figure 5.5), derived properties of the deformation fields were examined (Figure 5.6), including local expansion, contraction, or shearing effects recovered by the warping transformation. As was noted earlier, the Jacobian of the deformation field has been used as a local index of gender-specific shape differences in the corpus callosum (Davatzikos, 1996), while here it is used to indicate its growth. Other local vector field operators, including the gradient and divergence ($\nabla u(x)$, $\nabla^T \bullet u(x)$; see Thompson et al., 1998a) and the specialized norm × divergence operator ($\|u(x)\| . \nabla^T \bullet u(x)$; see Thirion and Calmon, 1997) can be applied to deformation fields. These operators are specifically designed to reveal and emphasize different aspects of growth or pathological processes, including their local magnitude and directional biases.

REGIONAL TOPOGRAPHY OF CALLOSAL GROWTH Figure 5.6 shows the complex patterns of growth detected in a young normal subject during the 4-year period from 7 to 11 years of age. Despite minimal changes in overall

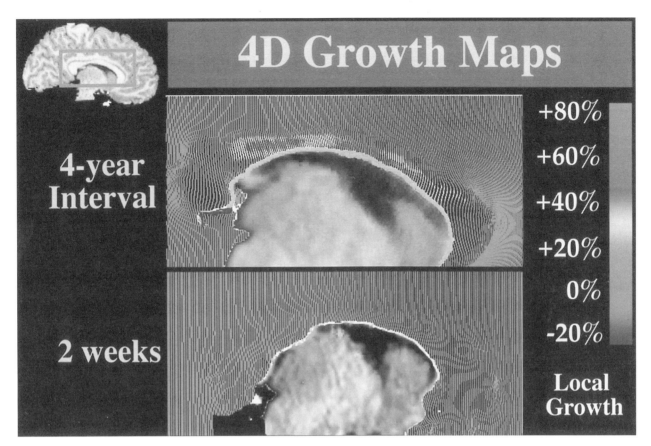

FIGURE 5.6. Local analysis of callosal growth patterns using vector field operators. Vector field operators help to emphasize patterns of contractions and dilations, emphasizing their regional character. Here, the color code shows values of the local Jacobian of the warping field, which indicates local volume loss or gain. Pronounced neuroanatomical growth is observed during the 4-year interval (upper panel). This contrasts sharply with the negligible change detected over a 2-week time span (lower panel). (See Color Plate 4.)

cerebral volume, striking regional growth is detected throughout the callosum, with peak values occurring at the isthmus (the same area that was found to degenerate preferentially in our dementia studies (see Thompson et al., 1998b). This pronounced pattern of growth contrasts with the near-zero maps of change observed over a 2-week interval (Figure 5.6, lower panel).

Warping algorithms hold tremendous promise in representing, analyzing, and understanding the extremely complex dynamic processes that affect regional anatomy in the healthy and diseased brain. Only with a four-dimensional approach will patterns of callosal growth or degeneration be recorded in their full spatial and temporal complexity.

Aging and the corpus callosum

The corpus callosum has been reported to maintain its shape and size during the third and fourth decades of life with a gradual decline in size during later years (Pujol et al., 1992). Ratio measurements of the corpus callosum as a proportion of midline internal skull surface area have been used to study aging effects while correcting for variations in head size (Laissy et al., 1993). Significant decreases were found in total callosal area without associated reductions in total brain size in subjects ranging in age from 12 to 74 years. Regional aging effects on callosal morphology are most prominent in anterior regions (genu, rostrum, and anterior body), while posterior regions have been found to remain stable with age (Parashos, Wilkinson, and Coffey, 1993; Weis, Kimbacher, and Wegner, 1993; Salat et al., 1997). However, age-related decreases have also been reported for midbody and posterior regions (Beigon et al., 1994). In addition, decreases in callosal width with age have been reported (Byne et al., 1988).

Fiber composition of the callosum has been studied to assess possible aging effects (Aboitiz et al., 1996). Age-related increases were found in the number of large-diameter myelinated callosal fibers, but no age-related increases in small-diameter fibers were seen. These results may suggest increases in myelin deposition during the later years. It was implied that increases in myelin deposition may serve as a compensatory mechanism for age-related decrements in efficiency of interhemispheric transfer.

Callosal T1 relaxation times, which describe the tissue-dependent decay of signals in MRI experiments, have been analyzed in an adult and elderly population (Doraiswamy et al., 1991). Positive correlations between age and callosal T1 relaxation times were found. Furthermore, a negative relationship between age and callosal area was seen. T1 relaxation values are sensitive to the environment of water in most tissues, and therefore longer callosal T1 relaxation times are suggestive of an increase in callosal hydrogen content.

Decreases in callosal size with age could have several functional consequences. One consequence might be a decline in the speed of interhemispheric information transfer. Since normal aging is associated with selective neurocognitive deficits, one possibility is that a decrease in callosal axon number can lead to a decline in performance in various cognitive tasks. Support for this theory comes from studies that have associated callosal atrophy with impaired information processing and delayed transfer of visual information (Roa et al., 1989).

Regional age effects in anterior callosal regions correspond well with aging effects seen in the cerebrum. Axons in the anterior callosum have been reported to connect homologous regions of the frontal lobe. Previous studies have suggested that frontal lobes may be disproportionately affected by age-related changes such as sulcal widening (Tomlinson, Blessed, and Roth, 1968), volume reductions (Coffey et al., 1992), and neuronal cellular alterations (Terry, de Theresa, and Hansen, 1987). These results are consistent with theories suggesting that phylogenetically newer regions of the brain may be more vulnerable to aging effects than visual and sensorimotor regions (Armstrong, 1990). In addition, functional imaging studies of aging show preferential decreases in blood flow in prefrontal regions, with little change in occipital and temporal cortex (Waldemar, 1995).

Alzheimer's disease and dementia

Alzheimer's disease (AD) is accompanied by a complex and distributed pattern of neuroanatomical change that is difficult to distinguish clinically from dynamic alterations in normal aging. Diagnosis of AD before death remains one of exclusion. Definitive diagnosis requires postmortem histological findings of diffuse neuronal and synaptic loss, accompanied by characteristic neuro-pathological lesions (McKhann et al., 1984; Khachaturian, 1985) such as β-amyloid plaques (Delaère et al., 1989), neurofibrillary tangles (Wilcock and Esiri, 1982), Hirano bodies (Katzman, 1986), and granulovacuolar degeneration (Di Patre, 1990).

Although definitive diagnosis of AD requires direct observation of autopsy or biopsy specimens with characteristic neuropathological lesions, the National Institute of Neurological and Communicative Disorders and Stroke/Alzheimer's Disease and Related Disorders Association (NINCDS-ARDRA) has defined criteria for probable AD (McKhann et al., 1984). These criteria include an acquired persistent decline involving at least three of the following cognitive domains: language, memory, visuospatial skills, cognition, emotion, and personality. The accuracy of these criteria has been evaluated at autopsy and has been demonstrated to be 80–85% (Blacker et al., 1994).

NEUROIMAGING IN DEMENTIA Structural neuroimaging is increasingly important in evaluating patients with probable AD (Davis, Mirra, and Alazraki, 1994). Computed tomography (CT) and magnetic resonance imaging (MRI) studies in AD reveal gross cerebral atrophy, starting in temporal and parietal areas (Kido et al., 1989; Erkinjuntti et al., 1993; Killiany et al., 1993). As the disease progresses, atrophy of the caudate, lenticular, and thalamic nuclei are observed (Jernigan et al., 1991), together with sporadic signs of sulcal and ventricular enlargement. Early damage occurs in the entorhinal cortex (Arnold et al., 1991; Braak and Braak, 1991; Gómez-Isla et al., 1996), the posterior aspect of the basal nucleus of Meynert (which has strong projections to the temporal lobe; see Whitehouse et al., 1981), the amygdaloid nuclei (Cuénod et al., 1993; Scott, 1993), and the CA1/subiculum zone of the hippocampal formation (West et al., 1994). These disease-induced changes in structure often escape detection because of the overlap between structural changes seen in normal aging and dementia (Friedland and Luxenberg, 1988). Controversy still exists as to whether aging and AD are dichotomous or represent a neuropathological continuum (Coleman and Flood, 1987; West et al., 1994).

CALLOSAL ANATOMY In view of the anatomically specific progression of cortical atrophy associated with AD, interest has focused on several questions that relate to the corpus callosum. The first question is whether local or diffuse atrophy of bilaterally connected brain regions might induce secondary effects on homotopically distributed fibers in the callosum. The second question is whether distinct regions of callosal anatomy undergo selective changes in different subtypes of dementia and whether these changes reflect observed patterns of neuronal loss at the cortex. The third major question is whether the pervasive callosal atrophy that is seen late in the course of AD is preceded by a more localized pattern of fiber loss at the onset of the disease.

In one of our recent studies (Thompson et al., 1998b), high-resolution three-dimensional structural MR images were acquired from 10 subjects diagnosed with AD according to NINCDS-ARDRA criteria (mean age: 71.9 ± 10.7 years, all 10 right-handed), and 10 elderly controls, matched for age (72.9 ± 5.6 years), gender, educational level, and handedness (all 10 right-handed). The AD patient group had a mean MMSE (Mini-Mental State Exam) score of 19.7 ± 5.7 (maximum score: 30), a rating that is comparable with values obtained in other dementia studies (Murphy et al., 1993), and characteristic of the early stages of the disease. The use of 1-mm-thick MRI slices, combined with a high in-plane pixel resolution ($0.9765 \text{ mm} \times 0.9765 \text{ mm}$) resulted in an improved resolution imaging matrix relative to earlier studies of aging and AD pathology (e.g., slices acquired every 5 mm (Cuénod et al., 1993) or every 6 or 7 mm [Murphy et al., 1993]).

To determine whether there was a regionally selective pattern of callosal change accompanying AD pathology, the morphology of the callosum at the midsagittal plane was analyzed by using a five-sector partition that is relatively simple to apply (Figure 5.1a; see Duara et al., 1991; Larsen, Høien, and Ödegaard, 1992). This resulted in an approximate segregation of callosal fibers belonging to distinct cortical regions. Since individual data were standardized by digital transformation into Talairach stereotaxic space (Talairach and Tournoux, 1988), regional cross-sectional areas of callosal subdivisions were determined both before and after stereotaxic transformation. When areas of specific sectors were compared between groups, the isthmus of the callosum was of particular interest, since fibers crossing in this area selectively innervate the temporoparietal regions that are at risk for early neuronal loss in AD (Brun and Englund, 1981).

LOCALIZED ATROPHY Consistent with this hypothesis, a severe and significant reduction in the area of the callosal isthmus was found in AD relative to controls, reflecting a dramatic 24.5% decrease from 98.0 ± 8.6 mm^2 in controls to 74.0 ± 5.3 mm^2 in AD ($p < 0.025$; see Figure 5.7b). By contrast, the terminal sectors (1 and 5) of the callosum, corresponding to fibers crossing in the rostrum and splenium, respectively, did not undergo a significant area reduction, with almost identical values in the control and patient group of 160.9 ± 9.6 mm^2 and 158.6 ± 14.3 mm^2, respectively, for the rostral

sector ($p > 0.1$) and 148.7 ± 8.6 mm^2 and 150.8 ± 6.8 mm^2, respectively, for the splenial sector ($p > 0.1$). An observed 16.6% mean area loss in AD for the central midbody sector showed only a trend toward significance ($p < 0.1$), and an apparent 13.4% depression in mean anterior midbody area was statistically insignificant ($p > 0.1$) because of substantial intergroup overlap in the values of these parameters in the early stages of AD.

AVERAGE BOUNDARY REPRESENTATIONS AND VARIABILITY MAPS Selective changes in the corpus callosum accompanying AD pathology were examined in more detail by partitioning midsagittal sector outlines into upper and lower sectors. Average boundary representations (Figure 5.7) and local variability maps (Figure 5.8) were then made for the callosum in both subject groups. In both control and AD subjects, sectors showed a distinctly heterogeneous profile of variability in stereotaxic space (Figures 5.8a and 5.8b), with confidence limits on two-dimensional variation at the midsagittal plane varying from a standard deviation of 2.0–3.3 mm at the inferior splenium, central midbody, and genu to 4.6–5.0 mm at the posterior aspect of the rostrum. Intriguingly, at the isthmus, where a significant area reduction was apparent in AD, the average callosal representations showed a slight reduction in thickness in AD relative to controls (Figure 5.7b). In addition, a pronounced inflection in shape was demonstrated toward the inferior limit. This feature can be seen in Figure 5.7b, at stereotaxic location (0.0, −25.0, 19.0). This morphology has also been observed in studies of callosal shape in schizophrenia (DeQuardo et al., 1996; Bookstein, 1997).

SYLVIAN FISSURE ASYMMETRIES In view of the severe reduction in size at the isthmus, perisylvian areas where fibers in the isthmus originate were examined to determine whether their patterns of three-dimensional variability and asymmetry were altered in the disease. Methods for mapping patterns of three-dimensional cortical variation and asymmetry are discussed in detail by Thompson and colleagues (1998b); analysis of digital anatomical maps in normal aging and AD suggested a range of global and local disease-related differences (Figure 5.9). Confidence limits on three-dimensional cortical variation in controls showed a marked increase from 2–4 mm at the callosum to a peak of 12–13 mm at the external cerebral surface. In AD, however, while variability was marginally higher than in controls at the callosal surface, the variability across the surface of the Sylvian fissure rose extremely sharply from a standard deviation of 6.0 mm rostrally to 19.6 mm caudally on the left and from 5.0 mm rostrally to 9.0 mm caudally on the right.

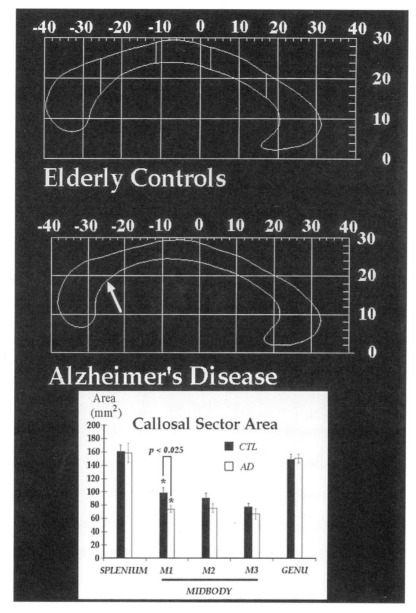

FIGURE 5.7. Average boundary representations of the callosum in (top panel) normal elderly subjects ($N = 10$) and (middle panel) Alzheimer's disease patients ($N = 10$). Average boundary representations of the midsagittal callosum in normal controls and patients with mild Alzheimer's disease (MMSE ∼ 19.7 ± 5.7) indicate a severe reduction in the area of the isthmus in AD relative to controls, accompanied by a pronounced inflection in shape (white arrow) in the neighborhood of stereotaxic location $(0.0, -25.0, 19.0)$. The overlying sector representing the isthmus (second of five, top panel) underwent a 24.5% reduction in area in AD compared with controls ($p < 0.025$).

Although there is a substantial literature on Sylvian fissure cortical surface asymmetries (Eberstaller, 1884; Cunningham, 1892; Geschwind and Levitsky, 1968; Davidson and Hugdahl, 1994; Galaburda, 1995) and their relationship to functional lateralization (Strauss, Kosaka, and Wada, 1983), handedness (Witelson and Kigar, 1992), language function (Davidson and Hugdahl, 1994), asymmetries of associated cytoarchitectonic fields (Galaburda and Geschwind, 1981), and their thalamic projection areas (Eidelberg and Galaburda, 1982), no prior studies had mapped the spatial profile of asymmetries in three-dimensional space. When Sylvian fissure asymmetries were mapped in three dimensions, the marked rostral and vertical extent asymmetries in controls (left posterior limit 9.7 mm more caudal than right; $p < 0.0005$) were severely increased in AD (left limit 16.6 mm more caudal than right; $p < 0.0002$), and between-hemisphere differences in the anterior-posterior position of the Sylvian fissure's posterior limit were also found to be significantly greater in AD than in matched controls ($p < 0.05$). Local maps (Figures 5.6 and 5.7) also revealed a sharp rise in three-dimensional asymmetry in AD, reaching 21.8 mm at the posterior limit of the left Sylvian fissure, compared with 15.4 mm in controls.

ASYMMETRIC PROGRESSION OF ALZHEIMER'S DISEASE
Greater variability of the left perisylvian surface and greater Sylvian fissure asymmetry in AD suggests that AD pathology asymmetrically disrupts the anatomy of temporoparietal cortex. In AD, Sylvian fissure CSF volume has also been shown to rise, relative to controls, more sharply on the left than on the right (left volume: 31.5% higher in AD than controls ($p < 0.02$, $N = 2$) but right volume only 20.4% higher ($p < 0.09$); see Wahlund et al., 1993). Underlying atrophy and possible left greater than right degeneration of perisylvian gyri may widen the Sylvian fissure, superimposing additional individual variation and asymmetry on that already seen in normal aging (Figure 5.9). Significant left greater than right metabolic dysfunction and cognitive impairment have been reported in both PET (Loewenstein et al., 1989; Siegel et al., 1996) and neuropsychiatric (Capitani, Della Sala, and Spinnler, 1990) studies of AD and in PET studies of related amnestic disorders (Corder et al., 1997). Recent PET studies have also examined cognitively normal subjects who are at risk for AD in the sense that they experience mild memory complaints and have at least two relatives with AD (Small et al., 1995). Left greater than right metabolic impairment also appears in these subjects, and the deficit has been shown to be significantly more asymmetric in at-risk subjects carrying the apolipoprotein type 4 allele (ApoEε4, a risk

factor for familial AD) relative to those subjects without ApoEε4 (Small et al., 1995). Accentuated patterns of structural asymmetry and variation found here in AD support these findings, suggesting either that the left hemisphere is more susceptible than the right to neurodegeneration in AD or that left hemispheric impairment results in greater structural change and lobar metabolic deficits (Loewenstein et al., 1989).

CALLOSAL DEFICITS IN ALZHEIMER'S DISEASE   An anatomically specific relationship was observed in this and other studies (Lyoo et al., 1997) between putative fiber loss in callosal regions and the dynamic progression of cortical and lobar atrophy that is characteristic of AD. Size reduction and shape inflection were observed in callosal regions that map association areas that are at risk of selective metabolic loss and incipient atrophy in early stages of AD (Figures 5.4 and 5.6). Greater resilience was observed in splenial sectors, which map the parieto-occipital and calcarine surfaces that are comparatively resistant to neuronal loss in AD (Pearson et al., 1985). Severe and regionally selective areal loss and focal shape inflection at the isthmus may reflect disease-related disruption of the commissural system connecting bilateral temporal and parietal cortical zones, since these regions are known to be at risk for early metabolic dysfunction, perfusion deficits, and selective neuronal loss in AD (DeCarli et al., 1996).

DIFFERENCES BETWEEN NORMAL AGING AND DEMENTIA
As was noted earlier, controversy exists over whether different callosal regions undergo selective changes in aging and dementia (Yoshii et al., 1990) and even whether effects in dementia are significant compared to age-matched controls (Biegon et al., 1994). Like Biegon and colleagues (1994), Black and colleagues (1996), and Kaufer and colleagues (1997), we did not find total callosal area to be significantly depressed in AD (mean ± S.D.: 525.9 ± 116.8 mm^2) relative to controls (575.4 ± 108.8 mm^2, $p > 0.05$). These values (determined before stereotaxic normalization) are in broad agreement with, but marginally higher than, previously determined callosal area values (Biegon et al., 1994) of 562 ± 98 mm^2 in elderly controls ($n = 13$; MR slice thickness: 10 mm; age: 64.8 ± 9.0 years) and 480 ± 133 mm^2 in AD ($p > 0.05$; $n = 20$; age: 70.1 ± 7.4 years, with slightly lower MMSE scores of 17 ± 7.2 and a range of 9–25). Both our data and those of Biegon and colleagues (1994), Black and colleagues (1996), and Kaufer and colleagues (1997) do not fully agree with earlier reports that total callosal area discriminated between AD and control subjects ($p < 0.05$; see Hofmann et al., 1995) and that combined callosal area was sig-

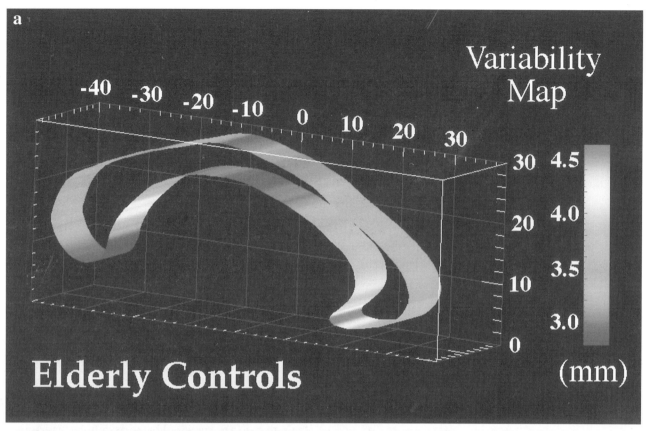

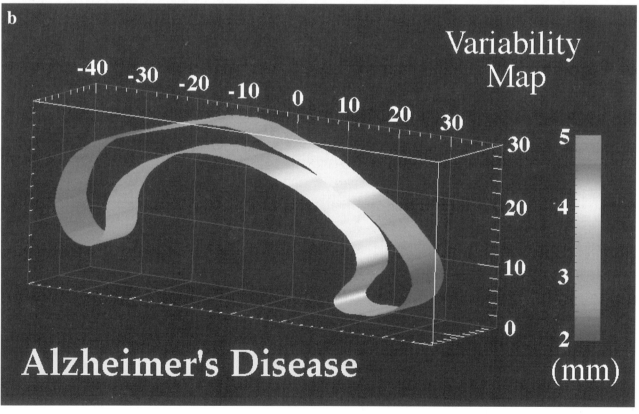

FIGURE 5.8. Maps of stereotaxic variability at the corpus callosum in patients with Alzheimer's disease and in elderly normal subjects. Separate maps of local variability were constructed for (a) Alzheimer's patients and (b) control subjects, expressing (in color) the r.m.s. variation of callosal points in each subject group around an average boundary representation of the callosum, at the midsagittal plane of Talairach stereotaxic space. Unlike the asymmetry and variability maps in Figure 5.9, these are strictly two-dimensional maps, since the midsagittal analysis of callosal morphology is conducted in a single vertical plane. Average boundary representations have therefore been thickened for visualization purposes only. Two trends are apparent. Although the variability measure peaks at the rostrum, this may be an artifact due to the difficulties of defining an unambiguous anatomical limit for the inferior aspect of the rostrum. Nevertheless, the pronounced rise in variability at the rostral midbody in AD (b) may reflect disease-related enlargement of the third ventricle, which forms its inferior boundary. (See Color Plate 5.)

←———————————————————————————

nificantly reduced in AD (by 7.0% relative to controls; $p < 0.05$; see Yoshii et al., 1990). If selective AD-related atrophy occurs in specific callosal sectors (Black et al., 1996), when areas of these sectors are pooled with those of other more robust regions, they may or may not be significantly reduced, depending on disease severity.

ALZHEIMER'S DISEASE AND SCHIZOPHRENIA The finding that the same highly circumscribed site at the callosum (Figures 5.8 and 5.10) shows a comparable shape inflection in schizophrenia (DeQuardo et al., 1996; Bookstein, 1997) is intriguing. Owing to differences in the etiology of the two diseases, fiber deficiency at this site in schizophrenia may be associated with a neurodevelopmental disruption of the sulcogyral organization of temporal lobe fibers that cross in this region (see Kikinis et al., 1994). In AD, however, a similarly localized fiber deficiency may result from temporoparietal neuronal loss, associated with the early perfusion and cognitive performance deficits in AD. As has been noted already, a massive perinatal loss of callosal axons, lasting from the thirty-fifth gestational week to the end of the first postnatal month (Clarke et al., 1989; LaMantia and Rakic, 1990) leads to a restricted pattern of adult callosal connections, but controversy exists over whether callosal area is further reduced in normal aging relative to young normal controls (Biegon et al., 1994; cf. Doraiswamy et al., 1991). Callosal area reductions in AD may have functional significance, as smaller partial callosal size often reflects a focal decrease in the number of small-diameter (<3 μm) fibers (Aboitiz et al., 1992a) or decreased myelin deposition associated with decreased conduction velocity and longer interhemispheric transmission times. These and other callosal studies, in-

terpreted in the context of (1) the temporoparietal perfusion deficits and temporal neuronal loss typical in early AD and (2) correlations between reduced association cortex metabolism and cognitive performance, suggest that neuronal loss and white matter abnormalities in AD may partially exert their effect through disruption of long corticocortical pathways (DeCarli et al., 1996). Earlier reports of CC alterations in clinically mild AD (Vermersch et al., 1994; Hoffman et al., 1995; Janowsky et al., 1996), support these observations and further highlight the selective vulnerability of callosal regions in AD.

OTHER DEMENTIA SUBTYPES Recent reports suggest that the pattern of callosal atrophy may differ in different subtypes of dementia, at least in the early stages of each disease. Using the Witelson (1989) partition (see Figure 5.1c), Lyoo and colleagues (1997) observed that mildly demented (MMSE > 21) subjects with AD exhibited significant area reductions at the posterior midbody, isthmus and splenium ($N = 49$; Figure 5.1c), while subjects with mild vascular dementia (according to DSM-III and Hachinski diagnostic criteria and with MMSE > 21, $N = 21$) had only a significantly smaller genu relative to normal controls ($N = 36$). This finding is consistent with prior reports that the anterior vasculature is preferentially affected in vascular dementia (Freedman and Albert, 1985; Ishii, Nishihara, and Imamura, 1986). Observed postmortem, patients with vascular dementia also have a reduced axon density specific to the anterior callosum ($N = 5$; see Yamanouchi, Sugiura, and Shimada, 1990). Nonetheless, all callosal sectors exhibit significant size reductions in the more severe stages of both diseases (MMSE < 21; see Lyoo et al., 1997). In view of the distinct etiologies of different types of dementia, further neuroimaging studies are required to clarify the relationship between structural and functional deficits throughout the dynamic course of each disease.

Schizophrenia

CALLOSAL MORPHOMETRY People with schizophrenia exhibit subtle and diffuse alterations in cerebral structure as revealed by evidence from postmortem and in vivo imaging studies. However, none of these neuroanatomical abnormalities have been shown to be requisite for diagnosis (Stevens, 1998). Nevertheless, technological advances in structural and functional imaging protocols and improvements in quantitative methods for measuring brain morphology and activation continue to increase the sensitivity with which deviation of neuroanatomical and functional norms can be detected. In spite of novel imaging techniques and applications, mor-

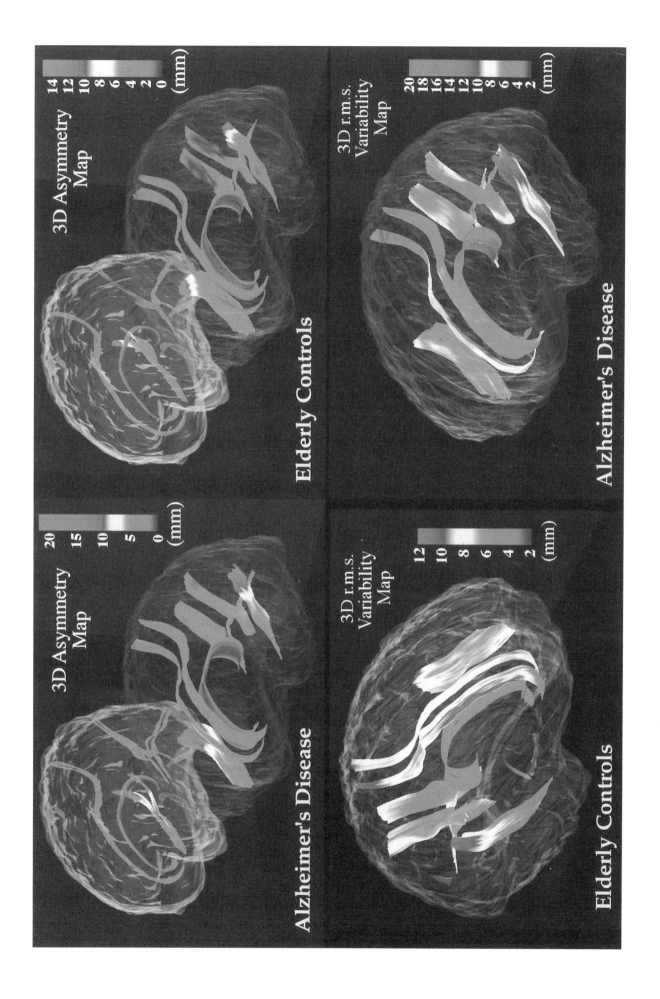

FIGURE 5.9. Population-based maps of three-dimensional structural variation and asymmetry. Statistics of three-dimensional deformation maps can be computed to determine confidence limits on normal anatomic variation. Three-dimensional maps of anatomical variability and asymmetry are shown for 10 subjects with Alzheimer's disease (age: 71.9 ± 10.9 years) and 10 normal elderly subjects matched for age (72.9 ± 5.6 years), gender, handedness, and educational level (Thompson et al., 1998). Normal Sylvian fissure asymmetries (right higher than left, $p < 0.0005$), mapped for the first time in three dimensions, were significantly greater in AD than in controls ($p < 0.0002$; top panels). In the three-dimensional variability maps derived for each group (lower panels), the color encodes the root mean square magnitude of the displacement vectors required to map the surfaces from each of the 10 patients' brains onto the average. Confidence limits on three-dimensional cortical variation (lower right panel), exhibited severe increases in AD from 2–4 mm at the corpus callosum to a peak standard deviation of 19.6 mm at the posterior left Sylvian fissure. (See Color Plate 6.)

◄—————————————————————

phometric findings in schizophrenic populations frequently lack consensus and fail to expose reliable patterns of structural variation within and across schizophrenia subtypes compared to normal. In fact, the reported morphometric differences appear to be as variable as patient symptomatology. Imaging studies designed to detect macroscopic alteration of callosal morphology have yielded mixed results. However, there is a fair amount of experimental evidence suggesting that transcallosal connectivity plays an important role in

the schizophrenia syndrome. Furthermore, schizophrenia fits the profile of a misconnection syndrome, reflecting dysfunctional callosal connections from homologous regions of cortex, especially those between the sometimes asymmetric areas of association cortex (Crow, 1998). In the following sections we will discuss (1) how maldevelopment of the callosum may relate to other structural neuropathology reported in schizophrenia, (2) theoretical issues that relate symptomatology in schizophrenia to callosal abnormality, (3) empirical evidence from neuroimaging and neuropsychological studies suggesting structural alterations of the callosum and related behavioral deficits, and finally (4) methodological issues related to detecting structural abnormalities of the callosum in this population.

CALLOSAL LINKS TO STRUCTURAL NEUROPATHOLOGY IN SCHIZOPHRENIA Diffuse structural abnormalities have been reported in neuroimaging, cytoarchitectural, epidemiological, and behavioral studies of schizophrenic populations. Converging evidence supports the idea of schizophrenia as a circuit disease, stemming from aberrant neurodevelopmental events (e.g., Carpenter et al., 1993; Pilowsky, Kerwin, and Murray, 1993; Waddington, 1993; Nopoulos et al., 1995; Weinberger, 1995; Buchanan, Stevens, and Carpenter, 1998). The disruption of neurodevelopmental events involving mechanisms such as abnormal neuronal migration, growth retardation, aberrant myelination, neuronal pruning, and/or apoptosis occurring prenatally or through

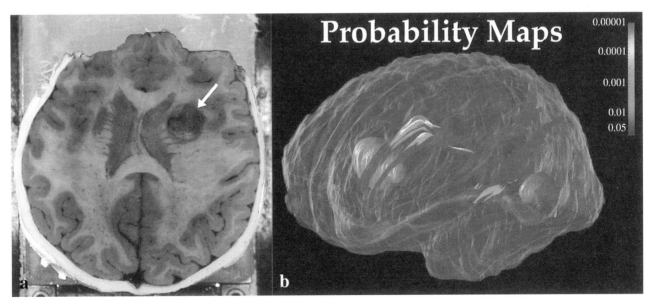

FIGURE 5.10. Distortions in brain architecture induced by tumor tissue: probability maps for ventral callosum and major sulci in both hemispheres. Color-coded probability maps (b) quantify the impact of two focal metastatic tumors (illustrated in red; see also cryosection blockface) (a) on the ventral callosal boundary, as well as the parieto-occipital and anterior and posterior calcarine sulci in both brain hemispheres. (See Color Plate 7.)

MAPPING STRUCTURAL ALTERATIONS OF THE CORPUS CALLOSUM   115 development are thought to account for the diversity of structural findings in schizophrenia (Waddington, 1993; Nopoulos et al., 1995). The fact that pruning and myelination in the corpus callosum continue into early adulthood and that interhemispheric coherence develops up until late adolescence may also have some relevance to the age of onset (Njiokiktjien et al., 1994). Furthermore, myelination begins prenatally and has been shown to be susceptible to malnutrition, asphyxia, exotoxins, and endotoxins of infectious origin (Njiokiktjien et al., 1994; Bishop and Wahlsten, 1997). It may be no coincidence that influenza epidemics or other viral infections during the second trimester, a critical period for neurodevelopment and obstetric complications, lead to an increase in schizophrenic births (Swayze et al., 1990; Waddington, 1993, Woodruff et al., 1995).

A clearer picture of callosal dysfunction in schizophrenia emerges by considering structural abnormalities in the context of their functional circuitry. After all, no brain region acts in isolation, and alterations in circuitry potentially lead to structural abnormalities and vice versa. In spite of primary confounding factors such as schizophrenia heterogeneity and different methodological approaches, there are some suggestive neurodevelopmental abnormalities that are frequently reported in schizophrenia populations involving neural systems linked by the callosal commissure. The major players include frontal, temporolimbic, and midline circuits (Cassanova et al., 1990; Andreasen et al., 1994, 1996; Bogerts, 1997; Goldman-Rakic and Selemon, 1998). As the primary channel of interhemispheric communication, the corpus callosum plays an important role in these systems by reciprocally connecting homologous regions of neocortex. This means that an abnormality in prefrontal or temporal cortices, for example, is likely to influence callosal morphology, and a disturbance in callosal development is likely to have reciprocal effects on these cortical regions.

CALLOSAL DEVELOPMENT IN SCHIZOPHRENIA As was noted earlier, the development of the corpus callosum and the neopallium occurs in parallel, with the embryonic callosum first connecting nonolfactory cortex, then extending anteriorly to connect frontal cortices and then posteriorly to join other lobes as they develop. Recent evidence, however, suggests that the callosum develops bidirectionally (Kier and Truwit, 1996). Nevertheless, there is no question that the corpus callosum develops in the hippocampal primordium in close relationship with the developing lobes.

Imaging studies indicate that median reductions in prefrontal cortex make these regions about 5.5% smaller in schizophrenic patients. Reductions are primarily due to a loss in gray rather than white matter (Lawrie and Abukmeil, 1998). Superior and rostral portions of the hippocampal formation also undergo regressive changes in association with callosal development. While findings regarding volume decreases in limbic structures remain equivocal in schizophrenic patients, results in homogeneous samples (males with positive symptoms) are more conclusive (Shenton et al., 1992; Flaum et al., 1995; Menon et al., 1995; Barta et al., 1997; Marsh et al., 1997). Morphological alteration of the superior temporal gyrus in schizophrenic patients has also been reported (e.g., Nestor et al., 1993). This gyrus has particular relevance to callosal circuitry because it has been identified as the approximate site of Wernicke's language area and marks the planum temporale on its superior banks (Geschwind and Galaburda, 1985; Galaburda et al., 1990). To focus on language-related cortex in schizophrenic patients, investigators have measured the asymmetry of the planum temporale and Sylvian fissure in MR images. Once again, results are mixed, with some studies reporting a decreased asymmetry in schizophrenic patients (Hoff et al., 1992; Kikinis et al., 1994; Petty et al., 1995) and others not (DeLisi et al., 1994; Kleinschmidt et al., 1994; Frangou et al., 1997). While corpus callosum morphometry and planum asymmetry have not been compared in the same schizophrenic sample, data from normal populations indicate that morphology in these areas are related (Aboitiz et al., 1992b). In summary, imaging studies examining temporal and limbic structures report a modest reduction in temporal lobe volume, with larger volume reductions in the hippocampus, amygdala, and superior temporal gyrus, and some reports of abnormal asymmetries of the planum temporale and Sylvian fissure.

Toward the end of embryonic callosal development, the area between the corpus callosum and the fornix becomes very thin and forms the septum pellucidum, where the cavum septi pellucidi may develop. MRI and postmortem studies have related presence of cavum septi pellucidi to psychosis. This developmental anomaly is especially prevalent in schizophrenia groups and relates to other schizophrenia structural abnormalities (Degreef et al., 1992; Nopoulos et al., 1996). In addition, the corpus callosum forms the rostral boundary and roof of the superior horn of the lateral ventricles. Cerebral ventricular enlargement is the most robust structural anomaly reported in schizophrenic patients. Median figures from many studies indicate the most substantial enlargement is in the ventricular body (Lawrie and Abukmeil, 1998). While finding no difference in corpus callosum area, thickness, or length in twins discordant for schizophrenia, Cassanova and colleagues (1990) used a statistical analysis of a Fourier expansion series to demonstrate differences in callosal shape between discordant twins. The shape difference was especially apparent in the middle and anterior segments of the callosum. The displacement of the corpus callosum in the vertical plane of schizophrenic patients, representing a shape difference between populations, has been replicated and reflects the increased size of the lateral ventricular body (Narr et al., unpublished findings). Finally, thalamic abnormalities along with other midline structure alterations such as cavum septum pellucidi (Nopoulos et al., 1996) and increased incidence of callosal agenesis (Swayze et al., 1990) suggest the role of neurodevelopmental abnormalities and the disruption of midline circuitry in schizophrenia.

CALLOSAL CONNECTIVITY IN SCHIZOPHRENIA Considering the major role the corpus callosum plays in hemispheric transmission, it is conceivable that the corpus callosum must be involved in schizophrenia neuropathology. Crow (1998) proposes that schizophrenic etiology arises from a component of callosal connectivity associated with the evolution of language, arguing that language and psychoses have a common evolutionary origin. He supports this view by pointing out that age of onset, relative constancy of incidence across societies, and affliction during reproductive and healthy phases of life are characteristics of schizophrenia, and this disease may not be selected out because of its association with language specialization. Although this misconnection hypothesis is difficult to test, evidence is cited of abnormalities in the "last to evolve" fiber pathways (for example, perisylvian temporal and dorsolateral prefrontal cortex) and reports of callosal morphological change over time in schizophrenic patients. Additionally, some studies have reported a link between schizophrenia and dyslexia, representing schizophrenia etiology as tied to language lateralization, and callosal connectivity (Stein, 1994; Horrobin, Glen, and Hudson, 1995). However, there are studies that directly dispute the misconnection hypothesis; for example, Bartley and colleagues (1993) found no evidence of altered asymmetry in language areas in monozygotic twins discordant for schizophrenia, and other studies have not found altered planum asymmetry in schizophrenic patients (DeLisi et al., 1994; Kleinschmidt et al., 1994; Frangou et al., 1997).

David (1994) discusses different views regarding how abnormal interhemispheric transmission accounts for typical schizophrenic phenomena, such as hallucinations and thought alienation. One view suggests that cognitive activity within the right hemisphere would be experienced as alien by the left hemisphere if the two hemispheres were not in full communication (Nasrallah, 1985). Another model of interhemispheric abnormality in schizophrenia assumes that excessive connectivity between the two hemispheres, perhaps due to insufficient pruning during development, causes confusion as to whether stimuli are of external or internal origin (Randall, 1983). Clinical studies have also reported cases of psychosis in patients with complete or partial callosal agenesis (David, 1994). As was mentioned above, callosal agenesis and other callosal abnormalities are thought to have increased incidence in schizophrenia (Swayze et al., 1990; Degreef et al., 1992; Nopoulos et al., 1996).

POSTMORTEM AND IMAGING STUDIES The most direct evidence of structural callosal abnormalities in schizophrenia comes from postmortem and imaging studies. Experimental neuropsychology also contributes with specific behavioral measures designed to assess impairments in interhemispheric communication implicating callosal abnormality. Findings of altered callosal morphology in schizophrenic patients appear complex and tempered by a number of variables, including sex, symptoms, disease course, and age of onset (DeLisi et al., 1997). In fact, there appears to be little consensus on whether the corpus callosum is larger or smaller in this population. In spite of conflicting evidence, a meta-analysis by Woodruff and colleagues (1995) found a modest reduction of callosal size across 11 studies with heterogeneous schizophrenic samples. To complicate matters further, structural differences are confounded by employment of different measurement techniques, making it difficult to compare results across studies. If one thing is clear from this body of research, it is that the story of callosal abnormality in schizophrenia is as complicated as other facets of the disease.

Early postmortem studies report an increase in callosal size in schizophrenia (Bigelow, Nasrallah, and Rausher, 1983), but this finding has not always been replicated (Brown et al., 1986). Advances in imaging procedures have made it easier to study the corpus callosum in vivo, but studies continue to report mixed results for different callosal parameters. For example, various studies have found total callosal area to be smaller (e.g., Rossi et al., 1989; Woodruff et al., 1993), larger (e.g., Nasrallah et al., 1986), or not significantly different (e.g., Uematsu and Kaiya, 1988) in schizophrenic patients compared to controls. Other studies measuring callosal thickness have similarly reported increases (e.g., Nasrallah et al., 1986), decreases (e.g., DeQuardo et al., 1996), and no difference across groups. As was discussed earlier, efforts have been made to parcellate the callosum into sections to isolate malformation of specific callosal channels (see Figure 5.1). Here again, results conflict, perhaps in part owing to variations in methods and the different schizophrenia subgroups that were tested. For example, roughly equivalent estimates of the anterior corpus callosum connecting frontal cortices have been reported as thicker or larger in area (Nasrallah et al., 1986; Uematsu and Kaiya, 1988), smaller in area (Woodruff et al., 1993, Jacobsen et al., 1997), or not different (Woodruff et al., 1997) in patients. Posterior and middle callosal regions in schizophrenic patients have also been found to be reduced (DeQuardo et al., 1996; Woodruff et al., 1993, Jacobsen et al., 1997), to be thicker (Nasrallah et al., 1986), or to have similar distributions with normal controls (Smith, Baumgartner, and Calderon, 1987; Uematsu and Kaiya, 1988; Woodruff et al., 1997).

GENDER INTERACTIONS Results mentioned above and elsewhere indicate an incredible range of callosal morphometric findings in schizophrenic populations. Although failure to replicate findings may be attributable to the heterogeneity of the patient groups examined, discrepancies may also result from structural differences between sexes in schizophrenic groups. As was noted earlier, there is an ongoing controversy concerning sex differences in callosal structure, and it appears that brain size has a larger influence over callosal morphology than does gender (see Rauch and Jinkins, 1994; Jäncke et al., 1997). Larger callosal size found in females relative to brain or skull size results directly from their smaller brain size, and this relative difference persists irrespective of sex. Even if no sex difference is present in normal callosal morphology (cf. Bishop and Wahlsten, 1997), this does not preclude sex effects from interacting with morphometric abnormalities in schizophrenic populations. Male and female schizophrenics may, in general, follow a different course of illness. There is typically a later age of onset in female schizophrenics, and hereditary factors may be unevenly distributed between the sexes (DeLisi, Dauphinais, and Hauser, 1989; Waddington, 1993). Callosal structural alterations in schizophrenic patients may therefore reflect gender differences or gender interactions. Hoff and colleagues (1992), for example, found that females with first episode schizophrenia had smaller total callosal area compared to controls. These findings partially replicated data from a study by Hauser and colleagues (1989) in which chronic female schizophrenic patients showed smaller anterior callosal widths compared to normals. In contrast, Nasrallah (1985) found increased thickness of the anterior and middle corpus callosum in females, while Raine and colleagues (1990) found increased thickness in the callosum of female schizophrenics compared to normal females and decreased callosal thickness in male patients compared to male controls. A similar trend toward a reversed sex difference in anterior and posterior callosal size was reported by Colombo and colleagues (1993).

CLINICAL VARIABLES Clinical and psychopathological heterogeneity in schizophrenic patients may account for inconsistencies in results when assessing structural morphology (Colombo et al., 1993). For example, patients with negative symptoms are shown to have smaller callosal sizes relative to patients with positive symptoms or to controls (Gunther et al., 1991; Woodruff et al., 1993). It has also been suggested, however, that patients with negative symptoms have thicker corpora callosa (Coger and Serafetinides, 1990; Jacobsen et al., 1997). Early onset schizophrenic patients have been shown to have larger total, anterior, and posterior callosal areas as compared to controls (Coger and Serafetinides, 1990; Jacobsen et al., 1997). These results are consistent with the postmortem data of Bigelow and colleagues (1983), which found early-onset chronic schizophrenic patients to have significantly greater callosal thickness than later-onset patients. In addition, auditory hallucinations have been related to callosal size (David et al., 1995). Finally, one study suggested that an elongated anterior callosum related to unfavorable prognosis, because large callosal size suggested poor heterosexual relationships, reduced numbers of hospitalizations, low academic grades, and mild anxiety-depression syndrome (Uematsu and Kaiya, 1988). Clearly, more information is needed to establish the role of these factors in relation to callosal morphometry in schizophrenia. Finally, almost all studies used solely right-handed subjects in their analyses or matched for handedness across groups. Controlling for handedness is important, since handedness appears to be a predictor of neuroanatomical asymmetry and bears a relationship to callosal morphology (Bartley et al., 1993; Clarke and Zaidel, 1994). Most studies also reported no influence of age in their findings of callosal pathology. Even though the effects of aging and callosal development are still under investigation, these results may not be surprising, as most studies controlled for age in some degree and used primarily adult samples.

STRUCTURE/FUNCTION CORRELATIONS To assess the relationship between callosal structure and function in schizophrenia, several investigators correlated measures of interhemispheric transfer and hemispheric specialization with callosal morphometry (Raine et al., 1990; Colombo et al., 1993; Woodruff et al., 1997). Tests of interhemispheric transfer include measures of visual, tactile, auditory, and cognitive transfer. Such tests have been derived from studies assessing the absence of callosal relay in split-brain patients. Patients with surgical transection of the corpus callosum exhibit impairments such as left-hand anomia in tactile tasks, inability to identify false speech sounds presented to the right ear, and deficits in matching stimuli across visual fields (Gazzaniga, 1995). Similar impairments in schizophrenic patients would therefore imply abnormalities in callosal relay. Raine and colleagues (1990) were one of the first groups to employ concurrent structural and functional callosal measures in a schizophrenia sample. Behavioral measures included verbal and nonverbal dichotic listening protocols and crossed versus uncrossed conditions in finger sequence repetition, tactile, and WAIS-R block design tasks. None of these tasks detected deficits in interhemispheric processing in patients, and attempts were not made to correlate scores with the sex interaction of callosal morphometry detected across groups. A neuropsychological battery with unilateral and bilateral conditions employed by Hoff and colleagues (1992) revealed an association of larger callosal size with better cognitive function, but no relationship was noted in female schizophrenic patients who exhibited significantly smaller callosal area or across genders in the schizophrenic group. Similar nonsignificant results of interhemispheric transfer have been reported in studies assessing behavioral measures alone (e.g., Schrift et al., 1986; Ditchfield and Hemsley, 1990). In another of the few studies simultaneously assessing structural and functional abnormality of the callosum in schizophrenic patients, no deficits were reported in interhemispheric transfer for an auditory comprehension task assessing transfer of speech information (Colombo et al., 1993). However, the degree of left versus right ear response in the monaural condition in this paradigm was significantly correlated with posterior callosal size in male schizophrenics.

COLOR NAMING AND MATCHING Although studies assessing interhemispheric transfer have yielded unpromising results in schizophrenic patients, more interesting results have stemmed from studies assessing color naming and matching. Here, patients show impairments in left visual field color naming, reflecting impairments in callosal transfer. Impairments are greater in across-field color matching relative to within-field matching (McKeever and Jackson, 1979; David, 1987). In a similar vein, a lateralized version of the color-word Stroop task administered to schizophrenic patients revealed that the reaction time difference across visual fields for congruent and incongruent color word pairs was increased (David, 1994). This suggests a hypoconnection of facilitation and/or interference between hemispheres. Using a version of the color-word Stroop task, Woodruff and colleagues (1997) found that bilateral facilitation was greater and interference less in schizophrenic patients. Furthermore, these investigators included simultaneous morphometric analysis of the corpus callosum in their sample. However, they found a positive correlation between facilitation and posterior callosal area and a com-

plimentary negative correlation between interference and posterior callosal area only when both patient and control groups were combined.

In general, tests of interhemispheric transfer in schizophrenic patients have yielded disappointing results as far as a misconnection hypothesis is concerned. Studies including morphometric measures and those assessing behavioral measures alone have so far yielded no consistent deficit in interhemispheric transfer specific to this population but instead have indicated a more particular left hemisphere deficit (Schrift et al., 1986; Ditchfield and Hemsley, 1990). Functional imaging studies, however, have revealed decreased activity in the corpus callosum in disorganized schizophrenic patients (Schroder et al., 1995). Evidence of different regional cerebral activation patterns in each clinically defined subgroup serves to emphasize the importance of studying homogeneous patient groups. Bilateral hyperactivation has also been reported in schizophrenic patients with primarily positive symptoms in a sensorimotor task, and this subgroup also exhibited increased callosal size (Gunther et al., 1991). However, many methodological problems occur in research assessing interhemispheric communication. Until more evidence is obtained, especially in regard to measuring structural and functional correlates, no solid conclusions can be drawn about interhemispheric impairment in schizophrenic patients.

METHODOLOGICAL ISSUES Morphometric analysis of structural differences in schizophrenic brains from postmortem and in vivo imaging studies is a relatively dirty task. That is, many extraneous variables interact to threaten the validity of results. Since the schizophrenia syndromes may arise from multiple pathophysiological mechanisms, it is not always clear how to reduce patient heterogeneity when examining particular and connected morphometric anomalies. As was indicated above, differences in sex, chronicity, symptomatology, age of onset, handedness, and age may all influence callosal morphology in schizophrenia groups. Other factors that may interfere with analysis include the incidence of perinatal insult, educational level, IQ, height, social status, premorbid adjustment, treatment history and response, and the duration and course of illness (Carpenter et al., 1993). Further difficulties arise from the large variability that is present in normal populations regarding callosal structure and the significant overlap with patient distributions. Interactions of these variables increasingly complicate the endeavor to examine structural alteration of the corpus callosum and its relationship with other neuroanatomical abnormalities in schizophrenia.

Some solutions to these problems may include the ability to compare images from individual patients with those of an appropriately matched average from normal brain archives. This is now becoming possible, as a probabilistic reference system for the human brain is being compiled whereby variables such as age, sex, and handedness may be matched (Mazziotta et al., 1995; Thompson et al., 1997, 1998b). Correcting for head size differences appears all-important when studying the nature of callosal structural neuropathology (Steinmetz et al., 1995; Jäncke et al., 1997), especially in view of sex differences in head size. Furthermore, while schizophrenic patients are shown to have decreased cranial and cerebral size, that does not necessarily hold true for other cerebral structures. To illustrate this point, no callosal structural abnormalities were revealed in childhood-onset schizophrenic patients (Jacobsen et al., 1997). However, after adjusting for the smaller cerebral volume of the schizophrenics, larger total, anterior, and posterior corpus callosum areas were detected in patients. Unfortunately, not all studies assessing callosal structure abnormalities in schizophrenia have adjusted for brain size. Transforming images into Talairach standardized space (Talairach et al., 1967; Talairach and Tournoux, 1988) or correcting for both measured cortical volumes and head positioning in the MR scanner is suggested to allow for proper morphometric comparison of neuroanatomical regions across populations.

PATIENT HOMOGENEITY   In a meta-analysis of heterogeneous schizophrenic patients, Woodruff and colleagues (1995) noted the huge variability in magnitude and direction of callosum size in the patient groups. To address the problem of patient heterogeneity, the simplest solution is to study homogeneous groups. Unfortunately, this has a trade-off with the ability to generalize results. Some investigators suggest that besides matching for demographic variables, either the type of course of illness or the evaluation of outliers should be used in assessing morphology in schizophrenia brains (Stevens, 1998). Others argue that neuroanatomy should be examined in the context of separate symptom complexes that may or may not alter regional anatomy (Carpenter et al., 1993). Furthermore, as was noted earlier in the chapter, large sample sizes are required to assess the relationships of structural brain abnormalities as exist in neural circuits, especially as callosal abnormality in schizophrenia appears to have a small to medium effect size (Woodruff et al., 1995).

Results are further complicated by different protocols used to divide the callosum into subregions (see Figure 5.1) and in the measures used to obtain maximal or minimal callosal thickness (see Figure 5.1d). Even though research in monkeys shows that the corpus callosum is organized by sensory modality (Pandya and Seltzer,

1986), there are no neuroanatomical landmarks by which to partition these areas. Although some investigators have studied how different partitioning protocols influence the validity of results (e.g., Allen et al., 1991), different methods make it difficult to compare results across studies. Furthermore, most analyses have looked only at traditional morphometric parameters that include midsagittal area and maximum and minimum width and length (Figure 5.1). More recent techniques allow the analysis of curvature, shape, and fractal complexity (Thompson et al., 1996a, 1996b). Methods that involve the creation of parametric meshes rendered from traces of regional surface anatomy enable the visualization of very local variability and group differences across the surfaces of individual structures (Thompson et al., 1996a, 1997). Additionally, even fewer studies have related callosal morphometric differences to data from other brain regions. Since callosal function depends on the integrity of the cortical regions it connects, it does not make sense to study this region in isolation. Tissue segmentation protocols indicate a gray matter volume loss in the cortices of schizophrenic patients (e.g., Lim et al., 1996; Sullivan et al., 1996). Considering the mixed findings of callosal abnormality, it is still not clear whether white matter sparing in schizophrenia includes the traversing callosal fibers or whether disconnection or misconnection occurs. Finally, only one study to our knowledge has looked at changes in callosal morphology in schizophrenic patients across time (DeLisi et al., 1995).

There are also difficulties in interpreting the nature of interhemispheric deficits in schizophrenic patients and their relationship to callosal structure. Part of the problem appears because even in normal people, many behavioral tests of interhemispheric transfer have often not been found to be related to measurements of callosal structure (Clarke and Zaidel, 1994). In postmortem studies, Aboitiz and colleagues (1992a) noted that only the numbers of small-diameter fibers that are thought to relay cognitive information across hemispheres relate to callosal size, while large-diameter fibers conducting sensory and motor information do not. Considering that most of the interhemispheric tasks employed in the schizophrenia studies reviewed involved mainly the transfer of sensory information (visual, tactile, and auditory transfer), it might not be surprising that these measures did not correlate well with callosal structural abnormalities, although abnormalities were detected in imaging activation tasks (Gunther et al., 1991; Schroder et al., 1995). Also, many trials are required to assess small differences in reaction time for stimuli presented within versus between hemispheres. In these types of behavioral paradigms, results may be compromised by patient distractibility. Finally, the fine temporal resolution of EEG studies augments the power to detect differences in processing time across the hemispheres, and these studies have reported abnormal interhemispheric transfer time in schizophrenic patients (e.g., Heidrich and Strik, 1997; Weisbrod et al., 1997).

The large body of research dedicated to studying callosal abnormality in schizophrenic patients at the structural and behavioral levels has thus far been unable to reach a consensus. As improvements in imaging analysis techniques provide enhanced detection of subtle differences, and as more is learned about callosal structure and function in normal populations, a clearer picture of callosal abnormality in schizophrenia is likely to emerge.

Atlas-based pathology detection

PROBABILISTIC ATLASING Probabilistic atlasing is a research strategy whose goal is to generate anatomical templates that retain quantitative information on intersubject variations in brain architecture (Mazziotta et al., 1995; Thompson et al., 1997; Thompson and Toga, 1998). A digital probabilistic atlas of the human brain, incorporating precise statistical information on positional variability of important functional and anatomical interfaces, may help to address many of the methodological difficulties that we have observed in detecting alterations in callosal anatomy. As the database of subjects on which probabilistic atlases are based increases in size and content, the digital electronic form of the atlas provides efficiency in statistical and computational comparisons between individuals or groups. In addition, the population on which probabilistic atlases are based can be stratified into subpopulations by age, gender, handedness, or other demographic factors; by stage of development; or to represent different disease types. A probabilistic framework for structural brain data solves many of the limitations of a fixed atlas in representing highly variable anatomy. A statistical confidence limit, rather than an absolute representation of neuroanatomy, may also be more appropriate for representing particular subpopulations.

WARPING ALGORITHMS CAN CREATE PROBABILISTIC ATLASES As was noted earlier, when applied to two different three-dimensional brain scans, a nonlinear registration or warping algorithm (Toga, 1998; Toga and Thompson, 1998) calculates a deformation map (Figures 5.2 and 5.3) that matches up brain structures in one scan with their counterparts in the other. The deformation map indicates three-dimensional patterns of anatomical differences between the two subjects. By defining probability distributions on the space of deformation trans-

formations that drive the anatomy of different subjects into correspondence (Grenander, 1976; Amit, Grenander, and Piccioni, 1991; Grenander and Miller, 1994; Davatzikosand and Prince,1996; Thompson and Toga, 1997; Thompson et al., 1997), statistical parameters of these distributions can be estimated from databased anatomical data to determine the magnitude and directional biases of anatomical variation. Encoding of local variation can then be used to assess the severity of structural variants outside of the normal range, which, in brain data, may be a sign of disease (Thompson et al., 1997).

ENCODING BRAIN VARIATION The random vector field approach is a general strategy to construct population-based atlases of the brain (Thompson and Toga, 1997; Thirion et al., 1998). Briefly, given a three-dimensional MR image of a new subject, a warping algorithm (Thompson and Toga, 1996) calculates a set of high-dimensional volumetric maps, elastically deforming this image into structural correspondence with other scans, selected one by one from an anatomical image database. Target scans are selected from subjects matched for age, handedness, gender, and other demographic factors (Thompson et al., 1997, 1998a). The resulting family of volumetric warps provides empirical information on patterns of local anatomical variation. A probability space of random transformations, based on the theory of anisotropic Gaussian random fields (Thompson et al., 1997), is then used to encode the variations. Specialized continuum-mechanical approaches are required to encode information on complex variations in gyral and sulcal topography from one individual to another (Thompson et al., 1997; Thompson and Toga, 1998). Confidence limits in stereotaxic space are determined, for points in the new subject's brain, enabling the creation of color-coded probability maps to highlight and quantify regional patterns of deformity.

CALLOSAL ANATOMY Although probabilistic systems are under development for the population-based analysis of callosal data (Thompson et al., 1998a), their ability to resolve callosal differences in small groups of subjects with dementia is indicated in Figure 5.7. In one validation experiment (Thompson et al., 1997) (Figure 5.10), probability maps were created to highlight abnormal deviations in the callosal anatomy of a specific subject. The medical history of the subject in question indicated the presence of lung cancer, which had spread to the brain. Two metastatic tumors were present, one in each hemisphere. The first, and larger, tumor (volume: 95.2 cm^3) was centered in the high putamen of the right hemisphere (see Figure 5.10), while a second tumor (volume: 24.6 cm^3) was located in the left occipital lobe. No other neuropathology was present, and the primary cause of death was cardiopulmonary arrest. The two regions of metastatic tissue induced marked distortions in the normal architecture of the brain. This effect was reflected both in the blockface imagery itself (Figure 5.10b) and in the values of the probability maps of structures proximal to the lesion sites (Figure 5.10a).

PATHOLOGY DETECTION   To identify differences in brain structure between two groups or between an individual subject and a database of demographically matched subjects, we define $W_{ij}(x)$ as the deformation vector required to match the structure at position x in an atlas template with its counterpart in subject i of group j, and we model the deformations as

$$W_{ij}(x) = \mu_j(x) + \Sigma(x)^{1/2}\varepsilon_{ij}(x)$$

Here, $\mu_j(x)$ is the mean deformation for group j, and $\Sigma(x)$ is a nonstationary, anisotropic covariance tensor field, which relaxes the confidence threshold for detecting abnormal structure in regions where normal variability is extreme, $\Sigma(x)^{1/2}$ is the upper triangular Cholesky factor tensor field, and $\varepsilon_{ij}(x)$ is a trivariate random vector field whose components are independent stationary Gaussian random fields.

A T^2- or F-statistic that indicates evidence of significant difference in deformations between the groups is calculated at each lattice location in a three-dimensional image or parameterized three-dimensional surface to form a statistic image (Thompson et al., 1997). Specialized algorithms, using corrections for the metric tensor of the underlying surface, are required to calculate these fields at the cortex (Thompson and Toga, 1998). Under the null hypothesis of no abnormal deformations, the statistic image is approximated by a T^2 random field. The global maximum of the random deformation field, or derived tensor fields (Thompson et al., 1998a), can be used to test the hypothesis of no structural change in disease (Worsley, 1994a, 1994b; Cao and Worsley, 1998). Similar multivariate linear models can be used to test for the effect of explanatory variables (e.g., age, gender, clinical test scores) on a set of deformation field images.

Probabilistic atlases based on random deformation fields and associated scalar fields derived by using operators that emphasize specific deformational characteristics have been used to assess gender-specific differences in the brain (Davatzikos, 1996; Cao and Worsley, 1998). These algorithms are currently being tested on databases of three-dimensional MRI and high-resolution cryosection volumes with the goal of detecting structural

abnormalities in schizophrenia (Moussai et al., 1998) and in neurodegenerative disorders such as AD (Figures 5.4–5.6) (Thompson et al., 1997, 1998b; Mega et al., 1998).

In summary, group-specific patterns of brain structure may go unnoticed in individual subjects or groups owing to extreme variations in anatomy between subjects. Population-based brain atlases, however, linked with appropriate warping algorithms can incorporate extensive regional information on structural variability and show great promise in identifying group trends and characteristics, especially in disease states.

Conclusion

Extreme variations in callosal anatomy are found in normal and diseased populations. These variations complicate the design of systems to detect callosal anomalies in disease and to clarify associations between callosal structure and sex, handedness, and a variety of behavioral and cognitive factors.

In this chapter we have reviewed the perplexing variety of methods that are available for analyzing callosal structure. In view of the controversy over callosal differences and their determinants, probabilistic reference systems based on large human populations may help to identify group-specific patterns of callosal structure, providing a sample size appropriate to investigate subtle effects. Anatomical models can be combined with anatomically driven elastic transformations that associate homologous brain regions in a database of anatomical data. These strategies provide the ability to perform morphometric comparisons and correlations in three dimensions between a given subject's MR scan and a population database or between population subgroups stratified according to relevant clinical and/or demographic criteria.

In many ways, static representations of brain structure are ill suited to analyzing the dynamic processes of brain development and disease. The inherently changing morphology complicates attempts to compare callosal anatomy across subjects and groups, and interaction effects between age, sex, and other demographic factors are also observed. The intense interest in brain development and disease mandates the design of mathematical systems to track anatomical changes over time and map dynamic patterns of growth or degeneration. In this chapter we introduced an approach to mapping patterns of growth at the callosum, emphasizing the regional complexity of growth patterns over a prolonged period.

In the near future, brain-mapping techniques will provide the ability to map growth and degeneration in their full spatial and temporal complexity. In spite of the logistic and technical challenges, these mapping approaches hold tremendous promise for representing, analyzing, and understanding the extremely complex dynamic processes that affect regional anatomy in the healthy and diseased brain.

ACKNOWLEDGMENTS Paul Thompson was supported by the U.S. Information Agency, under Grant G-1-00001, by a Fellowship of the Howard Hughes Medical Institute, and by a research grant from the U.S.-U.K. Fulbright Commission, London. Additional support was provided by research grants from the National Library of Medicine (LM/MH05639), the National Science Foundation (BIR 93-22434), and the NCRR (RR05956) and by a Human Brain Project grant to the International Consortium for Brain Mapping, which is funded jointly by NIMH and NIDA (P20 MH/DA52176). Special thanks go to our colleagues Michael Mega, Jay Giedd, Roger Woods, David MacDonald, Colin Holmes, Keith Worsley, Alan Evans, and John Mazziotta, whose advice and support have been invaluable in these investigations.

REFERENCES

ABOITIZ, F., E. RODRIGUEZ, R. OLIVARES, and E. ZAIDEL, 1996. Age-related changes in fiber composition of the human corpus callosum: Sex differences. *NeuroReport* 7:1761–1764.

ABOITIZ, F., A. B. SCHEIBEL, R. S. FISHER, and E. ZAIDEL, 1992a. Fiber composition of the human corpus callosum. *Brain Res.* 598 (1–2):143–153.

ABOITIZ, F., A. B. SCHEIBEL, R. S. FISHER, and E. ZAIDEL, 1992b. Individual differences in brain asymmetries and fiber composition in the human corpus callosum. *Brain Res.* 1992 598:154–161.

ALLEN, L. S., and R. A. GORSKI, 1990. Sex difference in the bed nucleus of the stria terminalis of the human brain. *J. Comp. Neurol.* 302 (4):697–706.

ALLEN, L. S., M. HINES, J. E. SHRYNE, and R. A. GORSKI, 1989. Two sexually dimorphic cell groups in the human brain. *J. Neurosci.* 9 (2):497–506.

ALLEN, L. S., M. F. RICHEY, Y. M. CHAI, and R. A. GORSKI, 1991. Sex differences in the corpus callosum of the living human being. *J. Neurosci.* 11 (4):933–942.

AMIT, Y., U. GRENANDER, and M. PICCIONI, 1991. Structural image restoration through deformable templates. *J. Am. Stat. Assoc.* 86 (414):376–386.

ANDREASEN, N. C., S. ARNDT, V. SWAYZE, T. CIZADLO, M. FLAUM, D. O'LEARY, J. C. EHRHARDT, and W. T. C. YUH, 1994. Thalamic abnormalities in schizophrenia visualized through magnetic resonance imaging. *Science* 266:294–298.

ANDREASEN, N. C., D. S. O'LEARY, T. CIZADLO, S. ARNDT, K. REZAI, L. L. PONTO, G. L. WATKINS, and R. D. HICHWA, 1996. Schizophrenia and cognitive dysmetria: A positron emission tomography study of dysfunctional prefrontal-thalamic-cerebellar circuitry. *Proc. of the Natl. Acad. Sci. U.S.A.* 93:18:9985–9990.

ARMSTRONG, E., 1990. *Evolution of the Brain: The Human Nervous System.* San Diego, Calif.: Academic Press.

ARNOLD, S. E., B. T. HYMAN, J. FLORY, A. R. DAMASIO, G. W. VAN HOESEN, 1991. The topographical and neuroanatomical distribution of neurofibrillary tangles and neuritic plaques in the cerebral cortex of patients with Alzheimer's disease. *Cereb. Cortex* 1:103–116.

ASHBURNER, J., P. NEELIN, D. L. COLLINS, A. C. EVANS, and K. J. FRISTON, 1997. Incorporating prior knowledge into image registration. *Neuroimage* 6 (4):344–352.

BARKOVICH, A. J., and B. O. KJOS, 1988. Normal postnatal development of the corpus callosum as demonstrated by MR imaging. *Am. J. Neuroradiol.* 9:487–491.

BARKOVICH, A. J., and D. NORMAN, 1988. Anomalies of the corpus callosum: correlation with further anomalies of the brain. *Am. J. Neuroradiol.* 9:493–501.

BARTA, P. E., R. E. POWERS, E. H. AYLWARD, G. A. CHASE, G. J. HARRIS, P. V. RABINS, L. E. TUNE, and G. D. PEARLSON, 1997. Quantitative MRI changes in late onset schizophrenia and Alzheimer's disease compared to normal controls. *Psychiatry Res.* 68:65–75.

BARTLEY, A. J., D. W. JONES, E. F. TORREY, J. R. ZIGUN, and D. R. WEINBERGER, 1993. Sylvian fissure asymmetries in monozygotic twins: A test of laterality in schizophrenia. *Biol. Psychiatry* 34:853–863.

BAUMGARDNER, T. L., H. S. SINGER, M. D. DENCKLA, B. S. RUBIN, B. A. ABRAMS, M. J. COLLI, and A. L. REISS, 1996. Corpus callosum morphology in children with Tourette syndrome and attention deficit hyperactivity disorder. *Neurology* 47:477–482.

BEATON, A. A., 1997. The relation of planum temporale asymmetry and morphology of the corpus callosum to handedness, gender and dyslexia: A review of the evidence. *Brain Lang.* 60:255–322.

BEIGON, A., J. L. EBERLING, B. C. RICHARDSON, M. S. ROOS, S. T. WONG, B. R. REED, and W. J. JAGUST, 1994. Human corpus callosum in aging and Alzheimer's disease: A magnetic resonance imaging study. *Neurobiol. Aging* 15 (4):393–397.

BELL, A. D., and S. VARIEND, 1985. Failure to demonstrate sexual dimorphism of the corpus callosum in childhood. *J. Anat.* 143:143–147.

BIGELOW, L. B., H. A. NASRALLAH, and F. P. RAUSHER, 1983. Corpus callosum thickness in chronic schizophrenia. *Arch. Gen. Psychiatry* 142:284–287.

BISHOP, K. M., and D. WAHLSTEN, 1997. Sex differences in the human corpus callosum: Myth of reality? *Neurosci. Biobehav. Rev.* 21:581–601.

BLACK, S. E., C. SZEKELY, J. P. SZALAI, D. KIDRON, D. YU, J. PARKER, B. BUCK, P. STANCHEV, and M. BRONSKILL, 1996. Can MRI brain measures distinguish Alzheimer's disease from normal aging?, Poster Presentation, Second International Conference on Functional Mapping of the Human Brain, June 17–21, 1996, Boston, MA, *NeuroImage* 3 (3):S476.

BLACKER, D., M. S. ALBERT, S. S. BASSETT, R. C. GO, L. E. HARRELL, and M. F. FOLSTEIN, 1994. Reliability and validity of NINCDS-ADRDA criteria for Alzheimer's disease. The National Institute of Mental Health Genetics Initiative, *Arch. Neurol.* 51 (12):1198–1204.

BLEIER, R., 1985. *Sex Differences Research in the Neurosciences: Science or Belief?* Society of Neuroscience Address, Dallas, Texas.

BOGEN, J. E., E. D. FISHER, and P. J. VOGEL, 1965. Cerebral

commissurotomy: A second case report. *J.A.M.A.* 194 (12):1328–1329.

BOGERTS, B., 1997. The temporolimbic system theory of positive schizophrenia symptoms. *Schizophr. Bull.* 23 (3):423–434.

BOOKSTEIN, F., 1989. Principal warps: Thin-plate splines and the decomposition of deformations. *IEEE Trans. Pattern Analysis and Machine Intelligence* 11 (6):567–585.

BOOKSTEIN, F. L., 1997. Landmark methods for forms without landmarks: Morphometrics of group differences in outline shape. *Med. Image Anal.* 1 (3):225–243.

BRAAK, H., and E. BRAAK, 1991. Neuropathological staging of Alzheimer-related changes. *Acta Neuropathol.* 82:239–259.

BROWN, J. W., and J. JAFFE, 1975. Hypothesis on cerebral dominance. *Neuropsychologia* 13:107–110.

BROWN, R., N. COLTER, J. CORSELLIS, T. J. CROW, C. D. FRITH, K. JANGOE, E. C. JOHNSTON, and C. MARSH, 1986. Postmortem evidence of structural brain changes in schizophrenia. *Arch. Gen. Psychiatry* 43:36–42.

BRUN, A., and E. ENGLUND, 1981. Regional pattern of degeneration in Alzheimer's Disease: Neuronal loss and histopathologic grading. *Histopathology* 5:549–564.

BUCHANAN, R. W., J. R. STEVENS, and W. T. CARPENTER, 1998. The neuroanatomy of schizophrenia: Editor's introduction. *Schizophr. Bull.* 23 (3):365–366.

BURKE, H. L., and R. A. YEO, 1994. Systematic variations in callosal morphology: The effects of age, gender, hand preference, and anatomic asymmetry. *Neuropsychology* 8:563–571.

BYNE, W., R. BLEIER, and L. HOUSTON, 1988. Variations in human corpus callosum do not predict gender: A study using magnetic resonance imaging. *Behav. Neurosci.* 102 (2):222–227.

CAO, J., and K. J. WORSLEY, 1999. The geometry of the hotelling's T-squared random field with applications to the detection of shape changes. *Ann. Statist.* 27:925–942.

CAPITANI, E., S. DELLA SALA, and H. SPINNLER, 1990. Controversial neuropsychological issues in Alzheimer's disease: Influence of onset-age and hemispheric asymmetry of impairment. *Cortex* 26 (1):133–145.

CARLSON, M., F. EARLS, and R. D. TODD, 1988. The importance of regressive changes in the development of the nervous system: Towards a neurobiological theory of child development. *Psychiatr. Dev.* 1:1–22.

CARPENTER, W. T., R. W. BUCHANAN, B. KIRKPATRICK, C. TAMMINGA, and F. WOOD, 1993. Strong inference, theory testing, and the neuroanatomy of schizophrenia. *Arch. Gen. Psychiatry* 50:825–831.

CASSANOVA, M. F., R. D. SANDERS, T. E. GOLDBERG, L. B. BIGELOW, G. CHRISTISON, E. F. TORREY, and D. R. WEINBERGER, 1990. Morphometry of the corpus callosum in monozygotic twins discordant for schizophrenia: A magnetic resonance imaging study. *J. Neurol. Neurosurg. Psychiatry* 53:416–421.

CHRISTENSEN, G. E., R. D. RABBITT, and M. I. MILLER, 1993. A deformable neuroanatomy textbook based on viscous fluid mechanics. In *Proceedings of the 27th Annual Conference on Information Sciences and Systems*, pp. 211–216.

CHRISTENSEN, G. E., R. D. RABBITT, and M. I. MILLER, 1996. Deformable templates using large deformation kinematics. *IEEE Trans. Image Processing* 5 (10):1435–1447.

CHUGANI, H. T., M. E. PHELPS, and J. C. MAZZIOTTA, 1987. Positron emission tomography study of human brain functional development. *Ann. Neurol.* 22:487–497.

CLARKE, J. M., and E. ZAIDEL, 1994. Anatomical-behavioral relationships: Corpus callosum morphometry and hemispheric specialization. *Behav. Brain Res.* 64:185–202.

CLARKE, S., R. KRAFTSIK, H. VAN DER LOOS, and G. M. INNOCENTI, 1989. Forms and measures of adult and developing human corpus callosum. *J. Neuropathol. and Exp. Neurol.* 280:213–230.

COFFEY, C. E., W. E. WILKINSON, I. A. PARASHOS, S. A. SOADY, R. J. SULLIVAN, L. J. PATTERSON, G. S. FIGIEL, M. C. WEBB, C. E. SPRITZER, and W. T. DJANG, 1992. Quantitative cerebral anatomy of the aging human brain: A cross-sectional study using magnetic resonance imaging. *Neurology* 42 (3):527–536.

COGER, R. W., and E. A. SERAFETINIDES, 1990. Schizophrenia, corpus callosum, and interhemispheric transfer: A review. *Psychiatr. Res.* 34:163–184.

COLE, M., and S. R. COLE, 1993. *The Development of Children.* New York: Scientific American Books.

COLEMAN, P. D., and D. G. FLOOD, 1987. Neuron numbers and dendritic extent in normal aging and Alzheimer's disease. *Neurobiol. Aging* 8:521–545.

COLOMBO, C., A. BONFANTI, S. LIVIAN, M. ABBRUZZESE, and S. SCARONE, 1993. Size of the corpus callosum and auditory comprehension in schizophrenics and normal controls. *Schizophr. Res.* 11 (1):63–70.

CORDER, E. H., V. JELIC, H. BASUN, L. LANNFELT, S. VALIND, B. WINBLAD, and A. NORDBERG, 1997. No difference in cerebral glucose metabolism in patients with Alzheimer disease and differing apolipoprotein E genotypes. *Arch. Neurol.* 54 (3):273–277.

CROW, T. J., 1998. Temporolimbic or transcallosal connections: Where is the primary lesion in schizophrenia and what is its nature. *Schizophr. Bull.* 23 (3):521–523.

CUÉNOD, C. A., A. DENYS, J. L. MICHOT, P. JEHENSON, F. FORETTE, D. KAPLAN, A. SYROTA, and F. BOLLER, 1993. Amygdala atrophy in Alzheimer's disease: An in vivo magnetic resonance imaging study. *Arch. Neurol.* 50:941–945.

CUNNINGHAM, D. J., 1892. Contribution to the surface anatomy of the cerebral hemispheres, Cunningham Memoirs. *R. Irish Acad.* 7:372.

DAVATZIKOS, C., 1996. Spatial normalization of 3D brain images using deformable models. *J. Comput. Assist. Tomogr.* 20 (4):656–665.

DAVATZIKOS, C., and J. L. PRINCE, 1996. Convexity analysis of active contour problems. In *Proceedings of CVPR, San Francisco*, June 17–20, 1996.

DAVATZIKOS, C., M. VAILLANT, S. M. RESNICK, J. L. PRINCE, S. LETOVSKY, and R. N. BRYAN, 1996. A computerized approach for morphological analysis of the corpus callosum. *J. Comput. Assist. Tomogr.* 20 (1):88–97.

DAVID, A. S., 1987. Tachistoscopic tests of colour naming and matching in schizophrenia: Evidence for posterior callosum dysfunction? *Psychol. Med.* 17 (3):621–630.

DAVID, A. S., 1994. Schizophrenia and the corpus callosum: Developmental, structural and functional relationships. *Behav. Brain Res.* 164:203–211.

DAVID, A. S., C. MINNE, P. JONES, I. HARVEY, and M. A. RON, 1995. Structure and function of the corpus callosum in schizophrenia: What's the connection? *Eur. Psychiatry* 10:28–35.

DAVIDSON, R. J., and K. HUGDAHL, 1994. *Brain Asymmetry.* Cambridge, Mass.: MIT Press.

DAVIS, P. C., S. S. MIRRA, and N. ALAZRAKI, 1994. The brain in older persons with and without dementia: Findings on

MR, PET and SPECT Images [Review Article]. *Am. J. Radiol.* 162:1267–1278.

DeCarli, C., C. L. Grady, C. M. Clark, D. A. Katz, D. R. Brady, D. G. Murphy, J. V. Haxby, J. A. Salerno, J. A. Gillette, A. Gonzalez-Aviles, and S. I. Rapoport, 1996. Comparison of positron emission tomography, cognition, and brain volume in Alzheimer's disease with and without severe abnormalities of white matter. *J. Neurol. Neurosurg. Psychiatry* 60 (2):158–167.

Degreef, G., B. Bogerts, P. Falkai, B. Greve, G. Lantos, M. Ashtari, and J. Leiberman, 1992. Increased prevalence of the cavum septum pellucidum in magnetic resonance scans and post-mortem brains of schizophrenic patients. *Psychiatry Res.* 45:1–13.

DeLacoste, M. C., J. B. Kirkpatrick, and E. D. Ross, 1985. Topography of the human corpus callosum. *J. Neuropathol. Exp. Neurol.* 44 (6):578–591.

DeLacoste-Utamsing, M. C., and R. L. Holloway, 1982. Sexual dimorphism in the human corpus callosum. *Science* 216:1431–1432.

Delaère, P., C. Duyckaerts, J. P. Brion, V. Poulain, and J. J. Hauw, 1989. Tau, paired helical filaments and amyloid in the neocortex: A morphometric study of 15 cases with graded intellectual status in aging and senile dementia of Alzheimer type. *Acta Neuropathol. (Berl.).* 77 (6): 645–653.

DeLisi, L. E., I. D. Dauphinais, and P. Hauser, 1989. Gender differences in the brain: Are they relevant to the pathogenesis of schizophrenia? *Comp. Psychiatry* 30:197–208.

DeLisi, L. E., A. L. Hoff, C. Neale, and M. Kushner, 1994. Asymmetries in the superior temporal lobe in male and female first-episode schizophrenic patients: Measures of the planum temporale and superior temporal gyrus by MRI. *Schizophr. Res.* 12:19–28.

DeLisi, L. E., M. Sakuma, W. Tew, M. Kushner, A. L. Hoff, and R. Grimson, 1997. Schizophrenia as a chronic active brain process: A study of progressive brain structural change subsequent to the onset of schizophrenia. *Psychiatry Res.* 74 (3):129–140.

DeLisi, L. E., W. Tew, S. Xie, A. L. Hoff, M. Sakuma, M. Kushner, G. Lee, K. Shedlack, A. M. Smith, and R. Grimson, 1995. A prospective follow-up study of brain morphology and cognition in first-episode schizophrenic patients: Preliminary findings. *Biol. Psychiatry* 38:349–360.

Demeter, S., J. L. Rongo, and R. W. Doty, 1985. Sexual dimorphism of the human corpus callosum? *Soc. Neurosci. Abstr.* 11:868.

Denenberg, V. H., A. Kertesz, and P. E. Cowell, 1991. A factor analysis of the human's corpus callosum. *Brain Res.* 548 (1–2):126–132.

DeQuardo, J. R., F. L. Bookstein, W. D. Green, J. A. Brunberg, and R. Tandon, 1996. Spatial relationships of neuroanatomic landmarks in schizophrenia. *Psychiatry Res.* 61:81–95.

Di Patre, P. L., 1990. Cytoskeletal alterations might account for the phylogenetic vulnerability of the human brain to Alzheimer's disease. *Med. Hypotheses* 34:165–170.

Diamond, A., 1990. The development and neural basis of higher cognitive functions. Annals of the New York Academy of Sciences, 608:267–317.

Ditchfield, H., and D. R. Hemsley, 1990. Interhemispheric transfer of information and schizophrenia. *Eur. Arch Psychiatry Neurol. Sci.* 239:309–313.

DiVirgilio, G., and S. Clarke, 1997. Direct interhemispheric visual input to human speech areas. *Hum. Brain Mapp.* 5 (5):347–354.

Doraiswamy, P. M., G. S. Figiel, M. M. Husain, W. M. McDonald, S. A. Shah, O. B. Boyko, E. H. Ellinwood, and K. R. R. Krishnan, 1991. Aging of the human corpus callosum: Magnetic resonance in normal volunteers. *J. Neuropsychiatry Clin. Neurosci.* 3:392–397.

Duara, R., A. Kushch, K. Gross-Glenn, W. W. Barker, B. Jallad, S. Pascal, D. A. Loewenstein, J. Sheldon, M. Rabin, and B. Levin, 1991. Neuroanatomic differences between dyslexic and normal readers on magnetic resonance imaging scans. *Arch. Neurol.* 48:410–416.

Eberstaller, O., 1884. Zür oberflachen anatomie der grosshirn hemisphaeren. *Wien. Med. Bl.* 7:479, 642, 644.

Eidelberg, D., and A. M. Galaburda, 1982. Symmetry and asymmetry in the human posterior thalamus: I. Cytoarchitectonic analysis in normal persons. *Arch. Neurol.* 39 (6):325–332.

Erkinjuntti, T., D. H. Lee, F. Gao, R. Steenhuis, M. Eliasziw, R. Fry, H. Merskey, V. C. Hachinski, 1993. Temporal lobe atrophy on magnetic resonance imaging in the diagnosis of early Alzheimer's disease. *Arch. Neurol.* 50 (3):305–310.

Evans, A. C., W. Dai, D. L. Collins, P. Neelin, and S. Marrett, 1991. Warping of a computerized 3D atlas to match brain image volumes for quantitative neuroanatomical and functional analysis. *SPIE Med. Imaging* 1445:236–247.

Feng, J. Z., and J. F. Brugge, 1983. Postnatal development of auditory callosal connections in the kitten. *J. Comp. Neur.* 214:416–426.

Ferrario, V. F., C. Sforza, G. Serrao, T. Frattini, and C. del Favero, 1996. Shape of the human corpus callosum in childhood: Elliptic Fourier analysis on midsagittal magnetic resonance scans. *Invest. Radiol.* 31 (1):1–5.

Flaum, M., V. W. Swayze, D. S. O'Leary, W. T. C. Yuh, J. C. Ehrhardt, S. V. Arndt, and N. C. Andreasen, 1995. Effects of diagnosis, laterality, and gender on brain morphology in schizophrenia. *Am. J. Psychiatry* 152:5704–5714.

Frangou, S., T. Sharma, T. Sigmudsson, P. Barta, G. Pearlson, and R. M. Murray, 1997. The Maudsley Family study: 4. Normal planum temporale asymmetry in familial schizophrenia: A volumetric MRI study. *Br. J. Psychiatry* 170:230–233.

Freeborough, P. A., R. P. Woods, and N. C. Fox, 1996. Accurate registration of serial 3D MR brain images and its application to visualizing change in neurodegenerative disorders, *J. Comput. Assist. Tomogr.* 20 (6):1012–1022, Nov. 1996.

Freedman, M., and M. L. Albert, 1985. Subcortical dementia. In *Handbook of Clinical Neurology: Neurobehavioral Disorders*, Vol. 46, J. A. M. Fredericks, ed. Amsterdam: Elsevier, pp. 311–316.

Friedland, R. P., and J. Luxenberg, 1988. Neuroimaging and dementia. In *Clinical Neuroimaging: Frontiers in Clinical Neuroscience*, Vol. 4, W. H. Theodore, ed. New York: Allan Liss, pp. 139–163.

Gaffney, G. R., S. Kuperman, L. Y. Tsai, S. Minchin, and K. M. Hassanein, 1987. Midsagittal magnetic resonance imaging of autism. *Br. J. Psychiatry* 151:831–833.

Galaburda, A. M., 1995. Anatomic basis of cerebral dominance. In *Brain Asymmetry*, R. J. Davidson and K. Hugdahl, eds. Cambridge, MA: MIT Press, pp. 51–73.

GALABURDA, A. M., and N. GESCHWIND, 1981. Anatomical asymmetries in the adult and developing brain and their implications for function. *Adv. Pediatr.* 28:271–292.

GALABURDA, A. M., G. D. ROSEN, and G. F. SHERMAN, 1990. Individual variability in cortical organization: Its relationship to brain laterality and implications to function. *Neuropsychologica* 28:529–546.

GAZZANIGA, M. S., 1995. Principles of human brain organization derived from split-brain studies. *Neuron* 14:217–228.

GEE, J. C., M. REIVICH, and R. BAJCSY, 1993. Elastically deforming an atlas to match anatomical brain images. *J. Comput. Assist. Tomogr.* 17 (2):225–236.

GEORGY, B. A., J. R. HESSELINK, and T. L. JERNIGAN, 1993. MR imaging of the corpus callosum. *Am. J. Radiol.* 160:949–955.

GESCHWIND, N., and A. M. GALABURDA, 1985. Cerebral lateralization: Biological mechanisms, associations and pathology. *Arch. Neurol.* 42:428–459.

GESCHWIND, N., and W. LEVITSKY, 1968. Human brain: left-right asymmetries in temporal speech region. *Science* 161:186.

GIEDD, J. N., F. X. CASTELLANOS, B. J. CASEY, P. KOZUCH, A. C. KING, S. D. HAMBURGER, and J. L. RAPAPORT, 1994. Quantitative morphology of the corpus callosum in attention deficit hyperactivity disorder. *Am. J. Psychiatry* 151:665–669.

GIEDD, J. N., J. M. RUMSEY, F. X. CASTELLANOS, J. C. RAJAPAKSE, D. KAYSEN, A. C. VAITUZIS, A. C. VAUSS, S. D. HAMBURGER, and J. L. RAPAPORT, 1996. A quantitative MRI study of the corpus callosum in children and adolescents. *Dev. Brain Res.* 91:274–280.

GOLDMAN-RAKIC, P. S., and L. D. SELEMON, 1998. Functional and anatomical aspects of prefrontal pathology in schizophrenia. *Schizophr. Bull.* 23 (3):437–458.

GÓMEZ-ISLA, T., J. L. PRICE, D. W. McKEEL, J. C. MORRIS, J. H. GROWDON, and B. HYMAN, 1996. Profound loss of layer II Entorhinal Cortex Neurons Occurs in Very Mild Alzheimer's disease. *J. Neurosci.* 16 (14):4491–4500.

GRENANDER, U., 1976. Pattern synthesis: Lectures in pattern theory. In *Applied Mathematical Sciences*, Vol. 13, New York: Springer-Verlag.

GRENANDER, U., and M. I. MILLER, 1994. Representations of knowledge in complex systems. *J. Roy. Statist. Soc. B*, 56 (4):549–603.

GUNTHER, W., R. PETSCH, R. STEINBERG, E. MOSER, P. STRECK, H. HELLER, G. KURTZ, and H. HIPPIUS, 1991. Brain dysfunction during motor activation and corpus callosum alterations in schizophrenia measured by cerebral blood flow and magnetic resonance imaging. *Biol. Psychiatry* 29:535–555.

HALLER, J. W., A. BANERJEE, G. E. CHRISTENSEN, M. GADO, S. JOSHI, M. I. MILLER, Y. SHELINE, M. W. VANNIER, and J. G. CSERNANSKY, 1997. Three-dimensional hippocampal MR morphometry with high-dimensional transformation of a neuroanatomic atlas. *Radiology* 202 (2):504–510.

HAUSER, P., I. D. DAUPHINAIS, W. BERRETTINI, L. E. DeLISI, J. GELERNTER, R. M. POST, 1989. Corpus callosum dimensions measured by magnetic resonance imaging in bipolar affective disorder and schizophrenia. *Biol. Psychiatry* 26:659–668.

HEIDRICH, A., and W. K. STRIK, 1997. Auditory P300 topography and neuropsychological test performance: Evidence for left hemispheric dysfunction in schizophrenia. *Biol. Psychiatry* 41:327–335.

HOFF, A. L., H. ROIDAN, D. O'DONNELL, P. STRITZKE, C. NEALE, A. BOCCIO, A. K. ANAND, and L. E. DeLISI, 1992. Anomalous lateral sulcus asymmetry and cognitive function in first-episode schizophrenia. *Schizophr. Bull.* 18 (2):257–270.

HOFMANN, E., T. BECKER, J. MEIXENSBERGER, M. JACKEL, M. SCHNEIDER, and H. REICHMANN, 1995. Disturbances of cerebrospinal fluid (CSF) circulation: Neuropsychiatric symptoms and neuroradiological contribution. *J. Neural Transm. Gen. Sect.* 99 (1–3):79–88.

HOLLOWAY, R. L., M. C. DE LACOSTE, 1986. Sexual dimorphism in the corpus callosum: An extension and replication study. *Human Neurobiol.* 5:87–91.

HORROBIN, D. F., A. I. GLEN, and C. J. HUDSON, 1995. Possible relevance of phospholipid abnormalities and genetic interactions in psychiatric disorders: The relationship between dyslexia and schizophrenia. *Med. Hypotheses* 45:605–613.

HUTTENLOCHER, P. R., 1990. Morphometric study of human cerebral cortex development. *Neuropsychologia* 28:517–527.

HYDE, T., M. STACEY, R. COPPOLA, S. HANDEL, K. RICKLER, and D. WEINBERGER, 1995. Cerebral morphometric abnormalities in Tourette's syndrome: A quantitative MRI study of monozygotic twins. *Neurology* 45:1176–1182.

HYND, G. W., J. HALL, E. S. NOVEY, R. T. ELIOPULOS, K. BLACK, J. J. GONZALEZ, J. E. EDMONDS, C. RICCIO, and M. COHEN, 1995. Dyslexia and corpus callosum morphology. *Arch. Neurol.* 52:32–38.

HYND, G. W., M. SEMRUD-CLIKEMAN, A. R. LORYS, E. S. NOVEY, D. ELIOPULOS, and J. LYYTINEN, 1991. Corpus callosum morphology in attention deficit hyperactivity disorder: Morphometric analysis of MRI. *J. Learn. Disabil.* 24:141–146.

INNOCENTI, G. M., 1994. Some new trends in the study of the corpus callosum. *Behav. Brain Res.* 64:1–8.

ISHII, N., Y. NISHIHARA, and T. IMAMURA, 1986. Why do frontal lobe symptoms predominate in vascular dementia with lacunes? *Neurology* 36:340–345.

IVY, G. O., and H. KILLACKEY, 1981. The ontogeny of the distribution of callosal projection neurons in rat parietal cortex. *Comp. Neurol.* 195:367–389.

JACOBSEN, L. K., GEIDD, J. N., J. C. RAJAPAKSE, S. D. HAMBERGER, A. C. VAITUZIS, J. A. FRAZIER, M. C. LENANE, and J. L. RAPAPORT, 1997. Quantitative magnetic resonance imaging of the corpus callosum in childhood onset schizophrenia. *Psychiatry Res.* 68:77–86.

JÄNCKE, L., J. F. STAIGER, G. SCHLAUG, Y. HUANG, and H. STEINMETZ, 1997. The relationship between corpus callosum size and forebrain volume. *Cereb. Cortex* 7:1047–3211.

JANOWSKY, J. S., J. A. KAYE, and R. A. CARPER, 1996. Atrophy of the corpus callosum in Alzheimer's disease versus healthy aging. *J. Am. Geriatr. Soc.* 44:798–803.

JERNIGAN, T. L., U. BELLUGI, E. SOWELL, S. DOHERTY, and J. R. HESSELINK, 1993. Cerebral morphological distinctions between Williams and Down syndromes. *Arch. Neurol.* 50:186–191.

JERNIGAN, T. L., D. P. SALMON, N. BUTTERS, and J. R. HESSELINK, 1991. Cerebral structure on MRI: Part I. Localization of age-related changes. *Biol. Psychiatry* 29:55–67.

JOHNSON, V. P., V. W. SWAYZE, Y. SATO, and N. C. ANDREASON, 1996. Fetal alcohol syndrome: Craniofacial and central nervous system manifestations. *Am. J. Med. Genet.* 61:329–339.

JOSHI, S., M. I. MILLER, and U. GRENANDER, 1998. On the

geometry and shape of brain sub-manifolds. *Int. J. Patt. Recogn. Artif. Intell.* 11:8.

KATZMAN, R., 1986. Alzheimer's disease. *N. Engl. J. Med.* 314:964.

KAUFER, D. I., B. L. MILLER, L. ITTI, L. A. FAIRBANKS, J. LI, J. FISHMAN, J. KUSHI, and J. L. CUMMINGS, 1997. Midline cerebral morphometry distinguishes frontotemporal dementia and Alzheimer's disease. *Neurology* 48 (4):978–985.

KHACHATURIAN, Z. S., 1985. Diagnosis of Alzheimer's disease. *Arch. Neurol.* 42:1097–1105.

KIDO, D. K., E. D. CAINE, M. LEMAY, S. EKHOLM, H. BOOTH, and R. PANZER, 1989. Temporal lobe atrophy in patients with Alzheimer disease: A CT study. *Am. J. Neuroradiol.* 7:551–555.

KIER, E. L., and C. L. TRUWIT, 1996. The normal and abnormal genu of the corpus callosum: An evolutionary, embryologic, anatomic and MR analysis. *Am. J. Neuroradiol.* 17:1631–1641.

KIKINIS, R., M. E. SHENTON, G. GERIG, H. HOKAMA, J. HAIMSON, B. F. O'DONNELL, C. G. WIBLE, R. W. MCCARLEY, and F. A. JOLESZ, 1994. Temporal lobe sulco-gyral pattern anomalies in schizophrenia: An in vivo MR three-dimensional surface rendering study. *Neurosci. Lett.* 182:7–12.

KILLIANY, R. J., M. B. MOSS, M. S. ALBERT, T. SANDOR, J. TIEMAN, and F. JOLESZ, 1993. Temporal lobe regions on magnetic resonance imaging identify patients with early Alzheimer's disease. *Arch. Neurol.* 50:949–954.

KLEINSCHMIDT, A., P. FALKAI, Y. HUANG, T. SCHNEIDER, G. FURST, and H. STEINMETZ, 1994. In vivo morphometry of planum temporale asymmetry in first-episode schizophrenia. *Schizophr. Res.* 12:9–18.

LAISSY, J. P., B. PATRUX, C. DUCHATEAU, D. HANNEQUIN, P. HUGONET, H. AIT-YAHIA, and J. THIEBOT, 1993. Midsagittal MR measurements of the corpus callosum in healthy subjects and diseased patients: A prospective study. *Am. J. Neuroradiol.* 14:145–154.

LAMANTIA, A. S., and P. RAKIC, 1990. Axon overproduction and elimination in the corpus callosum of the developing rhesus monkey. *J. Neurosci.* 10 (7):2156–2175.

LARSEN, J. P., T. HØIEN, and H. ÖDEGAARD, 1992. Magnetic resonance imaging of the corpus callosum in developmental dyslexia. *Cogn. Neuropsychol.* 9:123–134.

LAWRIE, S. M., and S. S. ABUKMEIL, 1998. Brain abnormality in schizophrenia. *Br. J. Psychiatry* 172:110–120.

LIM, K. O., E. V. SULLIVAN, R. B. ZIPURSKY, and A. PFEFFERBAUM, 1996. Cortical gray matter volume deficits in schizophrenia: A replication. *Schizophr. Res.* 20:157–164.

LOEWENSTEIN, D. A., W. W. BARKER, J. Y. CHANG, A. APICELLA, F. YOSHII, P. KOTHARI, B. LEVIN, and R. DUARA, 1989. Predominant left hemisphere metabolic dysfunction in dementia. *Arch. Neurol.* 46 (2):146–152.

LYOO, I. K., G. G. NOAM, K. L. CHANG, K. L. HO, B. P. KENNEDY, and P. F. RENSHAW, 1996. The corpus callosum and lateral ventricles in children with attention deficit hyperactivity disorder: A brain magnetic resonance imaging study. *Biol. Psychiatry* 40:1060–1063.

LYOO, I. K., A. SATLIN, C. K. LEE, and P. F. RENSHAW, 1997. Regional atrophy of the corpus callosum in subjects with Alzheimer's disease and multi-infarct dementia. *Psychiatry Res.* 74 (2):63–72.

MARSH, L., D. HARRIS, K. L. LIM, M. BEAL, A. L. HOFF, K. MINN, J. G. CSERNANSKY, S. DEMENT, W. O. FAUSTMAN, E. V. SULLIVAN, and A. PFEFFERBAUM, 1997. Structural magnetic resonance imaging abnormalities in men with severe chronic schizophrenia and an early are at clinical onset. *Arch. Gen. Psychiatry* 54:1104–1112.

MAZZIOTTA, J. C., A. W. TOGA, A. C. EVANS, P. FOX, and J. LANCASTER, 1995. A probabilistic atlas of the human brain: Theory and rationale for its development. *NeuroImage* 2:89–101.

MCKEEVER, W. F., T. L. JACKSON, JR., 1979. Cerebral dominance assessed by object- and color-naming latencies: Sex and familial sinistrality effects. *Brain Lang.* 17:175–190.

MCKHANN, G., D. DRACHMAN, M. FOLSTEIN, R. KATZMAN, D. PRICE, and E. M. STADIAN, 1984. Clinical diagnosis of Alzheimer's disease: Report of the NINCDS-ARDRA Work Group under the auspices of the Health and Human Services Task Force on Alzheimer's Disease. *Neurology* 34:939–944.

MEGA, M. S., P. M. THOMPSON, J. L. CUMMINGS, C. L. BACK, L. Q. XU, S. ZOHOORI, A. GOLDKORN, J. MOUSSAI, L. FAIRBANKS, G. W. SMALL, and A. W. TOGA, 1998. Sulcal variability in the Alzheimer's brain: Correlations with cognition. *Neurology* 50:145–151.

MENON, R. R., P. E. BARTA, E. H. AYLWARD, S. S. RICHARDS, D. D. VAUGHN, A. Y. TIEN, G. J. HARRIS, and G. D. PEARLSON, 1995. Posterior superior temporal gyrus in schizophrenia: Grey matter changes and clinical correlates. *Schizophr. Res.* 16:127–135.

MOUSSAI, J., B. A. ANVAR, K. L. NARR, A. F. CANNESTRA, P. M. THOMPSON, T. SHARMA, and A. W. TOGA, 1998. 3-dimensional analysis of lateral ventricles in schizophrenia. In *Proceedings of the 5th International Conference on Human Brain Mapping.* Abstract 505.

MURPHY, D. G. M., C. D. DECARLI, E. DALY, J. A. GILLETTE, A. R. MCINTOSH, J. V. HAXBY, D. TEICHBERG, M. B. SCHAPIRO, S. I. RAPOPORT, and B. HORWITZ, 1993. Volumetric magnetic resonance imaging in men with dementia of the Alzheimer Type: Correlations with disease severity. *J. Biol. Psychiatry* 34:612–621.

NASRALLAH, H. A., 1985. The unintergrated right cerebral hemispheric consciousness as alien intruder. *Comp. Psychiatry* 126:273–282.

NESTOR, P. G., M. E. SHENTON, R. W. MCCARLEY, J. HAIMSON, R. S. SMITH, B. O'DONNELL, M. KIMBLE, R. KIKINIS, and F. A. JOLESZ, 1993. Neuropsychological correlates of MRI temporal lobe abnormalities in schizophrenia. *Am. J. Psychiatry* 150:1849–1855.

NJIOKIKTJIEN, C., L. DE SONNEVILLE, and J. VAAL, 1994. Callosal size in children with learning disabilities. *Behav. Brain Res.* 64:213–218.

NOPOULOS, P., V. SWAYZE, and N. C. ANDREASEN, 1996. Patterns of brain morphology in patients with schizophrenia and large cavum septi pellucidi. *J. Neuropsychiatry Clin. Neurosci.* 8 (2):147–152.

NOPOULOS, P., I. TORRES, M. FLAUM, N. C. ANDREASEN, J. C. EHRHARDT, and W. T. C. YUH, 1995. Brain morphology in first-episode schizophrenia. *Am. J. Psychiatry* 152:1721–1723.

OPPENHEIM, J. S., J. E. SKERRY, M. J. TRAMO, and M. S. GAZZANIGA, 1989. Magnetic resonance imaging morphology of the corpus callosum in monozygotic twins. *Ann. Neurol.* 26 (1):100–104.

PAKKENBERG, H., and H. VOIGT, 1964. Brain weight of the Danes. *Acta Anat.* 56:297–307.

PANDYA, D. N., and B. SELTZER, 1986. The topography of commisural fibers. In *Two Hemispheres—One Brain: Functions of the Corpus Callosum*, F. Lepore, M. Ptito, and H. H. Jasper, eds. New York: Alan R. Liss, pp. 47–73.

PARASHOS, I. A., W. E. WILKINSON, and C. E. COFFEY, 1993. Magnetic resonance imaging of the corpus callosum: Predictors of size in normal adults. *J. Neuropsychiatry Clin. Neurosci.* 7:35–41.

PEARSON, R. C., M. M. ESIRI, R. W. HIORNS, G. K. WILCOCK, and T. P. POWELL, 1985. Anatomical correlates of the distribution of the pathological changes in the neocortex in Alzheimer disease. *Proc. Natl. Acad. Sci. U.S.A.* 82 (13):4531–4534.

PETERSON, B. S., J. F. LECKMAN, and J. S. DUNCAN, 1994. Corpus callosum morphology from magnetic resonance images in Tourette's syndrome. *Psychiatry Res. Neuroimaging* 55:85–99.

PETTY, R. G., P. E. BARTA, G. D. PEARLSON, I. K. McGILCHRIST, R. W. LEWIS, A. Y. TIEN, A. PULVER, D. D. VAUGHN, M. F. CASANOVA, and R. E. POWERS, 1995. Reversal of asymmetry of the planum temporale in schizophrenia. *Am. J. Psychiatry* 152:5:715–721.

PILOWSKY, L. S., R. W. KERWIN, and R. M. MURRAY, 1993. Schizophrenia: A neurodevelopmental perspective. *Neuropsychopharmacology* 9:83–91.

PIVEN, J., J. BAILEY, B. J. RANSON, and S. ARNDT, 1997. An MRI study of the corpus callosum in autism. *Am. J. Psychiatry* 154 (8):1051–1056.

POZZILLI, C., S. BASTIANELLO, A. PADOVANI, D. PASSAFIUME, E. MILLEFIORINI, L. BOZZAO, and C. FIESCHI, 1991. Anterior corpus callosum atrophy and verbal fluency in multiple sclerosis. *Cortex* 27 (3):441–445.

PUJOL, J., P. VENDRELL, C. JUNQUE, J. L. MARTI-VILALTA, and A. CAPDEVILA, 1992. When does human brain development end? Evidence of corpus callosum growth up to adulthood. *Ann. Neurol.* 34 (1):71–74.

RAINE, A., G. N. HARRISON, G. P. REYNOLDS, C. SHEARD, J. E. COOPER, and I. MEDDLEY, 1990. Structural and functional characteristics of the corpus callosum in schizophrenics, psychiatric controls, and in normals. *Arch. Gen. Psychiatry* 47:1060–1064.

RAJAPAKSE, J. C., J. N. GIEDD, J. M. RUMSEY, A. C. VAITUZIS, S. D. HAMBURGER, and J. L. RAPOPORT, 1996. Regional MRI measurements of the corpus callosum: A methodological and developmental study. *Brain Dev.* 18:379–388.

RAKIC, P., and P. I. YAKOVLEV, 1968. Development of the corpus callosum and cavum septi in man. *J. Comp. Neurol.* 26:100–104.

RANDALL, P. L., 1983. Schizophrenia, abnormal connection and brain evolution. *Med. Hypotheses* 1983;10:247–280.

RAO, S. M., L. BERNADIN, G. L. LEO, ET AL., 1989a. Cerebral disconnection in multiple sclerosis: Relationship to atrophy in the corpus callosum. *Arch. Neurol.* 46:918–920.

RAO, S. M., G. L. LEO, V. M. HAUGHTON, ET AL., 1989b. Correlation of MRI with neuropsychological testing in multiple sclerosis. *Neurology* 39:161–166.

RAUCH, R. A., and J. R. JINKINS, 1994. Analysis of cross-sectional area measurements of the corpus callosum adjusted for brain size in male and female subjects from childhood to adulthood. *Behav. Brain Res.* 64:65–78.

RILEY, E. P., S. N. MATTSON, E. R. SOWELL, T. L. JERNIGAN, D. F. SOBEL, K. L. JONES, 1995. Abnormalities of the corpus callosum in children prenatally exposed to alcohol. *Alcohol. Clin. Exp. Res.* 19 (5):1198–1202.

RIZZO, G., M. C. GILARDI, A. PRINSTER, F. GRASSI, G. SCOTTI, S. CERUTTI, and F. FAZIO, 1995. An elastic computerized brain atlas for the analysis of clinical PET/SPET data. *Eur. J. Nucl. Med.* 22 (11):1313–1318.

ROSSI, A., P. STRATTA, M. GALLUCCI, R. PASSARIELLO, and M. CASACCHIA, 1989. Quantification of corpus callosum and ventricles in schizophrenia with nuclear magnetic resonance imaging: A pilot study. *Am. J. Psychiatry* 146:99–101.

RUMSEY, J. M., P. ANDREASON, A. J. ZAMETKIN, T. AQUINO, A. C. KING, S. D. HAMBURGER, A. PIKUS, J. L. RAPOPORT, and R. M. COHEN, 1994. Failure to activate the left temporoparietal cortex in dyslexia: An oxygen-15 positron emission tomographic study. *Neurology* 49:527–534.

SAITOH, O., E. COURCHESNE, B. EGAAS, A. J. LINCOLN, and L. SCHREIBMAN, 1995. Cross-sectional area of the psoterior hippocampus in autistic patients with cerebellar and corpus callosum abnormalities. *Neurology* 45:317–323.

SALAT, D., A. WARD, J. A. KAYE, and J. S. JANOWSKY, 1997. Sex differences in the corpus callosum with aging. *Neurobiol. Aging* 18 (2):191–197.

SANDOR, S. R., and R. M. LEAHY, 1995. Towards automated labeling of the cerebral cortex using a deformable atlas. In *Information Processing in Medical Imaging*, Y. Bizais, C. Barillot, and R. Di Paola, eds. Dordrecht, The Netherlands: Kluwer Academic Press, pp. 127–138.

SCHAEFER, G. B., J. N. THOMPSON, J. B. BODENSTEINER, M. HAMZA, R. R. TUCKER, W. MARKS, C. GAY, and D. WILSON, 1990. Quantitative morphometric analysis of brain growth using magnetic resonance imaging. *J. Child Neurol.* 5:127–130.

SCHLAUG, G., L. JANCKE, Y. HUANG, J. F. STAIGER, and H. STEINMETZ, 1995. Increased corpus callosum size in musicians. *Neuropsychologia* 33 (8):1047–1055.

SCHRIFT, M. J., H. BANDLA, P. SHAH, and M. A. TAYLOR, 1986. Interhemispheric transfer in major psychoses. *J Nerv. Ment. Dis.* 174:203–207.

SCHRODER, J., M. S. BUCHSBAUM, B. V. SIEGEL, F. J. GEIDER, and R. NEITHAMMER, 1995. Structural and functional correlates of subsyndromes in chronic schizophrenia. *Psychopathology* 28:38–45.

SCOTT, S. A., 1993. Dendritic atrophy and remodeling of amygdaloid neurons in Alzheimer's disease. *Dementia* 4 (5):264–272.

SEMRUD-CLIKEMAN, M., P. A. FILIPEK, J. BIEDERMAN, R. STEINGARD, D. KENNEDY, P. RENSHAW, and E. BEKKEN, 1994. Attention-deficit hyperactivity disorder: Magnetic resonance imaging morphometric analysis of the corpus callosum. *J. Am. Acad. Child and Adolesc. Psychiatry* 33 (6):875–881.

SHENTON, M. E., R. KIKINIS, F. A. JOLESZ, S. D. POLLACK, M. LEMAY, C. G. WIBLE, H. HOKAMA, J. MARTIN, D. METCALF, M. COLEMAN, and R. McCARLEY, 1992. Abnormalities of the left temporal lobe and thought disorder in schizophrenia. *N. Engl. J. Med.* 327 (9):604–612.

SIEGEL, B. V., JR., L. SHIHABUDDIN, M. S. BUCHSBAUM, A. STARR, R. J. HAIER, and D. C. VALLADARES NETO, 1996. Gender differences in cortical glucose metabolism in Alzheimer's disease and normal aging. *J. Neuropsychiatry Clin. Neurosci.* 8 (2):211–214.

SMALL, G. W., J. C. MAZZIOTTA, M. T. COLLINS, L. R. BAXTER, M. E. PHELPS, M. A. MANDELKERN, A. KAPLAN, A. LA RUE, C. F. ADAMSON, L. CHANG, ET AL., 1995. Apolipoprotein E type 4 allele and cerebral glucose metabolism in relatives at risk for familial Alzheimer disease. *J.A.M.A.* 273 (12):942–947.

SMITH, R. C., R. BAUMGARTNER, and M. CALDERON, 1987. Magnetic resonance imaging studies of the brains of schizophrenic patients. *Psychiatry Res.* 20:33–46.

SOBIRE, G., F. GOUTIERES, M. TARDIEU, P. LANDRIEU, and J. AICARDI, 1995. Extensive macrogyri or no visible gyri: Distinct clinical, electroencephalographic, and genetic features according to different imaging patterns. *Neurology* 45:1105–1111.

STAIB, L. H., and J. S. DUNCAN, 1992. Boundary finding with parametrically deformable models. *IEEE Pattern Analysis and Machine Intelligence* 14 (11):1061–1075.

STEERE, J. C., and A. F. T. ARNSTEN, 1995. Corpus callosum morphology in ADHD. *Am. J. Psychiatry* 152 (7):1105.

STEIN, J. F., 1994. Developmental dyslexia, neural timing and hemispheric lateralization. *Int. J. Psychophysiology* 18:241–249.

STEINMETZ, H., J. F. STAIGER, G. SCHLAUG, Y. HUANG, and L. JANCKE, 1995. Corpus callosum and brain volume in women and men. *NeuroReport* 6 (7):1002–1004.

STEVENS, J. R., 1998. Anatomy of schizophrenia revisited. *Schizophr. Bull.* 23 (3):373–383.

STIEVENART, J. L., M. T. IBA-ZIZEN, A. TOURBAH, A. LOPEZ, M. THIBIERGE, A. ABANOU, and E. A. CABANIS, 1997. Minimal surface: A useful paradigm to describe the deeper part of the corpus callosum? *Brain Res. Bull.* 44 (2):117–124.

STRAUSS, E., B. KOSAKA, and J. WADA, 1983. The neurobiological basis of lateralized cerebral function. A review. *Hum. Neurobiol.* 2 (3):115–127.

STRAUSS, E., J. WADA, and M. HUNTER, 1994. Callosal morphology and performance on intelligence tests. *J. Clin. Exp. Neuropsychol.* 16 (1):79–83.

SULLIVAN, E. V., P. K. SHEAR, O. L. KELVIN, R. B. ZIPURSKY, and A. PFEFFERBAUM, 1996. Cognitive and motor impairments are related to gray matter volume deficits in schizophrenia. *Biol. Psychiatry* 39:234–240.

SWAYZE, V. W., N. C. ANDREASEN, J. C. EHRHARDT, W. T. YUH, R. J. ALLIGER, and G. A. COHEN, 1990. Developmental abnormalities of the corpus callosum in schizophrenia. *Arch. Neurol.* 47 (7):805–808.

SWAYZE, V. W., V. P. JOHNSON, J. W. HANSON, J. PIVEN, Y. SATO, J. N. GIEDD, D. MOSNIK, and N. C. ANDREASEN, 1997. Magnetic resonance imaging of brain anomalies in fetal alcohol syndrome. *Pediatrics* 99 (2):232–240.

TALAIRACH, J., G. SZIKLA, P. TOURNOUX, A. PROSALENTIS, M. BORDAS-FERRIER, L. COVELLO, M. IACOB, and E. MEMPHEL, 1967. *Atlas d'Anatomie Stereotaxique du Telencephale.* Paris: Masson.

TALAIRACH, J., and P. TOURNOUX, 1988. *Co-planar Stereotaxic Atlas of the Human Brain.* New York: Thieme.

TEMPLE, C. M., M. A. JEEVES, and O. O. VIARROYA, 1990. Reading in callosal agenesis. *Brain Lang.* 39 (2):235–253.

TERRY, R. D., R. DE THERESA, and L. A. HANSEN, 1987. Neocortical cell counts in normal human adult aging. *Ann. Neurol.* 21:530–539.

THIRION, J.-P., and G. CALMON, 1997. *Deformation Analysis to Detect and Quantify Active Lesions in 3D Medical Image Sequences.* INRIA Technical Report 3101.

THIRION, J.-P., S. PRIMA, and S. SUBSOL, 1998. Statistical analysis of dissymmetry in volumetric medical images. *Med. Image Anal.* 4(2):111–121.

THOMPSON, P. M., J. N. GIEDD, R. E. BLANTON, C. LINDSHIELD, R. P. WOODS, D. MACDONALD, A. C. EVANS, and A. W. TOGA, 1998a. Growth patterns in the developing human brain detected using continuum-mechanical tensor maps and serial MRI. Proc. 4th International Conference on Functional Mapping of the Human Brain, Montreal, Canada, June 1998.

THOMPSON, P. M., D. MACDONALD, M. S. MEGA, C. J. HOLMES, A. C. EVANS, and A. W. TOGA, 1997. Detection and mapping of abnormal brain structure with a probabilistic atlas of cortical surfaces. *J. Comput. Assist. Tomogr.* 21 (4):567–581.

THOMPSON, P. M., J. MOUSSAI, A. A. KHAN, S. ZOHOORI, A. GOLDKORN, M. S. MEGA, G. W. SMALL, J. L. CUMMINGS, and A. W. TOGA, 1998b. Cortical variability and asymmetry in normal aging and Alzheimer's disease. *Cereb. Cortex.* 8:492–509, Sept.–Oct. 1998.

THOMPSON, P. M., C. SCHWARTZ, and A. W. TOGA, 1996a. High-resolution random mesh algorithms for creating a probabilistic 3D surface atlas of the human brain. *NeuroImage* 3:19–34.

THOMPSON, P. M., C. SCHWARTZ, R. T. LIN, A. A. KHAN, and A. W. TOGA, 1996b. 3D statistical analysis of sulcal variability in the human brain. *J. Neurosci.* 16 (13):4261–4274.

THOMPSON, P. M., and A. W. TOGA, 1996. A surface-based technique for warping 3-dimensional images of the brain. *IEEE Trans. Med. Imaging* 15 (4):1–16.

THOMPSON, P. M., and A. W. TOGA, 1997. Detection, visualization and animation of abnormal anatomic structure with a deformable probabilistic brain atlas based on random vector field transformations [paper, with video sequences on CD-ROM with journal issue]. *Med. Image Anal.* 1 (4):271–294.

THOMPSON, P. M., and A. W. TOGA, 1998. *3D Brain Image Matching Using a Concept from General Relativity.* Technical Report, UCLA Laboratory of Neuro Imaging.

TOGA, A. W., 1998. *Brain Warping.* New York: Academic Press.

TOGA, A. W., and P. M. THOMPSON, 1998. An introduction to brain warping. In *Brain Warping,* Toga A. W., ed. New York: Academic Press.

TOGA, A. W., P. M. THOMPSON, and B. A. PAYNE, 1996. Modeling morphometric changes of the brain during development. In *Developmental Neuroimaging: Mapping the Development of Brain and Behavior,* R. W. Thatcher, G. R. Lyon, J. Rumsey, and N. Krasnegor, eds. New York: Academic Press.

TOMLINSON, B. E., G. BLESSED, and M. ROTH, 1968. Observations of the brains of nondemented old people. *J. Neurol. Sci.* 7:331–356.

UEMATSU, M., and H. KAIYA, 1988. The morphology of the corpus callosum in schizophrenia: An MRI study. *Schizophr. Res.* (1):391–398.

VERMERSCH, P., J. ROCHE, M. HAMON, C. DAEMS-MONPEURT, J. P. PRUVO, P. DEWAILLY, and H. PETIT, 1996. White matter magnetic resonance imaging hyperintensity in Alzheimer's disease: Correlations with corpus callosum atrophy. *J. Neurol.* 243 (3):231–234.

VON HOFSTEN, C., 1984. Developmental changes in the organization of prereaching movements. *Dev. Psychol.* 20:369–382.

WADDINGTON, J. L., 1993. Neurodynamics of abnormalities in cerebral metabolism and structure in schizophrenia. *Schizophr. Bull.* 19:55–58.

WAHLUND, L. O., G. ANDERSSON-LUNDMAN, H. BASUN, O. ALMKVIST, K. S. BJORKSTEN, J. SAAF, and L. WETTERBERG, 1993. Cognitive functions and brain structures: A quantitative study of CSF volumes on Alzheimer patients and healthy control subjects. *Magn. Reson. Imaging* 11 (2):169–174.

WALDEMAR, G., 1995. Functional brain imaging with SPECT in normal aging and dementia: Methodological, pathophysiological, and diagnostic aspects. *Cerebrovasc. Brain Metabolism Rev.* 7 (2):89–130.

WANG, P. P., S. DOHERTY, J. R. HESSELINK, and U. BELLUGI, 1992. Callosal morphology concurs with neurobehavioral and neuropathological findings in two neurodevelopmental disorders. *Arch. Neurol.* 40:407–411.

WEINBERGER, D. R., 1995. From neuropathology to neurodevelopment. *Lancet* 346:552–557.

WEIS, S., M. KIMBACHER, and E. WEGNER, 1993. Morphometric analysis of the corpus callosum using MR: Correlation of measurements with aging in healthy individuals. *Am. J. Neuroradiol.* 14:637–645.

WEISBROD, M., S. WINKLER, S. MAIER, H. HILL, C. THOMAS, and M. SPITZER, 1997. Left lateralized P300 amplitude deficit in schizophrenic patients depends on pitch disparity. *Biol. Psychiatry* 41:541–549.

WEST, M. J., P. D. COLEMAN, D. G. FLOOD, and J. C. TRONCOSO, 1994. Differences in the pattern of hippocampal neuronal loss in normal aging and Alzheimer's disease. *Lancet* 344:769–772.

WHITEHOUSE, P. J., D. L. PRICE, A. W. CLARK, J. T. COYLE, and M. R. DeLONG, 1981. Alzheimer's disease: Evidence for selective loss of cholinergic neurons in the nucleus basalis. *Ann. Neurol.* 10:122–126.

WILCOCK, G. K., and M. M. ESIRI, 1982. Plaques, tangles and dementia: A quantitative study. *J. Neurol. Sci.* 56:343–356.

WITELSON, S. F., 1985. The brain connection: The corpus callosum is larger in left-handers. *Science* 229 (4714):665–668.

WITELSON, S. F., 1989. Hand and sex differences in the isthmus and genu of the human corpus callosum: A postmortem morphological study. *Brain* 112:799–835.

WITELSON, S. F., 1991. Sex differences in neuroanatomical changes with aging. *N. Engl. J. Med.* 325 (3):211–212.

WITELSON, S. F., and D. L. KIGAR, 1992. Sylvian fissure morphology and asymmetry in men and women: Bilateral differences in relation to handedness in men. *J. Comp. Neurol.* 323:326–340.

WOODRUFF, P. W. R., I. C. McMANUS, and A. S. DAVID, 1995. Meta-analysis of corpus callosum size in schizophrenia. *J. Neurol. Neurosurg. Psychiatry* 58:457–461.

WOODRUFF, P. W. R., G. D. PEARLSON, M. J. GEER, P. E. BARTA, and H. D. CHILCOAT, 1993. A computerized imaging study of corpus callosum morphology in schizophrenia. *Psychol. Med.* 23:45–56.

WOODRUFF, P. W. R., M. L. PHILLIPS, T. RUSHE, R. C. WRIGHT, R. M. MURRAY, and A. S. DAVID, 1997. Corpus callosum size and inter-hemispheric function in schizophrenia. *Schizophr. Res.* 23:189–196.

WOODS, R. P., J. C. MAZZIOTTA, and S. R. CHERRY, 1993. Automated image registration. In *Quantification of Brain Function. Tracer Kinetics and Image Analysis in Brain PET*, K. Uemura et al., eds. New York: Elsevier Science Publishers, pp. 391–398.

WORSLEY, K. J., 1994a. *Quadratic Tests for Local Changes in Random Fields with Applications to Medical Images.* Technical Report 94-08, Department of Mathematics and Statistics, McGill University, Montreal, Quebec, Canada.

WORSLEY, K. J., 1994b. Local maxima and the expected Euler characteristic of excursion sets of chi-squared, F and t fields. *Adv. Appl. Probability* 26:13–42.

YAKOVLEV, P. I., A. R. LECOURS, 1967. *Regional Development of the Brain.* Oxford, Engl.: Blackwell.

YAMANOUCHI, H., S. SUGIURA, and H. SHIMADA, 1990. Loss of nerve fibres in the corpus callosum of progressive subcortical vascular encephalopathy. *J. Neurol.* 237 (1):39–41.

YOSHII, F., Y. SHINOHARA, and R. DUARA, 1990. Cerebral white matter bundle alterations in patients with dementia of Alzheimer type and patients with multi-infarct dementia: Magnetic resonance imaging study. *Rinsho Shinkeigaku* 30 (1):110–112.

EDITORIAL COMMENTARY 1
New Insights in Callosal Anatomy and Morphometry

ERAN ZAIDEL AND MARCO IACOBONI

The section on the anatomy of the corpus callosum is divided in two main parts: one devoted to anatomical studies of the corpus callosum in animals and humans and one devoted to morphometric studies of the human corpus callosum. The section opens with a chapter by Innocenti and Bressoud on development and computational properties of callosal axons. Innocenti and Bressoud look at callosal axon morphology in order to understand callosal computations. With the use of modern three-dimensional computerized reconstruction of axonal branching and simulations studies on conduction velocity, they provide data that are extremely useful to physiologists and psychologists interested in callosal transmission time. With their overview on corticotopic callosal mapping, they provide compelling evidence for a view of the corpus callosum that goes beyond the classical point-to-point intra-areal mapping. The coexistence of diverging and converging patterns of callosal axons suggests that information, whatever it is at the neural level, is thoroughly shuffled by callosal axons in the cortical areas receiving callosal input. This pattern is typically observed in diffuse networks of fairly homogeneous cells that are generally associated with associative memory and models the theory of cell assemblies (Palm, 1982; Braitenberg and Schuz, 1991). With their elegant overview of developmental changes in the corpus callosum, Innocenti and Bressoud indicate the extrinsic and intrinsic factors that are known to be effective on those changes. They also underline that much work needs to be done to better define the mechanisms producing the exuberance and retraction of callosal fibers during

ERAN ZAIDEL   Department of Psychology, University of California at Los Angeles, Los Angeles, California.
MARCO IACOBONI   Ahmanson Lovelace Brain Mapping Center, Neuropsychiatric Institute, Brain Research Institute, David Geffen School of Medicine, University of California at Los Angeles, Los Angeles, California.

development. Ptito's and Rosen's commentaries on Innocenti and Bressoud provide further insights into two such factors: early damage to the cortical plate and the absence of visual input.

Aboitiz and colleagues look also at temporal changes in the organization of callosal fibers. They study the effect of aging on callosal fibers in the two sexes and also propose an evolutionary theory on the role of the corpus callosum. Further, they look at the relationships between corpus callosum and laterality, studying hemispheric asymmetries in relation to callosal fiber composition. This has been done by assuming a rather precise topographical organization of callosal fibers in the human corpus callosum. This assumption is challenged by Stephanie Clarke in her commentary. She proposes that, with the exception of the splenium and rostrum, the topographical arrangement of callosal fibers is complex and not orderly.

Jäncke and Steinmetz explore the relationships between brain size and callosal morphology and morphometry. They find that the relationship between callosal size and brain size is best captured by a geometric rule. They interpret their findings as supporting the hypothesis of Ringo and colleagues, which suggests that hemispheric specialization arises in species with large brains because interhemispheric transfer in large brains would be too slow for online processing.

In his commentary, Jeffrey Clarke discusses the relation between morphometric measures and anatomical factors, such as neuronal density in the cortex or axonal density in the corpus callosum. Clarke underlines how still unclear are the relationships between gross morphological measures and finer anatomical details and how, without this information, it is difficult to understand the significance of some morphometric studies.

Finally, the chapters by Bookstein and by Thompson and colleagues demonstrate how modern imaging techniques can address aspects of variability across popu-

131

lations or statistical measurements of shape variations that were impossible with classic morphometric approaches.

We next turn to a more in-depth consideration of some issues associated with inferring callosal function from callosal structure in humans.

From anatomy to behavior

Our ultimate goal is to understand the function of the human corpus callosum. But the experimental arsenal for studying the microphysiology of the corpus callosum is still limited. The method of choice is still ERP (see the next section). The application of TMS methodology has been useful but limited (e.g., Pascual-Leone, Walsh, and Rothwell, 2000), recording from depth electrodes during behavior is still in its infancy (cf. Fried, MacDonald, and Wilson, 1997), and PET methodology still has crude spatial resolution that prevents a precise regional analysis.

One unique data set comes from recording electrical activity on the exposed cortex while stimulating different points on the midsagittal callosum area during callosal section for epilepsy (Chen, 1986). Behavioral methods for studying callosal function are better developed for sensorimotor integration through the corpus callosum (witness the Poffenberger paradigm) than for cognitive and control functions (see Part III). There remains the anatomy of the corpus callosum, visualized by ever improving methodology of brain imaging. But how do we analyze the structure of the corpus callosum? And how do we study its structure/function relationship? The standard approach has been to analyze the size and shape of the midsagittal cross-section of the corpus callosum. But analysis of the structure of the corpus callosum off the midsagittal plane and volumetric measures of the corpus callosum may have differential functional organizational significance. They are likely to receive increased morphometric attention in the next decade.

Consider the anatomical approach. Two questions immediately arise: what to measure and how to measure it.

The partitioning problem

It is natural to conceive of the corpus callosum as a collection of function-specific channels. But how do we define them? One logical way is by the cortical modules that the channels interconnect. In principle we can trace such cortico-cortical connections with retrograde degeneration staining methods, but such studies are scarce in humans (see S. Clarke's commentary in this section). A complementary source of data are behavioral discon-

nection effects associated with localized callosal lesions. Another approach is by the regional morphology of callosal fibers. This is the approach taken by Aboitiz and his associates. They classified callosal axons by their size and myelination and showed a differential distribution of different fiber types in different callosal regions, thus supporting the channel doctrine. Small-diameter fibers that interconnect association cortex predominate in anterior and posterior callosal regions, whereas large-diameter myelinated fibers predominate in the body of the callosum. This leaves open two critical questions. First, which fibers interconnect homotopic areas and which interconnect heterotopic areas? Aboitiz and colleagues focus their discussion on the functional significance of homotopic connections, but S. Clarke challenges this. Thus, she challenges the channel doctrine, with the possible exception of the genu and the splenium. Second, the anatomy does not tell us which callosal fibers serve to facilitate interhemispheric transfer and which serve to inhibit or modulate it.

A third approach to decomposition is by factor analysis of regional size differences in the corpus callosum. This has the advantage that the data themselves, rather than our preconceptions, generate the hypothesis. The rationale is that callosal regions that are functionally independent vary more across individuals than do regions that are functionally homogeneous. This, in turn, may reflect differential developmental trajectories for different callosal channels. This approach has been applied to callosal area but not yet to callosal shape, where points of maximum change may signal regional boundaries. Factor analysis of regional size has not been rewarding about function (cf. Cowell, this section; Clarke, 1990). Clarke (1990) partitioned 60 corpus callosum into 30 radial regions. Principal component analysis of absolute area measures revealed one main factor associated with overall callosum size. Principal component analysis of areas normalized for total callosum size revealed two main factors. The first factor includes the anterior half of the corpus callosum without the rostrum. This region contains fibers that originate primarily from the frontal lobes. It is surprising that the factor does not distinguish a subregion associated with motor functions from a subregion associated with prefrontal, executive functions. The second factor, including the posterior midbody, may be associated with somesthetic functions (Pandya, Dye, and Butters, 1971). Clarke studied the correlations of these two callosum factors with behavioral laterality effects observed in a set of multimodal tests that tap hemispheric specialization and callosal connectivity in vision, audition, somesthesis, and language. Out of 44 correlations, the only significant one (negative) was between the left-hand condition of a roughness discrimination test and the anterior callosal factor normalized for total callosal area (see below). Clarke also administered a battery of cognitive tests that measured handedness, visual, perception, verbal production, memory, and executive functions. There were no significant correlations between any of the cognitive measures and the two factors. Thus, this anatomical-behavioral approach to callosum partitioning was not successful.

Note that Clarke's factor analytic approach assumes that functionally unitary regions of the callosum form a continuous surface, with no holes. This might not be the case. For example, sensorimotor integration appears to be controlled by a frontal premotor-inferior parietal circuit, which has strong callosal connections (Iacoboni, Woods, and Mazziota, 1998). It is not known whether the interhemispheric connections of the circuit are implemented through a single channel that sends both homotopic and heterotopic projections to parietal and frontal areas or whether the connection consists of two or more noncontiguous channels.

A fourth approach is to partition the corpus callosum by its behavioral correlates. The idea is to obtain callosum morphometry and behavioral laterality measures tests for many subjects and intercorrelate them to find which behaviors are associated with which regions. There is a dual rationale for this approach. First, behavioral tests of transfer of information in a specific modality or a specific code should be associated with a specific callosum channel. Unfortunately, this assumption is not likely to be true, at least for sensorimotor fibers. That is because Aboitiz and his associates (see their chapter in this section) found that regional callosum size is not correlated with the number of large-diameter myelinated fibers that interconnect primary sensorimotor cortex. The assumption may be valid for small-diameter fibres and more abstract codes, although our understanding of abstract callosum channels is rudimentary.

The second rationale for the function/structure correlations is the hypothesis that anatomical-functional asymmetry of cortical modules is inversely related to the degree of connectivity of the callosal channels that interconnect the modules. This hypothesis was first articulated by Geschwind and Galaburda (e.g., Galaburda and Geschwind, 1980). It has received support from anatomical studies in animals (Rosen, Sherman, and Galaburda, 1989), from anatomical studies in humans (Aboitiz et al., 1992b, and chapter in this section), and from behavioral studies in humans (Clarke, 1990; Clarke and Zaidel, 1994). The chapter by Aboitiz and colleagues is distinguished by bringing an evolutionary perspective to bear on this issue. One particular hypothesis discussed by Aboitiz and colleagues and due to

Ringo and colleagues (1994) posits that as brain grows in size through phylogeny, callosal connectivity decreases owing to increased distance, and this, in turn, leads to increased hemispheric specialization. The chapter by Jäncke and Steinmetz in this section cites data in support of this hypothesis.

The standard partition

The most commonly used scheme for partitioning the human corpus callosum is due to Witelson: the anterior third (genu and rostrum), the anterior and posterior body (middle third), the isthmus (the anterior fifth of the posterior third), and the splenium (the remainder of the posterior third). This scheme defines callosal regions as proportions of linear length and is undoubtedly partly arbitrary. But on the basis of clinical partial disconnection syndromes, the visual function of the splenium, the auditory function of the isthmus, and the motor and somatosensory functions of the anterior and posterior midbody, respectively, are fairly well established (Bogen, 1993). The isthmus also seems to be associated with linguistic (lexical semantic) transfer (Clarke and Zaidel, 1994). Phonetic information may be transferred through more anterior callosum channels (Clarke and Zaidel, 1994; Berman, Mandelkern, Phan, and Zaidel, submitted). More abstract codes, such as generalization sets, may also be mediated by anterior callosal channels that interconnect frontal modules (Sidtis et al., 1981).

Aboitiz and colleagues (this section) analyze the morphological correlates of the standard partition. Jäncke and Steinmetz, in turn, analyze its psychometric features, especially its relationship to brain size. Let us approximate the midsagittal cross section of the corpus callosum in the cortex by a rectangle in circle, and let us approximate the cortex by a sphere. Then the area of the corpus callosum is proportional to r^2, and the volume of the brain is proportional to r^3. Thus, (1) $CC = c_1 r^2$ and (2) $V = c_2 r^3$, where CC = corpus callosum area, V = cortical volume, and c_1 and c_2 are constants. Solving for r in (2) and substituting in (1), we get $CC = c_3 V^{2/3}$, where c_3 is a constant. As the brain—that is, r—grows, the area of the corpus callosum grows more slowly than the volume of the cortex. Thus, the ratio of CC to V is larger in smaller brains, such as those of females. This confounding factor needs to be avoided in studies of individual differences or development and aging, in which brain size is known to vary.

The chicken and the egg

Is the size of the corpus callosum associated with interhemispheric connectivity and/or with hemispheric specialization? Some studies assume group differences in corpus callosum connectivity or behavioral asymmetry and seek morphometric confirmation in the corpus callosum. This is especially common with sex and handedness differences. While there is a consensus that handedness differences in hemispheric specialization are real, with left-handers showing decreased asymmetry and more bilateral functional representation, there is less information about handedness effects in callosal connectivity. The consensus is much less clear in the case of sex differences. While it is true that males are more likely to show lateral differentiation (interaction with lateralized sensory field in a behavioral laterality experiment) than females (Zaidel et al., 1995), they are not always more lateralized. Other studies find group differences in callosum morphometry and conclude that the groups differ in hemispheric specialization and/or callosal connectivity. This iterative mutual bootstrapping dance between group differences in behavioral asymmetries and in regional callosum morphometry is a valid scientific maneuver as long as we are aware of it.

Hemispheric specialization versus callosal connectivity

What possible relationships could exist between the asymmetry of cortical modules and the connectivity of the channels that interconnect them? We distinguish two general hypothesis:

1. The developmental/organizational hypothesis states that increased specialization is associated with decreased callosal connectivity as specified genetically and implemented perinatally through callosal pruning (cf. Geschwind and Galaburda, 1985). This hypothesis applies to direct-access tasks (Zaidel, 1983), that is, to behavioral tasks that are processed independently in the two hemispheres and thus admit of degrees of specialization.

2. The functional/activational hypothesis states that regional callosal size is related to implicit or explicit cognitive transfer (not sensory) or to callosal inhibition/shielding. The reason that regional callosal size is unlikely to be related to sensory transfer is that Aboitiz found no correlation between regional callosal size and the density of large-diameter myelinated fibers that mediate sensory/motor transfer (Aboitiz et al., 1992a, and this volume). When the callosal channel serves to facilitate the transfer of cognitive information, we expect a positive correlation between the anatomical size of the channel and the behavioral measure of transfer or a negative correlation with the behavioral laterality effect. When the callosal channel serves to shield one hemisphere from the other by inhibiting cognitive interhemispheric exchange, we may expect a positive correlation

between the anatomical size of the channel and the behavioral laterality effect.

ANATOMICAL ASYMMETRY VERSUS REGIONAL CALLOSAL MORPHOLOGY Aboitiz and colleagues (1992b) analyzed the regional fiber structure and Sylvian fissure asymmetry in 20 postmortem brains, 10 male and 10 female. There were no sex differences in either Sylvian fissure asymmetry or the regional fiber composition. However, there was a negative correlation between Sylvian fissure asymmetry and the total number of fibers (mostly small and unmyelinated) in the isthmus of males and in the anterior splenium of females. This suggests a sexual dimorphism in the relationship between hemispheric specialization and callosal connectivity.

BEHAVIORAL LATERALITY AND INTERHEMISPHERIC TRANSFER VERSUS REGIONAL CALLOSAL MORPHOMETRY Clarke (1990, Clarke and Zaidel, 1994) analyzed midsagittal callosal morphometry and behavioral laterality/interhemispheric transfer in 60 students, male and female, left- and right-handed. His behavioral measures included tasks differing in sensory modality (visual, auditory, tactile) and in level of cognitive processing: (1) lateralized shape (Vanderplas) discrimination, within and between VFs; (2) lateralized texture discrimination, within and between hands; (3) lateralized lexical decision with associative priming, where primes and targets occur in the same or opposite visual fields (VFs); and (4) dichotic listening to consonant-vowel syllables, which requires callosal relay of the left ear (LE) signal from the right hemisphere to the left hemisphere before phonetic analysis. Thus, each task includes intrahemispheric and interhemispheric components. Tasks 1, 2, and 3 are direct access, capable of being processed independently in each hemisphere, whereas task 4 is callosal relay, exclusively specialized in the left hemisphere.

The results are summarized in Table 1 on page 233. The shape discrimination task showed no laterality effect but yielded a positive correlation between the (insignificant) laterality effect (left–right) and the size of the callosal midbody. The texture discrimination task also showed no significant laterality effect but a positive correlation between the laterality effect and the anterior third as well as the midbody of the CC. The interhemispheric conditions of both tasks did not correlate with any callosal region. Clarke and Zaidel (1994) proposed that tasks that show weak specialization, such as these visual and tactile tests, are sensitive to individual attentional bias asymmetries mediated by the anterior corpus callosum. Left-hemisphere-biased individuals would tend to be associated with larger anterior callosa and right-biased individuals with smaller anterior callosa.

The dichotic listening test showed a right ear advantage (REA) but no correlation of this behavioral laterality effect and any callosal region. The right ear (RE) score, associated with callosal relay, did not correlate with regional callosal morphometry. However, the RE score correlated negatively with anterior third of the corpus callosum. This is consistent with both the developmental hypothesis and the inhibitory functional hypothesis.

The lexical decision task revealed a right visual field advantage (RVFA), which did not correlate with any region of the corpus callosum. Again, the interhemispheric priming condition did not correlate with any region of the corpus callosum. However, there was a negative correlation between the RVFA for associated prime-target pairs and the size of the isthmus, and this was significant only for males. This result parallels the anatomical findings of Aboitiz and colleagues (1992b, and this volume). It suggests a role for the isthmus in bilateral language processing.

In these data, the presence of a behavioral laterality effect (found only for the dichotic listening and lexical decision tasks) did not imply the presence of a correlation between that effect and callosal morphometry (found only for the visual shape and tactile tasks), arguing against a general version of the ontogenetic callosal-elimination hypothesis of Galaburda, Rosen, and Sherman (1990). Additionally, an individual difference (sex or handedness) in a behavioral laterality effect does not imply the same individual difference in callosal morphometry or in the relationship between anatomy and behavior. Finally, when significant correlations between behavioral laterality effects and callosal morphometry do occur, they can involve different corpus callosum regions for different tasks.

In sum, the absence of any significant relationships between callosal morphometry and performances on the interhemispheric conditions of our tasks suggests that corpus callosum size is not a reliable index of individual differences in interhemispheric transfer of sensory information. Instead, the behavioral laterality-callosal morphometry findings that were significant point to a relationship between corpus callosum size and higher-order "associative" functions of the corpus callosum. We have proposed that these functions may include (1) interhemispheric support of bilateral language representation, (2) interhemispheric inhibitory control, and (3) interhemispheric influences that contribute to hemispheric differences in arousal (Clarke and Zaidel, 1994).

BEHAVIORAL LATERALITY VERSUS INTERHEMISPHERIC TRANSFER Some behavioral laterality experiments incorporate both intrahemispheric and interhemispheric components. If a task is direct access, that is, can be pro-cessed independently in each hemisphere, the specialization-connectivity hypothesis may predict that these two components should be negatively correlated. This presupposes that transfer is cognitive, that is, between the hemispheric modules that identify the stimuli, rather than sensory, through different, "earlier," callosal channels. We have studied two tasks with evidence for a nonsensory transfer component so that they make good candidates for testing the hypothesis.

The first task is the "bilateral lexical decision," with lateralized targets and lexical distractors in the opposite VF (see above). Recall that the task is direct access and shows an RVFA. The task also shows an interhemispheric lexicality priming (LP) effect. We know that the LP effect is not due to sensory transfer because it does not occur intrahemispherically, when both targets and primes are in the same VF (Zaidel et al., 1998). Is there a relationship between the RVFA and LP? We define the LP effect as follows: Let $\underline{XY}$ be the latency or accuracy of lexical decision, where X denotes the LVF stimulus, Y denotes the RVF stimulus, the target is underlined, and $X, Y = $ Word (W^+) or nonword (W^-). Then LP $= (\underline{W^+}W^- - \underline{W^+}W^+) + (\underline{W^-}W^+ - \underline{W^-}W^-) + (W^-\underline{W^+} - W^+\underline{W^+}) + (W^+\underline{W^-} - W^-\underline{W^-})$. In one particularly large $(N = 85)$ and well-behaved data set, we found a significant negative correlation between LP and the RVFA in accuracy, Pearson r (LP, (R − L)/(R + L)) $= -0.31$, $p = 0.0037$. However, other, smaller data sets failed to find such a relationship, suggesting that it can be modulated by individual differences.

The second task involves the bilateral distribution advantage (BDA) in the lateralized Posner-Mitchell letter-matching task by shape and by name (see Commentary 9.2 by Banich and Editorial Commentary 3). Recall that the BDA refers to an advantage of comparing two stimuli *between* the two VFs compared to *within* either VF. We interpret the BDA as reflecting an advantage of parallel processing in the two hemispheres before exchanging an abstract decision code. We posit that the BDA exists for tasks (1) that require comparison of an abstract code that can be computed in both hemispheres and (2) in which these computations are carried out in modules that have direct interhemispheric callosal connections. We term these two prerequisites for the BDA (1) the *common hemispheric code* and (2) the *privileged callosal channel* conditions.

We ran a four-item display version of the letter comparison task (Copeland, 1995; Copeland and Zaidel, 1996). This equates the perceptual load in the two conditions (within and between comparisons) and in the two hemispheres. The two targets to be compared were indicated by peripheral cues (surrounding rectangular frames). The results showed no VFA for either shape or name matching. There was no latency BDA in the shape task, but there was a significant BDA in the name task, leading to a Task (shape, name comparison) × Distribution (within, between) interaction ($p = 0.01$). When we correlated the BDA with the (insignificant) VFA, we obtained Pearson $r = -0.205$, $p = 0.378$ ($N = 21$). Thus, we could not confirm the specialization-connectivity hypothesis. Why? Possibly because the BDA is due to inhibition of intermediate computations via an anterior callosal channel that is distinct from the phonological channel that interconnects the modules that compute the final code for comparing letters by name.

All in all, the first section of the book demonstrates how dynamic is the research on callosal functions today. Our contributors agree on some general concepts of the corpus callosum but also vigorously disagree on others. For instance, on the relative importance of homotopic and heterotopic callosal connections, Innocenti and Bressoud and S. Clarke emphasize the large heterotopic contingent, whereas Aboitiz and colleagues emphasize more classically the homotopic contingent. On the topographical arrangement of callosal fibers, Aboitiz and colleagues subscribe to the canonical view of an orderly arrangement, whereas Clarke challenges this view. Concerning possible interspecies differences in callosal transmission time due to interspecies differences in brain size, Innocenti and Bressoud and Aboitiz and colleagues invoke compensatory mechanisms (such as the presence of gigantic fibers in large-brained animals) that would make the interhemispheric transmission time through callosal fibers fairly stable across species. In contrast, Jäncke and Steinmetz support the hypothesis that large-brained animals have longer interhemispheric transmission times that determine increased laterality (Ringo et al., 1994). These unsettled questions will undoubtedly generate more studies on the anatomy of the corpus callosum in the future.

REFERENCES

ABOITIZ, F., A. B. SCHEIBEL, R. S. FISHER, and E. ZAIDEL, 1992a. Fiber composition of the human corpus callosum. *Brain Res.* 598:143–153.

ABOITIZ, F., A. B. SCHEIBEL, and E. ZAIDEL, 1992b. Morphometry of the Sylvian fissure and the corpus callosum, with emphasis on sex differences. *Brain* 115:1521–1541.

BERMAN, S., M. MANDELKERN, H. PHAN, and E. ZAIDEL, submitted. Complementary hemispheric specialization for word and accent identification.

BOGEN, J. E., 1993. The callosal syndromes. In *Clinical Neuropsychology*, 3rd edition, K. M. Heilman and E. Valenstein, eds. New York: Oxford, pp. 337–407.

BRAITENBERG, V., and A. SCHUZ, 1991. *Anatomy of the Cortex: Statistics and Geometry.* New York: Springer-Verlag.

CHEN, B. H., 1986. Selective corpus callosotomy for the treatment of intractable generalized epilepsy. *Chin. J. Neurosurg.* 1:197.

CLARKE, J. M., 1990. *Interhemispheric functions in humans: Relationships between anatomical measures of the corpus callosum, behavioral laterality effects and cognitive profiles.* Unpublished doctoral dissertation, Department of Psychology, University of California, Los Angeles.

CLARKE, J. M., and E. ZAIDEL, 1994. Anatomical-behavioral relationships: Corpus callosum morphometry and hemispheric specialization. *Behav. Brain Res.* 64:185–202.

COPELAND, S. A., 1995. *Interhemispheric interaction in the normal brain: Comparisons within and between the hemispheres.* Ph.D. dissertation, Department of Psychology, University of California at Los Angeles.

COPELAND, S. A., and E. ZAIDEL, 1996. Contributions to the bilateral distribution advantage. *J. Intl. Neuropsychol. Soc.* 2:29.

FRIED, I., K. A. MACDONALD, and C. L. WILSON, 1997. Single neuron activity in human hippocampus and amygdala during recognition of faces and objects. *Neuron* 18:753–765.

GALABURDA, A. M., and N. GESCHWIND, 1980. The human language areas and cerebral asymmetries. *Rev. Med. Suisse Romande* 100:119–128.

GALABURDA, A. M., G. D. ROSEN, and G. F. SHERMAN, 1990. Individual variability in cortical organization: Its relationship to brain laterality and implications to function. *Neuropsychologica* 28:529–546.

GESCHWIND, N., and A. M. GALABURDA, 1985. Cerebral lateralization. Biological mechanisms, associations and pathology. *Arch. Neurol.* 42:428–459.

IACOBONI, I., R. P. WOODS, and J. C. MAZZIOTTA, 1998. Bimodal (auditory and visual) left frontoparietal circuitry for sensorimotor integration and sensorimotor learning. *Brain* 121:2135–2143.

PALM, G., 1982. *Neural Assemblies: An Alternative Approach to Artificial Intelligence.* New York: Springer.

PANDYA, D. N., P. DYE, and N. BUTTERS, 1971. Efferent cortico-cortical projections of the prefrontal cortex in the rhesus monkey. *Brain Res.* 31:35–46.

PASCUAL-LEONE, A., V. WALSH, and J. ROTHWELL, 2000. Transcranial magnetic stimulation in cognitive neuroscience: Virtual lesion, chronometry, and functional connectivity. *Curr. Opin. Neurobiol.* 10:232–237.

RINGO, J. L., R. W. DOTY, S. DEMETER, and P. Y. SIMARD, 1994. Time is of the essence: A conjecture that hemispheric specialization arises from interhemispheric conduction delay. *Cereb. Cortex* 4:331–343.

ROSEN, G. D., G. F. SHERMAN, and A. M. GALABURDA, 1989. Interhemispheric connections differ between symmetrical and asymmetrical brain regions. *Neuroscience* 33:525–533.

SIDTIS, J. J., B. T. VOLPE, D. H. WILSON, M. RAYPORT, and M. S. GAZZANIGA, 1981. Variability in right hemisphere language function after callosal section: Evidence for a continuum of generative capacity. *J. Neurosci.* 1:323–331.

ZAIDEL, E., 1983. Disconnection syndrome as a model for laterality effects in the normal brain. In *Cerebral Hemisphere Asymmetry: Method, Theory, and Application*, J. Hellige, ed. New York: Praeger, pp. 95–151.

ZAIDEL, E., F. ABOITIZ, J. M. CLARKE, D. KAISER, and R. MATTESON, 1995. Sex differences in interhemispheric relations for language. In *Hemispheric Communication: Mechanisms & Models*, F. Kitterle, ed. Hillsdale, NJ: Erlbaum, pp. 85–175.

ZAIDEL, E., M. IACOBONI, K. A. LAACK, B. T. CRAWFORD, and J. RAYMAN, 1998. Implicit interhemispheric lexicality priming in lateralized lexical decision. *Brain Lang.* 65:102–105.

II PHYSIOLOGICAL ASPECTS OF CALLOSAL SENSORIMOTOR INTEGRATION

6 Functions of the Corpus Callosum as Derived from Split-Chiasm Studies in Cats

MAURICE PTITO

ABSTRACT The corpus callosum, referred to as the *great cerebral commissure*, is the major set of fibers connecting the two cerebral hemispheres. Since the pioneering work of Myers and Sperry in the early 1960s, the corpus callosum has been confirmed into its role in interhemispheric transfer of sensorimotor information. This led to the development of a surgical technique known as *commissurotomy* or *split-brain*, which is aimed at reducing the interhemispheric transmission of abnormal electrical discharges in epileptic patients. Over the years, animal research has proved to be useful in delineating other visual functions of the corpus callosum using not only split-brain preparations but also animals with a section of the optic chiasm. In this review, we report previous studies that indicate that the corpus callosum is indeed involved in the interhemispheric transfer of visual information in adult cats and that this commissure is plastic, in the sense that its neonatal section does not prevent interhemispheric transfer. The corpus callosum is also involved in the midline fusion of the visual information presented to each hemisphere, thus supporting the "zipper" theory. Finally, its contribution to stereoperception based on disparity cues concerns mainly coarse stereopsis, its role being different from that of the direct geniculostriate system concerned with fine stereopsis. Chemical studies suggest that the corpus callosum exerts its influence on postsynaptic targets through excitatory amino acids such as aspartate and glutamate.

The mammalian brain consists of two symmetrical hemispheres, connected by a set of commissural fibers that cross the midline. These interhemispheric connections ensure the integrated functioning of the brain by rendering the information reaching one hemisphere accessible to the other. Among the various direct telencephalic (e.g., the anterior and hippocampal commissures), diencephalic (e.g., the interthalamic and posterior commissures), and mesencephalic (e.g., the intertectal commissure) commissures that interconnect the two hemispheres, the corpus callosum is undoubtedly the most important, not only by virtue of its size but also because of the wealth of its neural connections. What are the functions subserved by this great cerebral commissure?

In the eighteenth century the corpus callosum was considered the site of the soul (Lancisi, 1739; de la Peyronie, 1741); in the early twentieth century it was assigned the mere role of preventing the cerebral hemispheres from collapsing onto each other (Lashley, in Lassonde et al., 1994). It was only in the 1950s that the corpus callosum, in the pioneering work of Myers and Sperry, was attributed a function in the interhemispheric transfer of visual information. This was followed by the development, in the early 1960s, of a surgical intervention aimed at reducing the interhemispheric transmission of abnormal electrical discharges in epileptic patients. This involved the sectioning of the corpus callosum and other neocortical commissures, or *commissurotomy* (see Bogen and Vogel, 1962).

The study of these patients by Sperry, Gazzaniga, and collaborators has greatly contributed to our knowledge of the functions of this midline structure and has led to the description of a set of interhemispheric deficits called the *disconnection syndrome* (reviewed by Geschwind, 1965; Bogen and Vogel, 1975) followed later by discussions on the nature of consciousness (Sperry, 1986) and the duality of the mind (Bogen, 1986).

The corpus callosum is still the focus of interest for many neuroscientists who study interhemispheric communication. The development of new methods of investigation in both animals and humans has led to major

MAURICE PTITO Ecole d'Optometrie, Université de Montréal, Montreal, Quebec, Canada.

discoveries regarding the various roles of this structure such as interhemispheric transfer of lateralized information (see reviews by Berlucchi, 1972, 1977, 1981, 1990), midline fusion (see the review by Lepore et al., 1994), and, more recently, depth perception (see reviews by Ptito et al., 1986, 1991). In this chapter we review some of our work on the role of the corpus callosum in the interhemispheric transfer of visual information in adult and neonate split-brain cats, in the midline fusion of the visual information presented to each hemisphere, and in stereoperception based on disparity cues.

Anatomical considerations

With the advent of modern tract-tracing techniques, it has been possible to determine precisely the sites of origin and termination of transcallosally projecting neurons (see Rosenquist, 1985; Innocenti, 1986) as well as the trajectory of their axons through the corpus callosum (Lomber, Payne, and Rosenquist, 1994). Briefly, each hemisphere projects callosal axons not only to homologous (homotopic) areas in the contralateral hemisphere but also to heterologous (heterotopic) areas. The callosal tract consists of myelinated and unmyelinated axons with a wide range of diameters (0.08–5 μm) and conduction velocities (1.4–30 m/s) (reviewed by Innocenti, 1986). The estimate of callosal axons has radically changed since the advent of electron microscopy, which can detect small unmyelinated fibers, undetected by light microscopy studies. In the cat, for example, electron microscopy studies have reported an estimate of 23 million callosal axons, compared to the 2 million previously reported with light microscopy analysis (Innocenti, 1986). In a previous study (Tremblay et al., 1987), we examined the pattern of callosal projecting neurons in all the visual cortical areas of the cat's brain by sectioning the posterior half of the corpus callosum and exposing the cut-end axons to the retrograde tracer HRP. The results, depicted in Figure 6.1, indicate that the labeled cellular bodies were absent in area 17 and were mainly focused in the 17/18 border corresponding to the representation of the vertical meridian. The extrastriate areas exhibit a high density of callosal projections. This overall topography of the distribution of callosal cells is similar to what has been reported by Seagraves and Rosenquist (1982). More recently, Lomber and colleagues (1994), using HRP exposition to discrete severed portions of the corpus callosum, have furnished the first description of the complete cortical field that gives rise to purely callosal axons. Moreover, these authors were able to link the functional divisions of the cerebral cortex to fiber trajectory through the corpus callosum. The motor cortex sends fibers through the

rostrum and genu of the corpus callosum. The adjacent somatosensory cortex projects fibers through the anterior half of the body, whereas axons arising from auditory regions course in the posterior two-thirds of the body and the dorsal splenium, where they match the distribution of axons originating in the limbic cortex. Finally, axons from visual cortices, which occupy the greatest single fraction of the cortical mantle, pass through the largest portion of the corpus callosum; the fibers are present throughout the splenium and extend well into the body and the anterior portion. These results also indicate the presence of unimodal and multimodal regions within the rostrocaudal extent of the corpus callosum.

The corpus callosum and the other commissures in interhemispheric transfer of visual information

The anatomical organization of the visual system is such that stimuli perceived by one eye are sent simultaneously to both hemispheres. This transfer of information is accomplished through the crossed thalamocortical pathway (via the optic chiasm) and the transcallosal route. One way to study the contribution of the corpus callosum to the interhemispheric transfer of visual information is to lateralize the stimuli to one hemisphere. This can be achieved by the surgical interruption of the chiasmatic decussation (the split-chiasm preparation). Myers (1956) has shown that a cat with a split chiasm that is trained to learn a pattern discrimination task with one eye (the other being occluded) can successfully transfer the acquired discrimination to the contralateral hemisphere. A section of both the optic chiasm and the corpus callosum (the split-brain preparation) prevents any form of interocular transfer of monocularly learned visual discriminations (Figure 6.2). That each hemisphere is capable of learning a visual task independently of the other was elegantly demonstrated by Myers (1962) in the cat and Trevarthen (1962) in the monkey. A split-brain animal can learn, without any conflict, opposite discrimination tasks presented to each eye. Since these early studies, numerous experiments carried out on a number of species have largely confirmed the role of the corpus callosum in interhemispheric transfer of visual information (reviewed by Berlucchi, 1990). However, the corpus callosum is not the only commissure allowing the exchange of information between the cerebral hemispheres (see the beginning of the chapter), and it is now well accepted that the interhemispheric transfer of visual information might depend on several factors (the nature of the task, its difficulty, the level and type of motivation, and the age at surgery). In one experiment (Lepore et al., 1985), we demonstrated that the amount

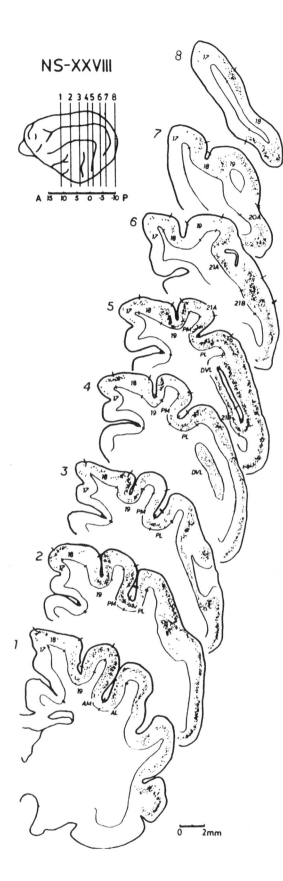

NS-XXVIII

FIGURE 6.1. Distribution of callosally transported retrograde label following the placement of horseradish peroxidase soaked gelfoam in the cut ends of the corpus callosum of a normal cat. Sections are taken at the levels indicated on the lateral view of the brain appearing in the upper left. Each black dot represents a labeled cell, and the single bars indicate the boundaries between the various visual cortical areas. AM: anteromedial; Al: anterolateral; PM: posteromedial; PL: posterolateral; DVL: dorsoventrolateral suprasylvian areas; (Adapted from Tremblay et al., 1987.)

of interhemispheric transfer of pattern discriminations in split-brain cats can be influenced by the nature of the training task (see Figure 6.3). We found that split-brain cats that were trained in a classic two-choice discrimination box with a food reward for correct responses showed no interhemispheric transfer, whereas those trained in a Lashley-type jumping stand demonstrated a rather good interocular transfer. If the type of incentive was changed (i.e., instead of a food reward for a correct response, the animals were administered a mild electric shock for an incorrect response), interhemispheric transfer was slightly improved (Figure 6.4). When the cerebral hemisphere are separated by the transection of

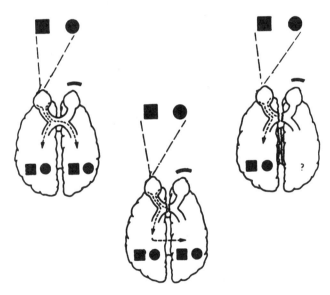

FIGURE 6.2. The split-chiasm preparation demonstrating the role of the corpus callosum in interhemispheric transfer of visual information. Left: The stimuli presented to the left eye in the split-chiasm cat (the other eye being occluded) are sent simultaneously to both hemispheres and the animal learns the discrimination. Center: When the animal is tested with the naive eye, learning is immediate; this indicates that the discrimination acquired in step 1 was probably transferred to the right hemisphere via the corpus callosum. Right: If the corpus callosum is sectioned in a split-chiasm animal (split-brain), the interocular transfer of lateralized visual presentation is abolished. (Adapted from Myers, 1962.)

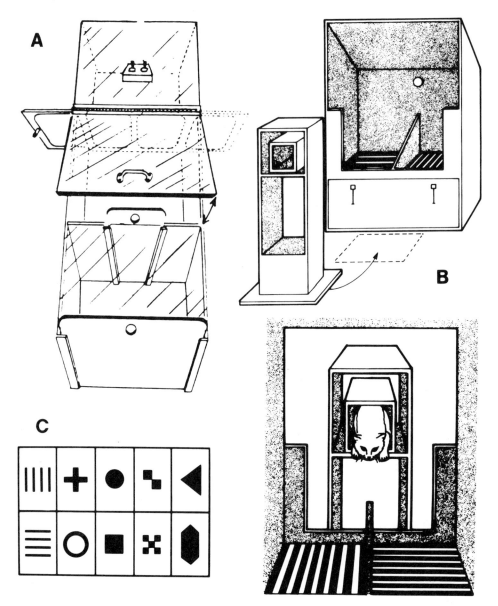

FIGURE 6.3. The two apparatus used in the experiments by Lepore and colleagues. (a) Two-choice discrimination box. The box consists of three compartments: a holding chamber, a decision corridor, and a reward chamber. The metal floor of the decision corridor is coupled with an electric shock generator. Once in the decision corridor, the animal makes its choice by pushing one of the doors on which the stimuli are affixed. A correct response leads to a food reward for animals in group 1, whereas an incorrect response is rewarded by a mild electric shock (0.4 mA for 0.5 s) for those in group 2. (b) Lashley jumping stand: The box contains two doors on which are placed the visual stimuli. The door with the correct stimulus is secured, whereas the one containing the negative stimulus gives way to the cat's weight. To make its choice, the animal has to jump from the platform onto the stimulus. An incorrect response induces the opening of the door and the fall of the animal into the underlying cavity. (c) Visual stimuli used in the various discriminations.

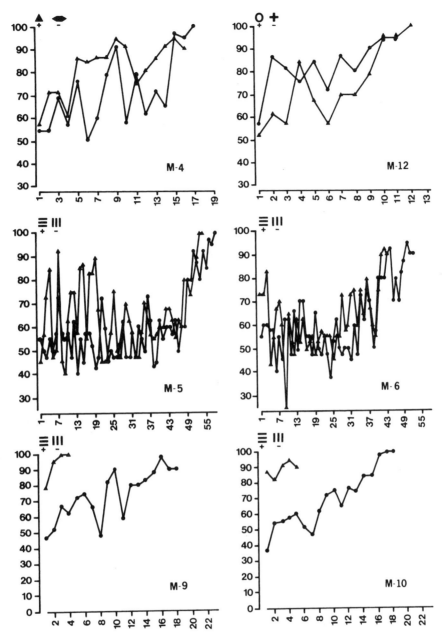

FIGURE 6.4. Learning and transfer pattern discrimination performance curves for two cats belonging to each of the three experimental groups. Solid dots: initial learning; solid triangles: transfer. Abscissa: blocks of 40 trials; Ordinate: percent of correct responses. The upper left of each figure shows the stimuli used in the discrimination, and the lower right shows the cat's number. Top: Tests carried out in the two-choice discrimination box with food reward, Center: Tests carried out in the two-choice discrimination box with aversive reward. Bottom: Tests carried out in a Lashley-type jumping stand.

both the optic chiasm and the corpus callosum, the only way for the information entering one eye to reach the contralateral hemisphere is through extracallosal commissures. The most likely candidate for such a transfer would be the intertectal commissure, although its section in otherwise intact animals does not affect interhemispheric transfer of monocularly acquired form discriminations (Berlucchi, Buchtel, and Lepore, 1978). The intertectal commissure originates in the deep layers of the superior colliculus and terminates in the same layers of the contralateral one (Edwards, 1977). Since these layers are not strictly visual in nature, they might have a role in eye and head movements. This could explain why the split-brain cats tested in the jumping stand could achieve a successful interhemispheric transfer. In this task the animals could easily perform, from the platform, eye and head movements to scan the stimuli and use the acquired bilateral oculomotor pattern as a cue to facilitate the interocular transfer. It is also possible that in the absence of the neocortical commissures, the anatomically demonstrated crossed corticotectal projections (Baleydier, 1983) could mediate the residual transfer abilities. In the split-brain monkey, an additional section of the intertectal commissure results in the abolition of any residual interhemispheric transfer (Tieman and Hamilton, 1973). In another experiment (Ptito et al., 1993), we tested the contribution of extracallosal pathways more directly using the following experimental approach: Cats first underwent the section of the left optic tract to limit the visual input to the right hemisphere. They were then tested in a two-choice discrimination box on a series of visual discriminations. Once learning criterion was achieved, the visual cortical areas of the right hemisphere were ablated (17, 18, 19, lateral suprasylvian cortex). If learning was still present, it had to be mediated by the hemisphere deafferented by the left optic tract section. This was the case in the sense that although learning was retarded, all operated animals learned the various discriminations. Finally, the corpus callosum was sectioned, and we predicted that if the animal could still learn new discriminations, the information would be conveyed to the intact hemisphere via extracallosal routes. Following this last surgery, all animals were able to learn the new discriminations (see Figure 6.5). Interestingly enough, an improvement in the learning and retention of the discriminations was also noticed. This paradoxical result can be explained by the increased use of the colliculocollicular pathway, which could convey the information from the retina to the intact visual areas of the left hemisphere. This alternative visual pathway is prevented from functioning at its optimal capacity by abnormal inputs from the lesioned right hemisphere; removal of this input through

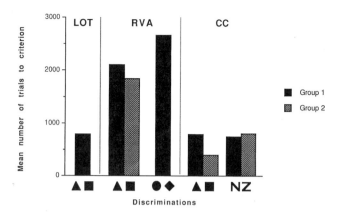

FIGURE 6.5. Bar charts illustrating the learning and retention performance for pattern discriminations following the various surgical interventions. LOT: Trials to criterion for learning a pattern discrimination following the left optic tract section in group 1. LOT + RVA: Trials to criterion after an additional lesion of the visual cortical areas of the right hemisphere for the relearning of the previously acquired pattern discrimination and learning of a new one (group 1) and for initial pattern discrimination learning (group 2). LOT + RVA + CC: Trials to criterion for the relearning of one pattern discrimination and learning of a new one following the additional section of the corpus callosum for both groups. Note the improved performance not only for the relearning of previously learned discriminations but also for learning a new one following the callosotomy. (Adapted from Ptito et al., 1993.)

callosotomy allows the left hemisphere to function more normally. In fact, the section of the intercollicular commissure in a similar surgical preparation abolishes pattern discrimination learning (Luybymov, 1965), and these latter results lend support to the involvement of extracallosal commissures in interhemispheric transfer.

Callosal plasticity and interhemispheric transfer

It is generally well accepted that cerebral lesions occurring early in life (before the so-called critical period) result in anatomical reorganization and consequently in functional recovery. Studies carried out in young patients who have undergone a callosotomy for intractable epilepsy or in patients with callosal agenesis have demonstrated the absence of the disconnection syndrome reported in commissurotomized adult patients (reviewed by Lassonde et al., 1990). The young callosotomized patients and those with callosal agenesis could perform tactile and visual interhemispheric tasks without any difficulty. These results suggest that in the absence of the corpus callosum in young individuals, extracallosal commissures could undergo anatomical reorganization and facilitate interhemispheric communication. We have tested (Ptito and Lepore, 1983) whether the interhemispheric transfer of visual information is possible

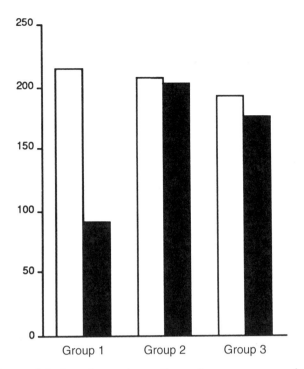

FIGURE 6.6. Learning and transfer performance curves obtained following the section of the corpus callosum in three age groups: 20 days, 45 days, and adulthood. Note that cats belonging to group 1 (20 days) show a good interocular transfer whereas those in the two other groups show no savings when tested with the naive eye, indicating the absence of interhemispheric transfer. (Adapted from Ptito and Lepore, 1983.) Abscissa: Mean number of trials to criterion; Ordinate: experimental groups (20 days, 45 days, and adults, respectively). White bars: learning; solid bars: transfer.

in callosotomized kittens. Three groups of animals were callosotomized at three different ages: group 1 at 20 days old (corresponding to the premyelinization period of the corpus callosum), group 2 at 45 days (corresponding to the postmyelinization period), and group 3 in adulthood. Subjects in groups 1 and 2 received an additional section of the optic chiasm at about 8 months of age, whereas those in group 3 were chiasmatomized at the same time as the callosotomy. All subjects were tested monocularly on various visual discriminations tasks in a two-choice discrimination box, and interhemispheric transfer was assessed. Results illustrated in Figure 6.6 indicate that cats belonging to group 1 demonstrated a good interocular transfer, although not immediate, whereas those in groups 2 and 3 did not show any savings when the nontrained eye was tested. The latter results are in agreement with many previous studies that reported a lack of interhemispheric transfer in adult split-brain animals. Moreover, the results obtained on the early callosotomized kittens support the assumption that the animals use extracallosal pathways to transfer infor-

mation from one hemisphere to the other, although it is not known at the moment which commissures are involved. The intertectal commissure, at least in cats, is for many the most likely candidate. In addition, the presence of interhemispheric communication is reminiscent of what has been reported in human subjects with callosotomy or agenesis of the corpus callosum (see Lassonde and Jeeves, 1994). This might suggest a similar process of anatomical reorganization (i.e., an increased use of extracallosal pathways also involving the anterior commissure in monkeys and humans).

Stereoperception

STUDIES ON NORMAL ADULT CATS   In the mid-nineteenth century, Wheatstone (1838), using a stereoscope, showed that not only do two bidimensional images viewed with each eye independently appear as a fused single image, but that the image is also seen in depth. This three-dimensional stereoscopic binocular vision appears to depend upon binocular retinal disparities along the horizontal axis. The neural mechanisms underlying stereoperception seem to be based on the convergence of information from the two eyes onto single cortical cells. This binocular convergence and subsequent binocular fusion are mediated by two pathways: the crossed retinothalamocortical pathway (via the optic chiasm) and the transcallosal route. Over the past few years we have carried out a series of behavioral and electrophysiological experiments to determine the contribution of each of these pathways to stereoperception (reviewed by Ptito et al., 1991). These studies were first done on normal cats to show that this species indeed possesses the neural substrates to mediate stereoperception and on cats with sections of the optic chiasm or/and the corpus callosum. A number of studies carried out on cats and monkeys (see reviews by Ptito et al. (1986, 1991) and Wang and Dreher (1996) for the cats and Poggio (1991) for the monkeys) have indicated the presence of cells in the visual cortex that are sensitive to binocular disparity. For example, using single-cell recording techniques, we have found four response profiles in area 17 of the cat that characterize cells that are differentially sensitive to stimulus disparities and that constitute 70% of all sampled neurons. The tuned excitatory disparity detectors (TEDD) and the tuned inhibitory disparity detectors (TIDD) represent cells that respond with excitation or inhibition to stimuli situated at or very close to the fixation plane (Figures 6.7a and 6.7c). The near or crossed disparity detectors and the far or uncrossed disparity detectors (UDD) are sensitive to disparities that would place the image farther in front of or behind the fixation plane (Figures 6.7b and 6.7d). It seems, moreover, that

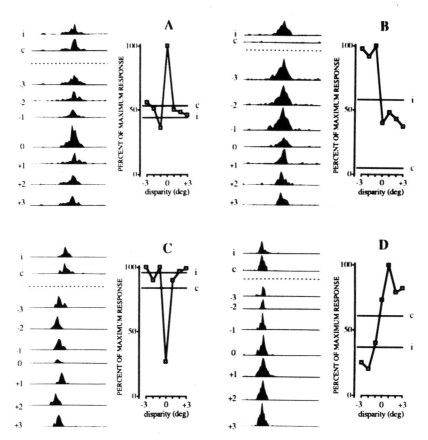

FIGURE 6.7. The four types of disparity-sensitive cells recorded in area 17–18 of normal cats. i: response of the ipsilateral only; c: response of the contralateral eye only. On the left are represented the peristimulus time histograms from which were derived the sensitivity profiles presented on the left. (a) Tuned excitatory. (b) Near cell. (c) Tuned inhibitory. (d) Far cell.

these disparity detectors are also present in area 19 of the normal cat, although more widely tuned and in lower proportion than in areas 17–18 (about 42%) (Lepore et al., 1992; Guillemot et al., 1993).

This first set of results confirmed that the cat has the necessary physiological substrates to ensure the perception of depth using fine spatial disparity as the principal cue to discrimination. At the behavioral level, the various methods used to assess this function offered only the assumption that cats could indeed have disparity-based stereopsis (since in some cases the discriminanda were not totally free of monocular cues and in others the stimuli had a configuration or form) (Ptito et al., 1986). To resolve this problem, we trained cats in visual discrimination tasks using random-dot stereograms that contained disparity cues only (Julesz, 1960). The stereograms consisted of a matrix of squares that were identical except that one of them had a rectangular region at its center in which all the elements were uniformly displaced to one side. When viewed through the appropriate filters, the rectangle appeared to float out in space in front of the background (crossed stereopsis). Two sets

of stereograms were built, one that would produce a vertical rectangle and the other a horizontal one (Figures 6.8a and 6.8b). For the animals to be able to extract the disparity information, they were equipped with special opaque lenses with a 7-mm hole in their centers on which the color filters were affixed (Figure 6.8c). The animals were trained in a two-choice discrimination box, first on a light-dark discrimination and then on two sets of pattern discriminations. One consisted of a vertical versus a horizontal bar on a white background, with dimensions equal to those of the bars of the stereograms.

The other set was made up of similar bars but drawn on a random dot surround (pseudo-stereoscopic condition). After the learning criterion was reached in each condition, the animals were subjected to the random-dot discrimination wearing the special lenses. Moreover, to ensure that the animals were using only disparity cues to perform the stereoscopic discrimination, two sets of controls were used: The stereopairs had a null disparity, and the animals were tested monocularly. Our results indicated that all cats were able to solve the random-dot problem (Figure 6.9a) and that they could extract the

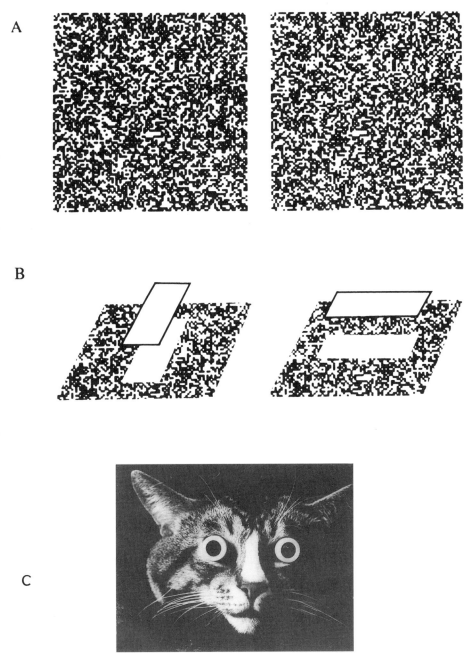

A

B

C

FIGURE 6.8. The random-dot stimuli used in the behavioral experiments. (a) Julesz random-dot stereograms the way they appear to the naked eyes. (b) Simulated effects of the virtual images in the crossed disparity condition. (c) Cat wearing the special scleral lenses. (Adapted from Ptito et al., 1991.)

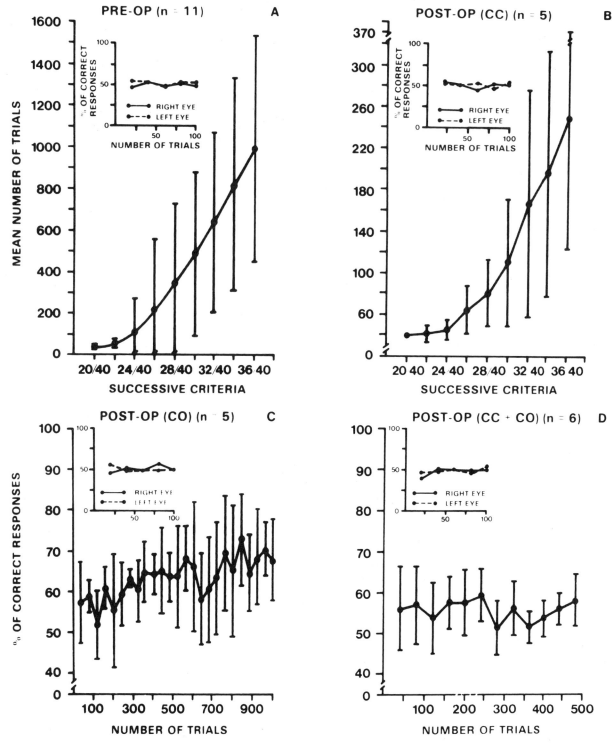

FIGURE 6.9. Performance of the cats in the random-dot discrimination task in the various experimental conditions. (a) Normal cats. (b) Following corpus callosotomy. (c) Following the transection of the optic chiasm. (d) The split-brain condition. Insets illustrate the monocular control trials. (Adapted from Ptito et al., 1986.)

figure from the background using only the disparity cues contained in the figures (inset of Figure 6.9a).

STUDIES ON SPLIT-CHIASM OR/AND SPLIT-CALLOSUM CATS
Two pathways can be used for stereopsis: (1) the crossed retinothalamocortical pathway decussating at the optic chiasm and (2) the transcallosal pathway that connects the two visual cortices. The relative contribution of these two pathways to stereopsis was measured by using cats with sections of the optic chiasm of the corpus callosum.

There are a number of indications in the literature that both systems are involved in depth perception. The absence of binocular cells, such as in strabismus, for example, leads to deficits in some forms of stereoperception. It has been shown that split-chiasm cats can still discriminate depth when tested in a jumping stand, although their performance was somewhat inferior to that of normal animals (Timney and Lansdown, 1989). Split-callosum cats were comparable to normal ones, and split-brain cats had results resembling those obtained under monocular testing. In humans, Blakemore (1970) examined a patient whose optic chiasm had been sectioned in a bicycle accident and found that this subject could still discriminate depth involving a 2° disparity. Presumably, the residual capacity is ensured by the corpus callosum. In support of this assumption, Mitchell and Blakemore (1970) found that coarse stereopsis was defective at the midline in a callosotomized subject. Similarly, Rivest and colleagues (1994) observed deficits in the estimation of the relative depth of various objects in both the central and peripheral visual fields of callosotomized and callosum-agenesis subjects. Random-dot discrimination of the crossed type was also examined in these as well as in one split-chiasm subject. All subjects showed some difficulty in extracting the pattern from the stimuli, including the split-chiasm subject, who was able to identify the stereo pattern at some of the larger disparity tested.

Because the stereodot patterns were used only in the human studies, we examined disparity-based discrimination in cats lacking one or both of these two sources of convergent inputs to determine their relative contribution to this function.

Ten normal cats that were able to solve the random-dot discrimination tasks were assigned to two groups of five subjects each. Those in the first group underwent section of the optic chiasm, and those in the second group were callosotomized. All animals were again subjected to all the steps of the preoperative training procedure: light-dark, horizontal versus vertical bars, pseudo-stereoscopic, and stereoscopic discriminations. The results illustrated in Figure 6.9b show that callosal

transection has little effect on the ability of the cats to relearn the random-dot discrimination and suggest that the corpus callosum is not involved in depth discrimination based on fine disparity cues. It might, however, as suggested by human studies, be involved in coarse stereopsis, which was not tested in the present experiment. The transection of the optic chiasm, on the other hand, had detrimental effects on the animal's ability to solve the random-dot problem. After 1000 trials, performance remained at 68%, and testing was discontinued, since there was no sign of improvement across sessions. Although the success criterion was not achieved, performance was significantly above chance, as revealed by trend analysis across the 25 blocks of 40 trials (Figure 6.9c). The deficit in performance in comparison to normal or split-chiasm cats cannot be accounted for by some eye misalignment induced by the chiasm section, since our measurements of eye alignment found it to be within normal ranges for individual subjects (Ptito et al., 1986). These results suggest that the corpus callosum can contribute to stereoperception to a limited extent and is less important than the crossed retinothalamic pathway in the resolution of fine spatial disparity.

When the animals were rendered split-brain by either the additional section of the corpus callosum in split-chiasm cats or the optic chiasm in split-callosal ones, performance in the random-dot task was completely at chance (Figure 6.9d). This confirmed the prediction that the elimination of binocular inputs to the appropriate cortical areas eliminates depth discrimination based on spatial disparity. Along the same line, our electrophysiological data on split-chiasm cats indicated that the number of binocular cells in primary visual cortex was drastically reduced, although disparity-tuned cells were still present (albeit in a reduced proportion). For example, cells sensitive to stimuli situated behind the fixation plane (far cells) were no longer found, given the fact that such stimuli would fall on the nasal hemiretinae that were deafferented by the chiasm transection. However, the proportion of the other types of disparity-sensitive cells (TEDD, TIDD, and UDD) was found to be about 22% compared to 71% in normal cats. The fact that split-chiasm cats are able to solve the random-dot discriminations can be explained by these residual disparity-sensitive cells in the primary visual cortex, although performance is rather poor given the reduced proportion of these units.

The midline fusion hypothesis

The pattern of anatomical projections of callosal neurons (see the section titled "Anatomical Considerations") suggests that one of the roles played by the

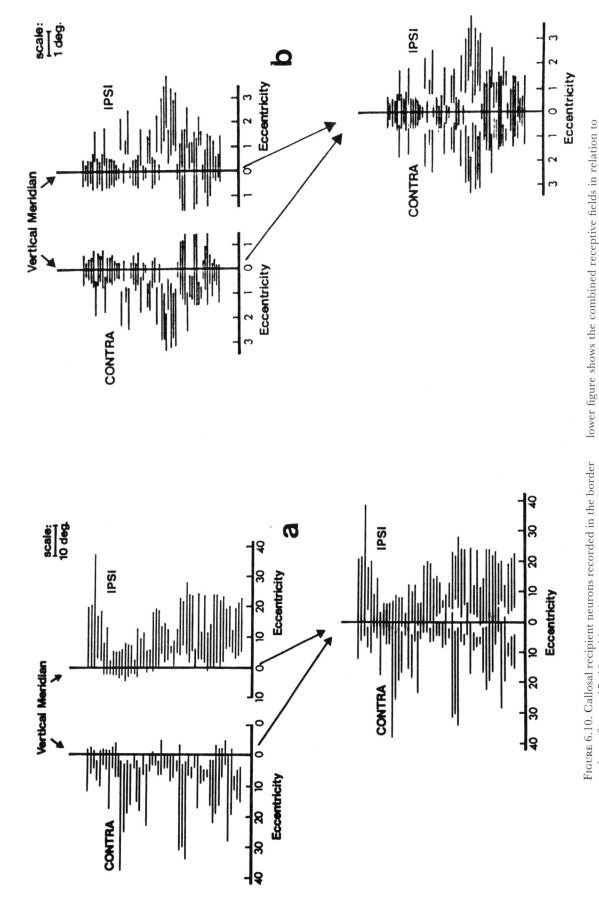

FIGURE 6.10. Callosal recipient neurons recorded in the border regions of areas 17–18 and lateral suprasylvian area and their relationship with the vertical meridian. Each horizontal line represents the mediolateral extent of each receptive field. (a) Areas 17–18. (b) Suprasylvian area. The upper figure illustrates the monocular fields of the binocular units, and the lower figure shows the combined receptive fields in relation to the vertical meridian. (Adapted from Lepore et al., 1986.) For the ectosylvian cortex the receptive fields are located at the same position in regards to the vertical meridian (not shown; see Ptito et al., 1987).

corpus callosum is the unification of both hemifields, thus ensuring the continuity of images through the midline. The cortical areas receiving (afferent) or sending (efferent) callosal inputs are those where the vertical meridian is represented. Electrophysiological studies have continuously supported the "midline fusion hypothesis" (reviewed by Lepore et al., 1986). By using the split-chiasm preparation, it is possible to record single units in the cortical areas where there is a representation of the vertical midline such as the 17/18 border (the suprasylvian cortex and the ectosylvian cortex) (see Figure 6.10). With this preparation, any unit which could still be activated through each eye (binocular cell) receives an ipsilateral geniculocortical input and a contralateral callosal input. In our laboratory we have previously shown that about 33% of the cells situated in the border region of areas 17/18 were binocularly activated in a split-chiasm preparation (Lepore and Guillemot, 1982). The receptive properties (RF) of these binocular units (such as orientation and directional selectivity, preferred velocity, size, and elevation in visual space) did not differ for each eye. The position of the median edge of the RF determined for each eye was close to the midline abutting or straddling the vertical meridian (VM). Figure 6.10a illustrates the relationship of callosal recipient neurons recorded at the 17/18 border with the vertical meridian. All binocular units have RFs whose medial borders for each eye either abut or cross the VM. The midline fusion hypothesis seems therefore to be confirmed for the primary visual cortex. This hypothesis also seems to hold true for higher-order areas, as demonstrated in the lateral suprasylvian cortex (Antonini et al., 1983). Single-unit recordings performed in this area in split-chiasm cats showed that although many units had very large RFs, the medial border of the RFs for each eye touched or straddled the VM (Figure 6.10b). In the ectosylvian cortex (EVA), which is very remote from the classically defined visual areas and has heavy reciprocal connections with the suprasylvian cortex, the same midline rule can be applied. We have found (Ptito, Tassinari, and Antonini, 1987) that visual cells recorded in EVA of split-chiasm cats had large RFs whose median borders also touched or straddled the VM. These results indicate that all cortical visual areas that are callosally connected have their RFs close to the vertical midline (touching or crossing it) and offer evidence that one of the principal functions of the corpus callosum is to unite the two visual hemifields to ensure continuity across the midline. Directly recording the activity of callosal axons also confirmed this hypothesis, since most of the RFs obtained were situated in the vicinity of the VM (Lepore et al., 1986). Studies carried out on other sensory systems (somatosensory and auditory) indicated that both the somatosensory and auditory callosal systems are closely associated with midline functions (reviewed by Lepore et al., 1994).

Conclusion and new perspectives in corpus callosum research

The large numbers of studies carried out on the corpus callosum since the pioneering work of Myers and Sperry in the mid-1950s have largely confirmed, in various animal species including humans, the functions of the corpus callosum reported in this chapter. There is little doubt that the corpus callosum is involved in interhemispheric transfer of lateralized information, although it might share this function with other secondary commissures. It is also generally accepted that another function of this great cerebral commissure is to ensure the continuity of lateralized stimuli across the midline (the midline fusion hypothesis). The implication of the corpus callosum in the fusion of three-dimensional objects is still a matter of debate, since the electrophysiological results on the preservation of disparity sensitive cells in split-chiasm cats do not always account for the behavioral deficits observed in the discrimination of random-dot stereograms. The various anatomical, electrophysiological, and behavioral results obtained on animals are parallel to those observed in human patients with callosal deficiencies and support the notion that the corpus callosum is involved in a number of sensory and cognitive functions (see reviews by Lassonde and Jeeves, 1994). The question, however, of how the corpus callosum exerts its influence on its target hemisphere remains to be investigated. Several hypotheses originating from electrophysiological and behavioral experiments have suggested that the corpus callosum has excitatory effects (e.g., Lassonde et al., 1986), whereas some have proposed, on the contrary, an inhibitory action (Cook, 1984). Neurochemical studies in recent years have emphasized a more complex chemical architecture that led to a reconciliation of ideas suggesting that the corpus callosum exerts both excitatory and inhibitory actions on neurons in the contralateral hemisphere (see Conti and Manzoni, 1994). Indeed, several studies have furnished evidence that a number of chemicals belonging to several classes (amino acids, amines, peptides, etc.) are directly associated with callosal transmission. It has been shown that excitatory amino acids are used by the corpus callosum, of which glutamate and aspartate are the most documented. For example, hemidecortication in rats induces a decrease in glutamate levels in the contralateral hemisphere (Peinado and Mora, 1986), whereas electrical stimulation of the cat's suprasylvian cortex increases dramatically the glutamate levels in the homotopic contralateral cortex (Hicks et al., 1985). The use of tritiated transmitter compounds injected into one side of the brain and retrogradely transported to the cell body and visualized by autoradiography allowed researchers to show that the injection of D-[^{3}H] aspartate in the cortex of one hemisphere resulted in a number of labeled neurons in the contralateral hemisphere (Barbaresi et al., 1987; Elberger, 1989). With the advent of immunohistochemical techniques, not only were the latter results confirmed, but it became possible to study the morphology, the laminar distribution, and the percentage of callosally projecting axons. In the somatosensory system of cats, for example, positive immunoreactive callosally projecting neurons to anti-aspartate or anti-glutamate sera represent about half of all retrogradely labeled neurons for each antibody (Conti, Fabri, and Manzoni, 1988a, 1988b). That aspartate- and glutamate-positive neurons do project to the corpus callosum is further supported by electron microscopy immunocytochemical studies that demonstrated that many axon terminals forming synapses in the cerebral cortex are indeed glutamate- and aspartate-positive and are distributed in the layers of termination of callosal axons (see Conti and Manzoni, 1994). At the electrophysiological level, intracellular recordings from several cortical neuronal populations have shown that postsynaptic cells develop both excitatory and inhibitory postsynaptic potentials (EPSP and IPSP) in response to electrical stimulation of the callosal input (reviewed by Conti and Manzoni, 1994). It is generally agreed that most of the transcallosal EPSPs are monosynaptic (Toyama et al., 1969), and there is little evidence that this is also the case for IPSPs.

Although the reported evidence seems to point to an excitatory influence of the corpus callosum, there are some suggestions derived from neurochemical and electrophysiological studies (see above) that some callosal-projecting axons could also have inhibitory effects. This seems to be true in the developing organism, since there is an agreement that in perinatal life, the majority of callosal-projecting neurons are GABAergic inhibitory neurons. In the adult animal the results are still conflictual (see Conti and Manzoni, 1994).

In conclusion, most studies (behavioral, anatomical, physiological, and chemical) support the suggestion that the corpus callosum exerts an excitatory influence on postsynaptic targets. Since the demonstration that a proportion, albeit small, of callosally projecting neurons have axons with inhibitory effects, the debate has been reopened on the nature of the action of the corpus callosum. In fact, many neuropsychologists, on the basis of work done on brain-damaged patients, have recently proposed an inhibitory action of the corpus callosum (e.g., Cook, 1984; Jeeves, 1986).

REFERENCES

ANTONINI, A., G. BERLUCCHI, and F. LEPORE, 1983. Physiological organization of callosal connections of visual lateral suprasylvian area in the cat. *J. Neurophysiol.* 48:902–921.

BALEYDIER, C., 1983. A bilateral cortical projection to the superior colliculus in the cat. *Neurosci. Lett.* 4:9–14.

BARBARESI, P., M. FABRI, F. CONTI, and T. MANZONI, 1987. D-[3H]aspartate retrograde labelling of callosal and association neurones of somatosensory areas I and II of cats. *J. Comp. Neurol.* 263 (2):159–178.

BERLUCCHI, G., 1972. Anatomical and physiological aspects of visual functions of the corpus callosum. *Brain Res.* 37:371–392.

BERLUCCHI, G., 1977. Interazioni interemisferiche cerebrali. In *Enciclopedia del Novecento*, Vol. 2. Rome: Istituto dell'Enciclopedia Italiana, pp. 476–499.

BERLUCCHI, G., 1981. Recent advances in the analysis of the neural substrate of interhemispheric communication. In *Brain Mechanisms of Perceptual Awareness and Purposeful Behavior*, O. Pompeiano and C. Ajmone-Marsan, eds. New York: Raven Press, pp. 133–152.

BERLUCCHI, G., 1990. Commissurotomy studies in animals. In *Handbook of Neuropsychology*, Vol. 4, F. Boller and J. Grafman, eds. Amsterdam: Elsevier, pp. 9–47.

BERLUCCHI, G., M. G. BUCHTEL, and F. LEPORE, 1978. Successful interocular transfer of visual pattern discrimination in split-chiasm cats with sections of the intertectal and posterior commissures. *Physiol. Behav.* 20:331–338.

BLAKEMORE, C., 1970. Binocular depth perception and the optic chiasm. *Vision Res.* 10:43–47.

BOGEN, J. E., 1986. One brain, two brains, or both? In *Two Hemispheres—One Brain*, F. Lepore, M. Ptito, and H. H. Jasper, eds. New York: Alan Liss.

BOGEN, J. E., and P. G. VOGEL, 1962. Cerebral commissurotomy in man: Preliminary case report. *Bull. Los Angeles Neurol. Soc.* 27:169–172.

BOGEN, J. E., and P. J. VOGEL, 1975. Neurological status in the long term following complete cerebral commissurotomy. In *Les Syndromes de Deconnexion Calleuse Chez l'Homme*, F. Michel and B. Schott, eds. Lyon: Presses de l'Imprimerie JP, pp. 227–254.

CONTI, F., M. FABRI, and T. MANZONI, 1988a. Glutamate-positive cortico-cortical neurons in the somatic sensory areas I and II of cats. *J. Neurosci.* 8:2948–2960.

CONTI, F., M. FABRI, and T. MANZONI, 1988b. Immunocytochemical evidence for glutamatergic cortico-cortical connections in monkeys. *Brain Res.* 462:148–153.

CONTI, F., and T. MANZONI, 1994. The neurotransmitters and post-synaptic actions of callosally projecting neurons. *Behav. Brain Res.* 64:37–53.

COOK, N. D., 1984. Homotopic callosal inhibition. *Brain. Lang.* 23:116–125.

DE LA PEYRONIE, M., 1741. Observations par lesquelles on tâche de découvrir la partie du cerveau où l'âme exerce ses fonctions. In *Histoire de l'Académie Royale des Sciences*. Paris, pp. 199–218.

EDWARDS, S. B., 1977. The commissural projection of the superior colliculus in the cat. *J. Comp. Neurol.* 173:23–40.

ELBERGER, A. J., 1989. Selective labeling of visual corpus callosum connections with aspartate in cat and rat. *Vis. Neurosci.* 2 (1):81–85.

GESCHWIND, N., 1965. Disconnection syndromes in animals and man. *Brain* 88:237–260.

GUILLEMOT, J. P., L. RICHER, M. PTITO, and F. LEPORE, 1993. Disparity coding in the cat: A comparison between areas 17–18 and area 19. *Prog. Brain Res.* 95:179–187.

HICKS, T. P., W. D. RUWE, W. L. VEALE, and J. VEENHUIZEN, 1985. Aspartate and glutamate as synaptic transmitters of parallel visual cortical pathways. *Exp. Brain Res.* 58:421–428.

INNOCENTI, G., 1986. General organization of callosal connections in the cerebral cortex. In *Cerebral Cortex*, Vol. 5, E. G. Jones and A. Peters, eds. New York: Plenum Press, pp. 291–353.

INNOCENTI, G., 1994. Some new trends in the study of the corpus callosum. *Behav. Brain Res.* 64:1–8.

JEEVES, M. A., 1986. Callosal agenesis: neuronal and developmental adaptations. In *Two Hemispheres—One Brain*, F. Lepore, M. Ptito, and H. H. Jasper, eds. New York: Alan Liss, pp. 403–421.

JULESZ, B., 1960. Binocular depth perception of computer generated patterns. *Bell Syst. Technol. J.* 39:1001–1020.

LANCISI, M., 1739. Dissertatio altera de sede cogitantis animae. *Opera Varia* 2:104–110.

LASSONDE, M., 1986. The facilitatory influence of the corpus callosum on intrahemispheric processing. In *Two Hemispheres—One Brain*, F. Lepore, M. Ptito, and H. H. Jasper, eds. New York: Alan Liss, pp. 385–402.

LASSONDE, M., M. PTITO, and F. LEPORE, 1990. La plasticité du système calleux. *Rev. Can. Psychol.* 44:166–179.

LASSONDE, M., and M. A. JEEVES, 1994. Callosal agenesis: A natural split-brain? In *Advances in Behavioral Biology*. New York: Plenum Press, pp. 275–284.

LEPORE, F., and J. P. GUILLEMOT, 1982. Visual receptive field properties of cells innervated through the corpus callosum. *Exp. Brain Res.* 46:413–424.

LEPORE, F., A. SAMSON, M. C. PARADIS, M. PTITO, and J. P. GUILLEMOT, 1992. Binocular interaction and disparity coding at the 17–18 border: contribution of the corpus callosum. *Exp. Brain Res.* 90 (1):129–140.

LEPORE, F., M. LASSONDE, P. POIRIER, A. SCHIAVETTO, and N. VEILLETTE, 1994. The midline fusion hypothesis. In *Callosal Agenesis: A Natural Split-Brain? Advances in Behavioral Biology*, M. Lassonde and M. A. Jeeves, eds. New York: Plenum Press, pp. 155–169.

LEPORE, F., M. PTITO, and J. P. GUILLEMOT, 1986. The role of the corpus callosum in midline fusion. In *Two Hemispheres—One Brain*, F. Lepore, M. Ptito, and H. H. Jasper, eds. New York: Alan Liss, pp. 211–230.

LEPORE, F., M. PTITO, C. PROVENÇAL, S. BÉDARD, and J. P. GUILLEMOT, 1985. Le transfert interhémisphérique d'apprentissages visuels chez le chat à cerveau divisé: Effets de la situation expérimentale. *Rev. Can. Psychol.* 39 (3):400–413.

LOMBER, S. G., B. R. PAYNE, and A. ROSENQUIST, 1994. The spatial relationship between the cerebral cortex and fiber trajectory through the corpus callosum of the cat. *Behav. Brain Res.* 64:25–35.

LUYBYMOV, N. N., 1965. Relay of visual information at midbrain level. *Fed. Proc.* 24 (6):1011–1014.

MITCHELL, D. E., and C. BLAKEMORE, 1970. Binocular depth perception and the corpus callosum. *Vision Res.* 10:49–54.

MYERS, R. E., 1956. Functions of the corpus callosum in interocular transfer. *Brain* 79:358–373.

MYERS, R. E., 1962. Commissural connections between the occipital lobes of the monkey. *J. Comp. Neurol.* 68:1–16.

PEINADO, J. M., and F. MORA, 1986. Glutamic acid as a putative neurotransmitter of the interhemispheric corticocortical connections in the rat. *J. Neurochem.* 47:1598–1603.

POGGIO, G., 1991. Physiological basis of stereoscopic vision. In *Binocular Vision*, Regan, D. ed., Basingstoke, Hampshire, United Kingdom, MacMillan, Houndmills, pp. 224–238.

PTITO M., and F. LEPORE, 1983. Interocular transfer in cats with early callosal transection. *Nature* 301:513–515.

PTITO, M., F. LEPORE, and J. P. GUILLEMOT, 1991. Stereopsis in the cat: Behavioral demonstration and underlying mechanisms. *Neuropsychologia* 29 (6):443–464.

PTITO, M., F. LEPORE, M. LASSONDE, C. DION, and D. MICELI, 1986. Neural mechanisms for stereopsis in cats. In *Two Hemispheres—One Brain*, F. Lepore, M. Ptito, and H. H. Jasper, eds. New York: Alan Liss, pp. 335–350.

PTITO, M., F. LEPORE, M. LASSONDE, and J. P. GUILLEMOT, 1993. Paradoxical improvement of residual vision following corpus callosotomy in brain damaged cats. *J. Hirnforsch.* 1:43–46.

PTITO, M., G. TASSINARI, and A. ANTONINI, 1987. Electrophysiological evidence of interhemispheric connections in the anterior ectosylvian sulcus in the cat. *Exp. Brain Res.* 66:90–98.

RIVEST, J., P. CAVANAGH, and M. LASSONDE, 1994. Interhemispheric depth judgement. *Neuropsychologia* 32 (1):69–76.

ROSENQUIST, A. C., 1985. Connections of visual cortical areas in the cat. In *Cerebral Cortex*, Vol. 3: *Visual Cortex*, A. Peters and E. G. Jones, eds. New York: Plenum Press, pp. 81–117.

SEAGRAVES, M. A., and A. C. ROSENQUIST, 1982. The distribution of the cells of origin of callosal projections in cat visual cortex. *J. Neurosci.* 2:1079–1089.

SPERRY, R. W., 1986. Consciousness, personal identity and the divided brain. In *Two Hemispheres—One Brain*, F. Lepore, M. Ptito, and H. H. Jasper, eds. New York: Alan Liss, pp. 3–20.

TIEMAN, S. B., and C. R. HAMILTON, 1973. Interocular transfer in split-brain monkeys following serial disconnection. *Brain Res.* 63:368–373.

TIMNEY, B., and G. LANSDOWN, 1989. Binocular depth perception, visual acuity and visual fields in cats following neonatal section of the optic chiasm. *Exp. Brain Res.* 74:272–278.

TOYAMA, K., S. TOKASHIKI, and K. MATSUNAMI, 1969. Synaptic action of commissural impulses upon association efferent cells in cat visual cortex. *Brain Res.* 14 (2):518–520.

TREMBLAY, F., M. PTITO, F. LEPORE, D. MICELI, and J. P. GUILLEMOT, 1987. Distribution of visual callosal projection neurons in the siamese cat: An HRP study. *J. Hirnforsch.* 5:491–503.

TREVARTHEN, C. B., 1962. Double visual learning in split-brain monkeys. *Science* 86:258–259.

WANG, C., and B. DREHER, 1996. Binocular interactions and disparity coding in area 21a of cat extrastriate visual cortex. *Exp. Brain Res.* 108:252–272.

WHEATSTONE, C., 1838. Contributions to the physiology of vision. I. On some remarkable, and hitherto, phenomena of binocular vision. *Philos. Trans. R. Soc. Lond.* 128:371.

COMMENTARY 6.1

The Midline Fusion Hypothesis Is All Right But Cannot Explain All Callosal Functions

GIOVANNI BERLUCCHI

ABSTRACT The corpus callosum links at the vertical midline motor and sensory maps in the two hemispheres. In addition to this major function, there are other known or suspected callosal functions that eschew the midline fusion interpretation. Examples of such functions are (1) an involvement of the corpus callosum in visual cortex reorganization in response to distortion of visual input, (2) a callosal participation in the interhemispheric synchronization of neuronal activities putatively implicated in the cerebral representation of complex objects and events, and (3) the dependence on the corpus callosum of changes in synaptic efficacy that are thought to underlie learning and memory.

Maurice Ptito's paper centers on the hypothesis of a major role of the corpus callosum in midline fusion and the resulting functional unification of sensory and motor maps of the two hemispheres, in accordance with Sperry's principle of supplemental complementarity (see Berlucchi, 1990). Although I can hardly be expected to take issue with him on that particular view of the corpus callosum, I would like to mention a few examples suggesting (at least to me) that the "midline fusion" generalization, comprehensive and cogent as it may be, is not wide enough to subsume some newly demonstrated or suspected callosal functions.

The first example comes from the visual domain, just where the midline fusion hypothesis has received the strongest support from the experimental evidence reviewed by Ptito. Sugita (1996) has recently described a major reorganization of the primary visual cortex in macaque monkeys that were submitted to a prolonged complete inversion of the visual field by means of optical prisms. Three months after the beginning of treatment, well after the monkeys had developed a good visuomotor adaptation to their distorted optic input, some visual cortex neurons appeared to have acquired an abnormal receptive field in the ipsilateral half of the visual field, lying in a mirror position with respect to a "normal" receptive field in the contralateral half field. The important point here is that the two mirror receptive fields of these neurons did not meet each other at the vertical midline, as is typical of the bilateral receptive fields with a callosal component found in animals with normal vision. Rather, the bilateral receptive fields observed in the prism-wearing monkeys lay in mirror right and left positions several degrees away from the vertical meridian and thus were separated by a distance quite incompatible with their fusion at the midline. According to Sugita (1996), the cortical reorganization underlying the appearance of the ipsilateral abnormal receptive fields would involve a callosally mediated remapping of the visual field in extrastriate cortical areas, which would then be relayed to striate cortex by means of intrahemispheric feedback corticocortical connections. He further believes that this cortical reorganization would parallel and perhaps account for the perceptual (as opposed to visuomotor) prism adaptation. It is known that in humans the two aspects of prism adaptation can indeed be dissociated, with the experiential component lagging behind the sensorimotor component by a considerable amount of time. The interpretation of these cortical changes as an adaptation to the optic input distortion was corroborated by the disappearance of the abnormal ipsilateral receptive fields shortly after the prisms had been removed to restore normal vision. These data and their interpretation are still too preliminary to allow firm conclusions; if replicated and sustained, they would justify the inference that the callosal connections of visual cortical areas possess at least the potential for breaking the midline fusion rule by interconnecting regions of the visual field totally unrelated to the vertical meridian.

GIOVANNI BERLUCCHI Dipartimento di Scienze Neurologiche e della Visione, Sezione di Fisiologia Umana, Università di Verona, Verona, Italy.

154

The second example refers to the recent interest in fine scale synchronization between activities of distant but anatomically and functionally related neurons as a possible code for representing sensory features, objects, and events in the brain (e.g., Engel et al., 1991; König, Engel, and Singer, 1995). Selective short and long interneuronal connections are of course required for ensuring the synchronization between the components of widely distributed cell assemblies. Theoretical consideration of putative transcortical cell assemblies spanning both hemispheres (Pulvermüller and Mohr, 1996) argues for an essential role of the corpus callosum in cross-midline synchronization within such assemblies, and Singer and coworkers (Engel et al., 1991) have found that severing the callosum does indeed suppress the synchrony between visually evoked oscillatory responses of neurons of the right and left primary visual cortices of the cat. These authors (König et al., 1995) have made an explicit distinction between the synaptically powerful visual callosal influences that contribute to building up receptive fields of cortical neurons, as revealed by the midline fusion phenomena reported by Ptito, and the subtler callosal modulatory influences that become expressed in the synchronization of firing, rather than in the actual receptive field structure, of contralateral visual cortical neurons. By a serial activation of local intra-areal connections, the modulatory callosal influences should be able to spread beyond the major site of callosal fiber termination at the vertical meridian representation and thus act on the entire cortical representation of the visual field. Bullier and his coworkers have confirmed that neurons in contralateral visual cortices of the cat tend to synchronize their discharges (Nowak et al., 1995) and that interhemispheric coupling is abolished by a callosal section (Munk et al., 1995) They found the most precise synchronization with contralateral neurons that had overlapping receptive fields, that is, neurons that must have been in the vertical midline representation and were possibly connected by monosynaptic callosal connections. By contrast, the synchronization of neurons with nonoverlapping receptive fields was less precise, being probably mediated by intracortical connections driven by callosal inputs. These results therefore suggest that bilateral synchronization of neurons with receptive fields close to the midline may be effected by the same callosal connections that take part in receptive field organization, whereas bilateral synchronization of neurons with receptive fields away from the midline is based on the modulatory, probably multisynaptic influences postulated by König et al. (1995).

The final example of callosal activities that are unlikely to be accommodated by the midline fusion concept bears on the possibility that the corpus callosum actively participates to reinforcement and the establishment, rather than the mere interhemispheric transfer, of learning and memories. The electrophysiological phenomena of long-term potentiation (LTP) and long-term depression (LTD) of synaptic transmission are thought by many to index learning-related modifications of neural pathways. It has now been shown that appropriate repetitive electrical stimulation of callosal fibers in slice preparations of the rat brain can induce LTP or LTD of the excitatory synapses between these fibers and their targets in limbic periarchicortex, that is, anterior ventral (Sah and Nicoll, 1991) and posterior cingulate cortex (Hedberg and Stanton, 1995). The synaptic effects thus induced display the canonical properties of cooperativity and heterosynaptic associativity. The latter property has been demonstrated for LTD in posterior cingulate cortex by alternate repetitive stimulation of corpus callosum and subiculocingulate tract (Hedberg and Stanton, 1995). LTP of callosal synaptic transmission in rat frontal or occipital neocortex in vivo, though impossible to obtain in acute or short chronic experiments, has been induced with multiple daily sessions of high-frequency callosal stimulation performed over several days (Racine et al., 1995). Excitatory synapses made by callosal fibers on their target neurons are glutamatergic (Conti and Manzoni, 1994) and act through both AMPA and NMDA receptors (Sah and Nicoll, 1991; Kawaguchi, 1992); the latter receptors are generally regarded as being instrumental for long-term effects of synaptic modification. Particularly relevant to the hypothesis of a direct contribution of the corpus callosum to reinforcement and learning effects is the finding of an in vitro excitation of neurons in nucleus accumbens by electrical stimulation of the corpus callosum in a slice preparation in the rat (Pennartz et al., 1991). The nucleus accumbens is an important component of the ventral striatum that lies at the functional interface between the motivational limbic system and the motor systems necessary for action (Mogenson, Jones, and Yim, 1980). Reinforcement and reward effects mediated by the nucleus accumbens seem to come about through an interactive convergence of glutamatergic limbic afferents and dopaminergic brain stem inputs to accumbens neurons (Robbins and Everitt, 1996). Pennartz and coworkers' finding (1991) suggests that the input to the nucleus accumbens from the contralateral limbic cortex is conveyed by heterologous, corticosubcortical fibers of the corpus callosum. In short, the anatomical and physiological heterogeneity of the callosal connections implicitly suggests that they are involved in the interhemispheric monitoring of information at all stages of cortical processing. This implies that in addition to the relatively simple categories of sensory signals that are interhemispherically transferred according to the midline fusion rule, highly digested information involved in learning processes, memory engrams, ideas, thoughts, emotions, and motivations must also be communicated between the hemispheres by the corpus callosum and the other forebrain commissures (Berlucchi, 1990). The codes used in these communications and the rules governing them are still largely unknown, and it is foreseeable that much time and effort will be necessary to understand them fully.

REFERENCES

BERLUCCHI, G., 1990. Commissurotomy studies in animals. In *Handbook of Neuropsychology*, Vol. 4, F. Boller and J. Grafman, eds. Amsterdam: Elsevier, pp. 9–47.

CONTI, F., and T. MANZONI, 1994. The neurotransmitters and postsynaptic action of callosally projecting neurons. *Behav. Brain Res.* 64:37–53.

ENGEL, A. K., P. KÖNIG, A. K. KREITER, and W. SINGER, 1991. Interhemispheric synchronization of oscillatory neuronal responses in cat visual cortex. *Science* 252:1177–1179.

HEDBERG, T. G., and P. K. STANTON, 1995. Long-term potentiation and depression of synaptic transmission in rat posterior cingulate cortex. *Brain Res.* 670:181–196.

KAWAGUCHI, Y., 1992. Receptor subtypes involved in callosally induced postsynaptic potentials in rat frontal agranular cortex in vitro. *Exp. Brain Res.* 88:33–40.

KÖNIG, P., A. K. ENGEL, and W. SINGER, 1995. Relation between oscillatory activity and long-range synchronization in cat visual cortex. *Proc. Natl. Acad. Sci. U.S.A.* 92:290–294.

MOGENSON, G. J., D. L. JONES, and C. Y. YIM, 1980. From motivation to action: Functional interface between the limbic system and the motor system. *Prog. Neurobiol.* 14:69–97.

MUNK, M. H. J., L. G. NOWAK, J. I. NELSON, and J. BULLIER, 1995. Structural basis of cortical synchronization: II. Effects of cortical lesions. *J. Neurophysiol.* 74:2401–2414.

NOWAK, L. G., M. H. J. MUNK, J. I. NELSON, A. C. JAMES, and J. BULLIER, 1995. Structural basis of cortical synchronization: I. Three types of interhemispheric coupling. *J. Neurophysiol.* 74:2379–2400.

PENNARTZ, C. M. A., P. H. BOEIJINGA, S. T. KITAI, and F. H. LOPES DA SILVA, 1991. Contribution of NMDA receptors to postsynaptic potentials and paired-pulse facilitation in identified neurons of the rat nucleus accumbens in vitro. *Exp. Brain Res.* 86:190–198.

PULVERMÜLLER, F., and B. MOHR, 1996. The concept of transcortical cell assemblies: A key to the understanding of cortical lateralization and interhemispheric interaction. *Neurosci. Biobehav. Rev.* 20:557–566.

RACINE, R. J., C. A. CHAPMAN, C. TREPEL, G. C. TESKEY, and N. W. MILGRAM, 1995. Post-activation potentiation in the neocortex: IV. Multiple sessions required for induction of long-term potentiation in the chronic preparation. *Brain Res.* 702:87–93.

ROBBINS, T. W., and B. J. EVERITT, 1996. Neurobehavioral mechanisms of reward and motivation. *Curr. Opin. Neurobiol.* 6:228–236.

SAH, P., and R. A. NICOLL, 1991. Mechanisms underlying potentiation of synaptic transmission in rat anterior cingulate cortex *in vitro*. *J. Physiol. Lond.* 433:615–630.

SUGITA, Y., 1996. Global plasticity in adult visual cortex following reversal of visual input. *Nature* 380:523–526.

7 Forebrain Commissures: Glimpses of Neurons Producing Mind

ROBERT W. DOTY

ABSTRACT   The nature of the information traversing the forebrain commissures is poorly understood but certainly shares in the complexity of cortical computations, as emphasized by ipsicortical collaterals of many callosal axons. In larger brains, or in time-critical functions, the slow velocity of most callosal axons makes intracortical processing more efficient than bilateral calculation, thus promoting functional specialization within a single hemisphere. The consistency with which the right or left hemisphere becomes superior to, or dominant over, the other in humans and certain animals for a given function remains puzzling, and an example is given for a macaque in which well-established dominance spontaneously reversed. While it is possible to produce unilateral engrams using electrical excitation of cortex as the input signal, the more common mode for vision is that limitation of input to a single hemisphere nonetheless produces a bilateral memory trace. When the forebrain commissures are absent (the split brain), significant subcortical modulation of the hemispheres remains and seems to unite into a single trace input that is received simultaneously by the two isolated hemispheres. Given the functional specialization of the hemispheres, some cost in time and efficiency can be expected when processing must be switched from one hemisphere to the other.

As multicellular organisms discovered the advantages of moving through space, presumably at first along a substrate, they inevitably encountered the problem of attractions and threats that lay to either side of the direction of motion. Turning thus became desirable, and laterality came into being, with receptors to detect what lay to right or left and muscular contractility and inhibition to provide appropriate steering. As a consequence, duplicate neuronal systems arose on each side of the body. With the singular exception of radial symmetry, a secondary overlay in echinoderms, this pattern persists from flatworms to humans.

Despite recent compelling evidence, it is not commonly appreciated how profound this duplication of

ROBERT W. DOTY   Department of Neurobiology and Anatomy, University of Rochester School of Medicine and Dentistry, Rochester, New York.

neuronal organization remains, even in human beings. There are two dramatic demonstrations that either cerebral hemisphere is unequivocally human: the now extensive literature on hemispherectomy, showing that individuals with a single surviving hemisphere can function in society, sometimes at quite high levels (e.g., Griffith and Davidson, 1966; Gott, 1973; Austin, Hayward, and Rouhe, 1974; Smith, 1974; Schepelmann et al., 1976; Patterson, Vargha-Khadem, and Polkey, 1989; Ogden, 1996), and the thoroughly studied cases in whom the forebrain commissures have been transected, resulting in two undeniably human entities within the single individual (e.g., Sperry, Zaidel, and Zaidel, 1979; Sperry, 1984). From the latter it must be concluded that the forebrain commissures somehow achieve the mental unity enjoyed by most normal, bihemispheric human beings.

There has in the past been some argument as to whether, for intact individuals, the left, "speaking" (linguistically talented) hemisphere is actually the only one that is truly conscious in the human sense. The evidence just alluded to clearly denies this, as does a huge body of data on localized lesions in either hemisphere, now extensively supported by imaging of differential blood flow in the active, thinking brain. Perhaps the latest evidence here is the most convincing, showing that contemplation of events unique to one's personal history yields distinct activation of areas in the right (nonlinguistic) hemisphere (Fink et al., 1996).

Three primary questions arise from these facts:

1. What is the nature of the exchange between the hemispheres provided by the corpus callosum that accounts for unity of conscious experience in the face of the potentially independent mental life of each hemisphere alone?

2. Why does this unification nevertheless leave each hemisphere with distinctly different propensities and skills?

3. By what process is the "decision" achieved as to which hemisphere will lead at any given moment; that is, "who is in charge?"

Interhemispheric signals

Very little is known about the neural signals that pass between the hemispheres. From anatomy and phylogeny it is apparent that most interhemispheric signaling arises from cortical elements downstream from the initial processing of sensory input. The clearest evidence for this is seen in primary visual cortex, which is essentially devoid of callosal connections in the cat (Lomber, Payne, and Rosenquist, 1994), the macaque (Innocenti, 1986), and the human (Clarke and Miklossy, 1990). This pattern is particularly significant in that it is also quite comparable in the rat and the opossum, despite the fact that the latter lacks a corpus callosum and instead achieves interhemispheric communication via a large anterior commissure (Granger, Masterton, and Glendenning, 1985). Indeed, these two species show highly comparable variation in density of interhemispheric neurons among the various cortical areas. For the rat, however, a high proportion of the interconnecting neurons arise from cortical layer 5, thus benefiting from the rich input provided to that layer from collaterals of fibers descending from the supragranular layers, whereas in the opossum most of the interhemispheric outflow originates from layers 2 and 3.

In the first study of the response of single cortical neurons to input from the corpus callosum, on cats under Nembutal anesthesia, neurons that were identified as projecting to the spinal cord (pyramidal tract cells) were almost uniformly inhibited, and cells projecting across the callosum could be activated by stimulation of the foreleg (Asanuma and Okamoto, 1959). The inhibition noted in this and other studies on anesthetized animals promoted the idea that the influence of one hemisphere on the other is predominantly inhibitory. However, in the ensuing 30 years, techniques have become far more sophisticated, and it is now clear that the callosal signal shares the complexity of most cortical processes.

An outstanding example of current analyses is provided by Mountcastle, Atluri, and Romo (1992). They recorded the activity of neurons in the motor cortex controlling the arm a macaque used to signal its discrimination between two highly similar cutaneous stimuli, a task in which the animal's performance equals that of a trained human observer. The stimuli were applied to the finger of one hand, and the animal responded with the other hand; hence, the information as to what response was required had to be transmitted from one hemisphere

to the other across the callosum. Control experiments demonstrated that this transfer was made directly into the motor cortex. A trial began upon contact of the mechanical stimulator with the skin of the finger, and previous work had shown that cells in the cortex of the sensing hemisphere began responding to this event within about 20 ms. The ensuing transcallosal signal began, at the earliest, some 15–20 ms after that. The average time for this transcallosal signal to begin in the arm region of the appropriate motor area was nearly 90 ms, and it continued for 100 ms or more. There is, of course, no direct way of determining whether this continued response, or even the initial discharges with longer latency, are being supported callosally or whether local excitation within the motor area simply produces this activity once triggered by the callosal input. Far more complicated is the signal that must be conveyed from the hemisphere analyzing the sensory input to instruct the responding hemisphere what movement is required for the correct choice of response. No clue as to the nature of this sensorial calculation appears in the callosally controlled discharge in the motor area. The great majority of the transcallosally identified signals here are excitatory in nature and, obviously, can convey information that is highly refined.

The visual systems of cats and primates present unique opportunities to study callosal signaling, since in these species the visual field is split quite precisely down the "middle" (the vertical meridian), half the scene being projected to one hemisphere and the other half to the other. There being, subjectively, no indication whatever of this division, it must be assumed that callosal mechanisms are highly efficient in welding the two halves of the visualized world together. As was noted above, this amalgamation proceeds not in the cortical area having the most direct input from the retina, but in adjacent cortex specialized in having rich (and fast) callosal interconnections.

Despite this specialization in cortex addressing the problem of the vertical meridian, the basic organization and characteristics of the processing elements are likely to be similar to those throughout callosally connected cortex. Swadlow (1991), working with unanesthetized rabbits (whose singular advantage is that their instinct is to remain motionless for long periods of time), has identified several types of neurons whose behavior is virtually the same in visual cortex and two different somesthetic areas. Neurons of cortical layers 3 and 5 that send an axon into the callosum are commonly silent, that is, discharge no spikes unless responding to sensory input, and have an axonal conduction velocity averaging 2.6 m/s, with many less than 1 m/s. These characteristics of slow conduction velocity and little background activity are shared with other neurons projecting intracortically and with those of layer 6 that project back into the thalamic relay nucleus. Some 20% of the neurons send an axon both within the ipsilateral cortex and across the callosum. Most striking is the comparison of callosal neurons in layer 5 with their neighbors, neurons projecting to the brain stem or spinal cord. The latter discharge at an average rate of about 6 Hz and have an average conduction velocity of around 12 m/s. These are the output neurons of the cortex, and it is of interest that 43% of them could be discharged by callosal input, whereas none of the callosal or intracortically or thalamically projecting neurons responded. An even higher number of suspected inhibitory interneurons, 78%, were fired via the callosum (and had a high rate, ~12 Hz, of spontaneous activity). From this it can be deduced that the callosal input operates primarily on the cortical output and its inhibitory control.

Time and its consequences

As was just noted, the conduction velocity of callosal axons is exceedingly slow. This arises, of course, from the fact that these axons are very small, probably as a price for there being so many of them! Aboitiz and colleagues (1992) confirm the earlier estimate of Tomasch that there are roughly 200,000,000 callosal axons in humans, and there are 40 times as many having an axon greater than 0.6 µm as with an axon greater than 1.5 µm in diameter. Interestingly, the human callosal axons are, on average, smaller than those of macaques (LaMantia and Rakic, 1990). Thus, it would seem, the trade-off between number of connections and rapidity of communication as brains increase in size is being decided in favor of number. As Ringo and colleagues (1994) noted, a trade-off is inevitable because of the compounding effect that increasing axon size will in turn increase conduction distance, and so on. In this regard, cetaceans seem simply to have given up, for while the brain of the dolphin is about 75% of that of the human, the size of its callosum is less than 20% of that of the human (Nieto, Nieto, and Pacheco, 1976). This paucity of hemispheric interconnection may underlie the remarkable ability of these creatures to sleep with one hemisphere at a time (e.g., Mukhametov, 1987).

In any event, it is clear that a one-way message across the human callosum will, on average, given the distances involved and the size of the fibers, require on the order of 25 ms (Aboitiz et al., 1992; Ringo et al., 1994); and, of course, with longer interhemispheric paths and the large number of smaller fibers, such communication in many instances may take 100 ms or more! Ringo and colleagues (1994) proposed that such long delays for a one-way passage essentially preclude repeated back-and-forth exchange between the hemispheres in neuronal computation. Thus, in the interest of time, each hemisphere must achieve most of its multistage synaptic arguments locally, and as a consequence, each hemisphere will develop its own modus operandi. While this hypothesis offers an explanation for hemispheric specialization in larger brains or where temporal demands are critical, it says nothing as to why the right and left hemispheres each have the same individual propensities for the great majority of human beings, for example, linguistic talent in the left hemisphere and visual perceptual skills in the right.

It must also be recognized that there are some large, fast fibers in the human callosum, some 160,000 >4.6 µm according to Aboitiz and colleagues (1992). Typical of these is a group probably connecting the cortices of the vertical meridian (Shoumura, Ando, and Kato, 1975). This small contingent of fast fibers is undoubtedly responsible for the brevity seen for interhemispherically evoked potentials or for reaction times to simple stimuli. Lest it be thought that a "mere" 80,000 fibers provides but a feeble and primitive input from one hemisphere to the other, it need but be recalled that this is roughly the population of fibers from the eye of the cat projecting to the forebrain (Illing and Wässle, 1981), a system that is undeniably capable of intricate signaling.

Hemispheric specialization

As extensively reviewed by Bradshaw and Rogers (1993), throughout the animal kingdom there are many behavioral processes that are supported better by one than the other cerebral hemisphere. Obviously, the time delay noted for intercommunication in larger brains is not the only factor contributing to this lateralization. The efficiency achieved by performing computations within closely adjacent neuronal populations likely provides further pressure in this direction, as does the fact that effective interhemispheric communication, rather than simply being slow, may be essentially lacking in certain instances (see Doty, 1989; Doty and Ringo, 1994; Ringo et al., 1994), thus encouraging or necessitating the local solution.

There is a variety of specializations, ranging from paw or hand preference to attention (see below) to very high levels of analysis, such as recognition of faces or species-specific calls. The more pertinent here are those that seem to adumbrate the human situation, where across the population there is a high degree of similarity as to which hemisphere is specialized for which function. Such uniformity is generally lacking for handedness in nonhuman species.

The left hemisphere in birds is strongly specialized for production and interpretation of species- and individual-specific song (see Bradshaw and Rogers, 1993); and the same seems to be true in mice of either sex responding to calls of pups (Ehret, 1987; Ehret and Koch, 1989). Two Japanese macaques (*Macaca fuscata*) likewise displayed a slight ($p < 0.05$) right ear, presumably left hemisphere, advantage in recognizing species-specific calls, in contrast with a *M. nemestrina* and a *M. radiata* that were equally accurate but showed no bias to one or the other ear (Petersen et al., 1984) for the *M. fuscata* calls.

The question of hemispheric specialization for analysis of visual material by macaques has received somewhat more attention. As far as discriminating and remembering a wide variety of patterned visual inputs is concerned, there appears to be no difference between the hemispheres (Doty, Ringo, and Lewine, 1988, 1994; Hamilton, 1990). Some of the data suggest that for particularly difficult tasks the left hemisphere may have an advantage (Hamilton and Vermeire, 1991; Lewine, Doty, Astur, and Provencal, 1994), but it is not yet clear whether such an effect is truly independent of the type of visual material or problem with which the animal must cope.

The important discovery is not only that the majority of macaques display hemispheric specialization for certain problems, but also that there is a complementarity— that each hemisphere is uniformly better at one type of problem than another (Hamilton and Vermeire, 1988, 1991; Vermeire, Hamilton, and Erdmann, 1998). In 25 split-brain animals (optic chiasm, anterior commissure, and corpus callosum all transected, allowing each hemisphere to be tested separately by closing one eye), they found only three that had a very slight right hemisphere superiority for discriminating the orientation of lines, the others all being better, commonly much better, when using the left hemisphere ($p < 0.001$). Correspondingly, in 22 of the same animals, 18 showed a generally robust superiority with the right hemisphere in categorizing the facial expression of their conspecifics, despite the fact that the stimuli were provided by different individuals (again $p < 0.001$). It could be shown that these specializations were independent in the two hemispheres, that is, that excelling with one type of material in one hemisphere had no significant effect on the presence or absence of type of superiority in the other. About three fourths of the animals, however, showed the full differentiation: left hemisphere best for line orientation, right for facial and emotional recognition. The differentiation was strongest in females.

One of the attractions of these data of Hamilton and Vermeire is that right hemispheric specialization for face recognition is congruent with human findings (e.g., Carey, 1981; Sobotka, Pizlo, and Budohoska, 1984; Diehl and McKeever, 1987; Barrett, Rugg, and Perrett, 1988; Sergent and Signoret, 1992; Mertens, Siegmund, and Grüsser, 1993). Although Overman and I (1982) failed in an attempt to show that macaques, as did human subjects, would find the right half of a face more representative of a face than the left, this is scarcely a crucial test. A bit more fundamental is the experiment of Heywood and Cowey (1992), although not directly addressed to the issue of hemispheric specialization. They performed a bilateral extirpation of the cortex in the macaque temporal lobe that has been repeatedly found to contain a substantial population of neurons specifically responsive to faces. However, the animals showed little or no problem with facial recognition, while human prosopagnosic patients had difficulty with many of the stimuli employed. This suggests that the homolog of the human cortical area that is most responsible for facial recognition has still to be identified in macaques.

With two split-brain macaques we (Doty et al., 1999) endeavored to confirm and extend the findings of Hamilton and Vermeire but using a more demanding mnemonic task. The animals were required to identify whether an item was new or had been seen previously (old) in the session of 142 trials, with up to three images intervening between the new and old items. Ocular fixation on a small target centered above the image signaled new, and fixation on a lower target signaled old. The laterality of fixations during examination of each image was used to indicate which hemisphere was in control of the viewing when both eyes were open. Initially, there was no significant difference between the hemispheres of either animal in remembering colored, nonobjective images or human faces, but both showed a right hemispheric superiority for remembering macaque faces, precisely as Vermeire, Hamilton, and Erdmann (1998) had shown.

The male animal was then eliminated, but work continued with the female. To our total surprise the hemispheric dominance, some 15 months after surgery and start of testing, shifted entirely to the left hemisphere, probably as a gradual shift, but its unexpectedness left us unprepared to define its progression. This change was true for superiority in remembering human faces and nonobjective images as well as the macaque faces that were originally better remembered by the right hemisphere. The left hemispheric superiority was reflected not only in the accuracy of performance but also in the pattern of eye fixations during examination of the presented item (Kavcic, Fei, Hu, and Doty, 2000). This unequivocal change in predominance of one hemisphere over the other cautions that one may not—in any case, with macaques—be dealing with hemispheric specialization per se. Rather, it may be a question of metacontrol (Levy and Trevarthen, 1976), that is, which hemisphere endeavors to assume behavioral control in a given situation. Hellige (1993), for instance, has demonstrated in human subjects that it is not always the most appropriately specialized hemisphere that controls the response. It is quite possible in the case of this reversal of hemispheric specialization just described that the only specialization is that of controlling the response, even when the now-dominant hemisphere is not viewing the to-be-remembered image. In other words, even when only one hemisphere is viewing an item, the other may intrude by endeavoring to control the response (see Chiarello and Maxfield, 1996). This possibility is indeed suggested by the fact that in the present case, reversing a superiority of performance from the right to the left hemisphere, the performance of the previously superior right hemisphere did, in fact, significantly diminish (Doty et al., 1999).

Memory: Making and finding the engram

Given that one hemisphere is better than the other at performing certain tasks, it might be expected that the memories related to these tasks would be associated with (stored in?) the more proficient hemisphere. There are, however, many complications in endeavoring to establish the relevant facts (see Doty and Ringo, 1994). In the first place, it is clear that in macaques, either hemisphere has access to the mnemonic store of the other via either the anterior commissure or the corpus callosum (e.g., Doty, Ringo, and Lewine, 1988, 1994). For some human patients the anterior commissure seems incompetent in this regard (e.g., McKeever, Sullivan, Ferguson, and Rayport, 1981), although this may reflect merely a sampling problem in that the physical size of the human anterior commissure has a sevenfold variation (Demeter, Ringo, and Doty, 1988).

Being able to forestall the creation or utilization of an effective memory trace in either hemisphere by tetanization of perihippocampal structures, Ringo (1993) has greatly clarified the situation. In animals with a transected optic chiasm and either of the forebrain commissures, it could be shown that visual input into one hemisphere established a memory trace in both; and when, by use of the tetanization, the trace was limited to the initially viewing hemisphere, it could subsequently be accessed via the other hemisphere. Because of the possibility that any input with the forebrain commissure intact might establish a bilateral engram, this was the first clear demonstration that in "normal" circumstances a unilaterally established engram could be activated via an "ignorant" hemisphere.

Unilateral engrams have been established in other circumstances. Perhaps the most interesting is that of Kucharski and Hall (1988), who established an olfactory discrimination via one nostril in rat pups. Before maturation of the anterior commissure the memory was inaccessible via the other nostril, but subsequently, it could be activated via this untrained side. Thus, a memory trace that is established even before the existence of effective interhemispheric connections could still be found and utilized once the appropriate fibers were functional. Such was not the case, however, when more complex behavior was involved. Rudy and Paylor (1987) found that young rats that were trained on a water maze with one eye open before maturation of the callosum did not benefit when tested with the other eye after the callosum was functional.

Doty, Negrão, and Yamaga (1973) used macaques having either anterior commissure or callosum cut before experimentation but with intact optic chiasm. When trained to respond to electrical excitation of striate cortex in one hemisphere, animals continued doing so to excitation of striate cortex in the other hemisphere only as long as the corpus callosum was intact, while continuing to respond to nontrained striate loci in the original hemisphere. Such unilaterality was not true in the case of the anterior commissure, in which responding continued unabated for stimulation of the untrained striate cortex after the commissure was cut (completing transection of both forebrain commissures). It is speculated that it is the continuing input to both striate cortices, both eyes being open and callosum intact, that produced the confinement of the engram to the stimulated hemisphere. Unlike the situation in the Ringo (1993) experiments with split chiasm, in which the nonviewing eye is occluded, the nontrained hemisphere here would be occupied by its normal visual processing and unavailable for further encoding. On the other hand, it is equally plausible that the absence of callosal connections between striate cortices might underlie the unilaterality. Ringo, Doty, and Demeter (1991) showed with split-chiasm macaques with intact forebrain commissures that if the two hemispheres concurrently viewed congruent images (superimposed so that the correct response could be obtained via either or both hemispheres), there was an advantage over viewing the same material by either hemisphere alone; but if the images were noncongruent, that is, different images were presented to each hemisphere, this advantage was lost. This is somewhat reminiscent of the above in that two greatly differing activities, electrical excitation and normal visual input, cannot be processed concurrently via the callosal path. However, also in line with the above, this was not true when only the anterior commissure was available. In that case binocular viewing was advantageous even though each hemisphere concurrently viewed a different image!

Perhaps even more surprising is the fact that binocular viewing held a slight advantage even with split-brain animals. This might simply arise because of absence of interference from the hemisphere that is literally kept in the dark on monohemispheric trials. However, there is evidence for participation of brain stem elements in mnemonic processing, such that there is a limited-capacity system shared by the two hemispheres (Lewine et al., 1994). The experiments on macaques are somewhat complicated, since they involved giving the animal a set of two to six target images that it had to remember temporarily and distinguish from nontarget items. Such a task is noted for the fact that the time required to reach a decision on a given item shows an increment that is linearly proportional to the number of target items. Accuracy of the decision also diminishes proportionally with the number of targets. The experiments sought to determine what happens, in split-chiasm animals with either the splenium of the corpus callosum or the anterior commissure intact, when some of the targets to be remembered are presented to one hemisphere and some to the other. The result was that either commissural system was effective in unifying mnemonic load, so that response via either hemisphere reflected the total number of targets regardless of how they had been distributed between the hemispheres initially. However, when the hemispheres were isolated from each other by completion of the commissural transection, the reaction time for each hemisphere reflected only the number of targets that it had been given; but the accuracy of the response depended on the total mnemonic load given to the two hemispheres together! Thus, even in the absence of the forebrain commissures, some subcortical system was unifying an aspect of the mnemonic processing.

We (Kavcic, Fei, Hu, and Doty, 2000) have recently derived further evidence, on two split-brain macaques, that processes are in play that endeavor to form a unified engram from images viewed simultaneously by the isolated hemispheres. First, if the two hemispheres viewed the same image, there was commonly better performance than if each hemisphere viewed an entirely different image. However, if both hemispheres had concurrently viewed different images and were then asked to recognize a repeat, simultaneous presentation of these same two images, performance was excellent. Indeed, as was noted above, it was significantly better than when either

hemisphere alone viewed an image on each occasion. The critical test arose when the two hemispheres at first viewed images simultaneously (parallel processing), and then only one of them alone was called upon subsequently to recognize the image that it had seen in conjunction with the other. Performance in such case was significantly worse than when either hemisphere worked alone on a single image. Thus, in sum, bihemispheric performance is excellent, showing that there is no deficiency arising from parallel processing per se, but when only half of the simultaneously experienced visual input is present, recognition is worse than if there was only a single input to a single hemisphere on each occasion. This strongly suggests that when the two isolated hemispheres view two images concurrently, there is some amalgamation of the separately derived memory traces, yielding a deficiency in recognition when only half of that scene is viewed (by either hemisphere).

Switching

While the above discussion of memory has emphasized its probable bilaterality in many instances, this is by no means a closed subject. Regardless of just where engrams may lie and how they are accessed, the human hemispheres display a pronounced and unequivocal specialization for different types of neuronal processing. This alone raises the issue as to how attention may be distributed between the hemispheres to deal with the differing modes of operation. There is a large literature on the focusing of attention, mostly involving, ultimately, location in space. This immediately harks back to the point made in the introductory paragraph of this essay: that duplication arose in nervous systems consequent to the desirability of making choices between right and left. It is thus rather surprising that the extensive research on attentive locus is couched purely in terms of space, without reference to hemispheric function.

As a general rule, both hemispheres cannot be attended to concurrently. This situation is particularly well illustrated in split-brain patients, in whom for most circumstances attention still needs to be directed to one or other hemisphere/visual field. Trevarthen (1974), for instance, reports that when such a patient was asked to mark with her left hand a large white square present on a black background, she protested that the square disappeared; that is, when the right hemisphere assumed control of the left hand, the attentive focus passed to that hemisphere, and perceptual processing in the left, speaking hemisphere was curtailed. Other work with split-brain patients confirms this general theme: that attention is primarily a process that is not readily divided and must thus be allotted sequentially, rather than concurrently, to each hemisphere (Holtzman, 1985; Levy and Trevarthen, 1976; Teng and Sperry, 1974).

If attention must then be switched between hemispheres, how long does it take? Although couched merely in terms of right and left visual fields, an ingenious experiment of Weichselgartner and Sperling (1987) suggests an answer, and it is surprisingly long. Their subjects, all normal, were required to watch for a particular letter in a stream of letters being displayed for 18 ms at a rate of 10–12.5 letters/s in the left visual field. When the target letter appeared, the subjects then had to switch attention to a similar stream of numerals in the right visual field and report the first numeral(s) that they could detect and remember. On 50% of the occasions the first remembered numeral occurred 300 ms after the signal to switch, the great majority lying between 200 and 400 ms. On the other hand, if the subject was already attending to the numeral stream and the signal to begin remembering was a brightening or highlighting of one of the numerals, either that numeral or the one immediately following it at 100 ms could be reported; that is, without the switch in visual field, the attentive process was engaged much more rapidly. Interestingly, in this second situation the later engagement of attention also occurred, for subjects then also had a peak of remembering in the 300-ms time frame found in the switching experiment.

A further feature of such engagement of attention is that once activated, it runs a course of 100–300 ms during which switching to other items is impaired (Duncan, Ward, and Shapiro, 1994).

We (Kavcic, Krar, and Doty, 2000) have endeavored to measure such temporal cost in a situation more clearly allied to switching between use of one hemisphere versus the other. Two types of stimuli were used, chosen to tap left and right hemisphere aptitudes, respectively: nonoffensive four-letter English words and complexly patterned multicolored images having no ready verbal descriptors. These items were intermingled pseudorandomly and presented on a computer monitor one at a time for 200 ms followed by a multicolored, patterned masking flash. The subject's assignment was to identify whether a given item had or had not been seen previously in the sequence, that is, a continuous recognition task. In the 240 trials 120 items were new and 120 old; on 20 occasions a word followed an image, and on 20 others a word preceded an image. These latter two conditions were the focus of the experiment, measuring the extra time it took in evaluating whether the item was new or old when a switch (in activation of one versus the other hemisphere?) occurred in comparison with when it

did not. With nine subjects, for an image following a word, the added time averaged 78 ms beyond the 850 ms when an image followed an image; and for a word following an image, the added time was 92 ms beyond the 792 ms for a word following a word. Thus, there was a very significant delay ($p \leq 0.001$ and 0.005, respectively) in switching between processing the one to the other type of stimulus.

To affirm whether this was indeed a switch between hemispheres, a putatively intrahemispheric switch was assayed between words and nonwords. The switching cost in such circumstance was only ~30 ms, thus being consonant with the idea that the comparable times for word/image switching might include an interhemispheric cost. However, such simplicity was dispelled by the next finding: that switching between stimuli, presumably both targeted at right hemispheric processes, human faces and colored images, exacted a switching time of 70–79 ms. Thus, to assign a credible cost to interhemispheric switching per se, rearrangement of the underlying neuronal processing will have to be more effectively limited to a selected hemisphere. It is of some interest that in no instance were any of the subjects aware that their reaction time was slowed on the switch trials.

An important factor that needs to be considered in such experiments is that attention may be a specialty of the right hemisphere. This is most strikingly illustrated by the fact that lesions of the right human hemisphere are prone to produce neglect of events occurring to the left, whereas the corresponding deficit following left hemisphere lesions is far less (e.g., Robertson and Marshall, 1993). The remarkable uniformity of this right hemispheric propensity for control of attention in the human population has been demonstrated by Spiers and colleagues (1990). In a series of 48 consecutive patients undergoing amobarbital infusion into right versus left carotid arteries, which briefly inactivates the respective hemisphere to test for sidedness of speech before neurosurgery, only injection on the right produced neglect (of events to the left). Surprisingly, this was also true of left-handed individuals, even of those in whom speech appeared to be a function of the right hemisphere! The effect was particularly marked by changes in the electroencephalogram of the right frontal cortex.

More subtle evidence of this right hemispheric prepotency for attentive activation appears in the study of Levy, Wagner, and Lu (1990). Using verbal stimuli presented randomly to one or the other visual field for ~200 ms in normal subjects, followed by a masking stimulus, they found the expected superiority of the right visual field. However, it was also clear that the trials that were preceded by presentation to the left visual field (right hemisphere), regardless of which hemisphere responded next, were consistently more accurate than when a right visual trial preceded. Thus, activation of the right hemisphere had a lingering effect, perhaps of sustaining a more alert state, leading to augmented performance by either hemisphere. Unfortunately, Levy and colleagues did not report measures of reaction time in these experiments.

Perhaps equally unexpected is the finding that this right hemispheric bias for attentive processes can be seen even in split-brain patients (Mangun et al., 1994). In this instance reaction time was the critical measure, and it was demonstrated that the right hemisphere allocated attention to either visual field (faster or slower response depending on field location of a cue preceding the target), whereas the left hemisphere dealt only with the right visual field. As they note, such findings clearly implicate the participation of subcortical systems in attentive processes, since the asymmetry and bilaterality demonstrated here survive callosotomy.

REFERENCES

ABOITIZ, F., A. B. SCHEIBEL, R. S. FISHER, and E. ZAIDEL, 1992. Fiber composition of the human corpus callosum. *Brain Res. (Amsterdam)* 598:143–153.

ASANUMA, H., and K. OKAMOTO, 1959. Unitary study on evoked activity of callosal neurons and its effect on pyramidal tract cell activity in cats. *Jpn. J. Physiol.* 9:473–483.

AUSTIN, G., W. HAYWARD, and S. ROUHE, 1974. A note on the problem of conscious man and cerebral disconnection by hemispherectomy. In *Hemispheric Disconnection and Cerebral Function*, M. Kinsbourne and W. L. Smith, eds. Springfield, Ill.: Charles C Thomas, pp. 95–114.

BARRETT, S. E., M. D. RUGG, and D. I. PERRETT, 1988. Event-related potentials and the matching of familiar and unfamiliar faces. *Neuropsychologia* 26:105–117.

BRADSHAW, J., and L. ROGERS, 1993. *The Evolution of Lateral Asymmetries, Language, Tool Use, and Intellect*. San Diego: Academic Press.

CAREY, S., 1981. The development of face perception. In *Perceiving and Remembering Faces*, G. Davies, H. Ellis, and J. Shepherd, eds. London: Academic Press, pp. 9–38.

CHIARELLO, C., and L. MAXFIELD, 1996. Varieties of interhemispheric inhibition, or how to keep a good hemisphere down. *Brain Cogn.* 30:81–108.

CLARKE, S., and J. MIKLOSSY, 1990. Occipital cortex in man: Organization of callosal connections, related myelo- and cytoarchitecture, and putative boundaries of functional visual areas. *J. Comp. Neurol.* 298:188–214.

DEMETER, S., J. L. RINGO, and R. W. DOTY, 1988. Morphometric analysis of the human corpus callosum and anterior commissure. *Hum. Neurobiol.* 6:219–226.

DIEHL, J. A., and W. F. McKEEVER, 1987. Absence of exposure time influence on lateralized face recognition and object naming latency tasks. *Brain Cogn.* 6:347–359.

DOTY, R. W., 1989. Some anatomical substrates of emotion, and their bihemispheric coordination. In *Experimental Brain Research Series 18-Emotions and the Dual Brain*, G. Gainotti, ed. Berlin: Springer Verlag, pp. 56–82.

DOTY, R. W., R. FEI, S. HU, and V. KAVCIC, 1999. Long-term reversal of hemispheric specialization for visual memory in a split-brain macaque. *Behav. Brain Res.* 102:99–113.

DOTY, R. W., N. NEGRÃO, and K. YAMAGA, 1973. The unilateral engram. *Acta Neurobiol. Exp.* 33:711–728.

DOTY, R. W., and J. L. RINGO, 1994. Hemispheric distribution of memory traces. In *The Memory System of the Brain*, J. Delacour, ed. Singapore: World Scientific, pp. 636–656.

DOTY, R. W., J. L. RINGO, and J. D. LEWINE, 1988. Forebrain commissures and visual memory: A new approach. *Behav. Brain Res.* 29:267–280.

DOTY, R. W., J. L. RINGO, and J. D. LEWINE, 1994. Interhemispheric sharing of visual memory in macaques. *Behav. Brain Res.* 64:79–84.

DUNCAN, J., R. WARD, and K. SHAPIRO, 1994. Direct measurement of attentional dwell time in human vision. *Nature* 369:313–315.

EHRET, G., 1987. Left hemisphere advantage in the mouse brain for recognizing ultrasonic communication calls. *Nature* 325:249–251.

EHRET, G., and M. KOCH, 1989. Recognition of communication sounds is lateralized in the mouse brain. *Behav. Brain Res.* 33:322.

FINK, G. E., H. J. MARKOWITSCH, M. REINKEMEIER, T. BRUCKBAUER, J. KESSLER, and W.-D. HEISS, 1996. Cerebral representation of one's own past: Neural networks involved in autobiographical memory. *J. Neurosci.* 16:4275–4282.

GOTT, P. S., 1973. Language after dominant hemispherectomy. *J. Neurol. Neurosurg. Psychiatry* 36:1082–1088.

GRANGER, E. M., B. MASTERTON, and K. K. GLENDENNING, 1985. Origin of interhemispheric fibers in acallosal opposum (with a comparison to callosal origins in rat). *J. Comp. Neurol.* 241:82–98.

GRIFFITH, H., and M. DAVIDSON, 1966. Long-term changes in intellect and behaviour after hemispherectomy. *J. Neurol. Neurosurg. Psychiatry* 29:571–576.

HAMILTON, C. R., 1990. Hemispheric specialization in monkeys. In *Brain Circuits and Functions of the Mind*, C. Trevarthen, ed. Cambridge: Cambridge University Press, pp. 181–195.

HAMILTON, C. R., and B. A. VERMEIRE, 1988. Complementary hemispheric specialization in monkeys. *Science* 242:1691–1694.

HAMILTON, C. R., and B. A. VERMEIRE, 1991. Functional lateralization in monkeys. In *Cerebral Laterality: Theory and Research*, F. L. Kitterle, ed. Hillsdale, N.J.: Erlbaum, pp. 19–34.

HELLIGE, J. B., 1993. *Hemispheric Asymmetry: What's Right and What's Left*. Cambridge, Mass.: Harvard University Press.

HEYWOOD, C. A., and A. COWEY, 1992. The role of the 'face-cell' area in the discrimination and recognition of faces by monkeys. *Phil. Trans. R. Soc. Lond. B: Biol. Sci.* 335:31–38.

HOLTZMAN, J., 1985. The integrity of attentional control following commissural section. In *Epilepsy and the Corpus Callosum*, A. G. Reeves, ed. New York: Plenum, pp. 357–368.

ILLING, R.-B., and H. WÄSSLE, 1981. The retinal projection to the thalamus in the cat: A quantitative investigation and a comparison with the retinotectal pathway. *J. Comp. Neurol.* 202:265–285.

INNOCENTI, G. M., 1986. General organization of callosal connections in the cerebral cortex. In *Cerebral Cortex, Vol. 5, Sensory-Motor Areas and Aspects of Cortical Connectivity,*

E. G. Jones and A. Peters, eds. New York: Plenum, pp. 291–353.

KAVCIC, V., R. FEI, S. HU, and R. W. DOTY, 2000. Hemispheric interaction, metacontrol, and mnemonic processing in split-brain macaques. *Behav. Brain Res.* 111:71–82.

KAVCIC, V., F. J. KRAR, and R. W. DOTY, 1999. Temporal cost of switching between kinds of visual stimuli in a memory task. *Cog. Brain Res.* 9:199–203.

KUCHARSKI, D., and W. G. HALL, 1988. Developmental change in the access to olfactory memories. *Behav. Neurosci.* 102:340–348.

LAMANTIA, A. S., and P. RAKIC, 1990. Cytological and quantitative characteristics of four cerebral commissures in the rhesus monkey. *J. Comp. Neurol.* 291:520–537.

LEVY, J., and C. TREVARTHEN, 1976. Metacontrol of hemispheric function in human split-brain patients. *J. Exp. Psychol. Hum. Percept. Perform.* 2:299–312.

LEVY, J., N. WAGNER, and K. LUH, 1990. The previous visual field: Effects of lateralization and response accuracy on current performance. *Neuropsychologia* 28:1239–1249.

LEWINE, J. D., R. W. DOTY, R. S. ASTUR, and S. L. PROVENCAL, 1994. Role of the forebrain commissures in bihemispheric mnemonic integration in macaques. *J. Neurosci.* 14:2515–2530.

LOMBER, S. G., B. R. PAYNE, and A. C. ROSENQUIST, 1994. The spatial relationship between the cerebral cortex and fiber trajectory through the corpus callosum of the cat. *Behav. Brain Res.* 64:25–35.

MANGUN, G. R., S. J. LUCK, R. PLAGER, W. LOFTUS, S. A. HILLYARD, T. HANDY, V. P. CLARK, and M. S. GAZZANIGA, 1994. Monitoring the visual world-hemispheric asymmetries and subcortical processes in attention. *J. Cog. Neurosci.* 6:267–275.

MCKEEVER, W. F., K. F. SULLIVAN, S. M. FERGUSON, and M. RAYPORT, 1981. Typical cerebral hemisphere disconnection deficits following corpus callosum section despite sparing of the anterior commissure. *Neuropsychologia* 19:745–755.

MERTENS, I., H. SIEGMUND, and O. J. GRÜSSER, 1993. Gaze motor asymmetries in the perception of faces during a memory task. *Neuropsychologia* 31:989–998.

MOUNTCASTLE, V. B., P. P. ATLURI, and R. ROMO, 1992. Selective output-discriminative signals in the motor cortex of waking monkeys. *Cereb. Cortex* 2:277–294.

MUKHAMETOV, L. M., 1987. Unihemispheric slow-wave sleep in the Amazonian dolphin, Inia geoffrensis. *Neurosci. Lett.* 79:128–132.

NIETO, A., D. NIETO, and P. PACHECO, 1976. Possible phylogenetic significance of the corpus callosum with special reference to the dolphin brain (*Stenella graffmani*). *Acta Anat.* 94:397–402.

OGDEN, J. A., 1996. Phonological dyslexia and phonological dysgraphia following left and right hemispherectomy. *Neuropsychologia* 34:905–918.

OVERMAN, W. H., JR., and R. W. DOTY, 1982. Hemispheric specialization displayed by man but not macaques for analysis of faces. *Neuropsychologia* 20:113–128.

PATTERSON, K., F. VARGHA-KHADEM, and C. E. POLKEY, 1989. Reading with one hemisphere. *Brain* 112:39–63.

PETERSEN, M. R., M. D. BEECHER, S. R. ZOLOTH, S. GREEN, P. R. MARLER, D. B. MOODY, and W. C. STEBBINS, W. C., 1984. Neural lateralization of vocalizations by Japanese macaques: communicative significance is more important than acoustic structure. *Behav. Neurosci.* 98:779–790.

RINGO, J. L., 1993. The medial temporal lobe in encoding, retention, retrieval and interhemispheric transfer of visual memory in primates. *Exp. Brain Res.* 96:387–403.

RINGO, J. L., R. W. DOTY, and S. DEMETER, 1991. Bi- versus monohemispheric performance in split-brain and partially split-brain macaques. *Exp. Brain Res.* 86:1–8.

RINGO, J. L., R. W. DOTY, S. DEMETER, and P. Y. SIMARD, 1994. Time is of the essence: A conjecture that hemispheric specialization arises from interhemispheric conduction delay. *Cereb. Cortex* 4:331–343.

ROBERTSON, I. H., and J. C. MARSHALL, Eds., 1993. *Unilateral Neglect: Clinical and Experimental Studies.* Hillsdale, N.J.: Erlbaum.

RUDY, J. W., and R. PAYLOR, 1987. Development of interocular equivalence of place learning in the rat requires convergence sites established prior to training. *Behav. Neurosci.* 101:732–734.

SCHEPELMANN, F., G. PRÜLL, A. FELLMANN, W. BECKER, and H. RÖSSING, 1976. Klinisches Bild, Verhalten der motorischen Aktivität, elektroenzephalographische, neuropsychologische und linguistische Befunde bei einem Fall von linksseitiger Hemisphärektomie. *Fortschr. Neurol Psychiatr* 44:381–432.

SERGENT, J., and J.-L. SIGNORET, 1992. Varieties of functional deficits in prosopagnosia. *Cereb. Cortex* 2:375–388.

SHOUMURA, K., T. ANDO, and K. KATO, 1975. Structural organization of 'callosal' OBg in human corpus callosum agenesis. *Brain Res. (Amsterdam)* 93:241–252.

SMITH, A., 1974. Dominant and nondominant hemispherectomy. In *Hemispheric Disconnection and Cerebral Function*, M. Kinsbourne and W. L. Smith, eds. Springfield, Ill.: Charles C Thomas, pp. 5–33.

SOBOTKA, S., Z. PIZLO, and W. BUDOHOSKA, 1984. Hemispheric differences in evoked potentials to pictures of faces in the left and right visual fields. *Electroencephalogr. Clin. Neurophysiol.* 58:441–453.

SPERRY, R. W., 1984. Consciousness, personal identity and the divided brain. *Neuropsychologia* 22:661–673.

SPERRY, R. W., E. ZAIDEL, and D. ZAIDEL, 1979. Self-recognition and social awareness in the deconnected minor hemisphere. *Neuropsychologia* 17:153–166.

SPIERS, P. A., D. L. SCHOMER, H. W. BLUME, J. KLEEFIELD, G. O'REILLY, S. WEINTRAUB, P. OSBORNE-SHAEFER, and M. M. MESULAM, 1990. Visual neglect during intracarotid amobarbital testing. *Neurology* 40:1600–1606.

SWADLOW, H. A., 1991. Efferent neurons and suspected interneurons in second somatosensory cortex of the awake rabbit: Receptive fields and axonal properties. *J. Neurophysiol.* 66:1392–1409.

TENG, E. L., and R. W. SPERRY, 1974. Interhemispheric rivalry during simultaneous bilateral task presentation in commissurotomized patients. *Cortex* 10:111–120.

TREVARTHEN, C., 1974. Functional relations of disconnected hemispheres with the brain stem, and with each other: Monkey and man. In *Hemispheric Disconnection and Cerebral Function*, M. Kinsbourne and W. L. Smith, eds. Springfield, Ill.: Charles C Thomas, pp. 187–207.

VERMEIRE, B. A., C. R. HAMILTON, and A. L. ERDMANN, 1998. Right-hemispheric superiority in split-brain monkeys for learning and remembering facial discriminations. *Behav. Neurosci.* 112:1048–1061.

WEICHSELGARTNER, E., and G. SPERLING, 1987. Dynamics of automatic and controlled visual attention. *Science* 238:778–780.

COMMENTARY 7.1

From the Physiology of Callosal Connections to the Understanding of the Mind: Still a Long Way to Go

GIOVANNI BERLUCCHI

ABSTRACT This commentary on Professor Doty's paper on the relationship between the corpus callosum and the mind discusses some aspects of the basic physiology of callosal connections and some newly reported effects of brain splitting on attention and memory functions. Specific consideration is given to (1) the physiological excitatory and inhibitory effects of callosal inputs on cortical neurons, as contrasted with massive psychological excitatory and inhibitory effects on one hemisphere that are thought to result from a callosal disconnection from the other hemisphere, (2) possible noncallosal interhemispheric interactions in learning and memory, and (3) left hemispheric dominance in visual attention tasks after brain splitting.

In the paper on which I am commenting, Professor Doty has once again exhibited his knack for discussing the corpus callosum from a daunting variety of viewpoints, ranging from the single-neuron level to the mind. Because of limitations of my competence and the space allotted to me, I will only touch on very few of the many aspects of callosal activities he has surveyed in his paper.

Cortical excitation and inhibition by the corpus callosum

Doty says that very little is known about the neural signals that pass between the hemispheres, and the same could be said of the effects of these signals on their target neurons in the human brain. In the analysis of interhemispheric interactions, it is often claimed that one hemisphere may wholly inhibit or facilitate the other hemisphere in a multitude of sensory, motor, and cog-

nitive activities. Apart from the unlikelihood that normal cerebral organization may include such massive and indiscriminate interhemispheric actions, the terms *facilitation* and *inhibition* are used in this connection in a very loose sense, simply to mean that a particular behavioral performance that is attributed to one hemisphere appears to be improved or worsened, respectively, when that hemisphere is freed from interhemispheric influences. There is still much confusion about how these gross inhibitory and facilitatory interhemispheric influences inferred from behavior can be related to precise physiological actions of the corpus callosum at the neuronal level. In experimental animals, classic electrophysiological techniques have succeeded in demonstrating synaptic facilitatory and inhibitory effects of callosal fibers onto single cortical neurons (e.g., Matsunami and Hamada, 1984). At present, the available electrophysiological evidence suggests that all callosal fibers are excitatory to their direct target neurons in the cortex. The presence of exceptional callosal fibers that may be directly inhibitory to their postsynaptic targets is inferred from anatomical findings of very few GABA-immunopositive neurons among the nonpyramidal neurons that project to the corpus callosum. In adult rats, GABA-immunopositive neurons that are presumed to be inhibitory have been estimated to account for at most 3–5% of callosally projecting neurons (Gonchar, Johnson, and Weinberg, 1995). By contrast, in rat pups 21% of callosal neurons were found to be GABA-positive, and 57% of callosal neurons were found to have an electrophysiologically demonstrable direct inhibitory action on their target neurons (Kimura and Baughman, 1997). Taken together, these findings in adult and fetal or neonatal rats indicate that a transient contingent of callosal inhibitory fibers, whose prenatal and perinatal functions are as yet unknown, is virtually eliminated during post-

GIOVANNI BERLUCCHI   Dipartimento di Scienze Neurologiche e della Visione, Sezione di Fisiologia Umana, Università di Verona, Verona, Italy.

166

natal development by the process of corpus callosum pruning discovered by Innocenti (1986).

In adult animals, inhibition of cortical neurons by the callosal input is assumed to be indirect insofar as it is predicated on callosal excitation of intracortical inhibitory neurons. As Doty mentioned, the findings of Asanuma and Okuda (1962) suggest that corticipetal callosal discharges set up highly organized spatial patterns of combined and concurrent excitatory and inhibitory effects in discrete cortical regions, rather than widespread inhibitions or facilitations of large cortical areas or even of an entire hemisphere. As can be expected, direct evidence of synaptic inhibitory and excitatory actions of the corpus callosum in humans is virtually nonexistent, but recent applications of the noninvasive transcranial magnetic stimulation technique for activating the cortex have provided suggestive indirect information. Appropriate magnetic stimulation of the motor cortex on one side produces electromyographic responses in the intrinsic muscles of the contralateral hand; callosal inhibition or excitation of motor cortex can be inferred from changes in the threshold for obtaining such responses as a result of conditioning stimuli applied to the motor cortex of the other side. Although some of these studies have reported that inhibition is the only consistent effect of such transcallosal stimulation (e.g., Ferbert et al., 1992), others have found that inhibition is systematically preceded by excitation (Ugawa, Hanajima, and Kanazawa, 1993; Salerno and Georgesco, 1996), in agreement with the notion that callosal excitation is monosynaptic while callosal inhibition is polysynaptic. However, the interpretation of these results is made difficult by the possible antidromic activation of callosal neurons, a confounding factor that has plagued the understanding of cortical responses to electrical callosal stimulation since the early electrophysiological experiments in animals. Like most corticofugal neurons, callosal neurons have axons with recurrent collaterals that project to intracortical neuronal pools on the side of the parent cell body, thus providing an anatomical basis for positive and negative feedback effects. The participation of antidromic callosal stimulation to cortical effects was first shown by Clare, Landau, and Bishop (1961), who cut the corpus callosum in cats, waited for the anterograde degeneration of callosal fibers, and then recorded surface cortical responses to electrical stimulation of the ipsilateral callosal stump. The evoked responses were remarkably similar to those evoked by electrical stimulation of the intact corpus callosum and such as to suggest that the latter stimulation always evokes nonsynaptic (purely antidromic) and synaptic responses. Clare and colleagues (1961) assumed that synaptic responses to callosal stimulation following anterograde degeneration

of callosal fibers must have been mediated via recurrent axonal collaterals of antidromically activated callosal neurons, and their assumption was later confirmed with single-neuron recordings by Feeney and Orem (1971). Although transcranial magnetic stimulation is supposed to act mainly on neurons rather than fibers, the possibility that callosal fibers are directly activated in an antidromic way by such stimulation is by no means excluded (Cracco et al., 1989), and in fact it is indirectly supported by a study of activation of corticospinal neurons by magnetic transcranial stimulation in monkeys (Edgley et al., 1997). In sum, the emphasis on cortical inhibition as a major effect of transcallosal magnetic stimulation in humans may be misplaced if intracortical inhibitory neuronal pools are brought into play via recurrent axonal collaterals of antidromically activated callosal fibers. Thus, transcranial magnetic stimulation may be useful for studying local inhibitory mechanisms in the human cortex (e.g., Meyer et al., 1995; Liepert, Tegenthoff, and Malin, 1996; Schnitzler, Kessler, and Benecke, 1996) but cannot clarify the normal physiological participation of the corpus callosum in such mechanisms unless the contribution of antidromic stimulation to the observed effects can be fully understood and measured.

Memory and hemispheric disconnection

As Doty mentions, the very interesting findings of Lewine and colleagues (1994) suggest that even though forebrain commissurotomy seems to create two independent and disconnected cognitive systems, one in each hemisphere, some aspects of mnemonic (as well as attentional) processing are in fact shared between the hemispheres, possibly at the brain stem level. I would like to mention a recent paper by Mascetti (1997) on interhemispheric transfer in split-brain cats, the results of which go along with the above suggestion. He trained two groups of cats with section of the optic chiasm and the forebrain commissures on two visual pattern discriminations. Training was monocular, and the eye used for training was changed from one session to the next in both groups. With each discrimination the contingencies of reinforcement were consistent for both eyes in one group, while the other group was reinforced for choosing one of the two discriminanda when using the right eye and the other discriminandum when using the left eye. The learning curves of the two eyes of the group with consistent contingencies of reinforcement were generally superimposable, in agreement with the notion of an independent, parallel acquisition of the discriminations by the two hemispheres. In the other group of cats, learning was much slower with either eye, presumably because both hemispheres were jointly handicapped by the conflict between their respective contingencies of reinforcement; and there were strong differences between the learning rates of the two eyes, presumably because the two hemispheres were differentially sensitive to the unfavorable influence of the conflictual pattern of reinforcement. Like the effect of mnemonic load in the split-brain monkeys of Lewine and colleagues (1994), the effect of conflictual reinforcement in Mascetti's (1997) split-brain cats appears to depend on an information-processing mechanism that acts on both hemispheres in spite of their anatomofunctional disconnection at the cortical level. Though insufficient by itself to ensure interhemispheric transfer of visual discriminations in split-brain cats, this mechanism would nonetheless participate in the learning processes of both hemispheres, presumably by allowing them to share task-related contextual information.

Monopolization of attentional resources by one hemisphere

In referring to visuospatial attention, Doty mentions possible relationships between hemispheric interactions and the mechanisms for the focusing of attention. I would like to discuss some evidence that a section of the corpus callosum upsets the interhemispheric balance in the control of visuospatial attention in some simple tasks of light detection. It may be argued that the detection of a simple light stimulus in a visual field region must be preceded by a shift of the focus of attention toward that region. Proverbio and colleagues (1994) found that normal observers were equally fast in detecting light stimuli in the right and left visual fields, whereas in the same task a callosotomy patient exhibited a striking superiority of the right field over the left. Concurrent electrophysiological findings of positive correlations between the P300 component of the stimulus or event-related potentials in the two hemispheres and the reaction time (RT) data suggested that the advantage for RT to right-field stimuli and the disadvantage for RT to left-field stimuli could be accounted for by a monopolization of attentional control by the left hemisphere. A significant overall advantage for the right visual field in simple RT was also found in three commissurotomy patients out of four by Clarke and Zaidel (1989). A recent study from my laboratory (Berlucchi et al., 1997a) has reported a strong rightward attentional bias in another callosotomy patient who was tested in a different RT task, involving a manual keypress to the second of two identical light stimuli presented at random in the right and left fields. The first stimulus (the cue) did not predict the location of the second stimulus (the target) but forewarned the

subject that the target would be presented within 0.2–4 s. Contrary to normal controls, who showed no interfield differences, RT of the callosotomy patient was longest when both cue and target went to the left field and the right hemisphere, intermediate when cue and target occurred in opposite fields, and shortest when both cue and target went to the right field and the left hemisphere. It was as if the patient's focus of attention was consistently shifted toward the right visual field during the presentation of both cue and target, even though we made sure that his direction of gaze was firmly held at the center on each trial. In yet another RT task, involving a covert orienting toward a visual location indicated by an arrow, Zaidel (1995, Fig. 17.12) found a massive advantage for RT to right-field targets compared to RT to left-field targets in one of two commissurotomy patients, regardless of whether the targets appeared at the cued location or elsewhere. All these findings of a rightward attentional bias, as well as other converging results obtained in more complex tasks (Corballis, 1995; Kingstone et al., 1995), seem to indicate that after interhemispheric disconnection the control of visuospatial attention is preferentially lateralized to the left hemisphere, at least when such control is voluntary rather than automatic (Gazzaniga, 1995; Berlucchi et al., 1997b). Since the rightward bias is not present in all tasks, and certainly is not apparent in normal daily life activities, we still need to arrive at an exact and exhaustive definition of the conditions in which attentional control is monopolized by the left hemisphere.

REFERENCES

ASANUMA, H., and O. OKUDA, 1962. Effects of transcallosal volleys on pyramidal tract cell activity of cats. *J. Neurophysiol.* 25:198–208.

BERLUCCHI, G., S. AGLIOTI, and G. TASSINARI, 1997a. Rightward attentional bias and left hemisphere dominance in a cue-target light detection task in a callosotomy patient. *Neuropsychologia* 35:941–952.

BERLUCCHI, G., G. R. MANGUN, and M. S. GAZZANIGA, 1997b. Visuospatial attention and the split brain. *News Physiol. Sci.* 12:226–231.

CLARE, M. H., W. M. LANDAU, and G. H. BISHOP, 1961. The cortical response to direct stimulation of the corpus callosum in the cat. *Electroencephalogr. Clin. Neurophysiol.* 13:21–33.

CLARKE, J. M., and E. ZAIDEL, 1989. Simple reaction times to lateralized light flashes: Varieties of interhemispheric communication routes. *Brain* 112:849–870.

CORBALLIS, M. C., 1995. Visual integration in the split brain. *Neuropsychologia* 33:937–959.

CRACCO, R. Q., V. E. AMASSIAN, P. J. MACCABEE, and J. B. CRACCO, 1989. Comparison of human transcallosal responses evoked by magnetic coil and electrical stimulation. *Electroencephalogr. Clin. Neurophysiol.* 74:417–424.

EDGLEY, S. A., J. A. EYRE, R. N. LEMON, and S. MILLER, 1997. Comparison of activation of corticospinal neurons and spinal motor neurons by magnetic and electrical transcranial stimulation in the lumbosacral cord of the anaesthetized monkey. *Brain* 120:839–853.

FEENEY, D. M., and J. M. OREM, 1971. Influence of antidromic callosal volleys on single units in visual cortex. *Exp. Neurol.* 33:310–321.

FERBERT, A., A. PRIORI, J. C. ROTHWELL, B. L. DAY, J. G. COLEBATCH, and C. D. MARSDEN, 1992. Interhemispheric inhibition of the human motor cortex. *J Physiol. Lond.* 453:525–546.

GAZZANIGA, M. S., 1995. Principles of human brain organization derived from split-brain studies. *Neuron* 14:217–228.

GONCHAR, Y. A., P. B. JOHNSON, and R. J. WEINBERG, 1995. GABA-immunopositive neurons in rat cortex with contralateral projections to SI. *Brain Res.* 697:27–34.

INNOCENTI, G. M., 1986. General organization of callosal connections in the cerebral cortex. In *Cerebral Cortex*, Vol. 5, E. G. Jones and A. Peters, eds. New York: Plenum Press, pp. 291–353.

KIMURA, F., and R. W. BAUGHMAN, 1997. GABAergic transcallosal neurons in developing rat cortex. *Eur. J. Neurosci.* 9:1137–1143.

KINGSTONE, A., J. ENNS, G. R. MANGUN, and M. S. GAZZANIGA, 1995. Guided visual search is a left hemisphere process in split-brain patients. *Psychol. Sci.* 6:118–121.

LEWINE, J. D., R. W. DOTY, R. S. ASTUR, and S. L. PROVENCAL, 1994. Role of the forebrain commissures in bihemispheric mnemonic integration in macaques. *J. Neurosci.* 14:2515–2530.

LIEPERT, J., M. TEGENTHOFF, and J.-P. MALIN, 1996. Changes of inhibitory interneurons during transcallosal stimulations. *J. Neur. Transm.* 103:917–924.

MASCETTI, G. G., 1997. Interaction between the hemispheres of split brain cats. *Neuropsychologia* 35:913–918.

MATSUNAMI, K., and I. HAMADA, 1984. Effects of stimulation of corpus callosum on precentral neuron activity in the awake monkey. *J. Neurophysiol.* 52:676–691.

MEYER, B.-U., S. RÖRICHT, H. GRÄFIN VON EINSIEDEL, F. KRUGGEL, and A. WEINDL, 1995. Inhibitory and excitatory interhemispheric transfers between motor cortical areas in normal humans and patients with abnormalities of the corpus callosum. *Brain* 118:429–440.

PROVERBIO, A. M., A. ZANI, M. S. GAZZANIGA, and G. R. MANGUN, 1994. ERP and RT signs of a rightward bias for spatial orienting in a split-brain patient. *NeuroReport* 5:2457–2461.

SALERNO, A., and M. GEORGESCO, 1996. Interhemispheric facilitation and inhibition studied in man with double magnetic stimulation. *Electroencephalogr. Clin. Neurophysiol.* 101:395–403.

SCHNITZLER, A., K. R. KESSLER, and R. BENECKE, 1996. Transcallosally mediated inhibition of interneurons within human primary motor cortex. *Exp. Brain Res.* 112:381–391.

UGAWA, Y., R. HANAJIMA, and I. KANAZAWA, 1993. Interhemispheric facilitation of the hand area of the human motor cortex. *Neurosci. Lett.* 160:153–155.

ZAIDEL, E., 1995. Interhemispheric transfer in the split brain: Long-term status following complete cerebral commissurotomy. In *Brain Asymmetry*, R. J. Davidson and K. Hugdahl, eds. Cambridge, Mass.: MIT Press, pp. 491–532.

8 Interhemispheric Visuomotor Activation: Spatiotemporal Electrophysiology Related to Reaction Time

CLIFFORD D. SARON, JOHN J. FOXE, GREGORY V. SIMPSON, AND
HERBERT G. VAUGHAN, JR.

ABSTRACT   Ipsimanual and contramanual simple reaction time (RT) responses elicited by unilateral visual stimuli (Poffenberger, 1912) are often conceptualized in terms of a fastest or critical route between initial visual system activation and generation of motor output. Quantitative indices of brain function based on this interpretive scheme, such as interhemispheric transmission time (IHTT), have often failed to consider the anatomical complexity of the pathways involved and the multiple activation routes possible. These realities are reflected interindividually as differing patterns of cortical activations across RT and intraindividually as RT variability due to trial-to-trial differences in the relative contributions of different pathways. These considerations suggest a need to empirically reevaluate methods for the assessment of interhemispheric communication to improve the explanatory power of behavioral and electrophysiological results from this paradigm. This chapter provides a theoretical and empirical background for exploring these issues by examining the spatiotemporal dynamics of visuomotor activation and relations between physiology and behavior using high-density multichannel event-related potential recordings. Data analyses involved spherical spline-interpolated scalp current density mapping on a per-subject basis by condition and RT. Exploratory spatiotemporal dipole analysis estimated the intracranial sources of activation foci. The data suggest that bilateral posterior and central activations occur even when the same hemisphere receives direct visual input and generates motor output, violating the intrahemispheric processing assumption for this condition underlying the behavioral estimation of IHTT. Further, it was found that RT is directly related to magnitude, as well as timing, of motor cortex activation. The findings are discussed in terms of alternative interpretations of the Poffenberger paradigm (e.g., Chapter 10 in this volume). In addition, a brief methodological tutorial provides background on basic techniques of high-density electroencephalograph recording and analysis.

Origins

The research that will be presented in this chapter takes as its motivating roots two complementary lines of work. The first was a series of studies using behavioral and electrophysiological methods to investigate interhemispheric visual communication in dyslexic boys. These were performed with Dr. Richard Davidson and colleagues at the State University of New York College at Purchase and then the University of Wisconsin–Madison beginning in the late 1970s. The second line has been a research program, conducted by Dr. Herbert Vaughan, Jr., and colleagues at the Albert Einstein College of Medicine over the past 35 years, focused on elucidating the brain electrical activity related to basic sensory and motor processes. A primary aim of these efforts, which involved both human and primate studies, was to increase the information derived from human scalp recordings to determine the neural basis for noninvasively recorded human brain potentials. The experimental work to be described here, which investigates interhemispheric visuomotor integration, has also taken advantage of recent methodological and technological advances. These tools enable visualization of the spatiotemporal dynamics of electrocortical activations during tasks that have been previously characterized both behaviorally

CLIFFORD D. SARON   Center for Mind and Brain, University of California at Davis, Davis, California.
JOHN J. FOXE   Cognitive Neurophysiology Laboratory, Program in Cognitive Neuroscience and Schizophrenia, The Nathan S. Kline Institute for Psychiatric Research, Orangeburg, New York; Departments of Neuroscience and Psychiatry, Albert Einstein College of Medicine, Bronx, New York.
GREGORY V. SIMPSON   Department of Radiology, University of California at San Francisco, San Francisco, California.
HERBERT G. VAUGHAN   Departments of Neurology and Neuroscience, Albert Einstein College of Medicine, Bronx, New York.

and electrophysiologically. The richness and complexity of these spatiotemporal data have suggested a reinterpretation of prior findings regarding these tasks, which is the focus of this chapter.

The chapter is broadly organized into four sections: an overview of early studies and issues regarding interhemispheric visuomotor integration, a description of an evolution in experimental technique that provides the rationale for the general analytic approach taken here, findings that illustrate theoretical and methodological points in the first two parts, and a discussion of provisional conclusions based on the initial analyses.

Early behavioral studies

We chose originally to investigate callosal function in dyslexia because of numerous reports of abnormal lateralization during cognitive tasks (e.g., Yeni-Komshian, Isenberg, and Goldberg, 1975; Hynd et al., 1979), impaired interhemispheric coordination during motor tasks (e.g., Badian and Wolff, 1977), and altered patterns of interhemispheric EEG coherence (Sklar, Hanley, and Simmons, 1972) in this population. An initial study in our laboratory (Dunaif, 1979) suggested that some dyslexic children might indeed have deficits in interhemispheric communication. Using methods developed by Sperry and Gazzaniga (Gazzaniga, 1985) to examine interhemispheric haptic recognition in callosotomy patients, Dunaif found that dyslexics differed from controls only in one cross-hand condition when recognizing felt objects that they could not see. If an object was felt first with the left hand and then the right hand was used to find the same object among other choices, dyslexics performed worse than controls. A second behavioral study (Nirenberg, 1980) replicated this effect intermodally with dihaptic, dichotic, and bilateral hemiretinal stimuli. These studies suggested that our samples of dyslexic boys had a right-to-left hemisphere information transfer deficit. The findings challenged us to relate difficulties in reading with problems in interhemispheric communication. The model we developed to account for this suggested that abnormal timing of the right-to-left transfer of visual information during reading results in disruption of left-hemispheric linguistic processing (see Davidson, Leslie, and Saron, 1990, for a fuller description of the model).

Poffenberger and the measurement of IHTT

On the basis of this model, we assessed interhemispheric transfer time (IHTT) in dyslexic and normal boys (Davidson, Leslie, and Saron, 1990). We used the behavioral task invented by Poffenberger (1912) to estimate

IHTT. Ipsimanual and contramanual simple reaction times (RTs) to unilateral visual stimuli are obtained. The basic experimental design is shown in Figure 8.1. The bidirectional arrows indicate schematically major intrahemispheric and interhemispheric pathways. Parallel horizontal arrows represent parietal, central, and frontocentral callosal pathways, while the diagonal solid arrows indicate the existence of heterotopic callosal connections (Hedreen and Yin, 1981; Kennedy, Meissirel, and Dehay, 1991; Di Virgilio and Clarke, 1997; Chapter 21 in this volume).

The ipsilateral hand/visual field conditions (e.g., left visual field (LVF) input/left hand response) are generally associated with faster RTs compared with the contralateral hand/visual field conditions (e.g., Berlucchi et al., 1971, 1995; Clarke and Zaidel, 1989; Iacoboni and Zaidel, 1995). The mean difference in RT between the crossed and uncrossed conditions (CUD) across studies in adults ranges from 2.5 ms (Bashore, 1981) to 4 ms (Marzi, Bisiacchi, and Nicoletti, 1991). This difference has classically been taken to be an estimate of the timing of transcallosal information transfer. This presumption is supported by the increase in IHTT that is seen when patients with total agenesis (e.g., Milner et al., 1985; Lassonde et al., 1988; Di Stefano et al., 1992; Aglioti et al., 1993; Tassinari et al., 1994 (CUD = 23 ms); Di Stefano and Salvadori, 1998; Chapter 15 in this volume) or complete transection of the corpus callosum (e.g., Sergent and Myers, 1985; Clarke and Zaidel, 1989 (CUD = 48 ms); Aglioti et al., 1993) have been tested in this paradigm. Further discussion of IHTT measurement methods and populations studied can be found in the work of Hoptman and Davidson (1994). Further conceptual and methodological criticisms of this paradigm emerge throughout this chapter (see also Saron et al., in press).

Our model predicted that dyslexics would differ from controls in the conditions that reflected transfer from the right to the left hemisphere (i.e., the LVF input/right-hand response conditions). However, the group comparison in our study did not support this prediction. There were no reliable differences in IHTT between dyslexics and controls. However, when we examined the correlations between IHTT derived from right-hand conditions and performance on measures of reading and related cognitive functions, we found that faster IHTT was associated with poorer performance (Davidson, Leslie, and Saron, 1990). The percentage of subjects who showed IHTT values in the direction of anatomical prediction across groups and conditions was only 57%. The fact that the percentages were so low underscores one major problem with the use of RT measures to make inferences about IHTT: Reliable intraindividual

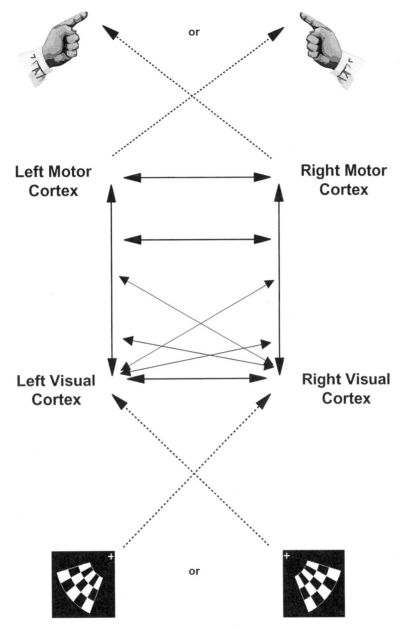

FIGURE 8.1. This diagram illustrates the design of the classic Poffenberger (1912) paradigm and includes schematic brain activation pathways. Hemiretinal stimuli are briefly presented in a simple reaction time (RT) task. Responses are made with the hand either ipsilateral or contralateral to the stimulated visual field. Ipsilateral task conditions have been thought to involve visuomotor integration within one hemisphere, while contralateral conditions require interhemispheric transfer (using either visual and/or motor routes) via the corpus callosum for response execution. The checkerboard wedges indicate the visual stimuli used in the reported experiments. Diagonal arrows indicate heterotopic callosal projections.

measurement requires thousands of responses per condition (St. John et al., 1987; Iacoboni and Zaidel, 2000). This is often an unrealistic constraint, given the time available to test subjects.

Visual event-related potentials and IHTT: Normals

The lack of reliability associated with RT measures of IHTT motivated our search for alternatives. On the basis of the underlying logic and anatomical assumptions of the Poffenberger task, we chose to apply electrocortical measures using event-related potentials (ERPs) to this paradigm. This approach was designed to circumvent what we took as one of the strongest methodological problems with the RT design of the task: the inability to measure responses from both sides of the brain simultaneously. Simultaneous measurement has been employed in animal studies of interhemispheric transfer beginning with Curtis (1940) and McCulloch and Garol (1941). An early ERP study by Andreassi, Okamura, and Stern (1975) demonstrated delayed ipsilateral compared with contralateral responses elicited with hemifield stimuli. In another early study, ERPs were used in a choice RT variant of the Poffenberger paradigm by Ledlow, Swanson, and Kinsbourne (1978), which also showed delayed ipsilateral compared with contralateral waveforms. Our simpler experimental design consisted of recording visual ERPs to hemiretinal presentations of checkerboard stimuli. Subjects were required to make a simple finger lift in response to each stimulus occurrence to maintain their involvement in the task and provide an independent behavioral measure. Brain electrical activity was recorded from occipital scalp regions, and ERPs were derived in response to left and right visual field (LVF, RVF) presentations. IHTT was inferred by comparing separately the latencies of the P100 and N160 components of the evoked response recorded over each hemisphere. It is important to note that as logical as this approach seemed, there was a great deal of skepticism at the time (the early 1980s) regarding the ability to record, in intact individuals, any electrocortical signs of callosally mediated interhemispheric transfer. This was due to the strong demonstration by Barrett and colleagues (1976) and further studies by Blumhardt and Halliday (1979) of the paradoxical lateralization of the visual evoked response. These studies used large hemifield stimuli (up to 16°) and produced greater magnitude responses over the ipsilateral, rather than the anatomically predicted contralateral, visual cortex. This finding was interpreted as reflecting, through volume conduction, potentials recorded over the ipsilateral hemisphere that were in fact generated in the contralateral hemisphere. This was thought to be due to the physical orientation of medial calcarine cortex stimulated by such a peripheral stimulus. However, when these same authors used smaller annular stimuli (Blumhardt et al., 1978), these effects greatly diminished, as the orientation of stimulated regions of visual cortex was more radial at the occipital poles. Careful examination of the published waveforms from this paper suggested interhemispheric delays in recordings that were not described in the text (Saron and Davidson, 1989a). The issue of volume conduction is critical and will be discussed below, as will further direct evidence in the intervening years of the callosal mediation of the delayed ipsilateral responses seen with appropriate hemifield stimuli. However, a number of reports using small lateralized stimuli did emerge by the mid-1980s, demonstrating clear ERP amplitude and latency shifts in accord with anatomical prediction (Lines, Rugg, and Milner, 1984; Rugg, Lines, and Milner, 1984, 1985a). See Brown, Larson, and Jeeves (1994) for a review of similar studies.

Before applying this method to our reading-disabled and normal reading sample of children, we needed to establish both the reliability and validity of visual ERP measures of IHTT. In a series of parametric studies on adults (Saron and Davidson, 1988a, 1988b, 1989a, 1989b), we found that a larger proportion of subjects had IHTT values consistent with anatomical prediction compared with simultaneously obtained RT measures. Grand average waveforms from 11 subjects (Saron and Davidson, 1989a), recorded from lateral occipital sites in the left-hand response condition, are shown in Figure 8.2. Responses to both LVF and RVF stimuli are earlier when recorded from electrodes contralateral to the stimulated visual field.

ERP IHTT values were in accord with this anatomical prediction for 91% of subjects in response to LVF stimulation and 100% of subjects in response to RVF stimulation. Moreover, the actual values obtained for IHTT

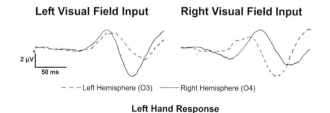

FIGURE 8.2. Grand mean ERPs from 11 subjects recorded from lateral occipital sites referred to linked ears in response to horizontal checkerboard hemiretinal stimuli during the left-hand response condition. The waveforms recorded from sites contralateral to the stimulated visual field show earlier P100 and N160 peaks, with larger interhemispheric delays in response to RVF input. The displayed ERP epoch is 0–200 ms poststimulus. (Modified from Saron and Davidson, 1989a.)

(10–15 ms) were more consistent with theoretical predictions of IHTT based on the distribution of conduction velocities derived for interhemispheric axons of known diameter and length than were RT measures (see Lamantia and Rakic, 1990, and Aboitiz et al., 1992a, for analyses of callosal fiber diameters). Further, the callosal mediation of the ipsilateral P1 has been demonstrated by recordings from individuals with agenesis of the corpus callosum (e.g., Rugg et al., 1985b; Saron et al., 1997; Brown, Bjerke, and Galbrait, 1998; Chapter 16 in this volume) and from those with complete or partial collosotomies (Tramo et al., 1995; Brown et al., 1999). Recently, Tootell and colleagues (1998) demonstrated extensive ipsilateral occipital activation during hemifield stimulation using functional magnetic resonance imaging (fMRI), effects that were interpreted as representing callosally mediated interhemispheric visual transfer.

Three additional findings from our early studies were (1) a suggestion of asymmetrical IHTT, (2) a dissociation between RT and evoked potential-based estimates of IHTT, and (3) an interaction of motor demand with interhemispheric communication. These will be considered in more detail below, in the sections entitled "Relationships Between RT and ERP Measures of IHTT," "Asymmetrical IHTT," and "Effect of Task Demand on IHTT."

Visual event-related potentials and IHTT: Dyslexics

When we returned to the original cohort of the reading study, we found that dyslexics *could* be differentiated from normal readers on the basis of ERP measures of IHTT (Davidson and Saron, 1992). Overall, the results that we obtained were consistent with our model. Dyslexics had faster IHTT from the right-to-left hemisphere and slower IHTT in the reverse direction compared with controls. Moreover, IHTT was correlated with measures of reading and other cognitive functions, as had been found in our RT study (Davidson, Leslie, and Saron, 1990). Faster right-to-left hemisphere transfer was associated with poorer performance on reading and cognitive measures, while faster left-to-right hemisphere transfer was associated with better performance on these measures. The pattern of results for IHTT computed on the basis of LVF stimulus presentations (reflecting right-to-left hemisphere transfer) was similar to our previous behavioral findings. Markee and colleagues (1996) have also differentiated dyslexic from normal readers using visual evoked potential estimates of IHTT, although they found overall slower transfer times for dyslexics. There are a number of factors that could account for the differences in findings between these two studies. Callosal function may differ significantly between our 9- to

12-year-old sample and the adult subjects of Markee and colleagues, since the myelination of the callosum continues through adolescence, the largest age-related changes being in splenial regions (Giedd et al., 1996). In addition, task differences between the studies may account for different ERP findings. Markee and colleagues (1996) used linguistic stimuli in a dual-letter matching choice RT task and preceded each trial with a warning tone. Our findings may reflect primarily visual interhemispheric transfer through splenial regions that have been found to be larger in dyslexics (Duara et al., 1991), while the linguistic nature of Markee and colleagues' study may additionally involve more anterior callosal regions that have been found to be smaller in dyslexic children (Hynd et al., 1995). Although it is beyond the scope of this chapter to review the current status of interhemispheric relations in dyslexia, several additional lines of evidence may relate to our model and are summarized by Saron (1999).

Relationships between RT and ERP measures of IHTT

There were three observations in the results from our initial ERP studies of IHTT (Saron and Davidson, 1989a) that have provided a foundation for our further studies in normal adult subjects. The first of these was our observation in a group of nine right-handed males that RT-IHTT and ERP-IHTT were *uncorrelated*. Recently, Hoptman and colleagues (1996) used methods nearly identical to those of Saron and Davidson (1989a) and obtained large differences between ERP and RT IHTT estimates for a much larger ($n = 45$) sex- and age-varied (19–87 years) population than was studied in Saron and Davidson (1989a). The mean RT-based CUD was 2.8 ms, while both P100 and N160 IHTT estimates based on peak latency differences were 23 ms (see also Potvin, Braun, and Achim, 1995).

One view of these findings is based on an insensitivity of RT measures of IHTT to manipulations of the visual stimulus (intensity or eccentricity), which has been interpreted to reflect primarily motor-related transfer (Berlucchi, 1972; Milner and Lines, 1982). The discrepancy between RT and visual ERP measures of IHTT, derived as they have been from occipital scalp regions, has been thought of as a contrast in IHTTs between motor and visual regions of the callosum. Initial ERP evidence for this came from short ERP estimates of IHTT recorded over central regions (Rugg et al., 1984, 1985a; Ipata et al., 1997). RTs also reflect a more complex final common output than visual ERPs because ERPs can be recorded from sensory cortex in the absence of motor output, while visuomotor integration is required with RT. The anatomical paths by which this integration takes place are varied and may involve both visual and motor interhemispheric transfer (Bisiacchi et al., 1994).

Asymmetrical IHTT

The second finding from Saron and Davidson (1989a) was a clear directional asymmetry in transfer times. Right-to-left transfer was faster than left-to-right transfer (10.0 ms versus 15.4 ms based on P100 peak latency differences). We replicated this asymmetrical pattern in a second study (Saron and Davidson, 1989b). The second study used more eccentric stimuli than in the prior study (5.1° versus 2.8°). We found LVF (right-to-left) IHTT = 16.0 ms and RVF (left-to-right) IHTT = 24.7 ms. The difference in IHTT across fields between studies may reflect the different stimulus eccentricities. The same pattern of directional asymmetry was found for both upper and lower visual field stimuli, suggesting retinotopic independence of the basic transfer asymmetry (Saron and Davidson, 1989c).

Asymmetrical transfer times have now been inferred from meta-analyses using RT (Marzi et al. 1991; Braun, 1993) and ERP methods (Brown et al. 1994). The additive factors of a right hemispheric superiority for the detection of brief visual stimuli or a left hemispheric advantage for unilateral motor output could contribute to, or wholly account for, this effect. However, both Marzi et al. (1991) and Brown et al. (1994) interpret the asymmetrical data as reflecting primarily callosal and not hemispheric asymmetries. Bisiacchi and colleagues (1994) addressed this question directly. These authors tested, in the same subjects, the classic Poffenberger design, a variant using unilateral visual stimuli and bilaterally controlled responses (chin drops), and a second variant using bilateral visual stimuli (foveal presentations) and unilateral responses (finger keypresses). The variant tasks produced neither visual nor motor evidence of hemispheric advantage. These results further support the existence of directional asymmetries in callosal transfer.

The anatomical basis of this asymmetry is unclear. Asymmetries in fiber number or in the distribution of axon diameters could both result in differences in effective IHTT. Increased numbers of large- and medium-diameter myelinated fibers could result in larger regions of callosal-recipient cortex receiving near-synchronous activation (see Houzel and Milleret, 1999). This in turn could be represented as faster response execution to callosally mediated inputs. Cerebral morphometry using high-resolution MRI has been applied to the question of gross anatomical brain asymmetries (e.g., Kertesz et al.,

1986, 1990; Myslobodsky et al., 1991b). These studies reveal complex yet consistent asymmetries in occipital cortex, with a tendency in right-handers toward larger left than right posterior brain regions. One possibility, based on the notion that axon survival during development is determined primarily by neurotrophic factors related to target availability (e.g., Henderson, 1996), is that larger left occipital regions would be more sparsely connected to their homologous regions of the right hemisphere than the converse. The increased probability of right-to-left axons surviving, given the initial exuberance of callosal development, could result in a standing asymmetry in the direction of callosal connections, which may be reflected in asymmetric IHTT.

Perhaps a more parsimonious explanation, at least for some splenial fibers, comes from the data of Murphy (1985) regarding volumetric asymmetry in human striate cortex. Murphy found that right striate cortex was larger than left in 24 of 31 brains examined. Given the clustering of callosal connections at the V1/V2 border (Van Essen, Newsome, and Bixby, 1982; Clarke and Miklossy, 1990; Chapters 1, 6, and 21 in this volume), larger cortical volume would translate into a longer border and hence more callosal originating and recipient zones in that section of the right hemisphere. A right-to-left hemisphere callosal connectional advantage could arise by larger numbers of originating fibers crossing the midline and successfully terminating homotypically.

Effect of task demand on IHTT

The third result from Saron and Davidson (1989a) was evidence suggesting that response hand influenced IHTT. Several subjects showed a striking pattern: When interhemispheric transfer was required to perform the task (e.g., LVF input, right-hand response), the time delay of visual responses between the hemispheres decreased. This suggested to us that there may be a facilitation of interhemispheric transfer under conditions of "obligatory" transfer, that is, when the transferred information is required for response execution. Intrahemispheric task conditions (e.g., LVF input, left-hand response) would, in this view, not require interhemispheric interaction, with less demand on cortical resources to selectively activate fast interhemispheric pathways. One potential cause of the lack of an overall hand effect may have been recording only from medial occipital sites. Such recordings have provided lower percentages of IHTT estimates consistent with anatomical prediction and overall shorter IHTT values than do recordings from lateral occipital sites.

When we made the same comparison using lateral occipital sites in the dyslexic and normal reader cohort, we did find robust effects in the expected direction, with interhemispheric conditions of the Poffenberger task resulting in shorter occipital ERP estimates than intrahemispheric conditions (Saron and Davidson, 1986). This effect was found for the control subjects but not the dyslexic subjects (Davidson and Saron, 1992). The basis of this group difference is unclear. It may be related to functional aspects of the anatomical differences in posterior callosal anatomy that have been shown in dyslexics (Duara et al., 1991; Rumsey et al., 1996).

The establishment of this effect in the control subjects strengthened our sense that the requirement for interhemispheric transfer influenced transfer time. It was not a large leap to consider that if motor demand altered IHTT, hemispheric specialization might also. That is, would facilitated interhemispheric transfer be seen when a task was presented to one hemisphere that is better performed by the other? We have developed a task optimized for ERP recording that used identical stimuli for left- and right-hemisphere tasks (Saron and Davidson, 1988b). It consisted of unilateral hemiretinally presented words. In the condition with demonstrated left-hemisphere superiority, the words were read as a semantic categorization task. In the condition with demonstrated right-hemispheric advantage, a randomly occurring font change was detected within the words. The electrophysiology of this task remains to be investigated.

Nowicka, Grabowska, and Fersten (1996) more recently completed a similar study using visual ERPs. Their putative left-hemispheric task was presentation of three-letter words; the right-hemispheric task was presentation of visual line grating patterns. While not allowing direct comparison between tasks using the same stimuli, their findings suggest that hemispheric specialization does interact with IHTT, with faster transfer times in the direction of the hemisphere specialized to perform a given task. However, these findings need to be considered tentatively in light of the lack of reported behavioral evidence for hemispheric specialization in task performance and the findings of Larson and Brown (1997). These latter authors found a right-to-left transfer speed advantage across putative left-hemispheric (letter-matching) and right-hemispheric (pattern-matching) tasks. However, in that study, only the pattern-matching task demonstrated a significant hemifield (left) performance advantage. Importantly, there was no significant difference in right-to-left versus left-to-right transfer time during this task. In contrast, the letter-matching task, which also failed to show evidence of hemispheric specialization, showed significant asymmetrical ERP-IHTT, with the pattern of faster right-to-left transfer that has been seen with nonlinguistic stimuli. The diminution of the directional asymmetry in the pattern-matching task

may therefore reflect a finding more similar to that seen by Nowicka and colleagues than discussed by Larson and Brown. Further studies using tasks that, in the tested sample, demonstrate clear patterns of hemispheric specialization will be required to clarify the interaction of hemispheric specialization and interhemispheric transfer.

An evolution in method

As we have argued, ERP IHTT measures were likely to provide anatomically predicted values much more in keeping with estimations of transcallosal fiber conduction times than behavioral estimates. However, these were more or less population statements. Some normal subjects had ERP waveforms that lacked clearly defined components or had negative or near zero IHTT values computed from well-defined ERPs. These difficult-to-interpret data may have reflected normal variations of cortical geometry given our recording methods at the time.

In a brief but remarkable paper, Brindley (1972) presented photographs of casts of six pairs of human cerebral hemispheres reassembled after sectioning, with the location of striate cortex marked with India ink. Seen in both the posterior and medial aspect, the variation between hemispheres and between brains is striking. An immediate conclusion reached on inspection of these images is that homotopic recording electrodes do not necessarily overlie homologous cortical regions. Further, a recording montage of few electrodes positioned with respect to bony fiduciary markers (as is the case in most EEG and ERP studies) could not be expected to serve as an adequate system for interindividual comparisons (see also Stensaas, Eddington, and Dobelle, 1974; Myslobodsky, Coppola, and Weinberger, 1991a; Kennedy et al., 1998). Therefore, we concluded that a whole-brain, case-study approach is required to move forward with reliably estimating interhemispheric visuomotor communication within single individuals. Recent advances in biological signal processing, lower costs of massive data storage, widely available computational power, and the development of appropriate software tools have made this approach feasible.

We have continued to record ERPs to hemiretinal stimuli (Saron et al., 1995a, 1995b, 1996, 1998, 1999; Saron, 1999) using electrophysiological and neuroimaging methodology that was not available for the earlier studies. Formally identical to the classic Poffenberger task, these experiments have included in their design and approach to data analysis, methods to increase the explanatory power of scalp-recorded electrophysiology (see Simpson et al., 1995a, 1995b). Described below are some of these techniques. Although specifically related here to a single task, these methods are also applicable to other experimental designs in sensorimotor and cognitive research.

DESIGN ELEMENTS

Control conditions Viewed in a physiological context, the Poffenberger task (simple RT with left or right visual field input and left- or right-hand responses; see Figure 8.1) suggests two additional control conditions: stimuli seen without the requirement for a motor response and motor responses made in the absence of stimuli. The no-response viewing condition allows examination of interhemispheric transfer of visual input without motor task demand. The most basic comparison possible with this condition concerns the role of motor demand on visual processing. That is, is there any activation of motor output regions when there is no need for a motor response (see Saron et al., 2001a)? Additionally, this condition relates to prior evidence for the interaction of interhemispheric task demand with transfer time. It would be expected that IHTTs for the view-only (no manual response) condition would be similar to those obtained for intrahemispheric task conditions (e.g., LVF input/left-hand response) if the interhemispheric transfer seen during intrahemispheric conditions reflects processing restricted to the input/output hemisphere. Conversely, longer IHTTs for the view-only condition compared to the intrahemispheric conditions would be expected if an active coordination between the hemispheres is required even with same-hemisphere initial input and final motor output. Support for this latter idea comes from findings of bilateral motor cortex activation associated with unilateral movements (see the section below entitled "Bilateral Motor Activation in an Intrahemispheric Condition") and the result, in patients with total section of the corpus callosum, of longer RTs during intrahemispheric task conditions compared to controls (Sergent and Myers, 1985; Clarke and Zaidel, 1989). Analytically, the view-only condition serves as a check for components of the visual response that may be due to movement-related activity, which, owing to volume conduction, may be seen in electrodes overlying posterior brain regions.

The self-initiated movement conditions allow comparisons to be made between visually and internally triggered movements. Analogous to the view-only condition, the motor-alone condition provides for the investigation of the dynamics of motor activation without temporally and potentially spatially overlapping visual activity. Furthermore, subtractions between the control and RT task conditions allow for potential isolation of paths of com-

mon input and output. Illustrative results from the RT and passive-view conditions will be presented in this chapter.

Stimuli: Location, type, and duration Many studies recording ERP measures of IHTT have used hemifield stimuli centered on the horizontal meridian (e.g., Andreassi et al., 1975; Rugg et al., 1984; Saron and Davidson, 1989a; Savage and Thomas, 1993; Hoptman et al., 1996; Ipata et al., 1997). This vertical placement adds complexity to the already complicated pattern of initial striate cortical activation (e.g., Foxe and Simpson, 2002). The contiguous upper and lower visual field portions of each stimulus activate noncontiguous regions of the upper and lower banks of calcarine cortex. (See Aine et al., 1996, for an investigation of individual differences in functional calcarine anatomy.) In addition, the upper and lower visual fields have been shown to differ in their pattern of extrastriate interhemispheric connectivity, which is of special concern in studies of interhemispheric visual transfer (Maunsell and Van Essen, 1987). In the studies presented in this chapter, lower visual field stimuli have been used exclusively. This choice of location was based on the increased callosal connectivity seen in brain regions representing the lower visual field (Maunsell and Van Essen, 1987) and human RT data in which faster responses are recorded for lower compared with upper visual field lateralized stimuli (Payne, 1967).

Within the lower visual field, dark-background perifoveal checkerboard wedges are presented (see examples in Figure 8.1). These stimuli have been designed to compensate in part for the effects of cortical magnification of the representation of visual space near the fovea and are oriented obliquely to avoid stimulation of either the horizontal or vertical meridians. The contrast and radial extent of the stimuli have been chosen to elicit a strong striate response in the directly stimulated hemisphere to aid in subsequent source localization of striate and extrastriate responses. Stimuli are presented as single computer screen refreshes and are approximately 6 ms in duration. Longer stimulus durations cause a stimulus-offset response, which adds to the ongoing activity evoked by pattern onset and may thus contribute unnecessary overlapping components to the initial pattern of cortical activation (Spekreijse, van der Twell, and Zuidema, 1973). Stimuli are presented in blocks for one location and response condition at a time. Randomized presentations have been found to produce large P300 responses compared to blocked presentations (Saron and Davidson, unpublished observations).

Trials: Timing and number The requirement for a behavioral response to each trial necessarily constrains the interstimulus interval (ISI) possible within a block of trials. Given the additional need to allow for a cessation of brain electrical activity due to the previous stimulus, stimuli are presented with a random ISI of 1–4 s. ISI has been shown to have a strong effect on the magnitude of visual cortical activations (Uusitalo, Williamson, and Seppa, 1996), and unintended priming effects of the previous stimulus have been documented in cognitive tasks (Iacoboni, Rayman, and Zaidel, 1997).

Competing with the requirement for a relatively leisurely trial rate is the need to collect very large numbers of trials. This need arises because of two concerns: First, high signal-to-noise ratios are desirable for the averages derived for the control conditions; second, the inherent variability of the behavioral response affords the opportunity to fractionate the data as a function of RT. The potential import of this approach is that it relates to a central question in studies of mental chronometry: the role of stimulus processing versus response execution in accounting for a given distribution of RTs (Saron, 1999; Saron et al., 2001b; Saron et al., in press; and see the section below entitled "Motor Activation Measures Predict Reaction Time"). Of special interest in the Poffenberger paradigm is the possibility that different RTs may be characterized by changes in the interhemispheric transfer routes that result in motor cortex activation.

It has long been known that RT differences affect the morphology of visual ERPs in simple RT tasks (Donchin and Lindsley, 1966; Morrell and Morrell, 1966; Vaughan, Costa, and Gilden, 1966; Bostock and Jarvis, 1970; Hartwell and Cowan, 1994; see Chalupa et al., 1976, for monkey data). Despite this evidence, few electrophysiological studies group responses by analog metrics of behavior. In addition to the data-intensive nature of such an analysis, the number of trials per condition would be multiplied by the number of behavioral response categories to be measured, quickly becoming unwieldy in multifactorial designs with large numbers of subjects. The approach taken here is to test few subjects in long-duration, repeated sessions. For some studies, approximately 1500 trials per simple RT condition were recorded, enabling derivation of at least 12 sets of ERPs for each condition, with RTs within a 10-ms range per set. The dependent measures that accompany these design changes are described in the following section.

Data Collection

Behavioral responses Forearm electromyographic activity (EMG) can be used as an adjunct behavioral response time measure. This long-established procedure (e.g., Vaughan et al., 1965; Kaluzny, Palmeri, and Wiesendanger, 1994) provides information regarding cortico-

muscular delay, RT switch latency, and an indication of movement duration that can be assessed as a function of RT. The most useful aspect of this measure in the present context is for anchoring the time at which a behavioral response begins. Combined with known corticomuscular conduction times (e.g., Salenius et al., 1997), EMG recordings allow identification of patterns of cortical activation associated with signs of motor output commands. This is important because postmovement reafferent activations appear before switch-indicated RTs (e.g., Praamstra et al., 1996).

High spatial density and temporal resolution recordings The basis of any approximation to a "whole-head" approach must be appropriately dense spatial sampling (Perrin et al., 1990; Koles, 1998), and the shortcomings of the standard 10–20 electrode position system for this purpose has been shown (e.g., Soong et al., 1993; Junghöfer et al., 1997). This requirement has been demonstrated in a variety of ways. Law, Nunez, and Wijesinghe (1993) used distributed arrays of 648 simulated neocortical potentials modeled on a spherical surface and examined the effects of various spatial sampling and interpolation methods in depicting the underlying spatial structure. Larger numbers of simulated electrodes provided more accurate representations of the spatial configuration of the underlying simulated neocortical sources. Yvert and colleagues (1997) also found increased accuracy of location of realistic simulations of intracranial sources with increased electrode number. Decreased susceptibility to spatial noise with increasing electrode number from 28 to 256 electrodes was demonstrated by Babiloni and colleagues (1995), consistent with the suggestion of Junghöfer and colleagues (1997) for use of more than 100 electrodes for a guarantee of reasonable accuracy in electrocortical mapping. The growth in information content in ongoing and event-related real EEG recordings as a function of number of electrodes has been systematically investigated (Pflieger and Sands, 1995, 1996) and has been found to grow as a constant times the square root of the number of channels up to at least 256 channels.

In the studies reported in this chapter, 62 channel recordings were made using custom electrode caps. These were designed to uniformly sample head and scalp in a hemispherical fashion (see Figure 8.3). Electrode locations for each subject are recorded by three-dimensional digitization (see Simpson et al., 1995a, 1995b). Data are recorded by using DC amplifiers that do not attenuate slow motor readiness potentials and are continuously digitized at 1 kHz. This relatively fast sample rate allows for precise timing measures of electrocortical activity to be compared with measures based on RT and captures

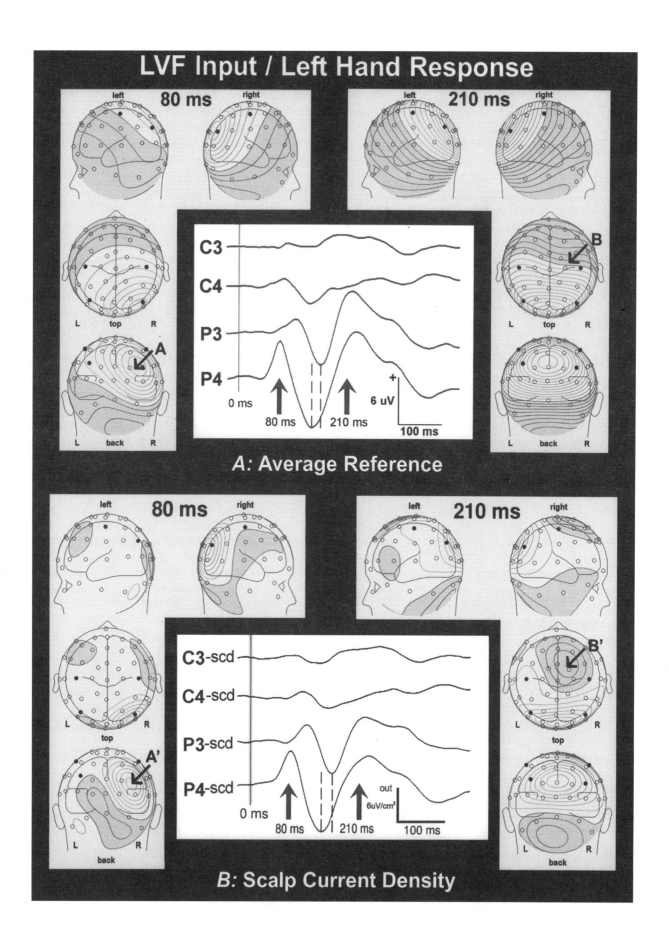

LVF Input / Left Hand Response

A: Average Reference

B: Scalp Current Density

FIGURE 8.3. (a) Average-referenced scalp isopotential contour maps with left and right central and parietal voltage waveforms (indicated as solid circles among the electrode locations drawn on the maps) from a 63-channel study using the Poffenberger task with LVF input and left-hand responses (grand mean of five subjects). The arrows indicate the times at which the map views are drawn. Stippled (blue) areas correspond to negative voltage (0.6 μV/line). Displayed ERP epoch is −25 ms to 425 ms poststimulus. Note the widespread positivity of the visual P1 shown at 80 ms, and the ill-defined motor response over right central regions. (b) SCD maps and Laplacian waveforms from the identical data as shown in part (a) plotted at equivalent sensitivity (0.6 μV/cm²). The activation at 80 ms is now restricted to the posterior regions of the right hemisphere, as expected, given LVF input. The 210-ms maps also now reveal a right central focus, in keeping with the execution of left-hand responses. The Laplacian waveforms show greater peak latency delays between left and right parietal regions and less early activity at C4 than seen in part (a). Stippled (blue) areas correspond to inward current, red areas correspond to outward current, both derived from scalp voltage. (See Color Plate 8.)

---

rapid transitions in the spatiotemporal pattern of cortical activation. The most important aspect of continuous recording for the present studies is the derivation of stimulus- *and* response-synchronized ERPs as a function of RT. Response-synchronized data afford direct comparison between self-initiated and visually triggered movements and limit the temporal dispersion in averaging movement-related events.

Large numbers of channels present a problem in the display of time-series data. The depiction of individual channel waveforms, characteristic of most ERP research, becomes infeasible here. For example, a displayed array of 128 waveforms, even if positioned within a head cartoon according to electrode location, would not allow visualization of scalp topography at any given time point and thus fails to convey the spatiotemporal dynamics of electrocortical activity. It is necessary then to conceptualize such a data set of derived waveforms in two complementary ways: (1) as a series of topographic maps that show event-related spatiotemporal patterns of brain activity recorded at the scalp and (2) as an input to further data analytic techniques that estimate the underlying brain electrical sources of the recorded surface potential. These two analytical approaches are further described in the following section.

DATA ANALYSIS, MODELING, AND DISPLAY

Interpolation and approximation Depicting ERP scalp topography requires a continuous surface mapping. Yet electrode locations represent a discrete spatial sampling. Therefore, estimates of scalp potential at nonelectrode locations need to be computed. One way to accomplish this interpolation is to map scalp potential at discrete points onto a spherical surface. Mathematical deformation of the sphere constrained to pass through the instantaneous potential measured at each electrode will then result in a smooth representation of scalp potential. The spherical spline interpolation approach used here is according to the methods of Perrin and colleagues (1989) as implemented in EEGFOCUS (MEGIS Corporation) software. By projecting the spherically interpolated values on a plane, voltage values for a given time sample are displayed as different point-of-view topographic maps using equipotential lines similar to the isocontours of geological survey maps.

The constraint that the spherical spline pass through the exact instantaneous value of each electrode can lead to erroneous interpolated values depending on the signal-to-noise ratio of the electrocortical data and the behavior of single electrodes (Perrin et al., 1989). To avoid this, the constraint is relaxed somewhat, and the resultant surface becomes an approximation, rather than a strict interpolation, of the spatial distribution of scalp potential. The factor that determines the degree of constraint is termed lambda (λ) and becomes an effective smoothing constant (Wahba, 1990; Babiloni et al., 1995, 1998).

Analysis of scalp current density The topographic display of scalp potential is of limited utility in relating scalp-recorded signals to their underlying electrocortical sources. There are two principal reasons for this. First, the apparent distribution of scalp potential is dependent on the reference electrode inasmuch as the voltage recorded by any pair of electrodes represents the difference between the voltage at each scalp electrode. Thus, activity picked up by the reference alters the absolute value of the voltage at each scalp site. Although the average reference has been advocated as a method that ameliorates the bias introduced by a single reference (Lehmann, 1987), this alternative is not entirely satisfactory unless the sum of voltages from all sites is zero, which is rarely the case. Of even greater importance, the conductive nature of the brain and its coverings disperses the volume currents generated within discrete brain areas, so the scalp potentials they generate are usually spatially and temporally overlapping. The widespread superposition of electrical fields generated by multiple intracranial sources greatly restricts the possibilities for differentiating and correctly identifying the contributions from each source using voltage mapping alone.

A simple analytic method that eliminates the influence of the reference electrode and emphasizes local contributions to the surface map, providing good visualization of approximate locations of intracranial generators, is provided by current source density (CSD) analysis. This technique, originally introduced by Stone and Freeman (1971) for the three-dimensional analysis of intracranially recorded field potentials, is based on the relationship between local current density and potential defined by Laplace's equation. CSD (or Laplacian) analysis involves the estimation of the second spatial derivative of the field potential, which is proportional to the current density at each point. The two-dimensional application of current density analysis to scalp recordings (scalp current density, or SCD) provides a method for estimating the component of current radial to the surface of the scalp, thus providing an estimate of local transcranial current flow (Perrin et al., 1987; Vaughan, 1987; Regan, 1989). SCD analysis mathematically eliminates the voltage gradients due to tangential current flows within the scalp, as well as the contribution of the reference. Thus, by sharpening the spatial resolution of scalp-recorded data, SCD facilitates the identification of activity generated by distinct intracranial sources.

Of particular significance for the present studies, SCD analysis may also improve temporal waveform differentiation by reducing the spatial overlap of waveforms generated by different sources. The importance of this feature of SCD analysis is illustrated in Figure 8.3, which depicts empirical differences between scalp potential and current density mapping. These are grand-average data from five subjects performing the LVF/LH simple RT task. Panel A depicts voltage waveforms (average referenced) from left and right central (C3 and C4, respectively) and parietal (P3 and P4) scalp locations, as well as topographic maps corresponding to the time points indicated by the red arrows. Red contours correspond to positive voltage, and blue stippled contours correspond to negative voltage. The open circles on the maps indicate all electrode locations, and the solid circles refer to the locations of the four waveforms. Panel B depicts the same data as scalp current density. Red contours correspond to outward scalp current, and blue contours to inward. At 80 ms there is a clear sharper right posterior activation focus for the SCD maps (see arrows A′ versus A). At 210 ms the SCD maps show a right central negativity that is not seen in the voltage maps (compare activation patterns at B′ and B).

In this illustration, differing timing of the voltage and SCD waveforms at the same electrode sites can result in differences in IHTT estimates. IHTT values computed from Laplacian waveform negative peak latencies appear to be longer compared with measures of scalp potential because the effects of volume conduction differ between the measures. The parallel dashed lines in panels A and B illustrate this. Such an effect may come about in the following manner: A voltage recording from an electrode overlying left occipital cortex, containing activity generated within the right hemisphere, could shift the apparent latency of the transcallosal activation of the left hemisphere to an earlier time. Conversely, this delayed crossed response may sum with the uncrossed response to increase the apparent duration of responses generated in the directly stimulated hemisphere. These effects, due to the superposition of potentials produced by left- and right-hemisphere sources, as well as noise and asymmetric source configurations, can result in a decreased peak latency differences in scalp potential. Shorter time delays between homotopic central compared with visual sites, as reported by Rugg and colleagues (1984), similar to those seen in Panel A have been used to suggest that measures of IHTT based on RT reflect motor, not visual transfer (e.g., Berlucchi et al., 1995; Ipata et al., 1997; Forster and Corballis, 1998). However, this interpretation is not supported by the Laplacian waveforms recorded over central cortex shown in Panel B. There is no well-defined early response in the C3 SCD waveform as compared to the voltage waveforms because the central voltage waveforms reflect volume conducted potentials generated in visual areas. This observation will be expanded upon in the section below entitled "Scalp Potential Versus Current Density Revisited II: Central Effects."

Adding time to space The spatial sampling of only two time points, as shown in Figure 8.3b, fails to depict the full spatiotemporal dimension of the data. Instead, the dynamic nature of the data has been further examined by using two related approaches. The first consists of creating linear arrays of sequential maps at 5-ms intervals. This allows graphical comparisons across subjects, conditions, or response times within a condition but is labor-intensive owing to the amount of graphical editing involved. A second approach is the creation of SCD animated time series maps, which will be referred to as ATSMs. These are created by using a procedure detailed by Saron (1999) that automatically creates movie frames from SCD maps. The finished animations are in standard video file formats and viewable without special software. These ATSMs allow the full temporal and spatial resolution of the recorded data to be dynamically displayed. The visual complexity and short real-time response duration require slowing the map display down by a factor of 100 to characterize spatiotemporal response patterns. In addition, the interactive nature of the display allows manual quantification of map features such as the latency and magnitude of map foci.

Laplacian waveforms derived from virtual electrodes The ability to portray the spatiotemporal dynamics of the electrocortical response in a manner such as the ATSMs or even as multiple discrete map time series creates the need for a selective form of data reduction that retains information regarding the distribution of brain regions active during performance of a given task. An approach to this problem that has proven extremely useful is the derivation of Laplacian waveforms from specific locations identified on the basis of activation foci visualized by SCD mapping. The spherical spline interpolation of the scalp potential allows computation of scalp current density at any point on the spherical surface. By using virtual electrodes (referred to as *virtrodes*) with the spherical coordinates of the identified activation foci, Laplacian waveforms are derived that portray the activation time course of identified activation foci, independent of the original locations of the recording electrodes. The principal benefit of this approach, provided that there is adequate spatial sampling (e.g., Junghöfer et al., 1997), is the ability to quantitatively characterize the likely activity of discrete brain regions as a function of experimental and behavioral variables. Virtrode-based waveforms were presented independently in a recent paper by Urbano and colleagues (1996).

Some caveats regarding SCD While recognizing the improved resolution afforded by SCD analysis, it is important to emphasize that measures of SCD, although reference-independent and more focused than scalp potential measures, are still also influenced by the dispersion of intracranial volume currents. These volume conduction effects, combined with the geometry of the intracranial sources, often lead to complex overlapping current distributions, particularly when adjacent cortical regions are coactive. This will be illustrated in the section below entitled "Source Localization Reveals Rate Effects." In addition, it is important to note that projecting real scalp potentials onto a sphere before computing the SCD will induce some geometric distortion of the actual scalp current density distribution (see Babiloni et al., 1996).

Brain electrical source analysis SCD maps provide important information about the large-scale pattern of brain region activation associated with our stimuli and task. As just reviewed, they do not do this unambiguously. Further, some map patterns represent active current sources or sinks, while others reflect passive current return to the brain through scalp and skull. The effects of superposition of temporally overlapping brain electrical sources also contributes to ambiguity in interpreting these surface maps in terms of their underlying cerebral sources.

The identification of the spatial and temporal configuration of activity generated within the brain is one instance of what is termed *the inverse problem*. As Helmholtz originally pointed out in 1853 (cited by Simpson et al., 1995a), there is no unique solution to the inverse problem based on measures obtained from the surface of a volume conductor because there are an infinite number of possible configurations of electrical sources that could produce a given surface potential distribution. Much effort has been expended over the past three decades to address the inverse problem as it applies to surface recorded electromagnetic data. These approaches have involved simplifying and constraining the parameters of the head and generator models and optimizing the amount of available data by increasing sensor density and enhancing signal-to-noise ratio, all of which serve to improve the inverse estimation of brain generators. There are many pitfalls and sources of error in the application of these methods, which are compounded by the lack of fully adequate methods for quantitative evaluation of results (e.g., Supek and Aine, 1993, 1997). Accuracy limitations in dipole localization due to the use of a spherical head model have been extensively studied (e.g., Murro et al., 1995; Yvert et al., 1997), and more realistic head models based primarily on boundary-element modeling (BEM) of the brain, skull, and scalp have been advocated (e.g., Cuffin, 1996; Yvert et al., 1996). A direct comparison between the accuracy of spherical and realistic BEM head models in source localization has recently been performed by using 32 known dipolar sources placed within a saline-gelatin filled human skull phantom (Leahy et al., 1998). EEG localization errors were actually quite similar for BEM and spherical head models, a finding that led these investigators to tentatively suggest that the concentric shell spherical model is adequate. Overall, the nonuniqueness of source solutions and the known methodological shortcomings of these procedures necessitates a large measure of caution in interpreting the results derived from currently available methods of source estimation. Nevertheless, anatomically and physiologically plausible solutions have been obtained in a number of circumstances (George et al., 1995; Simpson et al., 1995a, 1995b; Praamstra et al., 1996).

The illustration in this chapter of these methods (Figure 8.15) used brain electrical source analysis (BESA) (Scherg and Von Cramon, 1986; Scherg, 1990) to model the cortical sources underlying the surface potential distributions from a subset of the data described by Saron (1999). BESA models the scalp-recorded data as a linear superposition of potentials generated by sets of time-varying point dipoles within a four-shell concentric sphere, whose position and orientation are invariant across the time period of interest. The shells represent the volume conductive properties of brain, CSF, skull, and scalp. BESA iteratively adjusts dipole strength, location, and orientation over a specified interval to find a dipole configuration that minimizes the residual variance between the modeled and recorded data. BESA solutions provide source waveforms that characterize the time-varying strength of each dipole and the parameters of their location and orientation within the spherical head model. The specific application here of source estimation is presented in the section below entitled "Source Localization Reveals Rate Effects."

Initial findings

SCALP POTENTIAL VERSUS CURRENT DENSITY REVISITED I: POSTERIOR EFFECTS The grand-average data in Figure 8.3 do not allow a consideration of individual differences in comparing scalp potential to current density. Figure 8.4 presents data from a preliminary study (Saron et al., 1995a, 1995b) of six individuals (one per row) tested using the basic methods described previously in the section entitled "An Evolution in Method."

Figure 8.4 compares scalp ERP waveforms recorded from left- and right-hemisphere parieto-occipital sites with waveforms from the equivalent sites based on spherical spline-interpolated scalp current density from the full 62 channel data set. These sites were chosen on the basis of their proximity to the location of the SCD map foci that corresponded to the N160 ERP component. The left-hand response condition is shown here for both visual fields. The averages represent the trials associated with RTs that fell within the second and third quartiles of the RT distribution for each subject and condition. This range corresponds to the steepest portion of the cumulative probability distribution of RTs. This simple form of response latency jitter correction substantially improves definition of ERP components over inclusion of all trials.

Two main points are illustrated in Figure 8.4. The first concerns the decreased subject-to-subject variability seen in SCD waveforms compared to their corresponding voltage data. This is particularly striking for subjects 1–4 for both visual fields. The large intersubject variability seen in the voltage waveforms reflects the susceptibility of scalp potential to represent the superpositional effects, both additive and subtractive, of electrical activity generated simultaneously in widespread cortical regions. Variations in the cortical geometry and functional representations between subjects can therefore result in widely differing voltage waveforms, even if the basic pattern of visual activation in the brain is maintained across individuals.

The second and more crucial point from the perspective of measures of interhemispheric timing are the large differences in between-hemisphere component latencies for voltage and SCD waveforms. This effect is present for both P100 and N160 peaks, which will be considered in turn. Inspection of individual subjects' SCD maps (not shown) reveals that the early positivity for the directly stimulated hemisphere has a more medial distribution than later activation of visual areas. This suggests activation of early visual areas (V1 and V2; see Clark, Fan, and Hillyard, 1995; Foxe and Simpson, 2002) for the directly stimulated hemisphere, compared with the delayed P100 from the indirectly stimulated hemisphere (ipsilateral to the stimulus). This observation cautions against computing early positivity-based measures of IHTT from these data, since appropriate between-hemisphere components are often difficult to observe or select. For instance, the LVF SCD waveforms for subjects 3 and 4 (Figure 8.4) show inflections after the right-hemisphere P100 that likely represent subsequent extrastriate activations of the directly stimulated hemisphere and would thus be more comparable to the delayed response that is seen from the left hemisphere. Selection of appropriate time windows for peak latency measurement is complicated in the voltage waveforms by the apparent reasonableness of peak latency shifts. The LVF voltage data from subject 3 illustrates this well. The latency of the left-hemisphere P100 is 85 ms, suggesting a short (9-ms) delay with respect to the initial right-hemisphere positivity. The latency of this peak jumps to 119 ms in the SCD data, while the latency of the earliest positivity decreases from 76 to 73 ms. These latency shifts between waveform type are mainly due to the susceptibility of scalp potential measures to volume conduction of activity generated in the opposite hemisphere.

The N160 component is well defined for both the directly and indirectly stimulated hemispheres in these data for both waveform types. The most striking observation across subjects and visual fields is the smaller between-hemisphere latency shifts seen in the voltage data. Left- and right-hemisphere responses are of nearly identical latency for LVF data from subjects 2 and 3, as well as RVF data from subjects 2 and 6, whereas all subjects show clearly visible earlier responses from sites contralateral to the stimulated visual field in the SCD data. These differences are presented quantitatively in Figures 8.5a and 8.5b.

In this figure, N160 between-hemisphere peak latency difference values for all four RT conditions are presented by hand and visual field. The mean N160-based IHTT for voltage versus SCD measures across conditions is 9.5 versus 24.7 ms, respectively, a highly significant effect even in this small sample $F(1,5) = 80.1$,

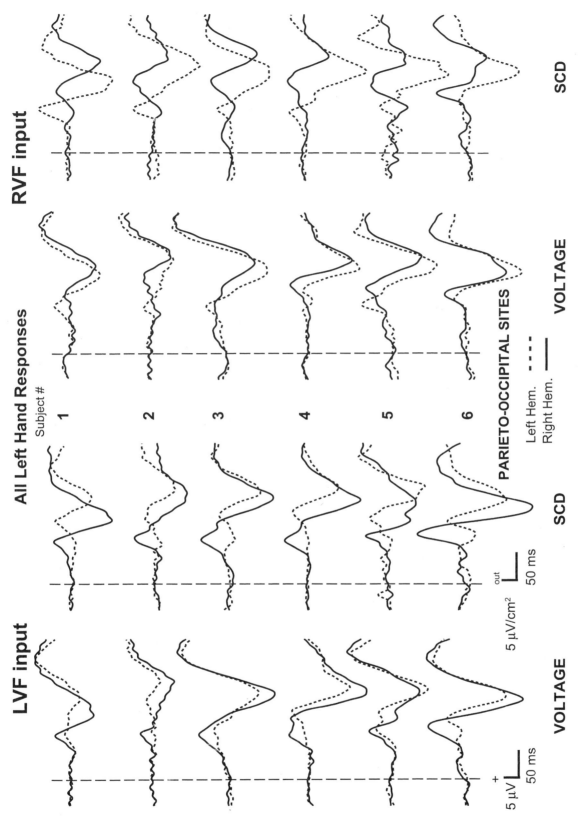

FIGURE 8.4. Scalp ERP (nose reference, −50 to +250 ms) and SCD waveforms from left- and right-hemisphere parieto-occipital sites (PO5/PO6) for six individual subjects (indicated by row number). Data are combined from quartiles 2 and 3 of the RT distribution within subject and condition (data for subject 4 include only second-quartile responses). The mean number of trials is 88. The stimulus onset time is indicated by the vertical dashed line. Note the decreased intersubject variability and increased interhemispheric delays seen in the SCD waveforms.

Mean N160 latency based IHTT

A: Voltage Referred to Nose

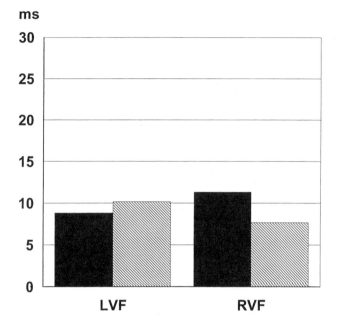

B: Scalp Current Density

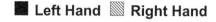
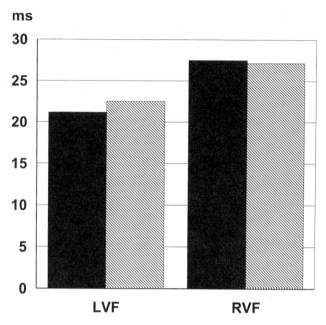

FIGURE 8.5. (a) IHTT estimates from scalp voltage N160 peak latency differences between hemispheres, presented by hand and visual field from the data shown in Figure 8.4. $N = 6$.

(b) SCD N160-based IHTT estimates presented as in part (a). The main effect for waveform type (9.5 versus 24.7 ms) is $F(1,5) = 80.1$, $p < 0.0003$.

$p < 0.0003$. The often-seen relative slowness of left-to-right transfer time is not significant here for either type of waveform. However, five of six subjects show slower left-to-right transfer in the passive view control condition (data not shown) for SCD measures (LVF SCD IHTT mean (S.D.) = 19.0 (8.3) ms, RVF SCD IHTT = 26.5 (6.41), while only one of six subjects showed this effect for voltage measures.

The difference between hands for the RVF voltage data is significant ($F(1,5) = 18.9$, $p < 0.01$). The complete absence of this effect in the SCD data suggests that rather than reflecting an interaction of motor demand on visual IHTT, as we originally thought, the voltage waveforms probably reflect differential effects of ipsilateral versus contralateral motor cortex activation on scalp voltage responses elicited by left versus right visual field stimuli. Overall, the larger values for SCD IHTT measures suggest that the modal visual transfer times that have been estimated in ERP studies using scalp potential measures (see Brown et al., 1994, for a meta-analysis) have, on aggregate, underestimated visual

transfer time. Such a finding further emphasizes the need to understand the basis for the discrepancy between methods of estimating IHTT based on RT and those based on ERPs.

SCALP POTENTIAL VERSUS CURRENT DENSITY REVISITED II: CENTRAL EFFECTS Recently, Ipata and colleagues (1997) examined the ERP voltage topography of both P100- and N160-based estimates of IHTT. They postulate the existence of two callosal "channels," in that P100- and N160-based IHTT have different values and distributions. They suggest that N1-based IHTT estimates, particularly recorded from left and right central locations reflect the interhemispheric transfer processes seen in behavioral measures. These authors base this suggestion on three factors: (1) that N1 IHTT is shorter overall than P1-based estimates (and hence closer to the values obtained with RT methods), (2) that only N1-IHTT from central sites demonstrated the slower left-to-right transfer seen in IHTT meta-analyses, and (3) the idea that N1 may be generated by higher-order

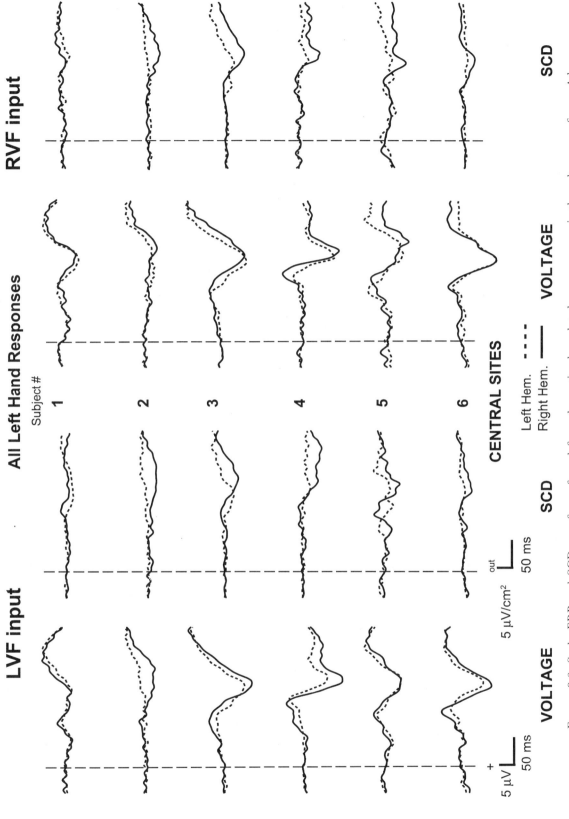

FIGURE 8.6. Scalp ERP and SCD waveforms from left- and right-hemisphere central sites (C3/C4) from the same subjects, conditions (left-hand responses), and trials as shown in Figure 8.4. The SCD waveforms generally fail to show the earlier stimulus-related responses seen in the voltage waveforms. Additionally, they do reflect left/right hemisphere differences consistent with the right-hemisphere motor output requirements of these task conditions.

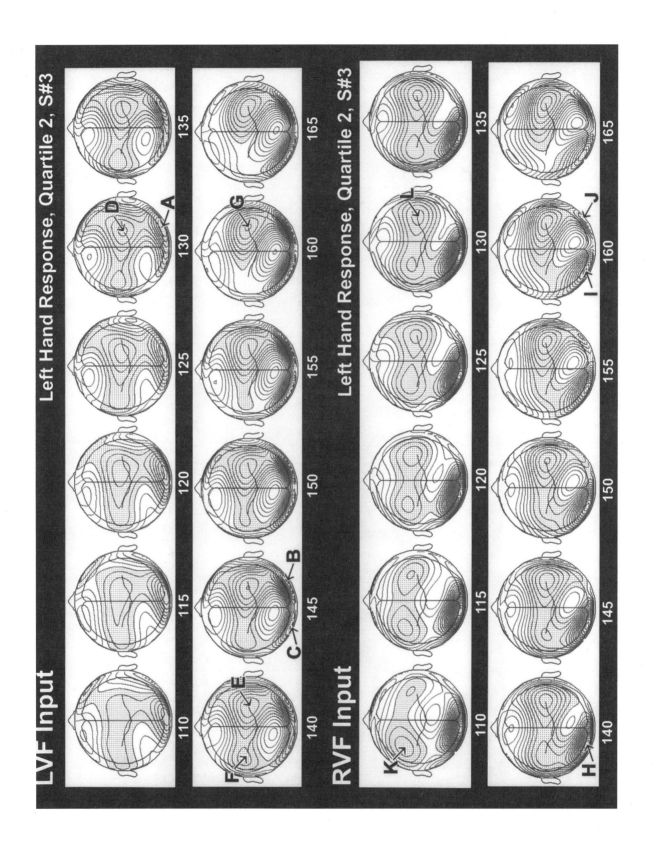

FIGURE 8.7. Top-view SCD maps at 5-ms intervals from 110 to 165 ms poststimulus, separately for LVF and RVF data from the second quartile of the left-hand RT distribution for subject 3. Stippled (blue) regions correspond to inward scalp current derived from scalp potential. Red isocontours correspond to outward scalp current. Plotted sensitivity is 0.5 μV/cm². Responses to LVF input reveal posteriorly the expected initial lateralization followed by callosally mediated bilateral activation. Central regions show an initial bilateral activation pattern that resolves into the unilateral right-hemisphere focus associated with the left-hand response. Posterior responses to RVF input are of opposite lateralization compared to those of LVF input, as expected. The central response pattern suggests a visuomotor routing of left-hemisphere visual-to-motor activation, followed by motor-related left-to-right interhemispheric transfer. See the text for details. (See Color Plate 9.)

---

extrastriate sources than P1 and may therefore reflect interhemispheric interaction associated with visuomotor integration. Occipital and temporal-occipital sites for both visual fields and medial central parietal sites for the right visual field did not, however, yield positive IHTT estimates in this study, suggesting that these voltage-based data may be reflecting some of the volume-conductive effects described above in Figure 8.4.

Differences between voltage and SCD waveforms from central sites (C3/C4) were examined in our study to specifically characterize the activation patterns in these regions within the time ranges of the P100 and N160 components seen more posteriorly. These waveforms are shown in Figure 8.6, plotted from the same subjects, left response hand, and at the same sensitivity as the data shown in Figure 8.4. The most striking feature of these data is that clearly defined ERP components in the voltage waveforms at central sites are greatly diminished or wholly absent in the SCD waveforms. In contrast to the preservation of amplitude and general shifts of latency seen in the parieto-occipital sites of Figure 8.4, visual responses seen at central sites in the voltage waveforms appear not to reflect processes occurring within central regions. Rather, the most consistent pattern of response seen in the SCD waveforms is an increased late negativity in the right, relative to the left, hemisphere, which is in accord with the left-hand response condition.

SIGNS OF MOTOR TRANSFER   To infer that potentials recorded from central regions reflect the interhemispheric transfer measured with RT methods, some evidence of interhemispheric delay should be visible in the SCD data from these sites. Such evidence might reflect a routing pattern of intrahemispheric visual-to-motor activation followed by interhemispheric motor-to-motor transfer. Only the data for subject 3 in Figure 8.6 show a

suggestion of interhemispheric delay of central activation in the SCD waveforms for the RVF/LH crossed RT condition. The basic spatiotemporal pattern of this response from subject 3 is displayed in Figure 8.7.

Top-view SCD maps are plotted at 5-ms intervals from 110 to 165 ms poststimulus, separately for LVF and RVF data from the second quartile (Q2) of the left-hand RT distribution (LVF Q2: RT mean = 221 ms, S.D. = 3.4 ms; RVF Q2: 225 (2.9) ms). The LVF data will be considered first. Red lines correspond to outward and blue (stippled) lines correspond to inward scalp current. Two parallel processes can be seen in these data. The first is initial unilateral posterior right-hemisphere activation due to direct visual input (A), followed by bilateral activation due to callosal transfer (B and C). This pattern corresponds to the N160 ERP component seen in Figure 8.4. The second process occurs centrally, with a large activation over right motor cortex that is associated with the left-hand response (e.g., D). What is most striking about these data is the pattern of central response between 125 and 155 ms. There appears to be bilateral central activity associated with activation of motor cortex (e.g., E and F) prior to the postmovement reafferent pattern which is seen by 160 ms (G). The suggestion from this overall electrocortical response profile is that bihemispheric movement-related activity occurs during intrahemispheric task conditions. This will be discussed further in the section below entitled "Bilateral Motor Activation in an Intrahemispheric Condition."

The spatiotemporal patterns elicited by RVF stimuli again depict separate visual and motor activation. Initial left-hemisphere posterior activation of the directly stimulated pathway (H) is followed at 155 ms by a bilateral response pattern (I and J). However, by 130 ms, before this posterior interhemispheric transfer, there is a clear activation of right central regions (L), following from prior left central activation (K). This response pattern strongly suggests a visuomotor routing of left-hemisphere visual-to-motor activation followed by left-to-right-hemisphere movement-related interhemispheric transfer. Figure 8.8 presents analogous data from subject 3 for right-hand response conditions. Independent of the visual field of input, as expected, the central response patterns reflect primarily left-hemisphere motor output (e.g., A and B). The stimulus-related posterior activations do not differ between Figures 8.7 and 8.8.

EFFECTS OF RT I   The pattern of interhemispheric motor transfer occurring before evidence of interhemispheric visual transfer seen in the RVF/LH condition of Figure 8.7 is particularly relevant to the issue of whether RT measures of IHTT reflect motor transfer. That is, with these data, both RT and physiological estimates of visual and movement-related IHTT may be obtained within the same individual. However, while the most basic features of the response pattern of Figure 8.7 were found across RT quartiles, there were nonetheless large differences in the pattern of movement-related activity as a function of RT. An example of changes in the electrocortical response as a function of RT is shown in Figure 8.9, which includes top-view SCD maps at 130 ms poststimulus from the RVF/LH condition of subject 3 for each quartile of the RT distribution. Stippled isocontours lines represent inward scalp current, corresponding to the blue lines of Figures 8.7 and 8.8.

This figure makes three points. First, note the consistency in the pattern of the visual response in left posterior regions across quartiles (Q1–4). This suggests that RT appears not to be a function of the magnitude or the timing of the sensory-related cortical activation in visual areas evoked by a particular stimulus. Second, although there are striking differences in the pattern of motor activation for the different quartiles, the activity in left-hemisphere central regions suggests left-visual to left-motor activation patterns independent of RT quartile (A–D). Third, the time at which the left-to-right motor transfer occurs is later for Q2 relative to Q1, but the interhemispheric central activation pattern is qualitatively different for Q3 and Q4. The third quartile (Q3) shows an activation pattern that is spatially similar to that of Q2 but with diminished amplitude. This observation suggests a relationship between activation magnitude over central regions and RT. The Q4 RTs fail to show a clear right central activation focus. These slowest responses include signs of right frontal activity (E). This may reflect a divergence in response execution from rapid, visually triggered movements to slower responses that include activation of motor regions via different pathways. A right central focus for Q4 does not appear to begin until 155 ms, which is after anterior spread of right posterior activity following the interhemispheric visual transfer. This pattern is depicted in Figure 8.10a, which shows top-view SCD maps from Q4 of subject 3 at 10-ms intervals beginning at 140 ms poststimulus.

The Q4 pattern suggests a rerouting, in contrast to the Q2 maps of Figure 8.7. That is, activation of right central regions effective for motor output occurs *after* stimulus-related information from the delayed, callosally mediated activation of right posterior regions (A–C). This observation suggests that right posterior regions contribute to activation of right motor cortex, a pattern that is not seen for faster RTs.

Figure 8.10b shows the same data synchronized with the manual response, optimally aligned with the spatiotemporal pattern in Panel A. This can be a useful way to minimize the effects of trial-to-trial differences in RT

that broaden response components when there is considerable variance in a population of reaction times. (The SD of Q4 was 37 ms for an *n* of 45.) While the pattern is quite similar to the data in panel A, there are three differences to note. First, at −130 ms (relative to the RT response) there is no evidence of right central activity compared with panel A (D versus D′). This is a consistent pattern. It begins at −155 ms (not shown), indicating that a persistent activation of left central regions did not result in apparent response-synchronized right central activation. Instead, the right frontal focus (E) is sustained during this time. Second, posterior spread of this right frontal activity seen at −120 ms (F), followed by the anterior spread of right posterior activity at −100 ms (G), suggests that a temporally offset, dual-pathway activation pattern of right central regions is associated with RTs in this slowest quartile. The major stimulus-related activation of motor output regions appears to occur via the interhemispheric activation of right visual cortex. The finding of a visual-to-visual, followed by visual-to-motor, transfer pattern represents a crucial point illustrated by the data from RVF stimulation in Figures 8.7 and 8.10: *Within an individual and within a given interhemispheric RT condition, different reaction times may be associated with different routes by which motor cortex becomes activated.* Finally, the greater degree of right central activity at −80 ms (H), relative to the 180-ms map in panel A (C), illustrates the enhanced visualization of movement-related activity with response-synchronized averaging. This is due to the diminution of the effects of temporal dispersion across the responding interval seen when time-locked to the stimulus.

Further studies

VISUAL VERSUS MOTOR INTERHEMISPHERIC TRANSFER TIME The existence of such large differences in response topography associated with differences in RT indicated a need to examine more closely the electrophysiological correlates of RT. In the subsequent experiment, described below (see Saron, 1999; Saron et al., in press), sets of ERPs were obtained with each average based on a small range of RTs. Sufficient trials were collected (~1500 per condition) to generate between 12 and 15 sets of ERPs, each from within nonoverlapping 10-ms-wide RT bins over the RT range (across subjects) of 190–380 ms. A comparison of left- and right-hemisphere SCD virtrode waveforms and associated SCD maps from the indicated peak latencies from the RVF/LH condition of the retest of subject 3 is presented in Figure 8.11a. Only trials with RTs in the second quartile of the RT distribution comprise these averages.

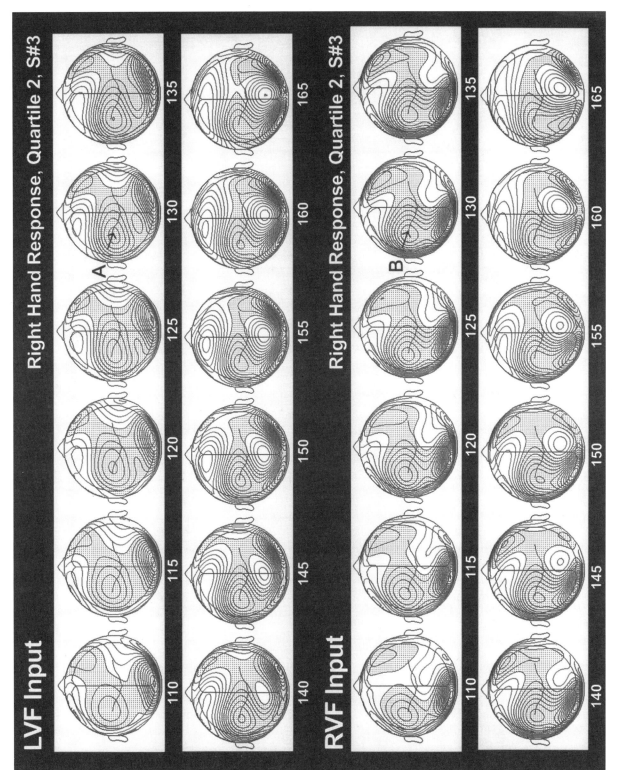

FIGURE 8.8. Top-view SCD maps at 5-ms intervals from 110 to 165 ms poststimulus, separately for LVF and RVF data from the second quartile of the right-hand RT distribution for subject 3. Stippled (blue) regions correspond to inward scalp current. The plotted sensitivity is 0.5 μV/cm². While the posterior activation pattern is nearly identical to that seen in Figure 8.7, the change of responding hand is clearly visible in the shift to left central activation independent of input visual field (A and B). (See Color Plate 10.)

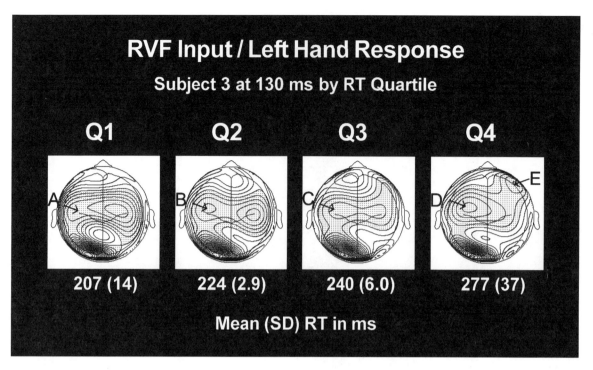

FIGURE 8.9. Top-view SCD maps at 130 ms poststimulus from the RVF/LH condition of subject 3 for each quartile of the RT distribution. The consistent pattern of left posterior responses across quartiles (Q1–4) suggests that RT in these data is not due to the strength of the sensory-related cortical activation. Large differences in the pattern of motor activation for the different quartiles are evident in right central regions. Left central responses suggest consistent initial left-visual to left-motor activation independent of RT. Stippled regions correspond to inward scalp current derived from scalp potential. Plotted sensitivity is 0.5 µV/cm². See the text for details.

The upper panel shows left and right posterior waveforms derived from the centers of left (A′) and right (B′) inward current maxima as seen in the back view SCD maps. Given the large n, these maps were plotted with a λ of 1×10^{-7}, which shows more spatial detail than is seen in the maps of the previous figures. The waveforms show the clear latency and amplitude advantage of the direct pathway. The posterior interhemispheric delay between the peaks of the SCD N160 (arrows A and B) is 38 ms (O1 = left hemisphere). The longer 48-ms interhemispheric delay between P1 peaks (1 and 2) likely reflects subtracting the peak latency of the initial striate and early extrastriate component of the left hemisphere visual response from the peak latency of later extrastriate activity from the callosally-mediated response of the right hemisphere.

The lower virtrode waveform row presents central responses obtained from the centers of left (C3) and right (C4) lateral activation foci (putative primary motor cortex, M1) seen at C′ and D′. The earlier activation of the left hemisphere for this condition replicates the pattern of the original testing seen in the RVF/LH data of Figure 8.7. The peak amplitude of the C4 waveform at 174 ms (D), 14 ms prior to the peak of the transferred visual response (B), again strongly suggests a within-left-hemisphere visual-to-motor activation followed by left-to-right motor-related transfer. The 36-ms estimated motor-related IHTT (difference of peak latencies at C and D) is within 2 ms of the visual IHTT estimate and stands in sharp contrast to RT results for this subject. Median LVF/LH RT ($N = 1326$) was 267 ms, and RVF/LH RT ($N = 1351$) = 264 ms, with an RT IHTT of −3 ms, an obviously implausible value of interhemispheric transfer time. This dissociation between physiological and behavioral data suggests that IHTT RT is not, in this instance, measuring motor transfer time even in the presence of a clear physiologic motor transfer pattern.

Additional central activations are notable in the top-view maps. The strong midline negativity seen at E and increasing in magnitude at F suggests supplementary motor area (SMA) involvement in movement generation. Given the medial location of SMA, midline central movement-related activations have been interpreted to represent bilateral SMA activity (Praamstra et al., 1996). Connections between left and right SMA likely subserve the central interhemispheric transfer suggested here, as these regions are richly callosally interconnected (Rouiller et al., 1994) and receive strong input from premotor regions (Luppino et al., 1993) that are interconnected

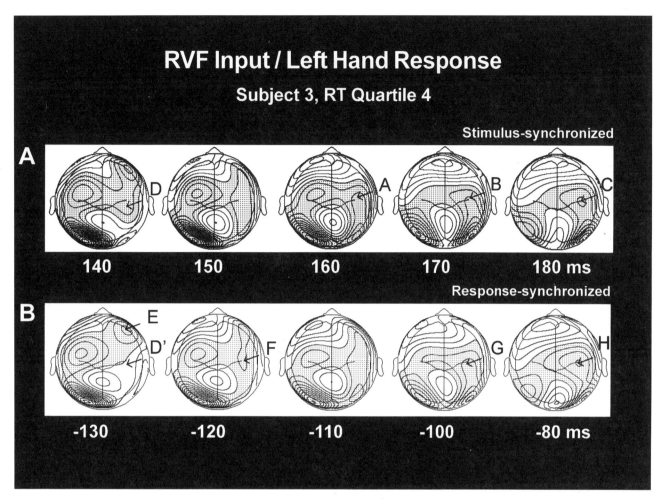

RVF Input / Left Hand Response

Subject 3, RT Quartile 4

FIGURE 8.10. (a) Stimulus-synchronized top-view SCD maps beginning at 140 ms poststimulus from the fourth quartile (Q4) of the RVF/LH task condition from subject 3. In contrast to the interhemispheric visuomotor routing pattern of Figure 8.7, activation of right central regions appears to occur after stimulus-related information from the interhemispheric activation of right posterior regions has resulted in activation of right motor regions. (b) Response-synchronized mapping of the same data as in part (a), beginning 130 ms prerespons. Posterior spread of this right frontal activity seen at −120 ms followed by the anterior spread of right hemisphere posterior activity suggests that a temporally offset, dual-pathway activation pattern of right central regions is associated with these slower responses. Stippled regions correspond to inward scalp current. Map sensitivity is 0.5 µV/cm². See the text for further details.

with parietal cortex (Wise et al., 1997). Since Rouiller and colleagues (1994) found weak callosal projections between the hand areas of left and right primary motor cortices, connections between SMA and primary motor cortex (Tokuno and Tanji, 1993; Tanji, 1994) are likely to provide additional pathways for central interhemispheric routes. The observation that SMA is among the regions of motor cortex that contain corticospinal projections that activate motor neurons of the contralateral hand (Dum and Strick, 1991, 1996) and its bilateral organization (Wiesendanger et al., 1996) suggests a general importance of central interhemispheric routes via SMA. The occurrence of movement-related activation of both putative SMA and M1 further suggests that multiple motor regions contribute to the corticospinal effer-

ence for finger lifts during this simple visuomotor RT task (Saron et al., 1998; Saron et al., in press).

VISUAL RESPONSES IN MOTOR REGIONS The steep negative-going portion of the C3 virtrode waveform peaking at C of Figure 8.11a begins approximately at 85 ms. This early activation, occurring during the first part of the visual response (1), suggests that the C3 activity reflects in part visual input to ipsilateral motor cortex. If this were the case, we might expect that a similar activation would occur even in the absence of a response requirement. Example data from such a condition are presented in Figure 8.11b. The early activation for C3 in the no-response, passive-view condition is nearly identical in timing to the left-hand response

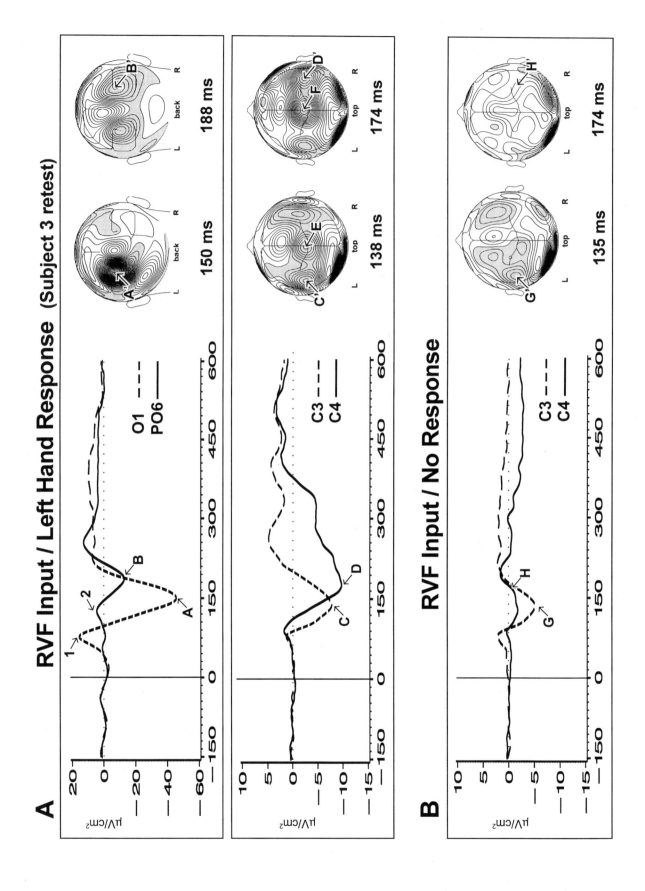

FIGURE 8.11. (a) Left- and right-hemisphere parieto-occipital (upper row) and central (lower row) virtrode SCD waveforms and back and top-view SCD maps from indicated time points from the retest of subject 3. Data are from the second quartile of the RT distribution (displayed $n = 416$, RT range 235–265 ms). The upper waveforms show the clear latency and amplitude advantage of the direct pathway (O1). The maps indicate initial left and then bilateral posterior activations associated with callosal transfer of the visual input. The motor activation pattern suggests an intra-left-hemisphere visual-to-motor activation followed by left-to-right motor-related transfer, including signs of midline (presumptive SMA) and lateral (presumptive M1) activation. (b) Left and right central SCD waveforms and top-view SCD maps in response to passive viewing of RVF stimuli for subject 3, $n = 740$. These data show similar onset times for C3 activity as in the left-hand response condition seen in part (a). This suggests the stimulus-related nature of this early left hemisphere central activation. As expected, the 174-ms SCD map shows the lack of motor activity associated with this no-response condition (D vs. H). Stippled regions correspond to inward scalp current derived from surface potential. The plotted sensitivity is 0.5 μV/cm², $\lambda = 1 \times 10^{-7}$. See the text for further details.

———◄———————————————

condition, with a peak latency that is 3 ms shorter than during the RT condition (C versus G, C′ versus G′), suggesting that this signal is related to visual input and not the motor response. The activation pattern of the motor output hemisphere, as expected, differs greatly between passive-view and RT conditions, as seen in the C4 waveforms from Panels A and B (D versus H) and the 174 ms SCD maps (D′ versus H′).

The similarity of early left-hemisphere central activations between no-response and RT conditions is in accord with recent advances in the understanding of visual inputs to premotor areas (e.g., Wise et al., 1997). These authors point to three major sources of visual input to dorsal premotor regions (PMd) based on anatomical studies in monkeys. A pathway from striate and extrastriate cortex to parieto-occipital visual areas (PO, also known as V6A), projects to PMd. Responses of PO neurons are characterized by a lack of foveal magnification and large peripheral receptive fields that are selective for orientation and direction (Wise et al. 1997). These authors suggest that such responses are important in ambient vision and for target detection and localization. A second pathway from PO to PMd is via medial intraparietal cortex (MIP). Both visual and somatosensory inputs activate cells in MIP. Their involvement in visuomotor integration is suggested by an increased responsiveness to visual stimuli presented within reaching distance (Colby and Duhamel, 1996) and larger response modulations when hand movements are made by the hemisphere receiving visual input (Colby and Duhamel, 1991). A third pathway from PO to PMd is

via the medial dorsal parietal region and area 7m (Wise et al., 1997). The functional role of PMd in visually elicited hand movements was demonstrated by Sasaki and Gemba (1986). In this experiment, the premotor cortex of macaques was reversibly inactivated by local cooling during a simple RT task to visually presented stimuli. Bilateral cooling resulted in disorganizing trained RT lever lifts into a pattern that bore little relationship to the light stimulus and that resembled self-paced, though apparently unimpaired, movements.

Sensory-related responses in M1 have also been investigated. Miller, Riehle, and Requin (1992) identified sensory-, sensorimotor-, and movement-related single-neuron responses recorded from contralateral M1 in a macaque during a go/no-go wrist flexion task. The central question of this experiment was whether motor preparation begins before complete analysis of the response signal. During no-go trials, sensory and sensorimotor cells identified during go trials were found to respond with identical latency as during go trials (within 150 ms) and with 77% of the peak amplitude recorded during go trials. Given the 307-ms RT for this task, these results demonstrate that sensory input contributes to response preparation prior to the decision to respond, consistent with the responses seen in Figure 8.11b. Recently, Endo and colleagues (1999) demonstrated a finding similar to that of Miller and colleagues (1992) in humans during a go/no-go task recording whole-head magnetoencephalography (MEG). Sensory responses were seen in motor regions during no-go trials. The sensory-related nature of these responses was additionally inferred from the observation of motor cortex activations with a constant delay from the visual go signal, independent of RT when subaverages based on RT were examined within subjects. Further, the topography of the evoked magnetic response over motor cortex was similar at 168 ms for both go and no-go conditions, a result that was interpreted as "automatic" activation to facilitate response preparation even before a decision is reached regarding executing the motor response.

An examination of the topography of early stimulus-related responses over motor cortex is presented in Figure 8.12. Here top-view SCD maps for all stimulus conditions are plotted at high sensitivity (0.1 μV/cm² versus 0.5 μV/cm² for all previous maps, $\lambda = 1 \times 10^{-5}$). These data from subject 3 use the full number of trials recorded ($N \approx 735$ for control conditions and $N \approx 1350$ for response conditions) and are presented at both 65 and 80 ms poststimulus. Red contours correspond to outward, and blue stippling to inward scalp current.

The posterior responses show the expected lateralization for each visual field. The growth of the visual P1 is indicated by the increased response magnitude from 65

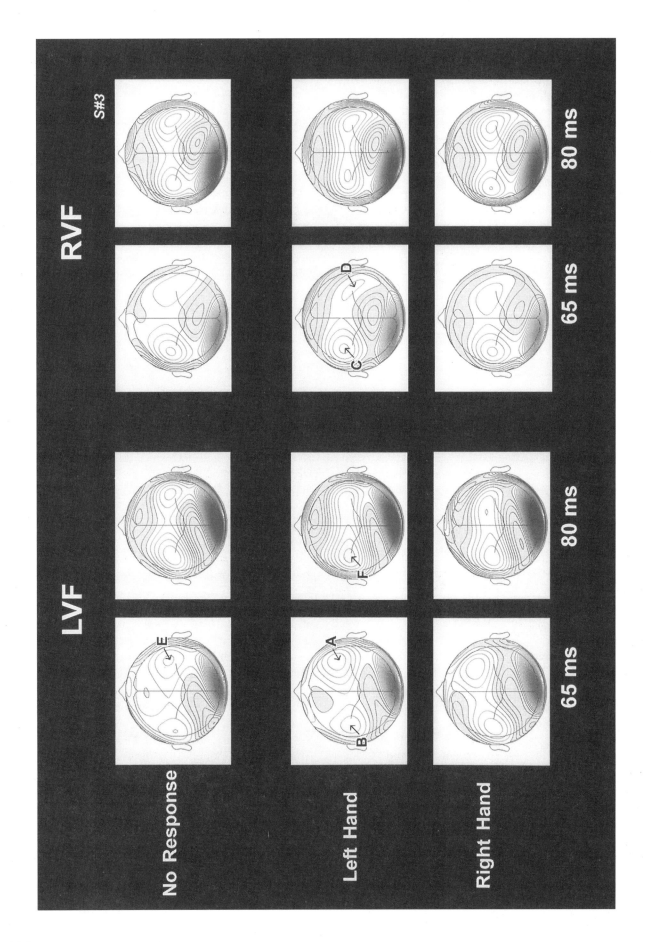

FIGURE 8.12. Top-view SCD maps for all stimulus and response conditions from the retest of subject 3 are plotted at high sensitivity $(0.1 \ \mu V/cm^2, \ \lambda = 1 \times 10^{-5})$ at 65 and 80 ms poststimulus. These across-RT data (120–600 ms) have $n \approx 1350$. $\mathcal{N} \approx 735$ for the passive view control conditions. Both LVF and RVF stimuli show a larger focus of activity over central regions ipsilateral to the hemisphere receiving visual input. The LVF data suggest that there may be an effect of response condition, with larger initial ipsilateral central activations seen in the reaction time conditions. At 80 ms, central regions contralateral to the hemisphere receiving visual input show equal or greater activity than seen ipsilateral to the stimulated hemisphere at 65 ms. This may reflect a very early visually generated central interhemispheric transfer. Stippled (blue) areas represent inward current flow. Red areas correspond to outward current. See the text for more details. (See Color Plate 11.)

◄─────────────────────────────────────

to 80 ms. Regarding the pattern of central activations, at 65 ms, for both visual fields, there is a larger focus of activity over central regions ipsilateral to the visual input (e.g., A versus B, C versus D). Within the LVF data there is a suggestion of an effect due to response condition, with larger activations seen in the RT conditions (e.g., A versus E). This observation would suggest that the need for subsequent motor output increases sensory input-related activation in these regions, consistent with a role in visuomotor integration. The location of these early activation foci slightly anterior to the strong movement-related focus generally seen 100 ms later is consistent with their overlying dorsal premotor cortex, based on current parcellations of human motor regions (Roland and Zilles, 1996). At 80 ms, for both input fields, the contralateral central regions show equal or greater activity than is seen ipsilateral to the stimulated hemisphere at 65 ms (e.g., B versus F). It is tempting to suggest that this reflects a very early sensory-related central interhemispheric transfer. Such an early activation of left and right central regions may facilitate subsequent bilateral activations of central regions prior to motor output, even within ipsilateral visual input and motor output conditions. (See Saron et al. (2001a) for further evidence of segregation of occipital and frontal cortex sensory-related activations.)

BILATERAL MOTOR ACTIVATION IN AN INTRAHEMISPHERIC CONDITION Numerous studies using a variety of methods have now demonstrated a pattern of bilateral activation before and during movements that appears to reflect more ipsilateral involvement in motor function than can be explained by the 5.9% of uncrossed corticospinal fibers that originate from primate primary motor cortex (Toyoshima and Sakai, 1982; see also Schoen, 1964; Porter and Lemon, 1995). Tanji, Okano, and Sato

(1988) examined single-neuron activity in macaque premotor, SMA, and M1 cortex during unilateral finger button presses to visual stimuli. Although activity in primary motor cortex was almost exclusively related to contralateral hand movements, 25% of SMA neurons and 17% of premotor neurons showed activity before ipsilateral movements. The bilateral organization of SMA has been suggested (Wiesendanger et al., 1996), and the rich callosal pathways that have been found between left and right distal forelimb representations in SMA (Rouiller et al., 1994) are likely to have mediated the responses observed by Tanji and colleagues (1988). Connections between SMA and primary motor cortex (Tokuno and Tanji, 1993; Tanji, 1994) and premotor regions (Luppino et al., 1993) likely provide the pathways for bihemispheric activation of multiple motor regions observed in human studies reviewed below. See Picard and Strick (1996) and Fink and colleagues (1997) for relations between monkey and human nonprimary motor areas.

Ikeda et al. (1995) have used intracranial recordings to examine human SMA activations during unilateral and bilateral movements. Bilateral premovement SMA activations were found for unilateral foot and thumb flexions of either side. Using whole-head (122 channel) MEG, Salmelin and colleagues (1995) also found a pattern of bilateral motor cortex activations for unilateral movements. Readiness fields (RFs) and movement-evoked fields (MEFs) were measured bilaterally for complex finger movements, while simple index finger flexions produced bilateral RFs and contralateral MEFs. This pattern for simple movements has been replicated by using combined whole-head MEG and ERP recordings by Gerloff and colleagues (1997), who report bilateral premotor cortex activations prior to unilateral M1 activation. Praamstra and colleagues (1996) have used spatiotemporal dipole modeling of ERPs and described bilateral activations before finger movement in putative locations corresponding to M1 and in SMA. The assumption of bilateral SMA activation is based on finding a radially oriented midline source dipole that could represent concurrent activity generated by left and right SMA. In support, a similar experiment using MEG data found bilateral premovement activity in dipoles located in left and right precentral cortex (Hoshiyama et al., 1997). One of the most sophisticated event-related electrocortical analyses of self-paced movement-related activity in humans has recently been performed by Urbano and colleagues (1996, 1998b). During brisk single-finger extensions similar to the movements performed in the RT task of the present studies, these investigators used 128-channel recordings and realistic head models obtained from the individual subjects' MRIs to compute

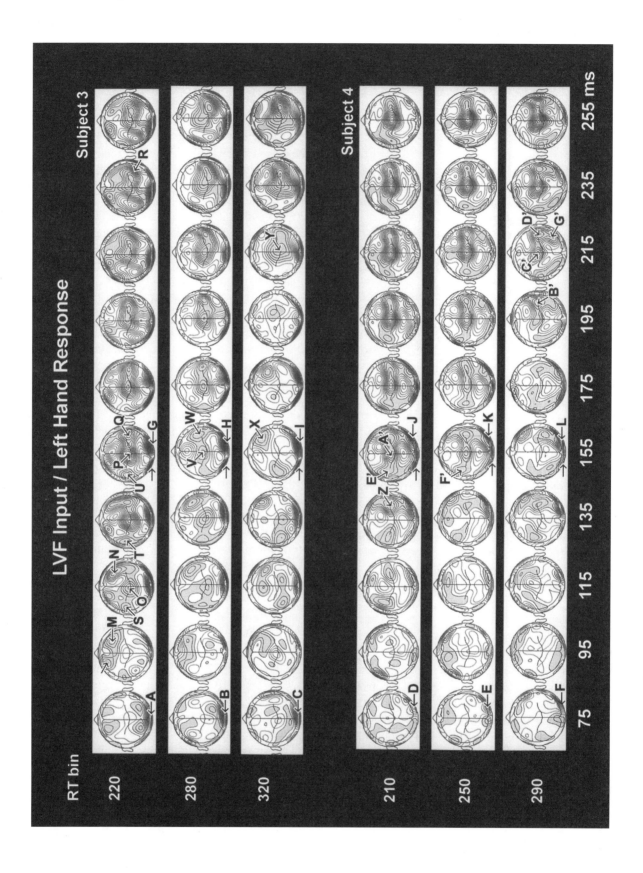

LVF Input / Left Hand Response

Subject 3

Subject 4

RT bin

the projection of the scalp-recorded Laplacian onto the cortical surface (see Babiloni et al., 1996, for EEG methods). Both left and right finger movements resulted in bilateral activation of nearly equal amplitude in left sensorimotor cortex (identified as M1-S1) during response preparation, movement initiation, and finger motion epochs. Right M1-S1 showed equal activations during response preparation and about one-half response amplitude during right (ipsilateral) compared with left finger movements. The authors interpret the ipsilateral responses as reflecting transcallosal activations mediated by the SMA–M1 interactions referred to above.

A more global measure of bilateral movement-related activation has been demonstrated by Stancák and Pfurtscheller (1996). These authors used event-related desynchronization (ERD) of EEG recorded in response to index finger movements. There was bilateral premovement ERD for both left and right responses, with equal degrees of left- and right-hemisphere desynchronization for left-handed movements. Urbano and colleagues (1998a) examined lagged cross-covariance measures of EEG between selected electrodes as an index of possible functional coupling between different cortical regions. Bilateral activation of motor cortex during right finger movements (the only hand that was tested) was also found using this technique.

Bilateral motor cortex activations have also been demonstrated using neuroimaging techniques. In a study using functional magnetic resonance imaging (fMRI) to investigate responses to finger movements, Kim and

colleagues (1993b) found a strong hemispheric asymmetry in bilateral motor cortex activation consistent with the ERD data of Stancák and Pfurtscheller and the ERP data of Urbano and colleagues (1998b) (see also Kim et al., 1993a). Particularly for right-handers, left-hemisphere motor regions showed nearly identical activations during left or right finger movements (contra/ipsi ratio = 1.3 versus 36.8 for the right hemisphere). This pattern of left-hemisphere activation in conditions of left-hand movement is found in the present data as well, though restricted to the premovement epoch. As such, the present data extend the findings from hemodynamic studies by suggesting temporal bounds for observed activations in neuroimaging studies. Boecker and colleagues (1994) also report ipsilateral activation of primary motor cortex during self-paced finger tapping in two of five subjects when using the right hand. Recently, Gordon and colleagues (1998) examined a variety of unimanual and bimanual typing tasks using high-field strength fMRI. While right-hand index finger sequenced key presses produced marked bilateral activation in M1, SMA, and cingulate cortex, even simple repetitive unidigit key strokes elicited ipsilateral activation in these regions in some subjects, a finding similar to that of Boecker and colleagues (1994).

Figure 8.13 displays top-view SCD map time series ($\lambda = 1 \times 10^{-7}$) from 75 ms to 255 ms poststimulus for the intrahemispheric LVF/LH condition for the retest of subject 3 and a second individual who was also tested in the large-trial-number version of the experiment, subject 4. The data are displayed as a function of RT, with each value the midpoint of a 10-ms range. The general pattern seen before of the stability of the posterior visual response across RT is evident. For example, both the initial lateralized positivity at 75 ms (A through F) and bilateral negativity seen at 155 ms (dual arrows at G–L) differ little by RT bin.

In contrast to the stability of the posterior responses across RT, the patterns of central activation for both subjects markedly differ by RT bin. For subject 3, the central activation patterns for the 220-ms RT bin are characterized by a bilateral frontal negativity at 95 ms (dual arrows at M) that shows a right-hemisphere increase by 115 ms (N). Midline central activation (presumptive SMA) is also visible by 115 ms (O), which increases in magnitude until 155 ms (P). Also at that time, right lateral-central negativity (presumptive M1 (Q)) is visible. The pattern of prior midline and frontal activations (O and N) suggest that M1 activation may be subsequent to sensory-related activations in these regions. The late posterior shift of the broad right central negativity by 235 ms (R) is suggestive of signs of somatosensory activation from postmovement reafference. Also

FIGURE 8.13. Top-view SCD map time series ($\lambda = 1 \times 10^{-7}$) from 75 to 255 ms poststimulus for the intrahemispheric LVF/LH condition for the retest of subjects 3 and 4. The data are displayed by RT bin, with each value the midpoint of a 10-ms range (n's for subject 3 were 86, 105, and 55 for RT bins 220, 280, and 320, respectively; n's for subject 4 were 49, 76, and 37 for RT bins 210, 250, and 290, respectively). The stability of the posterior visual response across RT is evident. The patterns of central activation for both subjects markedly differ, the faster two RT bins sharing similar overall activation patterns that are lower in magnitude for the middle RT bin. For both subjects, the slowest RTs show a delayed activation pattern. These data illustrate the multiplicity of motor regions of both hemispheres active during performance of intrahemispheric task conditions and highlight individual differences in spatiotemporal activation patterns during performance of simple RT. Stippled (blue) regions correspond to inward scalp current, red to outward current. Plotted sensitivity is 0.5 μV/cm^2 for subject 3 and 0.6 μV/cm^2 for subject 4. See the text for a detailed explanation of activation patterns. (See Color Plate 12.)

of note in earlier activations are the left lateral-central activations seen at S, T, and U. These foci, ipsilateral to the responding hand, are evidence of bilateral central involvement during this intrahemispheric task condition. The timing and topography of the central activation pattern for the 280-ms RT bin are similar to that seen for the 220-ms RT bin, though generally weaker in magnitude through 195 ms (see P and Q versus V and W). This observation further suggests that decreased magnitude of motor cortex activation, rather than timing of activation, may be related to slower RT.

It is important to point out that the early midline activations at 115 and 135 ms likely represent initial signs of corticospinal outflow for movement generation. This is because the 21-ms estimate of corticomuscular delay for the extensor indicus (Salenius et al., 1997) and lag in the optical response switch (70–80 ms) mean that a behaviorally measured RT may be as much as 100 ms after cortical initiation of the movement (Saron, 1999).

The 320-ms RT bin pattern differs markedly from that of the 220- and 280-ms RT bins and is more consistent with an association between this observed delay in the activation of motor cortex and the slowest RTs. For instance, the absence of central activation and presence of right frontal activation at 155 (X) is similar to features of earlier activation patterns for the faster RTs. A rapid increase in central negativity does not occur until after 195 ms, also consistent with a delayed activation pattern (Y).

The spatiotemporal patterns of central activation in subject 4 illustrate many of the same basic findings as subject 3, with some notable individual differences. For example, in this subject, activation of presumptive M1 (Z) precedes activation of presumed SMA (A′). However, the similar timing and topography of RT bins 210 and 250 replicate the observation of decreased magnitude of motor cortex activation as associated with slower RTs. In addition, the 290-ms RT bin data show a late onset of rapidly increasing central negativity beginning at 195 ms (B′–D′), a pattern that is consistent with delayed motor cortex activation for the slowest RTs. The left lateral-central negativities seen at 155 ms for RT bins 210 and 250 ms (E′ and F′) again demonstrate that bilateral motor cortex activations occur during unimanual intrahemispheric visuomotor simple RT tasks. The marked posterior spread of the right lateral central negativity at 215 ms (G′) suggests a basis for a secondary visuomotor activation of right motor regions by a reactivation of superior parietal cortex at this time.

MOTOR ACTIVATION MEASURES PREDICT REACTION TIME

SCD central magnitude effects Another way in which differences in movement-related activity as a function of RT have been examined is shown in Figure 8.14. In this approach, SCD virtrode waveforms calculated from the centers of presumed SMA and M1 activations were lag cross-correlated with the forearm EMG to estimate the corticomuscular delay (CMD) and to determine the primary location of motor output activations. The central region with lag values for the maximum correlations that most closely approximated the expected physiological CMD estimate for finger movements (21 ms; see Salenius et al., 1997) was taken as the appropriate location for further analysis of movement-related activations.

Figure 8.14a shows overlays of SCD waveforms for the LVF/LH condition of subject 3 for each of 12 RT bins. The waveforms are the difference between two activation foci located at FC2 and Cz, since the SCD maps showed a midline central activation pattern consistent with a tangentially oriented source configuration. The striking feature of these waveforms is the presence of a clearly defined stimulus-related positivity peaking near 85 ms, followed by a movement-related negativity that varies as a function of RT. This suggests the importance of this region in visuomotor integration. The amplitude of the early, presumed SMA activation is clearly variable as a function of RT, but this relation is not systematic. Measures of integrated amplitude between 50 and 110 ms (data not shown) demonstrate that the strongest activations are for RT bins 230–250, as can be seen from the waveforms. These differences may account in part for the magnitude and timing of subsequent movement-related activity in this region.

Three overall RT-related activation differences are present in the movement-related portion of these waveform overlays. The first, illustrated by the 220–250-ms RT bins, is characterized by a steep onset limb and similar amplitude of the movement-related negativity that is delayed 5–10 ms as RT slows. The second, illustrated by the 260- to 290-ms RT bins, are decreases in slope and magnitude of activation as RT slows, with onset times of the movement-related negativity similar to those for RT bins 220–250 ms. The third observation is of delayed activation onset that is best seen for the slowest RT bins, 320 and 330 ms. RT bins 300 and 310 ms show a transitional pattern of decreased initial activation slope and subsequent delayed reactivation. The importance of these observations is that RT differences are not simply due to graded differences in either the magnitude or timing of motor output activity but may constitute expression of different modes or classes of visuomotor activation pathways. The basic pattern of these magnitude and timing differences were consistently observed across subjects and for both intrahemispheric task conditions (Saron, 1999; Saron et al., in press).

LVF Input / Left Hand Response

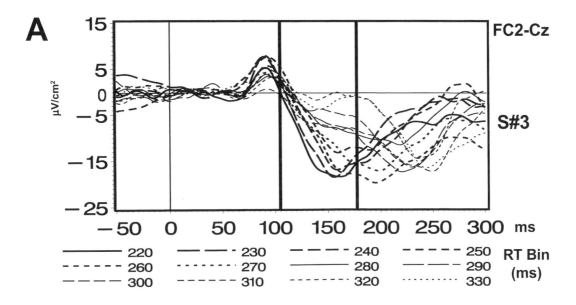

A

FC2-Cz

S#3

	RT Bin (ms)
—— 220	—— · 230	— — — 240	- - - - 250
- - - - 260	········ 270	—— 280	— — 290
— — — 300	— - - — 310	- - - - 320	········ 330

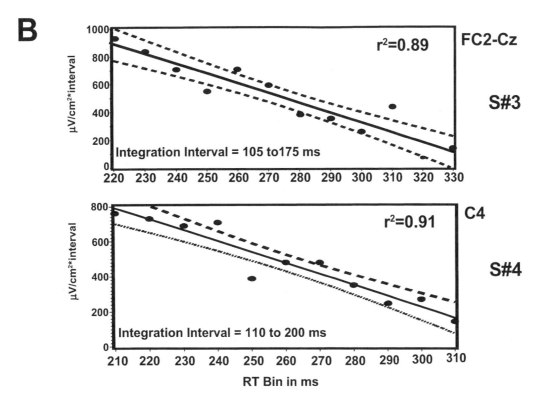

B

r^2=0.89 FC2-Cz

S#3

Integration Interval = 105 to175 ms

r^2=0.91 C4

S#4

Integration Interval = 110 to 200 ms

RT Bin in ms

FIGURE 8.14. (a) Overlays of SCD virtrode waveforms for the LVF/LH condition of subject 3 for each of 12 RT bins. The waveforms are the difference between two activation foci located at FC2 and Cz, since the SCD maps showed a midline (presumptive SMA) central activation pattern consistent with a tangentially oriented source configuration. The waveforms include a clearly defined stimulus-related positivity peaking near 85 ms, followed by a movement-related negativity that changes with RT. The differences in waveform shape by RT bin include both decreased slope and magnitude of movement-related activations, as well as patterns of delayed onsets for the slowest responses and are described in the text. (b) Segments of the waveforms described above were quantified by computing values of integrated amplitude for each RT bin within the interval indicated by the thick vertical lines in part (a) (and the indicated interval for the data from subject 4). Linear regressions by RT were performed on the integrated amplitude values obtained from these intervals. The dashed lines indicate the 95% confidence interval of the mean of predicted values. The results indicate a strong linear relation between decreasing initial activation magnitude of motor output regions and increasing RT.

Segments of the waveforms described above were quantified by computing values of integrated amplitude for each RT bin within the interval indicated by the thick vertical lines in Figure 8.14a. The onset time of the analysis interval was chosen to include the average onset of the movement-related negativity across conditions and subjects. The offset time was chosen to include the pattern of decreasing initial activation with increasing RT and to exclude the delayed activation associated with the slowest responses. Thus, the analysis provides a measure of the initial activations that resulted in movement for faster RTs and that failed to elicit rapid movement for slower RTs. Linear regressions by RT were performed on the integrated amplitude values obtained from the indicated intervals. These are plotted in Figure 8.14b for subjects 3 and 4. The dashed lines indicate the 95% confidence interval of the mean of predicted values. Each panel also indicates the r^2 for the analysis. The results indicate a strong linear relation between decreasing initial activation magnitude of motor output regions and increasing reaction time, despite differences in the RT ranges for different subjects ($F[1, 10] = 77.2$, $p < 0.0001$ for subject 3; $F[1, 10] = 80.4$, $p < 0.0001$ for subject 3). These results confirm the slope and magnitude observations of the virtrode waveforms.

The intriguing suggestion demonstrated by this finding is that, given the lack of difference in visual responses across RT shown in Figure 8.13, RT variability is likely not due primarily to variations in stimulus processing. More likely, it reflects the degree to which a given stimulus activates the motor system. This in turn may depend on moment-to-moment differences in the state of motor cortex at the time of input (Arieli et al., 1996). To put it another way, a behavioral response even in a simple RT task may reflect not only when motor regions become active, but also how much activation occurs. Thus, two identical response times could theoretically be generated by either early low-magnitude activation or later large-magnitude activations. These findings are further explored by Saron (1999) and Saron et al. (in press).

While an SCD analysis, as we have shown, greatly improves the visualization of electrocortical activation foci (see also Saron et al., 2001a), it does not eliminate the possibility of superposition effects from multiple brain regions. In addition, the waveforms overlaid here cannot capture the topographic shifts that were depicted in Figure 8.13. Accordingly, we have further examined these data, using the source estimation procedure BESA (see the section above entitled "Brain Electrical Source Analysis").

Source localization reveals rate effects The following strategy was adopted to examine the effect of RT on motor cor-

tex activation for subject 3 with BESA. The twelve 10-ms RT bins (210–330 ms) were collapsed into a set of six 20-ms bins to improve the ERP signal-to-noise ratio. Initial analyses fitting early occipital sources were conducted on the passive view control condition data (LVF alone) to minimize contributions from the motor response. Then, with these LVF-alone occipital sources in place, central dipoles were fit to the response-synchronized averages for each 20-ms RT bin. This approach minimized the temporal dispersion of the averages near the time of response execution. All sources were then optimized within each stimulus-synchronized average for each RT bin. Source locations and orientations were then averaged across bins, creating an overall model that was applied in turn to the original stimulus-synchronized data from each bin. This approach was used because inspection of the individual bin solutions revealed consistent source locations. The procedure resulted in a solution set of eight dipoles that accounted for an average of 97.95% variance in the data over the interval of 60–200 ms poststimulus, averaged across RT.

These dipoles are indicated in the three-view head cartoon of Figure 8.15a. The following descriptions of source locations represent reasonable hypotheses and not proven locations. Neither should location within the head cartoon signify analogous location within the subject's head, as the spherical head model of BESA may distort actual source locations, and the presented locations have not been coregistered with this subject's MRI. With these caveats in mind, Source 1 (S1) represents presumed striate/early extrastriate cortex of the directly stimulated hemisphere. Source 2 (S2) reflects subsequent activation of right hemisphere extrastriate regions. Source 3 (S3) corresponds to the transcallosal activation of extrastriate regions of the left hemisphere. Sources

FIGURE 8.15. (a) BESA dipole locations and orientations for the LVF input/left-hand response condition for subject 3. See the text for caveats and functional interpretations of each dipole. (b) Source waveform overlays based on the BESA solution depicted in part (a) and comparison with SCD waveforms from parieto-occipital sites. Across-RT data. (c) Waveforms from each of six 20-ms RT bins for source 6 are overplotted. Peak latencies reliably track RT for all bins; however, the response onset times do not. Note that responses from bins 225–285 begin within the same 15-ms period. This suggests that the slope/rate of motor-related cortical activation is reflected in RT. The slowest responses (bins 305 and 325) do not follow this pattern. There is a ~70-ms delay relative to the first four bins before a response is initiated, with a slope comparable to the faster responses. This suggests different routes of response-related activations for these reaction times compared with reaction times in the 215- to 295-ms range. See the text for further details. (See Color Plate 13.)

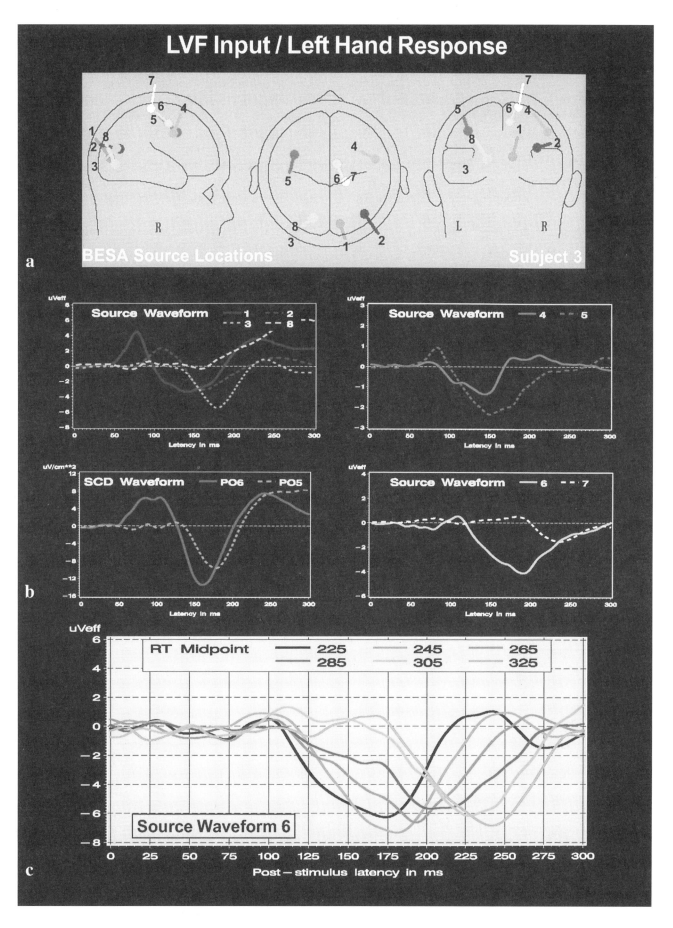

4 (S4) and 5 (S5) represent putative right and left premotor regions, respectively. The precentral location of source 6 (S6) suggests activation of motor output regions. The medial location of this source suggests a strong SMA contribution to motor output in these data. This finding is consistent with recent anatomical evidence demonstrating corticospinal efferents from SMA (e.g., Wise, 1996) and was suggested by examination of the SCD map data presented in Figures 8.11 and 8.13. The more posterior central source 7 (S7) suggests a postcentral somatosensory response representing postmovement reafference. The brain region and functional role of source 8 (S8) are unclear (see Figure 8.15b, upper left graph) but may represent late reactivation of left extrastriate visual areas.

In keeping with the general finding of consistent visual activations across RT, the source waveforms for sources 1, 2, 3, and 8 varied little among RT bins. Similarly, sources 4 and 5 were consistent across RT bin. Source 6 did indeed reflect the differing RTs of the six data sets, and source 7 reflected delayed and diminished activation associated with slower responses. Figure 8.15b presents the source waveforms for all dipoles derived from the full data set collapsed across RT ($N = 1366$). The solution accounted for 98.4% of the variance across the interval of 60–200 ms. Occipital sources are displayed in the upper left graph. The initial activation of S1 is clearly seen. The interhemispheric delay between the negative peaks of S2 and S3 is 16 ms in this condition. In this case this compares fairly well with the 19-ms IHTT estimate based on the N160 peak values of the PO5 and PO6 SCD waveforms shown in the lower left graph. A reasonable basis for a discrepancy between SCD waveform and source waveform estimates of IHTT is illustrated by comparison of these source and SCD waveform graphs. It is easy to see how the shape of the early positive deflection of the PO5 waveform represents a composite of the early activations of first S1 and then S2. Similarly, the PO5 N160 peak occurs roughly midway between the corresponding peaks of S1 and S2. Since S3 and PO6 share similar negative peak latencies, the earlier PO5 N160 peak relative to S2 results in the longer IHTT estimate. The cautionary point here is that electrophysiological estimates of interhemispheric delay might need to be computed on the basis of source waveforms to establish more accurate callosally mediated activations of specific cortical regions than are provided even by SCD measures.

The upper right graph of Figure 8.15b overlays S4 and S5. Although S4 paradoxically is of smaller amplitude than its contralateral counterpart, its earlier onset than S5 is consistent with the response pattern presented for this condition in Figure 8.13. The decreased ampli-

tude of S4 may result from differences between the hemispheres in the gyral pattern of the cortical regions generating these activations. Closed-field effects due to the electrical activity of opposing sheets of cortex canceling out components of their mutual activity can result in decreased scalp-recorded signals. The lower right graph displays S6 and S7. The delayed onset of S7 is consistent with an interpretation of this source as reflecting motor reafference.

Since S6 varied greatly as a function of RT, the source waveforms from each of the six RT bins are overplotted in Figure 8.15c. Although peak latencies reliably track RT for all bins, the negative-going waveform response onset times do not. These responses from bins 225–285 (RT range: 215–295 ms) all begin within the same 15-ms period. This suggests that the slope of motor output-related cortical activation, but not its activation onset time, may be reflected in RT. Notably, the slowest responses (bins 305 and 325) do not follow this pattern. There appears to be approximately a 70-ms delay relative to the first four bins before a response is initiated, with a slope comparable to the faster responses. This suggests different routes of response-related activations for these RTs compared with RTs in the 215- to 295-ms range.

These findings are generally consistent with the pattern of results obtained with the virtrode waveform analyses presented in Figure 8.14 and further suggest the importance of the slope/rate of motor cortex activation as a determinant of RT. This finding may represent a macroscopic confirmation in humans of the results of Hanes and Schall (1996) and Hanes, Patterson, and Schall (1998). These authors examined the behavior of single movement-related cells in macaque frontal eye fields during a saccade generation task. They found that RTs were highly linearly related ($r^2 = 0.97$) to the slope of the activation function of the recorded cells. The model of RT variability that they support involves a constant activation threshold to movement initiation. Different response times occur as activation functions of differing slope cross the threshold. Hanes and Schall conclude that the variability characteristic of RT distributions is "irreducible" and results from stochastic processes within response-generating or other neural circuits. The relative stability of the occipital and premotor source waveforms across a broad range of RTs supports the notion that variations in the state of motor output regions may account for much of the RT differences within a task condition. How differences in the time course and activation level of different cortical regions contribute to RT variability remains to be elucidated and is a question of central importance (Saron, 1999).

SEEING REACTION TIMES WITH ERPs If the electrophysiological measures reported here are to become useful in the interpretation of behavioral data concerning the timing and pathways of interhemispheric communication, there must be a demonstrated relation, in aggregate, between electrocortical signs of motor cortex output and RT. Two approaches have been taken to explore this issue. The first uses ERP motor activation patterns as an estimate of mean behavioral response time. This allowed direct comparison between motor-based ERP and RT IHTT estimates. Response-synchronized averages provided a template motor command pattern with a known relationship to the actual behavioral response. On the basis of comparison of EMG and response keypad signals, −70 ms relative to the RT was chosen as indicative of motor command generation. The time at which the same pattern occurs in stimulus-synchronized averages will then indicate the likely best estimate of when motor cortex activation patterns represent the motor command for a given condition. We restricted our analysis to data within the second quartile of the RT distribution for subject 3, given the large electrocortical differences that we have seen as a function of RT within a condition. Using this method, we measured the crossed minus uncrossed difference between hands separately for each visual field: LVF CUD = 7 ms (compared to 16 ms based on median RT), and RVF CUD = −17 ms (compared with −17 ms RT CUD).

The correspondence between these motor-based ERP and RT estimates of IHTT suggests that electrocortical signs of motor output relate directly to behavioral responses. This being the case, it is of note that while the RVF CUD was consistently −17 ms, the left-to-right motor-related IHTT with the RVF/left-hand condition was 36 ms as measured by peak latency differences between C3 and C4 SCD waveforms (see Figure 8.11). These analyses indicate that simultaneous measurement of physiological activity from both sides of the brain may be required to obtain anatomically predicted estimates of callosal function. In addition, the evidence for bilateral premovement motor system activation during unimanual tasks as simple as index finger flexions compromises the assumption that the behaviorally relevant processing occurring during intrahemispheric task conditions is restricted to the input/output hemisphere.

The second approach taken toward this issue is more direct. Laplacian waveforms derived from the centers of movement-related activation foci are directly compared with the rectified EMG waveforms using lagged cross-correlations. This method demonstrates the ongoing correspondence between electrocortical activity and behavior and provides estimates of corticomuscular delays.

The results of such analyses by subject are presented in Saron (1999) and Saron et al. (in press).

Preliminary conclusions and discussion

This chapter has represented two families of issues: methodological advances and caveats regarding electrophysiological research in humans and findings concerning interpretation of results from a long-standing experimental paradigm: the Poffenberger (1912) task. The emphasis regarding methodology has been to point out the utility of high spatial and fast temporal sampling when obtaining electrocortical measures during task performance. This facilitates undertaking a spatiotemporal analysis of visuomotor tasks that, in this context, can reveal activation patterns of visual and motor systems simultaneously. The need for data collection sufficient to group responses within a condition by small behavioral differences was demonstrated owing to the large effects of RT on cortical activation patterns. Problems with the interpretation of scalp potential versus scalp current density and source estimation measures were stressed owing to the susceptibility of scalp potential to volume conduction effects. Further, on the basis of individual differences in brain anatomy and functional organization, it has been argued that the development of a case study approach, in which subjects are extensively tested, even within the framework of simple tasks, is required to adequately investigate relations between electrocortical activity and behavior.

MOTIVATING QUESTIONS The initial intentions for the present studies were to follow up on earlier observations (Saron and Davidson, 1989a) that related to three areas: asymmetrical IHTT, differences between RT and ERP measures of IHTT, and the effects of task demand on IHTT. In the course of this work, the richness and complexity of the spatiotemporal data motivated a rethinking of some of the basic assumptions underlying the Poffenberger task. These can be stated as three questions:

1. It has been assumed that comparison of RTs for crossed versus uncrossed visuomotor responses provide an estimate of the fastest pathway for transcallosal transmission. This implies that only a single pathway for visuomotor activation contributes to the RT index of IHTT. Is this true?

2. Given the anatomical possibility for multiple intrahemispheric connections, as well as for homotopic and heterotopic interhemispheric connections, can the active pathways and their contributions to the motor response be physiologically defined?

3. The assumption that RT directly indexes a serial activation of motor cortex is confounded by the likeli-

hood that magnitude as well as timing of ongoing cortical activation contributes to RT. Can variation in RT within a subject and condition be used to examine the relative importance of physiological timing versus magnitude in determining RT?

POFFENBERGER IN EXTREMIS   Even on the basis of the preliminary data presented in this chapter, the assumption that IHTT can be inferred from the difference in RT for crossed versus uncrossed conditions does not appear correct. There is consistent bilateral activation of motor cortex with similar timing in intrahemispheric as well as interhemispheric conditions. *Thus, subtracting the uncrossed from the crossed RT may actually contrast one form of interhemispheric interaction with another, rather than the presence versus absence of callosal mediation.* Further, the assumption that interhemispheric versus intrahemispheric differences in RT represent the sum of activation delays from visual to motor cortex also appears to be problematic, inasmuch as changes in RT are closely related to the slope/rate of premovement activation of motor cortex, rather than the onset timing of this activation. Thus, it appears that RT is determined by the action of summed distributed inputs to motor cortex, the effects of which in turn depend on the current state of the motor system and, as such, cannot serve as a simple index of uncrossed versus callosally mediated activation.

Specific questioning of the assumptions underlying the RT subtraction method of computing IHTT is not new. More than 20 years ago, Swanson, Ledlow, and Kinsbourne (1978) disputed the approach on theoretical and empirical grounds. These authors, basing their argument on a model of lateral cerebral interactions put forward by Kinsbourne (e.g., Kinsbourne, 1974, and Chapter 10 in this volume) suggested that RT differences between crossed and uncrossed conditions do not reflect information transfer time across the corpus callosum, but rather reflect differential effects of response preparation due to the attentional bias produced by a unilateral stimulus. Two factors, independent of sensory relay via the corpus callosum, are seen to alter the speed with which visuomotor integration occurs for crossed and uncrossed conditions. The first, thought to facilitate response generation in uncrossed conditions, is a generalized activation of the hemisphere that initially receives the stimulus, which would then speed motor output via distributed activations of multiple cortical regions. The second is posited to be a complementary, callosally mediated, inhibitory influence of the activated hemisphere on the indirectly stimulated hemisphere, which would slow behavioral output in crossed conditions. Thus the processing speed effects of stimulus and response compatibility that are inherent in the design of

the Poffenberger paradigm are seen as an unavoidable confound in simple anatomical interpretations of the CUD. These authors presage the physiologically based conclusions stated in the present chapter: "In the context of the orientation model, either information is exchanged between the hemispheres in a time so short that it cannot reasonably or reliably be detected by RT methods, or *lateral processing takes place after interhemispheric integration of information and so a transfer time component is present in all response measures* [italics added]." (Swanson et al., 1978, p. 278). Recently, Kaluzny and colleagues (1994), using unilateral electrical stimulation of the finger and unimanual and bimanual RT, found highly inconsistent CUDs at the individual level and attribute this variability to potential individual differences in the routes of interhemispheric transfer and to attentional factors (Swanson et al. 1978; see also Braun, Collin, and Mailloux, 1997). Very recently, Kinsbourne (Chapter 10 in this volume) has interpreted the evidence of early intrahemispheric stimulus-related activations in motor regions contained in the present chapter as consistent with the activation processes posited in Swanson and colleagues (1978).

SPATIAL COMPATIBILITY EFFECTS   There is some support for both aspects of the Kinsbourne model: (1) attentional effects (in the form of stimulus-response spatial compatibility on IHTT) and (2) callosally mediated inhibitory effects. In a modification of the classic Poffenberger paradigm to include a go/no-go choice RT task, Ledlow and colleagues (1978) used two experimental factors to investigate S-R compatibility effects. The first was to vary the position of the responding hand to be either centrally located in front of the subject or positioned 15 cm lateral to the midline in the direction of the responding hand. The second factor was the predictability of the stimulus location. Half the trials were run with visual field blocked (known location), and the remaining trials were randomly distributed between the visual fields (unknown location). For the centrally located response button no significant interaction of hand and visual field was found, with overall CUDs of 2 ms. However, when laterally placed responses were made to stimuli randomly presented to the two visual fields (unknown location), a 20-ms CUD was found, due to markedly decreased RT to ipsilateral stimuli. These authors suggest that this effect is due to the generation of an orienting response (OR) by stimuli of unknown location that facilitates response generation and is absent when location is blocked.

The potentially large effect of spatial compatibility is further illustrated by a study of Anzola and colleagues (1977). Rather than compare central versus lateral response locations, this study used crossed versus uncrossed hand positions. Crossed hand positions were such that manual response positions were actually on the side of space opposite to a given shoulder. Uncrossed hand positions were analogous to the lateral positions of Ledlow and colleagues (1978). This study used a choice RT variant of the Poffenberger task requiring responses of either the hand ipsilateral or contralateral (in separate blocks) to randomly presented hemifield stimuli. RTs from the hand ipsilateral to the stimuli were consistently shorter than those of hands contralateral to the stimuli. That this effect held for the crossed hand conditions directly violates the anatomical assumptions of the Poffenberger paradigm. However, these same authors suggested, in another experiment also described by Anzola and colleagues (1977), that a simple RT version of Poffenberger paradigm was immune to these effects. In the earlier between-group study, crossed versus uncrossed hand positions did not interact with significant hand by visual field interactions, which were in the anatomically predicted directions. However, for RVF stimuli there was a shorter CUD for crossed versus uncrossed hands (1 versus 2 ms). These investigators view the lack of an interaction with hand position at the population level as indicative of the absence of S-R effects in the simple Poffenberger task. A contemporaneous study by Berlucchi and colleagues (1977) also shows that there is little effect of hand position in simple RT versions of the experiment. The presence of a spatial compatibility effect in choice RT experiments and the absence of the effect in simple RT led these authors to suggest that choice RT reflects hemispheric asymmetries in processing of lateralized stimuli and degradation of information via interhemispheric transfer. The complexity and increased duration of choice RT responses are seen to render these results more susceptible to attentional bias than the simple RT task, which is seen as "presumably a pure measure of interhemispheric transmission time" (p. 511). However, the lack of an overt spatial compatibility finding in the classic version of the Poffenberger paradigm is insufficient to claim the primacy of a structural (i.e., strict anatomical) view of positive CUDs. An interpretation of this dichotomy provided by Swanson and colleagues (1978) is not that choice RT *per se* results in susceptibility to attentional bias, but rather that knowledge of stimulus location is a critical variable. In conditions of randomized stimulus presentations, an orienting response elicited by a unilateral stimulus will speed output from the stimulated hemisphere or (owing to cross-hemisphere inhibition) slow output from the unstimulated hemisphere. When the stimulus location is known, OR generation is thought to be suppressed by the response preparation set governed by the task con-

dition, including (presumably for crossed conditions) a tonic inhibition of the responding hemisphere by the response preparation and repeated activations of the stimulated hemisphere. The prediction then from this view would be that IHTT estimates based on randomized stimulus presentations would be longer than those based on blocked presentations even in the case of simple RT. This is not the case. A tally of the simple RT Poffenberger-type studies used in Marzi and colleagues' (1991) meta-analysis yields an average IHTT of 3.7 ms for blocked stimuli ($n = 6$ studies) and 3.0 ms for randomized designs ($n = 9$ studies). Thus, the imposition of a decision component on the RT task appears critical to finding RT results consistent with the Kinsbourne model.

A modification of the Poffenberger task has recently been performed to specifically test the validity of structural versus asymmetrical activation interpretations of the CUD. Studying 138 normal individuals, Iacoboni and Zaidel (1998) embedded bilateral stimulus presentations on some trials of an SRT task to "equilibrate" hemispheric activation and compared the CUD obtained from lateralized stimuli to that found from conditions when only unilateral stimuli were presented. The CUD decreased from 3.0 to 0.3 ms when the embedded bilateral trials were added, consistent with results predicted by the Kinsbourne model. However, four of five patients with partial or complete callosal deficits failed to show a difference between the conditions, questioning the role of the callosum in equilibration of hemispheric activation. Yet the authors' structural interpretation of the 0.3-ms CUD as a physiologically plausible shift in active callosal fibers appears to require conduction velocities of 500 m/s (assuming an occipital interhemispheric pathway distance of 15 cm), which exceeds the conduction velocity of the largest 11-μm myelinated fibers seen by LaMantia and Rakic (1990) by a factor of 7.7 (Waxman and Bennett, 1972), discounting synaptic delays that would further add to the timing of interhemispheric neural transmission. Estimates of mammalian synaptic delays range from 0.15 ms for rat cerebellar synapses (Sabatini and Regehr, 1996) to 0.43 ms for rat trigeminal neurons to the V motor nucleus (Appenteng, Conyers, and Moore, 1989), and 0.7 ms measured in slice preparations of the anteroventral cochlear nucleus (Oertel, 1983). Considering a shorter motor-to-motor transcallosal route (~ 4–6 cm)—for example, via the callosal connections between left and right SMA (Rouiller et al., 1994)—a 0.3-ms CUD would also exceed the 66 m/s conduction times of large callosal fibers. These conflicting results further motivate a review of the spectrum of callosal function undertaken below.

Cellular evidence There is a variety of evidence supporting the existence of callosally mediated inhibition. There is, however, little question that the proximal actions of the bulk of callosal axons is excitatory. In a review of callosal organization, Innocenti (1986) cites numerous studies that show, across species, that callosal cells of origin are overwhelmingly pyramidal. Spiny stellate callosally projecting cells have also been found, particularly in cat visual cortex. More recent anatomical reports do include identification of other nonpyramidal callosal neurons within a much larger population of pyramidal cells of varying morphology. Analyzing adult rat striate cortex, Martinez-Garcia, Gonzalez-Hernandez, and Martinez-Millan (1994) found callosally projecting double bouquet cells in cortical layers II–III and V. The GABAergic nature of this cell type has recently been described on the basis of physiological and immunoreactive data in rat frontal cortex by Kawaguchi and Kubota (1997) and in cat visual cortex by Tamas, Buhl, and Somogyi (1997). A callosally projecting aspinous stellate cell type in layer V and a sparsely spiny stellate neuron type in layer IV were also found by Martinez-Garcia and colleagues (1994). These authors further describe for the first time large callosally projecting cells in layer I displaying long radiating dendrites that they interpret as corresponding to surviving Cajal-Retzius cells in the adult rat cortex. Imamoto and colleagues (1994) have immunohistochemically demonstrated the GABAergic nature of these cells. A study of the ultrastructure of the synapses formed by degenerating callosal axons after callosal lesions in rat visual cortex (Hughes and Peters, 1992) was consistent with the sparse distribution of inhibitory callosal cells of origin. This study examined 437 degenerating callosal axon terminals in layers II/III at the border of areas 17/18a. Symmetric (inhibitory, Peters and Jones, 1984) synapses were found with dendritic shafts and cell bodies of pyramidal cells, dendritic spines, and cell bodies of nonpyramidal cells. However, these synapses accounted for only 3.7% of the identified synaptic types, with the remaining seen as asymmetric (excitatory; Peters and Jones, 1984). Given the demonstrated small percentage of the callosal system that is directly inhibitory, how then might large-scale inhibitory actions be mediated by the callosum?

A review of the neurotransmitters and postsynaptic actions of callosally projecting neurons by Conti and Manzoni (1994) suggests two scenarios. The first is that transcallosal IPSPs are generated disynaptically by the action of inhibitory interneurons stimulated monosynaptically by excitatory callosal input. Evidence for this view comes from studies that analyze the timing of transcallosally stimulated EPSP and IPSP sequences. Toyama and colleagues (1974) recorded intracellularly from cells in cat visual cortex that exhibited an EPSP-IPSP sequence upon callosal stimulation. IPSP onset timing was determined by reversing IPSP polarity using current injection. IPSPs followed monosynaptic EPSPs consistently by 1 ms and were thus interpreted as a disynaptic feed-forward circuit. The involvement of inhibitory interneurons in callosally mediated IPSP generation has also been demonstrated pharmacologically in a slice preparation of rat frontal agranular cortex with preserved commissural inputs (Kawaguchi, 1992). In this study, two classes of IPSPs, early and late, corresponding to activation of $GABA_A$ and $GABA_B$ receptors were completely inhibited by application of excitatory amino acid (EAA) antagonists, an observation that was interpreted as reflecting the action of separate populations of inhibitory cells activated by EAAs from callosal terminals.

The second scenario follows from the claim by Hughes and Peters (1992) that one reason so few nonpyramidal cells have been labeled in tracer studies of callosal cells of origin is the poor uptake properties of thin long axons. Conti and Manzoni (1994) point out that this suggests that the relatively large population of small-diameter (0.08–0.6 μm, peaking at 0.1–0.2 μm for the rabbit) unmyelinated axons found in the callosum may, in fact, be inhibitory (for macaque and human fiber diameter data, see LaMantia and Rakic, 1990; Aboitiz et al., 1992a). The slow conduction rate of these fibers would be on the order of 0.3–0.4 m/s (Swadlow, Waxman, and Geschwind, 1980; Swadlow, 1985; Waxman and Bennett, 1972; see also related discussion by Innocenti, Aggoun-Zouaoui, and Lehmann, 1995). Taking cat visual cortex interhemispheric transfer as an example, Conti and Manzoni (1994) note that transcallosal responses mediated by such fibers would require 75–100 ms. Yet, they point out, numerous studies of cat visual transcallosal responses generally fail to find any interhemispheric delays greater than 20 ms. They suggest, following from previous suggestions in the literature, that a possible resolution to this disparity would be to regard the contributions en masse of the slow-conducting callosal fibers as modulatory, with punctate stimulations generally unable to initiate measurable postsynaptic responses.

Given that the function of the slow-conducting callosal fiber system is poorly understood, Conti and Manzoni (1994) leave the question open as to whether a significant portion of the entire callosal system (10–32%, based on the preponderance of small-diameter fibers) may be related to physiological functions, including direct inhibition, that differ from the excitatory inputs from the well-described pyramidal and spiny stellate callosal cells of origin.

Single-unit studies In keeping with this description of callosal organization, cortical responses to sensory input are both augmented and suppressed by callosal inputs. At the single-neuron level, evidence for callosally mediated inhibitory influences on V4 activity in the anesthetized monkey comes from Desimone and colleagues (1993). Recording responses contralateral to small hemiretinal color bars, these investigators examined the generation of "silent" surround suppression using larger color bars placed in the ipsilateral visual field. There were marked decreases in suppression following transection of the posterior half of the callosum. Further section of the anterior commissure or optic tract did not alter these effects, and recordings in V1 showed no difference between section and intact responses. These results were interpreted as callosally mediated inhibition through both direct activation of callosal inhibitory cells and indirectly through excitation of inhibitory interneurons in contralateral V4.

Several other speculations regarding callosal function and organization are offered by Desimone and colleagues (1993). The first is the conjecture that the wide distribution of callosal terminals in V4, including many in regions with classical receptive fields far from the vertical meridian, combined with the physiological evidence of callosal suppression, suggests that callosal function in this visual area is primarily suppressive. A second global point concerning callosal function considers areal variation in callosal function. These authors cite a split-chiasm lesion study (Seacord, Gross, and Mishkin, 1979) that showed interocular transfer of pattern discrimination learning in monkeys, demonstrating the efficacy of commissural connections in interhemispheric transmission of pattern information. Bilateral inferior temporal (IT) lesions abolished this transfer, suggesting IT as a center of interhemispheric visual integration, with the callosum and anterior commissure providing a rough equivalence, presumably via excitatory inputs, of visual input to each hemisphere. (A large number of related studies of effects of callosal section on visual memory in split-chiasm monkeys are summarized by Doty, Ringo, and Lewine, 1994; see also Chapter 7 in this volume.)

Such posited areal differences in callosal function also find support in the heterogeneity of population distributions of fiber diameters and degree of myelination described for different rostral-caudal sections in LaMantia and Rakic (1990). These data show greater proportions of large fibers interconnecting sensory cortices, where fast sensory relay may be most important in integrating sensory input across the midline. The smallest mean diameters and greatest proportion of unmyelinated fibers are in the genu, site of prefrontal interhemispheric connections, where multimodal processing within one hemisphere may exert more tonic influences on the other.

A highly controlled investigation of the specific effects of reversible blockade of interhemispheric transmission to the callosal recipient zone at the border of areas 17 and 18 in the cat was conducted by Payne, Siwek, and Lomber (1991). A cooling probe was used to inactivate homotopic regions of the left hemisphere while stimulus-evoked and spontaneous local field potentials were recorded in the right hemisphere. Neurons in layers II–VI of the right hemisphere evidenced both increases and decreases in activity. In layers II/III, spontaneous activity was increased as often as it was decreased, providing evidence of a callosally mediated tonic inhibitory influence for those cells that increased in activity. In layers IV and V/VI, only decreases in stimulus-evoked activity were found. Some evidence of increases in spontaneous activity was found for layers V/VI. These results were interpreted, again, as evidence for predominate excitatory callosal influences, with significant inhibition mediated by both direct callosal inhibition and via activation of inhibitory interneurons. Perhaps the most significant result in line with the present discussion is the evidence of increased spontaneous activity in layers II/III and V/VI upon callosal blockade.

A third approach to the study of callosal activity on units in the contralateral hemisphere is represented by Kitzes and Doherty (1994). Investigating auditory responses in anesthetized ferrets, these authors paired brief electrical stimulation of the right auditory cortex with concomitant monaural or binaural acoustic input to the left or right ears while recording single-unit activity in homologous left auditory cortex. The most common consequence of callosal stimulation was suppression of the acoustically elicited response (26% of 88 units). The suppression could be induced within 4 ms of stimulation of the contralateral cortex and the duration of this inhibitory influence often lasted >100 ms (assessed by manipulating the delay between stimulation and tone onset). The rapid onset of this response suggests callosal activation of inhibitory interneurons, and the long duration of the response is consistent both with IPSP classes found by Kawaguchi (1992) and with overlap with late-arriving direct inhibitory influences mediated by slow conducting callosal fibers. No evidence was found for callosal input facilitating acoustic responses, an unexpected finding given the preponderance of excitatory callosal input. However, excitation was observed in a subpopulation of cells that were responsive only to binaural stimulation. These cells were driven by callosal stimulation but silent with input to either ear alone in the absence of stimulation. Pairing left-hemisphere auditory cortex stimulation with right-ear input effectively mimicked binaural input. For some binaural cells, more complex patterns of mixed inhibitory and excitatory influences within a single cell's response to different combinations of auditory input were observed. In one case, callosal stimulation at 500 μA diminished the binaural response, while increasing the stimulation to 750 μA (all were 100-μs pulses) caused short latency excitation of this binaural cell within 4 ms, and complete suppression of the binaural response thereafter.

Human studies Helpful as these single-unit studies are in developing a view of callosal function that includes inhibition, their reliance on anesthetized preparations prompts caution in generalizing from their results. What of awake, behaving humans?

Over the past decade, an experimental paradigm has emerged that uses transcranial magnetic stimulation (TMS) to examine the effects of callosal stimulation on human motor cortex activation. Ferbert and colleagues (1992) used stimulating coils placed over the hand motor region of each hemisphere. One coil was used to elicit movements in the contralateral hand (the test stimulus), and the other coil was used to deliver a conditioning stimulus ipsilateral to the responding hand just prior to the test stimulation. Induced movements were measured by using the first dorsal interosseous muscle (FDI) surface EMG. Conditioning stimuli that were presented at least 5–6 ms before the onset of the test stimulus consistently resulted in attenuation of the movement evoked by the test stimulus. If the conditioning shock was set to be 10% above the threshold for eliciting movement in the contralateral hand, the inhibition effect lasted for conditioning-test (C-T) intervals up to 15 ms. Stronger conditioning stimuli (25% suprathreshold) produced inhibition for C-T intervals to 30 ms, suggesting additional activation of slower-conduction callosal fiber populations. The cortical interhemispheric mediation of these effects versus direct stimulation of pyramidal tract neurons was investigated, in part, by noting a lack of inhibitory effects of the conditioning stimulus using electrical stimulation that is known to directly stimulate neurons of the pyramidal tract. Single motor-unit studies were used to derive an approximate IHTT of 13 ms, a value consistent with ERP measures of IHTT and not with RT-based methods.

A validation of the callosal mediation of this effect is presented by Meyer and colleagues (1995). In this study, a transient inhibition of tonic maximal contraction of the FDI ipsilateral to the TMS-stimulated hemisphere

was measured in normal individuals and those with abnormalities of the corpus callosum. For normals, transcallosal inhibition had a mean onset time of 36 ms and a duration of 25 ms. This effect was absent or delayed in individuals lacking or with abnormalities in the anterior half of the corpus callosum, suggesting that the transcallosal fibers that mediated this effect obey the interhemispheric topography previously described (e.g., Pandya and Rosene, 1985; Pandya and Seltzer, 1986). The estimated transcallosal delay in this study was also 13 ms. Additional patient and control data in a similar paradigm are presented by Meyer, Roricht, and Woiciechowsky (1998).

The callosal mediation of these effects is further strengthened by comparison of eight normal and one acallosal individual in a study by Schnitzler, Kessler, and Benecke (1996). Using an experimental method that combined the approach of both Ferbert and colleagues (1992) and Meyer and colleagues (1995), these authors investigated the effects of a TMS conditioning stimulus that was presented ipsilateral to continuous FDI contraction. A test stimulus presented contralateral to that hand was used to elicit transient suppression (silent period, SP) of the ongoing contraction. Conditioning stimuli presented 10–20 ms before the test stimuli produced decreased SP durations. The authors attribute this effect to transcallosal inhibition of inhibitory interneurons activated by the test stimulus, an effect that was not observed in the acallosal individual. A replication of this effect in normals (Liepert, Tegenthoff, and Malin, 1996) found that SP durations were decreased by ipsilateral conditioning stimuli presented 20–30 ms before the test stimulus.

The original design of Ferbert and colleagues has now been used to systematically look at hemispheric asymmetries in the degree of transcallosal inhibition for both right- and left-handed individuals (Netz, Ziemann, and Homber, 1995). No systematic differences were found for left-handers, consistent with heterogeneous patterns of cerebral lateralization found in this population. However, for right-handers, 10 of 11 individuals showed greater inhibition of the FDI movements evoked by the test stimulus when the conditioning stimulus was given to the left hemisphere. These authors suggest that this left- to right-hemisphere transcallosal inhibitory advantage may relate to the interhemispheric transfer requirements of speech production due to left-hemisphere language dominance in right-handers and that it may be related to morphological asymmetries associated with longer Sylvian fissures and larger left-hemisphere planum temporale in right-handers (e.g., Steinmetz et al., 1995), which may alter interhemispheric connectivity. Aboitiz and colleagues (1992b) have investigated the specific relationship between morphological measures of brain asymmetry and callosum cross-sectional area. An inverse relation was found between degree of planum temporale asymmetry (independent of direction) and the size of the isthmus, only for males. However, the functional significance of this finding is unclear, given that fiber composition or number could account for the variation in cross-sectional area. In contrast to the hypothesis of Netz and colleagues (1995), a comprehensive review of handedness, planum temporale asymmetry, and morphology of the corpus callosum was undertaken by Beaton (1997), suggesting that asymmetry may be more related to handedness than to language lateralization (see also Shapleske et al., 1999). The functional utility of cross-hemisphere motor inhibition in the production of unimanual movements and consideration of the role of the corpus callosum in bimanual coordination was undertaken in a review by Geffen, Jones, and Geffen (1994).

Finally, functional evidence in humans interpreted as callosally mediated inhibition has been observed in a landmark study of ipsilateral visual activation elicited by hemifield moving gratings and other stimuli assessed by using 1.5T echo-planar fMRI (Tootell et al., 1998). These authors observed a mixed pattern of activation changes in the hemisphere ipsilateral to the stimulus. Increased activations were observed in a bifurcated pattern, from an origin lateral to the occipital pole. The superior branch of activation extended toward the parieto-occipital fissure, while the inferior region of activation ran anteroposteriorly along the inferior lateral occipital surface. Decreased activations were observed in the medial bank of calcarine cortex and related regions associated with V1 and V2, regions that corresponded to marked simultaneous increases in the hemisphere contralateral to the stimulus. These authors interpret these decreases as physiologically based inhibition of neural activity (citing Desimone et al., 1993) and not as hemodynamic artifacts.

TOWARD A VIEW OF CALLOSAL FUNCTION   Overall, the studies cited in this section provide convincing evidence of callosally mediated interhemispheric inhibition as one aspect of callosal function, supporting questioning of the assumptions underlying the Poffenberger paradigm and challenging a strict sensory-relay conception of callosal function. Several recent papers attempting to expand this view have reviewed theoretical frameworks and behavioral evidence for considering the callosum in terms of functional mechanisms of interhemispheric inhibition (Chiarello and Maxfield, 1998; Hellige et al., 1998), attention modulation (Banich, 1998), and as equilibrating activation between the hemispheres through coactiva-

tion (Chapter 10 in this volume). These views are summarized and critically discussed by Liederman (1998).

Given the heterogeneity of callosal cells of origin (Innocenti, 1986) and fiber diameters (LaMantia and Rakic, 1990), laminar distributions that suggest feedforward, horizontal, and feedback connectivity (Kennedy et al., 1991), variations in axon arborization patterns (Innocenti, 1994; Innocenti et al., 1995), patchy distribution of interhemispheric connections (e.g., Gould et al., 1986), regional differences in overlap with association neurons (Johnson et al., 1989), and heterotopicity (e.g., Hedreen and Yin, 1981; Di Virgilio and Clarke, 1997), there can be no monolithic statement of callosal function. This point is stressed in a review of the organization of callosal connections in primates by Kaas (1995), which describes the uneven and heterotopic distribution of callosal afferents. In this regard, it might be most fruitful to see the callosum as sharing the general organization and spectrum of diverse function as that subserved by intrahemispheric long-range connections, a view advocated by Kennedy and colleagues (1991) and originally proposed by Gross and Mishkin in 1977.

There is, however, very strong evidence that in some instances, a sensory relay model of callosal function is the most parsimonious view of the function of the highly prevalent excitatory callosal projections. For example, Tramo and colleagues (1995) summarize two-object visual discrimination experiments with patients who have undergone section of the corpus callosum. Within either visual hemifield, information regarding orientation, form, luminance, and position were reported nearly perfectly, while between-visual-field performance, when stimuli were constrained to the perifoveal region (2–6°), was at chance levels for orientation, form, and luminance. These findings held even with stimulus presentation times as long as 5 s (achieved with retinal image stabilization), demonstrating effective failure of subcortical commissures for transfer of these types of visual information. Such results seem difficult to conceptualize outside of viewing callosal connections as capable, in part, of relaying interhemispherically information of a nature similar to that received thalamocortically from the contralateral hemifield.

Evidence supporting this contention comes from a series of animal experiments using split-chiasm cats (Lepore et al., 1988). In the chiasm-sectioned animals, responses evoked through the contralateral temporal retina are presumed to be callosally mediated. By identifying binocular cells in visual cortex, thalamocortical versus callosal inputs can be directly compared. One result from these studies was that directional selectivity and orientation tuning were very similar for the callosally and thalamocortically determined fields of the same units recorded from the area 17/18 border, anterior ectosylvian, and lateral suprasylvian regions. Medial borders of the two receptive fields typically included the vertical meridian, consistent with the role of the corpus callosum in midline fusion (the so-called "midline rule"; see Innocenti, 1986). Subsequent section of the posterior third of the callosum abolished the contralaterally determined receptive fields. Additional split-chiasm studies (Leporé et al., 1992) have demonstrated some callosal mediation of near-focus binocular disparity tuning, prompting these authors to state: "that the callosal route is in part the transcortical extension of the thalamocortical pathway" (p. 137). This claim was explicitly not made to the exclusion of other possible nonspecific excitatory or inhibitory tonic modulatory callosal functions. A review of callosally mediated midline fusion in the somatosensory system by Manzoni and colleagues (1989) carefully considers the ways in which the organization of the somatosensory system parallels and diverges from visual system function.

One of these posited modulatory functions, mentioned briefly previously, is the equilibration of hemispheric activation via the callosum (see Chapter 10 in this volume), which could invoke both excitatory and inhibitory functions. The need for such a mechanism is postulated to counter wide swings in hemispheric activation posited to be induced by unilateral sensory inputs that activate subcortical reciprocally inhibitory mechanisms (see Doty, 1989). A callosal substrate for such an equilibrating mechanism is described by Manzoni and colleagues (1989). They detail a specific pattern of somatosensory callosal cells in SI of primates that synapse onto homotopic contralateral callosal cells, creating a bidirectional excitatory loop that also receives bilateral thalamocortical inputs from midline structures. Thus, through tight callosal interconnection, homologous cortical zones are hypothesized to act as a functionally coordinated unit despite location in opposite hemispheres. The generalizability of such a connectional pattern for other cortical areas is uncertain.

WHAT OF ERPs? This discussion has served to situate the canonical interpretation of the Poffenberger paradigm within the known complexity of interhemispheric cortico-cortical connectivity and to review evidence in support of alternative interpretations of RT-based indices of IHTT such as that expressed by Swanson and colleagues (1978) and elaborated recently by Kinsbourne (Chapter 10 this volume) and others. Further, it provides a context for the conceptual framework used in the interpretation of the data presented throughout this chapter. The physiological data have been described both intrahemispherically and interhemispherically in terms of sequential feed-forward excitatory patterns of activation that have more in common with a sensory- or local-activation-relay motif than with more diffuse claims of modulation or inhibition. The macroscopic nature of scalp recorded electrocortical measures, the similarities of the direct and indirect visual pathway activation time courses in response to visual input, the often tractable patterns of subsequent visuomotor activation, and similarities between the time courses of central activation and rectified forearm EMG during motor output (Saron et al., in press) lend themselves to this view. It is certainly likely that some of the functional consequences of the electrocortical foci described in this work reflect interhemispheric interactions beyond this heuristic.

A FIRST PHYSIOLOGICAL PICTURE Overall, the physiological data support contributions from both posterior and central transcallosal pathways to RT. From these initial analyses there appear to be no consistent differences in the timing of posterior transfer as a function of RT.

The relative prominence of particular visuomotor activation patterns does differ with RT. In one observed pattern, faster responses in crossed conditions were associated with a more prominent intrahemispheric visuomotor activation and central interhemispheric transfer. The slower responses, however, reflected an activation route via posterior interhemispheric transfer followed by intrahemispheric visual-to-motor cortex activation. To further complicate the picture, there are notable individual variations in the patterns of intrahemispheric and interhemispheric motor cortex activation. These variations in cortical activation patterns are well depicted in the SCD maps shown in Figure 8.13.

Finally, even the scalp current density method of ERP analysis does not permit a satisfactory spatial resolution of adjacent active intracranial regions, especially in posterior cortex, where the interhemispheric connections presumably differ both anatomically and functionally across visual regions. This is clearly illustrated in Figure 8.15b, which directly compares source estimation methods with SCD waveforms. However, the surviving utility of SCD measures is demonstrated by the basic pattern of findings detailed herein.

ACKNOWLEDGMENTS The authors wish to thank Dr. Seppo Ahlfors, Anna Brattson, Chester Freeman, Ed Geraghty, Dr. Jan Hrabe, Judy Kreuzer, James Long Company, Megis Software, and Neuroscan Corporation for technical support. We thank Dr. Diane Kurtzberg for helpful comments and crucial assistance. This research was supported in part by grants from the National Institutes of Health and Mental Health (NSRA 5T32MH15788-12 to C. D. S., NS27900 to G. V. S.,

MH11431 to J. J. F., and NIDCD 95261122 to H. G. V.), and the Human Frontier Science Program (GVS).

REFERENCES

ABOITIZ, F., A. B. SCHEIBEL, R. S. FISHER, and E. ZAIDEL, 1992a. Fiber composition of the human corpus callosum. *Brain Res.* 98:143–153.

ABOITIZ, F., A. B. SCHEIBEL, and E. ZAIDEL, 1992b. Morphometry of the Sylvian fissure and the corpus callosum, with emphasis on sex differences. *Brain* 115:1521–1541.

AGLIOTI, S., G. BERLUCCHI, R. PALLINI, G. F. ROSSI, and G. TASSINARI, 1993. Hemispheric control of unilateral and bilateral responses to lateralized light stimuli after callosotomy and in callosal agenesis. *Exp. Brain Res.* 95:151–165.

AINE, C. J., S. SUPEK, J. S. GEORGE, D. RANKEN, J. LEWINE, J. SANDERS, E. BEST, W. TIEE, E. R. FLYNN, and C. C. WOOD, 1996. Retinotopic organization of human visual cortex: Departures from the classical model. *Cereb. Cortex* 6:354–361.

ANDREASSI, J. L., H. OKAMURA, and M. STERN, 1975. Hemispheric asymmetries in the visual cortical evoked potential as a function of stimulus location. *Psychophysiology* 12:541–546.

ANZOLA, G. P., G. BERTOLONI, H. A. BUCHTEL, and G. RIZZOLATTI, 1977. Spatial compatibility and anatomical factors in simple and choice reaction time. *Neuropsychologia* 15:295–302.

APPENTENG, K., L. CONYERS, and J. A. MOORE, 1989. The monosynaptic excitatory connections of single trigeminal interneurones to the V motor nucleus of the rat. *J. Physiol. (Lond.)* 417:91–104.

ARIELI, A., A. STERKIN, A. GRINVALD, and A. AERTSEN, 1996. Dynamics of ongoing activity: Explanation of the large variability in evoked cortical responses. *Science* 273:1868–1871.

BABILONI, F., C. BABILONI, F. CARDUCCI, L. FATTORINI, P. ONORATI, and A. URBANO, 1996. Spline Laplacian estimate of EEG potentials over a realistic magnetic resonance-constructed scalp surface model. *Electroencephalogr. Clin. Neurophysiol.* 98:363–373.

BABILONI, F., C. BABILONI, L. FATTORINI, F. CARDUCCI, P. ONORATI, and A. URBANO, 1995. Performances of surface Laplacian estimators: A study of simulated and real scalp potential distributions. *Brain Topogr.* 8:35–45.

BABILONI, F., F. CARDUCCI, C. BABILONI, and A. URBANO, 1998. Improved realistic Laplacian estimate of highly-sampled EEG potentials by regularization techniques. *Electroencephalogr. Clin. Neurophysiol.* 106:336–343.

BADIAN, N. A., and P. H. WOLFF, 1977. Manual asymmetries of motor sequencing in boys with reading disability. *Cortex* 13:343–349.

BANICH, M. T., 1998. The missing link: The role of interhemispheric interaction in attentional processing. *Brain Cogn.* 36:128–157.

BARRETT, G., L. BLUMHARDT, A. M. HALLIDAY, E. HALLIDAY, and A. KRISS, 1976. A paradox in the lateralisation of the visual evoked response. *Nature* 261:253–255.

BASHORE, T. R., 1981. Vocal and manual reaction time estimates of interhemispheric transmission time. *Psych. Bull.* 89:352–368.

BEATON, A. A., 1997. The relation of planum temporale asymmetry and morphology of the corpus callosum to handedness, gender, and dyslexia: A review of the evidence. *Brain Lang.* 60:255–322.

BERLUCCHI, G., 1972. Anatomical and physiological aspects of visual functions of corpus callosum. *Brain Res.* 37:371–392.

BERLUCCHI, G., S. AGLIOTI, C. A. MARZI, and G. TASSINARI, 1995. Corpus callosum and simple visuomotor integration. *Neuropsychologia* 33:923–936.

BERLUCCHI, G., F. CREA, M. DI STEFANO, and G. TASSINARI, 1977. Influence of spatial stimulus-response compatibility on reaction time of ipsilateral and contralateral hand to lateralized light stimuli. *J. Exp. Psychol. Hum. Percep. Perf.* 3:505–517.

BERLUCCHI, G., W. HERON, R. HYMAN, G. RIZZOLATTI, and C. UMILTÀ, 1971. Simple reaction times of ipsilateral and contralateral hand to lateralized visual stimuli. *Brain* 94:419–430.

BISIACCHI, P., C. A. MARZI, R. NICOLETTI, G. CARENA, C. MUCIGNAT, and F. TOMAIUOLO, 1994. Left-right asymmetry of callosal transfer in normal human subjects. *Behav. Brain Res.* 64:173–178.

BLUMHARDT, L. D., G. BARRETT, A. M. HALLIDAY, and A. KRISS, 1978. The effect of experimental 'scotomata' on the ipsilateral and contralateral responses to pattern-reversal in one half-field. *Electroencephalogr. Clin. Neurophysiol.* 45:376–392.

BLUMHARDT, L. D., and A. M. HALLIDAY, 1979. Hemisphere contributions to the composition of the pattern-evoked potential waveform. *Exp. Brain Res.* 36:53–69.

BOECKER, H., A. KLEINSCHMIDT, M. REQUARDT, W. HANICKE, K. D. MERBOLDT, and J. FRAHM, 1994. Functional cooperativity of human cortical motor areas during self-paced simple finger movements: A high-resolution MRI study. *Brain* 117:1231–1239.

BOSTOCK, H., and M. J. JARVIS, 1970. Changes in the form of the cerebral evoked response related to the speed of simple reaction time. *Electroencephalogr. Clin. Neurophysiol.* 29:137–145.

BRAUN, C. M., 1993. Estimation of interhemispheric dynamics from simple unimanual reaction time to extrafoveal stimuli. *Neuropsychol. Rev.* 3:321–364.

BRAUN, C. M., I. COLLIN, and C. MAILLOUX, 1997. The "Poffenberger" and "Dimond" paradigms: Interrelated approaches to the study of interhemispheric dynamics? *Brain Cogn.* 34:337–359.

BRINDLEY, G. S., 1972. The variability of the human striate cortex. *J. Physiol (Lond.)* 225:1–3.

BROWN, W. S., M. D. BJERKE, and H. G. C. GALBRAIT, 1998. Interhemispheric transfer in normals and acallosals: Latency adjusted evoked potential averaging. *Cortex* 34:677–692.

BROWN, W. S., M. A. JEEVES, R. DIETRICH, and D. S. BURNISON, 1999. Bilateral field advantage and evoked potential interhemispheric transmission in commissurotomy and callosal agenesis. *Neuropsychologia* 37:1165–1180.

BROWN, W. S., E. B. LARSON, and M. JEEVES, 1994. Directional asymmetries in interhemispheric transmission time: Evidence from visual evoked potentials. *Neuropsychologia* 32:439–448.

CHALUPA, L. M., J. W. ROHRBAUGH, J. E. GOULD, and D. B. LINDSLEY, 1976. Cortical and subcortical visual evoked potential correlates of reaction time in monkeys. *J. Comp. Physiol. Psychol.* 90:119–126.

CHIARELLO, C., and L. MAXFIELD, 1998. Varieties of interhemispheric inhibition, or how to keep a good hemisphere down. *Brain Cogn.* 30:81–108.

CLARK, V. P., S. FAN, and S. A. HILLYARD, 1995. Identification of early visual evoked potential generators by retinotopic and topographic analyses. *Hum. Brain Mapp.* 2:170–187.

CLARKE, J. M., and E. ZAIDEL, 1989. Simple reaction times to lateralized light flashes: Varieties of interhemispheric communication routes. *Brain* 112:849–870.

CLARKE, S., and J. MIKLOSSY, 1990. Occipital cortex in man: Organization of callosal connections, related myelo- and cytoarchitecture, and putative boundaries of functional visual areas. *J. Comp. Neurol.* 298:188–214.

COLBY, C. L., and J. R. DUHAMEL, 1991. Heterogeneity of extrastriate visual areas and multiple parietal areas in the macaque monkey. *Neuropsychologia* 29:517–537.

COLBY, C. L., and J. R. DUHAMEL, 1996. Spatial representations for action in parietal cortex. *Brain Res. Cogn. Brain Res.* 5:105–115.

CONTI, F., and T. MANZONI, 1994. The neurotransmitters and postsynaptic actions of callosally projecting neurons. *Behav. Brain Res.* 64:37–53.

CUFFIN, B. N., 1996. EEG localization accuracy improvements using realistically shaped head models. *IEEE Trans. Biomed. Eng.* 43:299–303.

CURTIS, H. J., 1940. Intercortical connections of the corpus callosum as indicated by evoked potentials. *J. Neurophys.* 3:414–422.

DAVIDSON, R. J., S. C. LESLIE, and C. D. SARON, 1990. Reaction time measures of interhemispheric transfer time in reading disabled and normal children. *Neuropsychologia* 28:471–485.

DAVIDSON, R. J., and C. D. SARON, 1992. Evoked potential measures of interhemispheric transfer time in reading disabled and normal boys. *Dev. Neuropsychol.* 8:261–277.

DESIMONE, R., J. MORAN, S. J. SCHEIN, and M. MISHKIN, 1993. A role for the corpus callosum in visual area V4 of the macaque. *Vis. Neurosci.* 10:159–171.

DI STEFANO, M., and C. SALVADORI, 1998. Asymmetry of the interhemispheric visuomotor integration in callosal agenesis. *Neuroreport* 9:1331–1335.

DI STEFANO, M., H. C. SAUERWEIN, and M. LASSONDE, 1992. Influence of anatomical factors and spatial compatibility on the stimulus-response relationship in the absence of the corpus callosum. *Neuropsychologia* 30:177–185.

DI VIRGILIO, G., and S. CLARKE, 1997. Direct interhemispheric visual input to human speech areas. *Hum. Brain. Mapp.* 5:347–354.

DONCHIN, E., and D. B. LINDSLEY, 1966. Average evoked potentials and reaction times to visual stimuli. *Electroencephalogr. Clin. Neurophysiol.* 20:217–223.

DOTY, R. W., 1989. Schizophrenia: A disease of interhemispheric processes at forebrain and brainstem levels? *Behav. Brain Res.* 34:1–33.

DOTY, R. W., J. L. RINGO, and J. D. LEWINE, 1994. Interhemispheric sharing of visual memory in macaques. *Behav. Brain Res.* 20:79–84.

DUARA, R., A. KUSHCH, K. GROSS-GLENN, W. W. BARKER, B. JALLAD, S. PASCAL, D. A. LOEWENSTEIN, J. SHELDON, M. RABIN, B. LEVIN, ET AL., 1991. Neuroanatomical differences between dyslexic and normal readers on magnetic resonance imaging scans. *Arch. Neurol.* 48:410–416.

DUNAIF, A., 1979. *A behavioral investigation of interhemispheric communication in normal and dyslexic children.* Undergraduate thesis, State University of New York, Purchase College.

DUM, R. P., and P. L. STRICK, 1991. The origin of corticospinal projections from the premotor areas in the frontal lobe. *J. Neurosci.* 11:667–689.

DUM, R. P., and P. L. STRICK, 1996. Spinal cord terminations of the medial wall motor areas in macaque monkeys. *J. Neurosci.* 16:6513–6525.

ENDO, H., T. KIZUKA, T. MASUDA, and T. TAKEDA, 1999. Automatic activation in the human primary motor cortex synchronized with movement preparation. *Brain Res. Cogn. Brain Res.* 8:229–239.

FERBERT, A., A. PRIORI, J. C. ROTHWELL, B. L. DAY, J. G. COLEBATCH, and C. D. MARSDEN, 1992. Interhemispheric inhibition of the human motor cortex. *J. Physiol. (Lond.)* 453:525–546.

FINK, G. R., R. S. FRACKOWIAK, U. PIETRZYK, and R. E. PASSINGHAM, 1997. Multiple nonprimary motor areas in the human cortex. *J. Neurophys.* 77:2164–2174.

FORSTER, B., and M. C. CORBALLIS, 1998. Interhemispheric transmission times in the presence and absence of the forebrain commissures: Effects of luminance and equiluminance. *Neuropsychologia* 36:925–934.

FOXE, J. J., and G. V. SIMPSON, 2002. Flow of activation from V1 to frontal cortex in humans: A framework for defining "early" visual processing. *Exp. Brain Res.* 142:139–150.

GAZZANIGA, M. S., 1985. Some contributions of split-brain studies to the study of human cognition. In *Epilepsy and the Corpus Callosum*, A. G. Reeves, ed. New York: Plenum Press, pp. 341–348.

GEFFEN, G. M., D. L. JONES, and L. B. GEFFEN, 1994. Interhemispheric control of manual motor activity. *Behav. Brain Res.* 64:131–140.

GEORGE, J. S., C. J. AINE, J. C. MOSHER, D. M. SCHMIDT, D. M. RANKEN, H. A. SCHLITT, C. C. WOOD, J. D. LEWINE, J. A. SANDERS, and J. W. BELLIVEAU, 1995. Mapping function in the human brain with magnetoencephalography, anatomical magnetic resonance imaging, and functional magnetic resonance imaging. *J. Clin. Neurophys.* 12:406–431.

GERLOFF, C., N. UENISHI, T. NAGAMINE, T. KUNIEDA, L. G. COHEN, M. HALLETT, and H. SHIBASAKI, 1997. Bilateral premovement activation in the human motor system: Premotor cortex (PMC) or motor cortex (M1)? *Soc. Neurosci. Abstr.* 23 (2):1949.

GIEDD, J. N., J. M. RUMSEY, F. X. CASTELLANOS, J. C. RAJAPAKSE, D. KAYSEN, A. C. VAITUZIS, Y. C. VAUSS, S. D. HAMBURGER, and J. L. RAPOPORT, 1996. A quantitative MRI study of the corpus callosum in children and adolescents. *Dev. Brain Res.* 91:274–280.

GORDON, A. M., J. H. LEE, D. FLAMENT, K. UGURBIL, and T. J. EBNER, 1998. Functional magnetic resonance imaging of motor, sensory, and posterior parietal cortical areas during performance of sequential typing movements. *Exp. Brain Res.* 121:153–166.

GOULD, H. J., 3D, C. G. CUSICK, T. P. PONS, and J. H. KAAS, 1986. The relationship of corpus callosum connections to electrical stimulation maps of motor, supplementary motor, and the frontal eye fields in owl monkeys. *J. Comp. Neurol.* 247:297–325.

GROSS, C. G., and M. MISHKIN, 1977. The neural basis of stimulus equivalence across retinal translation. In *Lateralization in the Nervous System*, S. Harnad, R. W. Doty, L. Goldstein, J. Jaynes, and G. Krauthamer, eds. New York: Academic Press, pp. 109–122.

HANES, D. P., W. F. PATTERSON, 2ND, and J. D. SCHALL, 1998. Role of frontal eye fields in countermanding saccades: visual, movement, and fixation activity. *J. Neurophys.* 79:817–834.

HANES, D. P., and J. D. SCHALL, 1996. Neural control of voluntary movement initiation. *Science* 274:427–430.

HARTWELL, R. C., and J. D. COWAN, 1994. Covariability of visually evoked potentials and simple motor reaction times. *Electroencephalogr. Clin. Neurophysiol.* 92:487–490.

HEDREEN, J. C., and T. C. YIN, 1981. Homotopic and heterotopic callosal afferents of caudal inferior parietal lobule in Macaca mulatta. *J. Comp. Neurol.* 197:605–621.

HELLIGE, J. B., K. B. TAYLOR, L. LESMES, and S. PETERSON, 1998. Relationships between brain morphology and behavioral measures of hemispheric asymmetry and interhemispheric interaction. *Brain Cogn.* 36:158–192.

HENDERSON, C. E., 1996. Role of neurotrophic factors in neuronal development. *Curr. Opin. Neurobiol.* 6:64–70.

HOPTMAN, M. J., and R. J. DAVIDSON, 1994. How and why do the two cerebral hemispheres interact? *Psych. Bull.* 116:195–219.

HOPTMAN, M. J., R. J. DAVIDSON, A. GUDMUNDSSON, R. T. SCHREIBER, and W. B. ERSHLER, 1996. Age differences in visual evoked potential estimates of interhemispheric transfer. *Neuropsychology* 10:263–271.

HOSHIYAMA, M., R. KAKIGI, P. BERG, S. KOYAMA, Y. KITAMURA, M. SHIMOJO, S. WATANABE, and A. NAKAMURA, 1997. Identification of motor and sensory brain activities during unilateral finger movement: Spatiotemporal source analysis of movement-associated magnetic fields. *Exp. Brain Res.* 115:6–14.

HOUZEL, J. C., and C. MILLERET, 1999. Visual inter-hemispheric processing: Constraints and potentialities set by axonal morphology. *J. Physiol. Paris* 93:271–284.

HUGHES, C. M., and A. PETERS, 1992. Asymmetric synapses formed by callosal afferents in rat visual cortex. *Brain Res.* 583:271–278.

HYND, G. W., J. HALL, E. S. NOVEY, D. ELIOPULOS, K. BLACK, J. J. GONZALEZ, J. E. EDMONDS, C. RICCIO, and M. COHEN, 1995. Dyslexia and corpus callosum morphology. *Arch. Neurol.* 52:32–38.

HYND, G. W., J. E. OBRZUT, W. WEED, and C. R. HYND, 1979. Development of cerebral dominance: Dichotic listening asymmetry in normal and learning disabled children. *J. Exp. Child Psychol.* 28:445–454.

IACOBONI, M., J. RAYMAN, and E. ZAIDEL, 1997. Does the previous trial affect lateralized lexical decision? *Neuropsychologia* 35:81–88.

IACOBONI, M., and E. ZAIDEL, 1995. Channels of the corpus callosum: Evidence from simple reaction times to lateralized flashes in the normal and split brain. *Brain* 118:779–788.

IACOBONI, M., and E. ZAIDEL, 1998. Context effects in simple reaction times to lateralized flashes. *Soc. Neurosci. Abstr.* 25 (2):1263.

IACOBONI, M., and E. ZAIDEL, 2000. Crossed-uncrossed difference in simple reaction times to lateralized flashes: Between- and within-subjects variability. *Neuropsychologia* 38:535–541.

IKEDA, A., H. O. LUDERS, H. SHIBASAKI, T. F. COLLURA, R. C. BURGESS, H. H. MORRIS, 3RD, and T. HAMANO, 1995. Movement-related potentials associated with bilateral simultaneous and unilateral movements recorded from human supplementary motor area. *Electroencephalogr. Clin. Neurophysiol.* 95:323–334.

IMAMOTO, K., N. KARASAWA, G. ISOMURA, and I. NAGATSU, 1994. Cajal-Retzius neurons identified by GABA immunohistochemistry in layer I of the rat cerebral cortex. *Neurosci. Res.* 20:101–105.

INNOCENTI, G. M., 1986. General organization of callosal connections in the cerebral cortex. In *Cerebral Cortex*, Vol. 5: *Sensory-Motor Areas and Aspects of Cortical Connectivity*, E. G. Jones and A. Peters, eds. New York: Plenum Press, pp. 291–354.

INNOCENTI, G. M., 1994. Some new trends in the study of the corpus callosum. *Behav. Brain Res.* 64:1–8.

INNOCENTI, G. M., D. AGGOUN-ZOUAOUI, and P. LEHMANN, 1995. Cellular aspects of callosal connections and their development. *Neuropsychologia* 33:961–987.

IPATA, A., M. GIRELLI, C. MINIUSSI, and C. A. MARZI, 1997. Interhemispheric transfer of visual information in humans: the role of different callosal channels. *Arch. Ital. Biol.* 135:169–182.

JOHNSON, P. B., A. ANGELUCCI, R. M. ZIPARO, D. MINCIACCHI, M. BENTIVOGLIO, and R. CAMINITI, 1989. Segregation and overlap of callosal and association neurons in frontal and parietal cortices of primates: A spectral and coherency analysis. *J. Neurosci.* 9:2313–2326.

JUNGHÖFER, M., T. ELBERT, P. LEIDERER, P. BERG, and B. ROCKSTROH, 1997. Mapping EEG-potentials on the surface of the brain: A strategy for uncovering cortical sources. *Brain Topogr.* 9:203–217.

KAAS, J. H., 1995. The organization of callosal connections in primates. In *Epilepsy and the Corpus Callosum 2*, A. G. Reeves and D. W. Roberts, eds. New York: Plenum Press, pp. 15–28.

KALUZNY, P., A. PALMERI, and M. WIESENDANGER, 1994. The problem of bimanual coupling: A reaction time study of simple unimanual and bimanual finger responses. *Electroencephalogr. Clin. Neurophysiol.* 93:450–458.

KAWAGUCHI, Y., 1992. Receptor subtypes involved in callosally-induced postsynaptic potentials in rat frontal agranular cortex in vitro. *Exp. Brain Res.* 88:33–40.

KAWAGUCHI, Y., and Y. KUBOTA, 1997. GABAergic cell subtypes and their synaptic connections in rat frontal cortex. *Cereb. Cortex* 7:476–486.

KENNEDY, D. N., N. LANGE, N. MAKRIS, J. BATES, J. MEYER, and V. S. CAVINESS, JR., 1998. Gyri of the human neocortex: An MRI-based analysis of volume and variance. *Cereb. Cortex* 8:372–384.

KENNEDY, H., C. MEISSIREL, and C. DEHAY, 1991. Callosal pathways and their compliancy to general rules governing the organization of corticocortical connectivity. In *Vision and Visual Dysfunction*, Vol. 3: *Neuroanatomy of the Visual Pathways and Their Development*, B. Reher and S. R. Robinson, eds. (J. R. Cronly-Dillon, series ed.) Boca Raton, FL: CRC Press, pp. 324–359.

KERTESZ, A., M. POLK, S. E. BLACK, and J. HOWELL, 1986. Cerebral asymmetries on magnetic resonance imaging. *Cortex* 22:117–127.

KERTESZ, A., M. POLK, S. E. BLACK, and J. HOWELL, 1990. Sex, handedness, and the morphometry of cerebral asymmetries on magnetic resonance imaging. *Brain Res.* 530:40–48.

KIM, S. G., J. ASHE, A. P. GEORGOPOULOS, H. MERKLE, J. M. ELLERMANN, R. S. MENON, S. OGAWA, and K. UGURBIL, 1993a. Functional imaging of human motor cortex at high magnetic field. *J. Neurophys.* 69:297–302.

KIM, S. G., J. ASHE, K. HENDRICH, J. M. ELLERMANN, H. MERKLE, K. UGURBIL, A. P. GEORGOPOULOS, 1993b. Functional magnetic resonance imaging of motor cortex: Hemispheric asymmetry and handedness. *Science* 261:615–617.

KINSBOURNE, M., 1974. Lateral interactions in the brain. In *Hemispheric Disconnection and Cerebral Function*, M. Kinsbourne and W. L. Smith, eds. Springfield, IL: Charles C. Thomas, pp. 239–259.

KITZES, L. M., and D. DOHERTY, 1994. Influence of callosal activity on units in the auditory cortex of ferret (*Mustela putorius*). *J. Neurophys.* 71:1740–1751.

KOLES, Z. J., 1998. Trends in EEG source localization. *Electroencephalogr. Clin. Neurophysiol.* 106:127–137.

LAMANTIA, A. S., and P. RAKIC, 1990. Cytological and quantitative characteristics of four cerebral commissures in the rhesus monkey. *J. Comp. Neurol.* 291:520–537.

LARSON, E. B., and W. S. BROWN, 1997. Bilateral field interactions, hemispheric specialization and evoked potential interhemispheric transmission time. *Neuropsychologia* 35:573–581.

LASSONDE, M., H. SAUERWEIN, N. MCCABE, L. LAURENCELLE, and G. GEOFFROY, 1988. Extent and limits of cerebral adjustment to early section or congenital absence of the corpus callosum. *Behav. Brain Res.* 30:165–181.

LAW, S. K., P. L. NUNEZ, and R. S. WIJESINGHE, 1993. High-resolution EEG using spline generated surface Laplacians on spherical and ellipsoidal surfaces. *IEEE Trans. Biomed. Eng.* 40:145–153.

LEAHY, R. M., J. C. MOSHER, M. E. SPENCER, M. X. HUANG, and J. D. LEWINE, 1998. A study of dipole localization accuracy for MEG and EEG using a human skull phantom. *Electroencephalogr. Clin. Neurophysiol.* 197:159–173.

LEDLOW, A., J. M. SWANSON, and M. KINSBOURNE, 1978. Differences in reaction time and average evoked potentials as a function of direct and indirect neural pathways. *Ann. Neurol.* 3:525–530.

LEHMANN, D., 1987. Principles of spatial analysis. In *Handbook of Electroencephalography and Clinical Neurophysiology* (rev. ser.), Vol. 1: *Methods of Analysis of Brain Electrical and Magnetic Signals*, A. S. Gevins and A. Rémond, eds. New York: Elsevier Science Publishers, pp. 309–353.

LEPORÉ, F., M. PTITO, L. RICHTER, and J.-P. GUILLEMOT, 1988. Cortico-cortico callosal connectivity: Evidence derived from electrophysiological studies. *Prog. Brain Res.* 75:187–195.

LEPORÉ, F., A. SAMSON, M. C. PARADIS, M. PTITO, and J.-P. GUILLEMOT, 1992. Binocular interaction and disparity coding at the 17–18 border: Contribution of the corpus callosum. *Exp. Brain Res.* 90:129–140.

LIEDERMAN, J., 1998. The dynamics of interhemispheric collaboration and hemispheric control. *Brain Cogn.* 36:193–208.

LIEPERT, J., M. TEGENTHOFF, and J. P. MALIN, 1996. Changes of inhibitory interneurons during transcallosal stimulations. *J. Neural Transm.* 103:917–924.

LINES, C. R., M. D. RUGG, and A. D. MILNER, 1984. The effect of stimulus intensity on visual evoked potential estimates of interhemispheric transmission time. *Exp. Brain Res.* 57:89–98.

LUPPINO, G., M. MATELLI, R. CAMARDA, and G. RIZZOLATTI, 1993. Corticocortical connections of area F3 (SMA-proper) and area F6 (pre-SMA) in the macaque monkey. *J. Comp. Neurol.* 338:114–140.

MANZONI, T., P. BARBARESI, F. CONTI, and M. FABRI, 1989. The callosal connections of the primary somatosensory cortex and the neural bases of midline fusion. *Exp. Brain Res.* 76:251–266.

MARKEE, T. E., W. S. BROWN, L. H. MOORE, and D. C. THEBERGE, 1996. Callosal function in dyslexia: Evoked potential interhemispheric transfer time and bilateral field advantage. *Dev. Neuropsychol.* 12:409–424.

MARTINEZ-GARCIA, F., T. GONZALEZ-HERNANDEZ, and L. MARTINEZ-MILLAN, 1994. Pyramidal and nonpyramidal callosal cells in the striate cortex of the adult rat. *J. Comp. Neurol.* 350:439–451.

MARZI, C. A., P. BISIACCHI, and R. NICOLETTI, 1991. Is interhemispheric transfer of visuomotor information asymmetric? Evidence from a meta-analysis. *Neuropsychologia* 29:1163–1177.

MAUNSELL, J. H., and D. C. VAN ESSEN, 1987. Topographic organization of the middle temporal visual area in the macaque monkey: Representational biases and the relationship to callosal connections and myeloarchitectonic boundaries. *J. Comp. Neurol.* 266:535–555.

MCCULLOCH, W. S., and H. W. GAROL, 1941. Cortical origin and distribution of corpus callosum and anterior commissure in the monkey (*Macaca mulatta*). *J. Neurophys.* 4:555–563.

MEYER, B. U., S. RORICHT, H. GRAFIN VON EINSIEDEL, F. KRUGGEL, and A. WEINDL, 1995. Inhibitory and excitatory interhemispheric transfers between motor cortical areas in normal humans and patients with abnormalities of the corpus callosum. *Brain* 118:429–440.

MEYER, B. U., S. RORICHT, and C. WOICIECHOWSKY, 1998. Topography of fibers in the human corpus callosum mediating interhemispheric inhibition between the motor cortices. *Ann. Neurol.* 43:360–369.

MILLER, J., A. RIEHLE, and J. REQUIN, 1992. Effects of preliminary perceptual output on neuronal activity of the primary motor cortex. *J. Exp. Psychol. Hum. Percep. Perf.* 18:1121–1138.

MILNER, A. D., and C. R. LINES, 1982. Interhemispheric pathways in simple reaction times to lateralized light flashes. *Neuropsychologia* 20:171–179.

MILNER, A. D., M. A. JEEVES, P. H. SILVER, C. R. LINES, and J. WILSON, 1985. Reaction times to lateralized visual stimuli in callosal agenesis: Stimulus and response factors. *Neuropsychologia* 23:323–331.

MORRELL, L. K., and F. MORRELL, 1966. Evoked potentials and reaction times: A study of intra-individual variability. *Electroencephalogr. Clin. Neurophysiol.* 20:567–575.

MURPHY, G. M., JR., 1985. Volumetric asymmetry in the human striate cortex. *Exp. Neurol.* 88:288–302.

MURRO, A. M., J. R. SMITH, D. W. KING, and Y. D. PARK, 1995. Precision of dipole localization in a spherical volume conductor: A comparison of referential EEG, magnetoencephalography and scalp current density methods. *Brain Topogr.* 8:119–125.

MYSLOBODSKY, M. S., R. COPPOLA, and D. R. WEINBERGER, 1991a. EEG laterality in the era of structural brain imaging. *Brain Topogr.* 3:381–390.

MYSLOBODSKY, M. S., J. GLICKSOHN, R. COPPOLA, and D. R. WEINBERGER, 1991b. Occipital lobe morphology in normal individuals assessed by magnetic resonance imaging (MRI). *Vision Res.* 31:1677–1685.

NETZ, J., U. ZIEMANN, and G. V. HOMBER, 1995. Hemispheric asymmetry of transcallosal inhibition in man. *Exp. Brain Res.* 104:527–533.

NIRENBERG, L., 1980. *Interhemispheric and Intermodal communication in dyslexic and normal children.* Undergraduate thesis, State University of New York, Purchase College.

NOWICKA, A., A. GRABOWSKA, and E. FERSTEN, 1996. Interhemispheric transmission of information and functional asymmetry of the human brain. *Neuropsychologia* 34:147–151.

OERTEL, D., 1983. Synaptic responses and electrical properties of cells in brain slices of the mouse anteroventral cochlear nucleus. *J. Neurosci.* 3:2043–2053.

PANDYA, D. N., and D. L. ROSENE, 1985. Some observations on trajectories and topography of commissural fibers. In *Epilepsy and the Corpus Callosum,* A. G. Reeves, ed. New York: Plenum Press, pp. 21–40.

PANDYA, D. N., and B. SELTZER, 1986. The topography of commissural fibers. In *Two Hemispheres—One Brain: Functions of the Corpus Callosum,* F. Lepore, M. Ptito, and H. H. Jasper, eds. New York: Alan R. Liss, pp. 47–73.

PAYNE, B. R., D. F. SIWEK, and S. G. LOMBER, 1991. Complex transcallosal interactions in visual cortex. *Vis. Neurosci.* 6:283–289.

PAYNE, W. H., 1967. Visual reaction times on a circle about the fovea. *Science* 155:481–482.

PERRIN, F., O. BERTRAND, M. H. GIARD, and J. PERNIER, 1990. Precautions in topographic mapping and in evoked potential map reading. *J. Clin. Neurophys.* 7:498–506.

PERRIN, F., O. BERTRAND, and J. PERNIER, 1987. Scalp current density mapping: Value and estimation from potential data. *IEEE Trans. Biomed. Eng.* 34:283–288.

PERRIN, F., J. PERNIER, O. BERTRAND, and J. F. ECHALLIER, 1989. Spherical splines for scalp potential and current density mapping. *Electroencephalogr. Clin. Neurophysiol.* 72:184–187.

PETERS, A., and E. G. JONES, 1984. Classification of cortical neurons. In *Cerebral Cortex,* Vol. 1: *Cellular Components of the Cerebral Cortex,* A. Peters and E. G. Jones, eds. New York: Plenum Press, pp. 107–120.

PFLIEGER, M. E., and S. F. SANDS, 1995. Information growth in multichannel EEG [Abstract]. *Hum. Brain Mapp.* S1:99.

PFLIEGER, M. E., and S. F. SANDS, 1996. 256–channel ERP Information growth [Abstract]. *NeuroImage* 3:S10.

PICARD, N., and P. L. STRICK, 1996. Motor areas of the medial wall: A review of their location and functional activation. *Cereb. Cortex* 6:342–353.

POFFENBERGER, A. T., 1912. Reaction time to retinal stimulation with special reference to the time lost in conduction through nerve centers. *Arch. Psychol.* 23:1–73.

PORTER, R., and R. LEMON, 1995. *Corticospinal Function and Voluntary Movement: Monographs of the Physiological Society,* Vol. 45. Oxford, Engl.: Clarendon Press.

POTVIN, C., C. M. J. BRAUN, and A. ACHIM, 1995. Distinct functional channels in interhemispheric relay: Experimental evidence [Abstract]. *J. Int. Neuropsychol. Soc.* 1:184.

PRAAMSTRA, P., D. F. STEGEMAN, M. W. HORSTINK, and A. R. COOLS, 1996. Dipole source analysis suggests selective modulation of the supplementary motor area contribution to the readiness potential. *Electroencephalogr. Clin. Neurophysiol.* 90:468–477.

REGAN, D., 1989. *Human Brain Electrophysiology: Evoked Potentials and Evoked Magnetic Fields in Science and Medicine.* New York: Elsevier.

ROLAND, P. E., and K. ZILLES, 1996. Functions and structures of the motor cortices in humans. *Curr. Opin. Neurobiol.* 6:773–781.

ROUILLER, E. M., A. BABALIAN, O. KAZENNIKOV, V. MORET, X. H. YU, and M. WIESENDANGER, 1994. Transcallosal connections of the distal forelimb representations of the primary and supplementary motor cortical areas in macaque monkeys. *Exp. Brain Res.* 102:227–243.

RUGG, M. D., C. R. LINES, and A. D. MILNER, 1984. Visual evoked potentials to lateralized visual stimuli and the measurement of interhemispheric transfer time. *Neuropsychologia* 22:215–225.

RUGG, M. D., C. R. LINES, and A. D. MILNER, 1985a. Further investigation of visual evoked potentials elicited by lateralized stimuli: Effects of stimulus eccentricity and reference site. *Electroencephalogr. Clin. Neurophysiol.* 62:81–87.

RUGG, M. D., A. D. MILNER, and C. R. LINES, 1985b. Visual evoked potentials to lateralised stimuli in two cases of callosal agenesis. *J. Neurol. Neurosurg. Psychiatry* 48:367–373.

RUMSEY, J. M., M. CASANOVA, G. B. MANNHEIM, N. PATRONAS, N. DE VAUGHN, S. D. HAMBURGER, and T. AQUINO, 1996. Corpus callosum morphology, as measured with MRI, in dyslexic men. *Biol. Psychiatry* 39:769–775.

ST. JOHN, R., C. SHIELDS, P. KRAHN, and B. TIMNEY, 1987. The reliability of estimates of interhemispheric transmission times derived from unimanual and verbal response latencies. *Hum. Neurobiol.* 6:195–202.

SABATINI, B. L., and W. G. REGEHR, 1996. Timing of neurotransmission at fast synapses in the mammalian brain. *Nature* 384:170–172.

SALENIUS, S., K. PORTIN, M. KAJOLA, R. SALMELIN, and R. HARI, 1997. Cortical control of human motoneuron firing during isometric contraction. *J. Neurophys.* 77:3401–3405.

SALMELIN, R., N. FORSS, J. KNUUTILA, and R. HARI, 1995. Bilateral activation of the human somatomotor cortex by distal hand movements. *Electroencephalogr. Clin. Neurophysiol.* 95:444–452.

SARON, C. D., 1999. *Spatiotemporal electrophysiology of intra- and interhemispheric visuomotor integration: Relations with behavior.* Ph.D. dissertation, Albert Einstein College of Medicine, Bronx, N.Y.

SARON, C. D., and R. J. DAVIDSON, 1986. Response hand influences visual evoked potential estimates of interhemispheric transfer time in children [Abstract]. *Psychophysiology* 23:458.

SARON, C. D., and R. J. DAVIDSON, 1988a. Reliability of visual evoked response estimates of interhemispheric transfer time [Abstract]. *Psychophysiology* 25:479.

SARON, C. D., and R. J. DAVIDSON, 1988b. Verbal and spatial tasks matched on difficulty: Demonstration of hemispheric differences with identical stimuli [Abstract]. *J. Clin. Exp. Neuropsychol.* 10:55.

SARON, C. D., and R. J. DAVIDSON, 1989a. Visual evoked potential measures of interhemispheric transfer time in humans. *Behav. Neurosci.* 103:1115–1138.

SARON, C. D., and R. J. DAVIDSON, 1989b. Reliability of visual evoked response estimates of interhemispheric transfer time: further studies [Abstract]. *Psychophysiology* 26:S53.

SARON, C. D., and R. J. DAVIDSON, 1989c. Visual evoked potential estimates of interhemispheric transfer time in humans: Effects of vertical position within a hemifield. *Soc. Neurosci Abstr.* 15 (2):1061.

SARON, C. D., M. LASSONDE, H. G. VAUGHAN, JR., J. J. FOXE, S. P. ALFHORS, and G. V. SIMPSON, 1997. Interhemispheric visuomotor interaction in callosal agenesis: spatiotemporal patterns of cortical activation. *Soc. Neurosci. Abstr.* 23 (2):1949.

SARON, C. D., H. G. VAUGHAN, JR., G. V. SIMPSON, and J. J. FOXE, 1995a. Timing and spatial distribution of interhemispheric visuomotor communication [Abstract]. *Hum. Brain Mapp.* S1:289.

SARON, C. D., H. G. VAUGHAN, JR., G. V. SIMPSON, and J. J. FOXE, 1995b. Visual and motor interaction: Spatiotemporal patterns of intra- and interhemispheric cortical activation. *Soc. Neurosci. Abstr.* 21 (2):1423.

SARON, C. D., H. G. VAUGHAN, JR., G. V. SIMPSON, and J. J. FOXE, 1996. Effects of reaction time on visuomotor interaction: spatiotemporal patterns of intra- and interhemispheric cortical activation. *Soc. Neurosci. Abstr.* 22 (2):890.

SARON, C. D., H. G. VAUGHAN, JR., J. J. FOXE, and G. V. SIMPSON, 1998. Multiple visuomotor activation and motor output pathways in simple RT [Abstract]. *Neuroimage* 7:S960.

SARON, C. D., J. J. FOXE, G. V. SIMPSON, and H. G. VAUGHAN, JR., 1999. Electrophysiological evidence refutes the assumptions underlying reaction time measures of interhemispheric transfer. *Soc. Neurosci. Abstr.* 25 (2):1410.

SARON, C. D., C. E. SCHROEDER, J. J. FOXE, and H. G. VAUGHAN, JR., 2001a. Visual activation of frontal cortex: Segregation from occipital activity. *Cog. Brain Res.* 12:75–88.

SARON, C. D., J. J. FOXE, C. E. SCHROEDER, and H. G. VAUGHAN, Jr., 2001b. Magnitude of movement-related high-density ERP measures of cortical activation predicts reaction time [Abstract]. *Neuroimage*, 13, part 2, 1250b.

SARON, C. D., J. J. FOXE, C. E. SCHROEDER, and H. G. VAUGHAN, Jr., 2003. Complexities of interhemispheric interaction in sensorimotor tasks revealed by high-density event-related potential mapping. In *The Asymmetrical Brain*, K. Hugdahl and R. J. Davidson, eds. Cambridge, MA: MIT Press, pp. 341–408.

SASAKI, K., and H. GEMBA, 1986. Effects of premotor cortex cooling upon visually initiated hand movements in the monkey. *Brain Res.* 28:278–286.

SAVAGE, C. R., and D. G. THOMAS, 1993. Information processing and interhemispheric transfer in left- and right-handed adults. *Intl. J. Neurosci.* 71:201–219.

SCHERG, M., 1990. Fundamentals of dipole source potential analysis. In *Advances in Audiology*, Vol. 6, F. Grandori, M. Hoke, and G. L. Romani, eds. Basel, Switzerland: Karger, pp. 40–69.

SCHERG, M., D. VON CRAMON, 1986. Evoked dipole source potentials of the human auditory cortex. *Electroencephalogr. Clin. Neurophysiol.* 65:344–360.

SCHNITZLER, A., K. R. KESSLER, and R. BENECKE, 1996. Transcallosally mediated inhibition of interneurons within human primary motor cortex. *Exp. Brain Res.* 112:381–391.

SCHOEN, J. H. R., 1964. Comparative aspects of the descending fibre systems in the spinal cord. *Prog. Brain Res.* 11:203–222.

SEACORD, L., C. G. GROSS, and M. MISHKIN, 1979. Role of inferior temporal cortex in interhemispheric transfer. *Brain Res.* 167:259–272.

SERGENT, J., and J. J. MYERS, 1985. Manual, blowing, and verbal simple reactions to lateralized flashes of light in commissurotomized patients. *Percept. Psychophys.* 37:571–578.

SHAPLESKE, J., S. L. ROSSELL, P. W. R. WOODRUFF, and A. S. DAVID, 1999. The planum temporale: A systematic, quantitative review of its structural, functional and clinical significance. *Brain Res. Rev.* 29:26–49.

SIMPSON, G. V., M. E. PFLIEGER, J. J. FOXE, S. P. AHLFORS, H. G. VAUGHAN, JR., J. HRABE, R. J. ILMONIEMI, and G. LANTOS, 1995a. Dynamic neuroimaging of brain function. *J. Clin. Neurophys.* 12:432–449.

SIMPSON, G. V., J. J. FOXE, H. G. VAUGHAN, JR., A. D. MEHTA, and C. E. SCHROEDER, 1995b. Integration of electrophysiological source analyses, MRI and animal models in the study of visual processing and attention. *Electroencephalogr. Clin. Neurophysiol. Suppl.* 44:76–92.

SKLAR, B., J. HANELY, and W. W. SIMMONS, 1972. An EEG experiment aimed toward identifying dyslexic children. *Nature* 240:414–416.

SOONG, A. C., J. C. LIND, G. R. SHAW, and Z. J. KOLES, 1993. Systematic comparisons of interpolation techniques in topographic brain mapping. *Electroencephalogr. Clin. Neurophysiol.* 87:185–195.

SPEKREIJSE, H., L. H. VAN DER TWELL, and T. ZUIDEMA, 1973. Contrast evoked responses in man. *Vision Res.* 13:1577–1601.

STANCÁK, A., JR., and G. PFURTSCHELLER, 1996. Event-related desynchronisation of central beta-rhythms during brisk and slow self-paced finger movements of dominant and nondominant hand. *Cogn. Brain Res.* 4:171–183.

STEINMETZ, H., A. HERZOG, G. SCHLAUG, Y. HUANG, and L. JANCKE, 1995. Brain asymmetry in monozygotic twins. *Cereb. Cortex* 5:296–300.

STENSAAS, S. S., D. K. EDDINGTON, and W. H. DOBELLE, 1974. The topography and variability of the primary visual cortex in man. *J. Neurosurg.* 40:747–755.

STONE, J., and J. A. FREEMAN, 1971. Synaptic organisation of the pigeon's optic tectum: A Golgi and current source-density analysis. *Brain Res.* 27:203–221.

SUPEK, S., and C. J. AINE, 1993. Simulation studies of multiple dipole neuromagnetic source localization: Model order and limits of source resolution. *IEEE Trans. Biomed. Eng.* 40:529–540.

SUPEK, S., and C. J. AINE, 1997. Spatio-temporal modeling of neuromagnetic data. I: Multi-source location versus time-course estimation accuracy. *Hum. Brain Mapp.* 5:139–153.

SWADLOW, H. A., 1985. The corpus callosum as a model system in the study of mammalian cerebral axons: A comparison of results from primate and rabbit. In *Epilepsy and the Corpus Callosum*, A. G. Reeves, ed. New York: Plenum Press, pp. 55–74.

SWADLOW, H. A., S. G. WAXMAN, and N. GESCHWIND, 1980. Small-diameter nonmyelinated axons in the primate corpus callosum. *Arch. Neurol.* 37:114–115.

SWANSON, J., A. LEDLOW, and M. KINSBOURNE, 1978. Lateral asymmetries revealed by simple reaction time. In *Asymmetrical Function of the Brain*, M. Kinsbourne, ed. Cambridge, Engl.: Cambridge University Press, pp. 274–291.

TAMAS, G., E. H. BUHL, and P. SOMOGYI, 1997. Fast IPSPs elicited via multiple synaptic release sites by different types of GABAergic neurone in the cat visual cortex. *J. Physiol. (Lond.)* 500:715–738.

TANJI, J., 1994. The supplementary motor area in the cerebral cortex. *Neurosci. Res.* 19:251–268.

TANJI, J., K. OKANO, and K. C. SATO, 1988. Neuronal activity in cortical motor areas related to ipsilateral, contralateral, and bilateral digit movements of the monkey. *J. Neurophys.* 60:325–343.

TASSINARI, G., S. AGLIOTI, R. PALLINI, G. BERLUCCHI, and G. F. ROSSI, 1994. Interhemispheric integration of simple visuomotor responses in patients with partial callosal defects. *Behav. Brain Res.* 64:141–149.

TOKUNO, H., and J. TANJI, 1993. Input organization of distal and proximal forelimb areas in the monkey primary motor cortex: A retrograde double labeling study. *J. Comp. Neurol.* 333:199–209.

TOOTELL, R. B., J. D. MENDOLA, N. K. HADJIKHANI, A. K. LIU, and A. M. DALE, 1998. The representation of the ipsilateral visual field in human cerebral cortex. *Proc. Natl. Acad. Sci. U.S.A.* 95:818–824.

TOYAMA, K., K. MATSUNAMI, T. ONO, and S. TOKASHIKI, 1974. An intracellular study of neuronal organization in the visual cortex. *Exp. Brain Res.* 21:45–66.

TOYOSHIMA, K., and H. SAKAI, 1982. Exact cortical extent of the origin of the corticospinal tract (CST) and the quantitative contribution to the CST in different cytoarchitectonic areas: A study with horseradish peroxidase in the monkey. *J. Hirnforsch.* 23:257–269.

TRAMO, M. J., K. BAYNES, R. FENDRICH, G. R. MANGUN, E. A. PHELPS, P. A. REUTER-LORENZ, and M. S. GAZZANIGA, 1995. Hemispheric specialization and interhemispheric integration: Insights from experiments with commissurotomy patients. In *Epilepsy and the Corpus Callosum 2*, A. G. Reeves and D. W. Roberts, eds. New York: Plenum Press, pp. 263–295.

URBANO, A., C. BABILONI, P. ONORATI, and F. BABILONI, 1996. Human cortical activity related to unilateral movements: A high resolution EEG study. *Neuroreport* 8:203–206.

URBANO, A., C. BABILONI, P. ONORATI, and F. BABILONI, 1998a. Dynamic functional coupling of high resolution EEG potentials related to unilateral internally triggered one-digit movements. *Electroencephalogr. Clin. Neurophysiol.* 106:477–487.

URBANO, A., C. BABILONI, P. ONORATI, F. CARDUCCI, A. AMBROSINI, L. FATTORINI, and F. BABILONI, 1998b. Responses of human primary sensorimotor and supplementary motor areas to internally triggered unilateral and simultaneous bilateral one-digit movements: A high-resolution EEG study. *Eur. J. Neurosci.* 10:765–767.

UUSITALO, M. A., S. J. WILLIAMSON, and M. T. SEPPA, 1996. Dynamical organisation of the human visual system revealed by lifetimes of activation traces. *Neurosci. Lett.* 213:149–152.

VAN ESSEN D. C., W. T. NEWSOME, and J. L. BIXBY, 1982. The pattern of interhemispheric connections and its relationship to extrastriate visual areas in the macaque monkey. *J. Neurosci.* 2:265–283.

VAUGHAN, H. G., JR., 1987. Topographic analysis of brain electrical activity. *Electroencephalogr. Clin. Neurophys. Suppl.* 39:137–142.

VAUGHAN, H. G., JR., L. D. COSTA, L. GILDEN, and H. SCHIMMEL, 1965. Identification of sensory and motor components of cerebral activity in simple reaction time tasks. In *Proceedings of the 73rd Conference of the American Psychological Association*, Vol. 1, pp. 179–180.

VAUGHAN, H. G., JR., L. D. COSTA, and L. GILDEN, 1966. The functional relation of visual evoked response and reaction time to stimulus intensity. *Vision Res.* 6:645–656.

WAHBA, G., 1990. *Spline Models for Observational Data*. Philadelphia: S.I.A.M.

WAXMAN, S. G., and M. V. L. BENNETT, 1972. Relative conduction velocities of small myelinated and non-myelinated fibres in the central nervous system. *Nature New Biol.* 238:217–219.

WIESENDANGER, M., E. M. ROUILLER, O. KAZENNIKOV, and S. PERRIG, 1996. Is the supplementary motor area a bilaterally organized system? *Adv. Neurol.* 70:85–93.

WISE, S. P., 1996. Corticospinal efferents of the supplementary sensorimotor area in relation to the primary motor area. *Adv. Neurol.* 70:57–69.

WISE, S. P., D. BOUSSAOUD, P. B. JOHNSON, and R. CAMINITI, 1997. Premotor and parietal cortex: corticocortical connectivity and combinatorial computations. *Ann. Rev. Neurosci.* 20:25–42.

YENI-KOMSHIAN, G. H., P. ISENBERG, and H. GOLDBERG, 1975. Cerebral dominance and reading disability: Left visual field deficit in poor readers. *Neuropsychologia* 13:83–94.

YVERT, B., O. BERTRAND, J. F. ECHALLIER, and J. PERNIER, 1996. Improved dipole localization using local mesh refinement of realistic head geometries: An EEG simulation study. *Electroencephalogr. Clin. Neurophysiol.* 99:79–89.

YVERT, B., O. BERTRAND, M. THEVENET, J. F. ECHALLIER, and J. PERNIER, 1997. A systematic evaluation of the spherical model accuracy in EEG dipole localization. *Electroencephalogr. Clin. Neurophysiol.* 102, 452–459.

COMMENTARY 8.1

Interhemispheric Transfer of Visual Information as a Function of Retinal Eccentricity: Evidence from Event-Related Potentials

CARLO MINIUSSI, ANGELO MARAVITA, AND CARLO MARZI

ABSTRACT We measured behavioral interhemispheric transfer (IT) time in normal subjects while simultaneously recording event-related potentials (ERPs) to lateralized visual stimuli. There was no effect of the eccentricity of stimulus presentation (3° versus 30°) on behavioral IT and on ERP latency measures. In contrast, there was an effect of eccentricity on ERP amplitude measures of IT with a selective decrease of the commissural response at 30° versus 3°. Possible reasons for such a discrepancy are discussed.

Saron and colleagues' article demonstrates the complexity of interhemispheric visuomotor pathways in the normal brain. Here we address the issue of specific channel than subserves interhemispheric transfer (IT).

In a simple sensorimotor task such as that employed in the so-called Poffenberger paradigm (Poffenberger, 1912), when the responding hand is on the opposite side of the stimulated visual hemifield (crossed condition), an IT must occur at either the visual cortex level, the premotor cortex level, or both. Such is obviously not the case when hemifield and hand are on the same side (uncrossed condition), and this is witnessed by the typically shorter reaction time (RT) in comparison with the crossed condition (see Marzi et al., 1991, for a review). Following the pioneering study of Berlucchi and colleagues (1971), it has been assumed that IT does not

CARLO MINIUSSI   IRCSS S. Giovanni di Dio, Brescia, Italy.
ANGELO MARAVITA   Institute of Cognitive Neuroscience, University College London, London, United Kingdom.
CARLO MARZI   Department of Neurological and Visual Sciences, University of Verona, Verona, Italy.

occur at the visual level because manipulations of the eccentricity of stimulus presentation do not result in variation of IT. The rationale underlying such assumption is straightforward: In the primary visual cortex and in the immediately adjoining areas, the density of callosal connections decreases as one goes from areas representing the central portions of the visual field to those with more peripheral representations (see Marzi, 1986, for a review). Therefore, a stimulus presented within approximately 5° of the central vertical meridian will activate cortical areas full of callosally projecting neurons. By contrast, more peripherally presented stimuli will activate areas that are less rich in callosal connections. This would lead to a slower and less effective IT of visual information. In contrast to such a prediction, Berlucchi and colleagues (1971) and many others thereafter have found no lengthening of IT as a function of the eccentricity of stimulus presentation. Iacoboni and Zaidel (Chapter 12 in this volume; see also Iacoboni, Fried, and Zaidel, 1994) propose that in normals IT takes place at the premotor cortical level through the anterior portion of the CC, while in subjects lacking such a portion of the CC it occurs at the visual level through the splenium. In such patients there is evidence of a lengthening of IT as one increases the eccentricity of stimulus presentation (Iacoboni et al., 1994), and this is in accord with the above-mentioned neuroanatomical and neurophysiological data on the progressive reduction of the representation of the visual field in the callosal connections.

In this commentary we briefly report an event-related potential (ERP) experiment that attempted to cast fur-

TABLE 8.1

Mean reaction time (RT) for uncrossed and crossed hemifield-hand combinations for the two eccentricities of stimulus presentation. The mean crossed-uncrossed difference (CUD) in RT represents a measure of interhemispheric transfer. It is clearly not reliably different for the two eccentricities (see text).

Eccentricity	Uncrossed	Crossed	CUD
3°	249.9 ms	251.6 ms	1.7 ms
30°	270.3 ms	262.4 ms	2.4 ms

ther light on the problem of the effect of eccentricity manipulations on IT.

We tested 14 normal right-handed subjects on a Poffenberger paradigm and simultaneously recorded visual ERPs with a 32-channel computerized system; see Ipata and colleagues (1997) for details about the recording technique. The stimuli were presented along the horizontal meridian of the visual field at either 3° or 30° of eccentricity, and the subjects were asked to press a key as fast as possible with the right or the left hand in different blocks.

Behavioral results

Table 8.1 shows the behavioral results: In keeping with previous findings, the crossed-uncrossed difference (CUD) in RT, which is widely considered as a behavioral measure of IT (see Marzi et al., 1991, for a review), showed a small nonsignificant RT lengthening at 30° as compared to 3°. The overall mean CUD (2.0 ms) was within the well-established range in normals (Marzi et al., 1991).

ERP results

Figure 8.16 shows examples of grand-average ERPs at various electrode locations for stimuli presented at an eccentricity of 3° and 30°. We focused our analysis on the P1 and N1 components of the visual ERP; the former is a positive component peaking at about 100–130 ms from stimulus onset, and the latter is a negative component with a peak latency ranging between 150 and 220 ms from stimulus onset.

AMPLITUDE   Overall, the amplitude of all the main early components (P1 and N1) was larger for 3° than 30°. This comes as no surprise, given the progressively smaller density of retinal elements and the smaller cortical magnification factor as one goes from central to peripheral visual field locations. A potentially important new piece of evidence concerns the differential decrease

in amplitude of the two components. The P1 component decreased in its mean peak amplitude from 4.3 μv for stimuli at 3° to 1.57 μv for stimuli at 30°. A minuscule decrease was instead found for N1 (from 2.76 μv at 3° to 2.26 μv at 30°). Such a selective effect is in keeping with the P1 component having a generator in visual extrastriate areas while N1 is thought to be generated in multiple not strictly visual sites (see Mangun, 1995, for a review). More important for the present purposes, the effect of peripheral presentations on the amplitude of the two above components was greater for the indirect (commissural) than for the direct ERP responses. At 3° the differences in amplitude between indirect and direct responses were minimal and sometimes in the direction of a larger amplitude for the former. In contrast, at 30° the direct responses were generally of a higher amplitude than the indirect responses. Such an effect was larger for the N1 than for the P1 component, and this is in agreement with the notion that N1 can be considered a good functional landmark of IT. We recently found (Ipata et al., 1997) that for N1 the ERP measures of IT show a better fit with their behavioral counterparts than for P1. The N1 component not only yields a faster IT than P1 but also shows a shorter IT latency for the right-to-left hemisphere direction of IT, thus paralleling the behavioral results (Marzi et al., 1991; Braun, 1992; Brown, Larson, and Jeeves, 1994).

LATENCY   A somewhat different overall picture emerged from latency measurements: First, the mean latency for both P1 and N1 did not vary significantly with eccentricity of stimulus presentation (see Figure 8.16), and this is at odds with the behavioral data showing a robust lengthening of RT with eccentricity. Second, although there was a clear-cut overall latency advantage of the direct versus indirect responses such a difference was not related to eccentricity.

In other words, in keeping with the behavioral results, IT was unrelated to stimulus eccentricity.

Conclusions

Taken together, these findings show some discrepancy between two electrophysiological indices of IT: amplitude and latency of the early ERP components. Behaviorally, we found no interaction between eccentricity and CUD, and the same was true of ERP latency. In contrast, the amplitude of commissural ERP responses was clearly smaller than that of the direct responses at 30° but not at 3° of eccentricity. A possible speculation on the nature of such a dissociation is that amplitude and latency of ERPs rely on partially different aspects of the electrophysiological response. The amplitude of an

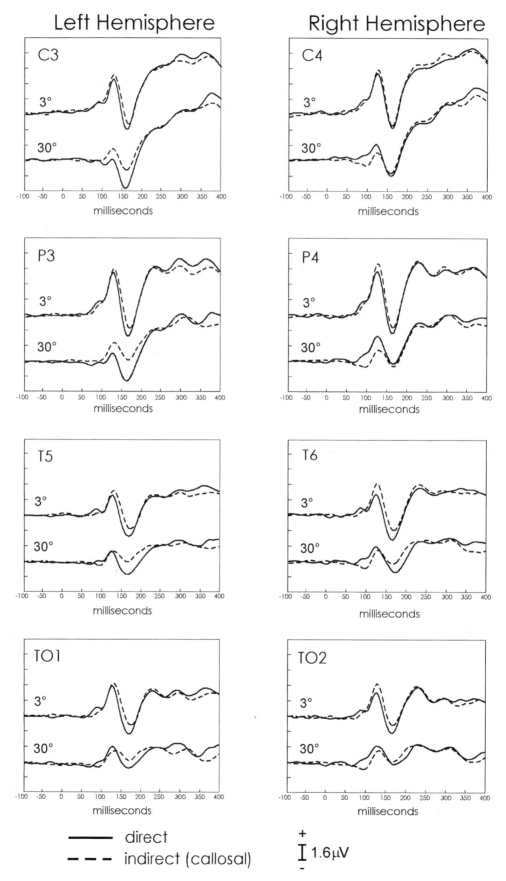

FIGURE 8.16. Event-related responses (ERPs) recorded at various electrode locations for direct and indirect hemifield-hemisphere combinations (see text).

ERP component is clearly dependent on the synchrony of the neuronal activity underlying that response and on the number of active neurons. Therefore, a stimulus that is presented to areas rich of callosally projecting neurons, such as those representing the centralmost portion of the visual field, will evoke a large transcallosal response. In contrast, a stimulus that is presented to peripheral visual field areas will activate less callosally projecting neurons in the visual cortex and a smaller response will be transmitted to the contralateral hemisphere. A different consideration applies to latency of the transcallosal ERP response, which we found to be unrelated to the eccentricity of stimulus presentation. It is reasonable to assume that the speed of IT, as measured by ERPs, depends upon the presence of a contingent of fast-conducting callosally projecting neurons in the visual cortical areas activated by a stimulus. A reasonable guess is that the proportion of fast-conducting callosal fibers does not show substantial variations among the visual areas representing central versus peripheral portions of the visual field. This would explain why the latency of direct versus indirect visual ERPs shows no reliable eccentricity-related differences in our present experiment. Such a consideration might apply to the behavioral results classically showing no relation between eccentricity of stimulus presentation and CUD, see above. Unfortunately, to our knowledge, it is not known whether in humans the proportion of large fast-conducting callosal fibers known to exist in the splenium (Aboitiz et al., 1992) varies according to the visuotopic organization of the cortical areas where they originate.

Such information would help to clarify the nature of the discrepancy between amplitude and latency ERP estimates of IT that we found in the present study.

REFERENCES

Aboitiz, F., A. B. Scheibel, R. S. Fisher, and E. Zaidel, 1992. Fiber composition of the human corpus callosum. *Brain Res.* 98:143–153.

Berlucchi, G., W. Heron, R. Hyman, G. Rizzolatti, and C. Umiltà, 1971. Simple reaction times of ipsilateral and contralateral hand to lateralized visual stimuli. *Brain* 94:419–430.

Braun, C. M., 1992. Estimates of interhemispheric dynamics from simple manual reaction time to extrafoveal stimuli. *Neuropsychol. Rev.* 3:321–365.

Brown, W. S., E. B. Larson, and M. Jeeves, 1994. Directional asymmetries in interhemispheric transmission time: Evidence from visual evoked potentials. *Neuropsychologia* 32:439–448.

Iacoboni, M., I. Fried, and E. Zaidel, 1994. Callosal transmission time before and after partial commissurotomy. *NeuroReport* 5:2521–2524.

Ipata, A., M. Girelli, C. Miniussi, and C. A. Marzi, 1997. Interhemispheric transfer of visual information in humans: The role of different callosal channels. *Arch. Ital. Biol.* 135:169–182.

Mangun, G. R., 1995. Neural mechanisms of visual selective attention. *Psychophysiology* 32:439–448.

Marzi, C. A., 1986. Transfer of visual information after unilateral input to the brain. *Brain Cogn.* 5:163–173.

Marzi, C. A., P. Bisiacchi, and R. Nicoletti, 1991. Is interhemispheric transfer of visuomotor information asymmetric? Evidence from a meta-analysis. *Neuropsychologia* 29:1163–1177.

Poffenberger, A. T., 1912. Reaction time to retinal stimulation with special reference to the time lost in conduction through nerve centers. *Arch. Psychol.* 23:1–73.

Commentary 8.2

Neuroimaging Patterns of Intra- and Interhemispheric Connectivity

Marco Iacoboni and Eran Zaidel

ABSTRACT Various imaging techniques have been used recently to map cortical activity during sensorimotor integration tasks requiring ipsilateral and contralateral unimanual responses to lateralized sensory stimuli. The picture that emerges is that even in simple sensorimotor transforms, the serial information processing model assumed by Poffenberger is probably too simplistic and that massive, parallel cortical architecture is engaged in these simple tasks. However, we believe that most of the evidence provided by neuroimaging studies is still consistent with the notion that the crossed-uncrossed difference in simple reaction times to lateralized flashes represents a conduction delay through callosal fibers.

When Poffenberger proposed the paradigm of simple reaction times to lateralized flashes as a behavioral estimate of interhemispheric conduction delay, he had in mind a very simple serial information-processing model of visuomotor integration (Poffenberger, 1912). This model has been previously challenged on both theoretical and empirical grounds (Ledlow, Swanson, and Kinsbourne, 1978; and see also Chapter 10 in this volume). The impressive data set of Cliff Saron and colleagues might at first look like the strongest challenge yet that the Poffenberger model has had to face. However, we believe that their data may be parsimoniously interpreted as suggesting that even though Poffenberger's simple serial information-processing model of simple visuomotor integration is probably wrong, the paradigm can still give us a parameter, the crossed-uncrossed difference (CUD), that is a valid estimate of interhemispheric conduction delay. In this commentary we will discuss neurophysiological and behavioral data that are relevant to the data of Saron and colleagues and to this issue.

MARCO IACOBONI Ahmanson Lovelace Brain Mapping Center, Neuropsychiatric Institute, Brain Research Institute, David Geffen School of Medicine, University of California at Los Angeles, Los Angeles, California.
ERAN ZAIDEL Department of Psychology, University of California at Los Angeles, Los Angeles, California.

It seems to us that a straightforward behavioral counterpart of the large trial-to-trial variability in activation maps shown by Saron and colleagues is the large variability in reaction times observed at the Poffenberger paradigm. We recently reported data on reaction times variability in this paradigm, collecting 40,000 trials of simple reaction times to lateralized flashes in three normal right-handers (Iacoboni and Zaidel, 2000). Among other results, there are some findings in our data set that are relevant to the question of whether the CUD is a reliable estimate of interhemispheric conduction delay. We observed that even though the CUD variability across several sessions in a single subject generally mimics the variability observed in a sample of subjects tested in a single session, the CUD variability was considerably reduced when the CUD was computed over at least 2400 trials per subject. Further, when CUDs were computed over 2400 trials or more, they tended to be extremely similar (about 2 ms) across subjects. Also, when reaction times were ordered from the fastest to the slowest and divided into bins, the observed CUD across bins was remarkably stable (from 1 to 4 ms) over the entire reaction time distribution. Taken together, these data suggest that the CUD computed over thousands of trials reflects hard-wired mechanisms of callosal transmission that must occur, *all the other things being equal*, at least one more time for crossed than for uncrossed responses.

Recently, another electrical scalp recording study has provided evidence for callosal transfer at a motor level (Thut et al., 1999), thus being consistent with previous behavioral data (Berlucchi et al., 1971; Iacoboni, Fried, and Zaidel, 1994; Iacoboni and Zaidel, 1995; Vallar, Sterzi, and Basso, 1988). Also, some positron emission tomography (PET) and functional magnetic resonance (fMRI) data are almost entirely consistent with the notion that the CUD represents interhemispheric conduction delay. A PET study has shown that, when crossed

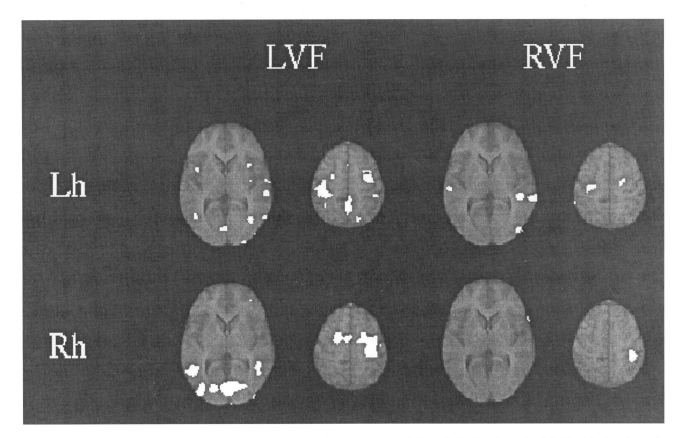

FIGURE 8.17. Activation maps for all four hand-field combinations during simple reaction times to lateralized flashes. Bilateral activations are seen in both premotor and visual areas in three conditions. Only the right visual field–right hand condition shows activations restricted to the left hemisphere.

responses were compared to uncrossed ones, blood flow increases were observed in the right occipital lobe and in the left superior parietal lobule (Marzi et al., 1999). This might represent the blood flow correlate of interhemispheric transfer. In fact, if there is an additional callosal transfer for crossed responses when compared to the uncrossed ones, then the axonal event associated with the additional callosal transfer is coupled with pre-synaptic and postsynaptic events that should in principle increase the cerebral blood flow. This study, however, also provided evidence for blood flow increases for uncrossed responses, compared to crossed ones, in the frontal lobe. This, obviously, is evidence that cannot be explained by the Poffenberger model. It is possible, however, that due to intrinsic features of PET scanning procedures, the frontal activations observed during uncrossed responses, compared to crossed ones, are due to spurious factors that have nothing to do with the task itself. PET data acquisition requires a steady state. This requires blocking of the experimental conditions under investigation. Thus, subjects must perform the same condition for several tens of seconds (in this study it was 1 minute). It is possible that subjects tend to think freely during very simple tasks as the blocked Poffenberger

paradigm, thus activating frontal lobe regions. Uncontrolled thoughts may be unbalanced across conditions and are more likely to occur more frequently during "easy" experimental conditions (such as the uncrossed ones), thus producing frontal activations that are intrinsically unrelated to the task.

To further define the cortical circuitry dedicated to simple visuomotor transforms, Iacoboni used fMRI and a single-trial design in eight normal right-handers (unpublished observations). With this approach, it is possible to observe the activation of cortical regions during a specific event, that is, left-hand responses to right flashes, without blocking the various experimental conditions. Given the duration of the hemodynamic response to single events (Menon and Kim, 1999), it is also possible to collect many more data points than in a canonical PET study (for instance, in this study more than twice as many data points per subject were collected than in the previous PET study). The results obtained suggest that simple reaction times to lateralized flashes are associated with bilateral activations even during uncrossed responses, and especially with the left hand, in line with the data of Saron and colleagues (Figure 8.17). They also suggest that the frontoparietal circuitry engaged

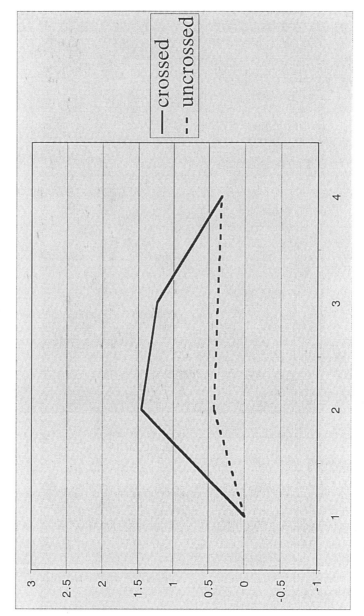

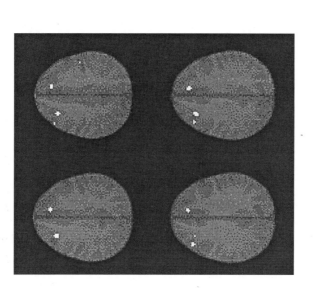

FIGURE 8.18. Left: Activation maps for crossed responses versus uncrossed responses in prefrontal cortex. Right: Time course of the averaged hemodynamic response for crossed and uncrossed responses in prefrontal cortex.

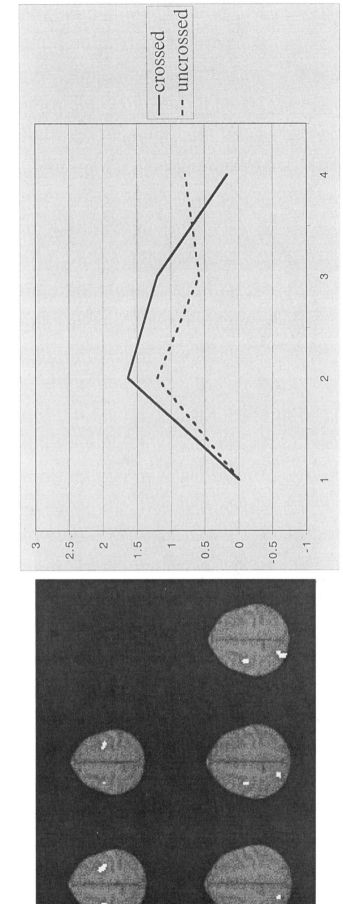

FIGURE 8.19. Left: Activation maps for crossed responses versus uncrossed responses in premotor and superior parietal cortex. Right: time course of the averaged hemodynamic response for crossed and uncrossed responses in premotor cortex.

227

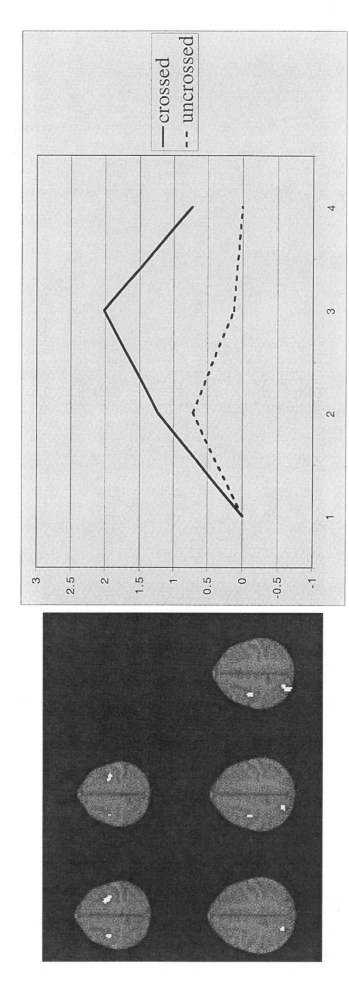

FIGURE 8.20. Left: Activation maps for crossed responses versus uncrossed responses in premotor and superior parietal cortex.

Right: time course of the averaged hemodynamic response for crossed and uncrossed responses in superior parietal cortex.

228

by complex sensorimotor transforms required by spatial compatibility and other visuomotor tasks (Iacoboni, 1999; Iacoboni et al., 1996, 1997, 1998) is also engaged by much simpler visuomotor transforms as simple reaction times to lateralized flashes. However, the results are also consistent with the notion that crossed responses require one extra callosal transfer, compared to uncrossed ones. In fact, when crossed responses were compared to uncrossed ones, activations were observed in dorsolateral prefrontal, dorsal premotor, and superior parietal regions (Figures 8.18–8.20). In contrast, uncrossed responses did not produce any additional activation when compared to crossed responses.

Taken together, the physiological data recently observed during simple reaction times to lateralized flashes call for a revision of Poffenberger's serial model of visuomotor integration but are still compatible with the notion that the CUD is a valid parameter for estimating interhemispheric conduction delay. In keeping with this, the CUD was recently measured in a split-brain patient during simple reaction times to visual and auditory stimuli. In this patient, the visual CUD was found to be abnormally long, whereas the auditory CUD was substantially zero, as predicted by the anatomical bilateral access of auditory fibers to both cerebral hemispheres (Iacoboni and Zaidel, 1999).

REFERENCES

BERLUCCHI, G., W. HERON, R. HYMAN, G. RIZZOLATTI, and C. UMILTÁ, 1971. Simple reaction times of ipsilateral and contralateral hand to lateralized visual stimuli. *Brain* 94:419–430.

COPELAND, S. A., and E. ZAIDEL, 1996. Contributions to the bilateral distribution advantage. *JINS* 2:29.

IACOBONI, M., 1999. Adjusting reaches: feedback in the posterior parietal cortex. *Nat. Neurosci.* 2:492–494.

IACOBONI, M., I. FRIED, and E. ZAIDEL, 1994. Callosal transmission time before and after partial commissurotomy. *NeuroReport* 5:2521–2524.

IACOBONI, M., R. P. WOODS, G. L. LENZI, and J. C. MAZIZIOTTA, 1997. Merging of oculomotor and somatomotor space coding in the human right precentral gyrus. *Brain* 120:1635–1645.

IACOBONI, M., R. P. WOODS, and J. C. MAZZIOTTA, 1996. Brain-behavior relationships: evidence from practice effects in spatial stimulus-response compatibility. *J. Neurophysiol.* 76:321–331.

IACOBONI, M., R. P. WOODS, and J. C. MAZZIOTTA, 1998. Bimodal (auditory and visual). Left frontoparietal circuitry for sensorimotor integration and sensorimotor learning. *Brain* 121:2135–2143.

IACOBONI, M., and E. ZAIDEL, 1995. Channels of the corpus callosum: evidence from simple reaction times to lateralized flashes in the normal and the split brain. *Brain* 118:779–788.

IACOBONI, M., and E. ZAIDEL, 1999. The crossed-uncrossed difference in simple reaction times to lateralized auditory stimuli is not a measure of interhemispheric transmission time: Evidence from the split brain. *Exp. Brain Res.* 128:421–424.

IACOBONI, M., and E. ZAIDEL, 2000. Crossed-uncrossed difference in simple reaction times to lateralized flashes: Between- and within-subjects variability. *Neuropsychologia.* 38:535–541.

LEDLOW, A., J. M. SWANSON, and M. KINSBOURNE, 1978. Differences in reaction times and average evoked potentials as a function of direct and indirect neural pathways. *Ann. Neurol.* 3:525–530.

MARZI, C. A., D. PERANI, G. TASSINARI, A. COLLELUORI, A. MARAVITA, C. MINIUSSI, E. PAULESU, P. SCIFO, and F. FAZIO, 1999. Pathways of interhemispheric transfer in normals and in a split-brain subject: A positron emission tomography. *Exp. Brain Res.* 126:451–458.

MENON, R. S., and S.-G. KIM, 1999. Spatial and temporal limits in cognitive neuroimaging with fMRI. *Trends Cogn. Sci.* 3:207–216.

POFFENBERGER, A., 1912. Reaction time to retinal stimulation with special reference to the time lost in conduction through nervous centers. *Arch. Psychol.* 23:1–73.

THUT, G., C.-A. HAUERT, S. MORAND, M. SEECK, T. LANDIS, and C. MICHEL, 1999. Evidence for interhemispheric motor-level transfer in a simple reaction time task: an EEG study. *Exp. Brain Res.* 128:256–261.

VALLAR, G., R. STERZI, and A. BASSO, 1988. Left hemisphere contribution to motor programming of aphasic speech: a reaction time experiment in aphasic patients. *Neuropsychologia* 26:511–519.

Commentary 8.3

The Use of Event-Related Potentials for Measuring Interhemispheric Transfer Time

STEVEN BERMAN

The chapter by Saron and colleagues describes a new thrust in use of averaged event-related scalp electrical potentials (ERPs) to trace the neural activation patterns that produce behavior across both time and space. While recent advances in functional brain imaging are speedily improving understanding of where in the brain a given task produces local activation, corresponding progress in clarifying when these activations occur and how they interact has lagged. Although delayed ERPs over the hemisphere ipsilateral to the visual field of a presented image were first described in the 1970s, the advances outlined by Saron and colleagues suggest that this paradigm is now ready to fulfill its early promise as a brain-behavior research tool with special benefits for the study of callosal communication.

Some of the advantages of ERPs over RTs in computation of interhemispheric transfer time (IHTT) are greater speed and reliability, better consistency with anatomical expectations and fiber conduction velocities, directionality, and the potential for teasing apart motor and sensory channels. The biggest problem comes from superimposition of the effects of multiple neural generators with differing locations/orientations on the scalp-recorded ERP at any given time point. By use of high spatial and temporal sampling, generation of both stimulus- and response-related averages, and mathematical transformations allowing better visualization of current flow and decomposition into underlying source waveforms, gratifying progress has been achieved by Saron and colleagues.

The chapter convincingly argues for several important points:

1. Crossed-uncrossed RT differences actually contrast different routes of interhemispheric interaction and therefore badly underestimate interhemispheric transfer time.

2. Previous ERP studies have also underestimated interhemispheric transfer time, owing to superimposition of effects of multiple generators.

3. Timing of posterior sensory ERPs is generally independent of RT, but careful analysis reveals that this is not true for ERP patterns recorded from frontocentral scalp.

4. Specifically, variation in reaction time is closely linked to the timing, magnitude, and rate at which a stimulus activates the motor system as indexed by current inflow over central motor areas.

The speculation that motor system state variables may be powerful predictors of RT is intriguing. Bauer and Nirnberger (1981) found faster learning and larger-amplitude ERPs when stimuli were presented during slow spontaneous negative as compared to positive EEG shifts. Combined with the present work, this suggests that EEG biorhythms may be explanatory for response timing through mediation of intrahemispheric and interhemispheric interaction. In fact, this may be one mechanism selecting between the two routes proposed by Saron and colleagues through which a visual sensory potential can initiate a contralateral motor process. The basic suggestion is that on trials associated with fast RTs quick intrahemispheric visuomotor activation is followed by interhemispheric motor-motor activation, whereas slower RTs reflect interhemispheric transfer of sensory information followed by intrahemispheric visuomotor activation. This dual-route model, while appealing, requires more direct evidence. Just as IHTT has long been related to lateralized visual ERP delays, bilateral motor preparation followed by contralateral motor execution has long been inferred from movement-related potentials (Deecke et al., 1984a, b). Since much brain processing involves parallel operations, temporally sequencing two

STEVEN BERMAN Neuropsychiatric Institute, University of California at Los Angeles, Los Angeles, California.

230

local activations does not necessarily indicate any communication between them. Motor activity is related to stimulus detection in simple RT paradigms but not in other paradigms, such as self-paced movements. When the sensory potentials do not temporally covary with the motor potentials and RTs, it is even more difficult to infer functional connectivity. Perhaps other physiological measures, such as EEG coherence, could assess the dependency component of the dual-route notion.

Although the progress demonstrated in this chapter is very impressive, few subjects were tested, and many of the presented data come from a single subject. The next step is to use these techniques to address some of the unresolved issues in the ERP/IHTT literature, such as the following: Is IHTT asymmetric, and, if so, under what conditions? How many callosal channels are there, and how can they be characterized? How does communication change in special populations (callosotomy patients, callosal agenesis, dyslexia, etc.)? Resolving these issues will require attention to paradigmatic sources of variance. For example, our laboratory has data from 10 subjects who made a choice RT button press in response to lateralized letters (H or S) under alcohol or placebo. Highly reliable IHTT measures for P1, N1, and P2 indicated at least two callosal channels because different ERP deflections were dissociated both by the effects of alcohol on transmission time and by directionality. While our untransformed posterior sensory potentials and their IHTT estimates look very similar to the Current Source Density (CSD) maps presented in Chapter 8, central motor effects were not apparent. Left-hand presses showed the expected C4 > C3 for N150, but the pattern was identical for right-hand presses. It is interesting to note that in all four conditions of Saron and colleagues' grand-mean and single-case data, the central CSD inward current flow from 130 to 150 ms extends more anteriorly on the right side, suggesting that both our data and those of Saron and colleagues indicate a right-lateralized frontocentral negativity independent of response hand at this latency. The lack of central motor potentials lateralized by response hand in our averages may be due to their lower sampling rates or super-imposition of far-field sources. However, they could also be due to our subjects' having little uncertainty about when the stimulus would occur but being uncertain about where it would occur, which letter would appear, and therefore which response would be required. In contrast, Saron and colleagues' subjects knew exactly where and what the stimulus would be and had only temporal uncertainty. This would greatly alter the strategic processing of the task. For example, subjects could unambiguously prepare a single motor response for release from inhibition.

While the small sample or an in-depth case study approach can be employed to address the callosal communication issues discussed above, results must be charted for enough single subjects to assess generalizability of the derived conclusions. In this respect, co-registration of EEG recordings with functional and structural images will be very useful in removing apparent disparities due to anatomical variation. Functionally active areas can be used to validate dipole mappings and weight them to improve anatomical precision of source potentials. The marriage of well-designed laterality paradigms, the fine spatial mapping of functional imaging, and the high temporal mapping of functional electrophysiology is now poised to deliver significant benefits to cognitive neuroscience.

REFERENCES

BAUER, H., and G. NIRNBERGER, 1981. Concept identification as a function of preceding negative or positive spontaneous shifts in slow brain potentials. *Psychophysiology* 18:466–469.

DEECKE, L., T. BASHORE, C. H. BRUNIA, E. GRUNEWALK-ZUBERBIER, G. GRUNEWALD, and R. KRISTEVA, 1984a. Movement-associated potentials and motor control. Report of the EPIC VI Motor Panel. *Ann. NY Acad. Sci.* 425:398–428.

DEECKE, L., B. HEISE, H. H. KORNHUBER, M. LANG, and W. LANG, 1984b. Brain potentials associated with voluntary manual tracking: Bereitschaftspotential, conditioned premotion positivity, directed attention potential, and relaxation potential. Anticipatory activity of the limbic and frontal cortex. *Ann. NY Acad. Sci.* 425:450–464.

EDITORIAL COMMENTARY 2

Current Directions in Physiological Studies of Callosal Functions

MARCO IACOBONI AND ERAN ZAIDEL

In this section of the book, animal and human studies on physiological properties of the corpus callosum are grouped together. The methodological approaches to the study of physiological properties of the corpus callosum reviewed here encompass more traditional techniques, such as lesion or single-unit approaches, as well as recently developed techniques, such as functional magnetic resonance imaging and high-density multichannel event-related potential recordings.

In his chapter, Maurice Ptito reviews three main aspects of callosal functions, studied in cats in his lab with a combination of lesion, behavioral, and single-unit approaches. The three aspects are (1) interhemispheric transfer of visual information, (2) stereoperception, and (3) the fusion of visual information at the midline. Taken together, the studies on interhemispheric transfer of visual information in cats show that the variety and richness of extracallosal routes may compensate for the loss of direct callosal connections from one hemisphere to the other. Another form of compensatory mechanism, even more powerful, is through plastic changes during development, and the studies reviewed by Ptito in callosotomized kittens clearly support this form. With regard to stereoperception, Ptito makes the point that binocular convergence and subsequent binocular fusion are necessary for it. Two pathways are possibly involved in binocular convergence: one is the crossed retinothalamocortical pathway, and the other is the cross-callosal pathway. The evidence reported by Ptito clearly suggests that the former is the critical pathway for appropriate binocular input to target cortical areas, whereas the

cross-callosal pathway plays only a minor role in it. In contrast, callosal neurons seem critical to the functional unification of visual inputs to the two hemifields, ensuring fusion of sensory percepts through the midline.

In his commentary on Ptito's chapter, Berlucchi emphasizes some other physiological callosal functions that Ptito did not address. For instance, the plastic reorganization of visual areas due to the use of optical prisms may be callosally mediated. Further, neuronal synchronization in distant visual areas belonging to the two cerebral hemispheres seems also to be callosally mediated. Finally, the possible role of callosal axons in the establishment and reinforcement of learning and memories through mechanisms of long-term potentiation were suggested by high-frequency callosal stimulation.

Doty's chapter deals mostly with callosal conduction delay and its consequences for hemispheric specialization, as well as with the effect of transection of callosal fibers in transfer of memory engrams. His argument is that the enlargement of the human brain, coupled with a very slow conduction velocity through callosal axons, facilitates hemispheric specialization. Thus, given that time is of the essence, local processing has a selective advantage over global processing, and each hemisphere develops its own computational capabilities. Doty also recognizes the existence of fast callosal fibers that could in principle transfer information very rapidly from one hemisphere to the contralateral one. However, given that these fibers are found in callosal regions that are thought to connect primary sensory and motor areas, Doty may be assuming that they play a little role in cognitive functions. With regard to memory functions in the two hemispheres and the role of callosal axons in their spreading, Doty suggests that, in fact, some aspects of mnestic processing may be shared between the two hemispheres even in the absence of callosal connections.

In his commentary on Doty's chapter, Berlucchi emphasizes that the gap from neurophysiological data on

MARCO IACOBONI   Ahmanson Lovelace Brain Mapping Center, Neuropsychiatric Institute, Brain Research Institute, David Geffen School of Medicine, University of California at Los Angeles, Los Angeles, California.
ERAN ZAIDEL   Department of Psychology, University of California at Los Angeles, Los Angeles, California.

TABLE 1

*Summary of anatomical-behavioral relationships indicating behavioral measures that correlated positively (pos), negatively (neg),
or did not correlate (—) with callosal morphometry measures*

	Laterality Effect	Laterality Index	Callosal Region	Interhem. Cond.	LH	RH
1. Visual discrimination	absent	pos	midbody, total	—	—	—
2. Texture discrimination	absent	pos	midbody, anterior 1/3	—	—	—
3. Dichotic listening	present	—	anterior 1/3	—	neg	—
4. Primed lexical decision	present	neg*	isthmus	—	—	—

LH and RH refer to left- and right-hemisphere conditions, respectively, based on side of stimulus presentation.
*Males only, for associated prime-target pairs.

callosal axons to complex behaviors, such as learning and memory processes, is still large. He also emphasizes that the complex geometry of callosal axons makes it somewhat difficult to infer the role of excitatory and inhibitory synapses when the behavior of neuronal systems is studied. Finally, Berlucchi briefly reviews data on attentional bias in split-brain patients that may be due to the lack of the corpus callosum.

The human studies of callosal functions presented in this section are composed of the work of Saron and colleagues using electrical scalp recordings and of Iacoboni using fMRI. The work of Saron and colleagues is presented in full for the first time here and represents one of the most remarkable data sets in the history of physiological studies of callosal functions of the human brain. Saron and colleagues have mapped the complex ever-varying neural dynamics during simple visuomotor processing, giving the full details of the richness of neural activity even in seemingly basic forms of human behavior. This work calls for a revision of feed-forward serial models of information processing in the human brain, even when dealing with very simple sensory stimuli and using very simple motor responses. Saron and colleagues further interpret their data as evidence against the possible use of simple reaction times to lateralized flashes for measuring interhemispheric transfer time. They suggest that subtracting RT in the uncrossed con-

dition from the crossed condition in the Poffenberger paradigm is just subtracting one type of callosal transfer from another type of callosal transfer.

Iacoboni and Zaidel think otherwise. In their commentary on Saron and colleagues' work, they present Iacoboni's fMRI data on simple reaction times to lateralized flashes that, by and large, are consistent with Saron and colleagues' electrical data. Using the single-trial fMRI technique, they show bilateral activations in visual, motor, and integrative cortical areas in three conditions out of four in the Poffenberger paradigm. The only condition that shows exclusively unilateral activation is the condition in which targets are presented to the right visual field and responses are given with the right hand. These data clearly support a model of feed-backwards neural processing during simple visuomotor behavior. However, Iacoboni and Zaidel also point out that the logic of the Poffenberger paradigm is a logic of subtraction of one condition from another. If one does this subtraction on the fMRI, the results are in line with the view that the crossed-uncrossed difference in simple reaction times to lateralized flashes is actually a reliable measure of interhemispheric transfer. In support of this view, Iacoboni and Zaidel also review briefly some chronometric data in normals and split-brain patients, preparing the ground for the following section of the book, which is mostly centered on behavioral studies.

III INTER-HEMISPHERIC SENSORI-MOTOR INTEGRATION: BEHAVIORAL STUDIES

9 The Evolution of the Concept of Interhemispheric Relay Time

CLAUDE M. J. BRAUN, ANDRÉ ACHIM, AND CAROLINE LAROCQUE

ABSTRACT   The idea of measuring interhemispheric transfer time dates back to Poffenberger, who in 1912 inferred that the 5-ms or so increment observed in reaction time in contralateral hand-stimulus relation over the ipsilateral relation is due to the requirement of interhemispheric relay in the former and not the latter experimental condition. This chapter reviews the fate of that inference after 90 years of investigation. The inference has appeared progressively very strained as researchers discovered marked variations of the index of relay time according to experimental conditions (direction of relay, stimulus eccentricity, motor preparation load, type of decision, RT versus evoked potentials, etc.) and handedness of subjects. Finally, analysis of omission errors has recently imposed a reconceptualization of asymmetric detection and response integration: high-speed contrateral and ipsilateral sensorimotor integration each comprise a distinct complex amalgamation of costs and benefits, among which interhemispheric relay time is only a small component.

Poffenberger (1912) developed one of the most intuitively palpable and appealing inferences in the history of neuropsychology. He reasoned that because the visual and motor projections are contralateral, the difference in reactions times (RT) between a contralateral (or crossed) and ipsilateral (uncrossed) stimulated-field/responding-hand relation (crossed-minus-uncrossed difference, or CUD) ought to be an accurate estimate of interhemispheric relay time (IHRT). Researchers are still conceptualizing interhemispheric dynamics in Poffenberger's terms. There have been close to a hundred published experiments investigating interhemispheric relay with simple reaction time (SRT), usually reporting a small lag of 1–5 ms attributable to IHRT (reviewed by Bashore, 1981; Braun, 1992; and Hoptman and Davidson, 1994). The validity of the IHRT inference has been further bolstered by the fact that callosal agenesics and callosotomized patients have greatly lengthened CUD (Jeeves, 1969; Sergent and Myers, 1985; Clarke and Zaidel, 1989; Aglioti et al., 1993; Iacoboni, Fried, and Zaidel, 1994; Tassinari et al., 1994b; Corballis, 1998).

The term IHRT is still used directly without caveat in many recently published articles exploring the Poffenberger paradigm, bypassing the inferential step from the surface phenomenon to the inference about the underlying mechanism. The objective of the present review is to demonstrate that there are substantial complications of attempts to estimate IHRT from CUDs and that, in fact, CUDs probably only very indirectly reflect IHRT. Ours is not a defeatist outlook. On the contrary, we hope that these considerations will help researchers who are interested in interhemispheric dynamics to develop more refined tools and less naïve concepts in such a manner as to eventually achieve success in the experimental deciphering of interhemispheric relations.

Complex behavioral paradigms are not amenable to strong inferences about IHRT

There are two basic reasons why complex reaction time paradigms do not yield very interesting information about interhemispheric relay time. First, complex reaction time paradigms, particularly response-choice paradigms, yield huge effects (field and/or hand effects and interactions between the two) that drown out estimates of IHRT (see Levy, 1984, for a discussion). The most obvious such contamination is the famous spatial compatibility effect (Wallace, 1971). In response-choice tasks, lateral emplacement of the responding hands, as opposed to emplacement on the vertical meridian, results in a huge RT advantage of ipsilateral over contralateral field-hand conditions. Furthermore, when the subject is required to cross his or her arms, the advantage of stimulus compatibility overrides the anatomical advantage of the direct route (in and out of a same hemisphere). Even when the hands are emplaced on the vertical me-

CLAUDE M. J. BRAUN, ANDRÉ ACHIM, AND CAROLINE LAROCQUE Centre de Neurosciences Cognitives, Université du Québec à Montréal, Montreal, Quebec, Canada.

ridian, the crossed-minus-uncrossed field-hand relation conditions yield an estimate of IHRT that is substantially longer than is the case in simple RT. It is assumed that this is the case because it is in the selection of the responding hand that spatial compatibility operates, including residually, when the responding hands are emplaced on the vertical meridian. A test of the spatial compatibility effect in simple RT, by means of using crossed (and uncrossed) hand emplacement, was negative. So contrary to complex (response-choice) RT, the inference of a cost in time due to interhemispheric relay in simple RT, and not spatial compatibility, best explained the results (Anzola et al., 1977; Berlucchi et al., 1977; Rizzolatti, 1979; Aglioti et al., 1993). There are innumerable other effects similar to spatial compatibility that have been obtained in response-choice RT experiments, falling into the general category of what is termed *stimulus-response compatibility* effects (direction of a finger movement, relative locus of the responding finger within the hand, and selection of fingers required to respond, etc.). Second, CUDs obtained from complex RT experiments are sometimes inordinately long (Filbey and Gazzaniga, 1969; McKeever, Gill, and VanDeventer, 1975; Amadeo, Roemer, and Shagass, 1977) or inordinately short, even to the extent of being significantly negative (Green, 1984). Furthermore, there seems to be no basis for an understanding of which specific conditions in complex reaction time paradigms yield large or small CUDs. For example, Braun and colleagues (1994b) found no relationship between global RT and the CUD in five different complex reaction time experiments. This suggests that task complexity is not (unequivocally) related to the CUD (see Figure 9.1).

Higher error frequencies and longer RTs in crossed than uncrossed conditions have frequently been reported in complex response-choice RT experiments (Zaidel et al., 1988), perhaps reinforcing in Zaidel and colleagues' minds the belief in degradation of the neural signal, and of the quality of information transported by it, during interhemispheric relay. However, complex RT paradigms, involving discriminative processing of patterned stimuli (e.g., words or faces) and subsequent instruction-driven selection of differential responses (e.g., "same-different," "yes-no," or even a choice among three keys), have not been able to provide any definitive evidence. As was explained above, the investigation of IHRT by means of complex (response-choice) RT paradigms is plagued by many methodological problems: huge stimulus-response compatibility artifacts (the simplest of which is the spatial compatibility artifact), complexity of experimental manipulation (Jäncke and Steinmetz, 1994), effects on CUDs of cognitive categorization (Filbey and Gazzaniga, 1969; McKeever et

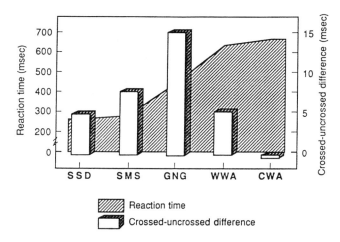

FIGURE 9.1. Absence of a relationship between global reaction time and the crossed-minus-uncrossed difference in five reaction time tasks. SSD = simple stimulus detection task, SMS = Sternberg memory scanning task, GNG = go/no-go task, WWA = word-word association task, CWA = color-word association task. (Reproduced with the publisher's permission from Braun et al., 1994b.)

al., 1975), and motor response (Hedge and Marsh, 1975; Simon, Sly, and Vilapakkam, 1981), and so on. All of the preceding produce accumulation of cognitive operations and constraints and extreme length of response intervals, sometimes over 1000 times longer than the typical CUD, all leading to extreme capriciousness and even unreplicability of CUD effects and inapplicability of the IHRT inference (see Bashore, 1981; Levy, 1984). Braun and colleagues (1994b) analyzed patterns of different types of errors in a two-response choice task (the Sternberg paradigm) implemented as a Poffenberger paradigm. They found that the patterns of omission and decision errors were wildly at odds (see Figure 9.2).

The same authors presented a similar analysis of a three-response choice task (a modified Stroop task) implemented as a Poffenberger paradigm. They again found that the error profiles (omission versus decision errors) were wildly at odds and that these were both quite different from the RT profile (see Figure 9.3).

This brief review of complex RT findings suffices to show that complex RT is not a good way to start trying to understand the extent to which the CUD is a valid (unequivocal) index of IHRT. In light of all of this, several authors have come to the conclusion that the few milliseconds observed by Poffenberger to be due to relay are not reliably measurable, except in simple RT (Bashore, 1981) or go/no-go tasks (Brysbaert, 1994) involving the simplest of motor decisions. Our own experience with complex RT paradigms leads us to the same conclusion. Consequently, the present review will deal only with research carried out in the SRT domain, with only a few references to the go/no-go domain.

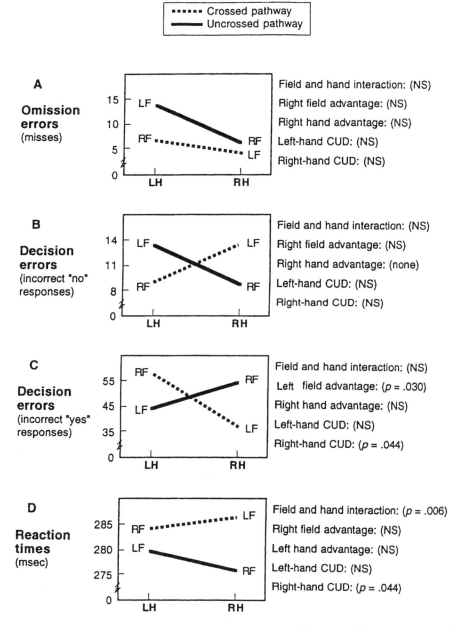

STERNBERG HIGH SPEED MEMORY SCANNING TASK

······ Crossed pathway
⎯⎯⎯ Uncrossed pathway

A
Omission errors (misses)

Field and hand interaction: (NS)
Right field advantage: (NS)
Right hand advantage: (NS)
Left-hand CUD: (NS)
Right-hand CUD: (NS)

B
Decision errors (incorrect "no" responses)

Field and hand interaction: (NS)
Right field advantage: (NS)
Right hand advantage: (none)
Left-hand CUD: (NS)
Right-hand CUD: (NS)

C
Decision errors (incorrect "yes" responses)

Field and hand interaction: (NS)
Left field advantage: ($p = .030$)
Right hand advantage: (NS)
Left-hand CUD: (NS)
Right-hand CUD: ($p = .044$)

D
Reaction times (msec)

Field and hand interaction: ($p = .006$)
Right field advantage: (NS)
Left hand advantage: (NS)
Left-hand CUD: (NS)
Right-hand CUD: ($p = .044$)

FIGURE 9.2. Differing reaction time, omission error, and decision error profiles as a function of the field stimulated and the hand used to respond in a two-choice rapid memory task (Sternberg paradigm) with special reference to crossed-minus-uncrossed differences. RF = right field, LF = left field, RH = right hand, LH = left hand, NS = nonsignificant. (Reproduced with the publisher's permission from Braun et al., 1994b.)

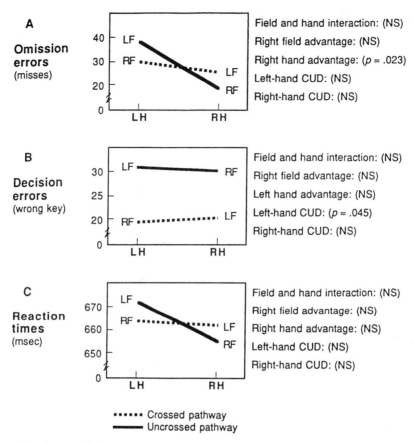

A

Omission errors (misses)

Field and hand interaction: (NS)
Right field advantage: (NS)
Right hand advantage: (p = .023)
Left-hand CUD: (NS)
Right-hand CUD: (NS)

B

Decision errors (wrong key)

Field and hand interaction: (NS)
Right field advantage: (NS)
Left hand advantage: (NS)
Left-hand CUD: (p = .045)
Right-hand CUD: (NS)

C

Reaction times (msec)

Field and hand interaction: (NS)
Right field advantage: (NS)
Right hand advantage: (NS)
Left-hand CUD: (NS)
Right-hand CUD: (NS)

•••••• Crossed pathway
———— Uncrossed pathway

FIGURE 9.3. Differing reaction time, omission error, and decision profiles as a function of the field stimulated and the hand used to respond in a three-choice color-word association task (modified Stroop paradigm) with special reference to crossed-minus-uncrossed differences. RF = right field, LF = left field, RH = right hand, LH = left hand, NS = nonsignificant. (Reproduced with the publisher's permission from Braun et al., 1994b.)

The single-cable metaphor

Several authors understandably continue to report results of simple RT experiments (and indeed of complex RT experiments) as if they assumed that the commissures of the animal and human brain are indeed simple systems of "transfer" or "relay," like an electrical wire in which no strand serves a function any different from that of another strand, in which relevant information travels in only one direction at a time, and that carries a binary signal of the type "lights on!" versus "lights off!" (see Jeeves, 1969, for explicit reference to a "pathway length" interpretation of CUDs). Rizzolatti (1979) even dared to go so far as to predict that no experimental manipulation of any kind would ever influence the CUD, its magnitude being nothing other than synaptic and conduction time of a passage of critical information along the length of the corpus callosum. The vast majority of authors who have attempted to falsify this prediction in SRT have failed (see Braun, 1992, for a review). CUDs of negative valence were observed in SRTs of a whole group of scotopically adapted normal right-handers

detecting near-liminal stimuli (Braun, Mailhoux, and Dufresne, 1996a), and similar conditions were probably the cause of a similar effect in the experiment by Clarke and Zaidel (1989). However, neither of these effects reached significance, such that these results can (but probably should not) be construed as a further argument for the single-cable metaphor (see Figure 9.4).

As a whole, manipulation of low-level (psychophysical) stimulus properties has not been apt to significantly modulate CUDs in behavioral experiments. For example, though stimulus duration (Kaswan and Young, 1965; Braun and Daigneault, 1994) and stimulus intensity (Raab and Fehrer, 1962; Clarke and Zaidel, 1989; Milner and Lines, 1982; Lines, Rugg, and Milner, 1984; Brysbaert, 1994) have a statistically significant impact on global RT, their proportionately greater impact on the CUD does not reach significance.

There have been equivocal findings regarding sex differences in CUDs. St. John and colleagues (1987) had found in five women and five men that women had CUDs six times longer than the men in a simple RT experiment. Dufresne and colleagues (1993) found that 22

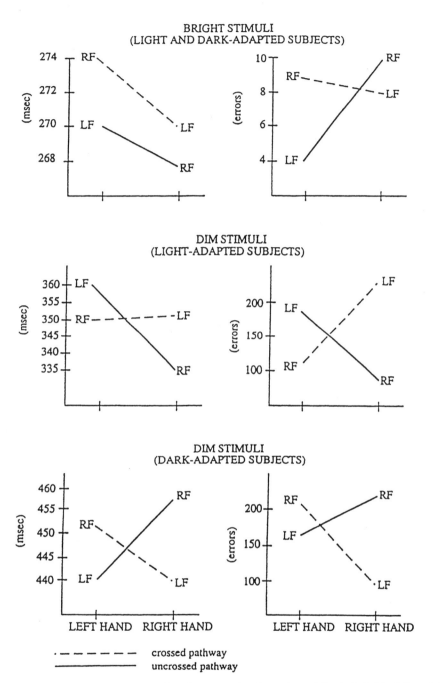

BRIGHT STIMULI
(LIGHT AND DARK-ADAPTED SUBJECTS)

DIM STIMULI
(LIGHT-ADAPTED SUBJECTS)

DIM STIMULI
(DARK-ADAPTED SUBJECTS)

$\cdot----$ crossed pathway
——— uncrossed pathway

FIGURE 9.4. Reaction times and omission errors as a function of the field stimulated and the hand used to respond in normal right-handed subjects required to detect a supraliminal or near-liminal target in conditions of scotopic or photopic reti- nal adaptation. LF = left field, RF = right field, LH = left hand, RH = right hand. Note that the effect mentioned in the text applies only to the conditions with dim targets. (See Braun et al., 1996a.)

women had a CUD 12 times longer than the 22 men. However, the majority of studies that have explored this issue have now failed to replicate this (McKeever and Hoff, 1979; Clarke and Zaidel, 1989; Aglioti et al., 1991; Savage and Thomas, 1993; Bisiacchi et al., 1994; Brizzolara et al., 1994). Women were found to have briefer CUDs in an evoked potential experiment, leading the authors to propose that EPs pick up sensory relay and that it is only in this respect that women have faster relay than men (Burnison, Larson, and Brown, 1993). However, an evoked potential experiment in our own laboratory failed to replicate this finding (Potvin, Braun, and Achim, 1994, 1995). In a more complex (go/no-go) experiment involving high-speed memorization of consonants (Sternberg paradigm), Braun, Dumas, and Collin (1994a) found that women had a longer CUD than men ($t(1, 14) = 3.01$, $p = .01$). The issue of sex differences in corpus callosum morphology is also controversial. Holloway and Delacoste (1986) claimed a larger (more bulbous) splenium in women. However, a recent meta-analysis of 49 studies published since 1980 did not find significant sex differences in the splenium, even when appropriate adjustments had been made for brain volume (Bishop and Wahlsten, 1997). Many successors reported greater overall volume of the corpus callosum in men; however, there has been controversy as to whether this difference is a mere artifact of greater overall brain volume of men or not. Finally, the studies have found that sex differences in corpus callosum morphology are not statistically significant unless other variables such as handedness are taken into account (Witelson, 1985; Habib et al., 1991). At any rate, since head width differences between men and women are so minute, and since attempts to find differences between the sexes in callosal histology have failed (Aboitiz et al., 1992a, 1992b), findings of large reliable sex differences in the CUD would have argued against the single-cable metaphor.

Experiments involving grafting of attentional demands on a simple reaction time task have also generally failed to significantly modulate the CUD. This has been the case for "hemispherically lateralized" concurrent tasks to be carried out during SRT (Milner et al., 1982; Rizzolatti, Bertoloni, and DeBastiani, 1982).

Finally, memory load in short-term memory (Braun et al., 1994a) was found to be linearly and positively related to the CUD, but the FIELD × HAND × LOAD interaction nevertheless failed to reach significance. Perhaps in this experiment, as in most other experiments having obtained meaningful and consistent but nonsignificant trends (e.g., studies of the eccentricity effect; see the next section), there is a problem of intrinsic variability of CUDs, making experimental predictions

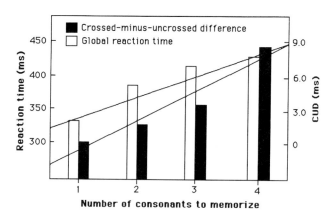

FIGURE 9.5. Effects of memory load in a high-speed scanning task (Sternberg paradigm) on the crossed-minus-uncrossed difference. (See Braun et al., 1994a.)

difficult to test. For example, as is depicted in Figure 9.5, the mean effect of memory load on the CUD has monotonic slope, as does the effect on global RT. However, the load effect on the CUD was not significant, whereas the load effect on global RT was highly significant ($F(3, 12) = 57$, $p = 0.0001$). See Figure 9.5.

As a consequence of all of the above, the perhaps dominant view of interhemispheric dynamics reflected in SRT-CUDs consists of a concept of passive relay of a binary signal (presence versus absence of a critical stimulus or respond versus do not respond) through a homogenous cable. However, there is a significant minority of findings demonstrating enough modulation of CUDs to invalidate the formula CUD = IHRT.

The two-cable metaphor

The role of the corpus callosum in midline fusion (including in the visual modality for binocular vision) is well established and rests on solid anatomical and physiological ground. Visual callosal neurons (Lepore et al., 1989) have most of their receptive fields on or near the body meridian. Consequently, several investigators have attempted to show that increasing eccentricity of stimuli ought to prolong CUDs in humans. We are aware of seven reports of such experiments (Berlucchi et al., 1971; Berlucchi et al., 1977; Harvey, 1978; Lines and Milner, 1983; St. John et al., 1987; Clarke and Zaidel, 1989; Iacoboni and Zaidel, 1995). However, though all the experiments obtained increasing CUDs as a function of increasing stimulus eccentricity, only the experiment of St. John and colleagues (1987) obtained a significant modulation of visual SRT-CUDs as a function of target eccentricity. Since all the experiments yielded trends in the expected direction, we take these results quite seriously, while realizing that the relatively great variability of the CUD index makes it difficult to bring such effects to significance.

Having failed to experimentally modulate the CUD in SRT via eccentricity of visual stimulation, Berlucchi and colleagues (1971) speculated that in the RT implementation of the Poffenberger paradigm, interhemispheric relay probably consists of relay of a motor signal. (For speculation about the same effect, see also Berlucchi et al., 1971; Berlucchi, 1978; Milner and Lines, 1982; Clarke and Zaidel, 1989; Aglioti et al., 1991; Iacoboni et al., 1994; Tassinari et al., 1994b.) There may be two types of interhemispheric relay, sensory and motor, and depending on the task, either route could be used to optimize interhemispheric integration of behavior. Lines and colleagues (1984) found, in a visual evoked potential experiment with normal humans, that occipital electrode sites yielded CUDs influenced by stimulus intensity, whereas central electrode sites yielded CUDs uninfluenced by stimulus intensity. The INTENSITY × SITE × FIELD × HEMISCALP interaction was significant. The authors proposed that central leads reflect motor relay, while occipital leads reflect visual relay. This idea has been echoed explicitly also by Burnison and colleagues (1993), who have stated that they believe RT CUDs reflect motor relay, whereas parietal CUDs from visual evoked potentials reflect sensory (visual) relay. These speculations introduce a slight complication of the initial metaphor but maintain the notion that CUDs are none other than a cable length effect.

Tassinari and colleagues (1994b) found that though complete callosotomy severely prolongs the SRT-CUD, section of only the anterior or posterior part of the corpus callosum does not change the CUD at all, a finding that is supportive of the proposal by Bisiacchi and colleagues (1994) of a horse race metaphor of interhemispheric relay, wherein relay will occur as fast as possible wherever it may, namely, in the anterior callosum or the posterior callosum. The horse race model of IHRT argues, of course, against the single-cable metaphor but fits nicely within the boundaries of a two-cable metaphor. The horse race effect could also reflect a mechanism of optimization of sensorimotor integration of the two body halves. Such a mechanism could consist of filtering, amplification, or routing devices on either side of the commissures or within the commissures. Functionally significant transcallosal inhibition (probably via interneurons) has been observed in the parietal lobe and in the frontal lobe in humans. Indeed, transcranial magnetic stimulation (interference) of the parietal lobe enhances ipsilateral somesthesia (Seyal, Ro, and Rafal, 1995), and transcranial magnetic stimulation (interference) of the frontal lobe enhances ipsilateral motor responding (Meyer et al., 1995).

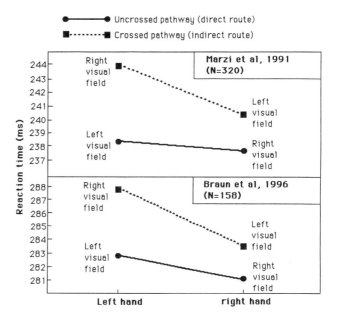

FIGURE 9.6. Reaction time profile as a function of the field stimulated and the hand used to respond in the meta-analysis of Marzi and colleagues (1991) and in the meta-analysis of Braun and colleagues (1996b).

Marzi, Bisiacchi, and Nicoletti (1991) found that the data from 16 previously published SRT experiments presented a left FIELD advantage and a right HAND advantage. They proposed that this pattern of results could be explained as slow IHRT from the left to the right hemisphere, and fast IHRT from the right to the left hemisphere. (For replications and extensions, see Braun, 1992; Bisiacchi et al., 1994.) Braun (1992) reviewed 49 SRT experiments, and the compilation of those results yielded the same pattern as described by Marzi and colleagues. Braun, Villeneuve, and Achim (1996b) compiled results from 135 of their own subjects tested in seven distinct experiments. They also obtained the same pattern as reported by Marzi and colleagues (see Figure 9.6).

The results of Bisiacchi and colleagues (1994) are particularly convincing in ruling out a second hypothesis of nothing other than hemispheric specialization (left hemisphere: motor advantage, right hemisphere: visual advantage). Brown, Larson, and Jeeves (1994) looked at asymmetry of CUDs in seven experiments in the evoked potential literature. They concluded that the most plausible interpretation of the ensemble of results was that interhemispheric relay is faster from the right hemisphere to the left. Braun, Achim, and Villeneuve (1999a) looked at more waveforms and covered more electrode sites, analyzed amplitudes, and also presented a visual evoked potential experiment of their own. They report that the highly dominant and significant asymmetry of CUDs supports the notion of faster relay from the right to the left hemisphere. However, they also found that amplitudes, as a whole, tend to support a notion of stronger relay from the left to the right hemisphere. In their own visual evoked potential experiment on normal right-handers, these authors obtained the same profile of asymmetries as described above. We point out, however, that a logical condition of inferring an asymmetry of interhemispheric relay in evoked potentials is that there must be a symmetry of direct routes (i.e., of measures taken at electrode sites purported to reflect processing occurring before interhemispheric transfer). Otherwise, a so-called asymmetry of interhemispheric relay cannot be distinguished from a simple hemisphere effect (i.e., asymmetry). An equivalent condition for the inference of asymmetry of transfer in SRT (as distinguished from a combination of independent field and hand effects) is that the two uncrossed conditions should not differ from each other (e.g., the solid lines in Figure 9.6).

If, then, interhemispheric relay is asymmetric and if, in addition, there is an interplay of asymmetries of signal velocity and signal strength, then another piece of the single-cable metaphor is challenged. It is not only a raw unequivocal signal that is relayed one way or the other by two identical hemispheres. The hemispheres do not seem to be perfectly identical in the manner in which they process the stimulus or decide upon or execute a response, even in a simple reaction time task. Braun (1992) proposed that IHRT asymmetry should result from asymmetry of early intrahemispheric stimulus-processing efficiency reflected in field effects. However, this idea has been disconfirmed (Brown et al., 1994). Furthermore, Braun and colleagues (1999a) have recently found that the CUD asymmetry occurs significantly in evoked potential latencies even when the direct routes have perfectly symmetrical latencies. This represents a fascinating and promising domain for future research, since nothing concrete is known about sources of interhemispheric relay asymmetries. Despite the fact that relay asymmetries seem to exist in several mammalian species (Bozhko and Shramm, 1990; Perez et al., 1990; Bianki and Makarova, 1994; Makarova and Bianki, 1994), we do not understand what might be the adaptive value of such asymmetries. Braun and colleagues (1999a) proposed that in the human there is an intrinsic overarching physiological mechanism, situated in the corpus callosum itself and its first-order synapses, ensuring that the right hemisphere will be able to send information to the left more quickly than the left to the right and that the left hemisphere will be able to relay more precise information to the right hemisphere (albeit more slowly) than the right to the left. This type of mechanism could apply, conceivably, to the simplest of tasks, such as simple reaction time. Alternatively, Now-

icka, Grabowska, and Fersten (1996) provide evoked potential evidence to the effect that when cognitive material must be relayed interhemispherically, the nonspecialized hemisphere relays initial processing more quickly to the opposite hemisphere. Di Stefano and Salvadori (1998) found that this asymmetry was markedly reversed in an acallosal subject, suggesting that it is indeed the corpus callosum that is the carrier of this basic asymmetry.

All of the above argues against the single-cable metaphor but not much against the notion according to which the CUD is nothing but a "cable" effect, whether comprising one, two, or several such cables.

The network-gradient metaphor

Berardi, Bisti, and Maffei (1987), Berardi and Fiorentini (1987), and Berardi and colleagues (1988) have found that interhemispheric relay is more efficient for high contrasts and low spatial and temporal frequencies of sinusoidal gratings. The effect was observed physiologically in photopically adapted cat and monkey and psychophysically in the normal human. Interhemispheric relay in their experiments favored the magnocellular contribution with regard to contrast and spatial frequency but the parvocellular contribution with regard to temporal frequency. The physiological mechanism(s) underlying these effects remain(s) unclear. We speculate that callosal neurons, which are primarily of the pyramidal glutamatergic type, have specific receptive field properties. In more theoretical terms, this would mean that the commissure(s) do not relay all types of information with equal efficiency, operating in some cases as a filter (when the stimulus type is suboptimal) and in other cases as an amplifier (when the stimulus type is optimal).

Along the same line of reasoning, Braun, Potvin, and Achim (1995b) speculated that CUDs obtained from visual evoked potentials might vary as a function of electrode site because of differing underlying density of callosal neurons. They observed in their own evoked potential experiment that the topography of CUDs derived from the N1 wave generally fitted with this idea (see Figure 9.7). Occipital and primary motor (hand area) electrode sites (sparse in callosal neurons) yielded much longer CUDs than sites located in the secondary visual association areas (temporal and parietal: densely populated with callosal neurons). However, the notoriously poor localizing quality of evoked potentials really allows this idea to stand only as a heuristic device. At any rate, we propose that the commissural system (especially the corpus callosum) is a topographically organized network of neurons and that CUD values obtained in

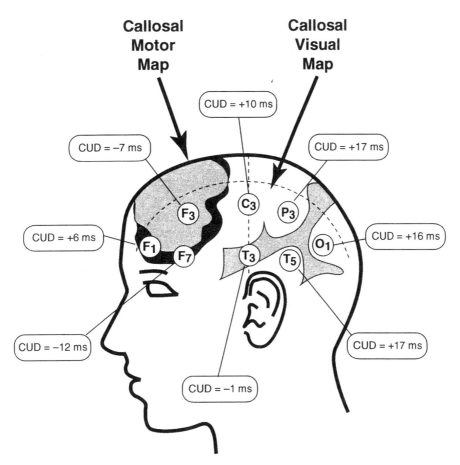

Callosal Motor Map

Callosal Visual Map

CUD = +10 ms

CUD = −7 ms

CUD = +17 ms

F₃   C₃   P₃

CUD = +6 ms

F₁   F₇   T₃   T₅   O₁

CUD = +16 ms

CUD = −12 ms

CUD = +17 ms

CUD = −1 ms

FIGURE 9.7. Schematization of cortical areas known to be sparsely (white) and densely (gray) packed with callosal neurons based on histological research on monkeys (Karol and Pandya, 1971; Van Essen, Newsome, and Bixby, 1982) and representation of N1 CUDs obtained by Braun and colleagues (1996a) from 10 normal right-handers by electrode site (10–20 system).

SRT experiments reflect this system property (albeit usually unreliably).

Finally, we are of the opinion that the stimulus-eccentricity effect on CUDs (consistent trends, one experiment out of six reaching significance) is a neural network effect and probably reflects a gradient in callosal input: The more eccentric a stimulus is, the less it directly contributes to the corpus callosum (see Braun, 1992, for a review).

The balance-of-cost metaphor

Our own understanding of CUDs derived from simple RT has evolved because we have been compelled to accommodate results that contradict any cable metaphor.

INDIVIDUAL DIFFERENCE EFFECTS   Individual differences in CUDs are enormous. In our own experiments in SRT, comprising a cumulative sample of 135 right-handed normal subjects, we have found the range of CUD estimates to extend from −42 ms to +105 ms

(Braun et al., 1996b). In short, the CUD is extremely variable. Some subjects present patterns of RTs that are in complete violation of the anatomy underlying Poffenberger's inference (CUD = IHRT). Various authors have responded in differing ways to this problem. Swanson, Ledlow, and Kinsbourne (1978) and Hasbroucq, Kornblum, and Osman (1988) simply dismissed the Poffenberger paradigm as unviable, that is, unable to provide any meaningful information about IHRT. The former group simply postulate that Kinsbourne's attentional model best explains CUDs, that is, that because the hand response is known in advance, this creates an asymmetry of attention, thus creating a CUD that has nothing to do with interhemispheric relay. Most of those who have published findings from within the Poffenberger paradigm have simply been content with a significant FIELD × HAND interaction as sufficient evidence for validity of the basic inference. Our own interpretation of the extreme variability of CUDs is that although there is assuredly an IHRT component embedded within the CUD, attentional effects (and other effects) in and between the hemispheres can easily surpass the small effect that is expected to occur due to the cost of interhemispheric relay, even in paradigms as simple as a keystroke-press response to raw detection of a supraliminal stimulus. The challenge, then, is to determine the exact nature of these attentional modulations (as well as modulations attributable to other sources such as individual differences, experimental conditions, etc.), so as to eventually be able to make the IHRT inference more confidently.

IHRT estimates vary as a function of the method used to estimate them even in simple reaction time. Saron and Davidson (1989) found that the behavioral CUD is not correlated with the latency CUD derived at posterior leads in evoked potentials. Potvin and colleagues (1995) and Savage and Thomas (1993) have since replicated this finding. In addition, CUD estimates from evoked potentials vary significantly as a function of the electrode site (Braun, Achim, and Villeneuve, 1999a; Lines et al., 1984). Estimates obtained at posterior sites tend to be very long (15–20 ms), incommensurate with CUDs obtained in SRT (1–5 ms), whereas estimates obtained at anterior electrode sites seem to be of shorter duration (−3 to 6 ms). Furthermore, Potvin and colleagues (1994) found that the CUD estimates based on the N1 wave did correlate significantly with CUD estimates obtained from RT, but only at frontal electrode sites. Recall that Lines and colleagues (1984) obtained a significant modulation of CUDs in visual evoked potentials as a function of stimulus intensity. CUDs were affected differently depending on the electrode sites (central versus occipital). Recall also that Burnison and colleagues (1993) and Rugg (1982) speculated that evoked potential estimates of IHRT at posterior electrode leads reflect visual components of interhemispheric relay, while RT estimates reflect motor components. The issue of whether in visual SRT it is a sensory signal (as Poffenberger had surmised) or a motor signal (Berlucchi et al., 1971) that constitutes the critical relay is still a matter of debate. However, we believe, as do Tassinari and colleagues (1994b), that CUDs obtained in SRT experiments reflect selective and adaptive processes that can enable either a sensory or motor signal to provide the critical interhemispheric relay, depending on individual characteristics of each subject's brain and particularities of each experimental montage. We know that SRT experiments consistently show briefer CUDs in left-handers than right-handers (especially left-handers who write with an inverted hand). Savage and Thomas (1993) investigated visual evoked potentials in right- and left-handers and analyzed the N1 wave. The CUDs did not differ as a function of handedness. So

here again, it seems that differing methods of investigating IHRT yield different values.

Even within the behavioral domain, estimates of CUDs may depend on the technique used. For example, Kleinman and colleagues (1976) found that CUDs drawn from simple vocal RT and CUDs drawn from simple unimanual RT to unpatterned light stimuli were incommensurable. However, the relevant interaction was not significant. A number of other details of experimental technique, within the behavioral (SRT) domain, are suspected to moderately influence the durations of CUD estimates obtained. Braun (1992) reviewed some of these details in a meta-analysis. He found that potentially significant modulation of CUDs seemed to result from several details of technique: emplacement of the responding hand on the vertical meridian rather than lateral hand emplacement favored larger CUDs (but recall that this effect of spatial compatibility did not stand up to experimental test; cf. Anzola et al., 1977)—and type of finger movement—a key release rather than press favored larger CUDs. Retinal size of stimuli had no relationship to CUDs at all.

NEGATIVE CUDs: FALSIFICATION OF POFFENBERGER'S INFERENCE? Average CUDs in simple reaction time experiments have usually been found to be disturbingly close to zero, especially in men (see Braun, 1992, for a review, and the section on individual differences). Even in Poffenberger's 1912 paper, the average CUD of all his subjects in all the experimental conditions (i.e., at all eccentricities) was very close to zero. We are aware of five experiments yielding group-average CUDs of negative valence in right-handers, though none significantly so (Rizzolatti, 1979; Milner and Lines, 1982; Lines et al., 1984; Clarke and Zaidel, 1989; Braun et al., 1996a). According to classical interpretation of the Poffenberger paradigm, this would mean that it takes less time for a neural impulse to cross the corpus callosum than not to cross, a conclusion that is patently absurd. We repeat that none of these five experiments produced a significantly negative CUD in SRT. We nevertheless believe that CUD estimates from RT are somewhat on the short side in general, probably reflecting an optimization process in intrahemispheric and interhemispheric dynamics working toward closely synchronized high-speed sensorimotor integration of the two body halves.

This issue becomes even more dramatic when hand dominance is taken into account. Jeeves (1969) and Jeeves and Dixon (1972) observed that their left-handers (mean CUD = 4.06 ms) had briefer CUDs than their right-handers (mean CUD = 4.71 ms). This difference was not submitted to statistical test. Two of three subsequent studies have shown that inverted left-handers have negative CUDs (McKeever and Hoff, 1979; Levy and Wagner, 1984; but see McKeever and Hoff, 1983, who found the CUD to be of 0.6 ms). The 65 inverted left-handers assessed in the three studies produced a mean CUD of −0.37 ms (with a 95% confidence interval of −1.23 to +0.50 ms). CUD differences between inverted left-handers and right-handers reached significance. In addition to the above SRT investigations, Moscovitch and Smith (1979) obtained a negative CUD of −8.7 ms in a go/no-go paradigm. Most subjects in the above-cited experiments were men. CUD differences between right- and left-handers could, in principle, be attributable to hemispheric specialization for motor control but are hard to reconcile with models relying only on the cable metaphor.

The accuracy domain argues against the single-cable metaphor. We are not aware of any author who has made a statement to the effect that interhemispheric relay may, should, or necessarily does entail cost in accuracy, specifically in SRT. However, McKeever and Huling (1971), Gross (1972), Berlucchi (1974), and Zaidel (1983, 1986) have stated, in a wider context, that interhemispheric relay does indeed suppose cost in accuracy. Their reasoning is simple and reasonable: An extra synapse may add noise to the signal or, in other words, is responsible for a "degradation" of the neural signal. Despite the fact that there are many very dynamic aspects to Zaidel's (1983, 1986) statements about interhemispheric communication, they proposed that interhemispheric relay always entails not only a cost in

time, but also a cost in accuracy, specifically expressed in terms of increased error rates.

Braun and colleagues (1996a) agreed that an error-CUD of positive valence in SRT would suggest a straightforward cost in accuracy associated with interhemispheric relay but considered that the opposite effect could also be explained. Normal right-handers ($N = 135$) gave 5815 omission errors in seven simple visual RT experiments previously reported. They recompiled all of the raw data and obtained the following result. The classical significant FIELD × HAND interaction (a CUD effect of 3.1 ms, ($F(1, 121) = 11.2$, $p = 0.001$) was obtained in the RTs. However, a significant FIELD × HAND interaction was obtained in the omission errors but of negative valence ($F(1, 121) = 4.6$, $p = 0.03$). In other words, subjects appeared to be making significantly fewer omission errors when interhemispheric relay was required than when it was not (see Figure 9.8).

We imagined three possible mechanisms, not necessarily mutually exclusive, which we thought could explain these surprising results: (1) Asymmetry of motor preparation for an individual response could generate neural noise within the responding hemisphere, interfering with signal detection; (2) processing resources could become tonically modulated over a large number of trials according to responding hand; and (3) the commissure(s) could have signal-to-noise enhancement properties.

Consideration of the strength of interhemispheric relay (interhemispheric relay strength, or IHRS) is beginning to take hold in the recent evoked potential literature. For example, Hoptman, Davidson, Gudmundsson, Schreiber, and Ershler (1996) recently reported that from adulthood to senescence, there is a decrement of IHRS but not of IHRT. They observed in a visual evoked potential investigation that although there is no decrement in CUD latencies, there is a significant decrement of CUD amplitudes. We see no reason why there should not exist a link between detection accuracy and amplitudes in the evoked potentials, as there is between speed of response to detection and latencies of evoked potentials. Furthermore, we see no reason why omission errors should continue to be neglected in the Poffenberger paradigm, especially considering that mechanisms of interhemispheric accuracy could, in principle, interact with mechanisms of minimization of interhemispheric relay time.

The Poffenberger paradigm reflects balance of costs more than interhemispheric relay effects. Anzola and Vignolo (1992) found that patients with unilateral cortical lesions had prolonged CUDs (mean = 20 ms) in the same order as callosal agenesics and concluded that

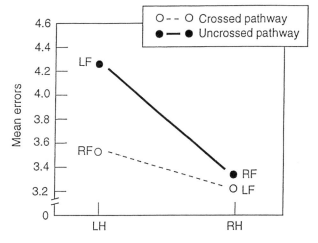

FIGURE 9.8. Crossed-minus-uncrossed differences in simple detection (omission errors) in normal right-handed subjects. LF = left field, RF = right field, LH = left hand, RH = right hand. (See Braun et al., 1996b.)

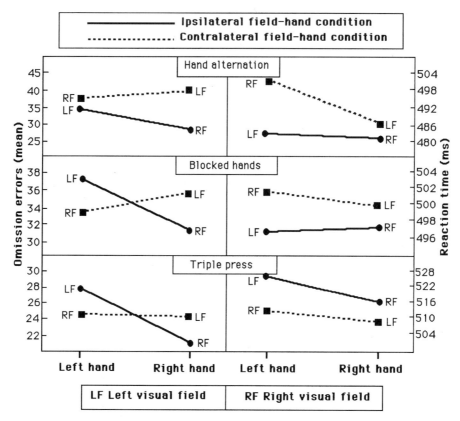

FIGURE 9.9. Effects of experimental manipulation of motoric load in the Poffenberger paradigm. (See Godbout et al., 1995.)

CUDs reflect intrahemispheric processing of an attentional nature. More specifically, they proposed that a lesion that prolongs the CUD selectively affects intrahemispheric relay of information from the posterior visual area first stimulated to the ipsilateral motor cortex or cortical-subcortical loops. We believe that the CUD is the net result of an ensemble of balancing of costs within and between the two hemispheres, of which IHRT is just one of the relevant factors.

To test this speculation in normal subjects, Godbout, Achim, and Braun (1995) manipulated response dimensions in a SRT implementation of the Poffenberger paradigm. Though all conditions of their experiment involved unimanual responses to simple detection, they devised a strategy to increase and decrease the asymmetry of the attentional effort required to produce the response. Their experiment comprised three conditions. Stimuli were presented randomly in one or the other field in all conditions. However, in a baseline condition they implemented a standard Poffenberger paradigm requiring a single key press to detection of stimulus off the vertical meridian. The same responding hand was used for blocks of 50 trials. The other hand was then used for another two blocks of trials, followed by a block from the previous hand (an ABBA sequence, completed twice). A second condition, devised to increase the motoric load (but not the decisional load), consisted of requiring of the subject three presses of the response key in rapid succession upon detection. A third condition, devised to alleviate the motoric load imbalance, required the subject to prepare for a response by placing his or her two index fingers on two response keys, producing the response to detection with one finger and then a response to the next oncoming stimulus with the other finger. In short, the subject alternated responding with the right and left hands in an ABAB sequence on a trial-by-trial basis. These conditions produced the following effects. The condition involving increased motoric load produced negative CUDs in the RTs and small CUDs in the omission errors. The condition involving alleviation of the motoric load imbalance (hand alternation) significantly prolonged the CUDs relative to the baseline condition (classical Poffenberger paradigm) and also significantly increased the omission error CUD. The interaction of FIELD × HAND × CONDITION, with regard to the RT domain was significant ($F(1,11) = 5.2$, $p = 0.039$). The interaction of FIELD × HAND × CONDITION, with regard to the omission error domain, was also significant ($F(1, 13) = 11.8$, $p = 0.003$, Greenhouse-Geiser adjustment). (See Figure 9.9.) The same authors (1995) have attempted to replicate their own findings. They obtained basically the same significant profile. In both studies, the blocked hand conditions produced the usual small CUD estimates, whereas the alternating hand condition produced significantly larger CUD estimates in both RTs and omission errors.

Iacoboni and Zaidel (1995) added motoric load to the blocked responding hand in a special implementation of the Poffenberger paradigm in normal subjects. They required that the subject respond with his or her index finger and major finger of the same hand in alternation from one trial to the next (in an ABAB sequence). The hand that was required to respond was blocked for sets of 40 trials. The finger alternation manipulation resulted in a significant decrease in the CUD. This finding is perfectly compatible with the findings of Godbout and colleagues. Indeed we consider that the finger alternation constraint (within the same hand) is a complexification of the output-processing stage of the task and an aggravation of the asymmetry of allocation of response preparation resources, as was the case for our triple press condition, which also had the effect of shortening the CUD.

Our interpretation of these effects once again calls into play the phenomenon of attention conceived of as task-dependent mechanisms of resource allocation or consumption. We believe that the balance of attentional demands on each of the two hemispheres is not the same when one hemisphere is required to take full responsibility for responding repetitively (especially in the case of a motorically demanding task) over a large number of trials, as opposed to when each hemisphere is alternatively solicited for a response (especially when the response required is as simple as can be, such as a simple key press). When one hemisphere assumes full responsibility for the entire response domain over extended time, we presume most plausible that the responding hemisphere becomes less susceptible to detect stimulus-driven signals received directly. In short, we believe that these results demonstrate clearly that CUDs are not just a reflection of IHRT, but are also a reflection of compensatory cost of processing the stimulus in the hemisphere carrying the burden of repetitive responding. These findings argue against the cable metaphor as well as the CUD = IHRT equation. This conclusion seems all the more tenable to us in light of the fact that we have been able to replicate these results in a new cohort of normal right-handers (Godbout, Braun, and Achim, 1996). Finally, we propose that the 15-ms CUD obtained in the hand alternation condition is probably a more accurate estimate of true interhemispheric relay time than the 4.03-ms CUD obtained in the classical version of the Poffenberger paradigm. Indeed, in the hand alternation condition we suppose that intrahemispheric processing is less biased by asymmetric compensating costs, thus leading to a less biased estimate of IHRT.

Braun and colleagues (1995a) obtained a statistically significant complex experimental modulation of the SRT-CUD as a function of lateral cueing of targets by means of a centrally emplaced arrow (80% valid and 20% invalid cues). There were three cueing experiments, each with a different cohort. In each experiment, valid cueing (a centrally emplaced warning arrow correctly predicted the hemifield in which the stimulus would appear) resulted in prolonged CUDs, and invalid cueing (a centrally emplaced warning arrow incorrectly predicted the hemifield in which the stimulus would appear) yielded negative CUDs. Unfortunately, this manipulation also greatly increased the variability of the CUD parameter, and the FIELD × HAND × CUE-TYPE interaction was not significant in two of the three experiments. We suspect that, to the extent to which the trend might reflect a real phenomenon, the effect probably consisted of an accentuation of hemispheric asymmetry of motoric processing resources (response preparation), that is, of the balance of cost of processing in each of the hemispheres (see Figure 9.10).

CUDs in Conditions of Bimanual Responding: An Anomaly for the Balance-of-Cost Model? Jeeves (1969) and Jeeves and Dixon (1972) provided data suggestive of modulation of CUDs as a function of whether the two hands were required to respond or only one.

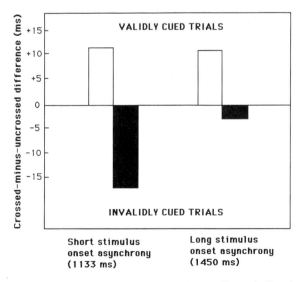

FIGURE 9.10. Summary depiction of the effect of directional cueing from a centrally emplaced arrow on the crossed-minus-uncrossed reaction time difference. (See Braun et al., 1995a.)

Though they did not test the effect statistically, they rather consistently found that unimanually obtained CUDs were longer (mean = 4.62 ms) than bimanually obtained CUDs (mean = 3.9 ms). Global unimanual RTs were, on the average, approximately 22 ms faster (mean = 228 ms) than the fastest of the two RTs in the bilateral condition (mean = 250 ms). We can imagine that the critical neural signal had enough time, in the bilateral condition, to cross the commissure(s) at least six times in the interim. Di Stefano and colleagues (1980) also found significant prolonged RT in bimanual conditions, but by only 1.45 ms. Kaluzny, Palmeri, and Wiesendanger (1994) obtained similar CUD results in the somesthetic modality (2.5 versus 0.5 ms), but bimanual global RTs were not slower than the unimanual ones. We propose that there are several dynamic mechanisms building up as a subject is preparing for a stimulus, processing the stimulus, preparing the response, and executing the response. Preparation for a unimanual response, we think, differentially (asymmetrically) affects the two hemispheres, creating a task-specific hemispheric asymmetry, on line, which changes sides when the responding hand is switched. This in turn probably affects the way in which each hemisphere processes the stimulus and relays visual information to the other hemisphere and/or receives information from the other hemisphere. Bimanual preparation for a response probably places the hemispheres in a more symmetric state of receptiveness to the stimulus but could also increase the cost of overall stimulus processing, depending on the task. For example, there is a unimanual advantage over simultaneous bimanual grip strength (Ohtsuki, 1981). There is always a highly significant cost of bimanual execution of such a task: Both hands become weaker when they are required to expend maximum effort simultaneously. The experimental technique used by Berlucchi and colleagues (1995), Jeeves (1969), Jeeves and Dixon (1972), and Kaluzny and colleagues (1994) consisted of having subjects press a key with each hand (both hands simultaneously) as fast as possible upon detection of a stimulus. According to the argument we developed above regarding the results of Godbout and colleagues (1995, 1996), removal of the asymmetry of response preparation (blocks of unimanual hand responses) makes response preparation hemispherically symmetrical, an effect that should redistribute hemispheric balance of cost, which in turn ought to result in a reliable prolongation of the CUD against a background of slightly briefer global RT. However, the results of Jeeves (1969), Jeeves and Dixon (1972), and Kaluzny and colleagues (1994) could be construed to represent an anomaly for this interpretation. Recall that bimanual responding had the effect of decreasing the CUD.

We suspect that a distinct mechanism is involved in simultaneous bimanual responding that would not compromise our basic account of balance of costs. For example, Aglioti and colleagues (1993) found that human subjects without a corpus callosum had tremendously prolonged unimanual CUDs but normal (very brief) CUDs under bimanual conditions. Berlucchi and colleagues (1995) replicated this finding and also found that SRT yields no CUD when axial responding is required instead of the usual distal finger response. In bimanual responding, the RTs at each hand are very close to each other and are very highly correlated (Kaluzny et al., 1994). Several authors have proposed that they are in fact released as a unity (Kelso, Southard, and Goodman, 1979; Al-Senawi and Cooke, 1985; Glickstein, 1990). Berlucchi, Aglioti, and Tassinari (1994) proposed a ventromedial reticulospinal system of this sort, and Kaluzny and colleagues (1994) proposed a contralaterally and ipsilaterally projecting cortical circuit as a basis for their own results.

Possible Physiological Mechanisms Underlying Balance of Cost Although our account of balance of asymmetric costs modulating the interhemispheric relay costs limits itself to a within-hemisphere mechanism, other mechanisms of balance of cost can be imagined. A similar effect on the CUD could result from any mechanism allowing relatively more efficient stimulus detection in the hemisphere that does not control the response, including, as was suggested earlier, cross-hemispheric (commissural) influences. Balance of cost can occur not only in timing of behavioral events, but also in performance accuracy (detection efficiency). Balance of cost of the type described above could result not only in longer RTs, but also in greater frequency of omission errors occurring in ipsilateral than in contralateral field-hand conditions or vice versa. Once this most basic challenge to the CUD = IHRT hypothesis is admitted, it then becomes necessary to recognize that any number of experimental variables could contribute to modulation of CUDs in SRT. Table 9.1 presents the main mechanisms that we think best present a challenge to the hypostasy of the CUD and the IHRT in simple reaction time investigations of interhemispheric dynamics.

Avenues for future research

Some of the ideas for future research that we have been nursing include the following:

1. In both experiments of Godbout and colleagues (1995, 1996) the prolongation of the classically obtained CUD by alternation of responding hand was highly sig-

TABLE 9.1
Putative mechanisms of modulation of interhemispheric relay

Neural signals can be amplified or accelerated via the interhemispheric commissure(s), perhaps benefiting from enhancement by lateral inhibition.

Neural signals can be filtered or decelerated via the interhemispheric commissure(s), perhaps owing to processing limits of the type of neurons (primarily pyramidal cells) forming the corpus callosum.

Tonic intrahemispheric allocation of *stimulus*-processing resources is asymmetric as a consequence of sustained asymmetry of response demands on the body, and this in turn influences interhemispheric relay.

Tonic intrahemispheric allocation of *response*-processing resources is asymmetric as a consequence of sustained asymmetry of response demands on the body, and this in turn influences interhemispheric relay.

Interhemispheric relay speed and accuracy are asymmetric, relay being apparently usually faster and more efficient from the right hemisphere to the left.

Receptive field and/or output specialization of commissural neurons define the limits of the stimuli or responses that are apt to be effectively relayed.

Interhemispheric relay expresses itself in the normal brain as an optimization process (selective and adaptable) for the most rapid and precise possible sensorimotor integration of the two body halves.

The balance of precision and speed of sensorimotor integration of the two body halves is itself subject to adaptive modulation.

nificant in both omission errors and RTs. Whether balance of cost(s) was just a trial-by-trial phenomenon or built up over a number of trials remains to be determined. Whether balance of costs can be interpreted as an effect of asymmetric hemispheric arousal remains at this time a matter of speculation. Pertinent tests of these ideas can be implemented by use of the evoked potential technique, as well as a breakup of analysis on a trial-by-trial basis. Furthermore, such experiments, comprising grafting of task demands onto the simple reaction time paradigm (cf. Godbout et al., 1995; Iacoboni and Zaidel, 1995) ought to be followed up in such a manner as to rule out the eventuality of a CUD effect being due to spatial compatibility. The experiments of Godbout and colleagues also comprised a condition designed to increase the asymmetry of response preparation (the three-tap condition). This condition did not always significantly reduce the CUD in errors and in RT. However, the eventuality of doing so is particularly exciting from a theoretical point of view. The reason is that CUDs could be predicted to become actually robustly or even significantly negative, at least according to the balance-of-costs model. This could perhaps be accomplished by adding more load to the response preparation (see Keele, Cohen, and Ivry, 1990; Rosenbaum, 1991). In fact, ideally, such a manipulation of motor load should be parametrized: A same subject could be tested under conditions of, say, one tap, two taps, three taps, four taps, and five taps.

2. There seems to exist a robust right-to-left hemisphere relay advantage in humans. More exploration of the eventuality of relay asymmetry would include cross-callosal intracerebral stimulation and recording experiments in animals and in those few epileptic patients with depth electrodes implanted bilaterally. The issue can also be addressed anatomically: A large, highly selective retrograde marker injection in the right hemisphere of monkeys, combined with recently developed histological enhancing preparations, could yield indication of more large-caliber callosal fibers than an identical injection in the left hemisphere.

3. We have speculated that there exists a right hemisphere advantage for magnocellular processing and a left hemisphere advantage for parvocellular processing (Braun et al., 1996a). This idea was previously presented by Kosslyn and colleagues (1992) and elaborated upon by Hellige (1996). Stomonyakov and Vassilev (1989) and Van Orden and House (1996) found that scalp evoked potential topography was compatible with left hemisphere superiority (greater amplitude) for processing of high spatial frequencies. Mecacci and Spinelli (1987) found a right-hemisphere dominance (greater amplitude of EPs) for processing fast temporal frequencies (checkerboard reversals) and the opposite for slow temporal frequencies. Finally, Proverbio and colleagues (1995) found a left-hemisphere EP advantage for high spatial frequencies and the opposite for low spatial frequencies in a split-brain patient. These patterns are all compatible with left-hemisphere parvocellular specialization and right-hemisphere magnocellular specialization. The psychophysical findings of Berardi and colleagues (1987, 1988) suggest filtering properties of commissural neurons along dimensions of spatial and temporal frequencies as well as spatial contrast. These properties dissociate in the magnocellular and parvocellular streams of the visual projection in humans, a construct that did not seem to preoccupy the authors. Such mechanisms would be compatible with faster relay from the right to the left hemisphere than from the left to the right hemisphere, as observed by several authors reviewed above. For example, interhemispheric transfer of magnocellular visual properties could be faster, or parvocellular visual properties could be filtered during interhemispheric relay. These ideas could easily be tested, for example, by im-

plementing a special version of the Poffenberger paradigm. The most effective way, we think, of making the demonstration (obtaining the predicted double dissociation of field effects and of relay effects in simple reaction time) would consist of creating an optimized magnocellular stimulus designed for simple detection (e.g., large moving eccentric fuzzy-contoured blue stimuli on an equichromatic background, set at the 80% detection threshold) and an optimized parvocellular stimulus for simple detection (e.g., small, stationary, near the vertical meridian, sharply contoured, green stimuli on an equiluminant red background, also set at the 80% detection threshold).

4. The balance of interhemispheric and intrahemispheric relations seems to vary in synchrony with the menstrual cycle in humans (Weekes and Zaidel, 1996; Weekes et al., 1999) and with pregnancy in animals (Bianki, Shramm, and Kharitonov, 1992). Central nervous system injection of serotonin in rats spectacularly reduces interhemispheric relay, by 50–90% (Read, Beck, and Dun, 1994), and serotonin is known to be modulated in synchrony with the menstrual cycle, the estrogen cycle in particular, in humans (Wirz and Chappuis-Arndt, 1976; D'Andrea et al., 1995), far more than is the case for the other amines such as dopamine (Lamprecht et al., 1974) or acetylcholine (Kawashima et al., 1987) and modestly more than is the case for noradrenaline (Collins, Eneroth, and Landgren, 1985; Davidson et al., 1985). The variation of interhemispheric dynamics along the menstrual cycle in humans has been investigated only with the dichotic listening method and with a Stroop paradigm and not with the more basic and limpid Poffenberger paradigm. In addition, steroid hormones were not assayed, the women were tested after the luteal-estrogenic peak, and the two menstrual periods (follicular and near-luteal) were sampled between subjects. It would be helpful to test women off the pill at the luteal and follicular peaks using an intrasubject design, sampling urine for LH, using a visual SRT implementation of the Poffenberger paradigm, and adding the dimension of evoked potentials.

5. The predominance of homotopic over heterotopic anatomical interhemispheric connectivity has been established in several mammalian species for most parts of the corpus callosum. However, it is still not clear whether this anatomical particularity is reflected in speed and accuracy of relay as indexed in behavior in humans. As would be expected from what we know about the predominance of callosal connectivity, simultaneous stimulation of one versus two visual fields (the Dimond paradigm; see Dimond, 1969) most often gives a bilateral advantage (or a reduced unilateral advantage) when stimuli are presented in a horizontal across-field display

than a diagonal across-field display. However, the "homotopic" advantage that has been found has been fragile and should perhaps not be generalized. For example, Brown and Jeeves (1993) found it to be significant only for accuracy and not for speed of decision making. Ludwig and colleagues (1993) found that decision latency was indeed significantly shorter for horizontal than for diagonal integration. These experiments comprised long stimulus displays and relatively complex discriminative decisions. A straightforward simple reaction time task, reported by Schieppati and colleagues (1984), comprised finger responses to cutaneous homotopic (finger) or heterotopic (shoulder) stimulation. CUDs were the same in the two conditions. Collin and Braun (1997) found an advantage of diagonal (heterotopic) over horizontal (homotopic) emplacement of interfield stimuli in a very simple visual discrimination task. Stimuli were presented for only 50 ms. These behavioral findings ought not necessarily be considered anomalous. Indeed, Cukiert and Timo-Iaria (1989) found that in certain conditions, intrahemispheric electrical stimulation yielded a faster and stronger electrical response in the contralateral hemisphere at heterotopic sites. Braun and colleagues (1999a) found that the early P1 wave of visual evoked potentials presented a topography more compatible with heterotopic than homotopic interhemispheric relay in the normal human. Berman and Payne (1988) state that "most visual cortical areas also send and receive connections from heterotopic areas of the opposite hemisphere," and these authors describe several cortical fields wherein heterotopic interhemispheric connection represents a large majority (75%) over homotopic interhemispheric connection. Similar predominantly heterotopic callosal neuron fields have been observed in motor cortex (of the macaque)—for example, in the hand area of the supplementary motor area (Rouiller et al., 1994). Tolchenova, Imankulova, and Schevchenko (1980) even claim to have observed more heterotopic than homotopic callosal connectivity for the parietal cortex as a whole in the cat. Bianki and colleagues have published, in Russian, a large number of anatomical and electrophysiological investigations on the subject of homotopic and heterotopic relay. Fortunately, one report in English (Bianki, Shramm, and Kharitonov, 1989) provides an overview: First, homotopic callosal fibers are in the top layers of cat parietal cortex, while heterotopic fibers (occipital-parietal) are in the lower layers; second, lower parietal cortical layers typically produce a positive-negative evoked potential (whether the fibers are callosal or not), whereas the opposite is true for upper layers; third, homotopic commissural fibers produce the negative-positive EP, while heterotopic commissural fibers produce the positive-negative EP;

fourth, the heterotopic EP has a shorter latency and a more focal postcallosal topography; fifth, the homotopic EP disappears after callosotomy, but the heterotopic EP is only attenuated, leading the authors to the conclusion that a fast subcortical component is also involved. The relative importance of specific heterotopic neuronal fields versus specific homotopic fields for sustaining the behavioral CUD is not known. However, we interpret the findings of Bianki and colleagues (1989, 1992, 1994) as clearly compatible with a fast focal heterotopic mechanism for very simple relay of a punctate critical signal (as in the Poffenberger paradigm) via its early excitatory phase and a massive slower diffuse homotopic inhibitory-excitatory mechanism for multimodal, ongoing, full-field interhemispheric integration. An important and yet-unresolved question, then, is whether behavioral estimation of interhemispheric relay can be made to reflect heterotopic properties of callosal connectivity. The Collin and Braun (1997) experiment was not designed specifically to test a relative advantage of homotopy or heterotopy *throughout* the visual fields, an experiment that obviously needs to be carried out. For such an experiment to be as physiologically relevant as possible, stimulus durations should be brief, displays should be small, and the entire visual field should be sampled systematically. There are two paradigms that are relevant for this experimentation: the Dimond paradigm, requiring comparison of two stimuli (one in each field) and discrimination for a "same" response or for a "different" response (go/no-go), or the noninformative cue (redundancy gain) paradigm (SRT can be facilitated or inhibited differently by an ipsilateral or contralateral noninformative cue) (Tassinari et al., 1987, 1989, 1994a; Tassinari and Berlucchi, 1993). Findings of facilitation by redundant homotopic stimulation in callosotomy patients (Reuter-Lorenz et al., 1995) suggest that the hemispheres are inhibited by response competition during unilateral stimulation, as occurs in the Poffenberger paradigm. This introduces the possibility that heterotopic integration may be less subject to such interhemispheric interference. Specifically, diagonality, or heterotopy, should be manipulated parametrically; for example, diagonality should be manipulated by varying eccentricity-off horizontality, and horizontality (homotopy) should also be manipulated with arrays presented at various levels of the upper and lower field. In both cases, interstimulus distances should also be manipulated experimentally (given that callosal relay is known to favor midline fusion, i.e., meridianal integration).

6. Cognitive data, we think, probably travel along fast large-caliber callosal neurons. What then are the small-caliber unmyelinated phylogenetically primitive callosal fibers for? We believe that they are for slow, diffuse, tonic (ultradian, circadian) interhemispheric distribution and balancing; sequencing and cycling of vigilance; arousal; and the like. Kolev and colleagues (1994) present a description of such cycling in the normal human. Oguni and colleagues (1994) have reported that bilateral slow-wave discharge synchrony in epileptics is disrupted following anterior callosotomy, a finding that has been reported by several research teams following complete callosotomy. It is possible to test ideas specifically concerning the role of small, unmyelinated, slow, phylogenetically primitive fibers in the corpus callosum: (a) Rats or cats should have the same low-level slow synchronization mechanisms as normal humans, and split-brain rats and cats should not; (b) patients with multiple sclerosis and atrophied callosi ought to manifest poor relay of cognitive information but less of a problem in those slow synchronisms that rely on unmyelinated slow callosal fibers, these being still intact in such patients.

7. Braun, Villeneuve, and Achim (2002) found in their SRT visual evoked potential experiment on 10 normal subjects that certain components of the "movement-related potential" were indeed compatible with an interhemispheric relay effect. The critical element of proof of a motor relay effect will come from an experiment with callosal agenesics or callosotomized subjects looking at both stimulus-related evoked potentials and movement-related potentials.

8. Disease and pathology may cause callosal degeneration and anomalies of interhemispheric relay. This is known to be the case in multiple sclerosis because this demyelinating disease cannot but seriously compromise the largest myelinated area of the brain: the corpus callosum (Moreau et al., 1998). The corpus callosum is also very sensitive to developmental insult, such that it is commonly found to be partially agenesic in developmental learning disorders (Njiokiktjien, de Sonneville, and Vaal, 1994), in fetal alcohol syndrome (Swayze et al., 1997), and even in maternal malnutrition during pregnancy (Galler, 1981). Chromosomal aberrations commonly severely inhibit the development of the corpus callosum. For example, callosal agenesis is observed in X aberrations, pseudotrisomy 13, partial 19 trisomy, chromosome 2 deletion, Klinefelter syndrome, deletion of the short arm of chromosome 17 (Miller-Dieker syndrome), Turner syndrome, translocation of chromosomes 4 and 5 and of chromosomes 4 and 15, and trisomies 4, 8, 9, 11, 13, 17, 18 and 21 (see Njiokiktjien, 1991). Hereditary disorders involving callosal agenesis include Varadi syndrome, PKU, Aicardi-Goutieres syndrome, Coffin-Lowry syndrome, Da Silva syndrome, and several others (see Njiokiktjien, 1991). The sensitivity of the corpus callosum to insult extends to adulthood, as is indicated

by the ability of prolonged alcohol abuse to cause severe callosal degeneration in Marchiafava-Bignami disorder (Ferracci et al., 1999) and head trauma to cause functional dysconnection (Levander and Sonesson, 1998). There is also evidence that because pyramidal cells are the most common in the corpus callosum and since this type of cell degenerates most in Alzheimer's disease (Lakmache et al., 1998), hemispheric disconnection is observed in that disease as well. It does not seem to be known why the hemispheric commissures are functionally and histologically abnormal in schizophrenia (Andreason et al., 1995). The field would gain from more thinking and research aiming at understanding why the corpus callosum is so sensitive to various kinds of insult. More subtle dysfunction of commissural systems, not visible with magnetic resonance imaging, may also contribute to certain behavioral anomalies in particular neuropsychological syndromes. Bipolar disorder may be the result of a genetic propensity for slow interhemispheric switching mechanisms that become "stuck" in one or the other state. Because slow switches are also "sticky" when compared with fast switches, the clinical manifestations of bipolar disorder may be explained by hemispheric activation being "stuck" on the left (mania) or on the right (depression) (Pettigrew and Miller, 1998). Dyslexia may well comprise, among other anomalies, right hemisphere interference on the left during reading in part owing to improper commissural relay (Robichon and Habib, 1998). Likewise, stuttering could be caused in part by inappropriate interference during speech from the right to the left premotor cortex (Nass, 1996; Webster, 1998). Alexithymia could be caused in some cases by a commissural insufficiency (Buchanan, Waterhouse, and West, 1980). It could be assumed that the right hemisphere superiority for emotional processing obtains impoverished verbal expression when the two hemispheres are disconnected. Finally, symptoms of Tourette's disease could be produced by the left hemisphere under an undue influence from the right limbic areas (Moriarty et al., 1997). These eventualities have hardly been explored at all and therefore deserve far more scrutiny.

REFERENCES

ABOITIZ, F., A. B. SCHEIBEL, R. S. FISHER, and E. ZAIDEL, 1992a. Fiber composition of the human corpus callosum. *Brain Res.* 598:143–153.

ABOITIZ, F., A. B. SCHEIBEL, R. S. FISHER, and E. ZAIDEL, 1992b. Individual differences in brain asymmetries and fiber composition in the human corpus callosum. *Brain Res.* 598:154–161.

AGLIOTI, S., G. BERLUCCHI, R. PALLINI, G. F. ROSSI, and G. TASSINARI, 1993. Hemispheric control of unilateral and bilateral responses to lateralized light stimuli after callosotomy and in callosal agenesis. *Exp. Brain Res.* 95:151–165.

AGLIOTI, S., R. DALL'AGNOLA, M. GIRELLI, and C. A. MARZI, 1991. Bilateral hemispheric control of foot distal movements: Evidence from normal subjects. *Cortex* 27:571–581.

AL-SENAWI, D., and J. D. COOKE, 1985. Matching of movements made independently by the two arms in normal humans. *J. Motiv. Behav.* 17:321–334.

AMADEO, M., R. A. ROEMER, and C. SHAGASS, 1977. Can callosal speed of transmission be inferred from verbal reaction times? *Biol. Psychiatry* 12:289–297.

ANDREASEN, N. C., V. SWAYZE, D. S. O'LEARY, P. NOPOULOS, T. CIZADLO, G. HARRIS, S. ARNDT, and M. FLAUM, 1995. Abnormalities in midline attentional circuitry in schizophrenia: Evidence from magnetic resonance and positron emission tomography. *Eur. Neuropsychopharmacol.* 5 (Suppl.): 37–41.

ANZOLA, G. P., G. BERTOLONI, H. A. BUCHTEL, and G. RIZZOLATTI, 1977. Spatial compatibility and anatomical factors in simple and choice reaction time. *Neuropsychologia* 15:295–302.

ANZOLA, G. P., and L. A. VIGNOLO, 1992. Interhemispheric communication following unilateral cerebrovascular lesions. *Ital J. Neurol. Sci.* 13:649–655.

BASHORE, T. R., 1981. Vocal and manual reaction time estimates of interhemispheric transmission time. *Psych. Bull.* 89:352–368.

BERARDI, N., S. BISTI, A. FIORENTINI, and L. MAFFEI, 1988. The transfer of visual information across the corpus callosum in cats, monkeys and humans: Spatial and temporal properties. *Progr. Brain Res.* 75:181–185.

BERARDI, N., S. BISTI, and L. MAFFEI, 1987. The transfer of visual information across the corpus callosum: Spatial and temporal properties in the cat. *J. Physiol.* 384:619–632.

BERARDI, N., and A. FIORENTINI, 1987. Interhemispheric transfer of visual information in humans: spatial characteristics. *J. Physiol.* 384:633–647.

BERLUCCHI, G., 1974. Cerebral dominance and interhemispheric communication in normal man. In *The Neurosciences, Third Study Program*, F. O. Schmitt and R. G. Worden, eds. Cambridge, Mass.: MIT Press.

BERLUCCHI, G., 1978. Interhemispheric integration of simple visuomotor responses. In *Cerebral Correlates of Conscious Experience*, P. A. Buser and A. Rougeul-Buser, eds. New York: North-Holland Biomedical Press, pp. 83–94.

BERLUCCHI, G., S. AGLIOTI, C. A. MARZI, and G. TASSINARI, 1995. Corpus callosum and simple visuomotor integration. *Neuropsychologia* 33:923–936.

BERLUCCHI, G., S. AGLIOTI, and G. TASSINARI, 1994. The role of the corpus callosum and bilaterally distributed motor pathways in the synchronization of bilateral upper limb responses to lateralized light stimuli. In *Interlimb Coordination: Neural, Dynamical and Cognitive Constraints*, S. P. Swinnen, H. Heuer, J. Massion, and P. Casaer, eds. San Diego: Academic Press, pp. 209–227.

BERLUCCHI, G., F. CREA, M. DI STEFANO, and G. TASSINARI, 1977. Influence of spatial stimulus-response compatibility on reaction time of ipsilateral and contralateral hand to lateralized light stimuli. *J. Exp. Psych. Hum. Percep. Perf.* 3:505–517.

BERLUCCHI, G., W. HERON, R. HYMAN, G. RIZZOLATTI, and C. UMILTA, 1971. Simple reaction times of ipsilateral and contralateral hand to lateralized visual stimuli. *Brain* 94:419–430.

BERMAN, N. E., and B. R. PAYNE, 1988. Development and plasticity of visual interhemispheric connections. In *Advances in Neural and Behavioral Development*, Vol. 3, P. G. Shinkman, ed. Norwood, N.J.: Ablex Publishing Corporation.

BIANKI, V. L., and I. A. MAKAROVA, 1994. Dinamika mezhpolusharnoi asimmetrii pri obrabotke transkallozal'nogo signala [The dynamics of interhemispheric asymmetry during the processing of a transcallosal signal]. *Fiziol. Zh.* 80:19–29.

BIANKI, V. L., V. A. SHRAMM, and E. V. KHARITONOV, 1989. Interhemispheric interzonal connections in the parietal cortex. *Int. J. Neurosci.* 47:333–350.

BIANKI, V. L., V. A. SHRAMM, and E. V. KHARITONOV, 1992. [The effect of pregnancy on transcallosal evoked potentials]. *Fiziol. Zh.* 78:10–20.

BISHOP, K. M., and D. WAHLSTEN, 1997. Sex differences in the human corpus callosum: Myth or reality? *Neurosci. Biobehav. Rev.* 21:581–601.

BISIACCHI, P., C. A. MARZI, R. NICOLETTI, G. CARENA, C. MUCIGNAT, and F. TOMAIUOLO, 1994. Left-right asymmetry of callosal transfer in normal human-subjects. *Behav. Brain Res.* 64:173–178.

BOZHKO, G. T., and V. A. SHRAMM, 1990. Mezhpolusharnaia asimmetriia vzaimodeistviia transkalloznal'nogo i voskhodiashchego potokov vozbuzhdeniia v zritel'noi kore koshki [Interhemispheric asymmetry in the interaction of the transcallosal and ascending flows of excitation in the cat visual cortex]. *Fiziol. Zh.* 76:3–11.

BRAUN, C. M. J., 1992. Estimation of hemispheric and interhemispheric dynamics from simple reaction time. *Neuropsychol. Rev.* 3:321–364.

BRAUN, C. M. J., A. ACHIM, and L. VILLENEUVE, 1999a. Topography of averaged electrical brain activity relating to interhemispheric dynamics in normal humans: Where does the critical relay take place? *Int. J. Psychophysiol.* 32:1–14.

BRAUN, C. M. J., and S. DAIGNEAULT, 1994. Effects of a right hemifield advantage on crossed-uncrossed differentials in simple reaction time: Toward a new model of interhemispheric relay. *Acta Psychol.* 85:91–98.

BRAUN, C. M. J., S. DAIGNEAULT, S. MILJOURS, and A. DUFRESNE, 1995a. Does hemispheric relay depend on attention? *Am. J. Psychol.* 108:527–546.

BRAUN, C. M. J., A. DUMAS, and I. COLLIN, 1994a. Effects of memory load on interhemispheric relay time. *Am. J. Psychol.* 107:537–549.

BRAUN, C. M. J., C. MAILHOUX, and A. DUFRESNE, 1996a. Left and right visual field advantages are a function of scotopic and photopic retinal adaptation respectively in simple reaction time to near-threshold targets. *Acta Psychol.* 91:3–14.

BRAUN, C. M. J., C. POTVIN, and A. ACHIM, 1995b. The relation of callosal synaptic density in cortex and electrode site in the estimation of interhemispheric relay time with evoked potentials [Abstract]. *J. Int. Neuropsychol. Soc.* 1:178.

BRAUN, C. M. J., A. SAPIN-LEDUC, C. PICARD, E. BONNENFANT, A. ACHIM, and S. DAIGNEAULT, 1994b. Zaidel's model of interhemispheric dynamics: Empirical tests, a critical appraisal, and a proposed revision. *Brain Cogn.* 24:57–86.

BRAUN, C. M. J., L. VILLENEUVE, and A. ACHIM, 1996b. Balance of cost in interhemispheric relay in the Poffenberger paradigm: Evidence from omission errors. *Neuropsychology* 10:565–572.

BRAUN, C. M. J., L. VILLENEUVE, and A. ACHIM, 2002. Topographical analysis of movement-related electrical scalp activity and interhemispheric dynamics in normal humans. *Int. J. Psychophysiol.* in press.

BRIZZOLARA, D., G. FERRETTI, P. BROVEDANI, C. CASALINI, and B. SBRANA, 1994. Is interhemispheric transfer time related to age: A developmental study. *Behav. Brain Res.* 64:179–184.

BROWN, W. S., and M. JEEVES, 1993. Bilateral visual field processing and evoked potential interhemispheric transmission time. *Neuropsychologia* 31:1267–1281.

BROWN, W. S., E. B. LARSON, and M. A. JEEVES, 1994. Directional asymmetries in interhemispheric transmission time: Evidence from visual evoked potentials. *Neuropsychologia* 32:439–448.

BRYSBAERT, M., 1994. Behavioral estimates of interhemispheric transmission time and the signal detection method: A reappraisal. *Percep. Psychophys.* 56(4):479–490.

BUCHANAN, D. C., G. J. WATERHOUSE, and S. C. WEST, 1980. A proposed neurophysiological basis of alexithymia. *Psychother. Psychosom.* 34:248–255.

BURNISON, D. S., E. B. LARSON, and W. S. BROWN, 1993. Hemispheric integration of visual information: Effects of gender and age. *J. Clin. Exp. Neuropsych.* 15:33.

CLARKE, J. M., and E. ZAIDEL, 1989. Simple reaction times to lateralized light flashes: Varieties of interhemispheric communication routes. *Brain* 112:849–870.

COLLIN, I., and C. M. J. BRAUN, 1997. The Poffenberger and Dimond paradigms: Neuropsychological effects and relations between the two paradigms. *Brain Cogn.* 34:337–359.

COLLINS, A., P. ENEROTH, and B. M. LANDGREN, 1985. Psychoneuroendocrine stress responses and mood as related to the menstrual cycle. *Psychosom. Med.* 47:512–527.

CORBALLIS, M. C., 1998. Interhemispheric neural summation in the absence of the corpus callosum. *Brain* 121:1795–1807.

CUKIERT, A., and C. TIMO-IARIA, 1989. Electrophysiological evidence for an L-shaped interhemispheric connection in the cat. *Arquivas Neuropsiquiatrica* 47:381–384.

D'ANDREA, G., L. HASSELMARK, A. R. CANANZI, M. ALECCI, F. PERINI, F. ZAMBERLAN, and K. M. WELCH, 1995. Metabolism and menstrual cycle rhythmicity of serotonin in primary headaches. *Headache* 35:216–221.

DAVIDSON, L., I. L. ROUSE, R. VANDONGEN, and L. J. BEILIN, 1985. Plasma noradrenaline and its relationship to plasma oestradiol in normal women during the menstrual cycle. *Clin. Exp. Pharm. Physiol.* 12:489–493.

DIMOND, S. J., 1969. Hemisphere functions and immediate memory. *Psychon. Sci.* 16:111–112.

DI STEFANO, M., M. MORELLI, C. A. MARZI, and G. BERLUCCHI, 1980. Hemispheric control of unilateral and bilateral movements of proximal and distal parts of the arm as inferred from simple reaction time to lateralized light stimuli in man. *Exp. Brain Res.* 38:197–204.

DI STEFANO, M., and C. SALVADORI, 1998. Asymmetry of the interhemispheric visuomotor integration in callosal agenesis. *Neuroreport* 9:1331–1335.

DUFRESNE, A., D. LAPIERRE, M.-J. CHOUINARD, S. DAIGNEAULT, and C. M. J. BRAUN, 1993. Are human callosi bigger and faster in men than women? Behavioral evidence [Abstract]. *J. Clin. Exp. Neuropsych.* 15:34.

FERRACCI, F., F. CONTE, M. GENTILE, R. CANDEAGO, L. FOSCOLO, M. BENDINI, and G. FASSETTA, 1999. Marchiafava-Bignami disease: Computed tomographic scan, 99mTc HMPAO-SPECT, and FLAIR MRI findings in a patient with subcortical aphasia, alexia, bilateral agraphia, and left-handed deficit of constructional ability. *Arch. Neurol.* 56:107–110.

FILBEY, R. A., and M. S. GAZZANIGA, 1969. Splitting the normal brain with reaction time. *Psychon. Sci.* 17:335–336.

GALLER, J. R., 1981. Visual discrimination in rats: The effects of rehabilitation following intergenerational malnutrition. *Dev. Psychobiol.* 14:229–236.

GLICKSTEIN, M. E., 1990. Brain pathways in the visual guidance of movement and the behavioral functions of the cerebellum. In *Brain Circuits and Functions of the Mind*, C. B. Trevarthen, ed. Cambridge, Engl.: Cambridge University Press, pp. 157–167.

GODBOUT, J. A., A. ACHIM, and C. M. J. BRAUN, 1995. Modulation motrice des dynamiques interhémisphériques dans le paradigme de Poffenberger [Abstract]. In *Comptes Rendus 18ième Congrès de la Société Québécoise de Recherche en Psychologie, Ottawa*.

GREEN, J., 1984. Effects of intrahemispheric interference on reaction times to lateral stimuli. *J. Exp. Psychol.* 10:292–306.

GROSS, M. M., 1972. Hemispheric specialization for processing of visually presented verbal and spatial stimuli. *Percep. Psychophys.* 12:357–363.

HABIB, M., D. GAYRAUD, A. OLIVA, J. REGIS, G. SALAMON, and R. KHALIL, 1991. Effects of handedness and sex on the morphology of the corpus callosum. *Brain Cogn.* 16:41–61.

HARVEY, L. O., Jr., 1978. Single representation of the visual midline in humans. *Neuropsychologia* 16:601–610.

HASBROUCQ, T., S. KORNBLUM, and A. OSMAN, 1988. A new look at reaction time estimates of interhemispheric transmission time. *Cahiers Psychol. Cogn.* 8:207–221.

HEDGE, A., and N. W. A. MARSH, 1975. The effect of irrelevant spatial correspondences on two-choice response-time. *Acta Psychol.* 39:427–439.

HELLIGE, J. B., 1996. Hemispheric asymmetry for visual information processing. *Acta Neurobiol. Exp.* 56:485–497.

HOLLOWAY, R. L., and M. C. DELACOSTE, 1986. Sexual dimorphism in the human corpus callosum: An extension and replication study. *Hum. Neurobiol.* 5:87–91.

HOPTMAN, M. J., and R. J. DAVIDSON, 1994. How and why do the two cerebral hemispheres interact? *Psych. Bull.* 116:195–219.

HOPTMAN, M. J., R. J. DAVIDSON, A. GUDMUNDSSON, R. T. SCHREIBER, and W. B. ERSHLER, 1996. Age differences in visual evoked potential estimates of interhemispheric transfer. *Neuropsychologia* 10:263–271.

IACOBONI, M., I. FRIED, and E. ZAIDEL, 1994. Callosal transmission time before and after partial commissurotomy. *Neuroreport* 5:2521–2524.

IACOBONI, M., and E. ZAIDEL, 1995. Channels of the corpus callosum: Evidence from simple reaction times to lateralized flashes in the normal and the split brain. *Brain* 118:779–788.

JÄNCKE, L., and H. STEINMETZ, 1994. Interhemispheric transfer time and corpus callosum size. *Neuroreport* 5:2385–2388.

JEEVES, M. A., 1969. A comparison of interhemispheric transmission times in acallosals and normals. *Psychon. Sci.* 16:245–246.

JEEVES, M. A., and N. F. DIXON, 1972. Hemisphere differences in response rates to visual stimuli. *Psychon. Sci.* 20:249–251.

KALUZNY, P., A. PALMERI, and M. WIESENDANGER, 1994. The problem of bimanual coupling: A reaction time study of simple unimanual and bimanual finger responses. *Electr. Clin. Neurophys.* 93:450–458.

KAROL, E. A., and D. N. PANDYA, 1971. The distribution of the corpus callosum in the rhesus monkey. *Brain* 94:471–486.

KASWAN, J., and S. YOUNG, 1965. Effect of luminance, exposure duration and task complexity on reaction time. *J. Exp. Psychol.* 69:393–400.

KAWASHIMA, K., H. OOHATA, K. FUJIMOTO, and T. SUZUKI, 1987. Plasma concentration of acetylcholine in young women. *Neurosci. Lett.* 80:339–342.

KEELE, S. W., A. COHEN, and R. IVRY, 1990. Motor programs: Concepts and issues. In *Attention and Performance*, Vol. 13: *Motor Representation and Control*, M. Jeannerod, ed. Hillsdale, N.J.: Lawrence Erlbaum Associates, pp. 77–110.

KELSO, J. A. S., D. L. SOUTHARD, and D. GOODMAN, 1979. On the nature of human interlimb coordination. *Science* 203:1029–1031.

KLEINMAN, K. M., R. CARRON, L. CLONINGER, and P. HALVACHS, 1976. A comparison of interhemispheric transmission times as measured by verbal and manual reaction time. *Int. J. Neurosci.* 6:285–288.

KOLEV, V., C. BASAR-EROGLU, F. AKSU, E. BASAR, 1994. EEG rhythmicities evoked by visual stimuli in three-year-old children. *Int. J. Neurosci.* 75:257–270.

KOSSLYN, S. M., C. F. CHABRIS, C. J. MARSOLEK, and O. KOENIG, 1992. Categorical versus coordinate spatial relations. Computational analyses and computer simulations. *J. Exp. Psychol. Hum. Percep. Perform.* 18:562–577.

LAKMACHE, Y., M. LASSONDE, S. GAUTHIER, J. Y. FRIGON, and F. LEPORÉ, 1998. Interhemispheric disconnection syndrome in Alzheimer's disease. *Proc. Natl. Acad. Sci. U.S.A.* 95:9042–9046.

LAMPRECHT, F., R. J. MATTA, B. LITTLE, and T. P. ZAHN, 1974. Plasma dopamine-beta-hydroxylase (DBH) activity during the menstrual cycle. *Psychosom. Med.* 36:304–310.

LEPORÉ, F., M. PTITO, L. RICHER, and J. P. GUILLEMOT, 1989. Cortico-cortical callosal connectivity: Evidence derived from electrophysiological studies. *Prog. Brain Res.* 75:187–195.

LEVANDER, M. B., and B. G. SONESSON, 1998. Are there any mild interhemispheric effects after moderately severe closed head injury? *Brain Inj.* 12:165–173.

LEVY, J., 1984. Can a reaction time paradigm simultaneously index arm position effects, spatial compatibility effects, and neural pathway effects? *Neuropsychologia* 22:95–97.

LEVY, J., and N. WAGNER, 1984. Handwriting posture, visuomotor integration, and lateralized reaction-time parameters. *Hum. Neurobiol.* 3:157–161.

LINES, C. R., and A. D. MILNER, 1983. Nasotemporal overlap in the human retina investigated by means of simple reaction time to lateralized light flash. *Exp. Brain Res.* 50:166–172.

LINES, C. R., M. D. RUGG, and A. D. MILNER, 1984. The effect of stimulus intensity on visual evoked potential estimates of interhemispheric transmission time. *Exp. Brain Res.* 57:89–98.

LUDWIG, T. E., M. A. JEEVES, W. D. NORMAN, and R. DEWITT, 1993. The bilateral field advantage on a letter-matching task. *Cortex* 29:691–713.

MAKAROVA, I. A., and V. L. BIANKI, 1994. Polovoi dimorfizm dinamiki mezhpolusharnoi asimmetrii pri obrabotke transkallozal'nogo signala [The sex dimorphism in the dynamics of interhemispheric asymmetry during the processing of a transcallosal signal]. *Fiziol. Zh.* 80:21–33.

MARZI, C. A., P. BISIACCHI, and R. NICOLETTI, 1991. Is interhemispheric transfer of visuomotor information asymmetric?

Evidence from a meta-analysis. *Neuropsychologia* 29:1163–1177.

McKeever, W. F., K. M. Gill, and A. D. VanDeventer, 1975. Letter versus dot stimuli as tools for "splitting the normal brain with reaction time." *Q. J. Exp. Psychol.* 27:363–373.

McKeever, W. F., and A. L. Hoff, 1979. Evidence of a possible isolation of left hemisphere visual and motor areas in sinistrals employing an inverted handwriting posture. *Neuropsychologia* 17:445–455.

McKeever, W. F., and A. L. Hoff, 1983. Further evidence of the absence of measurable interhemispheric transfer time in left-handers who employ an inverted handwriting posture. *Bull. Psychon. Soc.* 21:255–258.

McKeever, W. F., and M. D. Huling, 1971. Bilateral tachistoscopic word recognition as a function of hemisphere stimulated and interhemispheric transfer time. *Neuropsychologia* 9:281–288.

Mecacci, L., and D. Spinelli, 1987. Hemispheric asymmetry of pattern reversal visual evoked potentials in healthy subjects. *Int. J. Psychophysiol.* 4:325–328.

Meyer, B. U., S. Roricht, H. Grafin von Einsiedel, F. Kruggel, and A. Weindl, 1995. Inhibitory and excitatory interhemispheric transfers between motor cortical areas in normal humans and patients with abnormalities of the corpus callosum. *Brain* 118:429–440.

Milner, A. D., M. A. Jeeves, P. J. Ratcliff, and J. Cunnison, 1982. Interference effects of verbal and spatial tasks on simple visual reaction time. *Neuropsychologia* 20:591–595.

Milner, A. D., and C. R. Lines, 1982. Interhemispheric pathways in simple reaction time to lateralized light flash. *Neuropsychologia* 20:171–179.

Moreau, T., D. Sochurkova, M. Lemesle, G. Madinier, T. Billiar, M. Giroud, and R. Dumas, 1998. Epilepsy in patients with multiple sclerosis: Radiological-clinical correlations. *Epilepsia* 39:893–896.

Moriarty, J., A. R. Varma, J. Stevens, M. Fish, M. R. Trimble, and M. M. Robertson, 1997. A volumetric MRI study of Gilles de la Tourette's syndrome. *Neurology* 49:410–415.

Moscovith, M., and L. C. Smith, 1979. Differences in neural organization between individuals with inverted and non-inverted handwriting postures. *Science* 205:710–713.

Nass, R. D., 1996. Developmental stutter in a patient with callosal agenesis disappears during steroid therapy. *Pediatr. Neurol.* 15:166–168.

Njiokiktjien, C., 1991. Absence of the corpus callosum: Clinicopathological considerations. In *The Child's Corpus Callosum*, G. Ramaekers and C. Nijiokiktjien, eds. Amsterdam: Suyi Publications.

Njiokiktjien, C., L. de Sonneville, and J. Vaal, 1994. Callosal size in children with learning disabilities. *Behav. Brain Res.* 64:213–218.

Nowicka, A., A. Grabowska, and E. Fersten, 1996. Interhemispheric transmission of information and functional asymmetry of the human brain. *Neuropsychologia* 34:147–151.

Oguni, H., F. Andermann, J. Gotman, and A. Olivier, 1994. Effect of anterior callosotomy on bilaterally synchronous spike and wave and other EEG discharges. *Epilepsia* 35:505–513.

Ohtsuki, T., 1981. Decrease in grip strength induced by simultaneous exertion with reference to finger strength. *Ergonomics* 24:37–48.

Perez, H., S. Ruiz, A. Hernandez, and R. Soto-Moyano, 1990. Asymmetry of interhemispheric responses evoked in the prefrontal cortex of the rat. *J. Neurosci. Res.* 25:139–142.

Pettigrew, J. D., and S. M. Miller, 1998. A 'sticky' interhemispheric switch in bipolar disorder? *Proc. R. Soc. Lond. B Biol. Sci.* 265:2141–2148.

Poffenberger, A. T., Jr., 1912. Reaction time to retinal stimulation with special reference to the time cost in conduction through nerve centers. *Arch. Psychol.* 23:1–73.

Potvin, C., C. M. J. Braun, and A. Achim, 1994. VEP estimates of interhemispheric relay time. *Neurosci. Abs.* 20:1002.

Potvin, C., C. M. J. Braun, and A. Achim, 1995. Distinct functional channels in interhemispheric relay: Experimental evidence [Abstract]. *J. Int. Neuropsychological Soc.* 1:184.

Proverbio, A. M., A. Zani, G. R. Mangun, and M. Gazzaniga, 1995. *VEP evidence of hemispheric asymmetries for spatial frequency processing in a split brain patient.* Poster presented at the annual meeting of the Cognitive Neuroscience Society, San Francisco, Calif.

Raab, D., and E. Fehrer, 1962. Supplementary report: The effect of stimulus duration and luminance on visual reaction time. *J. Exp. Psychol.* 64:326–327.

Read, H. L., S. G. Beck, and N. J. Dun, 1994. Serotonergic suppression of interhemispheric cortical synaptic potentials. *Brain Res.* 643:17–28.

Reuter-Lorenz, P. A., G. Nozawa, M. S. Gazzaniga, and H. C. Hughes, 1995. Fate of neglected targets: A chronometric analysis of redundant target effects in the bisected brain. *J. Exp. Psych. Hum. Percep. Perform.* 21:211–230.

Rizzolatti, G., 1979. Interfield differences in reaction times to lateralized visual simuli in normal subjects. In *Structure and Function of the Cerebral Commissures*, I. S. Russell, M. H. Van Hof, and G. Berlucchi, eds. Dallas: University Park Press, pp. 390–399.

Rizzolatti, G., G. Bertoloni, and P. L. DeBastiani, 1982. Interference of concomitant tasks on simple reaction time: Attentional and motor factors. *Neuropsychologia* 20:447–455.

Robichon, F., and M. Habib, 1998. Abnormal callosal morphology in male adult dyslexics: Relationships to handedness and phonological abilities. *Brain Lang.* 62:127–146.

Rosenbaum, D. A., 1991. Programs for movement sequences. In *Bridges Between Psychology and Linguistics: A Swarthmore Festschrift for Lila Gleitmanpp*, D. J. Napoli and J. A. Kegl, eds. Hillsdale, N.J.: Lawrence Erlbaum Associates, pp. 19–33.

Rouiller, E. M., A. Babalian, O. Kazennikov, V. Moret, X. H. Yu, and M. Wiesendanger, 1994. Transcallosal connections of the distal forelimb representations of the primary and supplementary motor cortical areas in macaque monkeys. *Exp. Brain Res.* 102:227–243.

Rugg, M. D., 1982. Electrophysiological studies. In *Divided Visual Field Studies of Cerebral Organization*, J. G. Beaumont, ed. London: Academic Press, pp. 129–145.

Saron, C. D., and R. J. Davidson, 1989. Visual evoked potential measures of interhemispheric transfer time in humans. *Behav. Neurosci.* 103:1115–1138.

Savage, C. R., and D. G. Thomas, 1993. Information processing and interhemispheric transfer in left- and right-handed adults. *Int. J. Neurosci.* 71:201–219.

Schieppati, M., M. Musazzi, A. Nardone, and G. Seveso, 1984. Interhemispheric transfer of voluntary motor commands in man. *Electroencephalogr. Clin. Neurophysiol.* 57:441–447.

SERGENT, J., and J. J. MYERS, 1985. Manual, blowing, and verbal simple reactions to lateralized flashes of light in commissurotomized patients. *Percep. Psychophys.* 37:571–578.

SEYAL, M., T. RO, and R. RAFAL, 1995. Increased sensitivity to ipsilateral cutaneous stimuli following transcranial magnetic stimulation of the parietal lobe. *Ann. Neurol.* 38:264–267.

SIMON, J. R., P. E. SLY, and S. VILAPAKKAM, 1981. Effect of compatibility of S-R mapping on reactions toward the stimulus source. *Acta Psychol.* 47:63–81.

STOMONYAKOV, V., and A. VASSILEV, 1989. Hemispheric asymmetry of the harmonic components ot the visual potentials evoked by the onset-offset of spatially periodic stimuli. *Acta Physiol. Pharmacol. Bulg.* 15:63–69.

ST. JOHN, R., C. SHIELDS, P. KRAHN, and B. TIMNEY, 1987. The reliability of estimates of interhemispheric transmission times derived from unimanual and verbal response latencies. *Hum. Neurobiol.* 6:195–202.

SWANSON, J., A. LEDLOW, and M. KINSBOURNE, 1978. Lateral asymmetries revealed by simple reaction time. In *The Asymmetrical Function of the Brain*, M. Kinsbourne, ed. New York: Cambridge University Press, pp. 274–291.

SWAYZE, V. W., 2ND, V. P. JOHNSON, J. W. HANSON, J. PIVEN, Y. SATO, J. N. GIEDD, D. MOSNIK, and N. C. ANDREASEN, 1997. Magnetic resonance imaging of brain anomalies in fetal alcohol syndrome. *Pediatrics* 99:232–240.

TASSINARI, G., S. AGLIOTI, L. CHELAZZI, C. A. MARZI, and G. BERLUCCHI, 1987. Distribution in the visual field of the costs of voluntarily allocated attention and of the inhibitory aftereffects of covert orienting. *Neuropsychologia* 25:55–71.

TASSINARI, G., S. AGLIOTI, L. CHELAZZI, A. PERU, and G. BERLUCCHI, 1994a. Do peripheral non-informative cues induce early facilitation of target detection? *Vision Res.* 34:179–189.

TASSINARI, G., S. AGLIOTI, R. PALLINI, G. BERLUCCHI, and G. F. ROSSI, 1994b. Interhemispheric integration of simple visuomotor responses in patients with partial callosal defects. *Behav. Brain Res.* 64:141–149.

TASSINARI, G., and G. BERLUCCHI, 1993. Sensory and attentional components of slowing of manual reaction time to non-fixated visual targets by ipsilateral primes. *Vision Res.* 33:1525–1534.

TASSINARI, G., M. BISCALDI, C. A. MARZI, and G. BERLUCCHI, 1989. Ipsilateral inhibition and contralateral facilitation of simple reaction time to non-foveal visual targets from non-informative visual cues. *Acta Psychol.* 70:267–291.

TOLCHENOVA, G. A., C. S. IMANKULOVA, and N. I. SCHEVCHENKO, 1980. A complex approach to the study of interneuronal connections of cat associative cortex. *Nerv. Sys.* [Russian] 22:7–11.

VAN ESSEN, D., W. T. NEWSOME, and J. L. BIXBY, 1982. The pattern of interhemispheric connections and its relationship to extrastriate visual areas in the macaque monkey. *J. Neurophysiol.* 2:265–283.

VAN ORDEN, K. F., and J. F. HOUSE, 1996. Spatial frequency-dependant asymmetry of visual evoked potential amplitudes. *Percep. Mot. Skills* 82:1011–1018.

WALLACE, R. J., 1971. S-R compatibility and the idea of a response code. *J. Exp. Psychol.* 88:354–360.

WEBSTER, W. G., 1988. Neural mechanisms underlying stuttering: evidence from bimanual handwriting performance. *Brain Lang.* 33:226–244.

WEEKES, N. Y., and E. ZAIDEL, 1996. The effects of procedural variations on lateralized stroop effects. *Brain Cogn.* 31:308–330.

WEEKES, N. Y., L. CAPETILLO-CUNLIFFE, J. RAYMAN, M. IACOBONI, and E. ZAIDEL, 1999. Individual differences in the hemispheric specialization of dual route variables. *Brain Lang.* 67:110–133.

WIRZ, J. A., and E. CHAPPUIS-ARNDT, 1976. Sex specific differences in chlorimipramine inhibition of serotonin uptake in human platelets. *Eur. J. Pharmacol.* 40:21–25.

WITELSON, S. F., 1985. The brain connection: The corpus callosum is larger in left-handers. *Science* 229:665–668.

ZAIDEL, E., 1983. Disconnection syndrome as a model for laterality effects in the normal brain. In *Cerebral Hemisphere Asymmetry*, J. Hellige, ed. New York: Praeger, pp. 95–151.

ZAIDEL, E., 1986. Callosal dynamics and right hemisphere language. In *Two Hemispheres—One Brain: Functions of the Corpus Callosum*, F. Leporé, M. Ptito, and H. Jasper, eds. New York: AR Liss, pp. 435–459.

ZAIDEL, E., H. WHITE, E. SAKURAI, and W. BANKS, 1988. Hemispheric locus of lexical congruity effects: Neuropsychological reinterpretation of psycholinguistic results. In *Right Hemisphere Contributions to Lexical Semantics*, C. Chiarello, ed. New York: Springer-Verlag, pp. 71–88.

COMMENTARY 9.1

Does the CUD in SRT Measure IHTT? Or: Is the Crossed-Uncrossed Difference in the Simple Reaction Time Task a Pure Measure of Interhemispheric Transfer Time?

ERAN ZAIDEL AND MARCO IACOBONI

Braun, Achim, and Larocque (henceforth BAL) present an historical account of the crossed-uncrossed difference (CUD), arguing that its interpretation has evolved from a single-channel model to a model of a network of channels that can be modulated by task variables, show individual differences, and reflect factors other than callosal relay. In particular, BAL are impressed by the dependency of the CUD on hemispheric activation. But BAL's is a paradigm in transition: They cling to a concept of a single fixed-capacity callosal channel, without completely integrating it within a dynamic network model, which they also espouse. We have attempted such an integration in the introductory chapter of this volume. BAL's arguments include (1) theoretical, (2) methodological, and (3) substantive empirical claims. We will review these in turn from the vantage point of the introductory chapter.

Theoretical claims

THE CUD IN CHOICE RT TASKS DOES NOT MEASURE IHTT   It seems clear that the CUD in complex reaction time (CRT) tasks, which is typically ~30 ms or larger and is sometimes negative, does not measure simple sensory or motor relay through the corpus callosum

ERAN ZAIDEL   Department of Psychology, University of California at Los Angeles, Los Angeles, California.
MARCO IACOBONI   Ahmanson Lovelace Brain Mapping Center, Neuropsychiatric Institute, Brain Research Institute, David Geffen School of Medicine, University of California at Los Angeles, Los Angeles, California.

(CC). Rather, response hand × target visual hemifield (h × VF) interactions most likely reflect independent processing in each hemisphere (sensory isolation), resource dependence between the two hemispheres, and cognitive callosal relay (Zaidel et al., 1990). Such h × VF interactions are rare and can show either an ipsilateral h − VF advantage (a positive CUD, reflecting resource independence between the hemispheres, so that the same hemisphere can optimally control both the input and output stages of processing) or a contralateral h − VF advantage (a negative CUD, reflecting limited resources within the hemispheres and resource dependence between the hemispheres, so that segregating input and output processing to opposite hemispheres is advantageous). BAL are quite right that the CUD in CRT shows a spatial compatibility effect and that there is no linear relationship between task complexity (overall reaction time (RT)) and the size of the CUD. On the other hand, we and others have shown that increased task complexity leading to resource limitation can switch the CUD from positive to negative (Zaidel et al., 1988).

NEGATIVE CUD   BAL consider a negative CUD inconsistent with the single-channel concept of the CC. In fact, the CUD "algebra" shows that if callosal relay occurs through different channels from the right hemisphere (RH) to the left hemisphere (LH) and from the LH to the RH, then the CUD is not equal to interhemispheric transfer time (IHTT). Let V_R = latency of visual registration in the RH, D_R = latency of target detection in the RH, MP_R = latency of motor programming in the

RH, CR_{RL} = latency of callosal relay from the RH to the LH, M_R = latency of motor output in the RH, and so on. Suppose CR_{RL} is motor, following stimulus detection, but CR_{LR} is visual, prior to stimulus detection. Then the CUD = $[(D_R - D_L) + 2MP_R + (CR_{RL} + CR_{LR})] \div 2$ (see the introductory chapter). The value is negative if D_L is larger enough than D_R. Thus, if the task shows a robust RH specialization, then relay at different information-processing loci in the two directions can lead to a negative CUD. This does not challenge the anatomical model, but, of course, it presupposes a multiple-channel model.

BAL report five experiments that found a negative CUD, but none was significant. To this list we can add another experiment of our own with blocked response hand and visual field of target, using 4° target eccentricity. We obtained an average CUD of −3 ms, but it too was not significantly different from zero. That means that the condition of relay through sufficiently different channels is rarely met. However, BAL note that two of three experiments with "inverted" left-handers (angle between pencil and line on the written page is 790°) showed significant negative CUDs. BAL attribute this to a difference in hemispheric specialization for motor control. But as the CUD algebra shows, the CUD is independent of hemispheric specialization or of manual dominance, as long as the usual assumptions are met, including relay in both directions at the same information processing stage.

Of course, the most natural interpretation of a negative CUD is that ipsilateral motor control is faster than contralateral routes. It is easy to imagine conditions in which this would be the case, as when callosal channels are otherwise occupied.

How can we obtain CUDs that are not significantly different from zero? It could reflect a shift across channels between and within subjects, with some transfer in opposite directions occurring across channels that differ in speed. This would mean that relay channels can change dramatically within a task, as a function of shifts in attention, strategy, and skill.

ASYMMETRICAL IHTT   BAL note that Marzi, Bisiacchi, and Nicoletti's 1991 meta-analysis, Braun's own 1992 meta-analysis, and Braun and colleagues (1996a) all show a consistent pattern of a right-hand advantage (RhA) and a left visual field advantage (LVFA). They argue that this could be due to slower IHTT from the LH to the RH than vice versa. Suppose this corresponds to channels interconnecting homologous modules. In fact, the meta-analysis shows also that LVF-Rh < (is faster than) RVF-Lh. We can schematize the information-processing sequence from sensory registration to motor

response and estimate the response times in the four possible experimental visual fields by response hand conditions as follows:

(i)   LVF-Lh: $V_R + P_R + \phantom{CR_{RL} +} M_R$ (uncrossed)

(ii) LVF-Rh: $V_R + P_R + CR_{RL} + M_L$ (crossed)

(iii) RVF-Rh: $V_L + P_L + \phantom{CR_{RL} +} M_L$ (uncrossed)

(iv) RVF-Lh: $V_L + P_L + CR_{LR} + M_R$ (crossed)

where V_R is the latency of visual registration in the right hemisphere (LVF), V_L is the latency of visual registration in the left hemisphere (RVF), P_L is the latency of stimulus detection in the left hemisphere, P_R is the latency of stimulus detection in the right hemisphere, M_R is the latency of motor response with the Lh (right hemisphere), M_L is the latency of motor response with the Rh (left hemisphere), CR_{RL} is the latency of callosal relay from the right hemisphere to the left hemisphere, and CR_{LR} is the latency of callosal relay from the left hemisphere to the right hemisphere. We can incorporate next the hemispheric contributions to visual registration and stimulus detection into one component designated V, assuming that the same hemisphere that receives the visual stimulus makes the detection. Then equations (i)–(iv) simplify into

(i′)   LVF-Lh: $V_R + \phantom{CR_{RL} +} M_R$ (uncrossed)

(ii′) LVF-Rh: $V_R + CR_{RL} + M_L$ (crossed)

(iii′) RVF-Rh: $V_L + \phantom{CR_{RL} +} M_L$ (uncrossed)

(iv′) RVF-Lh: $V_L + CR_{LR} + M_R$ (crossed)

From these equations we can get

(v)   LVF − RVF = [i′] + [ii′] − [iii′] − [iv′]
$$= 2(V_R - V_L) + (CR_{RL} - CR_{LR})$$

(vi)   Lh − Rh = [i′] + [iv′] − [ii′] − [iii′]
$$= 2(M_R - M_L) + (CR_{LR} - CR_{RL})$$

(vii) uncrossed difference = [i′] − [iii′]
$$= (V_R - V_L) + (M_R - M_L)$$

(viii) crossed difference = [ii′] − [iv′]
$$= (V_R - V_L) + (CR_{LR} - CR_{LR})$$
$$+ (M_L - M_R)$$

From Marzi and colleagues' (1991) meta-analysis (Figure 9.11) we know that

(ix)   [v] < 0

(x)   [vi] > 0

(vi)   [vii] = 0

(vii) [viii] < 0

These conditions are consistent with either of the following two solutions: (1) CR_{RL} < (is faster than) CR_{LR}, as

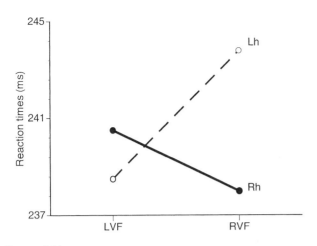

FIGURE 9.11.

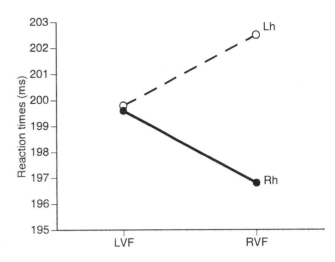

FIGURE 9.12.

suggested by BAL, including (1′) $V_L > V_R$ and (1″) $M_R > M_L$, or (2) $V_L > V_R$ and $M_R > M_L$ and, in particular, (2′) $CR_{LR} = CR_{RL}$. Thus, the meta-analysis need not imply asymmetry in relay. In particular, the asymmetry in hemispheric visual processing ($V_L > V_R$) need not be associated with asymmetrical transfer, as proposed by BAL. BAL argue that "an equivalent condition for the inference of asymmetry of transfer in SRT (as distinguished from a combination of independent field and hand effects) is that the two uncrossed conditions should not differ from each other." But our solution (2) above, yielding symmetric transfer, was in fact made assuming no difference between the uncrossed conditions, as dictated by the "meta-analytic" pattern (Bisiacchi et al., 1994).

Bisiacchi and colleagues (1994) offer circumstantial support for the argument that the meta-analytic response hand × visual field pattern reflects faster callosal relay from the RH to the LH than from the LH to the RH alone rather than RH specialization for visual processing ($V_R < V_L$) and LH specialization for motor programming/response ($M_L < M_R$) alone. Now, inequalities (ix)–(xii) have all of the following three solutions: (1) $CR_{RL} < CR_{LR}$, $M_L = M_R$, $V_L = V_R$, (2) $V_R < V_L$, $M_L < M_R$ ($V_L - V_R = M_R - M_L$), $CR_{RL} = CR_{LR}$, and (3) $V_R < V_L$, $M_L < M_R$, $CR_{RL} < CR_{LR}$. Bisiacchi and colleagues offer independent evidence that $V_L = V_R$ and $M_L = M_R$. If true, that would indeed show that only solution (1) is possible. It would then follow that $CR_{RL} < CR_{LR}$, as they claim.

The independent evidence comes from an SRT paradigm with central targets but unimanual responses and from another with lateralized targets but central (chin) responses. The experiment with central targets can be assumed to have enough of the target in both VFs to allow uncrossed responses, and it reduces conditions (i′)–

(iv′) to $V_R + M_R = V_L + M_L$, that is, $V_R - V_L = M_L - M_R$. As we showed above, this is consistent with solution (2), in which $V_R < V_L$, $M_L < M_R$, and $CR_{LR} = CR_{RL}$. Thus, the experiment with central targets shows neither equal hemispheric visual processing nor asymmetrical relay.

The experiment with central responses can be assumed to involve the same access to the response process in both hemispheres and also to allow uncrossed responses, so it reduces (i′)–(iv′) to $V_R + M = V_L + M$. This does suggest that $V_R = V_L$. It would then follow that $M_L = M_R$, so solution (1) obtains, and $CR_{RL} = CR_{LR}$ as argued by Bisiacchi and colleagues. But there is a difficulty here. Bisiacchi and colleagues' experiments with central targets and with central responses were interpreted here in light of the patterns (inequalities) observed in Marzi and colleagues' meta-analysis. Unfortunately, Bisiacchi and colleagues' own pattern of results in a standard SRT paradigm (Figure 9.12) diverges from the meta-analytic pattern (Figure 9.11).

The pattern in Figure 9.12 yields the following inequalities:

(xiii) $[v] = 0$

(xiv) $[vi] > 0$

(xv) $[vii] > 0$

(xvi) $[viii] < 0$

These inequalities have three solutions with different relationships between CR_{LR} and CR_{RL}: (1) $CR_{LR} = CR_{RL}$, $V_L = V_R$, $M_R > M_L$; (2) $CR_{LR} > CR_{RL}$, $V_R > V_L$; (3) $CR_{RL} > CR_{LR}$, $V_R < V_L$. All three solutions are inconsistent with the results from the experiments with central targets and central responses, which require that $V_L = V_R$ and $M_L = M_R$. Thus, Bisiacchi and colleagues' data are internally inconsistent. This may not be surprising. It may be unreasonable to assume that visual, decision, and motor processes bear the same interrelationships in the standard and the central paradigms.

In sum, Bisiacchi and colleagues' data are mutually inconsistent across experiments and do not support the conclusion that the SRT paradigm reflects asymmetrical transfer. However, if we accept only their central results in combination with the meta-analytic pattern and ignore their own standard SRT results, then there is evidence for asymmetrical transfer. The inconsistency across Bisiacchi and colleagues' experiments suggests that the assumption that some processes are shared between the central and the lateralized experiments may be oversimplified.

Event-related potentials (ERPs) can avoid many of these complications by measuring the asymmetry at any stage in the information-processing sequence, assuming adequate spatial localization from electrode sites. The ERP evidence cited by BAL for asymmetrical IHTT is more compelling than the argument from behavioral data. Further, a review of ERP experiments led BAL to conclude that latency measures show faster relay from the RH to the LH than from the LH to the RH but also, surprisingly, that amplitude measures show the opposite pattern: stronger relay from the LH to the RH than from the RH to the LH. BAL go on to posit the existence of a specific control mechanism that produces the asymmetry: Information transfer from the RH to the LH is faster, whereas information transfer from the LH to the RH is more precise. This is an intriguing idea, but just because we are ignorant about the origin of the effect, it does not follow that the effect is due to a specialized, dedicated callosally centered mechanism. More generally, the relationships between anatomical, physiological, and behavioral correlates of callosal channels remain largely unknown. In particular, the behavioral significance of asymmetrical ERP transfer measures is unclear.

PARALLEL CHANNELS   BAL, like much of the literature in the past 20 years, cogently argue that the CC does not consist of a single or several simple channels with a 1-bit channel capacity, but rather of multiple channels that differ in capacity and speed. Clarke and Zaidel (1989) outlined the behavioral characteristics of a parallel-channel model controlled by a horse race, and Aboitiz and colleagues (1992) provided an anatomical basis for it. Briefly, different cortical modules are interconnected by different (but overlapping) topographically organized callosal and subcallosal channels. Any computation activates multiple intrahemispheric and interhemispheric pathways, and the callosal channel associated with the fastest computation dominates the response. Sensorimotor modules are interconnected by large-diameter myelinated fibers that predominate in the posterior midbody and somewhat in the posterior splenium, whereas modules in association cortex interconnect through small-diameter unmyelinated fibers that predominate in the anterior callosum and in the middle of the splenium. Different cortical modules process information of different cognitive complexity, and they incorporate attentional effects. The capacity and speed of callosal channels of specific modules then reflect the cognitive complexity of the relayed information.

Thus, a long IHTT need not reflect extraneous components in addition to a true IHTT, as BAL would have it, but could rather reflect true cognitive relay. This also explains why different methods for eliciting the CUD (e.g., vocal versus unimanual responses) provide different estimates of IHTT and why the CUD can be modulated by manipulating motor and attentional variables. Thus, BAL have no cause for alarm on that score. In particular, it is not necessary to posit that task demands affect the properties of a single channel, and it is sufficient to posit instead that task demands determine the decision modules and that different modules engage different callosal channels.

BALANCE OF COST   BAL highlight the concept of balance of cost or relative hemispheric activation as a determinant of the CUD. They argue that task demands can change the degree of hemispheric involvement and consequently interhemispheric transfer. Changing the hemispheric balance of cost is tantamount to changing V, P, or M in the algebra underlying SRT. In the example above, equations (vii) and (viii) yield $CUD = CR_{RL} - CR_{LR} + 2(M_L - M_R)$. Thus, if the task activates motor cortex asymmetrically, the CUD can indeed change, but this change need not reflect a change in interhemispheric transfer. The CUD measures IHTT only if $M_L = M_R$.

Methodological claims

LATENCY VERSUS ACCURACY   BAL challenge the commonplace assumption that callosal relay results in loss of speed as well as in stimulus degradation and that, in principle, latency and accuracy should show similar effects on the CUD. This equivalence should actually apply to speed and sensitivity (d') but not necessarily to accuracy, which is sensitive to strategy effects. Consequently, observing a different pattern with different types of errors (accuracy) is not relevant. General rationales for dissociating speed and accuracy in behavioral analysis are weak. There is the special case of speed-accuracy trade-off when resources are limited (Norman and Bobrow, 1975). More generally, Mordkoff and Egeth (1993) argued that these two dependent variables index different components of the information-processing sequence: Accuracy measures the decision process, whereas speed measures also response programming. Indeed, behavioral laterality effects are not identical in both measures and are more common in accuracy (Zaidel, 1983).

But in the case of the CUD for SRT, BAL offer a particularly natural model for the dissociation between speed and sensitivity. They distinguish between signal velocity and signal strength. This model has a simple interpretation in the ERP: The latency differential of an appropriate component of the wave form indexes the velocity CUD, whereas the amplitude differential of the wave component indexes the strength CUD. Then relay asymmetries of the ERP suggest faster relay from right to left but more precise relay from left to right. Indeed, Hoptman and colleagues (1996) observed an aging-related decrease in relay strength but not speed as measured by the ERP.

ERP Versus Behavior With better techniques for spatial localization of the ERP dipole/generator, we can now associate frontotemporal leads with motor callosal relay, occipital leads with visual relay, and parietal leads with cognitive relay between temporoparietal association cortex. ERP evidence for asymmetry of IHTT in a callosal channel (Braun et al., 1996b) is more compelling than behavioral evidence because it involves fewer inferential steps, but one needs to first establish a strong concordance between ERP and behavioral measures of callosal relay before discrepancies between the two measures can be interpreted strongly. BAL report that CUDs measured from posterior sites (at what target eccentricity?) tend to be long (15–20 ms). This is in line with behavioral estimates for visual transfer at large eccentricities, not for short ones (Iacoboni et al., 1994). Estimates reported from anterior electrodes (1–5 ms) do fit behavioral estimates of motor relay. Braun and colleagues (1996b) also report that CUD estimates for the N1 wave at frontal sites correlate with CUD estimates from behavior. More generally, a discrepancy between the RT CUD and the ERP CUD is problematic only if it pertains to a dominant channel that controls the behavioral response. The ERP CUD at various sites may tap the IHTT through parallel but slower channels that do not affect the behavioral response. The picture is further complicated by Saron's observation (this volume) of ERP evidence for multiple motor/visual interhemispheric transfers before response in SRT.

Variability of the CUD BAL note that there are very large differences in the CUDs across individuals. In a sample of 135 right-handers they found CUDs ranging from −42 ms to 105 ms, but there is no information on the number of trials or on the reliability of the measure. What is the relationship between the variability of the CUD within an individual and across individuals? We analyzed the CUDs of three individuals over some 12,000 trials of an SRT task. The distribution of the CUDs within an individual was comparable to that across individuals in a group of 20 normal subjects (Iacoboni and Zaidel, 2000). This suggests again that the modules and channels subserving the SRT task vary with attentional shifts, with practice, and with strategy. The reliability of the CUD increases with target blocking and with focused attention (see Chapter 13 in this volume).

In view of the large variability in the CUD within and across subjects, it makes sense to use meta-analyses to study individual differences in the CUD. Meta-analyses use the more stable means of whole experiments and can be more reliable than individual experiments, provided that the inclusion criteria are coherent and consistent. But BAL report no meta-analytic data on sex or handedness effects on the CUD.

Empirical claims: Visual, attentional, and motor effects on the CUD

Visual Effects BAL note that of seven experiments investigating the effect of target eccentricity on the CUD, only one was significant (St. John et al., 1987). However, BAL also point out that all experiments obtained the same trend of increasing CUDs with increasing eccentricity and argue that the failure of the effect to be significant reflects the inherent noisiness of the CUD rather than the invalidity of the effect.

We recently administered to normal subjects an SRT task in which the visual targets consisted of images of a right hand, a left hand, or a neutral stimulus of a "cut and rearranged" hand (Aziz-Zadeh et al., 2002). Both neutral and hand stimuli showed negative CUDs that did not differ significantly from each other—so far, nothing new.

Subjects were also tested with the response hands in a crossed, unnatural position (i.e., right hand on the left, left hand on the right) to assess the possible effect of response arrangement on the CUD. The change in response arrangement (natural or uncrossed, unnatural or crossed) can be regarded as a motor manipulation of the experiment or, alternatively, as a manipulation of spatial attention. The CUD with hand stimuli was significantly sensitive to response arrangement, changing from −4 ms in the natural position to +4 ms in the unnatural position. By contrast, response arrangement did not have an effect on the CUD with neutral stimuli. Thus, a combination of meaningful stimuli and allocation of attention in motor space can affect the CUD.

The effect of hand stimuli may be attributed to a sensory-attentional-motor/parietal-prefrontal loop in which visual changes affect motor decision and consequently the motor transfer channel. It may be argued, on the other hand, that the effect of hand stimuli is due to an implicit choice RT task involving decision between left and right hand images, which is automatically engaged by the SRT task. In that case, part of the response hand × visual field interaction (the CUD) is due to the implicit choice rather than the explicit simple RT task.

Similar negative findings apply to the effects of target intensity on the CUD. BAL go on to summarize several new experiments that study the effects of motor and attentional manipulations on the CUD.

MOTOR EFFECTS Godbout, Achim, and Braun (1995) used an SRT task with random target presentation in the two VFs and with three response modes: (1) a standard blocked unimanual response, (2) a condition requiring three unimanual keypresses in a rapid succession upon detection, and (3) a condition requiring alternating response hands on sequential trials. The three taps condition resulted in a negative CUD (−8.27 ms), but this was not significantly different from the CUD in the standard condition. The alternating hands condition significantly prolonged the CUD (15 ms) relative to the standard condition (4.03 ms). This confirms the usual finding that motor manipulations affect the CUD (Table 9.2).

BAL review briefly the CUD obtained in an SRT task in which subjects were asked to respond with both hands simultaneously. This can be considered a motor manipulation of the SRT paradigm. They reason that bimanual responses should prime both hemispheres symmetrically and increase the CUD while decreasing overall RT. We carried out an SRT experiment with bimanual responses consisting of 160 trials and 32 subjects (Mooshagian et al., unpublished data). There was a slight decrease of overall RT from ∼253 ms to ∼249 ms. As far as the CUD is concerned, it is not altogether clear how to compute it, since each trial has a leading hand latency and a following hand latency. Should we use all trials? Leading hand trials only? Congruent trials only, that is, leading right-hand responses in the RVF and following left-hand responses in the RVF, leading left-hand responses in the LVF and following right-hand responses in the LVF? Each of these alternative measures has a reasonable rationale, and they all yield different CUDs. All trials combined yielded a CUD of 1.337 ms, leading hand trials yielded a CUD of −11.1 ms, and congruent trials yielded a CUD of 12.6 (positive by definition). This compares

TABLE 9.2
Summary of the effects of motor and attentional manipulations on the CUD

	RT	CUD
Motor		
Di Stefano et al. (1980) bimanual	+	+?
Iacoboni and Zaidel (1995) alternate fingers	−	+
Godbout et al. (1995) three presses	+	
Godbout et al. (1995) alternate hands		+
Attention		
Agliotti et al. (1993) VF blocking	+	−
Iacoboni and Zaidel spatial uncertainty	−	−
Iacoboni and Zaidel RG within hems.	+	−
Iacoboni and Zaidel RG between hems.	+	−
Braun et al. (1995)		
Valid cues	+	−
Invalid cues	+	−
Visual		
Berlucchi et al. (1971) Eccentricity	+	−
Berlucchi et al. (1977) Eccentricity	+	−
Milner and Lines (1982) Intensity	+	−
Lines et al. (1984) Intensity	+	−
St. John et al. (1987) Eccentricity		

with a CUD of 4.3 ms in the unimanual SRT (basic condition in Iacoboni and Zaidel, 1995). Thus, BAL's prediction is not uniformly supported.

Mooshagian and colleagues also administered this test to two commissurotomy patients (AA and NG; see Chapter 13 in this volume) but found the usual large CUDs when computed from all trials (AA = 37.1 ms, NG = 18 ms), unlike the results of Agliotti and colleagues (1993).

BAL believe that these changes in the CUD reflect factors other than IHTT, notably hemispheric activation. But as the algebra shows, hemispheric processing does not enter the computation of the CUD, assuming that the callosal relay channel remains the same. Our own interpretation of their findings, as well as of our own data (see Chapter 13 in this volume), is that the changes in the motor demands change the decision modules and thus also the channels that serve to interconnect them.

ATTENTIONAL EFFECTS BAL note that previous attempts to modulate hemispheric activation by using SRT with concurrent hemispherically specialized dual tasks failed to affect the CUD. Braun and colleagues (1995) combined an SRT task with a Posner-type spatial cuing paradigm. Each trial was preceded by a central arrow indicating the VF of the target. The cue was valid 80% of the time. There was a trend for valid cues to prolong the CUD ($\sim$10 ms) and for invalid cues to yield negative CUDs ($\sim$−10 ms), more so with shorter SOAs (1133 ms → $\sim$−17 ms CUD) than with larger SOAs (1450 ms → $\sim$−3 ms CUD), but these differences were not statistically significant, owing to a large variability in the CUD.

Conclusion

BAL's emerging concept of multiple callosal channels sensitive to hemispheric activation during SRT tasks is consonant with our own and others' view of the activation of parallel callosal and subcallosal channels during SRT—some sensory, some motor, and some cognitive. The dominant channel is determined by the detection modules, which shift as a function of task demand. An important remaining difference between our views is that BAL do not regard the CUD as a pure measure of IHTT, while we still do. Of course, the view that a callosal channel can be modulated by task demand is behaviorally, but not anatomically or physiologically, equivalent to the view that a callosal channel can be switched by those demands.

REFERENCES

ABOITIZ, F., A. B. SCHEIBEL, R. S. FISHER, and E. ZAIDEL, 1992. Fiber composition of the human corpus callosum. *Brain Res.* 598:143–153.

AGLIOTI, S., G. BERLUCCHI, R. PALLINI, G. R. ROSSI, and G. TASSINARI, 1993. Hemispheric control of unilateral and bilateral responses to lateralized light stimuli after callosotomy and in callosal agenesis. *Exp. Brain Res.* 95:151–165.

AZIZ-ZADEH, L., F. MAEDA, E. ZAIDEL, J. MAZZIOTTA, and M. IACOBONI. Lateralization in motor facilitation during action observations: a TMS study. *Ex. Brain Res.* 144:127–131.

BERLUCCHI, G., F. CREA, M. DI STEFANO, and G. TASSINAR, 1977. Influence of spatial stimulus-response compatibility on reaction time of ipsilateral and contralateral hand to lateralized light stimuli. *J. Exp. Psych. Hum. Percept. Perf.* 3:505–517.

BERLUCCHI, G., W. HERON, R. HYMAN, G. RIZZOLATTI, and C. UMILTA, 1971. Simple reaction times of ipsilateral and contralateral hand to lateralized visual stimuli. *Brain* 94:419–430.

BISIACCHI, P., C. A. MARZI, R. NICOLETTI, G. CARENA, C. MUCIGNAT, and F. TOMAIUOLO, 1994. Left-right asymmetry of callosal transfer in normal human-subjects. *Behav. Brain Res.* 64:173–178.

BRAUN, C. M. J., 1992. Estimation of hemispheric and interhemispheric dynamics from simple reaction time. *Neuropsychol. Rev.* 3:321–364.

BRAUN, C. M. J., S. DAIGNEAULT, S. MILJOURS, and A. DUFRESNE, 1995. Does hemispheric relay depend on attention? *Am. J. Psychol.* 108:527–546.

BRAUN, C. M. J., C. MAILHOUX, and A. DUFRESNE, 1996a. Left and right visual field advantages are a function of scotopic and photopic retinal adaptation respectively in simple reaction time to near-threshold targets. *Acta Psychologica* 91:3–14.

BRAUN, C. M. J., L. VILLENEUVE, and A. ACHIM, 1996b. Balance of cost in interhemispheric relay in the Poffenberger paradigm: Evidence from omission errors. *Neuropsychology* 10:565–572.

CLARKE, J. M., and E. ZAIDEL, 1989. Simple reaction times to lateralized light flashes: Varieties of interhemispheric communication routes. *Brain* 112:849–870.

DI STEFANO, M., M. MORELLI, C. A. MARZI, and G. BERLUCCHI, 1980. Hemispheric control of unilateral and bilateral movements of proximal and distal parts of the arm as inferred from simple reaction time to lateralized light stimuli in man. *Exp. Brain Res.* 38:197–204.

GODBOUT, J. A., A. ACHIM, and C. M. J. BRAUN, 1995. Modulation motrice des dynamiques interhémisphériques dans le paradigme de Poffenberger [Abstract]. *Comptes Rendus du 18ième Congrès de la Société Québécoise de Recherche en Psychologie, Ottawa*, p. 72.

HOPTMAN, M. J., R. J. DAVIDSON, A. GUDMUNDSSON, R. T. SCHREIBER, and W. B. ERSHLER, 1996. Age differences in visual evoked potential estimates of interhemispheric transfer. *Neuropsychology* 10:263–271.

IACOBONI, M., I. FRIED, and E. ZAIDEL, 1994. Callosal transmission time before and after partial commissurotomy. *Neuroreport* 5:2521–2524.

IACOBONI, M., and E. ZAIDEL, 1995. Channels of the corpus callosum: Evidence from simple reaction times to lateralized flashes in the normal and the split brain. *Brain* 118:779–788.

IACOBONI, M., and E. ZAIDEL, 2000. Crossed-uncrossed difference in simple reaction times to lateralized flashes: Between- and within-subjects variability. *Neuropsychologia* 38:535–541.

LINES, C. R., M. D. RUGG, and A. D. MILNER. The effect of stimulus intensity on visual evoked potential estimates of interhemispheric transmission time. *Exp. Brain Res.* 57:89–98.

MARZI, C. A., P. BISIACCHI, and R. NICOLETTI, 1991. Is interhemispheric transfer of visuomotor information asymmetric? Evidence from a meta-analysis. *Neuropsychologia* 29:1163–1177.

MILNER, A. D., and C. R. LINES, 1982. Interhemispheric pathways in simple reaction time to lateralized light flash. *Neuropsychologia* 20:171–179.

MORDKOFF, J. T., and H. E. EGETH, 1993. Response time and accuracy revisited: Converging support for the interactive race model. *J. Exper. Psych. Hum. Percept. Perf.* 19:981–991.

NORMAN, D. A., and D. G. BOBROW, 1975. On data limited and resources limited. *Cognit. Psychol.* 7:44–64.

ST. JOHN, R., C. SHIELDS, P. KRAHN, and B. TIMNEY, 1987. The reliability of estimates of interhemispheric transmission times derived from unimanual and verbal response latencies. *Hum. Neurobiol.* 6:195–202.

ZAIDEL, E., 1983. Disconnection syndrome as a model for laterality effects in the normal brain. In *Cerebral Hemisphere Asymmetry: Method, Theory and Application*, J. Hellige, ed. New York: Praeger, pp. 95–151.

ZAIDEL, E., H. WHITE, E. SAKURAI, and W. BANKS, 1988. Hemispheric locus of lexical congruity effects: Neuropsychological reinterpretation of psycholinguistic results. In *Right Hemisphere Contributions to Lexical Semantics*, C. Chiarello, ed. New York: Springer-Verlag, pp. 71–88.

Commentary 9.2

Interacting Hemispheres: A Means of Modulating Attention

MARIE T. BANICH

ABSTRACT Interaction between the cerebral hemispheres can serve to modulate attentional functioning of the human brain. We have found that interaction between the hemispheres is more advantageous to performance when tasks are computationally difficult rather than easy. We have also found that a division and subsequent reintegration of information across the hemispheres enhance selective attention. This phenomenon occurs both when selection is based on perceptual attributes and when selection is made at the level of a response. We interpret these findings as indicating that dividing processing across the hemispheres can increase the brain's computational capacity.

As this volume illustrates, researchers trying to understand the functioning of the corpus callosum are faced with a complex problem. Although we know the callosum to be the brain structure that is critically important for the transfer of information between the cerebral hemispheres, certain aspects of its functioning remain murky. Braun rightly suggests in his chapter that rather than conceptualizing the callosum as a single cable, we might better consider it as a network of connections—multiple channels, if you will. Such a notion is compatible with our knowledge that different sections of the callosum transfer different types of information (e.g., visual, motor, somatosensory, or tactual), suggesting specialized channels for differing representations of information. Evidence from neuroanatomy and electrophysiology also suggests the possibility of distinct temporal channels as well. For example, different regions of the callosum have varying degrees of myelination (see Aboitiz, this volume, and Aboitiz et al., 1992), and interhemispheric transfer times for different types of callosal signals appear to vary (e.g., see Chapter 8 in this volume and Rugg, Lines, and Milner, 1984). However, disentangling which channel we are measuring in any

given situation may prove to be somewhat difficult. This problem gets compounded as we move from trying to measure the transfer of basic sensory information (the onset of a light flash) to transfer about more complicated information, such as an object. For example, in the case of an object, information could be transferred in a multiplicity of ways: as a pattern of light and dark, as a description of geometric form, as a semantic description, and so forth.

There is, however, another question that we can ask with regards to callosal transfer. Rather than trying to determine what type of information is being sent across which section of the callosum at what time, we can ask the question of how the very fact of callosal transfer affects the information processing capacity of the human brain. Are there any emergent properties or functions of callosal transfer that occur because the callosum allows for integration between the specialized hemispheres? Work in our laboratory suggests, in fact, that interaction between the cerebral hemispheres via the corpus callosum has the ability to modulate the attentional capacity of the brain. We have found that under attentionally demanding conditions, mandatory interaction between the hemispheres actually improves task performance compared to situations in which interhemispheric interaction is not required. Our findings are robust, as we have demonstrated them across a variety of manipulations of attentional demands and across numerous modalities. Here I will just try to provide a flavor of those findings.

In our studies, we typically utilize a task in which an individual must decide whether a target item presented to one hemisphere matches either of two probes, each probe being directed to a different hemisphere. We have two types of trials. In one type, the target and matching probes are directed to opposite hemispheres, which necessitates that the hemispheres interact via the callosum if a decision is to be reached (across-hemisphere trials).

MARIE T. BANICH Departments of Psychology and Psychiatry, University of Colorado, Boulder, Colorado.

In the other type, the target and matching probes are directed to the same hemisphere and hence do not require interhemispheric interaction (within-hemisphere trials). The comparison between across- and within-hemisphere trials is critical for determining the effects of interhemispheric communication (for a larger discussion of this issue, see Banich and Shenker, 1994). We then typically have two conditions that vary in the attentional demands they impose upon the participant: one involving lesser attentional demands and one involving greater attentional demands.

We have examined how interaction between the hemispheres modulates attentional functioning from a variety of different perspectives. One theory of attention, multiple resource theory (e.g., Wickens and Liu, 1988) assumes that resources must be devoted to task performance, and because the brain has a limited processing capacity, those resources are limited. It has been suggested that each of the hemispheres has a separate and distinct resource pool, although the hemispheres may share a subcortical pool of resources (e.g., Herdman and Friedman, 1985). We have varied the attentional demands of a task by manipulating its computational complexity, that is, the number and kinds of operations that must be performed for a decision to be reached. In our less demanding task, we typically have individuals decide whether two items are physically identical, which merely requires a perceptual analysis of form and then a comparison. In our more demanding tasks, we ask individuals to make a decision that requires not only perceptual analysis of form and a comparison, but at least one additional step in processing. We have used a variety of tasks, including a name-matching task (e.g., A a) (Banich and Belger, 1990, Experiment 1) that requires the extraction of a name- or case-specific letter code, a summation task that requires two numbers to be added (Banich and Belger, 1990, Experiment 3), an ordinal task that requires the value of two numbers to be compared (Banich and Belger, 1990, Experiment 3), a spelling task that requires a comparison between a target word and two letters (Banich et al., 1990), and a form categorization task that requires the determination of whether two perceptually distinct forms (e.g., an isosceles triangle and equilateral triangle) belong to the same category (i.e., triangle) (Banich and Passarotti, unpublished manuscript). Invariably, we obtain a significant interaction between trial type (within-hemisphere, across-hemisphere) and condition (less attentionally demanding, more attentionally demanding). Typically, we obtain superior performance on across-hemisphere trials as compared to within-hemisphere trials for the more computationally complex and hence more attentionally demanding task, a pattern that is not observed for the less demanding task. The effect is linked to the computational complexity of the tasks, as it cannot be predicted solely on the basis of general task difficulty (e.g., predicted by mean RT; see Weissman and Banich, in press a; Weissman, Banich, and Puente, 2000). Thus, interaction between the hemispheres appears to be beneficial to task performance under demanding conditions.

We interpret these results in the following manner. When tasks are computationally simple, they can easily be performed by one hemisphere, and no advantage is derived from dividing processing across the hemispheres. In fact, the communication overhead required by interhemispheric integration actually makes interaction between the hemispheres disadvantageous. However, as tasks get more complex, the additional computational power gained by dividing processing across the hemispheres more than outweighs the overhead of communication costs between the hemispheres.

This phenomenon has a number of interesting aspects. In the studies described above, the trials were constructed to be of two types: one in which the hemispheres were forced to communicate and another in which they weren't. We simply observed which trial type yielded superior performance. What we have recently demonstrated is that the hemispheres can adaptively change their mode of processing, decoupling when tasks are relatively simple and coupling when they are more computationally complex (Weissman and Banich, 2000). Furthermore, Reuter-Lorenz, Stanczak, and Miller (1999) have demonstrated that relative to younger adults, older adults exhibit greater benefits from interhemispheric interaction in behavioral studies. They have suggested that having both hemispheres involved in processing may be a processing strategy that the aging brain employs to cope with diminished capacity.

We believe that these effects are general, rather than specific to transfer of visual information, because when we perform analogous studies in the auditory and somatosensory modality, we obtain similar results (Passarotti, Banich, Sood, and Wong, 2000). Information in each of these sensory modalities is likely to be transferred by different segments of the callosum (visual information via the splenium, auditory information via the anterior splenial region, and tactile information via the posterior section of the body of the callosum; e.g., DeLacoste, Kirkpatrick, and Ross, 1985). Hence, this convergence across modalities makes it more likely that we are observing a general overall function of the callosum, rather than a function of a particular callosal region.

Additional evidence that interhemispheric interaction can modulate attentional capacity comes from other experiments in which we modulate attention by asking an individual to pay attention to one specific attribute of an item while ignoring another. We have investigated this issue by using well-known selective attention paradigms such as the global-local paradigm and selective attention to form while ignoring color. In the global-local paradigm as initially popularized by Navon (1977), an individual sees a hierarchical figure, which is a large global figure made up of local elements (e.g., a large S composed of little Ss). In one condition, the individual is instructed to attend to the global shape and base a decision on an item's characteristics at that level. In another condition, the individual is instructed to attend to the local elements and base a decision on an item's characteristics at that level. Performance is examined for two types of trials. In one type, the overall shape and the component parts are identical (e.g., a large S composed of small Ss), which are referred to as compatible trials. In the other type, the overall shape of the item and the component parts lead to different decisions (e.g., a large S composed of small Hs). These are referred to as incompatible trials. Usually, responses to incompatible trials take longer than responses to compatible trials because information at the irrelevant level on incompatible trials must be ignored to avoid an incorrect response. We have found that interference engendered by incompatible trials is reduced on across-hemisphere trials as compared to within-hemisphere trials (Weissman and Banich, 1999).

We have also found that the more that irrelevant information must be filtered to reach a correct decision, the more interhemispheric interaction aids task performance. We have demonstrated such an effect with a shape-matching task in which individuals must decide whether a target shape matches either of two probes with regard to form. The shapes varied in color, which allowed color to provide either redundant information or conflicting information with regard to the decision about form. For example in some trials, color provided a redundant cue because the target and the probe that matched the target in form were the same color, while the probe that did not match the target was also distinct in color from the probe. In such cases, little suppression of information about color would be needed to reach a correct decision. On other trials, however, the target and matching probe were different colors, and the nonmatching probe was the same color as the target. On these trials, the demands on selective attention were much greater as color information had to be filtered out and ignored to reach the correct decision about form. The more that information about the unattended attribute, color, had to be filtered to reach a correct decision, the more interhemispheric interaction aided task performance (Banich and Passarotti, unpublished manuscript).

Our studies suggest that the callosum may help in selective attention both with regard to the selection of perceptual attributes and with regard to the selection of responses. For example, the way in which trials were constructed in our global-local paradigm was such that information at the irrelevant level would lead individuals to make the wrong response. Thus, in this paradigm, interhemispheric interaction probably modulates interference with regard to response selection. But we also have other evidence from this paradigm that interhemispheric interaction can modulate interference at the perceptual level. Kimchi and Palmer (1985) report that selection of either the global or local level of a display is more difficult when hierarchical figures are composed of few local elements as compared to many. They have proposed that in few-element displays the global and local levels are more integral and cannot be as easily separated (i.e., the local elements affect perception of the global form and vice versa). Our results indicate that interhemispheric interaction reduces interference more for the few-element than for the many-element displays. This finding indicates that interhemispheric interaction can aid in perceptual selection as well (Weissman and Banich, 1999). We have obtained similar evidence in a modified Stroop paradigm that the reduction of interference by interhemispheric interaction is linked to both perceptual and response factors (Shenker and Banich, unpublished manuscript). In all of these cases we believe that the need for increased attentional selection increases the computational complexity of the task and that interhemispheric interaction aids with ameliorating that increased load. For example, in the global-local paradigm, having the additional step of having to ignore task-irrelevant information increases computational demands compared to a situation in which task-irrelevant information need not be ignored.

In sum, our work has demonstrated, through a variety of attentional manipulations and in a variety of modalities, that the corpus callosum plays a role in influencing the attentional processing of the brain. This perspective is consistent with recent findings in other laboratories and other conceptualizations of interhemispheric interaction (see, for example, Sohn, Liederman, and Reinitz, 1996, and Chapter 10 and Commentary 10.1 in this volume). As such, it should be realized that although the callosum serves the important function of serving as a conduit of information transfer between the cerebral hemisphere, it has additional functions, such as modulating attentional selection, as well.

ACKNOWLEDGMENTS Preparation of this chapter was supported by NIMH grant R01 MH54217. I thank Kirk Erickson for comments on this manuscript.

REFERENCES

ABOITIZ, F., A. B. SCHEIBEL, R. S. FISHER, and E. ZAIDEL, 1992. Fiber composition of the human corpus callosum. *Brain Res.* 598:143–153.

BANICH, M. T., and A. BELGER, 1990. Interhemispheric interaction: How do the hemispheres divide and conquer a task? *Cortex* 26:77–94.

BANICH, M. T., S. GOERING, N. STOLAR, and A. BELGER, 1990. Interhemispheric processing in left- and right-handers. *International J. Neurosci.* 54:197–208.

BANICH, M. T., and A. PASSAROTTI, unpublished manuscript. Interhemispheric interaction aids task performance under conditions of selective attention.

BANICH, M. T., and J. I. SHENKER, 1994. Investigations of interhemispheric processing: Methodological considerations. *Neuropsychology* 8:263–277.

DELACOSTE, M. C., J. B. KIRKPATRICK, and E. D. ROSS, 1985. Topography of the human corpus callosum. *J. Neuropathol. Exp. Neurol.* 44:578–591.

HERDMAN, C. M., and A. FRIEDMAN, 1985. Multiple resources in divided attention: A cross modal test of independence of hemispheric resources. *J. Exp. Psychol. Hum. Percept. Perf.* 11:40–49.

KIMCHI, R., and S. E. PALMER, 1985. Separability and integrality of global and local levels of hierarchical patterns. *J. Exp. Psychol. Hum. Percept. Perf.* 11:673–688.

NAVON, D., 1977. Forest before trees: The precedence of global features in visual perception. Cognitive Psychology 9:353–383.

PASSAROTTI, A. M., M. T. BANICH, R. K. SOOD, and J. M. WONG, 2002. A generalized role of interhemispheric interaction under attentionally-demanding conditions: Evidence from the auditory and tactile modalities. *Neuropsychologia* 40:1082–1096.

REUTER-LORENZ, P. A., L. STANCZAK, and A. C. MILLER, 1999. Neural recruitment and cognitive aging: Two hemispheres are better than one, especially as you age. *Psychol. Sci.* 10:494–500.

RUGG, M. D., C. R. LINES, and A. D. MILNER, 1984. Visual evoked potentials to lateralized visual stimuli and the measurement of interhemispheric transmission time. *Neuropsychologia* 22:215–225.

SHENKER, J. I., and M. T. BANICH, unpublished manuscript. The modulation of attentional capacity in the Stroop task by communication between the cerebral hemispheres.

SOHN, Y. S., J. LIEDERMAN, and M. T. REINITZ, 1996. Division of inputs between the hemispheres eliminates illusory conjunctions: Evidence of hemispheric independence. *Neuropsychologia* 34:1057–1068.

WEISSMAN, D. H., and M. T. BANICH, 2000. The cerebral hemispheres cooperate to perform complex but not simple tasks. *Neuropsychology.* 14:41–59.

WEISSMAN, D. H., and M. T. BANICH, 1999, Global-local interference modulated by communication between the hemispheres. *J. Exp. Psychol. Gen.* 128:283–308.

WEISSMAN, D. H., M. T. BANICH, and E. I. PUENTE, 2000. An unbalanced distribution of inputs across the hemispheres facilitates interhemispheric interaction. *J. Int. Neuropsychol. Soc.* 6:313–321.

WICKENS, C. D., and Y. LIU, 1988. Codes and modalities in multiple resources: A success and a qualification. *Hum. Factors* 30:599–616.

10 The Corpus Callosum Equilibrates the Cerebral Hemispheres

MARCEL KINSBOURNE

ABSTRACT The corpus callosum equilibrates a neural system that subserves selection between lateralized cerebral processors. Subcortically mediated reciprocal inhibition enables unequivocal choice between orienting right and orienting left, between activating the left hemisphere and activating the right. The callosum stabilizes this positive (difference-amplifying) feedback opponent processor interaction. It coactivates the unengaged and therefore underactive hemisphere, maintaining it ready to respond and distributing attentional capacity between the hemispheres. Many consequences of callosal section may reflect lack of coactivation rather than blocked information transmission. Intrahemispheric corticocortical connections may also subserve equilibration, by coactivating their within-hemisphere cortical target areas. This model provides an alternative to disconnection for explaining neuropsychological syndromes. Evidence for these propositions is derived from functional neuroanatomy, split-brain symptomatology, and studies of the crossed-uncrossed difference in reaction time.

"Releasing forces acting on the brain from moment to moment shut out from activity whole regions of the nervous system, as they conversely call vast other regions into play. The resultant singleness of action from moment to moment is a keystone in the construction of the individual whose unity it is the specific office of the nervous system to perfect."
—Sherrington (1906, p. 234)

To ensure "singleness of action," the self-organizing nervous system selects one action system, suppressing other candidate systems. However, it has to hold them in readiness in case changing circumstances demand their instant intervention. Because of their parallel organization and ability to program divergent and even incompatible responses, the hemispheres offer the greatest challenge to singleness of action.

I present evidence that the corpus callosum is an integral component of a cortical/subcortical system that determines which lateralized processor or cerebral

MARCEL KINSBOURNE Department of Psychology, New School University, New York, New York

hemisphere assumes control of computing and directional orienting and responding. Split-brain symptoms have traditionally been attributed to disconnection of a callosal information highway. Instead, they may reflect a lapse in the callosum's role in holding the currently unengaged hemisphere ready for action.

Antecedents

Imamura and then Yoshimura (cited by Doty, 1973) first demonstrated the callosum's integrating role in Exner's laboratory in Vienna in the early twentieth century. They inflicted frontal lesions on dogs, generating contralateral neglect, from which the dogs recovered. Callosal section reinstated the neglect. The ipsilateral hemisphere had compensated for its frontal lesion, apparently by transcallosal activation from the intact hemisphere. In Leningrad, Pavlov's student Bykov (Bykov, 1924; Bykov and Speransky, 1924) discovered that a unilateral tactile eliciting stimulus (CS) for a conditioned reflex (salivation) to food reward irradiates across the midline in the intact but not the callosotomized animal. A further intriguing observation by Bykov (1924) has escaped attention. Even after callosal section, a very intense contralateral CS elicits salivation. So, whereas disconnected hemispheres usually fail to influence each other, this failure is not absolute. Bykov's findings are compatible with my proposal that after callosal section, the unstimulated hemisphere becomes underactivated and loses control of behavior. However, an intense CS might reactivate the contralateral hemisphere enough to reinstate its control over behavior. Apart from this special case, Bykov demonstrated that in contemporary terms (Zaidel, Clarke, and Suyenobu, 1990), callosal section transforms "hemispheric coupling" into "hemispheric independence." He could condition the callosally sectioned dog at one and the same time to respond to the identical stimulus with excitation when delivered to one side of the body (e.g., the shoulder) and with inhibition when it was applied to the opposite side (cf. Pavlov, 1927). Bykov's discoveries anticipated such findings as simultaneous incompatible actions performed by the right and left hands in the human split brain and alien hand syndromes and in split-brain baboons (Trevarthen, 1978).

Switchboard theory

By the mid-nineteenth century, investigators knew that some brain functions are localized. How do localized processors ("centers") interact? Lacking the necessary neurophysiological foundations, clinicians framed metaphors in terms of current technology. For Wernicke (1900), the task was to "find the route, the telegraph line, by which the telegram is conveyed": the brain as switchboard—(Kinsbourne, 1978). Sensory information converges on the receptor surfaces, from which it converges step by step into the brain. Why not extrapolate ("intrapolate"?) this convergence into the cerebrum itself? From the first cortical relays, input flows along private and specifically targeted connections to inform a privileged brain area such as the left temporal language area (Eccles, 1965) or the left angular gyrus (Geschwind, 1965), putative cross-modal integrators. Channels that diverge from the central point code the intended act in ever more specific detail. Convergence/divergence in a wasp-waisted "centered brain" has been superseded by evidence for central parallel processing and the non-existence of any point "where it all comes together" (Dennett and Kinsbourne, 1992). Fessard (1954) presciently confessed, "one may be tempted to admit the irrational statement that a heterogenous system of activities in the nervous system could form a whole in the absence of any identified liaison" (p. 208). But neuropsychologists still use unidirectional information transfer along predetermined channels as an explanatory device. Guiard (1980) characterized the application of switchboard theory as follows: "The corpus callosum is the critical integration structure transmitting information continuously from one cortex to the other." For instance, "a copy of the visual world as seen in one hemisphere is sent over to the other" through the callosum (Gazzaniga, 1967).

The application of switchboard theory to callosal lesions dates back to Dejerine (1892). When Myers and Sperry (1953) rediscovered callosotomy effects, switchboard theory was once more in vogue. For Geschwind and Kaplan (1962), the neuropsychological deficits in callosal lesions reflect interrupted information transfer.

Equilibration offers a more dynamic view of the callosum and of extrinsic cortical connections (ECCs) in general: coactivation that moderates competition between cerebral areas for control of output mechanisms, that is, of behavior. Though this view is new to the corpus callosum, it is in line with classical neurophysiology (e.g., Sherrington, 1906). Equilibration enables the potentially competing areas conjointly, and more adaptively, to control behavior. Disturbed equilibration may explain the types of deficit that are caused by callosal lesions.

Extrinsic corticocortical connections

The recursive network organization of the cortical gray matter (Pandya, Seltzer, and Barbas, 1988; Sutton and Anderson, 1995) discourages a switchboard model. Neither encapsulated modules nor dedicated channels visibly breach this continuous feltwork of neurons. Architectonic transitions are gradual and undramatic. Anatomically more specific, the ECCs are discrete fiber bundles that sweep through the cerebral medulla between distant loci in cortex. Are these the information-transmitting channels postulated by disconnection theory? Alternatively, does the unit of computation straddle ECCs? Or do the ECCs mediate modulating influences between processing units?

Glutamatergic projections of pyramidal cells (Braitenberg and Schuz, 1991), EECs are organized along three coordinates: anterior-to-posterior, between corresponding processing units in separate processing trends, for instance in prefrontal and parietal cortex; lateral within a hemisphere; and bilateral, coupling homologous units in the two hemispheres (Pandya, Seltzer, and Barbas, 1988), as the forebrain commissures, notably the corpus callosum. The ECCs have much in common in embryology and organization (Kennedy, Messirel, and Dehay, 1991): excitatory influence, two-way traffic, a pattern of spatial convergence and divergence, a pattern of connection by cortical layer, and discontinuous termination by multiple patches rather than point-to-point. Including the callosum, are the ECCs' various functions also fundamentally similar?

Reciprocal inhibition

According to the switchboard model, the disconnected hemispheres should be reliably able to process independently at the same time, as "double channels." The experimental evidence does not support this model (Guiard and Requin, 1978; Guiard, 1979, 1980).

Reciprocal inhibition (Sherrington, 1906) is implemented by positive (difference-amplifying) feedback loops between opponent processors. It is adapted to unequivocal (winner-takes-all) choice between mutually incompatible alternative acts, such as right versus left turning. Reciprocal inhibition occurs across species and even phyla (it occurs in the invertebrate echinoderm Octopus; Messenger, 1967). Reciprocal inhibition that alternates from side to side underlies the slithering of worms, the swimming of fishes (Horridge, 1965), and ambulating in humans. Reciprocal inhibition exists at all central nervous system segmental levels. Bilateral mirror-image synergisms compete in the spinal cord. Limb flexion inhibits the limb flexors on the opposite side and releases the contralateral extensors in the crossed extensor reflex. How is it implemented? The bidirectionality of commissures (lateral corticocortical projections connecting mirror-image loci) is consistent with their involvement in reciprocal inhibition. The need to turn flexibly right or left at a moment's notice, for pursuit or escape, is omnipresent. Commissures mediate this fundamental choice even in behaviorally primitive species (Kinsbourne, 1974a).

In the infant, not yet possessed of a functioning callosum, reciprocal inhibition is overt (Kinsbourne, 1993a). The asymmetrical tonic neck response (ATNR) offers the infant a binary choice, a coarse control, between extreme leftward and extreme rightward turning and orienting, rather than graduated directional orienting, except by reflex reaction to a stimulus. But most selection is graduated, blending in precise balance the vectors contributed by opponent processors. To accomplish this, the brain superimposes fine control in the form of equilibrating influences. Stabilizing negative (difference-minimizing) feedback modulates the underlying dichotomies of choice. As white matter matures, the ATNR becomes held in check by higher control levels. Analogously, does reciprocal inhibition prevail between the hemispheres? If so, is it mediated by cortical or subcortical commissures? When graduated response is called for, what holds an extreme swing in check?

Intrahemispheric extrinsic connections

The arcuate bundle, a prototypical intrahemispheric ("intrinsic") ECC, interconnects Wernicke's and Broca's area. It supposedly transmits auditory verbal input to the verbal output facility (by copy transfer). If the arcuate bundle is ruptured, the copy can no longer be transferred, and inability to repeat heard speech should result. Inability to repeat words indeed defines conduction aphasia, a syndrome caused by lesions of Wernicke's area and the arcuate bundle. However, like ECCs in general, the arcuate bundle conducts equally in both directions.

Kinsbourne (1972) studied two conduction aphasics. They could repeat one but not two successively spoken digit names correctly. They repeated the first one correctly but the second digit only about half the time, misidentifying or omitting the rest. The second word was repeated with longer latency. When two words were presented, latency for the first was greater than when one only was given. The patients could not repeat even common multisyllabic words or monosyllabic word pairs, such as letter names. Visual word presentation circumvents the deficit, exonerating the verbal response facility, but written response does not. The patients could perform same/different matching on word sequences that contained at least four words, showing that the deficient repetition was not due to short-term memory limitations.

If their lesion disconnects decoded speech signals from the speech-encoding area, why could the patients repeat even a single digit? Given that they could, why was their performance a function of verbal load? An alternative hypothesis is that the arcuate bundle mediates coactivation of the receptive and expressive language cortex, entraining them into a congruent joint state that facilitates repetition. When Wernicke's area is activated, it automatically induces activation in Broca's area. When the arcuate bundle is ruptured, the output area cannot sustain task-related activation, which soon falters. Failure to maintain coactivation is consistent with the metabolic (blood flow) results of Demeurisse and Capon (1991). They found that conduction aphasics' Broca's area does not maintain the normal task-related activation while the individual repeats words.

Generalizing from conduction aphasia, I propose that interrupting a corticocortical connection (intrahemispheric or interhemispheric) results in activation disparity unless the imbalance is corrected by other means. Geschwind and Kaplan's (1962) patient, who "behaved as if his two cerebral hemispheres were functioning nearly autonomously" (p. 683), perplexed the authors by his "retained ability ... to perform certain learned activities that require the cooperation of the two hands, such as threading a needle" (p. 684). These activities involve the two sides of the brain equally and therefore would not induce a disabling imbalance of activation.

Where is reciprocal inhibition mediated?

Reciprocal inhibition and coactivation would be particularly simple ways in which events in one hemisphere influence events in the other. Commissures are to be found at the cortical and subcortical levels. The levels at which reciprocal inhibition and coactivation are mediated are presumably distinct. Which are they?

Although most transcallosal fibers are excitatory (Innocenti, 1986), some are inhibitory, and some excitatory fibers activate inhibitory interneurons (reviewed by Saron et al., this volume). So the callosum could in theory mediate (reciprocal) inhibition or coactivation or both. These contrasting mechanisms generate contrasting predictions for the effects of callosal section.

When one hemisphere is transiently inactivated by electroshock (for depression), the specialized activities of the other may actually be enhanced (e.g., Deglin and Kinsbourne, 1996; Nikolaenko and Egorov, 1996). The unimpaired hemisphere presumably was transiently released from contralateral tonic inhibition. Repetitive transcranial magnetic stimulation of parietal cortex not only impaired detection in the contralateral visual field, but also enhanced attention ipsilaterally (Hilgetag, Theoret, and Pascual-Leone, 2001). Similarly, cooling a cortical area may result in increased activity in the mirror-image area (Payne, Siwek, and Lomber, 1991). The inhibition could be mediated cortically or subcortically. But certainly, callosal section is not known to enhance activities of the disconnected hemispheres. Also, if the callosum mediates reciprocal inhibition, then after it is sectioned, the coordinated ability to swing orientation right and left should be impaired. In fact, split-brain individuals orient and move to either side normally.

Alternatively, reciprocal inhibition is implemented subcortically, whereas the callosum superimposes fine tuning, dampens swings between hemispheres, and maintains the inactive hemisphere ready to respond. The callosum could also recruit contralateral hemisphere territory for computations for which the active hemisphere bears primary responsibility.

The equilibrating role of the callosum

The manifestations of the callosal syndrome reflect either interrupted transcallosal information flow to the uninformed hemisphere (the conventional explanation) or a lack of response of that hemisphere to information, when information does reach it, by a subcortical route. Kinsbourne (1974a, p. 253) suggested that the callosum equalizes hemispheric activity: "The corpus callosum minimizes disparities in the distribution of mental capacity ('attention') between the two hemispheres, so that both can be rapidly involved in any activity" (see also Kinsbourne, 1987).

If the callosum mediates equilibration, then transecting it should destabilize hemisphere equilibrium. At different times, a different hemisphere would be in control of behavior. This would not necessarily be obvious clinically. In everyday existence, enough stimulation affects both half-brains for them to be roughly equally active and ready for action. Hence the many ways in which callosal section impairs performance were long overlooked. They came to light in ecologically invalid experimental paradigms in which input was limited to one half-brain. Unilateral input would dramatically destabilize performance. Runs of trials controlled by one hemisphere would be interspersed with runs controlled by the other hemisphere. Only tasks that engage both hemispheres to an equal extent would maintain both hemispheres in comparable activation and response readiness. For instance, Trevarthen (1962) was able to teach split-brain monkeys contradictory discriminations simultaneously (cf. Bykov, 1924). Even slight differences in hemisphere activation, induced by asymmetrical external stimulation, a lateralized categorical mental set, or habituation of activation on one side, should switch hemisphere control (Kinsbourne, 1974b; Trevarthen, 1974). Callosal section would preclude the fine tuning between hemispheres, by which they could share, in graduated proportion, control of behavior.

Berlucchi (this volume) described effects in callosal agenesis that conform to the predictions outlined above. Kinsbourne (1974b) and Trevarthen (1974) first described hemisphere reciprocity. In collaboration, they studied three split-brain subjects. In one experiment, they used a visual search task, for a target letter among letters exposed either to one visual half-field or simultaneously to both (reported by Kinsbourne, 1974b). Subjects responded correctly to unilateral displays with the ipsilateral hand but could not simultaneously effectively search both visual half-fields. They neglected stimuli in the left field or responded nonspecifically when stimuli were also presented on the right. The patients could not attend simultaneously to both sides of visual space. By unopposed crossed inhibition, the activated left hemisphere preempted the attentional resource.

Circuits in which lower-level all-or-nothing reciprocal inhibition is modified by graduated higher-level fine tuning may be widespread. Sherrington (1906, pp. 284–285) observed that the reciprocal innervation of antagonistic muscle pairs, such as flexors and extensors at a limb joint, results from an interaction of these muscles' representations at a subcortical, not cortical, level. Absent cortical influence, as in decerebrate or decorticate rigidity, the disinhibited movements are no longer graduated but inhabit the extreme of the range (i.e., the joint is fully flexed or fully extended). It may be the cortex that graduates this reciprocity so as to offer the organism the choice of a wide range of possible states of relative activation of the antagonistic muscle groups. The callosum would offer a similar service in the special case of reciprocity between right and left lateralized cerebral functions.

That stimulation can maintain the disconnected hemispheres in balance, as shown by another of our experiments, described by Trevarthen (1974). The split-brain patients viewed briefly exposed simple geometric figures. These outline figures were incomplete on one side. Subjects named and drew what they saw. When the shape was presented in one half-field, so that its incomplete part abutted the midline, patients showed the completion effect that characterizes patients with unilateral parietal lesions (Kinsbourne and Warrington, 1962; Warrington, 1962). When figures or sketches of familiar objects are exposed laterally to fixation, their contralesional parts missing or overlapping a hemianopic field, the patient reports seeing the whole figure, intact. She has "completed" the figure on the basis of experience, not having observed the missing part. This is due to a bias of attention away from the contralesional extreme of the figures. Absent callosal equilibration, the stimulus activates a hemisphere, directing attention to the opposite side.

Next we combined pairs of shapes by their incomplete lateral borders so that one shape would be projected to one hemisphere and the other to the opposite hemisphere. Both would be missing their central component. For instance, an incomplete square with the left vertical side missing would be presented in the right visual field, together with a semicircle touching the free left ends of the square's horizontals and missing the other half of the circle. This first use of "chimeric" shapes elicited a novel phenomenon: double simultaneous completion. The right hand sketched a complete version of one shape (e.g., a complete square), and the left sketched a complete version of the other (e.g., a complete circle). In this paradigm, both hemispheres were concurrently active, in double simultaneous unilateral awareness, extrapolated contralaterally. This was possible because both hemispheres received an equally light stimulus load and the task, being unlateralized, did not throw off hemispheric balance by inducing unilateral task-specific activation. Nonetheless, the callosal section had divided the global activation pattern that underlies consciousness (Kinsbourne, 1988a) into two diminished patterns, each global within one hemisphere, subserving its inherently restricted awareness. Should stimulation from outside or endogenous lateralized mental set swing the activated hemisphere into ascendancy, then the other hemisphere becomes underaroused. A sudden heavy task

demand on one hemisphere channels activation to it, temporarily wresting control from the other (Kreuter, Kinsbourne, and Trevarthen, 1972). In the underactivated state, a hemisphere would respond only sluggishly to incoming signals. It might even lack sufficient activation to entrain stimulus attributes into coherent wholes (Liederman, 1995). This could explain the failure of the unstimulated hemisphere of a split-brain patient to respond to indirect stimulation rather than deficient information flow. The unstimulated hemisphere is unresponsive rather than uninformed.

If callosal section destabilizes interhemispheric equilibration, then each disconnected hemisphere would be released to exhibit its inherent contralateral attentional/orientational bias (Kinsbourne, 1970). In the split-brain individual, double simultaneous contralateral neglect should result. We (Trevarthen, 1974) and others (Teng and Sperry, 1974) have repeatedly observed this in laboratory settings, with the expected stronger rightward bias of the left hemisphere than leftward bias of the right hemisphere (Kinsbourne, 1993b).

The congenitally acallosal brain must have compensated to an extent for the lack of callosal equilibration, since split-brain symptoms are not apparent for simple matches across the median (e.g., Lassonde, Sauerwein, Chicoine, and Geoffroy, 1991). But deficiencies in more complex tasks, both linguistic and visuospatial, have been reported (Sauerwein, Nolin, and Lassonde, 1994). Tasks that are lateralized may induce hemisphere disequilibrium, to the detriment of performance.

Which subcortical mechanism distributes activation between hemispheres? Doty (1989) has nominated the serotonergic raphe system, in pons and mesencephalon, which on either side projects to both hemispheres. It is controlled by the habenulopeduncular system, which in turn receives projections from the hemispheres. For the visual system, Hilgetag (2000) offers a model that features bilateral competition between subcortical midbrain structures that derives from a classical study by Sprague (1966).

Poffenberger paradigm

A test case for callosal function is the interpretation of the difference between crossed and uncrossed reaction times (CUD). Poffenberger (1912) attempted to time a hypothesized event inside the brain, invading the "black box" by purely behavioral means. He assumed that the CUD measures interhemispheric transfer time (IHTT), extrapolating from the structural switchboard model (the only model then available). If stimulus-response processing traverses an inert medium along an invariant route, longer latency must indicate an extra stage, an extra (intercalated) neuron between hemispheres. This extra stage is now thought to be transfer between motor areas (Milner and Lines, 1982) accounting for IHTT. But can one study ECCs without acknowledging their coactivating influence?

Its oversimplified engineering approach to the brain may explain the IHTT measurement's perennial popularity. Swanson, Ledlow, and Kinsbourne (1978) remark, "The simple view that crossing a structural link (such as the corpus callosum) produces significant difference in RT can be held only when all other sources of variation (uncertainty of location, S-R compatibility, specialized cognitive processing, etc.) are held constant. Whether such factors can in fact be controlled is questionable" (p. 289). Indeed, the paradigm has been cumulatively stripped of all variables of psychological interest—expectancy, response conflict, stimulus-response compatibility—so as to render it as mechanical and psychologically arid as possible. The result is a measured time period of 1–4 milliseconds (ms). It continues to engage sustained psychological interest, even though the brain is a black box no longer and far more direct ways of timing brain processes have become available. The IHTT paradigm purports to isolate an automatic pathway that can be freed of contextual influence. Only if that were correct could one apply the subtractive method to so brief a time interval.

CUD operationalizing IHTT is open to an alternative interpretation. The stimulus engenders an orienting response in the stimulated hemisphere. The additional activation would carry that hemisphere to response threshold a few milliseconds earlier (Swanson et al., 1978). Degree of activation (Kinsbourne, 1970) had been strangely missing from neuropsychological theorizing, although it had long and extensive currency in neurophysiology. Single neurons do not automatically fire when stimulated, but only when they reach a threshold of excitation. This depends on both the stimulus and the neuron's base state. But neuropsychologists did not consider the activational base state or the arousing properties of the stimulation.

We suggested that "lateral processing takes place after interhemispheric integration of information, and so a transfer component is present in all response measures" (Swanson et al., 1978, p. 278). If the sequence of events were $V_d \rightarrow$ simultaneous activation of M_d and M_i, with more rapid rise in activation of M_d on account of ipsilateral stimulation, then the motor preparation time of M_d might be briefer. The CUD would reflect difference in time to activation threshold, and transcallosal conduction time would have nothing to do with the CUD. Because the CUD in three subjects was 2 ms, across

subjects and across trials within subjects, with comparable intersubject and intrasubject variability, Iacoboni and Zaidel (1999) considered it "hard-wired" IHTT. Can these conflicting accounts of the Poffenberger result be deconfounded electrophysiologically?

Evoked potential (EP) studies of the Poffenberger paradigm show that some of the evoked wave forms first appear in the directly stimulated hemisphere. They may not, however, be the earliest components. In a choice reaction time variant of the Poffenberger paradigm, Ledlow, Swanson, and Kinsbourne (1978) found different wave form latencies in the stimulated and the unstimulated hemispheres only beyond 120 ms. The time differentials at later EP stages are about five times greater than those in the behavioral paradigm. This finding is compatible with either model. Critical are the time relations of the visual and motor activation. Is the activation of the ipsilateral motor processor simultaneous with, but less steep than, that of the contralateral motor processor? If so, the CUD would reflect the faster response of the better-prepared motor processor (better prepared because it is housed in the stimulated and thereby aroused hemisphere). This would be predicted by the coactivation model. Does activation of the indirect (M_i) processor await transfer of visual information (i.e., transcallosal spread of the visual evoked potential)? This would favor IHTT. Or does M_i activation coincide with M_d activation, unrelated to, or even before, activation of V_i? That favors coactivation.

In a Poffenberger paradigm, Saron, Vaughan, Simpson, and Foxe (1996, this volume) observed bilateral activation in central leads earlier than transfer from the stimulated to the unstimulated visual cortex. The motor cortex activation was more robust on the directly stimulated side. Endo, Kizuka, Masuda, and Takeda (1999), using magnetoencephalography, also reported automatic bilateral motor areas activation, even when stimulus and response were within-hemisphere and even on no-go trials, without response. Both these findings had been predicted by Swanson and colleagues (1978). The minimally faster ipsilateral response is referred to more effective motor preparation, as indicated by a steeper rise in amplitude of the central evoked potential on the stimulated side. Saron, Foxe, Schroeder, and Vaughan (in press) summarize extensive physiological support for this concept. Thus, the reaction time was related to the *rate* of premovement activation rather than the *timing* of its onset. This finding supports the coactivation model.

The bilateral motor activation/preparation occurred even when Saron and colleagues' subjects did not respond (the "view-only" condition). This is a direct demonstration of coactivation. Not only is there an automatic (obligatory) link between input and a preferred output channel, but the mirror-symmetric output facility is coactivated, even without explicit or implicit response demands.

Further support for the activation interpretation of the CUD derives from Iacoboni and Zaidel (1998). They embedded occasional bilateral stimuli in a Poffenberger design to favor equilibration of hemisphere activation. As predicted by the activation account, the CUD decreased from 3.0 ms in the standard to a trivial 0.3 ms in the bilateral embedded condition.

Callosal microanatomy does not suggest the highly synchronized assault of action potentials implied by "hard-wiring" of transcallosal traffic. Most fibers arborize into contact with multiple contralateral columns: "The architecture of callosal axons is, in principle, suitable to promote the synchronous activation of multiple targets located across distant columns in the opposite hemisphere" (Houzel and Milleret, 1999, p. 271).

Imperfect callosal coactivation may explain the prolonged CUD in callosal agenesis (Lassonde, this volume) and in callosal section, especially if total. Absent transcallosal coactivation, the unstimulated hemisphere's motor strip is underactivated, unprepared for action, and slower to threshold in preparation for response. Deficient activation also explains two acallosal subjects' striking inverse relationship between their CUD duration and the luminance of the stimulus (Milner, Jeeves, Silver, Lines, and Wilson, 1985). (Note the analogy to the equilibration interpretation of Bykov's (1924) observation that callosally transected dogs would still transfer if the conditioned stimulus was intense.)

In summary, the view that a 2-ms CUD represents IHTT assumes incorrectly that all other pertinent physiological variables, including activation that affects motor preparation time (variables that Poffenberger could not have known about), are exquisitely matched between hemispheres. It is explicitly falsified by the Poffenberger ET findings of Marzi and colleagues (1999): unbalanced areas of activation, some in the stimulated and some in the unstimulated hemisphere. So the presuppositions for analysis by subtraction are lacking. Some factor advances ipsilateral relative to contralateral speed of reaction by roughly 2 ms. Nothing pinpoints IHTT as that variable.

Function of large and small callosal fibers (the Ringo hypothesis)

The primate callosum features a suite of fiber sizes, from few large, fast, conducting myelinated to many thin, slow, unmyelinated (Aboitiz, Scheibel, Fisher, and Zaidel, 1992; Aboitiz, this volume). Ringo, Doty, Demeter, and Sinard (1994) pointed out that for complex time-sensitive mental operations, the large and fastest fibers would be too few, and the smaller fibers would be too slow. They suggested that animals with relatively large brains, for whom the time factor would be most critical, solve the problem by lateralizing, confining time-sensitive computations to a single hemisphere. They predicted more lateralization in larger brains, specifically of time-sensitive processing. The underlying assumption was that bilateralization is the base state, from which deviations occur only under adaptive pressure.

However, non-time-sensitive computations such as cognitive style (e.g., Deglin and Kinsbourne, 1996), as well as relatively sluggish emotional states, are lateralized. Lateralization must have additional causes. Or is it bilateralization that needs to be explained, lateralization being the base state (Kinsbourne, 1974a)? Perhaps all cognitive computations are lateralized at base state unless they need to be bilateralized for adaptive reasons.

An oversized callosum distinguishes our species (Blinkov and Glezer, 1968). Referring to its equilibrating function, Kinsbourne (1974b) remarked, "Of all species, those that have greatest asymmetry of neurological representation have greatest need for such a stabilizing control system. Both because of the great repertoire of lateralized processors, and because of their ability to detach attention from their bisymmetric surroundings and internalize attention, humans have this need.... humans more than any other bisymmetric animals are likely to manifest grossly asymmetrical distributed activity at the highest neural level, and in them the stabilizing effect of the corpus callosum is particularly vital" (pp. 254–255).

Are small brains, then, not lateralized? To the contrary, they are, from behaviorally modest small-brained (e.g., mouse; Ehret and Koch, 1989) to sophisticated large-brained species (Hiscock and Kinsbourne, 1995). Lateralization is widespread or even the rule throughout at least the vertebrate phylum. Perhaps all complex computations are performed locally. If fewer processes are lateralized in mouse than human, this would be because the mouse has fewer such processes altogether, not because cognitive processes are disproportionately lateralized in humans. For behavior that is targeted to specific points in space, perhaps both hemispheres are equally adept (Zaidel et al.'s [1990] direct access variant). If there is no lateralization, that may merely mean that both hemispheres can individually control the computation in question. A more abstract computation may be entrusted to a single hemisphere (Kinsbourne, 1974b). Similar considerations apply to left-handed humans, many of whom are bilateralized for complex mental operations, notably linguistic. How do they span the small fiber temporal gap (estimated as averaging 25 ms by Ringo et al. [1994]) without loss of efficiency? Bilateralization is unlikely to impair efficiency, given many normative studies that have found no intellectual difference between right- and left-handers (Kinsbourne, 1988b). A possible solution again calls into question what it means functionally to be bilateralized. Does it mean using both hemispheres all the time or sometimes one and sometimes the other? The latter possibility, which would preserve the Ringo hypothesis, has not even been discussed.

Instead of time-sensitive computing, what do the small fibers do? Presumably, they can mediate tonic activation. By coactivating the contralateral hemisphere, they could prepare it for adaptively relevant contingencies and even anticipate them.

Could the Ringo argument be extended beyond the callosum? The ECCs that link prefrontal and posterior parietal cortex also have quite a distance to traverse. The factors that Ringo and colleagues suggest hold down fiber size in the callosa of animals with relatively large brains could equally be applied to their other ECCs. If so, the majority population of smaller fibers in ECCs also implements modulation rather than specific time-sensitive computations. We emerge with a picture of rapid local parallel computation, with mutual modulation into a momentary composite state of the global network, a vector in global state space.

Conclusions

Evidence from anatomy and physiology indicates that ECCs in general and the callosum in particular subserve coactivation. Split-brain symptoms would arise from failed hemisphere coactivation. The classical CUD in reaction time could arise from incomplete coactivation of the motor areas in the unstimulated hemisphere. I have applied the Ringo hypothesis to an argument for a coactivating role of the small-fiber majority complement in the callosum. There follows a summary of suggested mechanisms.

There is evidence for a control system for selection at the cerebral level that includes paired cortical and paired subcortical loci, as well as cortical and subcortical commissures. The subcortical commissures mediate the positive feedback that underlies reciprocal inhibition, permitting the individual an unequivocal choice in the direction of orienting. By their interaction across the forebrain commissures, cortical analyzers implement stabilizing negative feedback. Through coactivation, the callosum equilibrates the activation levels of the hemispheres in the face of greater activation of one of them. This allows for conjoint readiness of the hemispheres to collaborate, for both directing attention in a graduated fashion and supporting cognition. I have argued (Kinsbourne and Hicks, 1978) and illustrated experimentally (e.g., Kinsbourne and Byrd, 1985) that the two hemispheric networks, albeit the site of a jigsaw of specialized processors, also constitute a "multipurpose computational space," available for recruitment when increasing task difficulty calls for more neuronal units. Klingberg, O'Sullivan, and Roland (1997) have provided neuroimaging support for this concept. The callosum would recruit contralateral areas of cortex. After callosal section, this phasic coactivation and equilibration become unavailable, leaving the resting hemisphere sluggish in response. Also, the absence of bidirectional tonic activation might explain why our experiments show, in Trevarthen's (1974, p. 198) words, "that commissurotomy results in a marked deficit in readiness to perceive throughout the visual field, and a sluggishness or drop in attentional lability for orienting perception selectively."

Its role in selection does not exclude other functions of the forebrain commissure. Indeed, the fastest-conducting (most thickly myelinated) fibers may subserve urgent responding. Even in primitive vertebrates, the sluggish nerve net is supplemented by giant fibers for rapid response (especially withdrawal). As for information transmission, detailed copy transfer seems unlikely, since rather few fibers are available in the commissure (discussed by Cook, 1986). As Ringo and colleagues (1994) propose, computations probably do not straddle the callosum. Their outcomes influence one another but by entrainment rather than by movable representations (Kinsbourne, 1988a; Damasio, 1989). Manzoni, Barbaresi, Conti, and Fabri (1989) observed bidirectional excitatory loops constituted by homotopically interactive somatosensory callosal cells. Houzel and Milleret (1999) regard "the architecture of callosal axons ... suitable to promote the synchronous activation of multiple targets located across distant columns in the opposite hemispheres" (p. 271). Engel, Konig, Kreiter, and Singer (1991) have found neurons on either side of the callosum that entrain into synchronous firing. Are such coupled oscillators a microcosm of coactivation?

REFERENCES

ABOITIZ, F., A. B. SCHEIBEL, R. S. FISHER, and E. ZAIDEL, 1992. Fiber composition of the human corpus callosum. *Brain Res.* 598:143–153.

BLINKOV, S. M., and I. I. GLEZER, 1968. *The Human Brain in Figures and Tables*. New York: Plenum Press.

BRAITENBERG, V., and A. SCHUZ, 1991. *Anatomy of the Cortex*. New York: Springer.

BYKOV, K. M., 1924. Versuche an Hunden mit durchschneiden des Corpus Callosum. *Z. Neurol. Psychiat.* 39:199.

BYKOV, K. M., SPERANSKY, A. D., 1924. Observations upon dogs after section of the corpus callosum. *College Physiol., Labs I. V. Pavlov* 1:47–59 (in Russian, English translation by T. J. Hayek).

COOK, N. D., 1986. *The Brain Code: Mechanisms of Information Transfer and the Corpus Callosum*. London: Methuen.

DAMASIO, A. R., 1989. Time-locked multiregional retroactivation: A systems levels proposal for the neural substrates of recall and recognition. *Cognition* 33:25–62.

DEGLIN, V., and M. KINSBOURNE, 1996. Divergent thinking styles of the hemispheres: How syllogisms are solved during transitory hemisphere suppression. *Brain Cogn.* 31:285–307.

DEJERINE, J., 1892. Contribution à la étude anatomo-pathologique et cliniques des differentes varietés de cécité verbale. *C. R. Hebdomadaires Seances Memoires Soc. Biol. 9th Ser.* 44:61–90.

DEMEURISSE, G., and A. CAPON, 1991. Brain activation during a linguistic task in conduction aphasia. *Cortex* 27:285–294.

DENNETT, D., and M. KINSBOURNE, 1992. Time and the observer. *Behav. Brain Sci.* 15:183–247.

DOTY, R. W., 1973. Ablation of visual areas in the central nervous system. In *Handbook of Sensory Physiology*, Vol. 7: *Forebrain Commissures and Vision*, R. Jung, ed. Heidelberg, Germany: Springer.

DOTY, R. W., 1989. Schizophrenia: A disease of interhemispheric processes at forebrain and brainstem levels? *Behav. Brain Res.* 34:1–33.

ECCLES, J. C., 1965. *The Neurophysiological Basis of Mind*. Cambridge, Engl.: Cambridge University Press.

EHRET, G., and M. KOCH, 1989. Recognition of communication sounds is lateralized in the mouse brain. *Behav. Brain Res.* 33:222.

ENDO, H., T. KIZUKA, T. MASUDA, and T. TAKEDA, 1999. Automatic activation in the human primary motor cortex synchronized with movement preparation. *Cogn. Brain Res.* 3:229–239.

ENGEL, A. K., P. KONIG, A. K. KREITER, and W. SINGER, 1991. Interhemispheric synchronization of oscillatory neuronal responses in cat visual cortex. *Science* 252:1177–1179.

FESSARD, A. E., 1954. Mechanisms of nervous integration and conscious experience. In *Brain Mechanisms and Consciousness*, J. F. Delafresney, ed. Springfield, Ill.: Thomas, pp. 632–681.

GAZZANIGA, M. S., 1967. The split brain in man. *Scientific American* 27:24–29.

GESCHWIND, N., 1965. Disconnexion syndromes in animals and man. *Brain* 88:237–294.

GESCHWIND, N., and E. KAPLAN, 1962. A human cerebral deconnection syndrome. *Neurology* 12:675–685.

GUIARD, Y., 1979. Report of a severe accuracy deficit in the split-brain monkey performing a between-hand choice-RT task: Evidence for a unilateral functioning hypothesis. In *Structure and Function of Cerebral Commissures*, S. Russell et al., eds. New York: Macmillan, pp. 365–369.

GUIARD, Y., 1980. Cerebral hemispheres and selective attention. *Acta Psychol.* 46:44–61.

GUIARD, Y., and J. REQUIN, 1978. Between-hand and within-hand choice-RTs: A single channel of reduced capacity in the split-brain monkey. In *Attention and Performance*, Vol. 7, J. Requin, ed. Hillsdale, N.J.: Erlbaum, pp. 391–410.

HILGETAG, C. C., 2000. Spatial neglect and paradoxical lesion effects in the cat-A. *Neurocomputing* 32/33:793–799.

HILGETAG, C. C., H. THEORET, and A. PASCUAL-LEONE, 2001. Enhanced visual spatial attention ipsilateral to rTMS-induced "virtual lesions" of human parietal cortex. *Nature Neuroscience* 4:953–957.

HISCOCK, M., and M. KINSBOURNE, 1995. Phylogeny and ontogeny of cerebral lateralization. In *Brain Asymmetry*, R. Davidson, and K. Hugdahl, eds. Cambridge, Mass.: Bradford Books/MIT Press, pp. 535–578.

HORRIDGE, G. A., 1965. *Interneurons*. London: Freeman.

HOUZEL, J. C., and C. MILLERET, 1999. Visual interhemispheric processing: Constraints and potentialities set by axonal morphology. *J. Physiol. Paris* 93:271–284.

IACOBONI, M., and E. ZAIDEL, 1998. Context effects in simple reaction times to lateralized flashes. *Soc. Neurosci. Abstr.* 24 (2):1262.

IACOBONI, M., and E. ZAIDEL, 2000. Crossed-uncrossed difference in simple reaction times to lateralized flashes: Between- and within-subjects variability. *Neuropsychol.* 38: 535–541.

INNOCENTI, R. J., 1986. General organization of callosal connections in the cerebral cortex. In *Cerebral Cortex*, Vol. 5: *Sensory-Motor Areas and Aspects of Cortical Connectivity*, E. G. Jones and A. Peters, eds. New York: Plenum, pp. 291–354.

KENNEDY, H., C. MESSIREL, and C. DEHAY, 1991. Callosal pathways and their compliancy to general rules governing the organization of corticocortical connectivity. In *Neuroanatomy of the Visual Pathways and Their Development*, B. Reher and J. Cronly-Dillon, eds. Boca Raton, Fla.: CRC Press, pp. 324–359.

KINSBOURNE, M., 1970. The cerebral basis of lateral asymmetries in attention. *Acta Psychol.* 33:193–201.

KINSBOURNE, M., 1972. Behavioral analysis of the repetition deficit in conduction aphasia. *Neurology* 22:1126–1132.

KINSBOURNE, M., 1974a. Lateral interactions in the brain. In *Hemispheric Disconnection and Cerebral Function*, M. Kinsbourne and W. L. Smith, eds. Springfield, Ill.: Thomas, pp. 239–259.

KINSBOURNE, M., 1974b. Mechanisms of hemispheric interaction in man. In *Hemispheric Disconnection and Cerebral Function*, M. Kinsbourne and W. L. Smith, eds. Springfield, Ill.: Thomas, pp. 260–285.

KINSBOURNE, M., 1978. Biological determinants of functional bisymmetry and asymmetry. In *Asymmetrical Function of the Brain*, M. Kinsbourne, ed. Cambridge, Engl.: Cambridge University Press, pp. 3–16.

KINSBOURNE, M., 1987. The material basis of mind. In *Matters of Intelligence*, L. M. Vaina, ed. New York: Reidel, pp. 407–427.

KINSBOURNE, M., 1988a. Integrated cortical field theory of consciousness. In *Consciousness in Contemporary Science*, A. Marcel and E. Bisiach, eds. Amsterdam: Elsevier, pp. 230–256.

KINSBOURNE, M., 1988b. Sinistrality, brain organization and cognitive deficits. In *Brain Lateralization in Children*, D. L. Molfese and S. J. Segalowitz, eds. New York: Guilford Press, pp. 259–279.

KINSBOURNE, M., 1993a. Development of attention and metacognition. In *Handbook of Neuropsychology*, Vol. 7, I. Rapin and S. Segalowitz, eds. Amsterdam: Elsevier, pp. 261–278.

KINSBOURNE, M., 1993b. Orientational bias model of unilateral neglect: Evidence from attentional gradients within hemispace. In *Unilateral Neglect: Clinical and Experimental Studies*, I. H. Robertson and J. C. Marshall, eds. London: Erlbaum, pp. 63–88.

KINSBOURNE, M., and M. BYRD, 1985. Word load and visual hemifield shape recognition: Priming and interference effects. In *Attention and Performance 11*, M. I. Posner and O. M. Maier, eds. Hillsdale, N.J.: Erlbaum, pp. 529–546.

KINSBOURNE, M., and R. E. HICKS, 1978. Functional cerebral space: A model for overflow, transfer and interference effects in human performance: A tutorial review. In *Attention and Performance*, Vol. 7, J. Requin, ed. Hillsdale, N.J.: Erlbaum, pp. 345–362.

KINSBOURNE, M., and E. K. WARRINGTON, 1962. A variety of reading disability associated with right hemisphere lesions. *J. Neurol. Neurosurg. Psychiat.* 25:339–344.

KLINGBERG, T., B. T. O'SULLIVAN, and P. E. ROLAND, 1997. Bilateral activation of fronto-parietal networks by incrementing demands in a working memory task. *Cerebral Cortex* 7:465–471.

KREUTER, C., M. KINSBOURNE, and C. TREVARTHEN, 1972. Are deconnected cerebral hemispheres independent channels? A preliminary study of the effect of unilateral loading on bilateral finger tapping. *Neuropsychologia* 10:453–461.

LASSONDE, M., H. SAUERWEIN, A. CHICOINE, and G. GEOFFROY, 1991. Absence of disconnexion syndrome in callosal agenesis and early callosotomy: Brain reorganization or lack of structural specificity during ontogeny? *Neuropsychologia* 29:481–495.

LEDLOW, A., J. M. SWANSON, and M. KINSBOURNE, 1978. Differences in reaction times and averaged evoked potentials as a function of direct and indirect neural pathways. *Ann. Neurol.* 3:525–530.

LIEDERMAN, J., 1995. A reinterpretation of the split-brain syndrome: Implications for the function of corticocortical fibers. In *Brain Asymmetry*, R. C. Davidson and K. Hugdahl, eds. Cambridge, MA: MIT Press, pp. 451–490.

MANZONI, T., P. BARBARESI, F. CONTI, and M. FABRI, 1989. The callosal connections of the primary somatosensory cortex and the neural basis of midline fusion. *Exp. Brain Res.* 76:251–266.

MARZI, C. A., D. PERANI, G. TAESSINARI, A. COLLELUORI, A. MARAVITA, C. MINIUSSI, E. PAULESU, P. SCIFO, and F. FAZIO, 1999. Pathways of interhemispheric transfer in normals and in a split-brain subject: A positron emission tomography. *Exp. Brain Res.* 126:451–458.

MESSENGER, T. B., 1967. The effect on locomotion of lesions to the visuomotor system in Octopus. *Proc. R. Soc. Lond. Biol.* 167:252–281.

MILNER, A. D., M. A. JEEVES, P. H. SILVER, C. R. LINES, and J. WILSON, 1985. Reaction times to lateralized visual stimuli in callosal agenesis: Stimulus and response factors. *Neuropsychologia* 23:323–331.

MILNER, A. D., and C. R. LINES, 1982. Interhemispheric pathways in simple reaction times to lateralized light flashes. *Neuropsychologia* 20:171–179.

MYERS, R. E., and R. W. SPERRY, 1953. Interocular transfer of a visual form discrimination habit after section of the optic chiasm and corpus callosum. *Anat. Rec.* 115:351–352.

NIKOLAENKO, N. N., and I. I. EGOROV, 1996. Types of interhemispheric relations in man. *J. Evolut. Biochem. Physiol.* 32:278–286.

PANDYA, D. N., B. SELTZER, and H. BARBAS, 1988. Input-output organization of the primate cerebral cortex. In *Comparative Primate Biology*, Vol. 4: *Neurosciences*, H. D. Steklis and J. Erwin, eds. New York: Alan R. Liss, pp. 39–80.

PAVLOV, I. P., 1927. *Conditioned Reflexes*. Oxford, Engl.: Oxford University Press.

PAYNE, B. R., D. F. SIWEK, and S. G. LOMBER, 1991. Complex transcallosal interactions in visual cortex. *Vis. Neurosci.* 6:283–289.

POFFENBERGER, A. T., 1912. Reaction time to retinal stimulation with special reference to the time lost in conduction through nerve centers. *Arch. Psychol.* 23:1–73.

RINGO, J. L., R. W. DOTY, S. DEMETER, and P. Y. SINARD, 1994. Time is of the essence: A conjecture that hemispheric specialization arises from interhemispheric conduction delay. *Cereb. Cortex* 4:331–343.

SARON, C. D., J. J. FOXE, C. E. SCHROEDER, and H. G. VAUGHAN, in press. Complexities of interhemispheric communication in sensory-motor tasks revealed by high density event-related potential mapping. In *Brain Asymmetry*, 2nd edition, K. Hugdahl and R. J. Davidson, eds. Cambridge, Mass.: MIT Press.

SARON, C., H. G. VAUGHAN, G. V. SIMPSON, and J. J. FOXE, 1996. Effects of reaction time on visuomotor interaction: Spatiotemporal patterns of intra- and interhemispheric cortical activation. *Soc. Neurosci. Abstr.* 22 (2):890.

SAUERWEIN, H. C., P. NOLIN, and M. LASSONDE, 1994. Cognitive functioning in callosal agenesis. In *Callosal agenesis: A natural split brain?* M. Lassonde and M. A. Jeeves, eds. New York: Plenum, pp. 221–233.

SHERRINGTON, C. S., 1906. *Integrative Action of the Nervous System*. New Haven, Conn.: Yale University Press.

SPRAGUE, J. M. 1966. Interaction of cortex and superior colliculus in mediation of visually guided behavior in the cat. *Science* 153:1544–1547.

SUTTON, J. P., and J. A. ANDERSON, 1995. Computational and neurobiological features of a network of networks. In *Neurobiology of Computation*, J. M. Bower, ed. Boston, Mass.: Kluwer, pp. 317–322.

SWANSON, J., A. J. LEDLOW, and M. KINSBOURNE, 1978. Lateral asymmetries revealed by simple reaction time. In *Asymmetrical Function of the Brain*, M. Kinsbourne, ed. New York: Cambridge University Press, pp. 274–291.

TENG, E., and R. W. SPERRY, 1974. Interhemispheric rivalry during simultaneous bilateral task presentation in commissurotomized patients. *Cortex* 2:111–120.

TREVARTHEN, C. B., 1962. Double visual learning in split-brain monkeys. *Science* 136:258–259.

TREVARTHEN, C., 1974. Functional relations of disconnected hemispheres with the brain stem and with each other: Monkey and man. In *Hemispheric Disconnection and Cerebral Function*, M. Kinsbourne and W. L. Smith, eds. Springfield, Ill.: Thomas, pp. 187–207.

TREVARTHEN, C., 1978. Manipulative strategies of baboons and the origins of cerebral asymmetry. In *Asymmetrical Function of the Brain*, M. Kinsbourne, ed. Cambridge, Engl.: Cambridge University Press, pp. 329–391.

WARRINGTON, E. K., 1962. The completion of visual forms across hemianopic field defects. *J. Neurol. Neurosurg. Psychiatry* 25:208–217.

WERNICKE, C., 1900. *Grundriss der Psychiatrie in Klinischen Vorlesungen.* Leipzig, Germany: Thieme.

ZAIDEL, E., J. M. CLARKE, and B. SUYENOBU, 1990. Hemispheric independence: A paradigm case for cognitive neuroscience. In *Neurobiology of Higher Cognitive Function*, A. B. Scheibel and A. F. Wechsler, eds. New York: Guilford, pp. 297–355.

COMMENTARY 10.1

A Plan for the Empirical Evaluation of the Coactivation/Equilibration Model of Callosal Function

JACQUELINE LIEDERMAN

ABSTRACT   Kinsbourne emphasizes the role of the corpus callosum in mediating the coactivation of the two hemispheres so as to minimize arousal asymmetries and enable coherent hemispheric activation. Here, data reported by Yazgan and colleagues (1995) on the relationship between callosal size and performance is used to evaluate the predictions of three models of callosal function: the interhemispheric coactivation/ equilibration model, the interhemispheric inhibition model, and the interhemispheric information transfer model. For each paradigm, new experiments are proposed that enable one to further evaluate the differential predictions of the three models. It is concluded that the coactivation model best matches the data.

For the purposes of this commentary, I would like to review the following key points in Kinsbourne's paper. First, Kinsbourne points out the importance of viewing the corticocortical pathways (in general) and the corpus callosum (in particular) as mediating the same function: the coactivation of two hemispheres to minimize extreme arousal asymmetries and to permit their coherent conjoint activation. In accordance with many of his previous papers (e.g., Kinsbourne, 1982), he emphasizes the importance of moving away from the notion of grandmother cells and convergence zones as the means toward integration. He then emphasizes what I have termed "non-convergent temporal integration" (Liederman, 1995), which attributes the distribution and maintenance of activation between distant regions as the role of corticocortical fibers rather than information flow per se.

Kinsbourne suggests that two data sets have special relevance to his model. He claims that evoked potential recordings during the Poffenberger paradigm data manifest many of the characteristics predicted by Kinsbourne's model compared to the information flow model. Kinsbourne argues that what has been interpreted as an interhemispheric transfer time is simply the sluggishness of the unstimulated hemisphere in formulating and generating a response. When one hemisphere is activated by an input directed to it exclusively, the corpus callosum "compensates" by distributing activation to the opposite hemisphere. This distributed activation is less intense than the direct stimulation. It is this residual imbalance of activation (even after it has been minimized by the compensatory redistribution of activation by the corpus callosum) from which the delay in responding to the stimulated hemisphere by the ipsilateral hand derives. Kinsbourne also uses the data presented by Saron and colleagues (Chapter 8 in this volume) to argue that even in the nonmotor condition, when a response is not required of the ipsilateral hand, there is evidence of contralateral activation of the opposite hemisphere. Why should this second event be interpreted as transfer of information?

The second set of data that have special relevance to Kinsbourne's model are those that examine the relationship between callosal size and various interhemispheric functional interactions. He argues that one data set, which he was involved in collecting (Yazgan et al., 1995) confirms the predictions of a coactivation/equilibration model of callosal function over an information flow model.

The goal of this paper is to delineate the domains in which the coactivation/equilibration inhibition and in-

JACQUELINE LIEDERMAN   Brain, Behavior and Cognition Program, Boston University, Boston, Massachusetts.

TABLE 10.1
Effect of increased callosal size on performance of various laterality tasks according to three models of callosal function: A comparison to the outcome reported by Yazgan and colleagues, 1995

Task	Information Flow Model	Coactivation Model	Inhibition Model	Results Obtained by Yazgan et al., 1995
Line bisection bias	No prediction	Negative correlation	Positive correlation	Negative correlation
Turning bias	No prediction	Negative correlation	Positive correlation	Negative correlation
Dichotic listening bias	Negative correlation	Negative correlation	Positive correlation	Negative correlation
Verbal interference with right hand	No prediction	Negative correlation	No correlation	Negative correlation
Verbal interference with left hand	No prediction	Negative correlation	Negative correlation?	Negative correlation
Asymmetry of verbal manual interference	No prediction	Negative correlation	Positive correlation	No correlation
No. of predicted outcomes that match the results of Yazgan et al., 1995	1 match	5 or 6 matches	1 match	

formation models differ in their predictions. This will be done by using data from the dichotic listening paradigm and the verbal/manual interference paradigm of Yazgan and colleagues (1995). These patterns of predictions are summarized in Table 10.1. For each paradigm I suggest procedural variations that would enable one to evaluate the different predictions of the coactivation/equilibration models and the information flow models.

An evaluation of the models on the basis of the traditional dichotic listening paradigm

As can be seen in Table 10.1, for the traditional dichotic listening paradigm, both the coactivation/equilibration model and the information flow model predict the same outcome. Both models predict that increased callosal size should decrease the size of the right-ear advantage (i.e., the size of the right-ear advantage should be negatively correlated with callosal size).

On the basis of the coactivation/equilibration model, this effect would be predicted because as the size of the corpus callosum increases, the likelihood of both hemispheres being coactivated during either right- or left-ear presentation increases. Therefore, performance differences in response to right- versus left-ear presentation should decrease.

On the basis of the information transfer model, the same effect would be predicted because as the size of the corpus callosum increases, transfer of items from the left ear/right hemisphere to the left hemisphere should increase. Consequently, the relative superiority of direct right-ear/left-hemisphere presentation should decrease.

Hence, the dichotic listening experiments would have to be redesigned to differentiate between the predictions based on these theories. First, one would have to replace the fused word task of Wexler and Halwes (1983), which was used by Yazgan and colleagues (1995). The Wexler and Halwes (1993) paradigm does not provide one with separate right- and left-ear scores because only one response is recorded during each trial. Second, two additional experimental manipulations would help to dissociate the predictions of the coactivation/equilibration and information flow models. These new predictions are being generated within the context of a dichotic listening task, though in general, parallel experiments and predictions could be generated in other modalities.

Modifications of the dichotic listening task that would provide data that would be predicted differently by the models

EXPERIMENTAL VARIATION 1: VARY TASK DIFFICULTY
One experimental variation involves varying the difficulty level of the dichotic listening task. Only on the basis of the coactivation/equilibration model would one predict that there should be a positive correlation between size of the corpus callosum and right-ear performance, especially at high rather than low task difficulty. This is because as task difficulty increases, the left-hemisphere/right-ear performance asymptotes unless resources in the opposite hemisphere can be recruited to continue to match the increased demands of the task. The coactivation/equilibration model incorporates this as an essential role of the corpus callosum.

On the basis of the information transfer model, one would predict that oral word identification is what Zaidel, Clarke, and Suyenobu (1990) call "a callosal transfer task" because, irrespective of which hemisphere initially receives the task, the left hemisphere will ultimately be responsible for the computations. Thus, according to the information transfer model, right-ear performance should be unaffected by callosal size.

According to the information transfer model, only left-ear performance should be positively correlated with callosal size, so as to permit the task to be "transferred" to the left (language) hemisphere for processing.

EXPERIMENTAL VARIATION 2: VARY THE DIRECTION OF ATTENTION TOWARD THE RIGHT, LEFT, OR EITHER EAR Another experimental manipulation involves altering the direction of attention during the dichotic listening task. On the basis of the coactivation/equilibration model, one would predict a negative correlation between callosal size and the lateralized and central attentional conditions. This prediction would be based on the notion that as callosal size decreases, the ability to equilibrate attention after a lateralized signal decreases, and therefore attentional effects increase.

The information flow model might be able to accommodate the fact that there would be greater right-ear than left-ear performance during the "attend right" condition than during a central or left attention condition, but the difference between the lateralized and central attentional conditions should not be correlated with callosal size.

An evaluation of the models based on the traditional verbal manual interference paradigm

The second critical task employed by Yazgan and colleagues (1995) was a verbal manual interference task. This task measures the effect of a concurrent language task (which is presumed to require left-hemisphere mediation) on a timed unimanual task. The motor task required subjects to trace a path by connecting sequential numbers and letters. This language task required subjects to conjugate irregular verbs out loud.

This task is an interesting one because the three models make different predictions. The coactivation/equilibration model predicts that there should be less within-hemisphere dual task interference (i.e., disruption of right-hand maze performance by the simultaneous verbal task) as callosal size increases. This is because as the size of the corpus callosum increases, the extent to which the resources of the right hemisphere can be coactivated also increases, thereby distributing the workload.

Both the information flow and interhemispheric inhibition models would not predict that within-hemisphere interference would be affected by the size of the corpus callosum.

The theories also differ with reference to the between-hemisphere interference condition (i.e., disruption of left-hand maze performance by the simultaneous verbal task). The coactivation/equilibration model would predict that as task difficulty increases, callosal size becomes increasingly relevant. This is because the larger the corpus callosum, the greater the redistribution of the computational load and the less the amount of intertask interference. The information flow model would not predict differential interference effects contingent on callosal size. The inhibition model would predict that between-hemisphere interference would decrease as callosal size increases, because the corpus callosum serves to separate the activity of the two hemispheres from mutual interference.

Modifications of the verbal manual interference task

EXPERIMENTAL VARIATION 1: CREATE MORE SENSITIVE DEPENDENT MEASURES SO THAT INTERFERENCE EFFECTS CAN BE ASSESSED MORE ACCURATELY In the Yazgan report, interference is only examined for the effect of the verbal task on manual performance. Presumably, subjects preserved verbal performance at the expense of manual performance both because this is a general tendency (Hiscock, 1982) and because the task was paced. The dependent measure for the verbal task could be made more sensitive by using reaction time for conjugation of the verb as the dependent measure rather than accuracy.

EXPERIMENTAL VARIATION 2: VARY TASK DIFFICULTY FOR THE PRIMARY AND SECONDARY TASKS Task difficulty could be varied for the verbal task by systematically altering the rate of verb presentation. Task difficulty could be varied for the maze task by changing the number of times the maze requires one to cross over existing paths.

EXPERIMENTAL VARIATION 3: MANIPULATE TASK EMPHASIS Only the coactivation/equilibration model predicts that callosal size should influence within-hemisphere interference. The best way to test this model is to push performance to an extreme on one task and carefully measure its effect on the other task. Thus, when Ss are made to emphasize right-hand performance, only the coactivation/equilibration theory would predict that a larger corpus callosum would be associated with a smaller decrement in verbal performance. Similarly, when Ss are made to emphasize their speed of verb conjugation, only the coactivation/equilibration theory would predict that a larger corpus callosum would be associated with a smaller decrement in right-hand maze performance.

Well-established interhemispheric phenomena that can be differentially explained by the coactivation/equilibration and information transfer paradigms

In this section I would like to discuss two findings that have been repeatedly reported in the literature that could be interpreted differently by the information flow and coactivation/equilibration viewpoints. I will argue that the coactivation/equilibration model can account for more aspects of the findings than the information flow model.

FASTER INTERHEMISPHERIC TRANSFER TIMES FROM THE RIGHT HEMISPHERE TO THE LEFT HEMISPHERE THAN VICE VERSA   The first empirical observation is that interhemispheric transfer times differ in directionality, as inferred from reaction time paradigms. These paradigms examine the extent to which responding to a lateralized signal is faster using the contralateral as compared to ipsilateral hand. The ipsilateral versus contralateral difference in transfer time varies according to whether the signal was originally presented to the right or left hemisphere. (In other words, the so-called right-to-left-hemisphere transfer is faster than the so-called left-to-right-hemisphere transfer.) This has been reported both behaviorally and in terms of evoked potentials (see Chapters 9, 11, and 16 in this volume).

Information flow perspective   On the basis of the information flow model, one would likely seek a structural explanation for this effect. One would argue that there is literally faster transmission from the right hemisphere to the left hemisphere owing to an asymmetry within the fibers of the corpus callosum, permitting action potentials traveling to the left hemisphere to be conducted faster.

Coactivation perspective   On the basis of the coactivation/equilibration model, it would not be assumed that the effect is callosal because it would not necessarily be assumed that the crossed-uncrossed time difference merely represents the time that it takes for a signal to cross the corpus callosum. Instead, one would consider extracallosal factors to explain this effect. Claude Braun does a masterful job of reviewing such extracallosal factors (see Chapter 9 in this volume). In the current context, one such factor might be the greater tendency for right than left hemisphere to distribute activation both within and between hemispheres (Heilman and Van Abel, 1979).

NEGLECT BY SPLIT-BRAIN PATIENTS OF THE LEFTMOST ITEM WITH A PAIR OF IDENTICAL STIMULI DESPITE SUPRANORMAL REDUNDANCY GAINS IN RESPONSE SPEED   The other interhemispheric phenomenon that can be differentially explained by the coactivation/equilibration and information flow models has been reported in split-brain patients by Reuter-Lorenz and colleagues (1995). These patients detected a stimulus more rapidly when two identical or "redundant" stimuli were presented bilaterally (i.e., one to each hemisphere) than when a single stimulus was presented to just one hemisphere. In fact, the redundancy gain was supranormal in that the facilitation by redundant stimuli was greater than that seen in neurologically intact individuals. What makes this finding interesting is that the split-brain patients often did not consciously perceive that there were two stimuli. Thus, they manifested a supranormal redundancy gain to bilateral stimulation despite often being unaware that there were actually two stimuli.

Information flow model   One would not predict unilateral neglect on the basis of the information flow model unless the response was verbal (the stimulus appearing on the left side of space might not trigger a left-hemisphere verbal response, assuming that the occurrence of the stimulus has to be "transferred" to the left hemisphere before it an be verbally acknowledged). Because Reuter-Lorenz and colleagues (1995) did not require a verbal response, this was not a confound, and the information flow theory is at a loss to account for the neglect. In terms of the redundancy gain in response to bilateral stimuli, this would probably be interpreted by the information flow model as the level of information transfer capable of being communicated via a subcortical commissure in the absence of the cerebral commissures. However, the information flow model would not readily account for a supranormal redundancy gain.

Coactivation model   The coactivation/equilibration model can directly account for occurrence of neglect in a split-brain patient. The model assumes that reciprocal inhibition at a brain stem level, initiated by simultaneous bilateral stimulation, results in exaggerated arousal imbalances on a cortical level and lateral swings in attention (without the equilibratory influence of the corpus callosum).

From the coactivation/equilibration perspective, intrahemispheric arousal is abnormal in the split brain because of lack of callosal coactivation. Thus, contralateral activation from the unstimulated hemisphere may facilitate processing in the stimulated hemisphere by means of a thalamocortical and-gate as hypothesized by Payne (1994) and Lassonde (1986). Following this reasoning, the enhanced redundancy gain may be due to an exceptionally sluggish response to single stimuli rather than an exceptionally great response to bilateral stimuli.

Conclusion

The proposed experimental variations would permit evaluation of the three models of callosal function. Coupled with phenomena already reported in the literature, it is likely that a critical role for the corpus callosum is coactivation and distribution of activation between the two cerebral hemispheres. A more complete discussion of these ideas can be found in the work of Liederman (1995).

REFERENCES

HEILMAN, K., and T. VAN DEN ABEL, 1979. Right hemispheric dominance for mediating cerebral activation. *Neuropsychologia* 17:315–321.

HISCOCK, M., 1982. Verbal-manual time-sharing in children as a function of task priority. *Brain Cogn.* 1:119–131.

KINSBOURNE, M., 1982. Hemisphere specialization and the growth of human understanding. *Am. Psychol.* 37:411–420.

LASSONDE, M., 1986. The facilitory influence of the corpus callosum on intrahemispheric processing. In *Two Hemispheres–One Brain: Functions of the Corpus Callosum*, F. Lepore, M. Ptito, and H. H. Jasper, eds. New York: Alan R. Liss, pp. 385–401.

LIEDERMAN, J., 1995. A reinterpretation of the split brain syndrome: Implications for the function of cortico-cortical fibers. In *Brain Asymmetry*, R. Davidson and K. Hugdahl, eds. Cambridge, Mass.: MIT Press, pp. 451–490.

PAYNE, B. R., 1994. Neuronal interactions in cat visual cortex mediated by the corpus callosum. *Behav. Brain Res.* 64:55–64.

REUTER-LORENZ, P. A., G. NOZAWA, M. S. GAZZANIGA, and H. C. HUGHES, 1995. Fate of neglected targets: A chronometric analysis of redundant target effects in the bisected brain. *J. Exp. Psychol. Hum. Percept. Perform.* 21:211–230.

WEXLER, B. E., and T. HALWES, 1983. Increasing power of dichotic methods: The fused rhymed words test. *Neuropsychologia* 21:59–66.

YAZGAN, M. Y., B. WEXLER, M. KINSBOURNE, B. PETERSON, and J. LECKMAN, 1995. Functional significance of individual variations in callosal area. *Neuropsychologia* 33:769–779.

ZAIDEL, E., J. CLARKE, and B. SUYENOBU, 1990. Hemispheric independence: A paradigm case for cognitive neuroscience. In *UCLA Forum in Medical Sciences*, Vol. 29: *Neurobiology of Higher Cognitive Functioning*, A. B. Scheibel and M. D. Wechsler, eds. New York: Guilford Press, 1990, pp. 297–355.

11 Effects of Partial Callosal and Unilateral Cortical Lesions on Interhemispheric Transfer

CARLO A. MARZI, L. G. BONGIOVANNI, CARLO MINIUSSI, AND NICOLA SMANIA

ABSTRACT Partial lesions of the corpus callosum (CC) severely affect electrophysiological indices of interhemispheric transfer (IT), whereas they affect behavioral IT to a much lesser extent. A similar result has been found for unilateral lesions of the right hemisphere, presumably resulting in partial degeneration of the CC. In this paper we try to clarify such discrepancy in an attempt to cast light on the callosal mechanisms of IT of visuomotor information.

Individuals who lack the corpus callosum (CC) for surgical or genetic reasons are known to be impaired on a series of cognitive operations requiring interhemispheric transfer (IT) of information.

However, they can still perform various forms of IT. For example, they are able to respond unimanually to a light flash presented to the opposite visual hemifield. In such a condition the cortical sites of stimulus reception and of response initiation are in opposite hemispheres, and therefore an IT is required. The only difference from normals is represented by the consistently and substantially longer IT time as measured behaviorally with a reaction time (RT) paradigm originally devised by Poffenberger in 1912 (see Marzi, Bisiacchi, and Nicoletti, 1991, for a review). The behavioral estimate of IT, as assessed by subtracting the averaged RTs of the uncrossed hemifield-hand combinations from those of the crossed combinations (the so-called crossed-uncrossed difference, or CUD), ranges from 4 ms in normals to 18 ms in genetically acallosal subjects and to 55 ms in patients who underwent complete commissurotomy.

The lengthening of the CUD is clearly proportional to the amount of commissural fibers lost, given that it is less marked in agenetics who are known to have several commissural structures spared than in subjects with a complete commissurotomy. In spite of the role of the CC in IT, it is remarkable that commissurotomy patients remain able to transfer visuomotor information from one hemisphere to the other, albeit somewhat more slowly than normals. The few event-related potential (ERP) studies concerned with IT in patients lacking the CC (Rugg, Milner, and Lines, 1985; Tramo et al., 1995) found not just a lengthening but rather a complete disappearance of the early visual components of the ERP such as P1 and N1 from the hemisphere ipsilateral to the stimulated hemifield, that is, from the hemisphere receiving the commissural input. The discrepancy between electrophysiological and behavioral IT assessments may have interesting implications for a general understanding of the pathways of interhemispheric visuomotor integration. For example, it suggests that the early components of the visual ERP index a fast channel of IT that is absent in commissurotomy or agenesis patients. In contrast, response-related information can still cross interhemispherically via slower subcortical commissures. In subjects lacking the CC, waveforms such as P1, that is, a positive component peaking at about 100 ms from stimulus onset, and N1, that is, a negative component peaking at about 150 ms from stimulus onset (see Mangun, 1995, for a review), are absent from the ipsilateral (i.e., commissural) evoked response to a lateralized visual stimulus. As alluded to above, this suggests that whatever information is transferred from one hemisphere to the other following section or congenital absence of the CC must be concerned with response-related aspects of the visuomotor task rather than with visual aspects.

CARLO A. MARZI AND L. G. BONGIOVANNI Department of Neurological and Visual Sciences, University of Verona, Verona, Italy.
CARLO MINIUSSI IRCSS S. Giovanni di Dio, Brescia, Italy.
NICOLA SMANIA Rehabilitation Unit, Ospedale Civile Borgo Roma, Verona, Italy.

To try to cast light on such questions, we have studied patients with different cerebral lesions interfering with a normal callosal functioning. They include two patients with a partial callosal lesion and six patients with a unilateral hemispheric lesion. All these subjects have been studied by recording ERPs with a 32-electrode computerized system while performing the Poffenberger paradigm. A detailed description of our recording method and procedure can be found in the work of Ipata and colleagues (1997).

In addition to single stimuli, our task included presentation of randomly intermingled pairs of stimuli. These pairs were presented across the vertical meridian of the visual field so that the two stimuli fell into opposite hemifields. The purpose of introducing double stimuli was to test for the presence of a redundant target effect (RTE), that is, the speeding up of RT for multiple as compared with single stimuli. With bilaterally presented stimuli such an effect requires an IT for stimuli to be summated, and we thought it interesting to find out whether our callosum-lesioned patients might show a dissociation between different types of IT. There are two major interpretations of the RTE. One is based on a horse race model (Raab, 1962) and considers the RTE as related to probability summation. The other is represented by the coactivation model (Miller, 1982), which interprets the RTE as a neural summation phenomenon. The horse race interpretation requires that the two signals converge onto a hypothetical decision center where only the fastest stimulus of each pair triggers the motor response at the appropriate premotor and motor centers. In contrast, the coactivation account requires the two signals to access a common neuronal pool where they are summated according to "Sherringtonian" rules of neuronal summation. The effect of such a summation is to speed up the activation of the response-related centers.

Recently, we provided ERP evidence (Miniussi, Girelli, and Marzi, 1998) supporting a coactivation model operating at the level of the extrastriate visual cortex. We found that the early visual ERP components, namely, P1 and N1, were of shorter latency for bilateral stimuli than for the algebraic sum of two unilateral stimuli. This represents evidence that during bilateral presentations a neural summation between the stimuli has taken place with a consequent decrease in the latency of the evoked response.

Effects of partial callosal lesions

The patients studied were two males who suffered from closed head injury resulting from traffic accidents: S.M. was 35 years old at the time of testing (3 months after

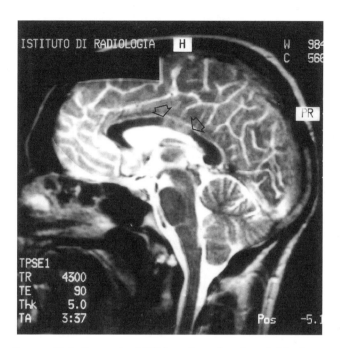

FIGURE 11.1. Parasagittal MRI section of patient S. M. showing between the arrows the lesioned part of the middle portion of the corpus callosum.

the trauma) and showed magnetic resonance imaging (MRI) evidence of damage in the middle third of the CC (see Figure 11.1). B.A. was 69 years old at the time of testing (22 months after the trauma) and showed computerized tomography (CT) evidence of a hemorrhagic lesion in the middle third of the CC.

Behavioral results

Figure 11.2 shows for S.M. (upper left panel) and B.A. (upper right) the cumulative distribution of RTs to patches of light (56 ms duration) presented at 8° to either the left (LVF) or the right (RVF) field or bilaterally (BVF). There were no interfield differences in RT to unilateral stimuli, while RTs to bilateral stimuli were consistently faster than those to unilateral stimuli, thus providing evidence for a normal RTE. This shows that some degree of interhemispheric integration is present in these subjects, given that during bilateral presentations the stimuli are projected initially to different hemispheres and therefore an IT is necessary for summation to occur. More important for the present purposes, both patients showed a lengthened CUD (S.M. = 11 ms; B.A. = 13 ms; usual value for normals: 4 ms; see Marzi et al., 1991).

The two bottom panels in Figure 11.2 show that the uncrossed responses are consistently faster than the crossed ones over practically the whole RT distribution for both S.M. (left) and B.A. (right). Thus, in these pa-

RTE

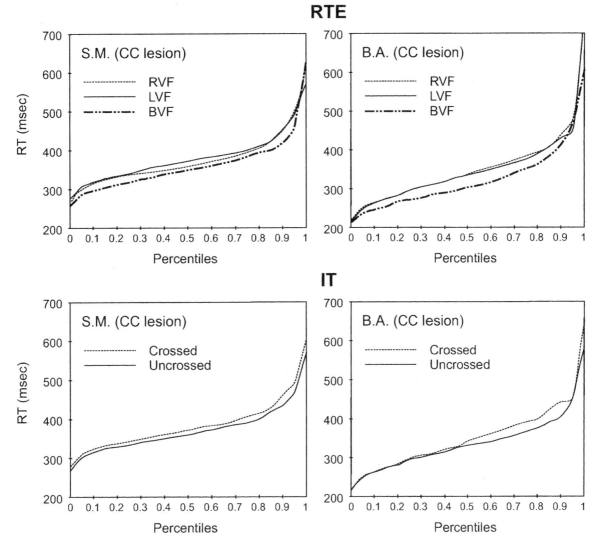

FIGURE 11.2. Cumulative frequency distributions (CFDs) of reaction times (RTs): At the top are reported RTs to unilateral stimuli presented to the right (RVF) or left (LVF) visual hemifield or bilaterally (BVF) across the vertical meridian for patient S.M. (left) and patient B.A. (right), both with a partial callosal lesion. At the bottom are reported for patients S.M. (left) and B.A. (right) the CFDs of RTs to stimuli presented either to the hemifield contralateral (crossed responses) or ipsilateral (uncrossed responses) to the responding hand. The left and right uncrossed and crossed combinations have been averaged together.

tients with a partial callosal damage, the pathways for interhemispheric integration of visuomotor responses are impaired, while those for the interhemispheric integration of the RTE seem to be spared.

Electrophysiological results

In keeping with the discrepancy discussed above for the commissurotomized patients, IT, as assessed by ERP, shows a more marked impairment than behavioral IT.

In patient S.M. a lack of an ipsilateral (commissural) response is evident in temporal, parietal, and anterior occipital areas (see the top trace in Figure 11.3 for recordings from electrode sites P3 and P5), while the con-

tralateral (direct) responses are preserved. The lack of ipsilateral responses concerns both P1 and N1 but is particularly evident in the latter; in contrast, the later ERP components do not differ in the direct and indirect conditions. A roughly similar picture is present in the other patient, B.A.; see Figure 11.4, where bilateral temporal and parietal and right occipital areas (see TO2 and O2) showed a lack of ipsilateral (commissural) response.

These results are of interest for two reasons: First, they show that a relatively restricted lesion in the CC can substantially abolish IT-ERP, as indexed by early visual components P1 and N1, in a relatively large area of the cortex. As is the case in complete commissuro-

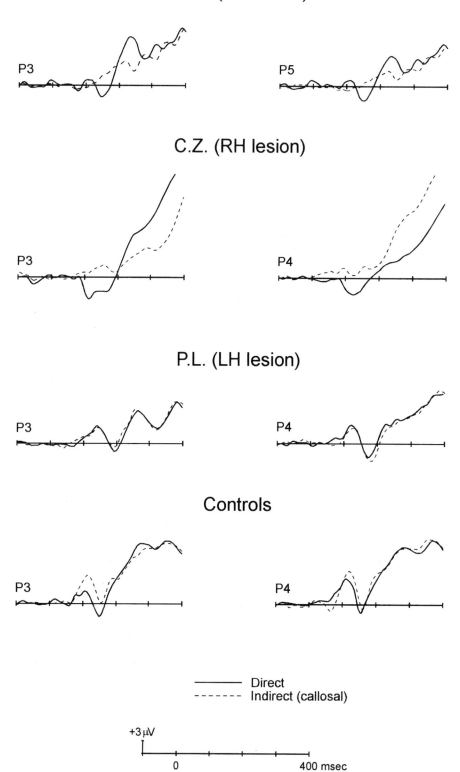

FIGURE 11.3. Event-related potential (ERP) direct (solid) or commissural (dashed) responses to lateralized visual stimuli for left (P3, P5) or right (P4) posterior parietal electrodes. The top trace is from a patient with a partial callosal lesion; the second and third traces are from patients with unilateral cortical lesions. The bottom trace is from a normal control.

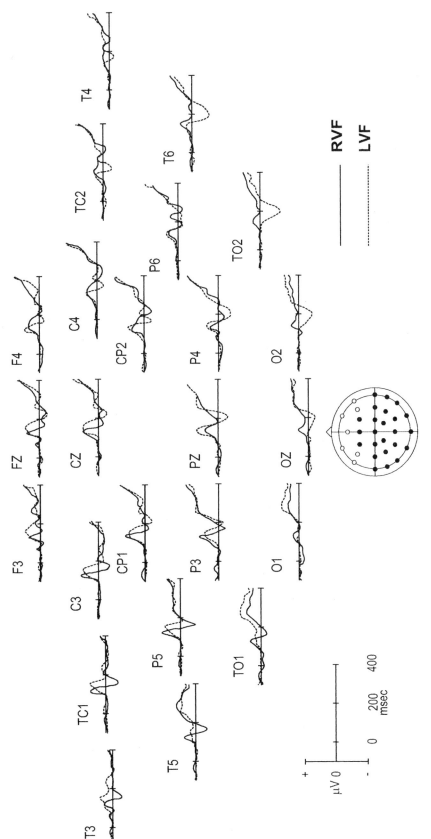

Figure 11.4. ERP traces for the recording sites of interest in patient B.A. with a partial callosal lesion. Responses to RVF stimuli: gray line; responses to LVF stimuli: black lines. Notice the missing ipsilateral responses in T5 and T6, TO1 and TO2.

tomized subjects or agenetics, the loss of the ipsilateral early visual ERP components is still compatible with an IT; in fact, in our patients, the CUD is only marginally lengthened relative to normals.

Second, both subjects show a normal interfield RTE, and this is evidence for the existence of different channels mediating IT in the two tasks.

Possible IT pathways in callosum-lesioned patients

An interesting question is whether the IT necessary for both visuomotor integration and the RTE takes place in the spared portions of the CC or via subcortical routes. The observation that patients with a resection of the anterior commissure in addition to the CC do not have a longer CUD than acallosal patients with a spared anterior commissure seems to rule out the importance of such a pathway for visuomotor IT (for a recent review, see Berlucchi et al., 1995). As to the callosal sites responsible for the CUD, there is converging evidence that partial lesions of the CC are compatible with a practically normal CUD whether they are located in the anterior or posterior portions of the CC (Berlucchi et al., 1995). Contrasting evidence has been provided by Di Stefano, Sauerwein, and Lassonde (1992), who found a lengthened CUD in a patient who underwent anterior callosotomy and by Iacoboni and Zaidel (1995), who found evidence of an abnormal CUD in a patient with a section of the anterior CC sparing the callosal splenium.

Our present results show that some lengthening of behavioral IT is indeed present in a patient with a lesion of the posterior third and in another one with a lesion of the middle third of the CC. However, such an effect is minimal, especially if one considers the absence in many areas of the ipsilateral (commissural) visual ERP response to lateralized stimuli. A more substantial behavioral effect of partial damage to the CC has been reported recently by Geschwind and colleagues (1995) in a patient with a vascular lesion of the middle and posterior portions of the CC. Unfortunately, ERP-IT measures are not available for this patient, whose lesion is probably larger than those of the two patients described above.

A different consideration applies to the RTE which is remarkably preserved in these patients and this is in keeping with the spared RTE of the complete split-brain cases described by Reuter-Lorenz and colleagues (1995) and that of Marzi and colleagues (1997). In light of a recent study by Tomaiuolo and colleagues (1997) showing a RTE for bilateral stimuli even in hemispherectomized patients, we believe that such an effect may be subserved by visual subcortical centers such as the superior colliculus. The IT necessary for a summation between the stimuli presented to different hemifields might

well take place via collicular or other subcortical commissures. It should be mentioned that the hypothesis of a subcortical IT in the absence of the CC is not shared by Reuter-Lorenz and colleagues (1995), who have proposed a model based on interhemispheric response competition to account for the RTE in split-brain subjects.

Summing up then, in our patients with a lesion of the middle part of the CC, behavioral IT is still present, albeit lengthened; in contrast, ERP-IT, as assessed by P1 and N1, is absent in many cortical areas. This suggests that the fast IT typical of normal subjects is subserved by the same neural processes that generate the P1 and N1 components of the ERP, while slower IT is indexed by longer-latency components such as the so-called lateralized readiness potential or P300 (see Coles and Rugg, 1995), which were similar for ipsilateral and contralateral responses, thus indicating a complete IT of these components.

Effects of unilateral cortical lesions on IT

Patients with large unilateral cortical lesions are likely to undergo a degeneration of callosal fibers as a consequence of the death of their cell bodies. By comparing patients with lesions in different cortical areas, one can hope to cast light on the callosal areas that are important for IT. Vallar, Sterzi, and Basso (1988) followed a similar line of reasoning in a study in which they found a lengthened CUD in paretic as compared to nonparetic patients with cortical unilateral lesions. Because prefrontal cortical areas are more likely to be affected in paretic than in nonparetic patients, it follows that such areas may be critical sites for visuomotor IT.

The problem with drawing conclusions on visuomotor IT from patients with unilateral motor cortical lesions is that if one uses only the nonparetic hand, there is an inevitable confound between CUD and hemifield asymmetries. Therefore, what appears to be a CUD lengthening may be related to an advantage of the ipsilesional hemifield in stimulus processing. To try to cast light on these problems, we have studied six patients with unilateral right ($n = 4$) or left ($n = 2$) hemispheric vascular lesions as well as age-matched normal controls in the same RT task as that described above, including both a Poffenberger and a RTE paradigm. ERP recording was carried out during performance of the task to have a measure of IT that is relatively free from a direct effect of the cortical lesion on hemispheric visuomotor processing.

Behavioral results

A common finding for all patients was that there was a marked overall lengthening of the CUD (R.P. = 63 ms,

C.Z. = 56 ms, L.G. = 21 ms, B.M. = 102 ms; mean for right hemisphere (RH) lesioned patients: 60.5 ms, mean for left hemisphere (LH) lesioned patients: 33 ms, controls mean: 2.2 ms). As was pointed out above, however, one should consider that only the ipsilesional hand could be used in the above patients, and therefore the CUD coincides with a difference in speed between the two visual hemifields (see the top two panels of Figure 11.5). In RH patients who used their normal right hand, there was a marked advantage of the RVF; conversely, in LH patients using the left hand, there was a less marked but still substantial advantage of the LVF.

Notice that no interfield differences were found, as is often the case in this task, in a normal control subject (see Figure 11.5, bottom panel).

To disentangle hemifield differences from IT, we tested two of the above patients (R.P. and C.Z.) and two other patients, F.D. (right parietal lesion) and P.L. (left parietal lesion), using a nonlateralized motor response such as a lowering of the chin. If the above differences depend on an impaired IT, they should diminish or disappear when using a response that can be initiated by either hemisphere.

The results were clear-cut: In all four patients there was a lengthening of the hemifield contralateral to the cortical lesion both when using the hand and when using the chin. In this experiment, the stimuli were presented at four different eccentricities in the two hemifields (10°, 20°, 30°, 40°), and the advantage of the ipsilesional hemifield was present for all eccentricities: RH patients ($n = 3$), right-hand response: CUD = 53.8 ms; chin response: RVF advantage over LVF = 61.0 ms. LH patient ($n = 1$), left-hand response: CUD = 24.2 ms; chin response: LVF advantage over RVF = 13.8 ms. Therefore, one can conclude that in our patients the advantage of the uncrossed versus crossed hand/field combinations may be related to an interfield difference favoring the hemifield ipsilateral to the lesion rather than to an increased CUD.

The reason why RTs are delayed when visual input is relayed to the contralesional hemisphere is not clear. The presence of a clinically ascertained field defect does not seem to be a necessary condition; presumably, intrahemispheric visuomotor connections are slower in the lesioned hemisphere.

In conclusion, the study of patients with unilateral lesions to assess IT with the Poffenberger paradigm requires testing of both hands to disentangle interfield differences from effects on IT. The use of a nonlateralized response has enabled us to ascertain that patients with a unilateral lesion centered on the parietal lobe show a delayed stimulus processing in the contralesional hemifield rather than an increased CUD.

As to the RTE, the results of our six patients were very consistent in showing a lack of an RTE (see Figure 11.5). This is not surprising, given the presence of strong interfield differences for unilateral stimuli. During bilateral presentations it is likely that the manual response is triggered by stimulation of the faster ipsilesional hemifield and therefore bilateral and ipsilesional presentations yield similar mean RTs.

Electrophysiological results and discussion

Figure 11.3 shows examples of ERP recordings for one RH and one LH patient with a unilateral lesion (second and third traces from top), for one of the patients with partial callosal damage (S.M.) referred to above, and two normal controls averaged together.

A puzzling, novel finding was that while the ipsilateral (commissural) response was lacking or reduced in patients with a RH lesion, such was not the case for LH patients (compare the second and third traces from top in Figure 11.3).

The reason for such a laterality difference is not clear, but it is tempting to relate it to a left-right asymmetry in callosal projections (Marzi et al., 1991). If, as has been hypothesized, callosally projecting neurons are more numerous in the right hemisphere than in the left hemisphere, it is reasonable to assume that a unilateral RH lesion will cause a greater loss of callosal fibers than a similar LH lesion. This speculation obviously awaits specific testing with a much larger number of cases than in the present study.

The results of an impaired callosal transmission in patients with a unilateral RH lesion (see also Marzi et al., 1997) can be related to the presence in our RH patients of unilateral extinction to contralesional stimuli, a frequent consequence of damage to the RH together with the more severe impairment known as hemineglect (Heilman et al., 1987). As is well known, extinction consists of the failure to perceive contralesional visual or tactile stimuli during bilateral presentations, while unilateral stimuli are normally perceived on both sides. We speculated elsewhere (Marzi et al., 1997) that the presence of a callosal impairment as a consequence of a unilateral RH lesion may cause unilateral contralateral extinction because the commissural input from the left visual field to the intact LH, which presumably mediates the task, given the impairment of the RH, is lacking or reduced. Under the more demanding conditions of bilateral stimulus presentation, the reduced callosal input from the contralesional left visual field may fail to be detected by the LH, and therefore contralesional extinction might ensue. Such would not be the case during unilateral stimuli because in the absence of competition with the

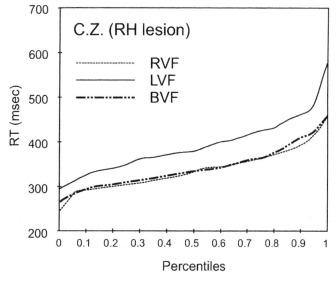

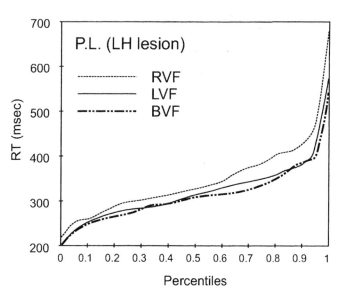

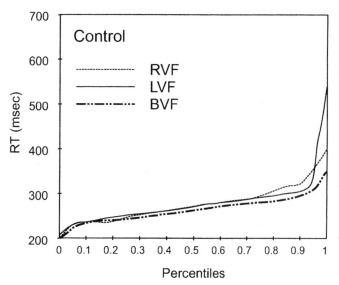

FIGURE 11.5. CFDs of RTs to unilateral or bilateral stimuli (see the caption for Figure 11.2) for two patients with a unilateral right (top) or left (middle) cortical lesion and an age-matched normal control (bottom).

other side, even a weak callosal input might be detected by the intact LH. According to our hypothesis unilaterally lesioned RH patients who do not present with extinction are those who do not have a (partial) degeneration of callosal fibers as a consequence of their lesion.

General conclusions

Taken together, our results show that by combined behavioral and ERP testing, it is possible to confirm the existence of a fast callosal channel, presumably subserved by the largest callosal axons, which is responsible for IT of visuomotor information. Its absence in split-brain or agenetic subjects results in a lengthening of behavioral IT, which, however, survives by virtue of slower-conducting subcortical commissural systems. Such a slow IT channel can be documented electrophysiologically in callosum-sectioned patients by the presence of ipsilateral (commissural) late components to lateralized stimuli that have latency and amplitude that are essentially similar to those of the corresponding contralateral late components. Partial callosal lesions tend to leave behavioral IT substantially unimpaired, presumably because they fail to remove all large axons from the CC. However, such lesions are sufficient to determine a loss of IT in the early components of the ERP response, notably N1, which is probably the best electrophysiological correlate of behavioral IT (Ipata et al., 1997). This is a puzzling discrepancy that clearly requires further studies.

REFERENCES

BERLUCCHI, G., S. AGLIOTI, C. A. MARZI, and G. TASSINARI, 1995. Corpus callosum and simple visuomotor integration. *Neuropsychologia* 33:923–936.

COLES, M. G. H., and M. D. RUGG, 1995. Event-related brain potentials: An introduction. In *Electrophysiology of Mind: Event-Related Potentials and Cognition*, M. D. Rugg and M. G. H. Coles, eds. Oxford, Engl.: Oxford Science Publishers, pp. 1–39.

DI STEFANO, M., H. C. SAUERWEIN, and M. LASSONDE, 1992. Influence of anatomical factors and spatial compatibility on the stimulus-response relationship in the absence of the corpus callosum. *Neuropsychologia* 30:177–185.

GESCHWIND, D. H., M. IACOBONI, M. S. MEGA, D. W. ZAIDEL, T. CLOUGHESY, and E. ZAIDEL, 1995. Alien hand syndrome: Interhemispheric motor disconnection due to a lesion in the midbody of the corpus callosum. *Neurology* 45:802–808.

HEILMAN, K. M., D. BOWERS, E. VALENSTEIN, and R. T. WATSON, 1987. Hemispace and hemispatial neglect. In *Neurophysiological and Neuropsychological Aspects of Spatial Neglect*, M. Jeannerod, ed. Amsterdam: Elsevier, pp. 115–150.

IACOBONI, M., and E. ZAIDEL, 1995. Channels of the corpus callosum: Evidence from simple reaction times to lateralized flashes in the normal and the split brain. *Brain* 118:779–788.

IPATA, A., M. GIRELLI, C. MINIUSSI, and C. A. MARZI, 1997. Interhemispheric transfer of visual information in humans: The role of different callosal channels. *Arch. Ital. Biol.* 135:169–182.

MANGUN, G. R., 1995. Neural mechanisms of visual selective attention. *Psychophysiology* 32:4–18.

MARZI, C. A., P. BISIACCHI, and R. NICOLETTI, 1991. Is interhemispheric transfer of visuomotor information asymmetric? Evidence from a meta-analysis. *Neuropsychologia* 29:1163–1167.

MARZI, C. A., A. FANINI, M. GIRELLI, A. E. IPATA, C. MINIUSSI, N. SMANIA, and M. PRIOR, 1997. Is extinction following parietal damage an interhemispheric disconnection phenomenon? In *Parietal lobe contribution to orientation in 3D space*, P. Their and H. O. Karnath, eds. Heidelberg: Springer-Verlag, pp. 431–445.

MILLER, J., 1982. Divided attention: Evidence for coactivation with redundant signals. *Cognit. Psychol.* 14:247–279.

MINIUSSI, C., M. GIRELLI, and C. A. MARZI, 1998. Neural site of the redundant target effect: Electrophysiological evidence. *J. Cogn. Neurosci.* 10:216–230.

POFFENBERGER, A. T., 1912. Reaction time to retinal stimulation with special reference to the time lost in conduction through nervous centers. *Arch. Psychol.* 23:1–73.

RAAB, D., 1962. Statistical facilitation of simple reaction times. *Trans. N.Y. Acad. Sci.* 24:574–590.

REUTER-LORENZ, P. A., G. NOZAWA, M. S. GAZZANIGA, and H. C. HUGHES, 1995. Fate of neglected targets: A chronometric analysis of redundant target effects in the bisected brain. *J. Exp. Psychol. Hum. Percept. Perform.* 21:211–230.

RUGG, M. D., A. D. MILNER, and C. R. LINES, 1985. Visual evoked potentials to lateralized stimuli in two cases of callosal agenesis. *J. Neurol. Neurosurg. Psychiatry* 48:367–373.

TOMAIUOLO, F., M. PTITO, C. A. MARZI, T. PAUS, and A. PTITO, 1997. Blindsight in hemispherectomized patients as revealed by spatial summation across the vertical meridian. *Brain* 120:795–803.

TRAMO, M. J., K. BAYNES, R. FENDRICH, G. R. MANGUN, E. A. PHELPS, P. A. REUTER-LORENZ, and M. S. GAZZANIGA, 1995. Hemispheric specialization and interhemispheric integration. In *Epilepsy and the Corpus Callosum II*, A. G. Reeves and D. W. Roberts, eds. New York: Plenum Press, pp. 263–295.

VALLAR, G., R. STERZI, and A. BASSO, 1988. Left hemisphere contribution to motor programming of aphasic speech: A reaction time experiment in aphasic patients. *Neuropsychologia* 26:511–519.

COMMENTARY 11.1

Interhemispheric Transfer of Visuomotor Inputs in a Split-Brain Patient: Electrophysiological and Behavioral Indexes

ALICE MADO PROVERBIO AND ALBERTO ZANI

ABSTRACT   Marzi and colleagues described the case of two partially acallosal patients, suggesting that their interhemispheric transfer in a Poffenberger paradigm could be mediated by slow subcortical routes. Some discrepancies between the CUD in RTs and visual event-related potentials (ERPs), along with a dishomogeneity in lesions locus, make it difficult to compare the data of the two patients and draw any straightforward conclusion. We present ERP data of a commissurotomized patient engaged in selective attention tasks to lateralized patterned stimuli. These data provide evidence of a delayed synchronized evoked response affected by stimulus eccentricity over the disconnected nonviewing hemisphere, probably mediated by collicular subcortical pathways.

Interhemispheric transfer in partial acallosals

In their chapter, Marzi and colleagues describe the case of two patients with a lesion in the middle third (patient B.A.) and posterior third (patient S.M.) of the corpus callosum (CC), respectively. Their performance in a Poffenberger paradigm was characterized by a slight lengthening of crossed-uncrossed difference (CUD), a practically normal redundant target effect (RTE), and a complete disappearance of their visual P1 and N1 early evoked responses to stimuli at the ipsilateral scalp sites. On the basis of these findings, the authors conclude that, in these patients, the interhemispheric transfer (IHT) could be mediated by slow subcortical routes involving the superior colliculus. Conversely, in commissure-intact subjects, the IHT would be based on fast callosal chan-

nels, as documented by the presence of early ipsilateral P1 and N1 evoked responses.

In our view, this is a reasonable and interesting hypothesis, which might actually account for IHT in patients who almost entirely lack the callosal commissure. However, we believe it should be used with caution for explaining the case of partial callosal patients, as also suggested by some recent interesting findings in neuropsychological literature (Aglioti et al., 1998). Patient B.A. is described as having an intact splenium, which is the portion of CC mostly devoted to visual transfer, and a strong RTE, along with an almost negligible CUD for fast responses (see the first five percentiles in Figure 11.2 of Marzi and colleagues' chapter). Unlike this pattern, his ERPs are described as having a clear CUD over visual areas. By contrast, patient S.M., suffering a lesion in the posterior third of the CC, had a slightly longer CUD, a smaller RTE, but apparently no CUD over visual areas for evoked responses. This discrepancy makes it difficult to compare the data of the two patients or to draw any straightforward conclusion.

With respect to this, it is important to underline that in their paradigm the authors made use of small patches of light, which have been shown to be mostly processed by the dorsal visual stream (scarcely sensitive to visual features but most sensitive to motion and spatial location) and to be conveyed by collicular-parietal pathways. Indeed, Iacoboni, Fried, and Zaidel (1994) have showed that for flashes of light presented at large eccentricities, in normal subjects IHT takes place at the level of anterior callosal fibers. This may explain why, in Marzi and colleagues' study, early components were larger over parietal areas. Conversely, when one stimulates visual cortex with luminance-modulated patterns of a given spatial frequency or orientation, in commis-

ALICE MADO PROVERBIO   Department of Psychology, University of Milano-Bicocca, Milano, Italy.
ALBERTO ZANI   Institute of Psychology, Consiglio Nazionale delle Ricerche, Rome, Italy.

sure-intact individuals responses have shown to be much larger over visual occipital areas. This is indexed by the focusing of early P1 and N1 components of sensory-evoked potentials at the latter areas (e.g., Proverbio and Zani, 1996; Proverbio, Zani, and Avella, 1996; Zani, Proverbio, and Avella, 1996; Anllo-Vento, Luck, and Hillyard, 1998).

Considering this evidence, we believe that the use of patterned stimuli may provide a useful mean of assessing the nature and efficiency of different interhemispheric pathways.

Visual evoked potential signs of visual IHT in normal subjects

In commissure-intact individuals, when a visual stimulus is restricted to one hemifield, it can be measured by an early evoked potential contralateral to the stimulus and a later ipsilateral potential in the nonviewing hemisphere. The difference in time between the contralateral and ipsilateral potentials roughly indicates the time it takes for information to cross the corpus callosum, that is, the interhemispheric transmission time. Collected evidence has shown that it may take from 8 to 15 ms for a signal to be transferred from one hemisphere to the other, depending on stimulus type, visual evoked potential component and brain area taken into account (Rugg, Lines, and Milner, 1984; Saron and Davidson, 1989; Proverbio et al., 1996; Zani et al., 1996). For example, if a 3-cpd grating is laterally presented in pattern onset in the LVF to a healthy individual, the first sign of cortex activity may appear at about 70 ms over the right lateral occipital (prestriate) area. The arising of an ipsilateral potential over the left prestriate area after only few milliseconds follows this contralateral activity. The ipsilateral potential gradually increases in amplitude until reaching its maximum value about 15 ms later than the contralateral potential.

This kind of callosal IHT is not observable in callosotomy patients who lack a normal ipsilateral evoked potential in the nonviewing hemisphere because of the absence of the splenium. Indeed, Rugg, Milner, and Lines (1985) have actually shown a lack of a normal N160 response to lateralized light flashes over the nonviewing hemisphere in two callosal agenesis patients. Although the patients' ipsilateral waveforms did show evidence of stimulus-evoked activity having a high degree of similarity with their contralateral counterparts, there was a lack of ipsilateral activity in the same latency range. On the basis of these findings, it was concluded that the ipsilateral early activity relies for its generation on the transcallosal transfer of information.

IHT in a split-brain patient

To investigate the mechanisms of visual IHT in a patient lacking the callosal commissure, we tested the split-brain patient J.W. This patient is a right-handed alert male. In his youth he underwent a two-stage callosotomy for therapeutical reasons. MRI scans documented the complete resection of corpus callosum with sparing of anterior commissure.

We had previously tested this patient in a Poffenberger paradigm to study visuomotor coordination using small patches of light laterally presented at two different eccentricities (4° and 7°). Both reaction times (RTs) and event-related potentials (ERPs) were recorded. The hand-hemifield uncrossed data demonstrated that CC plays an essential role in mediating the control of attention to locations in the extrapersonal space. In fact, compared to our neurologically intact controls, its surgical disconnection produced in our patient a strong attentional bias toward the rightmost space, along with a left-hemisphere neglect of the left space (Proverbio et al., 1994). This was true for both the RT and ERP indexes. Interestingly, the analysis of crossed responses showed the complete disappearance of the rightward bias, with no differences between the visual hemifields. Indeed, the CUD for RTs, which was of about 65 ms, was affected by retinal eccentricity. In the crossed condition the left hemisphere was more responsive to the ipsilateral space and not biased toward the rightmost stimuli. This pattern of results may be explained by assuming some kind of interhemispheric communication that is able to minimize the effects related to the functional isolation of both hemispheres in the uncrossed condition.

Visual evoked potential signs of subcortical transfer

To further investigate the mechanisms of interhemispheric communication, we carried out an electrophysiological and behavioral study using patterned stimuli that in normal controls have been shown to be actively processed by occipital visual areas, and transferred through the splenium. A selective attention task based on orientation discrimination was used to keep the patient attentive and alert. The patient was asked to press a button with the index finger of the ipsilateral hand to target stimuli (10% probability) presented at 4° or 7° of eccentricity in a given hemifield and to ignore all the other stimuli. He was instructed to maintain eye fixation on the center of the screen. His eye movements were controlled with an infrared videocamera and electro-oculogram recordings. ERPs were recorded from 61 scalp sites referenced to a noncephalic sternovertebral lead to avoid any possible ipsilateral activity generated

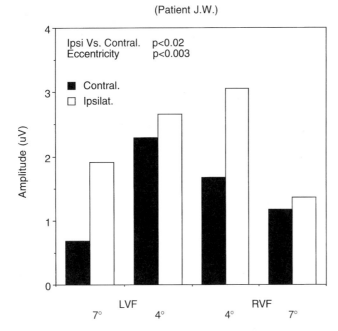

(Patient J.W.)

Ipsi Vs. Contral.   p<0.02
Eccentricity   p<0.003

■ Contral.
□ Ipsilat.

FIGURE 11.6. P1 mean amplitude values recorded at occipital sites as a function of visual field and stimulus eccentricity. Note that both contralateral (P90) and ipsilateral responses (P185) were affected by eccentricity.

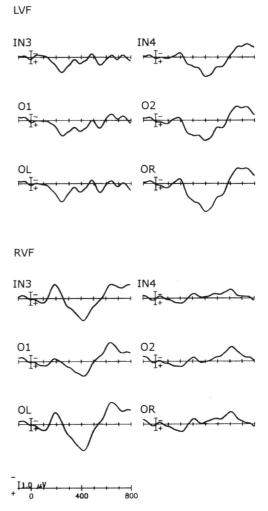

FIGURE 11.7. Event-related potentials (ERPs) to nontarget stimuli (vertical gratings) presented at 7° of eccentricity in the left and right visual fields. Recording electrodes were located at inion, mesial, and lateral occipital sites. Note the large and clear-cut early synchronized activity over the ipsilateral hemisphere.

at scalp reference sites. To get the best signal-to-noise ratio, a very high number of stimulus repetitions (over 600 trials per average) was adopted. Stimuli were spatial frequency gratings of 3 cpd presented at high contrast with two different orientations (vertical and horizontal). Quantification of sensory-evoked potentials over the posterior brain areas was accomplished by measuring peak amplitude and latency within the range of 60–120 ms over the contralateral and 90–200 ms over the ipsilateral hemisphere. Electrophysiological measures were analyzed by means of analyses of variance performed by subdividing all trials in random blocks, then using the blocks as random factor. (See Proverbio et al., 1994, for more details about this method.)

Figure 11.6 shows the amplitude of contralateral (P90) and ipsilateral (P185) as a function of stimulus field and hemisphere. Results indicated that both responses were affected by eccentricity, in that they were significantly larger to stimuli closest to the vertical meridian. Given that P185 did not show any sign of being either volume conducted or bilaterally generated (see Figure 11.7), we hypothesized that it might index a delayed synchronized activity of the ipsilateral hemisphere in response to visual stimuli. In principle, these data would indicate that the disconnected nonviewing hemisphere is provided with some kind of low-level visual information at relatively early stages of information processing.

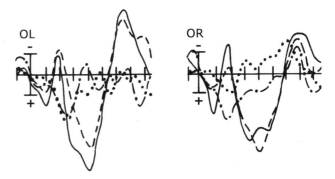

FIGURE 11.8. Event-related potentials (ERPs) to nontarget stimuli (vertical gratings) as a function of visual field of stimulation and cerebral hemisphere. Superimposed are waveforms recorded simultaneously over the contralateral (solid = 4°, dashed = 7°) and ipsilateral (dotted/dashed = 4°, dotted = 7°) hemisphere at occipital locations OL and OR.

It is worthy of note that, although late components were completely absent in the ipsilateral hemisphere in response to nontarget stimuli, ERP to targets (see Figure 11.8) showed P300s of normal amplitude and latency in both hemispheres. Quite interestingly also, the early N1 component to targets showed a less interhemispheric delay and a reasonable morphology. Both ERP and RT measures confirmed the pattern found in the Poffenberger paradigm (Proverbio et al., 1994) of a left-hemisphere bias toward the rightmost location in the uncrossed condition (see Figures 11.9 and 11.10).

Conclusions

It is well established that in intact brains, ipsilateral visual sensory-evoked responses within an early latency range rely on callosal transfer. Overall, the present findings in a complete callosotomy patient provided robust evidence that the appearance of a delayed synchronized activity over the disconnected nonviewing hemisphere might be an index of a lower level of interhemispheric

transfer of information through subcortical pathways that somehow functionally compensate for the lack of the CC commissure. Recent data indicating that the absence of cortical commissures does not completely preclude the transfer of visual information, allowing for object identification, also supports this hypothesis.

Indeed, it has been demonstrated that split-brain patients are able to make perceptual judgments, such as matching of nonsense shapes, across the vertical meridian (Zaidel, 1995). Support for this hypothesis has also come from neuropsychological findings of greater IHT deficits in partial agenesis than in complete callosal agenesis (Aglioti et al., 1998).

ACKNOWLEDGMENTS The authors are deeply indebted to Dr. G. R. Mangun and Dr. M. S. Gazzaniga for allowing the testing of patient J.W.

REFERENCES

AGLIOTI, S., A. BELTRAMELLO, G. TASSINARI, and G. BERLUCCHI, 1998. Paradoxically greater interhemispheric transfer deficits in partial than complete callosal agenesis. *Neuropsychologia* 36:1015–1024.

ANLLO-VENTO, L., S. LUCK, and S. A. HILLYARD, 1998. Spatiotemporal dynamics of attention to color: Evidence from human electrophysiology. *Hum. Brain Mapp.* 6:216–238.

IACOBONI, M., I. FRIED, and E. ZAIDEL, 1994. Callosal transmission time before and after partial commissurotomy. *NeuroReport* 5:2521–2524.

PROVERBIO, A. M., and A. ZANI, 1996. Differential activation of multiple current sources of foveal VEPs as a function of spatial frequency. *Brain Topogr.* 9:59–68.

PROVERBIO, A. M., A. ZANI, and C. AVELLA, 1996. Spatiotemporal mapping of visual evoked responses to hemi-foveal gratings. *Neuroimage* 3:295.

PROVERBIO, A. M., A. ZANI, M. S. GAZZANIGA, and R. G. MANGUN, 1994. ERP and RT signs of a rightward bias for spatial orienting in a split brain patient. *NeuroReport* 5:2457–2461.

RUGG, D. M., C. R. LINES, and A. D. MILNER, 1984. Visual evoked potentials to lateralized visual stimuli and the measurement of interhemispheric transmission time. *Neuropsychologia* 2:215–225.

RUGG, D. M., A. D. MILNER, and C. R. LINES, 1985. Visual evoked potentials to lateralized stimuli in two cases of callosal agenesis. *J. Neurol. Neurosurg. Psychiatry* 48:367–373.

SARON, C. D., and R. J. DAVIDSON, 1989. Visual evoked potential measures of interhemispheric transfer time in humans. *Behav. Neurosci.* 103:1115–1138.

ZAIDEL, E., 1995. Interhemispheric transfer in the split brain: Long-term status following complete cerebral commissurotomy. In *Brain Asymmetry*, R. J. Davidson and K. Hugdahl, eds. Cambridge, Mass.: MIT Press, pp. 491–532.

ZANI, A., A. M. PROVERBIO, and C. AVELLA, 1996. Contribution of the foveal strip at the visual vertical meridian to sensory-evoked responses to spatial frequency gratings. *Neuroimage* 3:303.

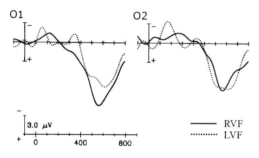

FIGURE 11.9. Event-related potentials (ERPs) to target stimuli (horizontal gratings) as a function of visual field of stimulation and cerebral hemisphere. Superimposed are waveforms recorded simultaneously over the contralateral (solid) and ipsilateral (dashed) hemisphere at occipital locations O1 and O2.

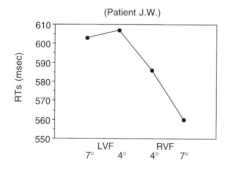

FIGURE 11.10. Reaction times to target stimuli (horizontal gratings) as a function of stimulus eccentricity and visual field. Responses were emitted with the ipsilateral hand. Note the strong advantage for the rightmost stimuli.

12 Stable and Variable Aspects of Callosal Channels: Lessons from Partial Disconnection

MARCO IACOBONI AND ERAN ZAIDEL

ABSTRACT It is argued that the investigation of interhemispheric transmission time in partial callosotomy patients is critical for understanding the nature of callosal channels. Through the systematic manipulation of visual and motor parameters in simple reaction times to lateralized flashes, it is possible to overcome the large variability in the distribution of callosal fibers and the complexity of human callosal connections and to demonstrate a behavioral dissociation between motor and visual component of callosal transfer. Partial split-brain patients showing such dissociation are useful in understanding more general mechanisms of sensorimotor integration through the corpus callosum.

Callosal channels and the CUD

There is a general consensus that the main function of the corpus callosum, the largest cerebral commissure in humans, is to allow interactions between the two cerebral hemispheres and transfer of information from one hemisphere to the other. To estimate the time that this interhemispheric transfer of information takes, Poffenberger (1912) proposed a simple behavioral paradigm (see Introduction). Normal subjects tend to have a CUD around 3 or 4 ms, whereas patients who are born with callosal agenesis tend to have a longer CUD, generally around 15 ms. Much longer CUDs, from 30 to 60 ms, are typically observed in patients with complete commissurotomy due to otherwise intractable epilepsy (Clarke and Zaidel, 1989; Marzi, Bisiacchi, and Nicoletti, 1991; Iacoboni and Zaidel, 1995). This is evidence for a major role of the corpus callosum in a fast

transfer of information from one cerebral hemisphere to the contralateral one.

Although in the paradigm proposed by Poffenberger auditory stimuli and somatosensory stimuli can be used as well (Moscovitch and Smith, 1979), in most published studies, visual stimuli have been used. Since motor responses are also required, it follows that both visual and motor cortical areas in the two cerebral hemispheres must be involved in the task. Anatomical studies have at first suggested a rather precise topographical arrangement of callosal axons according to their origin and termination. These studies were based on the fundamental assumption that callosal pathways are largely homotopic, that is, connecting homologous (corresponding) cortical areas (see the review in Chapter 2 in this volume). According to this model of callosal connections, callosal transfer of motor and visual information should be subserved by largely separate callosal channels in which fibers connecting motor and visual areas are separately funneled. Studies in monkeys and humans have suggested that motor fibers are restricted to the anterior region of the body of the corpus callosum, whereas visual fibers are contained in the splenium. This model predicts that motor and visual transfer of information can be easily dissociated and that the Poffenberger paradigm, if applied to patients with partial sections of the corpus callosum with selected lesions sparing, in a double dissociation fashion, anterior body containing motor fibers in some patients and splenium containing visual fibers in some other patients, can be used to measure the ITT of motor and visual information, respectively. To test whether in such patients with partial callosotomy the transfer is truly motor or visual, respectively, one might manipulate systematically motor and visual parameters of the task (Berlucchi et al., 1971). If the manipulation of motor parameters affects the CUD but the manipu-

MARCO IACOBONI Ahmanson Lovelace Brain Mapping Center, Neuropsychiatric Institute, Brain Research Institute, David Geffen School of Medicine, University of California at Los Angeles, Los Angeles, California.
ERAN ZAIDEL Department of Psychology, University of California, Los Angeles, California.

lation of visual parameters does not, then the transfer should be motor. By contrast, if the manipulation of motor parameters does not affect the CUD but the manipulation of visual parameters does, then the transfer should be visual.

Note that this anatomical model of callosal channels assumes also that the manipulation of motor and visual parameters can be effectively used in normal subjects, with only one exception. In principle, if the two ITTs of motor and visual information are completely equivalent and they can occur in parallel, then the manipulation of motor and visual parameters performed separately in normal subjects would not reveal any change in the CUD, because the "unaffected" channel (visual during the manipulation of motor parameters, motor during the manipulation of visual parameters) would still subserve interhemispheric transfer at its best efficiency. Only the simultaneous manipulation of motor and visual parameters would, in this case, affect the CUD.

In contrast, if the two ITTs of motor and visual information are not equivalent in the normal corpus callosum and one ITT is faster than the other, then the separate manipulation of motor and visual parameters should reveal which is the faster transfer, motor or visual, because one manipulation should affect the ITT of the most efficient transfer and, consequently, given that the other, less efficient transfer cannot fully compensate, affect also the CUD.

Recent anatomical data, however, challenge the most traditional account of a precise topographical arrangement of callosal pathways that are largely homotopic and underline that fibers originating from the same cortical area can show a widespread distribution in different callosal regions, especially in the body, and that the corpus callosum is composed of large contingents of heterotopic callosal connections, that is, callosal fibers connecting different cortical areas of the two cerebral hemispheres (Kennedy, Meissirel, and Dehay, 1991; Lomber, Payne, and Rosenquist, 1994; Clarke et al., 1995; see also Chapter 21 in this volume). This model predicts that a large number of patients with different partial sections of the corpus callosum would show a very similar CUD, regardless of the location of the section, because the widespread distribution of fibers in different callosal regions might prevent a partial section of the corpus callosum from interrupting all the callosal fibers subserving the most efficient transfer of information required by the Poffenberger paradigm. The only exception to this prediction might occur if the most efficient transfer were exclusively visual, given that the notion that visual callosal fibers are largely contained in the splenium has not been challenged by the new anatomical data. Moreover, the presence of hetero-

topic callosal connections that show the typical patterns of feedforward and feedback connections (Kennedy et al., 1991) suggests that the manipulation of motor and visual parameters might not be effective in normals in changing the CUD. Indeed, these connections are thought to subserve extremely flexible look-ahead and backtracking processes that might compensate for the effects of the manipulation of motor and visual parameters on ITT, leaving the CUD unaltered.

With regard to the type of fibers that subserve interhemispheric transfer in the Poffenberger paradigm, a CUD of only 3–4 ms in normal subjects is compatible only with callosal transfer through large-diameter, myelinated fibers with fast conduction velocity. Indeed, regardless of their origin and termination, their homotopicity or heterotopicity (unless heterotopic fibers connecting extremely anterior with extremely posterior cortical regions are considered), callosal fibers have to connect cortical areas at an approximate distance of 100–130 mm (considering also the convolution of the fiber tract) (see Chapter 2 in this volume). Assuming a constant mm/ms per millimeter of diameter for myelinated fibers, a CUD of 3–4 ms is compatible only with callosal fibers having fast conduction velocity and a diameter of 3 μm or larger. In humans this population of large-diameter callosal fibers is represented mostly in the posterior portion of the body of the corpus callosum, although three other callosal regions—the central portion of the body, the isthmus, and the posterior portion of the splenium—show a relatively high density of this large-diameter fiber population (Aboitiz et al., 1992). This predicts that patients with partial sections of the corpus callosum encompassing the callosal regions displaying high density of large-diameter fibers should show abnormally long CUDs. In normals, however, CUD variability is quite large, ranging from 1 ms to 10.3 ms in the 16 published studies that were included in Marzi and colleagues' (1991) meta-analysis on the Poffenberger paradigm. A CUD between 7 and 10 ms might even be compatible with interhemispheric transfer through 1-μm-diameter callosal fibers. These fibers show a relatively constant density across the whole corpus callosum (Aboitiz et al., 1992), and this would, of course, predict again that any partial section of the corpus callosum would leave the CUD unchanged for ITT between 7 ms and 10 ms.

To address these issues, we will review, in the next section of this chapter, data published in the literature and data collected in our lab that are relevant to the role of different callosal channels in the interhemispheric transfer of information that takes place in the Poffenberger paradigm and that determines the CUD. At first sight, some of these data seem to support the nontopographic model of callosal pathways, and some other data are consistent with the topographic model of callosal connections. We will attempt to reconcile these apparent inconsistencies.

Interhemispheric transfer in simple reaction times to lateralized flashes: Motor, visual, or both channels?

In an early attempt to differentiate between motor and visual transfer in the Poffenberger paradigm in normal subjects, Berlucchi and colleagues (1971) proposed that if the transfer is visual, then it should be sensitive to the experimental manipulation of visual parameters, and this should be reflected by a change in the CUD. Berlucchi and colleagues manipulated the retinal eccentricity of the visual stimulus, presenting it at 5°, 20°, and 35° of eccentricity to two groups of normal volunteers. Although overall reaction times increased with more peripheral retinal eccentricities, the results of this experiment showed very similar CUDs in the two groups for all three retinal eccentricities (2.5 ms, 4.5 ms, and 3 ms, respectively, in the first group and 3 ms, 0.5 ms, and 3 ms, respectively, in the second group). This was taken as evidence that the CUD in the Poffenberger paradigm is not determined by visual transfer but rather by motor transfer. These results, however, are also consistent with the hypothesis of a parallel, equivalently efficient transfer of motor and visual callosal connections. The manipulation of the retinal eccentricity of the light stimulus may not show any effect on the CUD because the unaffected motor channel would still allow a fast transfer of information from one hemisphere to the other.

A more direct evidence in favor of the hypothesis of a more efficient motor transfer in the Poffenberger paradigm was later provided by Vallar, Sterzi, and Basso (1988). The authors divided 24 aphasic patients with left-hemisphere lesions into two groups, one group (paretic) consisting of patients having motor deficits and the other group (nonparetic) consisting of patients without motor deficits. On the Poffenberger paradigm, the paretic group showed an abnormally long CUD of 23.32 ms, whereas the nonparetic group showed a CUD of 1.87 ms. Note that the overall RT of the paretic group was slightly, albeit not significantly, faster than the nonparetic group, showing once again that overall reaction times and CUD are two independent parameters in simple reaction times to lateralized flashes.

Taken together, the results of Berlucchi and colleagues (1971) and of Vallar and colleagues (1988) strongly suggest that the most efficient transfer in the Poffenberger paradigm occurs at the level of callosal fibers connecting cortical areas of motor significance. Given the large

contingent of premotor callosal connections and the relatively less important contingent of primary motor callosal connections, one would be tempted to conclude that the transfer occurs in callosal channels containing premotor fibers.

The evidence from the partial split-brain literature concerning the differential role of callosal channels in the transfer of information producing the CUD in the Poffenberger paradigm seems, at least at first sight, quite conflicting. Some data seem to support the general conclusion drawn from experimental data obtained in normal subjects and neurological patients with hemispheric lesions: that the CUD in simple reaction times to lateralized flashes reflects interhemispheric transfer through motor callosal channels (here and henceforth, the term "motor" is intended to include also premotor fibers), whereas other data seem to conflict with this conclusion. As we saw in the previous section of this chapter, however, the interpretation of data from partial split-brain patients may rely on two diverging anatomical models of callosal connections, which might lead to very different conclusions with regard to the callosal channel subserving the ITT reflected by the CUD.

Di Stefano, Sauerwein, and Lassonde (1992) have studied ITT with the Poffenberger paradigm in a patient with partial surgical section of the corpus callosum sparing the splenium, described in a previous report. The patient showed an abnormally large CUD of 58.3 ms. The data from this study are clearly in line with the previously mentioned evidence suggesting that interhemispheric transfer in the Poffenberger paradigm is dominated largely by motor transfer and that visual callosal fibers, funneled in the splenium, subserve a much less efficient ITT. However, Di Stefano and colleagues (1992) did not vary the retinal eccentricity or the brightness of the light stimulus, which was presented at 10° from the vertical meridian. Therefore, their data cannot support the hypothesis of Berlucchi and colleagues (1971) that the manipulation of visual parameters should affect the CUD if the transfer is mediated by visual callosal fibers.

A later report apparently challenged the notion that a fast ITT in the Poffenberger paradigm is subserved exclusively by motor callosal channels exclusively located in anterior or middle regions of the corpus callosum (Tassinari et al., 1994). These authors have studied eight patients with partial callosal lesions. Seven of these patients underwent surgical sections of the anterior and/or middle corpus callosum due to intractable epilepsy. The remaining patient had an intracerebral arterovenous malformation associated with agenesis of the posterior third of the corpus callosum, obviously including the splenium. The authors investigated the ITT in this series of patients by means of the Poffenberger paradigm. Although the experimental design was somewhat different across different patients participating in the study, all the observed CUDs were interpreted as being within the normal range in all patients. However, two patients showed a CUD of 14.5 ms and 11.8 ms, values that are often observed in acallosal patients. Moreover, the retinal eccentricity of the visual stimulus seemed not to have any effect on the CUD. Tassinari and colleagues (1994) concluded that both anterior and posterior regions of the corpus callosum subserve an equally fast ITT.

This conclusion, however, should be regarded with caution. Indeed, in their report, Tassinari and colleagues present the midsagittal magnetic resonance (MR) images of six of the eight patients. From these midsagittal MR images, it is evident that in four of the six patients the surgical procedure spared large portions of the midbody of the corpus callosum, where fibers connecting motor cortical areas are located, according to both the topographical and nontopographical anatomical models of callosal connections. Therefore, a normal CUD in these four patients cannot be considered as inconsistent with the findings of Berlucchi and colleagues (1971), of Vallar and colleagues (1988), and especially of Di Stefano and colleagues (1992).

Of the remaining two patients, in one case (F.P.) the callosal fibers spared by the surgery certainly encompass the isthmus, but it is not clear whether the end portion of the posterior body is spared or not. In the other patient (I.D.), only the splenium seems to be clearly visible after the surgery. Findings from these two patients seem, at first sight, to challenge the conclusions from the previous studies. There are still three considerations to be made, however, before we can dismiss the previous evidence. The first is a general consideration. Given that some of the patients in Tassinari and colleagues' series were particularly slow, only RTs that were longer than 700 ms were rejected from data analysis. This is an unusually high cutoff point compared to what is usually used in the literature. Although it seems to us valid to modify the cutoff point according to the overall RT of a given patient or a series of patients, it is unfortunate that F.P. and I.D. are among the fastest patients in the Tassinari series, F.P. having overall RT shorter than 400 ms and I.D. having overall RT around 300 ms. The unusually high cutoff point used in Tassinari and colleagues' study may have allowed too many outliers in the data analysis of fast patients such as F.P. and I.D., and this may have affected the computation of the CUD.

The second consideration concerns I.D., the patient having only the splenium spared. This is a patient who received a total of only 120 trials: 30 trials per visual field-response hand condition. This number of trials would be considered much too small to produce a reliable CUD even in a study with normal subjects (Iacoboni and Zaidel, 2000; St. John et al., 1987). In neurological patients, the variability of reaction times across trials is higher than in normal controls (Milner, 1986), and if anything, a greater number of trials should be used in these patients.

The last consideration concerns F.P. In this patient, some caudalmost fibers of the posterior portion of the body of the corpus callosum might have been spared (one midsagittal MR image cannot be considered completely reliable to assess the extent of the surgical section of the callosal fibers). As was previously mentioned, recent anatomical evidence clearly suggest that throughout the whole body of the corpus callosum, and possibly even in the isthmus, fibers originating from a variety of cortical areas can be found (see Chapter 21 in this volume). In this patient, some motor fibers located caudally in the body of the corpus callosum or in the isthmus may have subserved a fast ITT, resulting in a normal CUD. Indeed, in F.P., as in all the other patients of the Tassinari series in whom the retinal eccentricity was manipulated (some patients, such as I.D., were tested with the light stimulus at a fixed retinal eccentricity), the CUD was unaffected by the retinal eccentricity of the light flash. The absence of effect of retinal eccentricity on the CUD is compatible with only two explanations:

1. Berlucchi's hypothesis that the manipulation of any visual parameter should affect the CUD if the interhemispheric transfer is subserved by visual callosal fibers is not correct.

2. The transfer in the Tassinari series is motor, at least in the patients in which retinal eccentricity was varied.

Patient D.W.

To further investigate the issues raised by the previously mentioned papers, we measured the ITT by means of the Poffenberger paradigm in a patient (D.W.) who underwent partial callosotomy sparing the splenium of the corpus callosum and a few fibers of the rostralmost portion of the rostrum (Iacoboni, Fried, and Zaidel, 1994). The patient was tested before and after the surgery, and retinal eccentricity was varied from 4° to 8° from the vertical meridian in preoperative and postoperative testing sessions. We found that before the surgery the ITT was not affected by manipulation of the retinal eccentricity of the light stimulus, with a CUD of 5.1 ms at 4° of eccentricity and a CUD of 3.5 ms at 8° of retinal eccentricity. The difference between the two CUDs was not significant. After the surgery the patient showed a CUD of 5.8 ms when responding at light flashes located at 4° from the vertical meridian and a CUD of

20.6 ms when responding at light flashes located at 8° of retinal eccentricity from the vertical meridian. This difference was statistically significant ($p < 0.001$).

Our study demonstrated three things. First of all, we see that the manipulation of visual parameters can modify the CUD in partial split-brain patients having only the splenium. Previous studies had demonstrated the effectiveness of varying visual parameters in modifying the CUD only in complete commissurotomy patients and in patients born with agenesis of the corpus callosum (Clarke and Zaidel, 1989; Milner et al., 1985). In those studies, the involvement of extracallosal pathways containing visual interhemispheric fibers was invoked. Second, we see that visual transfer is generally slower than motor transfer. The postoperative CUD of our patient was 20.6 ms at 8° of eccentricity, consistent with the very large CUD observed by Di Stefano and colleagues (1992) in a partial split-brain patient with the splenium spared and tested with a light flash at 10° of retinal eccentricity from the vertical meridian. Third, we see that when the retinal eccentricity of the light flash is close to the vertical meridian, the visual callosal fibers may yield an ITT that is comparable to the ITT through motor fibers. This fast ITT might be subserved by a contingent of large-diameter myelinated fibers located in the caudalmost portion of the splenium, according to Aboitiz and colleagues (1992).

The effectiveness of the manipulation of the retinal eccentricity in modifying the CUD in our patient with an intact splenium of the corpus callosum after partial callosotomy clearly supports the notion that in this patient the postoperative CUD is largely subserved by visual fibers. What we needed at this point was to demonstrate that some motor manipulation might significantly affect the CUD in the normal brain with an intact corpus callosum but not in our patient. This would provide a double dissociation between the partial split-brain patient and normal subjects that would represent more convincing evidence that a fast motor transfer masks the effects of any manipulation of visual parameters in the normal brain.

We performed just such an experiment using 75 normal subjects, two patients with complete commissurotomy (L.B. and N.G.), and D.W. (Iacoboni and Zaidel, 1995). Normal volunteers were divided into three groups of 25 subjects, and each group had a different version of the Poffenberger paradigm. The two versions of the paradigm that are relevant to this chapter were the basic one and the motor one. In the basic task, subjects were asked to press a response key with the index finger in response to lateralized light flashes that were always presented on the horizontal meridian and at a fixed retinal eccentricity from the vertical meridian (4°). In the motor task,

subjects were asked to press the response key with the index finger on odd trials and with the middle finger on even trials, alternating the finger used for motor response, while the lateralized light flashes were still presented at the same fixed locations on the horizontal meridian as in the basic task.

The prediction here is the following: If the most effective transfer in the normal brain is subserved by callosal motor fibers, then the motor manipulation in the motor task should modify the CUD in normals. The very same manipulation might or might not be ineffective in complete commissurotomy patients, depending on whether or not they rely on subcallosal motor channels. With regard to D.W., the hypothesis that he has some motor fibers traveling in the splenium that subserve his CUD (already unlikely, given that his CUD is sensitive to eccentricity manipulation) must be ruled out if the motor manipulation in the motor task fails to modify the CUD.

The results of our experiment were as follows: Normal subjects showed a significant task by CUD interaction, with a significant advantage for uncrossed responses compared to crossed responses in the basic task (CUD = 4.3 ms) but not in the motor task (CUD = 1.0 ms). L.B. showed no task by CUD interaction, with a significant advantage for uncrossed responses compared to crossed responses in both the basic task (CUD = 27.3 ms) and the motor task (CUD = 28.45 ms). N.G. showed also no task by CUD interaction, with a significant advantage for uncrossed responses compared to crossed responses in both the basic task (CUD = 40.6 ms) and the motor task (CUD = 50.9 ms). Finally, D.W. showed the same lack of task by CUD interaction that is seen in complete commissurotomy patients, with an insignificant advantage for uncrossed responses compared to crossed ones, both in the basic task (CUD = 4.05 ms) and in the motor task (CUD = 9.4 ms). However, the main effect of response condition was significant ($p < 0.007$), with faster uncrossed responses compared to crossed responses and an overall CUD of 6.7 ms.

Taken together, the results of Berlucchi and colleagues (1971), Iacoboni and colleagues (1994), and Iacoboni and Zaidel (1995) provide a double dissociation between normal subjects and D.W., in that the manipulation of retinal eccentricity does not modify the CUD in normals but does modify the CUD in D.W., whereas the manipulation of motor response parameters does not modify the CUD in D.W. but does modify the CUD in normals. Note that the motor manipulation in normals produced a faster CUD than in the basic task. This is probably why we were able to observe a change in the CUD in normals. As was noted above, the data from D.W. suggest that a contingent of visual fibers can subserve a fast ITT at stimulus retinal eccentricity of 4°

from the vertical meridian. Any motor manipulation that would slow down the ITT carried out by motor fibers in normals would be masked by the ITT of these fast visual callosal fibers, thus leaving the CUD unchanged. This, of course, can be prevented by using large retinal eccentricities.

We conclude that motor fibers, wherever they are located in the corpus callosum, yield the fastest ITT in normal subjects performing the Poffenberger paradigm, whereas visual fibers yield the fastest ITT in D.W. Partial split-brain patients who do not show the effect of the manipulation of retinal eccentricity on their CUD must be considered patients in whom visual fibers do not determine the fastest ITT. If a partial split-brain patient with a normal CUD and a midsagittal MR image that shows that only the splenium is spared by the surgical section has a very fast CUD, the patient must be tested with an acceptable number of trials (Milner, 1986) and at large retinal eccentricities before it can be concluded that this patient (1) shows signs of callosal reorganization or that (2) the patient's CUD is determined by ITT subserved by splenial fibers that are not visual or (3) by visual fibers that subserve a very fast ITT.

REFERENCES

ABOITIZ, F., A. B. SCHEIBEL, R. S. FISHER, and E. ZAIDEL, 1992. Fiber composition of the human corpus callosum. *Brain Res.* 598:143–153.

BERLUCCHI, G., W. HERON, R. HYMAN, G. RIZZOLATTI, and C. UMILTÀ, 1971. Simple reaction times of ipsilateral and contralateral hand to lateralized visual stimuli. *Brain* 94:419–430.

CLARKE, J. M., and E. ZAIDEL, 1989. Simple reaction times to lateralized flashes: Varieties of interhemispheric communication routes. *Brain* 112:849–870.

CLARKE, S., D. C. VAN ESSEN, N. HADJIKHANI, H. DRURY, and T. A. COOGAN, 1995. Understanding human area 19 and 37: Contribution of two-dimensional maps of visual callosal afferents [Abstract]. *Hum. Brain Mapp.* (Suppl.) 1:33.

DI STEFANO, M., H. C. SAUERWEIN, and M. LASSONDE, 1992. Influence of anatomical factors and spatial compatibility on the stimulus-response relationship in the absence of the corpus callosum. *Neuropsychologia* 30:177–185.

IACOBONI, M., I. FRIED, and E. ZAIDEL, 1994. Callosal transmission time before and after partial commissurotomy. *Neuroreport* 5:2521–2524.

IACOBONI, M., and E. ZAIDEL, 1995. Channels of the corpus callosum: Evidence from simple RT to lateralized flashes in the normal and the split brain. *Brain* 118:779–788.

IACOBONI, M., and E. ZAIDEL, 2000. Crossed-uncrossed difference in simple reaction times to lateralized flashes: Betweeen- and within-subjects variability. *Neuropsychologia* 38:535–541.

KENNEDY, H., C. MEISSIREL, and C. DEHAY, 1991. Callosal pathways and their compliancy to general rules governing the organization of corticocortical connectivity. In *Vision and Visual Dysfunction*, Vol. 3: *Neuroanatomy of the Visual Pathways and Their Development*, B. Reher and S. R. Robinson, eds. (J. R. Cronly-Dillon, series ed.). Boca Raton, Fla.: CRC Press, pp. 324–359.

LOMBER, S. G., B. R. PAYNE, and A. ROSENQUIST, 1994. The spatial relationship between the cerebral cortex and fiber trajectory through the corpus callosum of the cat. *Behav. Brain Res.* 64:25–35.

MARZI, C. A., P. BISIACCHI, and R. NICOLETTI, 1991. Is interhemispheric transfer of visuomotor information asymmetric? Evidence from a meta-analysis. *Neuropsychologia* 29:1163–1177.

MILNER, A. D., 1986. Chronometric analysis in neuropsychology. *Neuropsychologia* 24:115–128.

MILNER, A. D., M. A. JEEVES, P. H. SILVER, C. R. LINES, and J. WILSON, 1985. Reaction times to lateralized visual stimuli in callosal agenesis: Stimulus and response factors. *Neuropsychologia* 23:323–331.

MOSCOVITCH, M., and L. C. SMITH, 1979. Differences in neural organization between individuals with inverted and non-inverted handwriting postures. *Science* 205:710–713.

POFFENBERGER, A. T., 1912. Reaction time to retinal stimulation, with special reference to the time lost through nerve centers. *Arch. Psychol.* 23:1–73.

ST. JOHN, R., C. SHIELDS, P. KRAHN, and B. TIMNEY, 1987. The reliability of estimates of interhemispheric transmission times derived from unimanual and verbal response latencies. *Hum. Neurobiol.* 6:195–202.

TASSINARI, G., S. AGLIOTI, R. PALLINI, G. BERLUCCHI, and G. F. ROSSI, 1994. Interhemispheric integration of simple visuomotor responses in patients with partial callosal defects. *Behav. Brain Res.* 64:141–149.

VALLAR, G., R. STERZI, and A. BASSO, 1988. Left hemisphere contribution to motor programming of aphasic speech: A reaction time experiment in aphasic patients. *Neuropsychologia* 26:511–519.

Commentary 12.1

Attentional Modulation of Interhemispheric Transfer: A Two-Channel Threshold Model

KENNETH HUGDAHL

ABSTRACT In this commentary I will present an argument for a sensory nonspecific, diffuse, transfer function across the corpus callosum involving the shift of attention to either side in space. The modality nonspecific transfer may follow a threshold function, in the sense that it is recruited only in situations in which the cognitive load is increased, as when involving simultaneous inputs from different sources (the cocktail party phenomenon). I will illustrate my arguments with data from auditory laterality, specifically dichotic listening performance.

Introduction

Studies in humans with magnetic resonance imaging (MRI) techniques have revealed differences in corpus callosum size between males and females and between young and old individuals (Cowell et al., 1994; see Chapter 5 in this volume for a recent update). Cowell and colleagues (1992) found that area size and axis length of the callosum in general increase up to the age 20 and then start declining. Interestingly, the onset of decline in area size occurs earlier in males than in females, depending on the specific sector studied.

Another variable that seems to interact with callosal size is handedness, with larger callosal size with consistent non-right-handedness (e.g., Witelson, 1989; Habib et al., 1991; Cowell, Kertesz, and Denenberg, 1993; Denenberg, Kertesz, and Cowell, 1991). Moreover, some studies have indicated that language lateralization is related to callosal size, with larger callosal size in left-hemisphere language individuals (e.g., Zaidel, Clarke, and Suyenobu, 1990). These latter studies have typically used dichotic listening to assess language function in the two hemispheres.

In their chapter, Iacoboni and Zaidel discuss the specific role of callosal channels dedicated to integrating sensorimotor information. In this commentary I discuss the role of callosal channels dedicated to attentional modulation of auditory interhemispheric transfer.

Dichotic listening and auditory pathways

In anatomical terms, an auditory stimulus activates neurons in the cochlear nucleus at the level of the vestibulocochlear nerve. Among the subdivisions of the cochlear nucleus, the ventral acoustic stria enters a second level, the superior olivary complex. From here, both inhibitory and excitatory impulses are projected within the lateral lemniscus to the dorsal nucleus and ventral nucleus of the lateral lemniscus, which make up a third-level relay station. Up to the level of the nuclei of the lateral lemniscus, the auditory system projects bilaterally, to both sides. However, from the nuclei of the lateral lemniscus, projections are mainly contralateral, projecting to a fourth relay station, the inferior colliculus in the tectum. The contralateral fibers then innervate the medial geniculate body in the pulvinar thalamus, which is the fifth relay station, sending its axons to neurons in the auditory cortex in the posterior superior temporal gyrus (Price et al., 1992). Thus, although auditory signals from one ear reach both auditory cortices in the temporal lobes, the contralateral projections are stronger and more preponderant.

Dichotic listening (DL) is a noninvasive technique to study lateralized information processing in the two hemispheres of the brain (see Bryden, 1988; Hugdahl, 1995; for reviews). In a more general sense, dichotic listening is a measure of temporal lobe function (Spreen and Strauss, 1991), attention, and stimulus-processing speed, in addition to being a measure of hemisphere language asymmetry (Hugdahl, 1995).

Over the last 15 years, our laboratory has been using the DL technique to study aspects of brain laterality for auditory stimuli and the interaction of laterality with cognitive processes, such as attention (see Hugdahl,

KENNETH HUGDAHL Department of Biological and Medical Psychology, University of Bergen, Bergen, Norway.

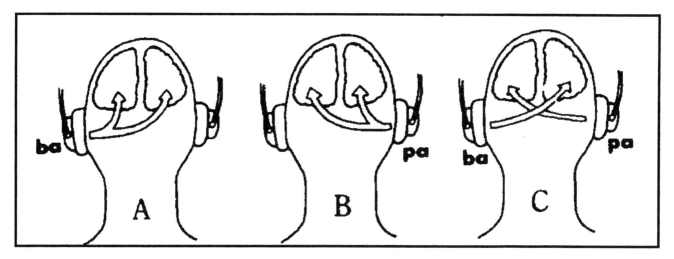

FIGURE 12.1. Schematic outline of the dichotic listening situation. A = monaural left-ear presentation of the syllable /ba/; note the ipsilateral and contralateral projections. B = monaural right-ear presentation of the syllable /pa/; note the ipsilateral and contralateral projections. C = dichotic presentation of the syllables /ba/ and /pa/; note that the stronger contralateral projections block out the weaker ipsilateral projections. See the text for further details. (Data from Hugdahl et al., 1999b.)

1991, 1995, 1999, for reviews, and see Asbjørnsen and Hugdahl, 1995; Asbjørnsen, Hugdahl, and Bryden, 1992; and Hugdahl and Andersson, 1986; for selected aspects of our work). We have also applied the DL technique to the study of patients with brain lesions (e.g., Hugdahl and Wester, 1992), neurodegenerative diseases (e.g., Hugdahl, Wester, and Asbjørnsen, 1990), and developmental disorders (e.g., Cohen, Hynd, and Hugdahl, 1992; Hugdahl et al., 1995; Hugdahl et al., 1999b).

Typically, two different consonant-vowel (CV) syllables are presented to the subject on each trial, one in each ear. The task is to report which syllable the subject perceives best. The CV-syllables are of the format /ba/, /da/, /ga/, and so on. The situation is shown in Figure 12.1.

The DL technique that we use was validated against the Wada procedure (Wada and Rasmussen, 1960), in which DL performance was compared preoperatively and postoperatively with the results from intracarotid injections of amobarbital in epileptic patients (Hugdahl et al., 1997). The DL results showed 92% correct classification of side of language dominance when compared with the results from the Wada test.

A critical issue is whether the DL technique actually taps cognitive processes related to temporal lobe function, particularly language processes related to the planum temporale (PT) anatomical area in the posterior part of the superior temporal gyrus (cf. Jäncke and Steinmetz, 1993). This was studied with the ^{15}O-PET technique (Hugdahl et al., 1999a). The subjects listened to either CV syllables, musical instruments, or simple

tones (baseline) in three different scans. PET subtraction images were obtained by subtracting activity during the tones condition from activity during the CV syllable and musical instrument conditions. Figure 12.2 shows the main findings from this study, and it reveals significant activations ($p < 0.001$, corrected for multiple comparisons) in the planum temporale area in the superior temporal gyrus. Interestingly, there was a left-sided asymmetry for the CV syllables and a right-sided asymmetry for the musical instrument stimuli.

With regard to reliability, Hugdahl and Hammar (1997) found reliability coefficients to vary between 0.61 and 0.86 for repeated presentations of the same CV syllables within 2 weeks. This is in agreement with most other studies of dichotic listening reliability for verbal stimuli.

Procedure: Empirical data

The data presented in this chapter were based on the standard DL technique used in our laboratory (see Hugdahl, 1995). The dichotic stimuli consisted of the six stop consonants paired with the vowel /a/ to form six CV syllables (/ba/, /da/, /ga/, /pa/, /ta/, and /ka/). The syllables were paired with each other in all possible combinations, thus giving 36 different syllable pairs. The homonymic pairs (/ba/-/ba/, etc.) were included as a perceptual control to ensure that the subjects did perceive the various stimuli. They were not included in the statistical analyses.

The 36 dichotic pairs were recorded three times on tape with three different randomizations. There were 36

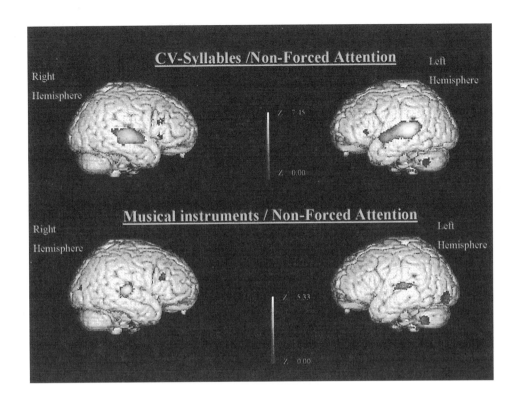

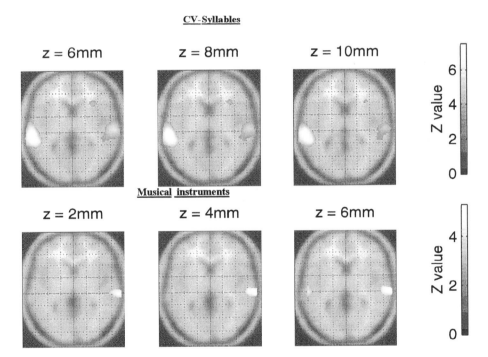

FIGURE 12.2. ¹⁵O-PET activation images after presentation of CV syllables (upper row in both panels), and musical instruments (lower row in both panels). The upper panel shows significant clusters of activation plotted onto lateral views of a brain template. The lower panel shows the same data plotted on axial slices. (Data from Hugdahl et al., 1999a.) (See Color Plate 14.)

trials for each attentional instruction. Thus, a maximum correct score was 30 (excluding the six homonyms). The syllables were originally read by a male voice, with intonation and intensity held constant. The syllables were digitized before computerized editing and temporal alignment of stimulus onset. The syllables were originally recorded on a REVOX B-77 reel-to-reel tape recorder. To facilitate testing of the subjects, the reel-to-reel tape was copied to a chrome-dioxide cassette and replayed from a Sony Walkman WMDD-II minicassette recorder with plug-in-type miniheadphones. The output from the cassette player was calibrated at a level of 75 dB.

On arrival to the laboratory, all subjects were instructed about the purpose of the study. They also filled out the handedness questionnaire and were screened for hearing acuity. Subjects who did not fulfill the criteria were excused; the other subjects were seated in a sound attenuated chamber in the laboratory. The earplugs were attached, and the subjects were given the specific instructions regarding direction of attention.

In the standard, divided, or nonforced (NF) attention condition, the subjects were told that they would be presented with a list of CV syllables. Their task was to answer with the syllable that they heard on each trial. Thus, one response for each trial was emphasized. If they were able to identify both syllables on a trial, they were nevertheless told to report only the one they "heard best." Thus, in trials in which subjects gave two correct responses, only the first response was used in the analysis, since the first response is highly correlated with the overall ear advantage.

In the forced-right (FR) attention condition, the subjects were told to pay close attention to the right-ear syllables and to report only what they heard in the right ear. Otherwise, the procedure was identical to that for the NF condition.

In the forced-left (FL) attention condition, the subjects were told to pay close attention to the left-ear syllables and to report only what they heard in the left ear. Otherwise, the procedure was identical to that for the NF condition.

A typical dichotic listening experiment thus involves three different attentional instructions: nonforced (NF), forced-right (FR), and forced-left (FL). In the NF condition, the subject is told that he or she will hear repeated presentations of the six CV syllables (/ba/, /da/, /ga/, /pa/, /ta/, and /ka/) and that after each trial the subject should report which one he or she heard. The subjects are instructed not to think about the syllables but to give the answer that spontaneously comes to mind after each presentation. In the FR and FL attention conditions, the subjects are instructed to focus attention to the right (or left) ear throughout the session and to report only what they hear from this ear.

The right-ear advantage (REA)

The typical finding in dichotic listening is the right-ear advantage (REA), which stands for superior identification of items presented in the right ear compared to items presented in the left ear (see Hugdahl, 1995, for further explanation).

The classic structural model (Kimura, 1967) argues that the REA is caused by several interacting factors:

1. The auditory input to the contralateral hemisphere is more strongly represented in the brain.

2. In most individuals, the left hemisphere is specialized for language processing.

3. Auditory information that is sent along the ipsilateral pathways is suppressed, or blocked, by the contralateral information.

4. Information that reaches the ipsilateral right hemisphere has to be transferred cross the corpus callosum to the left hemisphere language processing areas.

See Figure 12.3 for an illustration of the basic REA effect in a large sample of normal subjects.

The last point is nicely illustrated in the case of the split-brain patient who has undergone surgical disconnection of the two hemispheres through splitting the corpus callosum. These patients typically show a dramatic left-ear extinction effect (Sparks and Geschwind, 1968; Zaidel, 1976, 1983; Clarke, Lufkin, and Zaidel, 1993), which is caused by the absence of left-ear transfer across the cut callosum.

Attentional modulation of the REA

The REA is a fairly stable and robust empirical finding, but it can easily be modified by instructing the subject to attend to either the right or the left side in auditory space (Bryden, Munhall, and Allard, 1983; Hugdahl and Andersson, 1986). Thus, in the FR condition, the REA is typically increased, whereas it is decreased, or sometimes even switched to a left-ear advantage (LEA), in the FL condition. The effect of attentional modulation through instructions to attend either to the left or right ear is seen in Figure 12.4 for adult subjects and for children ages 8–9 years (data from Hugdahl and Andersson, 1986; see also Asbjørnsen and Hugdahl, 1995).

PET studies of the effect of attention in DL have provided mixed results. In the original study by O'Leary and colleagues (1996), it was found that blood flow increased in the temporal lobe opposite to the ear to which attention was focused. In a more recent study from our laboratory (Hugdahl et al., 1999c) we found decreased

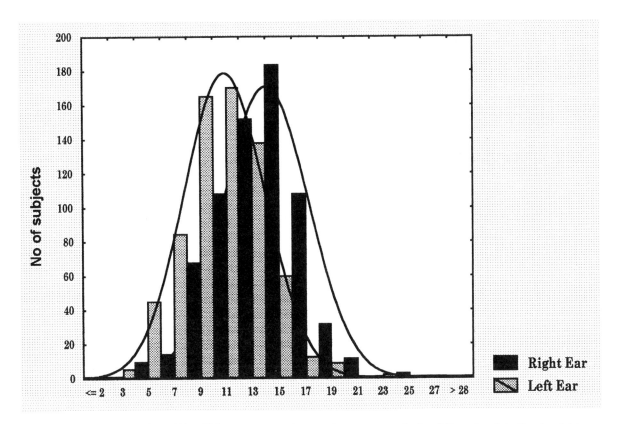

FIGURE 12.3. Distribution of subjects ($N = 692$) across scores in the dichotic listening test, separated for the right and left ears. Note the normal distributions for both ears and the right-ear advantage seen in the shift to the right for the right-ear scores (black bars). (Data from Hugdahl et al., 1999b.)

activity in the primary and secondary auditory cortices during focused attention, compared to divided attention, possibly indicating facilitation of callosal transfer during focused attention. This is illustrated in Figure 12.5.

Callosal transfer: Bottom-up versus top-down

The structural model of DL performance is silent with regard to attentional modulation of the REA, and it is therefore without predictive power to explain the effects of instructing the subject to switch attention to either side in auditory space. This is reminiscent of arguing that the structural model is a bottom-up model that does not take into account the top-down modulation that occurs when focusing attention to either side in auditory space. Hemispheric asymmetry is perhaps best understood as a dynamic interaction between bottom-up, or stimulus-driven, processes and top-down, or instruction-driven, processes. By default, a verbal stimulus that is presented in the right ear in the dichotic listening situation will be more efficiently processed in the left hemisphere, compared to the left-ear stimulus. This is the bottom-up or stimulus driven laterality effect. However, when the subject is instructed to attend to the left- or right-ear stimulus, the attentional, top-down effect will be either congruent or in conflict with the stimulus effect, depending on whether the subject is instructed to attend to the right- or left-ear stimulus, respectively. Thus, the dichotic listening situation is ideal for the study of how cognitive factors such as attention may affect the basic stimulus-driven laterality effect, possibly by altering the transfer across the corpus callosum.

The left-ear score

Second, and more important for the present argument, the structural model predicts that the left-ear score should be positively correlated with efficiency of callosal transfer (cf. Clarke et al., 1993). This means that size of callosal area should correlate with left-ear performance, particularly for the posterior sectors of the corpus callosum. As was explained above, the reason is that the left-ear stimulus has to be transferred across the corpus callosum from the right to the left hemisphere to be processed (Pollmann et al., 2002). (Space does not allow a discussion of the special situations in which the left-ear score may actually be processed in the right hemisphere; see Hugdahl and Wester, 1992.)

The prediction of callosal transfer in dichotic listening was tested in the study by Clarke and colleagues (1993)

ADULTS

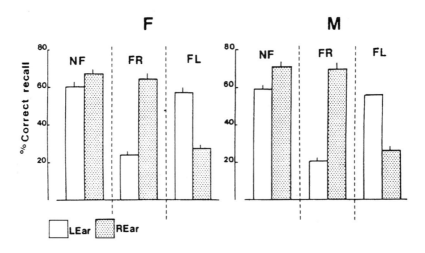

CHILDREN 8-9

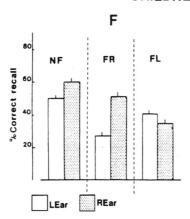
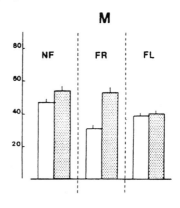

FIGURE 12.4. Percentage of correct reports from the left and right ears in the standard CV syllables dichotic listening paradigm with divided and focused attention. NF = nonforced attention, FR = forced-right attention, FL = forced-left attention, F = females, M = males, REar = right-ear scores, LEar = left-ear scores. (Data from Hugdahl and Andersson, 1986.)

in 60 normal adults. Callosal area size was determined from magnetic resonance images (MRI), in which the callosum was sectioned into five different areas in the rostral-caudal axis. The dichotic listening procedure involved manual identification (pointing) of left- and right-ear presentations of the CV syllables /bee/, /dee/, /gee/, /pee/, /tee/, and /kee/. Clarke and colleagues (1993) included only a nonforced attention (divided attention) condition, with no specific instructions to focus attention to either side in space. The results showed the expected significant right-ear advantage, with about 55% correctly identified items from the right ear and 45% correctly identified items from the left ear.

However, callosum area did not correlate with left-ear performance, that is, the expected positive correlation between larger callosal area size and better left-ear reports was not found. Instead, they found that right-ear performance was negatively correlated with callosum size, which was explained with reference to functional interhemispheric inhibition.

A two-channel model of callosal transfer

I will use some recent data from our laboratory to further explore the issue of interhemispheric transfer and callosal size, making an argument for a two-channel

**NF Attention:
"Attend both ears"**

**FR Attention:
"Attend right ear"**

**FL Attention:
"Attend left ear"**

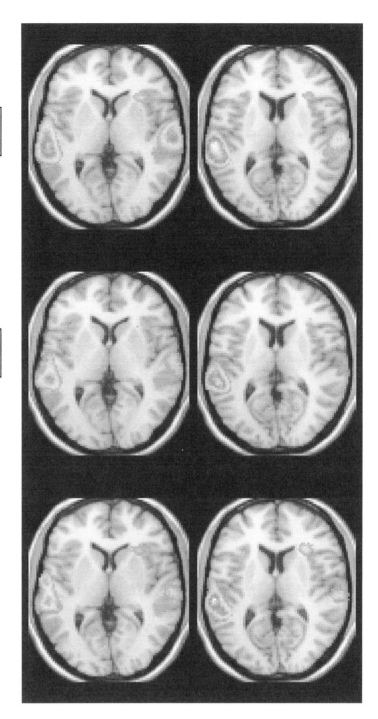

FIGURE 12.5. ^{15}O-PET activation images during the NF, FR, and FL attention conditions plotted onto axial slice brain templates across the superior temporal gyrus and planum temporale. The left column is 2 mm above the AC-PC mid-line; the right column is 8 mm above the AC-PC midline. Note the relative attenuation of activation during the FR and FL conditions compared to the NF attention condition. (Data from Hugdahl et al., 2000.) (See Color Plate 15.)

TABLE 12.1

Correlations between left- and right-ear scores in dichotic listening from normal healthy subjects split into four different age groups.

Age (years)	NF-RHanders	FR-RHanders	FL-RHanders	NF-LHanders	FR-LHanders	FL-LHanders
<15	−0.098 (n = 2859)	−0.394 (n = 270)	−0.537 (n = 270)	−0.475 (n = 136)	−0.022 (n = 11)	−0.358 (n = 11)
20–30	−0.353 (n = 260)	−0.774 (n = 140)	−0.626 (n = 140)	−0.366 (n = 23)	−0.903 (n = 20)	−0.806 (n = 20)
31–50	−0.306 (n = 46)	−0.827 (n = 32)	−0.876 (n = 32)	−0.692 (n = 6)	−0.595 (n = 6)	−0.627 (n = 6)
>50	−0.389 (n = 76)	−0.524 (n = 41)	−0.513 (n = 41)	—	—	—

NF = nonforced attention, FR = forced-right attention, FL = forced-left attention.

threshold model of callosal transfer that also includes transfer of attentional resources and the gating of sensory transfer by attention.

The starting point for my argument is the findings from our laboratory, reported by Reinvang, Bakke, Hugdahl, Karlsen, and Sundet (1994), on the relationship between callosal sector size and left-ear performance in multiple sclerosis (MS) patients. The corpus callosum often show atrophic changes in MS patients, and measures of the corpus callosum are also often included in the diagnosis of this disease (cf. Chapter 17 in this volume). The study by Reinvang and colleagues (1994) was similar to Clarke and colleagues' (1993) study in that it was based on dichotic presentations of CV syllables. Reinvang and colleagues (1994) also had MRI measures of callosal size (dividing the corpus callosum into four different sectors along the rostral-caudal axis).

However, in addition to the nonforced (NF) attention condition, Reinvang and colleagues (1994) also manipulated attention to the right (FR) and left (FL), thus including attention as a factor in the study. The results showed a significant REA in both the MS patients and a healthy control group during the NF condition. Table 12.1 lists the correlations between the left- and right-ear scores and callosal sector (marked 1–4, anterior to posterior) for each of the three attentional conditions (NF, FR, FL). The findings for the left-ear scores during the NF condition were quite similar to the findings of Clarke and colleagues (1993), that is, the absence of a significant correlation between the left-ear scores and callosal size. However, when subjects were instructed to focus their attention to the left ear during the session (FL condition), the correlations between left-ear performance and callosal size were clearly significant, particularly for the three posteriormost sectors (including the auditory

sector anterior to the splenium). The details are presented in Table 12.2.

It thus seems as though an attention-gating factor is needed to enhance callosal transfer of the left-ear score. This may indicate the existence of a two-channel threshold model of callosal transfer with a sensory modality-specific channel involving the large-diameter myelinated fibers and a diffuse sensory nonspecific channel involving the small-diameter nonmyelinated fibers that are responsible for transfer of cognitive information (cf. Aboitiz et al., 1992, and Chapter 2 in this volume). The model may act in a threshold mode in the sense that in most normal instances the recruitment of the cognitive channel is not necessary; the sensory channel is enough for efficient transfer. However, in situations of increasing cognitive load (as in the cocktail party situation) or when the callosum may be degenerated (as in the case of the MS patient), attention may be recruited to facilitate or amplify the sensory transfer. The point is that attention may be recruited only when the sensory transfer falls below a threshold value that defines the interaction between different ways of information transfer across the callosum (cf. Kinsbourne, 1974, for a discussion of cognitive factors in callosal functioning).

Callosal connectivity, dichotic listening, and age

An empirical test of some of the predictions of the model is seen in Table 12.1 and Figure 12.6. Table 12.1 shows correlations between the right- and left-ear scores in the standard NF condition in dichotic listening.

Although the table lists correlations for both right- and left-handers, I will base my arguments on the right-handed subjects, since there are rather few left-handers in the sample, which makes comparisons unreliable. The

TABLE 12.2

Correlations between callosum sector area and left- and right-ear scores in dichotic listening in MS patients. (Data from Reinvang et al., 1994.)

Dichotic Listening Condition	Callosal Sector 1	Callosal Sector 2	Callosal Sector 3	Callosal Sector 4
Left ear, NF	0.05	0.13	0.29	0.00
Left ear, FR	−0.09	−0.18	−0.17	−0.11
Left ear, FL	0.14	0.48*	0.61**	0.47*
Right ear, NF	0.11	−0.18	−0.28	−0.13
Right ear, FR	0.09	0.06	0.17	0.11
Right ear, FL	−0.06	−0.52*	−0.50*	−0.44

NF = nonforced attention, FR = forced-right attention, FL = forced-left attention.
*$p < 0.05$.
**$p < 0.01$.

two-channel threshold model would predict that the better the left-ear score is transferred during the FL condition, the more negative the correlation between the left and right ear should become (left-ear scores go up while the right-ear score is unaffected or goes down). As can be seen in Table 12.1, the correlation coefficients increase with increasing age up to the oldest age group, when the correlation decreases again.

This may be related to callosal connectivity in the sense that callosal fiber myelination is not completely established in the youngest age group (cf. Cowell et al., 1992). Similarly, in the oldest age group, a degeneration process may have been initiated. Interestingly, the corresponding correlation coefficients during the FR atten-

tion condition also show a similar increasing-decreasing trend with increasing age, which means that there also may be increase in the right-ear score changes with age, although to a lesser degree than for the left-ear score during the FL condition.

In a similar way, Figure 12.6 shows the actual left-ear performance on the dichotic listening test as a function of age, separated for males and females, based on a large sample of subjects. The upper panel shows the NF condition, and as predicted by the model, performance does not change as a function age. Basically the same relationship between performance and age is seen during the FR condition (middle panel in Figure 12.6). However, in the FL condition, performance increases with age, up through the twenties, and then it starts to decline. Interestingly, the decline is faster for males than females. Thus, the DL performance curve across age seen in the lower panel in Figure 12.6 has a striking resemblance to the callosal size curve as a function of age reported by Cowell and colleagues (1992). They found an increase with age, peaking at 20 years in males and then declining, while the females had a delayed decline in callosal size with increasing age. The DL data presented in Figure 12.6 were substantiated by the findings of Cowell and Hugdahl (2000) with decreasing DL performance with increasing age.

Using the same DL test, Beaton, Hugdahl, and Ray (2000) compared three age groups (20, 40, and 60 years) on both the nonforced and forced attention conditions. In the NF attention condition, the largest REA was seen in the youngest group, followed by the 40 group, and the 60 group. Thus, the size of the REA declined with in-

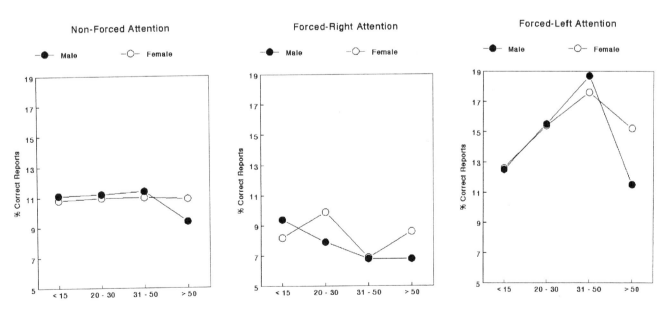

FIGURE 12.6. Number of correct reports for the left ear only in the standard CV syllables dichotic listening paradigm, separated for the three attentional conditions, for males and females, and for the three different age groups studied.

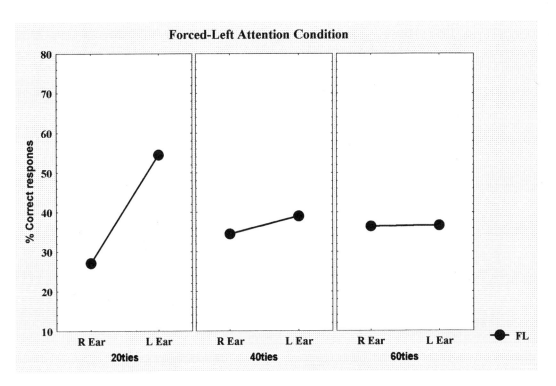

FIGURE 12.7. Percentage of correct reports for the left ear only during the forced-left (FL) attention condition. Data were collected from three different age groups (20, 40, 60). REar = right-ear score, LEar = left-ear score. (Data from Beaton, Hugdahl, and Ray, 2000.)

creasing age. Of perhaps greater interest for the present argument was that when the groups were compared during the forced-left attention condition, only the youngest group showed a significant LEA, with the 40 group showing a tendency toward an LEA, while the 60 group showed no ear advantage at all (see Figure 12.7). Thus, the ability to use attention to facilitate callosal transfer of the left-ear signal from the right to the left hemisphere was significantly reduced in the oldest group.

These preliminary arguments may be put to further empirical tests by corecording dichotic listening performance and MRI indices of callosal size in subjects differing in age. Thus, dichotic listening and callosal size should be correlated across the entire age span.

Summary and conclusions

Taken together, the data in Table 12.2 and Figures 12.6 and 12.7 suggest that left-ear performance in dichotic listening reflects callosal efficiency, particularly when attention is focused to the left side in auditory space. This would argue for a relay function of the corpus callosum in the processing of language-specific materials, the right-hemisphere input being transferred across the

callosum for processing. It is argued that callosal transfer of sensory and cognitive information follows a two-stage function, sensory information being transferred through the larger fibers in the designated callosal sector. However, in situations with increasing cognitive load, callosal transfer may be amplified through cognitive (attentional) gating that has a more diffuse anatomical sector specificity. The model predicts that callosal function may act in a threshold mode way with recruitment of the diffuse fibers only in situations of increasing demands for interhemispheric coactivation, when the callosum is degenerated (as in certain neurodegenerative diseases), or in children (in whom the corpus callosum is still developing). The point is that attention will be recruited only when the sensory transfer falls below a threshold value, which defines the interaction between different methods of information transfer across the callosum. Dichotic listening to CV syllables may be an important vehicle to empirically test a two-stage or two-channel model of callosal transfer, since the left-ear (but not the right-ear) stimulus input is transferred across the callosum for further processing in the left hemisphere. The change in left-ear performance as a function of (a) attentional instruction, (b) age, and (c) callosal size may thus be an interesting way of looking at the function of the corpus callosum.

ACKNOWLEDGMENTS The research presented in this chapter was financially supported by a grant from the Norwegian Research Council–Medical Branch. The author wants to acknowledge the contributions of Ian Law, Rikshospitalet, Copenhagen, Denmark; Alan Beaton, University of Wales, U.K.; and Patricia Cowell, University of Sheffield, U.K., for valuable discussions and data collection.

REFERENCES

ABOITZ, F., A. SCHEIBEL, and E. ZAIDEL, 1992. Morphometry of the sylvian fissure and the corpus callosum with emphasis on sex differences. *Brain* 115:1521–1541.

ASBJØRNSEN, A., and K. HUGDAHL, 1995. Attentional effects in dichotic listening. *Brain. Lang.* 49:189–201.

ASBJØRNSEN, A., K. HUGDAHL, and M. P. BRYDEN, 1992. Manipulations of subjects' arousal in dichotic listening. *Brain Cogn.* 19:183–194.

BEATON, A., K. HUGDAHL, and P. RAY, 2000. Lateral asymmetries and inter-hemispheric transfer in aging: a review and some new data. In *Side-bias: A Neuropsychological Perspective*, M. Mandal and G. Tiwian, eds. Dordrecht, The Netherlands: Klüwer Academic Publishers, pp. 101–152.

BRYDEN, M. P., 1988. Dichotic studies of the lateralization of affect in normal subjects. In *Handbook of Dichotic Listening: Theory, Methods, and Research*, K. Hugdahl, ed. Chichester, U.K.: Wiley and Sons, pp. 1–44.

BRYDEN, M. P., K. MUNHALL, and F. ALLARD, 1983. Attentional biases and the right-ear effect in dichotic listening. *Brain Lang.* 18:236–248.

CLARKE, J. M., R. B. LUFKIN, and E. ZAIDEL, 1993. Corpus callosum morphometry and dichotic listening performance: Individual differences in functional interhemispheric inhibition? *Neuropsychologia* 31:547–557.

COHEN, M., G. W. HYND, and K. HUGDAHL, 1992. Dichotic listening performance in subtypes of developmental dyslexia and a left temporal lobe brain tumor contrast group. *Brain Lang.* 42:187–202.

COWELL, P. E., L. S. ALLEN, N. S. ZALATIMO, and V. H. DENENBERG, 1992. A developmental study of sex and age interactions in the human corpus callosum. *Devel. Brain Res.* 66:187–192.

COWELL, P. E., and K. HUGDAHL, 2000. Individual differences in structural and behavioural measures of laterality and interhemispheric function. *Dev. Neuropsychol.* 18:95–112.

COWELL, P. E., A. KERTESZ, and V. H. DENENBERG, 1993. Multiple dimensions of handedness and the human corpus callosum. *Neurology* 43:2353–2357.

COWELL, P. E., B. I. TURETSKY, R. C. GUR, R. I. GROSSMAN, D. L. SHATSEL, and R. E. GUR, 1994. Sex differences in aging of the human frontal and temporal lobes. *J. Neurosci.* 14:4778–4755.

DENENBERG, V. H., A. KERTESZ, and P. E. COWELL, 1991. A factor analysis of the human's corpus callosum. *Brain Res.* 548:126–132.

HABIB, M., D. GAYRAUD, A. OLIVA, J. REGIS, G. SALAMON, and R. KHALIL, 1991. Effects of handedness and sex on the morphology of the corpus callosum: A study with brain magnetic resonance imaging. *Brain Cogn.* 16:41–61.

HUGDAHL, K., 1991. Considerations in the use of dichotic listening in children. In *Advances in Child Neuropsychology*, Vol. 1, M. Tramontana and C. Hooper, eds. New York: Springer-Verlag, pp. 137–168.

HUGDAHL, K., 1995. Dichotic listening: Probing temporal lobe functional integrity. In *Brain Asymmetry*, R. J. Davidson and K. Hugdahl, eds. Cambridge, Mass.: MIT Press, pp. 123–156.

HUGDAHL, K., 1999. Brain lateralization: Dichotic listening studies. In *Elsevier's Encyclopedia of Neurosciences*, 2nd ed. New York: Elsevier, pp. 276–279.

HUGDAHL, K., and L. ANDERSSON, 1986. The "forced-attention paradigm" in dichotic listening to CV-syllables: A comparison between adults and children. *Cortex* 22:417–432.

HUGDAHL, K., K. BRØNNICK, I. LAW, S. KYLLINGSBÆK, and O. B. PAULSON, 1999a. Brain activation during dichotic presentations of consonant-vowel and musical instruments stimuli: A ¹⁵O-PET study. *Neuropsychologia* 37:431–440.

HUGDAHL, K., G. CARLSSON, P. UVEBRANT, and A. J. LUNDERVOLD, 1997. Dichotic listening performance and intracarotid amobarbital injections in children/adolescents: Comparisons pre- and post-operatively. *Arch. Neurol.* 54:1494–1500.

HUGDAHL, K., and Å. HAMMAR, 1997. Test-retest reliability of the consonant-vowel syllables dichotic listening paradigm. *J. Clin. Exp. Neuropsychol.* 19:667–675.

HUGDAHL, K., E. HEIERVANG, H. NORDBY, A. I. SMIEVOLL, H. STEINMETZ, J. STEVENSON, and A. LUND, 1999b. Central auditory processing and brain laterality: Applications to dyslexia. *Scand. J. Audiol.* 27:26–34.

HUGDAHL, K., T. HELLAND, M. K. FÆREVÅG, E. T. LYSSAND, and A. ASBJØRNSEN, 1995. Absence of ear advantage on the consonant-vowel dichotic listening test in adolescent and adult dyslexics: Specific auditory-phonetic dysfunction. *J. Clin. Exp. Neuropsychol.* 17:833–840.

HUGDAHL, K., I. LAW, S. KYLLINGSBÆK, K. BRØNNICK, A. GADE, and O. B. PAULSON, 2000. Effects of attention on dichotic listening: An ¹⁵O-PET study. *Hum. Brain Mapp.* 10:87–97.

HUGDAHL, K., and K. WESTER, 1992. Dichotic listening studies of hemispheric asymmetries in brain damaged patients. *Int. J. Neurosci.* 63:17–29.

HUGDAHL, K., K. WESTER, and A. ASBJØRNSEN, 1990. The role of the left and right thalamus in language asymmetry: Dichotic listening in Parkinson-patients undergoing stereotactic thalamotomy. *Brain Lang.* 39:1–13.

JÄNCKE, L., and H. STEINMETZ, 1993. Auditory lateralization and planum temporale asymmetry. *NeuroReport* 5:169–172.

KIMURA, D., 1967. Functional asymmetry of the brain in dichotic listening. *Cortex* 3:163–168.

KINSBOURNE, M., 1974. Mechanisms of hemispheric interaction in man. In *Hemispheric disconnection and cerebral function*, M. Kinsbourne and W. L. Smith, eds. Springfield, Ill.: Thomas Publishers.

O'LEARY, D. S., N. C. ANDREASEN, R. R. HURTIG, R. D. HICHAWA, L. WATKINS, L. L. BOLES PONTO, M. ROGERS, and P. T. KIRCHNER, 1996. A positron emission tomography study of binaurally and dichotically presented stimuli: Effects of level of language and directed attention. *Brain Lang.* 50:20–39.

POLLMANN, S., M. MAERTENS, D. VON CRAMON, J. LEPSIEN, and K. HUGDAHL, 2002. Dichotic listening in patients with splenial and nonsplenial callosal lesions. *Neuropsychology* 16:56–64.

PRICE, C., R. WISE, S. RAMSAY, K. FRISTON, D. HOWARD, K. PATTERSON, and R. FRACKOWIAK, 1992. Regional response differences within the human auditory cortex when listening to words. *Neurosci. Lett.* 146:179–182.

REINVANG, I., S. BAKKE, K. HUGDAHL, N. R. KARLSEN, and K. SUNDET, 1994. Dichotic listening performance in relation to callosal area on the MRI scan. *Neuropsychology* 8:445–450.

SPARKS, R., and N. GESCHWIND, 1968. Dichotic listening in man after section of neocortical commissure. *Cortex* 4:3–16.

SPREEN, O., and E. STRAUSS, 1991. *A Compendium of Neuropsychological Tests.* New York: Oxford University Press.

WADA, J., and T. RASMUSSEN, 1960. Intracarotid injections of sodium amytal for the lateralization of cerebral speech dominance. *J. Neurosurg.* 17:266–282.

WITELSON, S. F., 1989. Hand and sex differences in the isthmus and genu of the human corpus callosum: A postmortem morphological study. *Brain* 112:799–835.

ZAIDEL, E., 1976. Language, dichotic listening and the disconnected hemispheres. In *Conference on Human Brain Function*, D. O. Walter, L. Rogers, and J. M. Finzi-Fried, eds. Los Angeles: BRI Publications Office, UCLA, pp. 103–110.

ZAIDEL, E., 1983. Disconnection syndrome as a model for laterality effects in the normal brain. In *Cerebral Hemisphere Asymmetry: Method, Theory and Application*, J. Hellige, ed. New York: Praeger, pp. 99–151.

ZAIDEL, E., J. CLARKE, and B. SUYENOBU, 1990. Hemispheric independence: A paradigm case for cognitive neuroscience. In *Neurobiological Foundations of Higher Cognitive Function*, A. Scheibel and A. Wechsler, eds. New York: Guilford Press.

13 Sensorimotor Integration in the Split Brain

ERAN ZAIDEL AND MARCO IACOBONI

ABSTRACT Patients who had complete cerebral commissurotomy retain the ability to integrate sensorimotor information across the midline. There are a variety of subcortical channels, both visual and motor, and they may show compensatory development following loss of normal commissural connections. All commissurotomy patients can perform the simple reaction time task of Poffenberger, that is, respond with a unimanual button press to lateralized unpatterned light flashes in both the ipsilateral and contralateral visual hemifields. The crossed-uncrossed difference (CUD) in the split brain (~40 ms) is an order of magnitude longer than that in the normal brain (~3 ms).

In the normal brain, the CUD is not affected by primary visual parameters of the target (intensity, eccentricity), but it *is* affected by motor parameters of the response (alternating finger responses, alternating hand responses, three presses, bimanual responses). The normal CUD is also unaffected by attentional parameters (stimulus blocking, spatial uncertainty, redundancy gain, spatial compatibility). Target meaningfulness ("hand stimuli"—a visual/cognitive parameter?) does not affect the CUD but it does make it sensitive to attentional modulation (spatial compatibility). This may be mediated by a parietal-prefrontal sensory-attentional motor loop (Aziz-Zadeh et al., 2000b).

By contrast, the CUD in the split brain may be affected by some visual parameters (eccentricity), by some motor parameters (bimanual responses), and by some attentional parameters (spatial compatibility), but the effects are subject to strong individual differences. These different CUDs likely reflect interhemispheric transfer through different subcallosal channels.

Redundant copies of the target in the opposite visual hemifield speed up responses in simple reaction time by statistical summation, but in the split brain the corresponding redundancy gain can be much greater, showing neural co-activation. Although this bilateral hyperredundancy gain does not affect the CUD in the split brain, it does represent enhanced interhemispheric activation. Thus, the normal corpus callosum serves to modulate and inhibit large attentional effects of subcallosal interhemispheric transfer.

Introduction: Disconnection syndrome

Patients with complete cerebral commissurotomy (split brain) exhibit cortically disconnected but subcortically connected cerebral hemispheres. Their corpus callosum, anterior commissure, and hippocampal commissure are surgically sectioned, but a variety of connecting subcallosal pathways in the cerebellum, midbrain, pons, and both hypothalamus and subthalamus remain intact (Zaidel et al., in press). In particular, the midbrain contains a phylogenetically archaic visual system, mediated by the superior colliculus (retina → superior colliculus → pulvinar → V2 → ···) and separate from the geniculostriate system (retina → lateral geniculate → V1 → ···). This system can relay simple visual features, such as movement, luminance, position, and orientation, as well as high-contrast patterns ipsilaterally from the left visual field (LVF) to the left hemisphere (LH) and from the right visual field (RVF) to the right hemisphere (RH) (LVF → right superior colliculus → intercollicular commissure → left superior colliculus → LH, etc.). The brain stem may also contain subcortical interhemispheric routes. An ipsilateral corticospinal motor pathway, in turn, permits ipsilateral motor control of the right hand (Rh) by the RH and of the left hand (Lh) by the LH, especially for movements of proximal joints (e.g., Brinkman and Kuypers, 1973). Since normal subjects appear capable of modulating their interhemispheric interaction via callosal traffic (Zaidel et al., 1990a), the split brain defines the scope and limits of normal hemispheric independence.

ACUTE DISCONNECTION When the corpus callosum, anterior commissure, and hippocampal commissure are surgically sectioned in a right-handed patient with LH

ERAN ZAIDEL Department of Psychology, University of California at Los Angeles, Los Angeles, California.
MARCO IACOBONI Ahmanson Lovelace Brain Mapping Center, Neuropsychiatric Institute, Brain Research Institute, David Geffen School of Medicine, University of California at Los Angeles, Los Angeles, California.

dominance for speech, she or he is unable to compare visual stimuli across the vertical meridian or somatosensory stimuli across the two hands, to name visual stimuli seen in the LVF or felt by the Lh, or to verbally identify sounds presented to the left ear (LE) in a dichotic listening paradigm (this signal normally reaches the LH from the RH via the isthmus of the corpus callosum) (Zaidel, Zaidel, and Bogen, 1999). There is no interhemispheric transfer for touch, pressure, and proprioception. Hand postures that are impressed on one unseen hand by the examiner cannot be mimicked in the opposite hand, and a brief flash of a hand form to one visual hemifield (VF) cannot be copied by the contralateral hand. There is loss of intermanual point localization, that is, loss of the ability to identify exact points stimulated on the other side of the body, especially on distal parts, such as the fingertips. In all of these cases intrahemispheric comparisons are intact.

Bimanual coordination of motor skills acquired before surgery remains intact. New bimanual tasks consisting of fine finger movements or parallel hand movements are also normally executed, but bimanual interdependent antagonistic control remains severely impaired.

Soon after surgery there are episodes of intermanual conflict, in which the hands act at cross-purposes. Patients sometimes complain that their left hand behaves in a "foreign" or "alien" manner, and they routinely express surprise at apparently purposeful left-hand actions (autocriticism) (Zaidel et al., in press).

CHRONIC DISCONNECTION In general, failure of communication between the two disconnected hemispheres persists. There is some progressive compensation with time, including a variety of noncallosal transfer mechanisms. This includes cross-cuing, ipsilateral sensory/motor projections, and a number of routes for subcallosal communication. Individual differences emerge in the degree to which patients can verbalize simple stimuli in the left sensory field or make same-different judgments about simple stimuli in the two visual hemifields (see below).

Failure of comparisons across the midline or of naming stimuli in the left sensory field in specific cases might not be sufficient to establish disconnection. Potential pitfalls or confounds need to be considered and excluded. Furthermore, no single sign is a sufficient index for disconnection. In fact, some apparent interhemispheric disconnection effects may be attributable to intrahemispheric disconnection in either hemisphere. For example, it is theoretically conceivable that LVF stimuli are available to LH processes that are disconnected from language centers in the same side. Cases of implicit knowledge or memory may be examples of intrahemi-

spheric disconnection from language (Zaidel, 1994). Similarly, LVF extinction may result in the inability to compare stimuli across the vertical meridian—a classic disconnection symptom (cf. J.W. from the Dartmouth series; see Proverbio, 1993). Thus, failure to name LVF stimuli may be insufficient to establish interhemispheric disconnection. (In this case, a possible way to demonstrate absence of disconnection may be to show that RVF stimuli cannot be named either.)

Cross-integration Trevarthen and Sperry (1973) distinguished between (1) a crossed geniculostriate cortical "focal" visual system, parafoveal, dedicated to object identification by form and demonstrating no ipsilateral VF → H transfer following callosal section, and (2) an uncrossed subcortical "ambient" (second) visual system that is peripheral, dedicated to space perception through movement, to relative size and brightness and to crude identification, and demonstrating ipsilateral VF → H transfer via the superior colliculus and pulvinar. Ipsilateral transfer extends to simple features of form, such as curved versus straight, elongated versus square, or unitary versus bipartite. Holtzman (1984) showed that location but not shape cues in one hemifield could direct eye movements to targets in the other hemifield in callosotomized subjects. Sergent (1987) showed and Corballis and Trudel (1993) confirmed bilateral integration of location and orientation information in various alignment tasks. Corballis (1995) reviewed the evidence and concluded that split-brain patients can integrate, subcortically, information about location, orientation, and movement but not form, though with some loss of spatial and temporal resolution.

Ramachandran, Cronin-Golomb, and Myers (1986) found more or less normal apparent motion with sequential lights in opposite hemifields of complete commissurotomy patients L.B., N.G., and A.A. from the Los Angeles series, concluding that the effect was mediated by the second visual system. Although the patients reported transition from apparent motion to temporal succession with increased interstimulus intervals, Gazzaniga (1987) argued that they infer motion rather than perceive it. He reported no apparent motion in callosotomized patient J.W. when the patient did not expect it. However, Corballis (1995) did obtain apparent motion in L.B. and in splenium-sectioned patient D.K., using Gazzaniga's parameters.

Directing attention to one ear during dichotic listening to nonsense CV syllables in split-brain patients yields unusual and variable results (Zaidel, Zaidel, and Bogen, 1990b) suggesting that the usual effects of attention are callosally mediated. This may help to explain why the patients do not spontaneously engage in activities that require (interhemispheric?) shifts of attentions, such as reading.

Naming stimuli in the left sensory field Occasionally, split-brain patients can name stimuli that are seen in the left hemifield (LVF) or palpated with the Lh (Butler and Norsell, 1968; Levy, Nebes, and Sperry, 1971; Teng and Sperry, 1973; Johnson, 1984; Myers, 1984). Excluding improper lateralization and cross-cuing, this could reflect (1) ipsilateral projection of sensory information from the LVF or Lh to the LH, where verbalization occurs, (2) subcortical transfer of cognitive information sufficient to identify the stimulus to the LH following recognition by the RH, or (3) RH speech. Mere naming of stimuli in the left sensory field in the absence of cross-field matching could simply be attributed to (4) neglect without disconnection. Similarly, cross-matching may fail because of a tendency to neglect one hemifield with bilateral presentation. Verbalization of stimuli in the left sensory hemifield is less likely to reflect RH speech if there is good nonverbal Rh identification of these stimuli. More generally, if LVF naming correlates with nonverbal Lh identification, then it is likely to reflect RH speech, whereas if it correlates with Rh nonverbal identification, then it is likely to reflect LH speech. Alternatively, if LVF naming is unaffected by RVF distractors, then it is likely to reflect RH speech, whereas if LVF naming is reduced by RVF distractors, then it is likely to reflect LH speech (see below).

Baynes and colleagues (1995) report a systematic series of experiments attempting to demonstrate RH speech in callosotomy patient J.W. from the Dartmouth series. However, the evidence is mixed. We have data from patient L.B. of the Los Angeles series, showing better partial naming of geometric shapes following Lh than LVF exposure, even though in both cases RH recognition was very high and equal in the two modalities (Zaidel, 1998). This argues (1) that naming of stimuli from the left sensory hemispace often reflects ipsilateral sensory projection that is better in somesthesis than vision, rather than subcallosal RH to LH transfer of more abstract stimulus features, and (2) that the naming reflects LH rather than RH speech. However, we now have evidence from naming of LVF words by L.B. that is unaffected by RVF distractors (Zaidel and Seibert, 1997a; Zaidel, 1998), arguing for authentic RH speech.

Interfield visual comparisons versus left hemifield naming: A double dissociation

PATIENT N.G. It is easy to conceive of intact same-different judgments of stimuli in the two visual hemifields together with failure to verbalize stimuli in the LVF. This could mean that the code that transferred between the hemispheres is relatively primitive, limited to the level of initial representation, or Marr's primal sketch, allowing figure-ground and contour discrimination without specifying the identity of the stimulus. (Patients with associative visual agnosia have similar symptoms; they can copy and compare shapes without being able to identify them.) That is why failure of verbal identification in the presence of intact comparison of shapes is insufficient grounds for establishing implicit (unconscious) knowledge (cf. Farah, 1991). But this is precisely the interhemispheric transfer pattern that was observed in patient N.G. The pattern is surprising because the visually transferred code is at once richer, or later in the microgenesis of the visual percept, than the simple features that are believed to be mediated by the second visual system and yet more impoverished, or earlier in the microgenesis of the visual percept, than the abstract connotative features that are believed to be mediated by subcortical pathways and shared midline structures of the autonomic system.

Specifically, N.G. was able to decide whether two nonsense geometric shapes (vanderplas figures) projected to opposite hemifields were same or different (89.7% correct, either hand) just as well as she could compare these shapes within either VF (LVF: 85%, RVF: 72.5%) (Clarke, 1990; Clarke and Zaidel, 1994). These shapes are not easily verbalizable. It is not clear whether N.G. has a particularly efficient superior collicular system for projecting, say, RVF stimuli to the RH or whether RVF stimuli are first processed in the LH and then transferred subcallosally to the RH.

Another task required N.G. to match uppercase and lowercase letters for shape or for name (the Posner-Mitchell paradigm) within or between the two hemifields (for example, "A" and "a" have the same name but not the same shape; "B" and "B" have the same shape). N.G. could match letter shapes between the hemispheres (Lh: 69% correct, Rh: 75%) just as well as within the hemispheres (LVF-Lh: 78%, RVF-Rh: 69%), but she could compare letter names only within the hemispheres (LVF-Lh: 72%, RVF-Rh: 87.5%, bilateral-Lh: 52%, bilateral-Rh: 61%; the last two are not significantly above chance) (Eviatar and Zaidel, 1994). In this case, then, N.G. was able to transfer a lower visual code but not a higher phonological or name code ipsilaterally or between the disconnected hemispheres (Eviatar and Zaidel, 1992).

More recently, Weems et al. (unpublished data) found that N.G. could match primary colors both within her LH and between the two VFs, with the right hand responding, presumably reflecting RH → LH transfer. She could also match shades of the same primary color in either hemisphere, as well as between the two VFs with the left hand responding, presumably reflecting LH → RH transfer. However, when color stimuli were equated for luminance, N.G. could match them in either hemisphere but not between the VFs, suggesting that luminance transfer via the superior colliculus mediated interhemispheric color matching. Surprisingly, N.G. could match colors for name (Do the two shades belong to the same color category, e.g., red?) in either hemisphere as well as between the two VFs, with either hand responding, suggesting that the color category could transfer between her disconnected hemispheres. N.G. could also match identical views of faces across the VFs, but she could not match different views of the face of the same individual.

In sum, N.G. is able to transfer some visual attributes, such as shape and luminance, but not others, such as color hue, and she seems unable to transfer more abstract linguistic or perceptual codes, such as letter name or person identity. Surprisingly, she can also transfer color category, and one wonders what interhemispheric code she uses for accomplishing that.

PATIENT L.B. What about the opposite dissociation: the ability to name LVF stimuli without the ability to compare LVF and RVF stimuli? We examined L.B.'s ability to name LVF words as a function of the presence and type of distractors in the RVF. We reasoned that if his LH controlled LVF naming, then LVF naming performance should drop when the LH is simultaneously occupied by a distractor in the RVF. Further, the drop should be greater for word than for figural distractors because then the distractor would engage more of the resources necessary for naming the LVF stimulus. Conversely, if L.B.'s RH controlled LVF naming, then the presence of distractors in the RVF should have no effect, or it could even improve LVF naming by removing LH inhibition.

In one experiment (Zaidel and Seibert, 1997a), we presented two lists of 96 LVF words each, half of each with and half without graphic distractors, consisting of nonsense geometric shapes, in the RVF. The first list showed significantly better prompt and correct naming of LVF words without distractors (33.3%) than with distractors (20.8%). This pattern is consistent with LH naming of LVF words. The second list, however, showed no difference between naming of LVF words with (40%) and without (35%) distractors. This could mean that the LH has enough resources to name the LVF words in spite of the RVF distractors, but it is more consistent with RH speech.

In the next experiment (Zaidel and Seibert, 1997b), we presented 12 lists of 96 words each. Half of each list consisted of target words (underlined) in the LVF, and the other half consisted of targets in the RVF. Half of the targets were unilateral, and half had distractors in the other VF. Half of the distractors were words, and half were nonwords. This experiment was administered twice, four months apart. In the first administration there was no difference in prompt and correct naming of LVF targets with (33%) and without (32%) distractors. Again, this could mean that the LH has enough resources to name LVF targets without interference from verbal distractors in the RVF. In that case, LH resources must fluctuate widely so that it is sometimes not affected by verbal distractors and other times it is affected by them. But the pattern is more consistent with RH naming of LVF targets. In the second administration of the experiment, there was significantly better naming of LVF targets without (43%) than with (27%) distractors $(F(1, 11) = 25.4, p = 0.0004)$. This supports the LH naming hypothesis. Furthermore, both administrations disclosed a frequency effect (better ability to read frequent than infrequent words), but only the second administration disclosed a regularity effect (better ability to read words with regular spelling-to-sound correspondence, such as "home"). This is consistent with the observations (1) that L.B.'s disconnected LH has access to a nonlexical route, which is characterized by a regularity effect, whereas his RH does not (Zaidel, 1998), and (2) that both his hemispheres have access to a lexical route, which is characterized by a frequency effect.

In sum, there is a great variability in L.B.'s LVF naming strategies both within and between sessions. Naming of LVF stimuli frequently fails. When it succeeds it sometimes reflects LH naming via cross-cuing, ipsilateral sensory projection, or subcallosal cognitive transfer. On other occasions it does appear to reflect true RH naming.

Together, the double dissociation between perceptual integration (N.G.) and verbal awareness (L.B.) can serve as an anatomical model for a double dissociation between implicit and explicit knowledge. The midbrain system that apparently underlies interhemispheric sensory transfer in N.G. may be the same system that mediates other forms of implicit cognition, such as blindsight. This system can be used to define the information-processing locus of attention in perception, that is, codes that can be mediated by the superior colliculus-pulvinar interhemispheric pathways do not require attention.

Simple reaction time to lateralized light flashes

Consider a simple reaction time (SRT) experiment a là Poffenberger. Subjects are required to press a button with one hand (h) as soon as an unpatterned light occurs in one or the other VF. We can measure the difference between reaction time (RT) to crossed VF-h conditions (RVF-Lh, LVF-Rh) that require interhemispheric transfer for sensorimotor integration and to uncrossed VF-h conditions (RVF-Rh, LVF-Lh) that do not require interhemispheric transfer. Under some simplifying assumptions (see Introduction) the crossed-uncrossed difference (CUD) (divided by 2) is independent of manual or hemispheric dominance and can estimate interhemispheric transfer time.

Recall the argument that if callosal relay in the simple reaction time task (SRT) is motor, then it (i.e., the CUD) should be sensitive to motor but not to visual parameters and, similarly, that if callosal relay is visual it should be sensitive to visual but not to motor parameters (Berlucchi et al., 1971, and see the Introduction). We will consider, in turn, the effects of visual, attentional, and motor manipulations on the CUD in the split brain. The visual manipulations include (1) brightness and (2) eccentricity. The attentional manipulations include (1) the number of copies of the target (one or two, within or between the hemifields), (2) the spatial uncertainty of the target position, and (3) the effect of spatial compatibility on the CUD. The motor manipulations include (1) alternating finger responses and (2) bimanual responses. These will be compared with the standard unimanual, index finger responses.

VISUAL EFFECTS

Brightness and eccentricity In the normal brain, intensity and eccentricity affect overall RT but not the CUD (Berlucchi et al., 1971, 1977; Milner and Lines, 1982; Lines, Rugg, and Milner, 1984; Clarke and Zaidel, 1989). A liberal meta-analysis did reveal significant, but very small, correlations between luminance (−0.29) or eccentricity (+0.2) and the CUD (Braun, 1992). The fact that these correlations are so low in spite of the power of the meta-analysis suggests that these data should be interpreted with caution. In the split brain, Sergent and Myers (1985) found no effect of stimulus intensity on the CUD in complete commissurotomy patients N.G. and L.B. from the Los Angeles series, but their manipulation had no effect on overall RT either, suggesting that it was not effective. By contrast, Clarke and Zaidel (1989) found significant effects of intensity and of eccentricity on overall RT as well as significant effects of at least one of these on the CUD in three out of four patients with complete cerebral commissurotomy from the Los Angeles series (L.B., N.G., A.A., and R.Y.) (Table 13.1).

Two of the four commissurotomy patients had RTs within the range (less than 2 standard deviations from the mean) of the normal control group. All of them had very large CUDs, ranging from 35 to 96 ms, all at least 8

standard deviations from the normal mean. L.B.'s reaction times were within the normal range. He displayed a Rh and RVF advantage, and his abnormally large CUDs (35 and 44 ms) were unaffected by changes in stimulus intensity or eccentricity, despite significant effects of these parameters on overall reaction times. N.G.'s reaction times were within normal limits, at least for those trials that did not require interhemispheric transfer. She had a RVF advantage and no consistent hand advantage. The CUD did not significantly differ for the two stimulus light intensities ($M = 42$ ms) but was significantly larger for stimuli at 10° eccentricity (67 ms) than at 4° eccentricity (45 ms). A.A.'s reaction times were unusually long and variable. There was no consistent hand or visual hemifield advantage across the two experiments. As for patient N.G., the CUD was not significantly affected by stimulus intensity ($M = 60$ ms) but was larger for stimuli at 10° (96 ms) than at 4° (40 ms) eccentricity. R.Y. had an idiosyncratic pattern of results. His reaction times were unusually long in comparison to the student controls but were probably within the normal limits for someone his age and medical condition (chronic medication for epilepsy). He had problems responding to stimuli in the RVF when he used his left but not right hand, at least for stimuli presented at 4° eccentricity. This resulted in a Rh advantage and a LVF advantage across the two experiments. The CUD was paradoxically larger for bright (89 ms) than for dim (51 ms) light flashes. A larger CUD was found for stimuli at 10° (83 ms) than at 4° (68 ms) eccentricity, consistent with the results from N.G. and A.A.

Thus, different patients apparently rely on different subcortical pathways for sensorimotor integration across the midline. The CUDs that are observed in commissurotomized patients L.B. (35 and 44 ms) and N.G. (42 and 56 ms) are similar to values obtained by Sergent and Myers (1985) when they tested the same subjects (29 and 50 ms for L.B. and N.G., respectively). For both commissurotomized patients N.G. and A.A., the CUD was larger (by 22 ms and 56 ms, respectively) for 10° than for 4° light flashes, while the CUD was not significantly affected by changes in stimulus intensity. However, the stimulus intensity manipulation had a greater effect on overall reaction times than did the eccentricity manipulation. Therefore, the magnitude of the CUD is not simply proportional to the overall reaction time. Interhemispheric transmission was probably occurring along visual pathways that are more sensitive to stimulus eccentricity than to intensity. As all of the cortical commissures have been transected surgically in the commissurotomized patients tested, subcortical commissures are probably responsible for the CUD in N.G. and A.A.

TABLE 13.1

Effects of visual, attentional, and motor manipulations on the CUD in split-brain patients

Patients	Visual — Sergent and Myers (1985) — Luminance RT	CUD	Visual — Clarke and Zaidel (1989), Aglioti et al. (1993) (M.E.) — Intensity RT	CUD	Eccentricity RT	CUD	Attentional — Aglioti et al. (1993) — VF Blocking RT	CUD	Attentional — Iacoboni and Zaidel (1994) — Spatial Uncertainty RT	CUD	Attentional — Iacoboni and Zaidel (unpublished) — RG Within RT	CUD	RG Between RT	CUD	Motor — Iacoboni and Zaidel (1995) — Alternate Fingers RT	CUD	Motor — di Stefano et al. (1980), Aglioti et al. (1993), Mooshagian et al. (unpublished) — Bimanual Responses RT	CUD
Normals	+	+?	+	−	+	−	+	−	−	−	+	+	+	−	−	+	+?	+
L.B.	−	−?	+	−	+	−			+	−	−	−	+	−	−	−		
N.G.	−	−?	+	−	+	+			+	−	−	−	+	−	+	−		
M.E.					+	−	+	+									+?	+
A.A.			+	−	+	+												
R.Y.			+	+	+	+											−	−

RT = reaction time, CUD = crossed-uncrossed difference, RG = redundancy gain.

Unit recordings within the superior colliculus of the monkey demonstrate a retinotopic organization (Schiller and Koerner, 1971; Goldberg and Wurtz, 1972), which may account for the eccentricity effect in N.G. and A.A. As this region receives both retinal and visual cortical neural inputs (Sprague et al., 1973), theoretically there are at least two neural routes that could account for the visual transfer. The first is a direct ipsilateral visual projection in which midline transfer, presumably via the superior colliculi, occurs before cortical processing. The second possible route involves an interhemispheric sub-callosal pathway, in which sensory articulation is reached in the contralateral cerebral hemisphere prior to sub-cortical transfer. A third, motor, route is discussed below.

The brain stem visual system may also be important for blindsight, in which patients with striate lesions demonstrate visual perceptual abilities in the blind field in the absence of visual awareness (see Weiskrantz, 1986, for a review). Patients with blindsight presumably have the ipsilateral visual pathway available to them, yet they report that they are not aware of having seen the visual stimuli. By contrast, the commissurotomized patients were fully aware of the presence of light flashes presented in either visual hemifield. Hence, response with awareness, as occurs in the commissurotomized patients, could not use only an ipsilateral visual pathway. Furthermore, unlike the blindsight patients, the commissurotomized patients have intact striate cortices. Thus, striate cortical processing appears to be necessary before full cognitive awareness of a visual stimulus can be achieved and before a response can be freely initiated. Commissurotomized patients N.G. and A.A. are therefore probably responding in the crossed condition by means of a subcortical interhemispheric route rather than by an ipsilateral visual pathway. Moreover, the corticofugal projections to the superior colliculus are probably retinotopically organized (Kawamura, 1974; Updyke, 1977), possibly accounting for the eccentricity effect in these commissurotomized patients.

Like N.G. and A.A., R.Y. showed an effect of eccentricity on the CUD. R.Y. was the only subject whose CUD was significantly affected by changes in stimulus light intensity. The CUD was paradoxically 38 ms larger for bright than for dim light flashes because of unusual responses in the RVF-Lh condition. Both the accuracy and the reaction time data suggest an asymmetry in interhemispheric subcortical transfer in this patient. Clarke and Zaidel (1989) speculate that there was a lesion, not visualized by MRI, within R.Y.'s left visual association area, that affected the transfer of visual information from the left to the right cerebral hemisphere.

For commissurotomized patient L.B., neither intensity nor eccentricity manipulations significantly affected the CUD. Therefore, unlike the other commissurotomized patients, subcortical interhemispheric transfer of visual information is probably not responsible for the CUD. L.B. may be responding in the crossed condition by means of ipsilateral corticospinal motor pathways that are not quite as effective as the contralateral connections. Compared with other commissurotomized patients, he appears to have unusually effective ipsilateral motor control of both hands (Bogen, 1969; Sperry, Gazzaniga, and Bogen, 1969; Zaidel and Sperry, 1977).

Aglioti and colleagues (1993, experiment 1) studied the effect of eccentricity on SRT in patient M.E. with complete callosotomy due to intractable epilepsy. M.E. had removal of a right frontal subdural hematoma and a partial right frontal polectomy at age 8 following a car accident and a further resection of the right frontal lobe at age 19 due to intractable seizures. At that time he also had a longitudinal section of the anterior third of the corpus callosum, followed four months later by sectioning of the rest of the callosum. Following surgery, the patient showed classic disconnection symptoms: a severe left-hand ideomotor apraxia to verbal command but not on imitation, a left-hand anomia, and alexia in the left hemifield. Subsequent MRI confirmed the completeness of the callosal section, the integrity of the anterior commissure, and the presence of a large right prefrontal lesion spanning the premotor and motor cortices, the basal ganglia and the internal capsule.

Target VF was in turn blocked and random. Targets occurred at $10°$, $35°$, and $75°$ of visual angle and eccentricity was held constant in each of 12 blocks of 50 trials. Each h × VF combination yielded only 25 RTs for each stimulus eccentricity in each of the two conditions (blocked and random), so the data may not be reliable (Iacoboni and Zaidel, 2000). There was a main effect of eccentricity on overall RT and an interaction between eccentricity and VF due to a larger increase in RT with eccentricity in the LVF than in the RVF, but the CUD did not vary with eccentricity (Table 13.1). Thus, M.E. behaved like L.B. but unlike N.G., A.A., and R.Y.

Effect of stimulus meaningfulness Aziz-Zadeh and colleagues (2000a) and Aziz-Zadeh and colleagues (2000b) administered an SRT task in which the targets were images of the backs of a left or a right hand. Control targets consisted of scrambled versions of the same stimuli. The rationale was that the image of a hand similar to the responding hand will facilitate a prefrontal-parietal sensorimotor loop and speed up RTs. We also asked whether this format will make the SRT paradigm susceptible to spatial compatibility effects. We tested this by having the subject respond with the hands in a "natural" (left hand on the left side, right hand on

TABLE 13.2
Effects of redundancy gain on the CUD

Subject	Reaction Time in Normal Range?				RG Effect on					Size of RG			Size of CUD			
	Focused			Divided	Overall RT?			CUD?		Focused		Divided	Focused			Divided
					Focused		Divided	Focused								
	S_F	W	B	S_D	W	B		W	B	W	B		S_F	W	B	S_D
Normals	+	+	+	+	+	+	+	−	−	3.2	4.1	9.2	−1.02	.12	1.1	1.8
L.B.	−	−	+	−	−	++[1]	++[2]	−	−	−4.4	25.8	31	43.2	39.5	22.2	36
N.G.	−	−	+	NA	−	++[2]	NA	−	−	−1.0	39	NA	9	20.5	18.5	NA

+ = presence of an effect; − = absence of an effect; ++ = hyper redundancy gain; NA = data not available.

RG = redundancy gain; CUD = crossed-uncrossed difference; S_D = single target, divided attention experiment; S_F = single target, focused attention experiment; W = within-field redundant target, focused attention experiment; B = between-field redundant target, focused attention experiment.

[1] Hyper RG in the right hemisphere.

[2] Hyper RG in both hemispheres.

the right side) or "unnatural" (left hand on the right side, right hand on the left side) response conditions. The critical question is whether the hand stimuli will affect the CUD and whether the CUD will be sensitive to spatial compatibility.

Normal subjects who were tested with scrambled targets disclosed a significant response hand × VF (negative CUD of −3 ms) and no spatial compatibility effect, that is, an insignificant condition (natural, unnatural) × response hand (left, right) interaction ($p = 0.1449$). However, normal subjects who were tested with hand images as targets disclosed a significant stimulus hand (left, right) × VF (left, right) interaction ($p = 0.0133$), with faster responses to left-hand images in the LVF and to right-hand images in the RVF. The response hand × VF interaction was not significant, but the three-way interaction condition × response hand × VF was significant ($p = 0.0154$), as was the four-way interaction condition × stimulus hand × response hand × VF ($p = 0.0058$). The CUD across the four condition × stimulus hand combinations varied from 7 ms (unnatural, left-hand stimulus) and 1.5 ms (unnatural, right-hand stimulus) to −7.5 ms (natural, left-hand stimulus) and −1.5 ms (natural, right-hand stimulus). Thus, the meaning of the stimulus and spatial attention together affected the CUD.

The effect of stimulus meaning on the CUD could be mediated by a sensorimotor loop that is activated for specific intrahemispheric sensorimotor relationships (when stimulus and response share action elements), and the effect on the CUD could then be via a motor rather than a visual callosal channel. It may be objected that the introduction of left- and right-hand images as targets may have turned the test into an implicit choice RT task and that this accounts for the effect of spatial attention.

But RTs to the hand images were similar to RTs to the scrambled images, and the stimulus hand × response hand × VF interaction was not significant.

Commissurotomy patient N.G. received the same test with hand images as targets. Her latency data showed faster responses with the left hand and faster responses to RVF targets. The two-way interaction response hand × VF was not significant ($p = 0.943$), and neither was the three-way stimulus hand × response hand × VF interaction ($p = 0.8892$), but as in normals, the three-way interaction condition (natural, unnatural) × response hand × VF interaction was significant ($p = 0.0003$), with a CUD of 47.5 ms in the unnatural position and of −45.5 ms in the natural position (Table 13.2). Thus, the test showed a strong effect of spatial attention on the CUD. The large negative CUD in the natural position contrasts with large positive CUDs obtained for N.G. with SRT tests with unpatterned targets.

ATTENTIONAL EFFECTS

Spatial uncertainty

Blocked versus random target visual hemifield Aglioti and colleagues (1993) studied the effect of blocking of target VF among normal subjects and found faster overall RTs in blocked than in random presentations but no difference in the CUDs. Braun's (1992) meta-analysis reveals that blocking of target VF yields larger CUDs, but this again must be considered weak data. Marzi, Bisiacchi, and Nicoletti's (1991) meta-analysis notes that blocking of target VF insignificantly shortens overall RT and does not affect the CUD.

Experiment 1 by Aglioti and colleagues (1993) manipulated blocking of target VF in complete collosotomy patient M.E. Half of the 12 blocks of 50 trials each were administered with VF of target changing randomly across the block. In the other six blocks, the first half (25 trials) included targets in one VF, and the second half included targets in the opposite VF. In the blocked condition, the subject was informed about the target VF before each block of 25 trials. The results showed faster overall RTs in the blocked than in the random condition, but this difference was significant only in the RVF. Uncrossed responses in the LVF were paradoxically faster in the random condition than in the blocked condition. There was a significant response hand × VF × condition (random, blocked) interaction, reflecting the absence of a CUD in the blocked LVF condition. Thus, there was a much larger CUD in the random condition (130.4 ms) than in the blocked condition (30 ms), and the CUD in the blocked condition was not significant. The difference between the CUDs was apparently significant.

Fixed versus variable target location Iacoboni and Zaidel (1995) compared a spatially fixed and a spatially variable version of the SRT in normals and in splits. In the fixed version, targets occurred at 4° eccentricity along the horizontal meridian, randomly either in the LVF or in the RVF. In the variable version, targets were randomly presented in nine different locations (three imaginary rows and three imaginary columns) in each VF, at 4°, 8°, and 12° from the vertical meridian, and on the horizontal meridian, 8° above and 8° below the horizontal meridian. Thus, neither version had blocked targets; both versions varied the VF of the target from trial to trial, but only the variable version varied the location of the target within a VF from trial to trial.

Normal subjects had a CUD of 4.3 ms in the fixed version and of 3.65 ms in the variable version. This difference was not significant. Neither version yielded a main effect of response hand. There was no VF advantage in the fixed version, but there was a LVF advantage in the variable version. The two versions did not differ in overall RT.

Patient L.B. had a CUD of 27.3 ms in the fixed version and a CUD of 25.1 ms in the variable version. Overall, RT in the fixed version was faster than in the variable version, but the difference between the CUDs in the two versions was not significant.

Patient N.G. had a CUD of 40.6 ms in the fixed version and a CUD of 75.9 ms in the variable version. In this case overall RT in the variable version was faster than in the fixed version, but again, the difference between the CUDs in the two versions was not significant. There was an RVF advantage in the fixed version but no VF advantage in the variable version.

Covert orienting of spatial attention The Posner paradigm with valid and invalid cues of lateralized targets can be considered an attentional manipulation of the CUD. We have administered several versions of this task to complete commissurotomy patients L.B. and N.G. (cf. Zaidel, 1994). The following experiment (conducted by A. Passarotti) illustrates the effects on the CUD. Four square boxes (2.5° × 2.5°) were positioned at the four corners of a square, with each corner 8° from the fixation cross. The peripheral cue that was used for covertly directing attention was a brightening of one of the boxes. The target was a square appearing in the cued box (valid condition, 80% of cued trials) or in an uncued box (invalid condition, 20% of cued trials). There were also catch trials (23% of total trials). Invalid trials equally often (1) crossed the horizontal meridian but in the same VF as the target, (2) crossed the vertical meridian only, and (3) crossed both meridians. The 50-ms cue came on 225 ms before the target appeared, and the target lasted 50 ms. Neutral cues consisted of cuing all four boxes.

Both patients showed the usual large CUDs in the neutral condition (L.B. = 40 ms, N.G. = 90 ms). Valid cues reduced the CUDs dramatically and invalid cues in the same VF resulted in a negative CUD. An analysis of variance (ANOVA) of L.B.'s latencies with condition (neutral, valid, invalid horizontal, invalid vertical, invalid diagonal), response hand (left, right), and VF (left, right) yielded main effects of condition and of hand and a significant interaction condition × hand but no three-way interaction. (The CUD is represented by a response hand × VF interaction.) However, this failure of the change in the CUD to be significant is undoubtedly due to the relatively small number of trials.

Redundant target effects

Consider a simple reaction time experiment with blocked target VF, in which some trials contain single targets, other trials contain a redundant copy of the target in the same VF, and yet other trials contain a redundant copy of the target in both VFs. How would redundant targets affect the CUD? We distinguish two conditions of *bilateral* targets: (1) focused attention, in which the subject attends to targets in one VF throughout a block of trials, and (2) divided attention, in which the subject attends to both VFs simultaneously. In general, we expect redundant copies to reduce overall RT. This is the well-known redundant target effect (RTE), and it can reflect a horse race (statistical summation) made possible by parallel processing of the target with unlimited resources. On other occasions the gain surpasses a horse race (violation of the horse race inequality), and it then reflects some multiplicative coactivation (neural summation) or priming (Miller, 1982). Statistical summation reflects a late interaction between the two target detection processes during response programming, whereas neural summation presumably reflects an earlier interaction during target detection. An fMRI experiment showed that neural summation was associated with activation in medial and lateral right extrastriate regions (Iacoboni et al., 2000). We interpreted this as cortical modulation of collicular activity.

We ran two versions of the experiment. In one version (focused attention, mixed stimuli), attention was focused on one VF, but trials changed randomly from single targets to redundant targets with copies in the same VF and to redundant targets with copies in the opposite VF. In a second version (divided attention, blocked stimuli), attention was always divided between the two VFs, but stimuli were blocked: one block with single targets in the LVF, another block with single targets in the RVF, and another block with redundant targets in both VF.

Focused attention/mixed stimuli In this experiment we consider in turn the within-field and between-field redundant conditions.

Within-field redundant targets Will the within-field RTE affect the CUD? It can be expected to accelerate target processing in some hemispheric module and consequently perhaps also to reduce callosal relay through callosal channels that interconnect the module with its symmetric homologue in the other hemisphere. If these channels dominate the multiple-channel race, then the CUD will be reduced. In fact, while overall RT in normal subjects was significantly faster with redundant targets, the CUD was not significantly different (Table 13.2) (Iacoboni and Zaidel, unpublished data).

Complete commissurotomy patient L.B. from the Los Angeles series showed no redundancy gain in either hemisphere. The within-field redundant target condition *reduced* the CUD (39.5 ms) relative to the single-target condition (43 ms) but not significantly so (Table 13.2). Complete commissurotomy patient N.G. from the Los Angeles series showed a redundancy gain only in the RH (LVF-Lh), but it did not violate the horse race inequality. The within-field redundant targets *increased* the CUD (20.5 ms) relative to the single-target condition (9 ms) but not significantly so (Table 13.2). N.G.'s CUD in the single-target condition is surprisingly small, much smaller than her CUD in Clarke and Zaidel's (1989) study (42–56 ms). This suggests that her effective subcortical channels vary with task as a function of the modules that are engaged in the detection.

Thus, both patients show a small or no redundancy gain in both hemispheres, without evidence for neural summation and with no effect on the CUD.

Between-field redundant targets In this case all responses represent uncrossed hand–visual field combinations, but attention is directed to one VF. Thus, RVF-Rh and LVF-Lh trials reflect interhemispheric redundant target effects. In turn, RVF-Lh and LVF-Rh trials reflect either (1) interhemispheric transfer, that is, the usual CUD, together with an interhemispheric redundant target effect, or else (2) an attentional shift to the other VF, followed by an uncrossed RT, perhaps together with a subsequent interhemispheric redundant target effect.

Normal subjects showed a slightly larger redundancy gain in the between-field redundant target condition (4.1 ms) than in the within-field redundant target condition (3.2 ms), but again the CUD in the between-field condition (1.1 ms) was not significantly different than the CUD in the within-field redundant condition (0.125 ms) or than the CUD in the single-target condition (−1.02 ms) (Table 13.2). (Although these CUDs are not significantly different from each other, it is interesting that there is a trend for *faster* overall RT to be associated with *larger* CUDs! This is counter to the small negative correlation between luminance and CUD ($r = -0.29$) found in Braun's (1992) meta-analysis.) It is surprising that redundant copies in the other VF facilitate RT as much as, or more than, copies within the target VF do. This is most dramatic for RVF-Rh responses, in which a redundant copy in the LVF confers a 6.6-ms advantage over a single RVF target, compared with a significantly smaller, 3.3-ms, advantage conferred by a redundant copy in the RVF. This implicates callosal relay in the redundant target effect and may be due to the fact that the two copies followed each other within a critical time window due to interhemispheric transfer.

Patient L.B. showed a very large and significant redundancy speed gain in the between-field condition (25.8 ms) compared with a redundancy loss (4.4 ms) in the within-field redundant condition (Table 13.2). The gain violated the horse race inequality in the RH (LVF-Lh). Nonetheless, the CUD in the between-field condition (22.2 ms) was not significantly smaller than that in the single-target condition (43.2 ms).

Patient N.G. also showed a very large and significant gain in the between-field condition (39 ms) relative to the single-target condition, as compared with a redundancy loss (−1 ms) in the within-field redundant condition. The gain violated the horse race inequality in both hemispheres (LVF-Lh and RVF-Rh). Again, the CUD in the between-field condition (18.5 ms) was not significantly different from the CUD in the within-field condition (20.5 ms) or in the single-target condition (9 ms) (Table 13.2).

Thus, both split-brain patients showed dramatic and selective redundancy gains from copies in the VF opposite the target, further implicating interhemispheric delay in the effect. This confirms the results, though not the interpretation, of Reuter-Lorenz and colleagues (1995) in patient J.W. of the Hanover series. On the basis of the redundant target effects in simple reaction time in patients with extinction due to right parietal damage, Marzi and colleagues (1996) also concluded that the RTE involves removal of callosal inhibition.

Divided attention   Recall that this experiment is different from the focused attention in two main respects. First, target VF was blocked in both experiments, but in the divided attention experiment, the same stimulus occurred throughout the block (stimulus blocking), whereas in the focused attention experiment, stimuli switched randomly between a single target, a target with a redundant copy within the same field, and a target with a redundant copy in the opposite field (attentional blocking). Although the target position was fixed throughout the block, there may have resulted a more diffuse distribution of attention for single targets in the focused attention experiment, because of the varying stimuli within a block, with a resulting cost in overall RT. Second, in the divided attention experiment, *bilateral* trials were all identical, without explicitly directing attention to either side. In the focused attention experiment, by contrast, attention on bilateral trials was directed to one side throughout the block, and bilateral trials alternated randomly with single targets and with same-field redundant trials. It is plausible that in the divided attention experiment, attention in bilateral trials was automatically directed to the visual hemifield ipsilateral to the response hand. In sum, unilateral targets may be expected to be detected faster in the divided attention experiment, owing to stimulus blocking, and bilateral targets faster in the focused attention experiment, because of directed attention, so the redundancy gain should be smaller in the divided attention experiment.

In this experiment, targets were presented at 8° eccentricity, and subjects responded unimanually with the index finger. Targets were blocked either in the LVF, in the RVF, or bilaterally with attention divided between both fields.

Normal subjects had faster overall RTs in the divided attention experiment. The CUD in the single-target condition was 1.8 ms. The redundancy gain for congruent response hands (right hand with RVF targets, left hand with LVF targets) was 9.2 ms.

Patient L.B. had a somewhat faster overall RT in the single-target condition of the divided attention experiment (325 ms) than of the focused attention experiment (341 ms), but this may reflect his usual variability range. The CUD in the single-target condition in the divided attention experiment was 36 ms, compared with 43.2 ms in the focused attention experiment (Table 13.2). The redundancy gain for corresponding hands was 31 ms. The gain violated the horse race inequality in either hand. This difference in redundancy gain between conditions is consistent with that observed in normals: In both normal subjects and L.B., the divided attention condition resulted in about twice the redundancy gain observed in the focused attention condition.

Summing up the redundancy gain experiments, we see first that normals show a similar modest RTE from redundant copies within and between the VFs, whereas splits show no RTE within hemispheres but a very large neural summation from redundant copies between the two VFs. Second, the gain in overall RT did not significantly affect the CUD either in the normal subjects or in the split-brain patients. Thus, the RTE is not correlated with the CUD. The pattern of results actually suggests an increase in CUD with increasing redundancy gain in the normal brain and a decrease in CUD with increasing gain in patient L.B. It is possible that the failure of the decrease in CUD with increasing gain in L.B. to reach significance merely reflects the low power of an ANOVA based on trials as a random factor. But accepting the failure of the gain to affect the CUD in L.B., the data are consistent with the failure of the other visual parameters—intensity and eccentricity—to affect his CUD, supporting the conclusion that he does not rely on a visual channel for sensorimotor integration in the simple reaction time task. By contrast, patient N.G. whose CUD had been shown to be sensitive to eccentricity, is not sensitive to the visual target redundancy. This illustrates that the failure of one visual parameter to affect the CUD does not mean that other visual parameters will fail as well. Further, we really need to better understand the locus of the effect of a particular variable in the information processing sequence before inferring its modality-specific status. Thus, it is quite plausible that the RTE is attentional and cognitive rather than strictly visual.

Our data suggest that the redundant target effect in simple reaction time is inherently interhemispheric. It is absent in the within-hemisphere condition in split-brain patients, and it is enhanced in the between-hemisphere condition in the split brain relative to the normal brain. This suggests that the redundancy gain is not due to sensorimotor transfer but to the removal of some inhibitory cross-callosal effects. These two functions are presumably subserved by different callosal channels.

Iacoboni and colleagues (2000) examined the RTE in two patients with complete commissurotomy (L.B. and N.G.), two patients with complete callosotomy (D.T. and G.C.), three patients with anterior callosal section

TABLE 13.3
Spatial compatibility effects on the CUD in SRT

| | Mooshagian et al. | | | | Aziz-Zadeh et al. | | | |
| | Unimanual Responses | | Bimanual Responses | | Hands vs. Neutral Targets | | Spatial Compatibility w/Hand Images | |
Patients	RT	CUD	RT	CUD	RT	CUD	RT	CUD
Normals	+	−	−	−	−	−	−	+
N.G.	−	−	+	−	−	−	+	+
A.A.	−	+	−	+				

+ = effect present, − = effect absent.

(B.M., J.P., and D.W.), and two patients with agenesis of the CC (M.M. and J.L.). The occurrence of a hyper RTE (violation of the horse race inequality) signaling neural summation was not associated with a specific callosal pathology: Two patients with complete commissurotomy, one patient with complete callosotomy, and one patient with agenesis of the CC all exhibited a hyper RTE. Instead, the hyper RTE was associated with long CUDs, exceeding 15 ms. This must be the time window that permits neural coactivation.

Spatial compatibility effects

Hand images as targets Since the pioneering experiments of Berlucchi and colleagues (1977), it has become dogma that the CUD in SRT experiments is not susceptible to spatial compatibility. Choice RT experiments, on the other hand, in which both stimuli and responses have a binary spatial dimension, show ubiquitous spatial compatibility (or Simon) effects. We have already described the dramatic experiment of Aziz-Zadeh and colleagues (2000a,b), in which unpatterned SRT targets were replaced by stimuli consisting of left- or right-hand images. This made the CUD of both normal subjects and a split-brain patient susceptible to spatial compatibility (i.e., placement of each response hand on the same or the opposite side as the associated target) (Table 13.3). Spatial compatibility reduces the CUD in the incompatible condition because it speeds up crossed responses and slows down uncrossed responses. But is the spatial compatibility effect visual, motor, or attentional? It deals with *spatial attention* (Rubichi et al., 1997) and thus blurs the distinction between the three types of callosal channels. One could still ask which physiological interhemispheric pathways mediate the effect, and we now know that it can be mediated subcallosally.

Bimanual responses Instead of requiring subjects to make unimanual responses in SRT, we can require simulta-

neous bimanual index finger responses. One hand invariably leads, and we can therefore compute a CUD in several ways. This can be regarded as motor manipulation of SRT. We found that measures of the bimanual CUD (e.g., uncrossed = trials with leading-hand responses to targets in the ipsilateral VF, crossed = trials with following-hand responses to targets in the contralateral VF) lead to an enlarged CUD in normals (∼10 ms), but as with the unimanual CUD, it is not susceptible to spatial compatibility (Mooshagian et al., in preparation). Two complete commissurotomy patients, N.G. and A.A., showed opposite effects of spatial compatibility on the CUD. In N.G. but not A.A. the unnatural position increased overall RT (Table 13.3). In N.G. the unnatural condition reduced the CUD from 39 ms to 29 ms, and the change was not significant. In A.A. the unnatural condition changed the CUD from 51 ms to −13 ms and the change was significant. This suggests that subcallosal channels for interhemispheric sensorimotor integration requiring bimanual synchrony can be sensitive to spatial attention. Is it the case that the CUD in unimanual SRT by commissurotomy patients is also susceptible to spatial compatibility?

Both patients were also tested in the unimanual SRT paradigm with blocked response hand/random target VF trials in the natural and unnatural positions (Mooshagian et al., in preparation). N.G. showed a CUD of 40 ms in the natural position, and it reduced to 3 ms in the unnatural position owing to a selective slowing down of the left-hand responses to LVF targets. A.A. showed a CUD of 58 ms in the natural position, and it changed to 24 ms in the unnatural position. The three-way condition (natural, unnatural) × response hand × VF interaction in A.A. was significant ($p = 0.0032$) (Table 13.3). This shows that the unimanual SRT in split-brain patients is affected by spatial attention and cannot be taken as a context-free measure of anatomic sensorimotor subcallosal interhemispheric transfer.

MOTOR EFFECTS We know that simple visual parameters do not affect the CUD, but is there evidence that motor parameters do? There are clinical data consistent with motor transfer in SRT. Patients suffering from a motor deficit as a result of a unilateral anterior cortical lesion show a longer transmission time compared with patients who have unilateral cortical lesions in similar areas but without motor symptoms (Vallar, Sterzi, and Basso, 1988). If the effective interhemispheric transfer is indeed motor, then we should be able to modulate it with manipulation of the motor programming component of the task. Braun (1992) carried out a meta-analysis of 49 SRT experiments with unimanual responses and found that the use of the index finger rather than the thumb weakly prolonged the CUD. But this result still awaits confirmation from an experiment that manipulates the response finger within the same subjects in both normal subjects and split-brain patients. Braun and colleagues (Chapter 9 in this volume) also report that alternating response hand on sequential trials significantly affects the CUD in normal subjects but that requiring three unimanual key presses instead of the usual one does not significantly change the CUD in these subjects. We will consider two motor manipulations: alternating finger responses and bimanual responses.

Alternating finger responses Iacoboni and Zaidel (1994) used an SRT paradigm with a fixed response hand but with random LVF or RVF target presentations within a block. In the standard experiment, responses were made with the index finger only; in the motor version of the task, responses alternated between index finger on odd trials and middle finger on even trials. Presentation of stimuli in the LVF or RVF was counterbalanced for odd and even trials. In both versions, flashes were presented on the horizontal meridian at 4° eccentricity either in the RVF or in the LVF in a random but counterbalanced fashion.

Normal subjects had a significant CUD of 4.3 ms in the standard version but an insignificant CUD of only 1 ms in the motor version. The two versions did not differ in overall RT (Table 13.1). The standard version had the classic response hand × VF pattern, with no response hand advantage or VF advantage. By contrast, the motor version showed a Rh advantage and a LVF advantage. There were significant task version (motor, standard) × response hand × VF and task version × congruity (crossed [LVF-Rh, RVF-Lh], uncrossed [LVF-Lh, RVF-Rh]) interactions. Thus, the motor manipulation affected the CUD (Table 13.1).

Patient L.B. had a CUD of 27.3 ms in the standard task and 28.45 in the motor version. The two tasks were not significantly different in overall RT. Both tasks showed Rh advantages and RVF advantages. Thus, the motor manipulation did not significantly affect the CUD (Table 13.1).

Patient N.G. had a CUD of 40.6 ms in the standard task and 50.9 in the motor task, but the difference was not significant. The standard task (488 ms) was significantly faster overall than the motor task (513 ms). Both tasks had RVF advantages, and neither had a response hand advantage. Thus, in N.G. too, the motor manipulation did not affect the CUD (Table 13.1).

In sum, the hypothesis that motor callosal channels dominate the normal CUD in SRT in normals is supported by our data. Motor manipulation affects callosal relay in normals but does not affect subcallosal relay in all splits, although it is likely to affect the CUD in some (like R.Y.) who use subcallosal motor pathways for the task.

Bimanual responses, Italian style Consider an SRT experiment with random presentations of targets in the two VFs and with bimanual responses. The subject is required to respond by pressing, say, both index fingers simultaneously. However, perfect synchrony does not occur, and one hand typically leads by about 10 ms. In this paradigm, each trial has an uncrossed sensorimotor connection, so in principle, no CUD need emerge. Nonetheless, both normals and agenetics show a significant CUD, *reduced* by 40–60% relative to the unimanual condition. That is, blocked RVF targets result in faster responses with the Rh, whereas blocked LVF targets result in faster responses with the Lh. The crossed and uncrossed RTs were highly correlated (Jeeves, 1969). The existence of a CUD suggests that bimanual synchrony is maintained by an interhemispheric pathway that relays postdecision cognitive codes from the hemisphere opposite the target VF to the other hemisphere. The hemispheric modules that mediate the requirement for bimanual responses must be interconnected by faster interhemispheric channels (reduced CUD), both callosal and subcallosal, than the usual motor channels.

Di Stefano and colleagues (1980) applied this paradigm to 12 normal right-handed males, with targets changing randomly between the VFs and appearing at 15° of eccentricity. Unimanual responses showed no response hand advantage and no VF advantage and yielded a CUD of 2.2 ms. Bimanual responses also showed no response hand advantage and no VF advantage. They significantly prolonged overall RT but reduced the CUD to 0.71 ms (Table 13.1). Aglioti and colleagues (1993) applied the same paradigm to collosotomy patient M.E. Stimuli were blocked at two eccentricities: 10° and 70°. Unimanual responses showed a CUD of 69.6 ms, whereas bimanual responses showed a CUD of 37.9 ms (Table 13.1). Berlucchi and colleagues (1995) noted that the reduction in the CUD occurred because of slowing down of uncrossed responses and inferred that bimanual synchrony is maintained in a central mechanism by retarding the faster, uncrossed response. In that case the bimanual CUD is not an accurate measure of interhemispheric transfer. However, this account fails to explain why complete synchrony is not achieved and why the CUD in M.E. is still so much larger than normal yet so much smaller than the usual unimanual CUD in this patient.

Eccentricity had no effect on the bimanual CUD. Thus, there is a (nonvisual?) subcallosal channel that mediates the synchrony code, and it is faster than the motor subcallosal channel that mediates crossed responses in the unimanual condition. Again, we see that varying the motor parameters of the task affects the CUD, consistent with transfer through motor channels.

Since the CUD of callosotomy patient M.E. with a spared anterior commissure is comparable to that of complete commissurotomy patients L.B. and N.G., Berlucchi, Aglioti, and Tassinari (1993) conclude that the anterior commissure does not play a role in interhemispheric integration in SRT. What about the possibility that the CUD in split-brain patients reflects ipsilateral motor control rather than interhemispheric transfer? Milner and colleagues (1985) argue that if the same motor system in the hemisphere opposite the target initiates motor responses on either side through ipsilateral and contralateral descending pathways, then the correlation between crossed and uncrossed responses to a given target should be higher in splits than in normals because of a stronger intrasystem than intersystem coupling. However, Berlucchi and colleagues (1993) found that these correlations are similar in M.E., callosal agenetics, and normals, implying interhemispheric transfer rather than ipsilateral motor control in crossed responses.

Aglioti and colleagues (1993) suggest that the role of the corpus callosum in bilateral coordination is in diversifying rather than equalizing bilateral responses. Thus, the absence of the corpus callosum induces an inability to suppress symmetry of concurrent bimanual movement (Preilowski, 1972).

Bimanual responses, California style Mooshagian and colleagues (unpublished data) administered an SRT task with bimanual responses. Subjects were required to press with both index fingers simultaneously. Targets measured $2° \times 2°$ of visual angle and were presented with the edge closest to fixation at $3°$ off the vertical meridian, along the horizontal meridian. Visual field of targets was blocked. Each response hand $\times$ VF block contained 80 trials. To assess the effect of spatial compatibility, responses were made in the natural position (right hand on the right side, left hand on the left side) and in an unnatural position (hands crossed: right hand on left side, left hand on the right). This paradigm permits several plausible measures of a CUD: (1) median responses of all trials by a given hand to targets in a given VF, (2) median latency of leading-hand responses to targets in the ipsilateral VF (uncrossed) and median latency of following-hand responses to targets in the contralateral VF (crossed), and (3) median latency of leading-hand trials by a given hand to a given VF. Here we will describe the results using the second measure, which provides a positive measure of the CUD by definition.

Normal subjects revealed a significant response hand $\times$ target visual field interaction ($p \leq 0.0001$), reflecting a CUD of about 10 ms, as contrasting with the standard unimanual CUD of about 3 ms. The longer CUD suggests that the bimanual responses engage a different, slower callosal channel than the unimanual responses. Could this channel be subcallosal? We administered the bimanual task to two complete commissurotomy patients, N.G. and A.A. A.A. showed the expected large CUD in the natural position (41 ms), and it was not significantly different than the CUD in the unimanual condition (27.2 ms) (Table 13.1). N.G. was slower overall, with bimanual than with unimanual responses. She also showed the expected large CUD in the natural position (39 ms) (Table 13.1). Thus, neither patient showed an effect of bimanual responses on the CUD.

Summary and conclusions

SUMMARY At first, manipulation of visual parameters in the SRT in normal subjects appeared to affect overall RT but not the CUD, whereas manipulation of motor parameters affected the CUD but not necessarily overall RT (Table 13.2). This supported the conclusion that interhemispheric transfer in SRT in normal subjects reflects motor relay. Of course, negative data here are inconclusive. The failure of visual parameters to affect the CUD so far does not exclude the possibility that a new visual manipulation will show such an effect in the future. This is just what we found with hand images serving as targets. We interpreted the effect on the CUD as being mediated by an interhemispheric sensorimotor loop, which enables visual changes in the targets to result in motor changes and thus affect motor interhemispheric transfer. Further, the failure of the CUD to change between conditions does not exclude the possibility that different modules are engaged in the detection tasks and that different callosal channels dominate the relay in the different conditions. Indeed, an apparent visual manipulation may in fact engage different non-visual, cognitive, or even motor modules and channels. This is especially likely if the stimuli and responses engage the sensorimotor parietal-prefrontal loop where visual stimuli affect motor responses and vice versa. There is particular reason to believe that varying the attentional demands of the SRT task may change the effective callosal channel (Zaidel et al., 1996). Thus, the modularity hypothesis in its strict form (visual parameters affect only visual relay, etc.) appears to be wrong. Refuting data can consist of normal subjects showing changes in the CUD in response to both visual and motor manipulation or of partial callosotomy patient whose section spares only the splenium yet whose CUD is affected by motor parameters. But so far, the available data are consistent with the channel doctrine and the modularity hypothesis. Our "escape clause" was the sensorimotor loop, which allegedly translates visual changes into motor ones.

Different split-brain patients show sensitivity variously to visual, motor, and attentional manipulation of the task, presumably reflecting a large individual difference in the subcallosal channels engaged by the task (Table 13.4). Data from the split-brain patients often show large absolute differences in the CUDs that are not significant in ANOVAs based on trial as a random variable (Table 13.4). These ANOVAs must be considered weak statistical tests, and the results should therefore be interpreted with caution.

PARALLEL CHANNELS   The following information-processing model is proposed to account for the apparent variety of interhemispheric transfer routes (Clarke and Zaidel, 1989). Visual information reaches both hemispheres through direct contralateral as well as indirect ipsilateral projections. However, full awareness of a visual stimulus can be achieved only via the contralateral visual system. Moreover, visual information transfers interhemispherically across the corpus callosum, ante-

TABLE 13.4
Summary of effects on the CUD in the split brain

Patient	Visual	Attentional	Motor
L.B.	−		−
N.G.	+	−	−
A.A.	+	+[1]	
M.E.		+[2]	+[3]
Normals	−	−	+

+ = effect present, − = effect absent.
[1] Spatial compatibility with unimanual responses.
[2] VF blocking.
[3] Bimanual.

rior commissure, and subcortical commissures. Following visual analysis, information undergoes cognitive elaboration, and again abstract cognitive information transfers, perhaps across more anterior parts of the corpus callosum. Finally, information flows into the motor programming stage, and motor commands again transfer between the two hemispheres via cortical and/or subcortical commissures. In addition, each hemisphere has direct contralateral and indirect ipsilateral motor control systems.

In this model, all possible connections are activated simultaneously and result in multiple parallel processes, often terminated horse race fashion by the one that completes processing first. Sometimes priority is established by control from above rather than by speed. Moreover, response may be delayed until several parallel processes are completed and their results have been compared.

An earlier model assumed modularity. Thus, visual parameters such as intensity, eccentricity, and visual complexity should affect only visual transfer. Furthermore, transfer along a particular visual pathway may be sensitive to one visual parameter (e.g., eccentricity) but not another (e.g., intensity). Similarly, decision complexity should affect the transfer of cognitive/abstract information but not visual or motor transfer, whereas the complexity of the motor response pattern should affect motor transfer exclusively. Of course it is possible that modularity does not always occur. Then visual parameters may affect decision or even motor transfer, and later stages of processing may affect earlier stages through feedback loops. We now have evidence that modularity may be circumvented. The CUD in the SRT paradigm is dominated by motor transfer, but visual and attentional variables may affect motor modules via a parietal-frontal sensory-attentional-motor loop.

The present results from commissurotomized subjects suggest that midbrain commissural fibers transfer information related to the spatial positioning of a stimulus, whereas previous evidence from acallosal subjects indicates that the anterior commissure transfers information associated with stimulus light flux. Similar tests in patients with selective lesions of the corpus callosum (e.g., the splenium versus the body of the corpus callosum) and patients with complete forebrain commissurotomy sparing the anterior commissure would further clarify the functions of the cerebral commissures in the SRT task.

ANATOMICAL SUBSTRATES   Alternative pathways for supporting interhemispheric sensorimotor integration in the split brain exist. In principle, a number of commissural pathways could transfer information from one side of the brain to the contralateral one. The anatomy and physiology of most of these alternative pathways are still unclear, and a challenge for future research is to elucidate the role of these pathways in preserving functional communication between the separated hemispheres of split-brain patients.

Among hypothetical alternative interhemispheric routes, we can enlist the hippocampal commissure, the posterior commissure, Ganser's or Meynert's commissure, Guddens' commissure, Forel's commissure, and the interhabenular commissure. The hippocampal commissure was thought to be vestigial and nonfunctional in primates on the basis of its phylogenetic shrinkage. In humans, however, EEG data have demonstrated that seizure activity can actually spread through this commissure, thus suggesting that this pathway is functional in the human brain (Gloor et al., 1993).

The functional role of the posterior commissure in sensory transfer is better established. Lesion studies have shown that this commissure is relevant to visual transfer (Hemsley and Savage, 1987, 1989) but not to tactile transfer (Hunter, Ettlinger, and Maccabe, 1975). Although these studies were not performed in humans, the anatomical location of the posterior commissures makes the application of these lesion data highly plausible to the human brain as well. Indeed, this commissure connects the lateral geniculate bodies and the superior colliculi, as well as visual neurons of the pulvinar (Nakamura and Kawamura, 1988, cited in Braun, 1992).

Pretectal and/or collicular processing and relay of extrafoveal stimulation in visual and visuomotor transfer is a plausible alternative to the callosum. There is reciprocal visual and motor innervation of the superior colliculi via the intercollicular commissure (Baleydier et al., 1983, cited in Braun, 1992). Further, each hemiretina projects to both superior colliculi (Antonini et al., 1979). Also, receptive fields of collicular neurons are extrafoveal (Antonini et al., 1979, cited in Braun, 1992). Indeed, there is a strong contribution of the tectum to visual orienting responses. The collicular system is activated preferentially by intense light stimuli, a property consistent with its pupillary role.

It is very likely, however, that in the absence of the corpus callosum, interhemispheric transfer in sensorimotor tasks, and in particular in visuomotor tasks, occurs in the primate through corticopontocerebellar loops. Corticosubcortical pathways connecting visual and motor areas have been clearly identified, and functional imaging data in the primate brain have supported the hypothesis that the cerebellum is critical for sensorimotor integration in the split brain (Glickstein, 2000). Thus, deoxyglucose maps obtained during reaching tasks to visual targets in monkeys with surgical sections of the forebrain commissures and of the optic tract show that the "blind" motor cortex is active during the task by means of activation of the cerebellar hemispheric extensions of vermina lobules V, VI, and VIII.

Conclusions SRT data support the channel doctrine of the corpus callosum, qualified by cross-talk between some of the channels via a sensory-attentional-motor loop. The data also support the thesis of parallel activation of interhemispheric channels, both callosal and subcallosal. Motor channels through the middle corpus callosum dominate callosal relay in normals, whereas visual, superior-collicular channels dominate subcallosal relay in splits. Both the corpus callosum and subcallosal pathways also subserve cognitive channels. The subcallosal channels can be selectively modulated by attention. Thus, the corpus callosum also has inhibitory channels that potentiate hemispheric independence in the normal brain.

The data reported here are consistent with the serial information-processing model of SRT. Distinct information-processing stages are processed in distinct cortical "modules," which may have dedicated callosal and subcallosal channels interconnecting them. But SRT is highly context-dependent, and this requires the serial model to proliferate modules and commissural channels. Even within this "simple" model, we still do not understand the mechanism of bimanual synchronous responses or the role of ipsilateral motor control. But there are neurophysiological data casting doubt on the prima facie validity of the serial model itself (cf. Chapter 8 in this volume).

REFERENCES

AGLIOTI, S., G. BERLUCCHI, R. PALLINI, G. F. ROSSI, and G. TASSINARI, 1993. Hemispheric control of unilateral and bilateral responses to lateralized light stimuli after callosotomy and in callosal agenesis. *Exp. Brain Res.* 95:151–165.

AZIZ-ZADEH, L., J. RAYMAN, and E. ZAIDEL, 2000a. Kinesthetic imagery and laterality. *J. Int. Neuropsych. Soc.* 6:119.

AZIZ-ZADEH, L., I. GIZER, J. RAYMAN, M. IACOBONI, and E. ZAIDEL, 2000b. Stimulus type affects simple reaction time: Evidence for a sensory-motor loop. *Soc. Neurosci. Abstr.* 26:1846.

BAYNES, K., C. M. WESSINGER, R. FENDRICH, and M. S. GAZZANIGA, 1995. The emergence of the capacity to name left visual field stimuli in a callosotomy patient: Implications for functional plasticity. *Neuropsychologia* 33:1225–1242.

BERLUCCHI, G., S. AGLIOTI, and G. TASSINARI, 1993. The role of the corpus callosum and bilaterally distributed motor pathways in the synchronization of bilateral upper-limb responses to lateralized light stimuli. In *Interlimb Coordination: Neural, Dynamics, and Cognitive Constraints*, S. Swinnen, H. Heuer, J. Massion, and P. Caesaer, eds. San Diego, Calif.: Academic Press, pp. 209–227.

BERLUCCHI, G., S. AGLIOTI, C. A. MARZI, and G. TASSINARI, 1995. Corpus callosum and simple visuomotor integration. *Neuropsychologia* 33:923–936.

BERLUCCHI, G., F. CREA, M. DI STEFANO, and G. TASSINARI, 1977. Influence of spatial stimulus-response compatibility on reaction time of ipsilateral and contralateral hand to lateralized light stimuli. *J. Exp. Psychol. Hum. Percept. Perform.* 3:505–517.

BERLUCCHI, G., W. HERON, R. HYMAN, G. RIZZOLATTI, and A. C. UMILTÀ, 1971. Simple reaction time of ipsilateral and contralateral hand to lateralized visual stimuli. *Brain* 94:419–430.

BOGEN, J. E., 1969. The other side of the brain. I: Dysgraphia and dyscopia following cerebral commissurotomy. *Bull. Los Angeles Neurol. Soc.* 34:73–105.

BOGEN, J. E., 1993. The callosal syndromes. In *Clinical Neuropsychology*, 3rd ed., K. M. Heilman and E. Valenstein, eds. Oxford: New York: Oxford University Press, pp. 337–407.

BRAUN, C. M. J., 1992. Estimation of interhemispheric dynamics from simple unimanual reaction time to extrafoveal stimuli. *Neuropsychol. Rev.* 3:321–364.

BUTLER, S. R., and U. NORRSELL, 1968. Vocalization possibly initiated by the minor hemisphere. *Nature* 220:793–794.

BRINKMAN, J., and H. G. KUYPERS, 1973. Cerebral control of contralateral and ipsilateral arm, hand and finger movements in the split-brain rhesus monkey. *Brain* 96:653–674.

CLARKE, J. M., 1990. *Interhemispheric functions in humans: Relationships between anatomical measures of the corpus callosum, behavioral laterality effects and cognitive profiles.* Unpublished doctoral dissertation, University of California, Los Angeles.

CLARKE, J. M., and E. ZAIDEL, 1989. Simple reaction times to lateralized flashes: Varieties of interhemispheric communication routes. *Brain* 112:849–870.

CLARKE, J. M., and E. ZAIDEL, 1994. Anatomical-behavioral relationships: Corpus callosum morphometry and hemispheric specialization. *Behav. Brain Res.* 64:185–202.

CORBALLIS, M. C., 1995. Visual integration in the split brain. *Neuropsychologia* 33:937–959.

CORBALLIS, M. C., and C. I. TRUDEL, 1993. The role of the forebrain commissures in interhemispheric integration. *Neuropsychology* 7:306–324.

DI STEFANO, M., M. MORELLI, C. A. MARZI, and G. BERLUCCHI, 1980. Hemispheric control of unilateral and bilateral movements of proximal and distal parts of the arms as inferred from simple reaction time to lateralized light stimuli in man. *Exp. Brain Res.* 38:197–204.

EVIATAR, Z., and E. ZAIDEL, 1992. Letter matching in the hemispheres: Speed-accuracy tradeoffs. *Neuropsychologia* 30:699–710.

EVIATAR, Z., and E. ZAIDEL, 1994. Letter matching within and between the disconnected hemispheres. *Brain Cogn.* 25:128–137.

FARAH, M. J., 1991. Patterns of co-occurrence among the associative agnosias: Implications for visual object representation. *Cogn. Neuropsychol.* 8:1–19.

GAZZANIGA, M. S., 1987. Perceptual and attentional processes following callosal section in humans. *Neuropsychologia* 25:119–133.

GLICKSTEIN, M., 2000. How are visual areas of the brain connected to motor areas or the sensory guidance of movement? *Trends Neurosci.* 23:613–617.

GLOOR, P., V. SALANOVA, A. OLIVIER, and L. F. QUESNEY, 1993. The human dorsal hippocampal commissure. *Brain* 116:1249–1273.

GOLDBERG, M. E., and R. H. WURTZ, 1972. Activity of superior colliculus in behaving monkey. II: The effect of attention on neuronal responses. *J. Neurophysiol.* 35:560–574.

HEMSLEY, J. P., and G. E. SAVAGE, 1987. Interocular transfer of shape discrimination in the goldfish: A reassessment of the role of the posterior commissure. *Exp. Neurol.* 98:664–672.

HEMSLEY, J. P., and G. E. SAVAGE, 1989. Interocular transfer of preoperatively trained visual discriminations in goldfish (*Carassius auratus*) following selective commissure transections. *Behav. Brain Res.* 32:297–304.

HOLTZMAN, J. D., 1984. Interactions between cortical and subcortical visual areas: Evidence from human commissurotomy patients. *Vision Res.* 24:801–813.

HUNTER, M., G. ETTLINGER, and J. J. MACCABE, 1975. Intermanual transfer in the monkey as a function of amount of callosal sparings. *Brain Res. Brain Res. Rev.* 93:223–240.

IACOBONI, M., A. PTITO, N. Y. WEEKES, and E. ZAIDEL, 2000. Parallel visuomotor processing in the split brain: corticosubcortical interactions. *Brain* 123:759–769.

IACOBONI, M., and E. ZAIDEL, 1995. Channels of the corpus callosum: Evidence from simple reaction times to lateralized flashes in the normal and the split brain. *Brain* 118:779–788.

IACOBONI, M., and E. ZAIDEL, 2000. Crossed-uncrossed difference in simple reaction times to lateralized flashes: between– and within–subjects variability. *Neuropsychologia* 38:535–541.

JEEVES, M. A., 1969. A comparison of interhemispheric transmission times in acallosal and normals. *Psychonomic Sci.* 16:245–246.

JOHNSON, L. E., 1984. Vocal responses to left visual stimuli following forebrain commissurotomy. *Neuropsychologia* 22:153–166.

KAWAMURA, S., 1974. Topical organization of the extrageniculate visual system in the cat. *Exp. Neurol.* 45:451–461.

LEVY, J., R. D. NEBES, and R. W. SPERRY, 1971. Expressive language in the surgically separated minor hemisphere. *Cortex* 7:49–58.

LINES, C. R., M. D. RUGG, and A. D. MILNER, 1984. The effects of stimulus intensity on visual evoked potential estimates of interhemispheric transmission time. *Exp. Brain Res.* 57:89–984.

MARZI, C. A., P. BISIACCHI, and R. NICOLETTI, 1991. Is interhemispheric transfer of visuomotor information asymmetric? Evidence from a meta-analysis. *Neuropsychologia* 29:1163–1177.

MARZI, C. A., N. SMANIA, M. C. MARTINI, G. GAMBINA, G. TOMELLERI, A. PALAMARA, F. ALESSANDRINI, and M. PRIOR. Implicit redundant-targets effect in visual extinction. *Neuropsychologia* 34:9–22.

MILLER, J., 1982. Divided attention: Evidence for coactivation with redundant signals. *Cogn. Psychol.* 14:247–279.

MILNER, A. D., M. A. JEEVES, P. H. SILVER, C. R. LINES, and J. WILSON, 1985. Reaction times to lateralized visual stimuli in callosal agenesis: Stimulus and response factors. *Neuropsychologia* 23:323–331.

MILNER, A. D., and C. R. LINES, 1982. Interhemispheric pathways in simple reaction time to lateralized light flash. *Neuropsychologia* 20:170–179.

MYERS, J. J., 1984. Right hemisphere language: Science or fiction? *Am. Psychol.* 39:315–320.

PREILOWSKI, B. F. B., 1972. Possible contribution of the anterior forebrain commissures to bilateral motor coordination. *Neuropsychologia* 10:267–277.

PROVERBIO, A. M., 1993. *Left and right hemisphere role for selective and sustained attention: An electrophysiological approach.* Doctoral Thesis of the University of Padua, Padua, Italy.

RAMACHANDRAN, V. S., A. CRONIN-GOLOMB, and J. J. MYERS, 1986. Perception of apparent motion by commissurotomy patients. *Nature* 320:358–359.

REUTER-LORENZ, P. A., G. NOZAWA, M. S. GAZZANIGA, and H. C. HUGHES, 1995. Fate of neglected targets: a chronometric analysis of redundant target effects in the bisected brain. *J. Exp. Psychol. Hum. Percept. Perform.* 21:211–230.

RUBICHI, S., C. IANI, R. NICOLETTI, and C. UMILTÀ, 1997. The Simon effect occurs relative to the direction of an attention shift. *J. Exp. Psychol. Hum. Percept. Perform.* 23:1353–1364.

SCHILLER, P. H., and F. KOERNER, 1971. Discharge characteristics of single units in superior colliculus of the alert rhesus monkey. *J. Neurophysiol.* 5:920–936.

SERGENT, J., 1987. A new look at the human split brain. *Brain* 110:1375–1392.

SERGENT, J., and J. J. MYERS, 1985. Manual, blowing, and verbal simple reactions to lateralized flashes of light in commissurotomized patients. *Percept. Psychophys.* 37:571–578.

SPERRY, R. W., M. S. GAZZANIGA, and J. E. BOGEN, 1969. Interhemispheric relationships: The neocortical commissures; syndromes of hemisphere disconnection. *Handbook Clin. Neurol.* 4:273–290.

SPRAGUE, J. M., G. BERLUCCHI, and G. RIZZOLATTI, 1973. The role of the superior colliculus and pretectum in vision and visually guided behavior. In *Handbook of Sensory Physiology.* Berlin: Springer-Verlag, pp. 7:27–101.

TENG, E. L., and R. W. SPERRY, 1973. Interhemispheric interaction during simultaneous bilateral presentation of letters or digits in commissurotomized patients. *Neuropsychologia* 11:131–140.

TREVARTHEN, C., and R. W. SPERRY, 1973. Perceptual unity of the ambient visual field in human commissurotomy patients. *Brain* 96:547–570.

UPDYKE, B. V., 1977. Topographic organization of the projections from cortical areas 17, 18 and 19 onto the thalamus, pretectum and superior colliculus in the cat. *J. Comp. Neurol.* 173:81–122.

VALLAR, G., R. STERZI, and A. BASSO, 1988. Left hemisphere contribution to motor programming of aphasic speech: A reaction time experiment in aphasic patients. *Neuropsychologia* 26:511–519.

WEISKRANTZ, L., 1986. *Blindsight.* Oxford: Clarendon Press.

ZAIDEL, D., and R. W. SPERRY, 1977. Some long-term motor effects of cerebral commissurotomy in man. *Neuropsychologia* 15:193–204.

ZAIDEL, E., 1994. Interhemispheric transfer in the split brain: Long-term status following complete cerebral commissurotomy. In *Brain Asymmetry*, R. H. Davidson and K. Hugdahl, eds., Cambridge: MIT Press, pp. 491–532.

ZAIDEL, E., 1998. Stereognosis in the chronic split brain: Hemispheric differences, ipsilateral control, and sensory integration across the midline. *Neuropsychologia* 36:1033–1047.

ZAIDEL, E., J. M. CLARKE, and B. SUYENOBU, 1990a. Hemispheric independence: A paradigm case for cognitive neuroscience. In *Neurobiology of Higher Cognitive Function*, A. B. Scheibel and A. F. Wechsler, eds. New York: Guilford Press, pp. 297–355.

ZAIDEL, E., and L. SEIBERT, 1997a. Speech in the disconnected right hemisphere? JINS 3:45.

ZAIDEL E., and L. K. SEIBERT, 1997b. Speech in the disconnected right hemisphere. *Brain Lang.* 60:188–192.

ZAIDEL, E., D. W. ZAIDEL, and J. E. BOGEN, 1990b. Testing the commissurotomy patient. In *Neuromethods*, Vol. 17: *Neuropsychology*, A. A. Boulton, G. B. Baker and M. Hiscock, eds. Clifton, N.J.: Humana Press.

ZAIDEL, E., D. W. ZAIDEL, and J. E. BOGEN, 1999. The split brain. In *Encyclopedia of Neuroscience*, 2nd ed., G. Adelman and B. Smith, eds. Amsterdam: Elsevier, pp. 1930–1936. (Also on CD-ROM.)

ZAIDEL, E., N. Y. WEEKES, M. IACOBONI, I. FRIED, and J. E. BOGEN, 1996. Two modes of functional reorganization following partial callosotomy in humans. *Soc. Neurosci. Abst.* 22:434.

Commentary 13.1

Water Under the Bridge: Interhemispheric Visuomotor Integration in a Split-Brain Man

MICHAEL C. CORBALLIS AND BETTINA FORSTER

ABSTRACT Interhemispheric transfer time was measured in a split-brain man (L.B.) using reaction time to crossed and uncrossed hand-field combinations. The crossed-uncrossed difference in reaction time did not depend systematically on variations in luminance of the signals but was increased slightly when the response was contingent on color. There was also evidence that L.B. was unable to transfer color interhemispherically. These results confirm previous evidence that it is response information, not stimulus information, that is transferred in tasks requiring interhemispheric visuomotor integration.

Introduction

Zaidel and Iacoboni argue that visuomotor integration in the split-brain subject L.B., like that in normal subjects, does not depend on a sensory channel connecting the hemispheres, on the grounds that the difference in his reaction time (RT) between crossed and uncrossed hand-field combinations (the crossed-uncrossed difference, or CUD) does not depend on either the luminance or the eccentricity of the visual stimuli. In this respect, L.B. differs from the three other split-brain subjects Zaidel and Iacoboni discuss. Since variations in the motor component of the task also fails to influence the CUD in L.B. (as in the other split-brain subjects), Zaidel and Iacoboni suggest that L.B. may have been responding in the crossed condition by means of ipsilateral corticospinal pathways, while the other three subjects relied on a subcortical visual route, presumably via the superior colliculus.

In our own studies with L.B., we have also varied luminance and eccentricity but have further tested the role of stimulus variables by using stimuli that are equilu-

minant with the background. We have also examined L.B.'s ability to make unimanual responses to contralateral stimuli on the basis of color or shape, attributes that are thought not to transfer subcortically between hemispheres. In all experiments, the stimuli were presented in one or other visual field, at an eccentricity of 2.5°, while the subject, L.B., maintained fixation on a central cross.

Simple reaction time

EFFECTS OF ECCENTRICITY AND LUMINANCE   In the first part of this study (Forster and Corballis, 1998), we varied the luminance of the stimuli, presented against a dark background, from 3.1 to 64.9 cd/m^2. As in previous studies, the RTs were longer to crossed than to uncrossed hand-field combinations, and the resulting CUDs were considerably longer than those obtained from neurologically intact individuals. The CUD was independent of luminance but jumped from an average of 35 ms at a 2.5° eccentricity to an average of 79 ms at a 5.0° eccentricity. This suggests that the CUD may in fact be sensitive to eccentricity. However, the picture is complicated by a reverse trend when the stimuli were equiluminant against the background.

EFFECT OF EQUILUMINANCE   To achieve equiluminant displays, we presented the stimuli in low-level blue light against a bright yellow background so that they actually appeared light gray against the yellow. This method of achieving equiluminance was proposed and verified by Cavanagh, Adelson, and Heard (1992). Equiluminant displays are thought to register only in the parvocellular division of the geniculocortical visual system and not in the evolutionarily more primitive magnocellular system (Livingstone and Hubel, 1987). It is also reasonable to suppose that the relatively primitive subcortical visual system, involving the superior colliculus, would be largely

MICHAEL C. CORBALLIS   Department of Psychology, University of Auckland, Auckland, New Zealand.

BETTINA FORSTER   School of Psychology, Birkbeck College, London, United Kingdom.

if not completely impervious to equiluminant displays. The technique of presenting gray stimuli against a yellow background also minimizes edge artifacts that might otherwise be transmitted by an achromatic system (Cavanagh et al., 1992).

Although L.B.'s overall RT was substantially increased with equiluminant stimuli, his CUD was unaffected overall. However, it was 78 ms for the 2.5° eccentricity and only 32 ms for the 5.0° eccentricity, reversing the trend for displays involving luminance contrast. We suspect that these variations in the CUD do not reflect the systematic effects of stimulus parameters so much as a seemingly random variation between blocks of trials. In any event, the fact that L.B. could even respond to contralateral equiluminant stimuli, and with no overall increase in CUD, suggests that the information transfer was nonsensory.

Color- and shape-contingent response

In a further series of studies, we presented stimuli to one or the other visual field and made responses contingent on the color or shape of the stimuli (Forster and Corballis, 2000). Previous research has shown that split-brain people, and L.B. in particular (Corballis, 1996; Johnson, 1984), are virtually at chance in judging the sameness or difference of shapes or colors flashed in opposite visual fields, suggesting that information about shape or color cannot be transferred subcortically. If L.B. is able to respond unimanually to contralateral stimuli on the basis of these attributes, it should therefore follow that the information transferred is not sensory information but rather represents the decision or the response to be made.

GO/NO-GO CONDITION In the color version of this task, the disks were either red or green, and L.B. was told to press a key only when the disk was red. He was 100% accurate to stimuli in either visual field, regardless of hand, indicating perfect transmission of information. Since other evidence suggests that color information is not transmitted interhemispherically in this subject, it follows again that the information transmitted was decisional or response information, rather than color information. On the same task, normal subjects produced CUDs that were not significantly different from those in simple RT. L.B.'s CUD was 73 ms, within the bounds of his CUD for simple RT.

In the shape version of the task, the stimuli were either circles or squares, and the task was to press a key only when the stimulus was a circle. L.B. missed 8% of targets when responding with his left hand to stimuli in

the right visual field (RVF) but was otherwise perfectly accurate. His CUD was 45 ms, again within the bounds of his values for simple RT.

These results provide additional evidence that the information transmitted is not stimulus information.

TWO-CHOICE REACTION TIME Here, the stimuli were the same as in the previous conditions, but this time L.B. was required to make binary choices. In the color version he was to press one key if the stimulus was red and the other if it was green; in the shape version he was to press one key if the stimulus was a circle and the other if it was a square. In both cases he used the forefinger and middle finger of the same hand. In the case of the color discrimination, L.B.'s accuracy dropped, especially under the crossed condition, in which the mean percentage of correct responses was 78.5%, which may raise doubts about whether the CUD, which was 132 ms, is a valid measure of transfer time. Under the shape condition, the corresponding values were 78% and 168 ms.

Again we see that L.B. was able to perform the task reasonably well, but the added information load caused some deterioration in interhemispheric transfer.

THREE-CHOICE REACTION TIME Here, there were three different stimuli, and L.B. was asked to discriminate among them by pressing one of three keys, using the forefinger, middle finger, and ring finger of the same hand. In the color condition, the stimuli were red, green, or blue disks; in the shape condition, they were circles, squares, or triangles. In this case response accuracies under the crossed conditions, especially for left-hand responses to RVF stimuli, were too low for RTs to be meaningful.

For both tasks, L.B. was more accurate in responding with his right hand to left visual field (LVF) stimuli (for colors, 84% correct; for shapes, 83% correct) than with his left hand to RVF (73% and 75%, respectively), indicating more accurate transfer from the right to the left hemisphere than vice versa. He was nevertheless significantly above chance in all conditions. We also assessed performance in terms of the amount of information transmitted between stimulus and response. This is measured in binary digits (bits), such that the choice of one stimulus from two equiprobable stimuli represents 1 bit (Garner and Hake, 1951). Perfect performance in the case of the three-choice tasks would represent the transfer of 1.58 bits.

Table 13.5 shows the information transmitted in the three-choice task. L.B. always transmitted more than 1 bit of information under the uncrossed conditions but less than 1 bit under the crossed conditions. This

TABLE 13.5
*Amount of information transferred, in bits, in the three-choice
discrimination tasks*

Task	Left Hand		Right Hand	
	LVF	RVF	LVF	RVF
Color	1.33	0.27	0.95	1.33
Shape	1.58	0.24	0.69	1.06

is consistent with previous suggestions that interhemispheric transfer may be limited to no more than binary information.

Conclusions

These studies reinforce the conclusion that in the split-brain subject L.B., sensorimotor integration in simple reaction time tasks is not achieved by means of a sensory interhemispheric channel. Interhemispheric transfer time, as estimated by the CUD, was largely unaffected by luminance. Although there may have been some effect of eccentricity, this did not appear to be systematic: The CUD was longer for the greater eccentricity for nonequiluminant displays but longer for the smaller eccentricity for equiluminant ones. The more compelling evidence that transfer was nonsensory came from the equiluminant displays themselves. Although equiluminance should in principle restrict, if not eliminate, subcortical visual transfer, the CUD was within the range of that for nonequiluminant stimuli, even though RT itself was significantly increased.

However, when the task itself was complicated by requiring the discrimination of color, the CUD was clearly longer. Given that L.B. appears unable to transfer information about color itself (Corballis, 1996), it is likely that the transferred signal concerned the response to be made, not the stimulus. Indeed, when the number of colors to be discriminated was increased to three, performance in the crossed conditions fell away. Zaidel and Iacoboni suggest that L.B. responds in the crossed conditions by means of ipsilateral corticospinal pathways

and that he is unusual among split-brain subjects in this respect. If this is so, the ability of each hemisphere to select among different responses of the ipsilateral fingers is nevertheless clearly limited. The alternative interpretation is that L.B.'s responses in the crossed conditions do depend on interhemispheric transfer but that the information transferred is based on decisional or response information. Again, this transfer appears to be informationally limited.

A final point is that the three-choice RT study, in particular, suggests that L.B. is better able to respond with the right hand to LVF information than with the left hand to RVF information. This may reflect a more general asymmetry of interhemispheric transfer, for which there is evidence also in normals (Marzi, Bisiacchi, and Nicoletti, 1991). Or it could mean that L.B.'s left hemisphere is more adept at interpreting diffuse signals from the right than the right hemisphere is at interpreting signals from the left.

REFERENCES

CAVANAGH, P., E. H. ADELSON, and P. HEARD, 1992. Vision with equiluminant color contrast. 2: A large-scale technique and observations. *Perception* 21:219–226.

CORBALLIS, M. C., 1996. A dissociation in naming digits and colors following commissurotomy. *Cortex* 32:515–525.

FORSTER, B. A., and M. C. CORBALLIS, 1998. Interhemispheric transmission times in the presence and absence of the forebrain commissures: Effects of luminance and equiluminance. *Neuropsychologia* 36:925–934.

FORSTER, B. A., and M. C. CORBALLIS, 2000. Interhemispheric transfer of colour and shape information in the presence and absence of the corpus callosum. *Neuropsychologia* 37:32–45.

GARNER, W. R., and H. W. HAKE, 1951. The amount of information in absolute judgments. *Psychol. Rev.* 58:446–459.

JOHNSON, L. E., 1984. Bilateral visual cross integration by human forebrain commissurotomy subjects. *Neuropsychologia* 22:167–175.

LIVINGSTONE, M. S., and D. H. HUBEL, 1987. Psychophysical evidence for separate channels for perception of form, color, movement and depth. *J. Neurosci.* 7:3416–3468.

MARZI, C., P. BISIACCHI, and R. NICOLETTI, 1991. Is interhemispheric transfer of visuomotor information asymmetric? Evidence from a meta-analysis. *Neuropsychologia* 29:1163–1177.

14 Parallel Processing in the Bisected Brain: Implications for Callosal Function

PATRICIA A. REUTER-LORENZ

ABSTRACT   Can the separated hemispheres function as independent parallel cognitive processors? To answer this question, I review split-brain evidence from the redundant signal paradigm, studies of dual-task performance, and studies of visual attention. The evidence from a variety of basic sensorimotor tasks indicates that the separated hemispheres can perform concurrent stimulus selection, encoding, decision making, and response selection. I propose that apparent limitations in the parallel processing abilities in the bisected brain result from a subcortical gating mechanism that enables one hemisphere to strategically inhibit the response output of the other. Transection of the corpus callosum does indeed produce two separate minds within the same cranium.

Introduction and overview

The right hemisphere of a typical split-brain patient cannot verbally describe a picture that is flashed to the left visual field. Nevertheless, the left hand, which is controlled by the right hemisphere, can accurately select the depicted item from a set of palpable options (Gazzaniga, Bogen, and Sperry, 1962). This simple demonstration raises one of the most intriguing questions in neuropsychology (Sperry, 1968): Does severing the corpus callosum produce two independent spheres of cognition?

Over the past four decades, this question has been pondered in the scientific, philosophical, and public arenas. Yet the answer remains uncertain. This uncertainty stems largely from the fact that, rather than exhibiting highly disassociated and disconnected behaviors in their day-to-day lives, many split-brain patients function quite effectively and in a seemingly unified manner. In the early stages of recovery, some patients show

PATRICIA A. REUTER-LORENZ   Department of Psychology, University of Michigan, Ann Arbor, Michigan.

intermanual conflict. For example, there are reports of one patient who, while shopping in the supermarket, would place an item in a cart with one hand but then return the item to the shelf with the other hand. Nevertheless, in most cases these conflicting behaviors resolve to the point at which split-brain patients can hold steady jobs, drive cars, and successfully perform the routine behaviors of daily living. There must, then, be limits on the extent to which the separated hemispheres operate independently. The primary objective of this chapter is to sketch where these limits might be and, by so doing, to define a domain of interhemispheric operations for which the corpus callosum is *not* responsible.

Toward this objective, I examine evidence concerning the ability of the separated hemispheres to process information in parallel. By definition, parallel processing involves the execution of multiple mental operations simultaneously. For the present purposes we want to understand the extent to which each separated hemisphere can execute an entire sequence of processing operations, including stimulus selection and encoding, decision making, response selection, response initiation, and movement execution, at the same time as the other hemisphere does too.

This chapter is organized as follows. I begin by reviewing results from my investigation of parallel processing in the bisected brain conducted with colleagues while I was at Dartmouth College (Reuter-Lorenz et al., 1995). Our results are strikingly counterintuitive and suggest that a response-gating mechanism mediates independent decisions generated by the separated hemispheres. Next I consider dual-task studies conducted with split-brain patients, including some that show parallel processing and others that show a cost associated with concurrent processing by the separated hemispheres. I propose that strategic response gating tailored to satisfy prevailing task requirements may help to explain the differences between results from these studies. With this idea in mind, I then review studies of visual attention in split-brain patients, including some that likewise support the hypothesis of independent, parallel processors and others that do not. Once again, by considering the strategic and response requirements of these different tasks, some sense can be made of such divergent outcomes. My conclusion is that the separated hemispheres can, by and large, execute perceptual, decision-making, and response-selection operations in parallel. When apparent limitations in parallel processing arise, they can be attributed to a response-gating mechanism that functions at a relatively late point in the information-processing stream and modulates response initiation for strategic purposes.

Parallel processing of redundant signals after callosotomy

THE REDUNDANT-SIGNALS PARADIGM Researchers have used the redundant-signal paradigm extensively (e.g., Miller, 1982, 1986; Marzi et al., 1986; Hughes, Reuter-Lorenz, Nozawa, and Fendrich, 1994; Tomaiuolo et al., 1997) in the study of human perception and cognition to examine parallel-processing capabilities and to clarify how information is combined from separate sensory channels (e.g., left and right eyes, left and right visual fields, eyes and ears). In this paradigm there is a detection task that requires an observer to respond as quickly as possible when he or she detects a target signal. The detection task involves two trial types. On single-signal trials the signal is presented individually to either of two channels. On redundant-signal trials both channels receive a signal. For both trial types, the observer simply presses a single response key when a target signal is detected. Not surprisingly, observers are typically faster on redundant-signal trials than on single-signal trials. This facilitation is called the "redundancy gain" or the "redundant-signal effect."

At least two mechanisms could mediate the redundant-signal effect (see also Chapters 11 and 12 in this volume). First, if the processing time associated with detection on each individual channel is independent of processing time on the other channel, and if these processing times are random variables, then the redundancy gain can be explained probabilistically (e.g., Raab, 1962). At any given moment, the likelihood of detecting a signal on redundant-signal trials is greater than the likelihood on single-target trials because there are two distinct opportunities for detection. Indeed, for a given observer, if we know the distribution of detection latencies associated with each channel on the single-target trials, then we can

predict the probability that a signal would be detected at each moment in time following the start of a redundant-target trial. This prediction is based on a model of probability summation, also known as the horse race model. The term "horse race" derives from the idea that the signals are being transmitted along separate, parallel, and independent channels or tracks and whichever signal crosses the finish line first wins the race and triggers a response (Miller, 1982, 1986; Townsend and Ashby, 1983; Meyer et al., 1988).

An alternative explanation for the redundant-signal effect is that simultaneous signals on two channels are combined (e.g., additively or multiplicatively) at some stage of processing, increasing the effective overall signal strength. This is the idea of neural summation (e.g., Miller, 1982, 1986; Hughes et al., 1994). It can be shown mathematically that with plausible ancillary assumptions, neural summation produces greater redundancy gain than probability summation does (Nozawa, 1993). On redundant-signal trials, performance that is faster than the prediction derived from probability summation may therefore suggest neural summation instead. Once indicated, additional analyses are required to identify the locus where signals are combined, and this locus could indeed vary depending on the task demands or the altered neural architecture of the patient (Marzi et al., 1996; Miniussi, Girelli, and Marzi, 1998; Cavina-Pratesi et al., 2001). This framework provides a basis to test for the presence or absence of parallel processing by the two hemispheres.

RESULTS FROM PATIENT J.W. Within this framework we have studied the effects of redundant signals presented to the separated hemispheres of callosotomy patient J.W. (Reuter-Lorenz et al., 1995). Our studies were designed to answer several related questions: Would a split-brain patient process such signals in parallel? Would there be any redundancy gain? Do the "horses" that run down the tracks of the separated left and right hemispheres compete in the same race and cross the same finish line, yielding probability summation? Or is the neural summation hypothesis somehow correct for split-brain patients?

As a preliminary step toward answering these questions, we determined whether J.W.'s left hemisphere could report verbally when a signal appeared in the left visual field at the same time as a signal also occurred in the right visual field (Reuter-Lorenz et al., 1995, Experiment 1). Our rationale for this step was straightforward. If the speaking left hemisphere can report accurately the occurrence of both signals, then it would not be surprising that J.W. shows a redundant-signal effect as neurologically intact observers do. On the other hand, if the speaking left hemisphere cannot make such reports, then we might expect J.W. to show reduced benefits from redundant signals for simple speeded responses. However, what we actually found was more interesting and unexpected than either of these two plausible possibilities, thereby setting the stage for further instructive studies.

In particular, during our first study (Reuter-Lorenz et al., 1995, Experiment 1), J.W. viewed brief flashes from light-emitting diodes (LEDs) that were positioned 7° to the left and right of a central fixation point. He reported whether he saw the left LED, the right LED, or both of them. We found that his likelihood of reporting the left signal plummeted when the right signal was presented simultaneously (i.e., 79% correct reports of the left signal presented alone versus 49% correct when it was accompanied by a right signal). J.W.'s extinction of the left LED implies that information from the left visual field is less useful or less available to the left hemisphere for at least some types of tasks when the left hemisphere must process other information concurrently. By itself, this result might suggest that the effects of redundant signals would be minimized in the bisected brain.

However, the effects of redundant signals on J.W.'s reaction times were surprising and paradoxical. In absolute terms, J.W. was always slower than normal controls (Figure 14.1). Still, despite his neglectful verbal reports, he had more redundancy gain than the control observers did! (Recall that the measure of redundancy gain is obtained by comparing an observer's reaction times for single signals with those for redundant signals.)

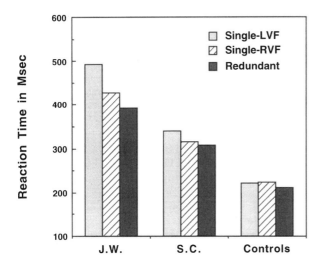

FIGURE 14.1. Average reaction times in each of three signal conditions for complete callosotomy patient J.W., partial callosotomy patient S.C., and two neurologically intact control observers. S.C. and controls show a small reduction in reaction time for the redundant signal condition. For J.W. this redundancy gain is greatly enhanced, and, unlike those of the other observers, its magnitude exceeds the prediction of probability summation (see also Reuter-Lorenz et al., 1995).

This is evident from the bar graph depicting the mean reaction times for J.W. and two control observers. (Although a comparison of the mean reaction times is really inadequate to evaluate redundant target effects, the basic pattern of results is evident in Figure 14.1; see Reuter-Lorenz et al. (1995) for more extensive and detailed analyses of these data.) The graph also presents the mean reaction times for patient S.C., who had only the anterior two-thirds of his callosum sectioned, thereby sparing the splenium and the interhemispheric transmission of visual information. By comparing the reaction times for the redundant-signal trials to those for the two single-target trial types, we see that J.W.'s redundancy gain is more than eight times greater than those of patient S.C. and the controls.

In a follow-up experiment, we showed that with brighter signals, the magnitude of redundancy gain increased for J.W. but not for the control observers. This result indicates that J.W.'s enhanced redundancy gain is not caused simply by his general tendency to respond more slowly than controls; otherwise, the redundancy gain should have decreased with J.W.'s faster responses to brighter signals. In a further experiment that displayed redundant signals within the same visual field, J.W.'s performance pattern was essentially the same as that of the control observers (Reuter-Lorenz et al., 1995, Experiment 3). Thus, J.W.'s enhanced redundancy gain depended specifically on the presentation of redundant signals to the left and right hemispheres, respectively. This result implies that J.W.'s redundancy gain enhancement is mediated by interhemispheric interactions that do not require the corpus callosum.

DISINHIBITION AND ENHANCED REDUNDANCY GAIN   The enhanced redundancy gain of J.W. greatly exceeds what probability summation predicts and is far greater than that observed for neurologically intact control subjects. Iacoboni and Zaidel (Chapter 12 in this volume) report similar results for other split-brain patients (see also Corballis, 1998; Iacoboni et al., 2000), and Pollman and Zaidel (1999) have replicated these basic effects in patient L.B. using a visual search procedure. In the normal brain, such facilitation would be clearly consistent with neural summation. However, this interpretation seems less plausible in the bisected brain because there are far fewer interhemispheric connections whereby information from the left and right hemispheres could be combined.

Thus, as an alternative, we hypothesized instead that a disproportionate slowing or inhibition of J.W.'s responses may occur on the single-target trials but not on redundant-target trials. According to our hypothesis, on single-target trials, one hemisphere perceives a signal

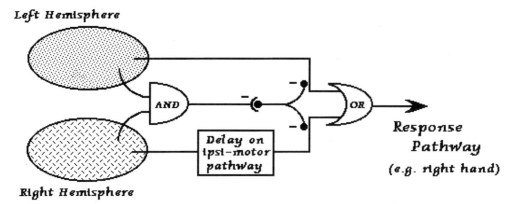

Left Hemisphere

AND

Delay on
ipsi-motor
pathway

OR

Response
Pathway

(e.g. right hand)

Right Hemisphere

FIGURE 14.2. An illustration of the And-Or model proposed to account for the enhanced redundant targets effect in J.W. The model depicts two parallel output pathways from each of the separated hemispheres. Each hemisphere has one input to an And-Gate. These inputs can be thought of as readiness signals indicating that the hemisphere is preparing a response. Thus, the And-Gate is true only when both hemispheres generate a response. The other pathways carry a motor command that serves as input to an Or-Gate. The Or-Gate is true when either hemisphere generates a motor command. However, the output of the And-Gate modulates the efficiency of the inputs to the Or-Gate. This modulation is achieved by disinhibition. The output of the And-Gate inhibits a node whose output chronically inhibits the motor command pathways. When this node is inhibited, the inhibitory influences on these pathways are attenuated. The disinhibition occurs when the And-Gate is true, a condition that arises on redundant signal trials. On single-signal trials the conditions of the And-Gate are not met, and as a result the inputs to the Or-Gate are inhibited. Because this illustration depicts the circuitry proposed for right-hand responses, the pathway originating in the right hemisphere (i.e., the ipsilateral pathway) is associated with a motor delay. Similar circuits may exist to modulate left-hand and verbal responses.

and the other does not, so they reach different decisions. The hemisphere that does not receive a signal maintains a tonic inhibitory influence on response generation mechanisms, while the hemisphere that detects the signal attempts to initiate a response. As a result, the commands that are sent to the effector then conflict. However, on redundant-signal trials, both hemispheres may reach the same decision within a critical window of time, so there is no response conflict and no inhibition. The details of this process are described more fully in our And-Or model of split brain performance for the redundant-signals paradigm (Figure 14.2; see also Reuter-Lorenz et al., 1995).

A further critical test of the And-Or model involves showing that one hemisphere can indeed slow the other's responses. We therefore next designed an explicit-stop task, in which either unilateral or bilateral flashes of red, green, or yellow LEDs were presented. The task required saying the word "go" as rapidly as possible in response to the onset of the green light under some but not other conditions. On unilateral trials J.W. was instructed to say "go" only when the LED was green and not when it was red or yellow. On the bilateral-flash trials, the colors of the LEDs could be different (i.e., a red on the left and a green on the right). If a red or yellow LED appeared, go responses had to be inhibited even when a green LED appeared simultaneously in the opposite visual field.

The data from this experiment are summarized in Figure 14.3 for split-brain patient J.W. Whenever a no-go signal appeared in either visual field, his responses were withheld. Because this occurred even when his right hemisphere viewed a no-go signal and his left hemisphere viewed a go signal, we have evidence that even J.W.'s right hemisphere can stop the left hemisphere from generating a verbal response, supporting our And-Or model and its account of J.W.'s enhanced redundancy gain in the redundant-signal paradigm (cf. Figure 14.1).

Evidence from several of our other studies indicates that color information does not transfer subcortically (Hughes et al., 1992; Seymour et al., 1994; Reuter-Lorenz et al., 1995). So J.W.'s success at withholding responses when the hemispheres received conflicting signals suggests that each hemisphere interprets the meaning of its respective stimuli and appropriately prevents response generation. Perhaps such inhibition is mediated by a response "gating mechanism" that both hemispheres can access and that is the locus of strategic response competition between them.

What implications does the study of redundant-signal effects in the separated hemispheres have for understanding parallel processing and its limits after brain bisection? At least two conclusions now seem warranted. First, the separated hemispheres can simultaneously interpret the significance of simple visual events and reach

Explicit-Stop Experiment

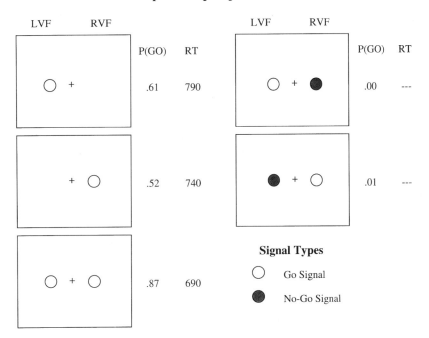

FIGURE 14.3. Sample stimulus displays along with the accuracy and reaction time data for J.W. in the explicit-stop experiment. This experiment required J.W. to say the word "go" when a go signal (i.e., a green LED) appeared alone or with another go signal. If a no-go signal (i.e., a red or yellow LED) appeared simultaneously with a go-signal, J.W. was to withhold his response. The P(GO) indicates the probability that J.W. responded in each condition. When a go signal went to one hemisphere and a no-go signal went to the other, J.W. successfully refrained from responding, regardless of which hemisphere received the no-go signal. This result is consistent with a subcortical response-gating mechanism by which one hemisphere can inhibit the output of the other.

independent decisions about appropriate responses. Second, one limit on parallel independent processing may arise through a gating mechanism that modulates response initiation and has subcortical components. Strategic control of it by one hemisphere (as in the explicit-stop experiment) and the channeling of conflicting response tendencies through it modulates the hemispheres' ability to respond independently and in parallel, particularly when they both must respond via the same effector (e.g., the right hand or vocal tract).

Dual-task studies in the split-brain patient

The studies reviewed in this section investigate the extent to which the separated hemispheres can perform two relatively distinct tasks simultaneously. From our previous results with the redundant-signals paradigm, it might be expected that as independent cognitive processors, the separated hemispheres would do better at dual-task performance than do the connected left and right hemispheres in normal individuals. However, as we shall see, this expectation is not always confirmed.

THE PSYCHOLOGICAL REFRACTORY PERIOD AND RESPONSE GATING   Further evidence for a response-gating mechanism comes from two recent studies of the psychological refractory period (PRP) effect in split-brain patients. In the typical PRP paradigm, the participant is instructed to perform two different tasks in a fixed sequence. For example, Task 1 might require a discrimination judgment about a visual stimulus together with a manual response by the left hand. The stimulus for Task 2 would be presented at some moment after the onset of the Task 1 stimulus, and a second response, made with the right hand or vocally, would be required for Task 2. Typically, the reaction time for Task 2 increases as the interval (i.e., the SOA) between the onsets of the Task 1 and Task 2 stimuli decreases. This is the PRP effect. Various results suggest that the PRP effect stems from postponement of either response selection or movement production stages for Task 2 (Pashler and Johnston, 1989; Schumacher et al., 2001). Practice and individual differences in participants' strategies can change the PRP effect (Meyer et al., 1995). In particular, strict or lax adherence to task priorities imposed by the instructions for the PRP procedure may affect the extent to which Tasks 1 and 2 are performed sequentially or in parallel (Meyer and Kieras, 1997a).

To the extent that the separated hemispheres are independent parallel processors, we might expect at first blush that the PRP effect would be greatly attenuated in split-brain patients. Specifically, this might be expected when the Task 1 and Task 2 stimuli go to the left and right hemispheres, respectively, and each hemisphere responds via its preferred, contralateral hand. However, two studies have yielded a markedly different result. Pashler and colleagues (1994) found a very large PRP effect (as measured by the difference between Task 2 reaction time at SOA 50 and SOA 1000) in patient J.W. when each hemisphere performed consecutive spatial discrimination tasks and responded using the contralateral hand. Ivry, Franz, Kingstone, and Johnston (1998) confirmed the PRP effect in patient J.W. using two tasks that were more distinct in their processing demands. Their Task 1 involved the presentation of a spatial configuration that required a discrimination response by the right hemisphere with the left hand, whereas Task 2 involved a lexical (word-nonword) decision by the left hemisphere with a right-hand response in one condition and a vocal response in another. In each case, J.W.'s PRP effect was robust and approximated the PRP effect observed for age-matched controls.

In a second experiment, both tasks required a spatial discrimination, and Ivry and colleagues (1998) varied the compatibility of the response mappings for Tasks 1 and 2. The left hand always used a spatially compatible stimulus-response mapping, such that pressing an upper button indicated that a target stimulus was above a reference figure and pressing a lower button indicated that the target stimulus was below the reference figure. In separate blocks, the stimulus-response mapping for the right hand was likewise compatible, or it was incompatible (upper button presses indicated an inferior target location; lower button presses indicated a superior location). Age-matched control subjects showed a marked effect of consistency between the S-R mapping for the two hands: The PRP effect was greater when the right-hand mapping differed from the left-hand mapping. This did not occur for J.W., who tended to show the opposite pattern.

As Ivry and colleagues point out, the absence of a consistency effect in the split-brain patient has two implications: (1) The separated hemispheres can maintain distinct rules for mapping stimuli onto responses, and (2) each hemisphere can select the appropriate response without interference from the other hemisphere (see also Franz et al., 1996; Kennerly et al., 2002). However, J.W.'s PRP effect implies a form of response gating that

seems specifically to influence when the hemispheres initiate responses. We may understand the nature of this gating by recalling that the PRP paradigm explicitly requires participants to perform Tasks 1 and 2 in a fixed order. Given this requirement, perhaps the gating mechanism is used strategically for making the outputs of the two hemispheres have the proper serial order. It is possible, therefore, that if the separated hemispheres are instructed to perform both tasks simultaneously, the PRP effect and the contribution of this response-gating mechanism would be reduced (Meyer and Kieras, 1997b).

CONCURRENT DUAL-TASK PERFORMANCE AFTER BRAIN BISECTION Two earlier experiments did indeed find evidence that hemispheric disconnection can produce superior performance of two concurrent tasks. In one experiment by Gazzaniga and Sperry (1966), subjects performed two different visual discrimination tasks simultaneously. The RVF task required a red-green discrimination and a right-hand response, while the LVF task required a bright-dark discrimination and a left-hand response. Normal subjects and callosotomy patients tested preoperatively were slower and less accurate on each of the tasks when they performed them concurrently than when the tasks were performed alone. This was not the case when the patients were tested postoperatively. Patients who had a complete callosal section and section of the anterior commissure performed the dual tasks as efficiently as they performed each of the tasks alone. Ellenberg and Sperry (1980) report similar results from a tactile sorting task performed either unimanually or bimanually without visual guidance. The performance of commissurotomized subjects was equivalent in the unimanual and bimanual conditions even when opposite sorting rules applied for the two hands. Normal control subjects performed much worse in the bimanual conditions, particularly when the sorting rules conflicted. These studies reveal that each of the separated hemispheres can process perceptual information, make decisions, and execute appropriate motor commands simultaneously without any detrimental effects on processing in the other hemisphere. Furthermore, two of the studies discussed (Ellenberg and Sperry, 1980; Ivry et al., 1998) indicate that the separated hemispheres can select responses using opposite decision rules without any performance decrement (see Franz et al., 1996, for an analogous effect in a drawing task).

How can we reconcile these results with the PRP effects reviewed above in which the split-brain patient J.W. did suffer dual-task decrements when each of his hemispheres performed different tasks? Perhaps the answer may be found in the instructions given to the participants. The procedures that yielded PRP effects required the participants to perform the tasks sequentially, and to abide by this instruction, responses may have been gated. That split-brain patients can follow these instructions on the one hand and still show the PRP effect on the other is consistent with a strategic subcortical response-gating mechanism whose operations do not depend on the corpus callosum (see Ivry et al., 1998, for a similar suggestion).

These considerations may even account for seemingly contrary results from two other studies that have reported impaired performance by commissurotomized patients in dual tasks. For example, Teng and Sperry (1973, 1974) required patients to identify a single alphanumeric character presented unilaterally or a pair of alphanumeric characters presented bilaterally, one in each visual field. Performance on unilateral trials was more accurate than that on bilateral trials. However, omissions were the predominant errors on bilateral trials. Most patients simply did not respond to one of the two stimuli on a large percentage of trials (e.g., 79% LVF omissions on bilateral trials versus 2% omissions on unilateral trials). Typically, the response to the left item was omitted. Perhaps the complexity of the response requirements played an important role here. To make their responses, patients had to search an array of various alphanumeric characters and locate and point to an item there that matched the stimulus. On bilateral trials they had to do this twice. During the time required to generate the first response, the other stimulus may have been forgotten. Also, even on unilateral trials, some patients were confused about which hand to use, manifesting some degree of response rivalry. Apparently, on bilateral trials, the left hemisphere often may have assumed control of performance, thereby gating the output of the right hemisphere.

Indeed, in a follow-up study, Teng and Sperry (1974) suggest that an all-or-none gating mechanism appeared to be operating and that the hemisphere with the processing advantage dominated (as also suggested by Levy, Trevarthen, and Sperry, 1972). Here again we see that limitations in parallel processing may arise from the strategic engagement of a response-gating mechanism. Consistent with this view, the following section examines studies of visual selective attention that implicate a similar gating mechanism.

Visual attention and limits on parallel processing

Selective visual attention involves preferentially processing a chosen subset of all the information present in the sensory milieu at any given moment. Human observers can selectively attend to a region of space and effectively filter out information from surrounding loca-

tions even while gazing elsewhere. This ability to direct or orient attention covertly has been likened to a movable spotlight that selectively illuminates regions of space. The characteristics of such an attentional spotlight have been the subject of some debate. However, in neurologically intact observers, there is considerable evidence that attention cannot be allocated to two spatially separate, noncontiguous locations (see Van der Heijden, 1992, for a review).

Numerous investigations with a wide range of experimental techniques have studied covert attention in the separated hemispheres of split-brain patients as well (e.g., Corballis, 1995). One goal of the latter studies has been to determine whether, after brain bisection, the separated hemispheres can operate independent attentional "spotlights" or whether they must compete for a unitary attentional focus. At present, there is evidence for each of these possibilities. Do such divergent outcomes arise from variations in patient samples, testing procedures, and experimental noise, or do they reflect important limitations in the degree of independence between the disconnected left and right hemispheres? Careful consideration of the evidence suggests the latter. The next section discusses these varying results with respect to the strategic engagement of a response-gating mechanism in the bisected brain.

INDEPENDENT SPOTLIGHTS? To assess the ability of the separated hemispheres to encode complex visual displays in parallel, Holtzman and Gazzaniga (1985) tested callosotomy patient J.W. and normal control observers in a visual-matching task. Two grids, each containing nine cells in a 3×3 arrangement, were positioned on either side of a visual fixation point (see Figure 14.4). On every trial, a target sequence of four X's appeared in each grid, followed by a probe sequence. The probe sequence occurred randomly in either the right or left visual field. The observer had to indicate with a unilateral manual response whether or not the probe sequence matched either one of the target sequences. There were two conditions: redundant and mixed. For the redundant condition, the same target sequence was presented in both visual fields, whereas for the mixed condition, the two target sequences were different. On positive trials of the mixed condition, the probe sequence could match either the LVF or the RVF target sequence, so the observer had to encode both target sequences as they appeared simultaneously in the two fields. In the redundant condition, control performance was almost 90% correct, whereas J.W. averaged 75% correct. J.W. was also 75% correct in the mixed condition, but controls' performance fell to chance there. This shows that the separated hemispheres of the bisected brain can attend

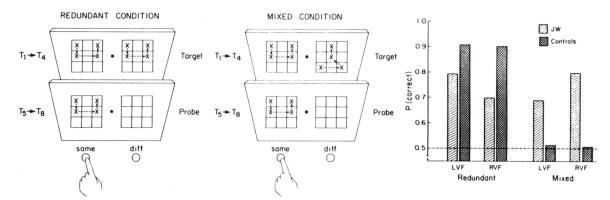

FIGURE 14.4. Example of redundant and mixed conditions from the experiment by Holtzman and Gazzaniga (1985). On redundant trials a bilaterally displayed target X moved among four homologous cells in the two matrices. A tone sounded, and a unilateral probe sequence was presented. The observer indicated whether the probe sequence matched the probed field's target sequence. In this example the bilateral trials sequences began at T1 in the upper left corners of the two matrices and concluded at T4 in the upper right corners, and the unilateral probe sequence was presented from T5 to T8. All X's appeared for 150 ms with a 500-ms interstimulus interval, and the probe and target sequences were separated by 1.5 s. In the mixed condition, illustrated in the middle diagram, different target sequences were presented to the two visual fields. The rightmost diagram displays the proportion correct for the left (LVF) and right (RVF) visual field trials in the redundant and mixed conditions. Data are presented separately for callosotomy patient J.W. and the average performance of the control observers.

to, encode, and retain two spatially disparate stimulus sequences. Holtzman and Gazzaniga (1985) clearly demonstrate parallel visual processing capabilities of the separated hemispheres.

Several more recent investigations echo these same conclusions based on evidence from different attention paradigms. Using a visual search task such as the conjunction-search procedure developed by Treisman and colleagues (e.g., Treisman and Gelade, 1980), Luck and colleagues (1989, 1993) showed that split-brain patients could search a display nearly twice as fast when the items were displayed bilaterally across the two visual fields rather than being displayed within a single hemifield. These results are consistent with the operation of two independent visual spotlights that can be deployed simultaneously by the two hemispheres (see also Kingstone et al., 1995). In contrast, search rates of control observers were essentially the same for unilateral and bilateral displays, suggesting that they used a single attentional spotlight.

DISCREPANT RESULTS FROM PRECUING STUDIES The results from visual search and visual matching tasks reveal a capacity for independent attentional processing in the separated hemispheres. However, studies with a spatial-precuing procedure (e.g., Posner, 1980) paint a more complicated picture. In this procedure a few locations are predesignated as potential target locations. Before the onset of the target, one of the locations is cued. Theoretical conclusions may be drawn from comparing the reaction times to detect or identify the target when it appears in the cued location and when it appears in a noncued location. Responses to cued targets are typically faster and more accurate than responses to noncued targets. The facilitation provided by an accurate or valid cue (relative to a neutral condition) is called "attentional benefit." These benefits are thought to result because attention is aligned with the cued location, facilitating target detection and identification there. The decrement in performance when the target occurs in a noncued location, called "attentional cost," is thought to result because attention must be realigned or shifted to the target location (Posner, 1980).

Although the spatial-precuing paradigm is relatively simple, seemingly minor changes in the visual stimuli, the response requirements, the temporal parameters, and even instructions can invoke different neurocognitive mechanisms (e.g., Rafal and Henik, 1994). It therefore should not be surprising that various investigations of split-brain patients with this general procedure have yielded different results.

In particular, one important characteristic of the spatial-precuing procedure is the type of cue used to direct attention (Jonides, 1981; see Rafal and Henik, 1994, for a review). Attention can be drawn automatically to a peripheral location by a transient change in luminance there. This form of cuing is called "peripheral" or "exogenous" cuing. Exogenous cues can summon attention even when they do not enable the target location to be predicted. Their effects are relatively fast acting and evident within the first 50–200 ms after cue onset. Attention can also be directed to a location voluntarily in response to a symbolic cue, such as an arrow, that points to the probable location of an upcoming target. For this type of central or endogenous cuing to be effective, the cues must provide valid information so that the observer develops an accurate expectancy about the upcoming target location. The effects of endogenous cues take somewhat longer to emerge (i.e., 150-ms SOA) than exogenous cuing effects, and they can be sustained for well over 1000 ms. Some variations of the outcomes from cuing studies in split-brain patients seem to stem from whether endogenous or exogenous cuing was used (Corballis, 1995; Reuter-Lorenz and Fendrich, 1990; Zaidel, 1995). However, as we shall see, response requirements, such as whether responses are made unimanually or bimanually, also influence the extent to which the hemispheres can operate independently and in parallel during attentional cuing studies.

Precuing evidence for unitary attention   In 1990 Robert Fendrich and I reported that split-brain patients are substantially slower than normal control subjects at shifting attention across the vertical meridian. Our results suggest that the separated hemispheres may compete for a single attentional spotlight. The experiment that revealed this was designed to compare costs of within-field and between-field attention shifts. For such purposes, four small boxes were arranged along the horizontal meridian, with two boxes in each visual field. A single location was cued on every trial by brightening one of the boxes, after which a target signal appeared either there or in one of the other boxes (see Figure 14.5). Although the cue was presented peripherally, the long SOAs (700 ms) and highly predictive nature of the cue make it likely that attentional allocation was mediated endogenously. On invalid trials, when the cue and target appeared at different locations in the same hemifield, costs were the same for split-brain patients and the control subjects. However, when the cue appeared in one visual field and the target appeared in the other (between-field invalid trial) patients showed substantially more costs than did control subjects (see Figure 14.6). We also showed that these results were indeed specific to the vertical meridian, because no additional costs occurred for shifting attention across the horizontal meridian. At the very least, these results therefore suggest that the attentional expectancy of one hemisphere affects the performance of the other hemisphere. This conclusion seems inconsistent with evidence that the hemispheres can operate independent attentional spotlights and suggests instead that the hemispheres compete for control of a unitary selective process.

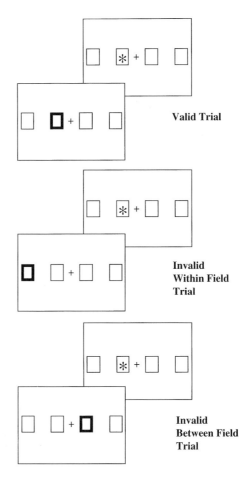

FIGURE 14.5. Sample displays indicating valid, invalid within-field, and invalid between-field trials used by Reuter-Lorenz and Fendrich (1990) to compare the efficiency of allocating attention within and between visual fields in callosotomized patients. The interval between the cue and the target was different in different experiments (see text for details).

However, in our study (Reuter-Lorenz and Fendrich, 1990), the attentional cost for between-field trials depended on the predictive value of the cue. In a further control experiment, we used the same physical cue but shortened the SOAs to 50 and 350 ms while making the cue uninformative about the target location. As a result, the attentional cost for between-field trials relative to within-field trials then dropped substantially, suggesting that intentional or endogenous allocation of attention caused the previous extra costs for between-field trials. More interhemispheric competition occurred when attention was controlled endogenously.

Further evidence against the hypothesis of dual, independent attentional spotlights comes from a study of J.W. by Holtzman, Volpe, and Gazzaniga (1984). They used a spatial-precuing procedure with two boxes, one in each visual field. On each trial an arrow cue appeared

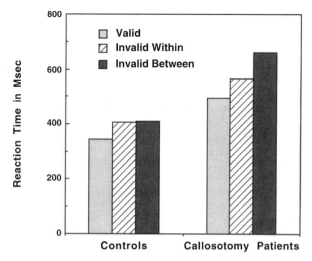

FIGURE 14.6. Average simple response times for callosotomy patients J.W. and V.P., along with neurologically intact control observers in the three spatial cuing conditions used by Reuter-Lorenz and Fendrich (1990). For patients and controls, valid trials are faster than invalid trials. Callosotomy patients show additional costs when the cue appears in one visual field and the target appears in the other. This result suggests that under some conditions the hemispheres compete for control of performance.

in each visual field to indicate the likely location of an upcoming target. The arrows pointed either to the same box (focused attention) or to opposite boxes (divided attention). A neutral condition was also included in which two noninformative X's appeared on either side of the fixation point. Fifteen hundred milliseconds after the cue, a digit appeared in one of the boxes (usually the one that was cued), and the subject indicated whether the digit was odd or even by responding manually.

This experimental design had a simple rationale. It was expected that the focused-attention condition would yield faster performance on trials with valid cuing than on trials with invalid cuing. Thus, if the two hemispheres have independent spotlights, then performance in the divided-attention condition should approximate performance with valid cues under the focused condition. However, if the attentional spotlight is unitary, then performance should be similar in the divided attention and neutral-cue conditions.

Holtzman and his colleagues found results consistent with the latter (unitary spotlight) implication. Responses were appreciably faster in the focused-attention condition than in the divided-attention condition. Performance under the latter condition did not differ from that under the neutral-cue condition. On the basis of these results, it appears that the attentional system remains

unified even in the bisected brain (see also Holtzman et al., 1981; Gazzaniga, 1987).

Precuing evidence for independent spotlights Nevertheless, two more recent precuing studies suggest that attention can be divided in the bisected brain. For example, a study by Mangun and colleagues (1994) provides evidence for independent spotlights. Their visual display had two boxes, one on either side of a central fixation mark. As in the previous study by Holtzman and colleagues (1984), there were three different experimental conditions. First, in a focused-attention condition, one box was cued by a brief brightening of its perimeter, which provided valid information about the location of the upcoming target signal on 80% of the trials. The interval between the cue and target (i.e., the SOA) varied between 150 and 600 ms, so at the shorter SOAs, the cuing effects probably involved an automatic or exogenous component. Second, in a divided-attention condition, both boxes brightened, and the target was equally likely at either location. Third, in a diffuse-cue condition, pixels brightened all over the display screen, so the observer was warned about the upcoming target event but received no specific location information. The observer indicated which of two color combinations made up the target by making a unimanual choice response. For the split-brain patients, the divided-attention condition yielded the same beneficial effect on performance as did the focused-attention condition, suggesting that the two hemispheres can deploy attention separately to different locations simultaneously.

This conclusion has been corroborated for a different group of callosotomy patients in a study by Arguin and colleagues (2000). Their procedure differed from that of Mangun and colleagues (1994) in two notable ways. Arguin and colleagues used symbolic arrow cues and a 500-ms SOA, so their parameters probably evoked endogenous attentional processes. Also, their patients responded bimanually, pulling a lever held with both hands when they detected the onset of the target. Nevertheless, the focused-valid cue condition and the divided-cue condition both yielded significantly faster responses than did the neutral and invalid-cue conditions, again indicating dual attentional mechanisms implemented in the two separate hemispheres.

A reconciliation The results from these different spatial-precuing experiments lead to markedly different conclusions regarding the extent of independent processing in the bisected brain. Is there a way to reconcile them in light of the strategic and response factors that may have come into play? Indeed, there is. When attention is allocated automatically via a peripheral luminance change, the results tend to suggest independent parallel processing (Holtzman and Gazzaniga, 1985; Reuter-Lorenz and Fendrich, 1990, Experiment 4; Mangun et al., 1994). In contrast, when attention is allocated via strategic or endogenous control mechanisms, the results suggest that attention cannot be divided and the separate hemispheres must compete for a unitary focus (Holtzman et al., 1984; Reuter-Lorenz and Fendrich, 1990, Experiment 1; see also Corballis, 1995).

Supplementing these generalizations are the results from the aforementioned study by Arguin and colleagues (2000). There the cues were symbolic and the SOA was sufficiently long for cuing to have been endogenously mediated, but clear evidence of dual attentional foci emerged. Arguin and colleagues' use of a bimanual response may be fundamental to this outcome. Perhaps bimanual responding allowed each hemisphere to assume strategic control over different effectors, thereby minimizing competitive interactions and maximizing the number of processing operations that could proceed in parallel.

The implication here is that the bisected brain may have independent attentional spotlights even when attention is controlled endogenously. Perhaps this capacity is evident only with bimanual responding because unimanual responses evoke strategic response competition. I hypothesize that when a hemisphere is endogenously cued to expect a target, it also takes control of the requisite effector system. If so, then when the noncued hemisphere gets the target signal, it would have to compete for access to this system. So the apparent limitation on parallel attentional selection with endogenous cuing may, in actuality, stem from competition for control of the response pathway.

These conclusions fit nicely with the results on visual search and visual-matching results reviewed in an earlier section of this chapter. During the visual-matching study by Holtzman and Gazzaniga (1985), a probe was equally likely to occur in the left or right visual field. Thus, even though responses were unimanual in their study, there was no reason for one hemisphere to take strategic control over the designated effector. The same is true for the studies by Luck and colleagues (1989, 1993). The target stimuli there were equally likely to occur in the left or right visual field. Moreover, Luck and colleagues used bimanual responses, which may maximize the number of parallel processing operations when attention is controlled strategically (endogenously).

I therefore infer that the limitations in parallel processing associated with attentional precuing tasks are related to the strategic control of response initiation and

that each hemisphere can do separate visual selection and encoding operations without between-hemispheric interference.

EXTINCTION EFFECTS: EVIDENCE FOR LIMITS IN PARALLEL PROCESSING? I have argued that a variety of evidence for limits in parallel processing in split-brain patients can be attributed to strategic response gating. In this section I will briefly review evidence for visual extinction that suggests additional constraints on parallel processing by the separated hemispheres. Again, such evidence is directly relevant to the response gating account developed thus far.

As Joynt (1977) pointed out, genuine extinction and inattention effects are relatively rare in the daily life of split-brain patients. This fact alone reveals the effective parallel-processing abilities of the separated hemispheres. Moreover, when visual extinction does occur under laboratory studies of these patients, it reveals further important clues about the nature of parallel processing in the bisected brain.

For example, consider the extinction effect that my colleagues and I observed with redundant signals and discussed earlier in this chapter (Reuter-Lorenz et al., 1995). This effect involved comparing the ability of J.W.'s left hemisphere to report verbally a left-visual-field signal when it appeared with or without a right-visual-field signal. J.W. showed clear evidence for extinction. Our proposal is that this effect stems from competition within the left hemisphere between the representation of the right- and left-field signals (Reuter-Lorenz et al., 1995).

Specifically, we suggest that the left hemisphere has access to a response-initiation command generated by the right hemisphere when a target occurs in the left visual field. According to this proposal, the left hemisphere bases its report of left-visual-field signals on this response-initiation command. When a right-visual-field signal occurs simultaneously, the salience of this sensory signal in the left hemisphere is likely to overwhelm the motor-based representation (i.e., the response-initiation command) of the left-visual-field signal resulting in apparent left-visual-field extinction (see Reuter-Lorenz et al., 1995, for a more detailed account). Thus, our evidence for left-visual-field extinction actually corroborates the occurrence of parallel sensory processing in the separated hemispheres. The processing of left-visual-field signals by the right hemisphere happens despite the simultaneous perception of right-visual-field signals by the left hemisphere.

Other extinction effects in split-brain patients, such as those reported originally by Levy, Trevarthen, and

Sperry (1972), are also consistent with the strategic response-gating mechanism described above. In a classic demonstration of hemispheric dominance, Levy and colleagues showed that when split-brain patients matched pictures of objects based on the object's function, the patients attended to the right half of the display and tended to ignore the left. To the extent that the left hemisphere is superior in determining an object's function, it dominates performance and prevents the right hemisphere from accessing response pathways. However, when the match was based on visual similarity rather than functionality, the right hemisphere assumed control of performance, and left-hemisphere responses were inhibited by the gating mechanism. One need not assume that the perceptual encoding, decision-making, or response selection operations of the "gated" hemisphere suffer from parallel processing by the other hemisphere (see also Levy, 1977).

Furthermore, the research of Levy and colleagues (1972) reveals important information about when response gating will occur and which hemisphere will assume control of performance. In their work, the hemisphere specialized for the cognitive demands of the task appeared to gate the output of the other hemisphere. Likewise, in various attentional or sensorimotor tasks, gating may be mediated by the hemisphere that is "dominant" for the particular instructional, strategic, or even representational demands of the task. For example, the left hemisphere may be superior to the right hemisphere in controlling guided, or strategic, visual search (Kingstone et al., 1995). Thus, when guided search is required to meet the task demands, the left hemisphere may gate the output of the right hemisphere. Whichever hemisphere is specialized for the task at hand can control the patient's output by strategically gating the output of the other hemisphere.

Response gating: Summary and conclusions

The research reviewed in this chapter leads to the conclusion that the separated hemispheres can function independently and in parallel, with minimal interference on a variety of basic sensorimotor tasks. Apparent limitations on parallel processing can be traced to strategic response gating that inhibits response initiation. While each hemisphere may gate the output of the other, perhaps subsequent research will discover asymmetries in this ability that are, for example, associated with lateralized executive or strategic processes.

Observed properties of the proposed response-gating mechanism in split-brain patients indicate that it does not require the corpus callosum. Instead, the basal ganglia and cerebellum are likely to be part of this mecha-

nism. The basal ganglia are known to modulate the speed of response initiation (Banich, 1997). Callosotomy would sever connections between the left and right basal ganglia as well as efferent projections to the basal ganglia from the contralateral hemisphere (e.g., Houk, Davis, and Bieser, 1994). Nevertheless, even after callosotomy, the basal ganglia may contribute to response gating by way of the thalamus, which also receives projections from the cerebellum. And the cerebellum may contribute to response gating because it receives both ipsilateral and contralateral projections from the cortical hemispheres by way of the pons (Glickstein, 1990). Indeed, some investigators (Ivry and Hazeltine, 1999) have attributed the temporal coupling that persists between left- and right-limb movements by split-brain patients (e.g., Preilowski, 1972; Zaidel and Sperry, 1977) to the timing functions of the cerebellum. This is consistent with my suggestion that the cerebellum mediates strategic response gating.

Of course, it should be acknowledged that most of the experiments reviewed in this chapter have used very basic sensorimotor tasks that make minimal demands on the cognitive system. The conclusions that I have offered regarding the extent of parallel processing in the bisected brain may be limited to performance of such tasks (cf. Kreuter, Kinsbourne, and Trevarthen, 1972; Holtzman and Gazzaniga, 1982; Commentary 9.2 in this volume). Future research on dual-task performance and resource utilization after callosotomy will determine when competition for cognitive resources poses limits on parallel processing in the separated hemispheres.

Further research is also needed to elaborate the properties of the proposed gating mechanism and to clarify the circumstances that evoke gating. Variations of the explicit-stop experiment designed by Reuter-Lorenz and colleagues (1995) and described earlier in this chapter would be useful to examine possible hemispheric differences in strategic gating, as well as their relative control over different response pathways. This paradigm could also be used to study temporal properties of the gating mechanism by varying the relative onsets of the go and no-go signals.

In conclusion, the answer to the long-debated question raised at the start of this chapter seems inescapable: Severing the corpus callosum does indeed produce two independent spheres of cognition. Taken all together, a vast number of studies reveal that the separated hemispheres can perform concurrent stimulus selection, encoding, decision making, and response selection. Clearly, then, for the intact brain the integrative functions of the corpus callosum unify the operations of two potentially autonomous cognitive systems (Reuter-Lorenz and Miller, 1998). In the bisected brain, potentially harmful consequences of this autonomy are circumvented strategically at relatively late stages of response initiation by a subcortical response-gating mechanism that precludes dissociated and conflicting behaviors.

ACKNOWLEDGMENTS The preparation of this chapter was supported by a grant from the National Institute on Aging and by an award from the International Institute of the University of Michigan. Thanks are due to David E. Meyer for many helpful discussions of this work.

REFERENCES

ARGUIN, M., M. LASSONDE, A. QUATTRINI, M. DEL PESCE, N. FOSCHI, and I. PAPO, 2000. Divided visuo-spatial attention systems with total and anterior callosotomy. *Neuropsychologica* 38:283–291.

BANICH, M. T., 1997. *Neuropsychology: The Neural Bases of Mental Function.* Boston: Houghton Mifflin.

CAVINA-PRATESI, C., E. BRICOLO, M. PRIOR, and C. A. MARZI, 2001. Redundancy gain in the stop-signal paradigm: Implications for the locus of co-activation in simple reaction time. *J. Exp. Psychol. Hum. Percept. Perform.* 27:932–941.

CORBALLIS, M. C., 1995. Visual integration in the split brain. *Neuropsychologia* 33:937–959.

CORBALLIS, M. C., 1998. Interhemispheric neural summation in the absence of a corpus callosum. *Brain* 121:1795–1807.

ELLENBERG, L., and R. W. SPERRY, 1980. Lateralized division of attention in the commissurotomized and intact brain. *Neuropsychologia* 18:411–418.

FRANZ, E. A., J. C. ELIASSEN, R. B. IVRY, and M. S. GAZZANIGA, 1996. Dissociation of spatial and temporal coupling in the bimanual movements of callosotomy patients. *Psychol. Sci.* 7:306–310.

GAZZANIGA, M. S., 1987. Perceptual and attentional processes following callosal section in humans. *Neuropsychologia* 25:119–133.

GAZZANIGA, M. S., J. E. BOGEN, and R. W. SPERRY, 1962. Some functional effects of sectioning the cerebral commissures in man. *Proc. Natl. Acad. Sci. U.S.A.* 48:1765–1769.

GAZZANIGA, M. S., and R. W. SPERRY, 1966. Simultaneous double discrimination response following brain bisection. *Psychonomic Sci.* 4:261–262.

GLICKSTEIN, M. E., 1990. Brain pathways in the visual guidance of movement and the behavioral functions of the cerebellum. In *Brain Circuits and Functions of the Mind: Essays in Honor of R. W. Sperry,* C. Trevarthen, ed. Cambridge, Engl.: Cambridge University Press, pp. 157–167.

HOLTZMAN, J. D., and M. S. GAZZANIGA, 1982. Dual-task interactions due exclusively to limits in processing resources. *Science* 218:1325–1327.

HOLTZMAN, J. D., and M. S. GAZZANIGA, 1985. Enhanced dual task performance following corpus commissurotomy in humans. *Neuropsychologia* 236:315–321.

HOLTZMAN, J. D., J. J. SIDTIS, B. T. VOLPE, D. H. WILSON, and M. S. GAZZANIGA, 1981. Dissociation of spatial information for stimulus localization and the control of attention. *Brain* 104:861–872.

HOLTZMAN, J. D., B. T. VOLPE, and M. S. GAZZANIGA, 1984. Spatial orientation following commissural section. In *Varieties of Attention,* R. Parasuraman and D. R. Davies, eds. New York: Academic Press, pp. 375–394.

HOUK, J. C., J. L. DAVIS, and D. G. BEISER, 1994. *Models of Information Processing in the Basal Ganglia.* Cambridge, Mass.: MIT Press.

HUGHES, H. C., P. A. REUTER-LORENZ, R. FENDRICH, and M. S. GAZZANIGA, 1992. Bidirectional control of saccadic eye movements by the disconnected cerebral hemispheres. *Exp. Brain Res.* 91:335–339.

HUGHES, H. C., P. A. REUTER-LORENZ, G. NOZAWA, and R. FENDRICH, 1994. Visual-auditory interactions in sensory-motor processing: Saccades versus manual responses. *J. Exp. Psychol. Hum. Percept. Perform.* 20:131–153.

IACOBONI, M., A. PTITO, N. Y. WEEKES, and E. ZAIDEL, 2000. Parallel visuomotor processing in the split brain: Cortico-subcortical interactions. *Brain* 123:759–769.

IVRY, R. B., E. A. FRANZ, A. KINGSTONE, and J. C. JOHNSTON, 1998. The PRP effect following callosotomy: Uncoupling of lateralized response codes. *J. Exp. Psychol. Hum. Percept. Perf.* 24:463–480.

IVRY, R. B., and E. HAZELTINE, 1999. Subcortical locus of temporal coupling in the bimanual movements of a callostomy patient. *Hum. Move. Sci.* 18:345–375.

JONIDES, J., 1981. Voluntary versus automatic control over the mind's eye's movement. In *Attention and Performance,* Vol. 9, J. Long and A. Baddeley, eds. Hillsdale, N.J.: Erlbaum.

JOYNT, R. J., 1977. Inattention syndromes in split-brain man. In *Advances in Neurology,* Vol. 18, E. A. Weinstein and R. P. Friedland, eds. New York: Raven Press, pp. 33–39.

KENNERLY, S. W., J. DIEDRICHSEN, E. HAZELTINE, A. SEMJEN, and R. B. IVRY, 2002. Callostomy patients exhibit temporal coupling during continuous bimanual movements. *Nat. Neurosci.* 5:376–381.

KINGSTONE, A., J. T. ENNS, G. R. MANGUN, and M. S. GAZZANIGA, 1995. Guided visual search is a left-hemisphere process in split-brain patients. *Psychol. Sci.* 6:118–121.

KREUTER, C., M. KINSBOURNE, and C. TREVARTHEN, 1972. Are deconnected cerebral hemispheres independent channels? A preliminary study of the effect unilateral loading on bilateral finger tapping. *Neuropsychologia* 10:453–461.

LEVY, J., 1977. Manifestations and implications of shifting hemi-inattention in commissurotomy patients. In *Advances in Neurology,* Vol. 18, E. A. Weinstein and R. P. Friedland, eds. New York: Raven Press.

LEVY, J., C. TREVARTHEN, and R. W. SPERRY, 1972. Perception of bilateral chimeric figures following hemispheric disconnexion. *Brain* 95:61–78.

LUCK, S. J., S. A. HILLYARD, G. R. MANGUN, and M. S. GAZZANIGA, 1989. Independent hemispheric attentional systems mediate visual search in split-brain patients. *Nature* 342:543–545.

LUCK, S. J., S. A. HILLYARD, G. R. MANGUN, and M. S. GAZZANIGA, 1993. Independent attentional scanning in the separated hemispheres of split-brain patients. *J. Cogn. Neurosci.* 6:83–90.

MANGUN, G. R., S. A. HILLYARD, S. J. LUCK, T. HANDY, R. PLAGER, V. P. CLARK, W. C. LOFTUS, and M. S. GAZZANIGA, 1994. Monitoring the visual world: Hemispheric asymmetries and subcortical processes in attention. *J. Cogn. Neurosci.* 6:267–275.

MARZI, C. A., M. SMANIA, M. C. MARTINI, G. GAMBINA, G. TORMERELLI, A. PALAMARA, F. ALESSANDRINI, and M. PRIOR, 1996. Implicit redundant target effects in visual extinction. *Neuropsychologia* 34:9–22.

MARZI, C. A., G. TASSINARI, S. AGLIOTI, and L. LUTZEMBERGER, 1986. Spatial summation across the vertical meridian in hemianopics: A test of blindsight. *Neuropsychologia* 24:749–758.

MEYER, D. E., and D. E. KIERAS, 1997a. A computational theory of executive cognitive processes and multiple-task performance. 1: Basic mechanisms. *Psychol. Rev.* 104:3–65.

MEYER, D. E., and D. E. KIERAS, 1997b. A computational theory of executive cognitive processes and multiple-task performance. 2: Accounts of psychological refractory-period phenomena. *Psychol. Rev.* 104:749–791.

MEYER, D. E., D. E. KIERAS, E. LAUBER, E. H. SCHUMACHER, J. GLASS, E. ZURBRIGGEN, L. GMEINDL, and D. APFELBLAT, 1995. Adaptive executive control: Flexible multiple-task performance without pervasive immutable response-selection bottlenecks. *Acta Psychol.* 90:163–190.

MEYER, D. E., D. E. IRWIN, A. M. OSMAN, and J. KOUNIOS, 1988. The dynamics of cognition and action: Mental processes inferred from speed-accuracy decompostion. *Psychol. Rev.* 95:183–237.

MILLER, J. O., 1982. Divided attention: Evidence for coactivation with redundant signals. *Cognit. Psychol.* 14:247–279.

MILLER, J. O., 1986. Time course of coactivation in bimodal divided attention. *Perception and Psychophysics*, 40:331–343.

MINIUSSI, C., M. GIRELLI, and C. A. MARZI, 1998. The neural site of the redundant target effect: Electrophysiological evidence. *J. Cogn. Neurosci.* 10:216–230.

NOZAWA, G., 1993. Stochastic models of human information processing. *Dissertation Abstracts International* 53 (7-A):2303.

PASHLER, H., and J. C. JOHNSTON, 1989. Chronometric evidence for central postponement in temporally overlapping tasks. *Q. J. Exp. Psychol.* 41A:19–45.

PASHLER, H., S. L. LUCK, S. A. HILLYARD, G. R. MANGUN, S. O'BRIEN, and M. S. GAZZANIGA, 1994. Sequential operation of disconnected cerebral hemispheres in split-brain patients. *Neuroreport* 5:2381–2384.

POLLMAN, S., and E. ZAIDEL, 1999. Redundancy gains for visual search after complete commissurotomy. *Neuropsychology* 13:246–258.

POSNER, M. I., 1980. Orienting of attention. *Q. J. Exp. Psychol.* 32:3–25.

PREILOWSKI, B. F. B., 1972. Possible contribution of the anterior forebrain commissures to bilateral motor coordination. *Neuropsychologia* 10:267–277.

RAAB, D., 1962. Statistical facilitation of simple reaction times. *Trans. N.Y. Acad. Sci.* 24:574–590.

RAFAL, R. D., and A. HENIK, 1994. The neurology of inhibition: Integrating controlled and automatic processes. In *Inhibitory Processes in Attention Memory and Language*, D.

Dagenbach and T. H. Carr, eds. New York: Academic Press.

REUTER-LORENZ, P. A., and R. FENDRICH, 1990. Orienting attention across the vertical meridian: Evidence from callosotomy patients. *J. Cogn. Neurosci.* 2:232–238.

REUTER-LORENZ, P. A., and A. MILLER, 1998. The cognitive neuroscience of human laterality: Lessons from the bisected brain. *Current Directions in Psychological Science* 7:15–20.

REUTER-LORENZ, P. A., G. NOZAWA, M. S. GAZZANIGA, and H. C. HUGHES, 1995. The fate of neglected targets in the callosotomized brain: A chronometric analysis. *J. Exp. Psychol. Hum. Percept. Perf.* 21:211–230.

SCHUMACHER, E. H., T. L. SEYMOUR, J. M. GLASS, D. E. FENCSIK, E. J. LAUBER, D. E. KIERAS, and D. E. MEYER, 2001. Virtually-perfect time sharing in dual-task performance: Uncorking the central cognitive bottleneck. *Psychol. Sci.* 12:101–108.

SEYMOUR, S., P. A. REUTER-LORENZ, and M. S. GAZZANIGA, 1994. The disconnection syndrome: Basic findings reaffirmed. *Brain* 117:105–115.

SPERRY, R. W., 1968. Mental unity following surgical disconnection of the cerebral hemispheres. In *Harvey Lectures*, Vol. 62. New York: Academic Press, pp. 293–323.

TENG, E. L., and R. W. SPERRY, 1973. Interhemispheric interaction during simultaneous bilateral presentation of letters or digits in commissurotomized patients. *Neuropsychologia* 11:131–140.

TENG, E. L., and R. W. SPERRY, 1974. Interhemispheric rivalry during simultaneous bilateral task presentation in commissurotomized patients. *Cortex* 21:249–260.

TOMAUIOLO, F., M. PTITO, T. PAUS, C. MARZI, and A. PTITO, 1997. Residual visual functions in hemispherectomized patients revealed by visual spatial summation across the vertical meridian. *Brain* 120:795–803.

TOWNSEND, J. T., and F. G. ASHBY, 1983. *Stochastic Modeling of Elementary Psychological Processes*. Cambridge, Engl.: Cambridge University Press.

TREISMAN, A., and G. GELADE, 1980. Feature-integration theory of attention. *Cognit. Psychol.* 12:97–136.

VAN DER HEIJDEN, A. H. C., 1992. *Selective Attention in Vision*. New York: Routledge.

ZAIDEL, D., and R. W. SPERRY, 1977. Some long-term motor effect of cerebral commissurotomy in man. *Neuropsychologia* 15:193–204.

ZAIDEL, E., 1995. Interhemispheric transfer in the split-brain: Long-term status following complete cerebral commissurotomy. In *Brain Asymmetry*, R. J. Davidson and K. Hugdahl, eds. Cambridge, Mass.: MIT Press, pp. 491–532.

COMMENTARY 14.1

In Search of Lost Time: Functional Significance of Crossed-Uncrossed Differences in Callosal Patients

MARCO IACOBONI AND ERAN ZAIDEL

ABSTRACT In this commentary we argue that the cortical modulation on subcortical activity is a critical parameter in determining the amplitude of the redundant target effect in patients with callosal lesions. Chronometrical and functional neuroimaging evidence in support of this proposal are briefly reviewed.

Reuter-Lorenz asks whether the separated hemispheres can function as independent parallel processors. To address this question empirically, she uses the redundant target paradigm. This paradigm compares human performance when multiple copies of the same stimulus are presented to performance when a single stimulus is presented. In a variety of sensorimotor tasks and, relevant to this book, in simple reaction time (RT) to lateralized flashes, RTs are faster when two or more copies of the light stimulus are presented, compared to the single-flash presentation. This phenomenon, called redundancy gain, can be explained by the summation of the independent probability of detecting each copy of the sensory stimulus, such that a motor response can be initiated by multiple independent channels (horse race model) or, alternatively, by a reciprocal potentiation of the neural activation produced by each copy of the sensory stimulus, such that the threshold for motor response can be reached earlier (coactivation model). Miller (1982) proposed a simple method based on the cumulative distribution functions of RT under the single-stimulus or multiple-copies condition. With this approach, it is pos-

sible to estimate the limit of the performance that can be accounted for by the probability summation of independent channels. If the actual performance under the multiple-copies condition exceeds this limit, then a "violation of race inequality" is observed, and neural coactivation must have occurred.

Recently, Reuter-Lorenz and colleagues (1995) have reported a paradoxical observation. In a simple reaction time task to lateralized flashes, two normal subjects, a partial split-brain patient with a surgical resection of the anterior two thirds of the corpus callosum, and a patient with complete callosotomy showed a typical redundancy gain, that is, faster RTs to two lateralized flashes presented simultaneously in the two visual hemifields than to a single lateralized flash, even when the single flash was presented to the visual hemifield ipsilateral to the responding hand. Paradoxically, the complete callosotomy patient showed a greater redundancy gain than the normal subjects and partial split-brain patient. Even more paradoxically, RTs to redundant flashes in the complete callosotomy patient exceeded the boundary of the horse race model and could not be accounted for by probability summation mechanisms. Thus, a neural coactivation in the complete callosotomy patient must have taken place. In contrast, the redundancy gain in normal subjects and in the partial split-brain patient did not violate the "horse race inequality." In her chapter, Reuter-Lorenz proposes that this paradoxical observation might be explained by a subcortically mediated gating mechanism. She assumes that in the normal brain, under the single-flash condition and for both uncrossed and crossed response conditions, the visual information is efficiently transferred through the corpus callosum to the contralateral hemisphere, and a release from a tonic inhibition to motor response is achieved in each hemi-

MARCO IACOBONI Ahmanson Lovelace Brain Mapping Center, Neuropsychiatric Institute, Brain Research Institute, David Geffen School of Medicine, University of California at Los Angeles, Los Angeles, California.

ERAN ZAIDEL Department of Psychology, University of California at Los Angeles, Los Angeles, California.

sphere. In complete callosotomy patients, visual transfer is prevented, and such tonic inhibition is not removed in either hemisphere. Only when two lateralized flashes are simultaneously presented in the two visual hemifields can the complete callosotomy patient release this tonic inhibition to motor responses to sensory stimuli. In partial split-brain patients, given that performance is typically similar to that of normal subjects, an efficient callosal visual transfer is assumed.

The model put forward by Reuter-Lorenz makes two interesting assumptions that are relevant to callosal channels and the Poffenberger paradigm. First, it is assumed that even during the uncrossed response condition a visual transfer of information to the contralateral hemisphere normally occurs before a motor response is delivered. Such an assumption seems to be substantiated by recent neurophysiological evidence (Chapter 8 in this volume). Note that this assumption does not invalidate the logic of the Poffenberger paradigm in tapping interhemispheric transmission time. Crossed responses always require an extra crossing of information from one hemisphere to the other, compared to uncrossed responses, before the visual information can reach motor areas controlling motor responses (see Commentary 8.2 in this volume). Second, the efficiency of the transfer that allows visual information to be shared between the two hemispheres such that a release from tonic inhibition of motor response is obtained should be inversely correlated with the redundancy gain and with overall RTs in the single-flash condition. The reader must keep in mind that in the canonical single-flash condition, if visual information is not shared between the two hemispheres, a tonic inhibition is assumed and the model predicts a general slowing down of RT. Thus, the model predicts that callosal patients should show a greater redundancy gain when their crossed-uncrossed difference (CUD) gets longer.

To test these predictions, we studied a series of nine patients with various callosal pathology using the redundant target paradigm. What we observed was that some patients had large redundancy gains violating probability models and that some other patients had smaller redundancy gains not violating probability models. The presence or absence of probability model violation was not associated with a specific callosal lesion. When we looked at the CUDs observed in these patients, however, we noticed that the patients with large redundancy gains violating probability models had CUDs longer than

15 ms, whereas the patients with smaller redundancy gains not violating probability models had CUDs shorter than 15 ms (Iacoboni et al., 2000). We hypothesized that long CUDs are associated with violation of probability models because of lack of synchronization between visual areas of the two hemispheres. Callosal fibers are important for interhemispheric synchronization of cortical activity, and this synchronization is best achieved among distant neuronal systems that are reciprocally connected if the conduction delays between the neuronal systems do not exceed one-third of the oscillatory cycle time. Cortical oscillations belong to the gamma band (30–70 Hz), and a CUD longer than 15 ms would interfere even with the slowest oscillation cycle.

This hypothesis predicts different neural activation pattern at extrastriate level in patients with long CUDs and large redundancy gains, compared to patients with short CUDs and small redundancy gains. That is exactly what we observed in a functional magnetic resonance imaging study of two patients with callosal agenesis. The patient with a large redundancy gain and long CUDs had large activations in the extrastriate cortex of the right hemisphere during a redundant target task, whereas the patient with short CUDs and a small redundancy gain did not (Iacoboni et al., 2000).

Taken together, these behavioral and fMRI data suggest that even though subcortical structures may be important for parallel visuomotor processing, their activity critically depends on cortical modulation. Thus, the subcortical gating mechanism postulated by Reuter-Lorenz might not play a critical role in parallel visuomotor processing. Rather, the disruption of complex cortical interactions determined by the lack of callosal fibers may be the determining factor in the paradoxical facilitation observed in some split-brain patients during parallel visuomotor processing.

REFERENCES

IACOBONI, M., A. PTITO, N. Y. WEEKES, and E. ZAIDEL, 2000. Parallel visuomotor transforms in the split brain: Cortico-subcortical interactions. *Brain* 123:759–769.

MILLER, J., 1982. Divided attention: Evidence for coactivation with redundant signals. *Cognit. Psychol.* 14:247–279.

REUTER-LORENZ, P. A., G. NOZAWA, M. S. GAZZANIGA, and H. C. HUGHES, 1995. Fate of neglected targets: A chronometric analysis of redundant target effects in the bisected brain. *J. Exp. Psychol. Hum. Percept. Perform.* 21:211–230.

15 Agenesis of the Corpus Callosum

MARYSE C. LASSONDE, HANNELORE C. SAUERWEIN, AND FRANCO LEPORE

ABSTRACT Agenesis of the corpus callosum, a congenital malformation of midline structures in the brain, has sometimes been referred to as a natural model of the split brain. Although this anomaly is often associated with other malformations, there are sporadic reports of acallosal patients without gross concomitant cerebral pathology. Cognitive assessment of the latter has revealed that individuals born without a corpus callosum can have normal intellectual abilities. Most experimental work has emphasized the absence of disconnection deficits in agenesis of the corpus callosum. However, this notion is increasingly challenged. Recent studies point to limitations of the putative compensatory pathways of interhemispheric transfer and integration in agenesis of the corpus callosum. Thus, acallosal individuals are consistently slower in simple reaction time experiments, and they have difficulties cross-integrating more complex material. Furthermore, they show deficits similar to those of split-brain patients in a variety of midline functions in the visual and tactile modalities. They are also impaired on tasks requiring visuospatial analysis and interhemispheric transfer of motor and tactuomotor learning. Nevertheless, they appear to have access to a number of compensatory mechanisms, and some of these may be privileged over others in certain patients, suggesting that there are individual variants of cerebral organization in agenesis of the corpus callosum.

Agenesis of the corpus callosum, a congenital malformation of midline structures in the brain, has sometimes been referred to as a natural model of the split brain. First described by Reil in 1812, this anomaly has since been reported by several investigators. However, it remained nothing more than a curiosity for the pathologist until interest in this malformation was revived in the 1960s following the now-classic studies in split-brain animals (Sperry, 1961) and commissurotomized patients (Bogen and Vogel, 1962; Sperry, Gazzaniga and Bogen, 1969) and the subsequent findings by Sperry (1970) that individuals born without a corpus callosum do not display the typical disconnection deficits found in split-brain patients. Since this seminal work, the bulk of neuropsychological research on callosal agenesis has focused on the

MARYSE C. LASSONDE, HANNELORE C. SAUERWEIN, AND FRANCO LEPORE Groupe de Recherche en Neuropsychologie Expérimentale, Département de Psychologie, Université de Montréal, Montréal, Québec, Canada.

particulars of interhemispheric transfer and integration. An ever-growing literature has emerged on the subject attempting to specify the extent and limits of neural plasticity in a nervous system that has evolved in the absence of the most important interhemispheric pathway.

While callosal agenesis proves to be an excellent model of cerebral plasticity, it has to be pointed out that this anomaly is often associated with other malformations and neurological diseases that may result in different degrees of mental retardation or selective cognitive and sensorimotor deficits. Neurological research on callosal agenesis has concentrated on the description of various syndromes associated with this pathology as well as on the attempt to specify its neurobehavioral manifestations (Geoffroy, 1994; Wisniewski and Jeret, 1994). There are, however, sporadic reports of acallosal patients without gross concomitant cerebral pathology. The study of these individuals allows for the identification of patterns of functioning that are characteristic of callosal agenesis per se. The purpose of this chapter is to provide an overview of the clinical and behavioral manifestations of this malformation.

What is callosal agenesis?

The development of the corpus callosum and the anterior commissure begins early during fetal life (Loeser and Alvord, 1968). By the twelfth week of gestation the first callosal fibers can be found in its anterior portion, the genu. The corpus callosum then develops along an anteroposterior axis with the splenium being formed by the eighteenth week. The rostrum, the most anterior portion of the corpus callosum, appears last between the eighteenth and twentieth weeks. Various insults to the fetus may result in total or partial absence of structures that are under development at the time of the noxious event. Thus, damage occurring around the seventh week may prevent the formation of both the corpus callosum and the anterior commissure. An injury between the seventh and twelfth weeks might result in total absence of the corpus callosum without interfering with the formation of the anterior commissure. An insult occurring

357

between the twelfth and twentieth weeks would not prevent the development of the genu but might result in the absence of other portions of the corpus callosum causing various degrees of partial callosal agenesis.

The first description of agenesis of the corpus callosum was based on an autopsy report (Reil, 1812). While the postmortem exam remains a major source of detecting this malformation, especially in asymptomatic cases, the development of more sophisticated techniques in neuroimaging has allowed for the detection of the anomaly during the individual's lifetime. In this context, Davidoff and Dyke (1934) were the first to describe a case of callosal agenesis diagnosed by pneumoencephalography. Since the advent of less invasive techniques, an increasing number of callosal agenesis patients have been detected by either computerized tomography, magnetic resonance imaging, or prenatal and postnatal ultrasonography (e.g., Rauch and Jinkins, 1994). Neuroradiological images of the acallosal brain typically show a marked separation of the lateral ventricles and an enlargement of the third ventricle and the posterior part of the lateral ventricles (Figure 15.1). Some of the images also show the so-called Probst's bundle, two parallel bands of white matter formed by callosal fibers that failed to cross the midline during fetal development that are usually visualized along either side of the interhemispheric fissure.

As for the epidemiological distribution of this malformation, callosal agenesis is far from being an isolated phenomenon. It has been described throughout the world, but its frequency may vary from one country to another. The incidence of this malformation depends on both the population studied and the diagnostic technique employed. Thus, among all children, the incidence is 0.0005–0.7%, and among developmentally disabled children it is 2.2–2.4% (see Wisniewski and Jeret, 1994). The number of new cases being reported is highest in centers that routinely use prenatal sonographic examination.

As was mentioned earlier, agenesis of the corpus callosum may be clinically asymptomatic and can occur as an isolated phenomenon that is discovered accidentally at autopsy or by neuroimaging. However, more often, it is associated with other developmental anomalies. Five disease entities have been described that are most frequently associated with agenesis of the corpus callosum. These are the Aicardi, Andermann, Shapiro, and acrocallosal syndromes and Menkes disease (see Geoffroy, 1994; Wisniewski and Jeret, 1994). The fact that callosal agenesis is often part of one of these syndromes suggests the presence of a genetic factor. Indeed, chromosomal aberrations are found in a relatively large number of cases (Serur, Jeret, and Wisniewski, 1988). Most of these involve X-linked de novo mutations (e.g., Donnenfeld et al., 1989; Baranzini et al., 1997). Others are associated with various types of trisomies (Atlas et al., 1988; Serur et al., 1988). Familial forms of callosal agenesis of both dominant and recessive autosomal inheritance have also been identified (e.g., Andermann et al., 1972; Lynn et al., 1980; Inbar et al., 1997).

Agenesis of the corpus callosum has also been observed in association with a variety of clinical entities, such as hydrocephaly, fetal alcohol syndrome, postradiation encephalopathy, and even schizophrenia. Symptomatic acallosal patients may manifest mental retardation, hydrocephaly, epileptic seizures, motor impairment, or ocular anomalies. These findings are usually nonspecific and occur in association with numerous other pathologies of the central nervous system.

Cognitive abilities in callosal agenesis

It is now recognized that individuals who are born without a corpus callosum can have normal cognitive abilities, but the majority of those who are diagnosed during their lifetime tend to function at the lower end of the normal range (see Sauerwein and Lassonde, 1994, for a review). Mental retardation may also be present, especially when other structural anomalies of the central nervous system coexist. Nevertheless, it should be pointed out that the cases reported in the clinical literature are biased toward a neurological population. In-

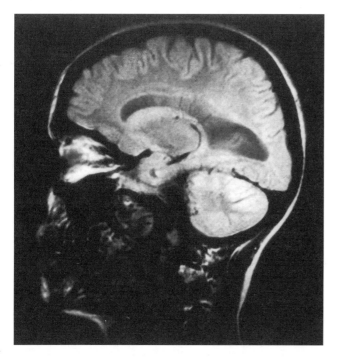

FIGURE 15.1. Midsagittal MRI view of an acallosal brain.

dividuals with normal or superior mental abilities may go undetected. Some of these inconspicuous cases are discovered when an autopsy is performed for unrelated clinical reasons. Others may be detected accidentally when a neuroradiological exam for an acute condition is indicated. In this context, a highly intelligent individual with a frontal cyst was recently diagnosed and examined by our team (see below). Finally, an increasing number of isolated cases of callosal agenesis are diagnosed by routine prenatal and postnatal sonography (Cioni et al., 1994).

Earlier studies of callosal agenesis patients suggested that verbal skills may develop at the expense of perceptual skills in these individuals (Sperry, 1970). However, an analysis of the intellectual quotient (IQ) obtained from 46 reviewed cases (Sauerwein and Lassonde, 1994) reveals that this is a misconception. When a discrepancy of 1 standard deviation between verbal and performance IQ was used to distinguish verbal and perceptual advantages, respectively, the proportion of cases that showed no imbalance in these skills was equal to or higher than that showing an advantage for either function. The distribution of IQ in this study also indicates that a large proportion (42.5%) of the acallosals fall in the low average range of cognitive functioning. Again, one has to keep in mind that these patients were diagnosed because of some neurological complaint and that asymptomatic cases may never come to attention of the clinician. Nevertheless, the fact remains that approximately 20% of the acallosals in these surveys fell in the high-to-superior range of mental abilities. These data suggest that agenesis of the corpus callosum per se is not the cause of the cognitive deficits that sometimes accompany this malformation. The data also disconfirm an earlier hypothesis put forth by Cook (1986) stating that absence or reduction of interhemispheric cross-talk would result in lower intelligence.

Other studies have concentrated on more specific cognitive domains, such as language (e.g., Dennis, 1977, 1981). The question of how language is organized in the acallosal brain is of particular interest in view of the hypothesis that the corpus callosum may be crucial for the development of hemispheric specialization (Doty, Negrao, and Yamaga, 1973; Moscovitch, 1977; Corballis and Morgan, 1978). According to this view, the hemisphere that is predisposed to take charge of a certain function supposedly suppresses the development of this function in its counterpart via the callosal pathway. Consequently, in the absence of transcallosal inhibition, language that is processed predominantly in the left hemisphere would be bilaterally represented in the acallosal brain. However, this hypothesis has not been borne out by empirical evidence (see Jeeves, 1986; Sauerwein

and Lassonde, 1994). One reason for rejecting this hypothesis derives from dichotic listening research. This technique consists of simultaneously presenting two stimuli (for instance, two words), one to each ear. Neurologically normal, right-handed subjects usually report the word that has been presented to the right ear, presumably because the contralateral connections (right ear/left hemisphere) are stronger than the ipsilateral (left ear/left hemisphere) connections in a situation of competitive input. Dichotic studies in acallosal subjects have yielded small but reliable ear asymmetries (evidence of hemispheric superiority), although, according to Chiarello's review of 29 cases, the side of the preferred ear is less consistent in acallosals than in normal subjects (Chiarello, 1980). In a more recent study carried out by our team (Lassonde, Bryden, and Demers, 1990), we have found the expected left-hemisphere superiority for verbal stimuli in the majority of our acallosal subjects. Interestingly, with respect to the magnitude of the asymmetry, the acallosal group ranked between the high-IQ and the IQ-matched control group by displaying smaller asymmetries than the high-IQ group but larger asymmetries than the low-IQ group. We take this finding as suggesting that the corpus callosum, by allowing continuous flow of information between the hemispheres, may in fact reduce possible asymmetries. In contrast to the prevailing view, this would suggest that the absence of interhemispheric cross-talk in the acallosal brain would favor a greater expression of such asymmetries.

Further evidence against the hypothesis of bilateral language representation in the acallosal brain comes from studies involving the injection of sodium amytal. This procedure is used to determine language lateralization in epileptic patients who are candidates for therapeutic brain surgery. When injected in the carotid artery, sodium amytal anesthetizes the hemisphere ipsilateral to the site of injection. If the injection reaches the hemisphere that is dominant for speech, the patient becomes temporarily mute. Of several cases of callosal agenesis that have been tested with this method, evidence of normal lateralization of speech in the left hemisphere has been found in all but two (see Sauerwein and Lassonde, 1994). Both of them were left-handed. Besides, one documented case of unilateral representation of speech suffices to discredit the hypothesis of bilateral organization of linguistic functions in acallosals.

Interhemispheric communication in callosal agenesis

Since the pioneer work of Sperry in the 1950s and early 1960s, a large body of knowledge has accumulated confirming the callosal involvement in interhemispheric transfer of lateralized information. The necessity of having a structure that ensures communication between the two half-brains derives from the fact that sensory and motor functions are essentially lateralized and from the observation that some higher-order processes, such as language, appear to be controlled primarily by one hemisphere. The interruption of this interhemispheric link through surgical intervention performed to alleviate uncontrollable epilepsy results in a number of modality-specific disconnection deficits (Sperry et al., 1969). Typically, these patients have difficulties carrying out bimanual comparisons of tactile stimuli placed in each hand out of their view. Furthermore, they are unable to compare visual stimuli that are briefly presented in different visual hemifields. They also show diminished abilities to transfer the locus of touch applied to the fingers of one hand to the unstimulated hand. Finally, when left-specialized for language, they cannot verbally identify stimuli that are conveyed to the right, non-speaking hemisphere, either through manipulation by their left hand or through presentation to their left visual hemifield. Although partial recovery has been reported in some of these functions, most of the deficits in interhemispheric communication appear to persist in the long term following the surgery (Bogen and Vogel, 1975; Goldstein and Joynt, 1975).

Because callosal agenesis may be considered a natural model of the split brain, experimental investigations have concentrated on evaluation of the capacities of acallosal subjects to perform tasks involving interhemispheric communication (for reviews, see Milner and Jeeves, 1979; Jeeves, 1994; Milner, 1994). Most of the early work emphasized the fact that individuals born without the corpus callosum do not show the disconnection syndrome that is observed after surgical section of the callosal commissure. For instance, acallosal subjects reportedly have no difficulties comparing objects, shapes, or other stimuli placed in each hand out of view, and they show no impairments in tachistoscopic tasks requiring interfield comparisons. A similar pattern of results has been reported for tasks involving recognition and verbal identification of material presented unilaterally to either hemisphere. Thus, with a few exceptions (e.g., Ettlinger et al., 1972; Donoso and Santander, 1982; Berlucchi, Aglioti, Marzi, and Tassinari, 1995), acallosals, unlike callosotomized patients, can read letters or words that are tachistoscopically projected to the left visual hemifield and have no difficulties naming objects palpated by their left hand (e.g., Milner and Jeeves, 1979; Sauerwein et al., 1981; Sauerwein and Lassonde, 1983).

The absence in acallosal subjects of the typical disconnection deficits reported after surgical division of the hemispheres has often been attributed to the fact that the acallosal brain had the opportunity to start early in life, probably before birth, to make use of neural plasticity to compensate for the lack of the principal commissure. In this context, several compensatory mechanisms have been postulated to account for the absence of the disconnection syndrome in acallosal subjects (see Jeeves, 1986, 1994; Lassonde et al., 1991).

It has often been argued that the preserved capacity of acallosal patients to name items presented to the left visual hemifield or the left hand could be attributed to the presence of bilateral representation of speech (Sperry, 1968). While bilateral organization of linguistic functions has been found in some cases, the reviews discussed above indicate that this is not the norm. Furthermore, although bilateral organization of speech, if present, could account for the ability of acallosal subjects to name lateralized stimuli, it could hardly explain patients' proficiency in carrying out interhemispheric comparisons. With regard to visual cross-matching, the early discussions of compensatory mechanisms in callosal agenesis speculated about the possible role of the anterior commissure and/or subcortical commissures, such as the intertectal or posterior commissure (Jeeves, 1965; Milner, 1994).

The anterior commissure, which connects visual areas of the inferior temporal lobes, has often been considered the most likely candidate for compensation, especially since its embryological development precedes that of the corpus callosum. Earlier case reports have in fact suggested that an enlarged anterior commissure might be present in acallosal patients (see Jeeves, 1994). However, although the anterior commissure seems to be present in most cases of callosal agenesis, magnetic resonance studies suggest that it is usually not hypertrophied (Rauch and Jinkins, 1994). Regardless of its size, the anterior commissure may nonetheless play an important role in interhemispheric transmission of particular kinds of visual information. A report comparing the abilities of two acallosal boys of normal intelligence, in one of whom the anterior commissure was also absent, has indeed shown that the patient lacking the anterior commissure was impaired on visual interhemispheric tasks, while the other patient, whose anterior commissure was enlarged, performed normally on these tasks (Fischer, Ryan, and Dobyns, 1992). Although the anterior commissure may be adequate to transfer visual pattern information, it appears to be limited in carrying visuospatial information (Martin, 1985). It has been convincingly argued that this type of visual information, as well as luminance and motion, may be more effectively transferred via subcortical commissures (Holtzman, 1984; Milner, 1994).

With regard to interhemispheric transfer of tactuo-motor information, the involvement of the anterior commissure is unlikely, given that this commissure has few, if any, anatomical connections between the somatosensory areas (Pandya, Karol, and Lele, 1973). On the basis of electrophysiological and behavioral studies, an enhanced proficiency of the ipsilateral connections of the spinothalamic pathway has so far been the most plausible explanation for this type of cross-integration in callosal agenesis (Dennis, 1976; Sauerwein et al., 1981; Jeeves, 1986, 1994; Vanasse, Forest, and Lassonde, 1994). It is conceivable that acallosal subjects use these connections in such a manner that intermanual comparisons are achieved through intrahemispheric integration of input reaching each hemisphere from both hands via ipsilateral and contralateral connections. However, the compensatory mechanisms used by acallosal patients are not unlimited.

One major limitation that has been confirmed by several authors concerns the speed of transfer: Response times for interhemispheric tasks in acallosal patients are consistently longer when compared to those of controls (Jeeves, 1969; Lassonde et al., 1988). Acallosal subjects have also been found to be less efficient than controls in transferring complex or multiple visual stimuli (Gott and Saul, 1978; Karnath, Schumacher, and Wallesch, 1991). Other impairments have been observed on tasks requiring asynchronous, distal movements, suggesting poor interhemispheric integration of bimanual activities (e.g., Jeeves, Silver, and Jacobson, 1988). Several studies have reported deficits in the transfer of tactuomotor learning (Ettlinger et al., 1972; Gott and Saul, 1978; Sauerwein and Lassonde, 1994) as well as deficits in cross-localization of finger stimulation (Geffen et al., 1994b).

Acallosal patients have also been found to manifest difficulties on tasks requiring the participation of only one hemisphere. These deficits, however, can be interpreted within the general framework of a mild disconnection syndrome, especially for higher functions. This assumes that one hemisphere is incapable of carrying out an analysis in the absence of communication with the other that is more proficient in processing a given kind of information. In this context the impaired performance of the right hand in the right hemispace reported by Temple and Ilsley (1994) in a visual neglect task has been attributed to the dissociation between the left and right hemispheres, the latter being more involved in attentional processes. The right visual field impairments for judgment of stimulus location and word orientation reported by Martin (1985) and the right-hand deficits in spatial processing observed in the tactile part of the De Renzi Rod Test (Meerwaldt, 1983; Jeeves

and Silver, 1988) are other examples of such interhemispheric disconnection. In both cases the patients' left hemisphere is not as proficient as the right in analyzing the spatial information.

Acallosal subjects display other problems that are more difficult to interpret in the context of interhemispheric disconnection. The visuoconstructive deficits occasionally reported in acallosals (Temple and Ilsley, 1994; Berlucchi et al., 1995), as well as impairments on auditory verbal learning tasks (Geffen et al., 1994a), fall into this category. Similarly, Temple and Ilsley (1994) have reported visuoperceptual problems and deficits in phonological processing in their patients that still need to be explained. Furthermore, our own findings indicate that acallosal subjects are as impaired as split-brain patients on a task that requires judgment of the relative distance between objects (Lassonde, 1986). In the latter task the estimation of distance was deficient in both the intrahemispheric or interhemispheric conditions. This observation had led us to postulate a facilitatory or modulating influence of the corpus callosum on the activity of both hemispheres (Lassonde, 1986), a hypothesis that gains support from the electrophysiological studies of Bremer (1966, 1967). More specifically, we hypothesized that the presence of unilateral and bilateral symptoms following agenesis or section of the corpus callosum may be explained by the absence of transcallosal enhancement of cortical activity. Specific cognitive impairments, such as the visuoconstructive deficits described by Temple and Ilsley (1994), may be explained likewise.

Midline sensory integration in callosal agenesis

Data derived from animal studies have ascribed yet another important function to the corpus callosum. Essentially, these findings indicate that the corpus callosum is involved in a number of midline functions, including fusion of the two hemispaces or hemibodies. Just as for mediation in interhemispheric communication, the need for the corpus callosum in midline fusion can be related to the fact that higher-order sensory analysis is essentially lateralized. Thus, in superior mammals, somatosensory experience from each half-body projects to the contralateral hemisphere, as does visual information from each half-field. In the auditory system the separation of the projections coming from the two ears is less precise. However, the crossed connections appear to dominate the ipsilateral connections in a proportion of approximately 2:1 (Barr, 1972).

When information is presented to one side of the body or in one half of the visual or auditory field and then crosses the midline, it excites structures first in one hemisphere and then in the other. Similarly, when a stimulus is presented around the midline, some portions project to one hemisphere and some to the other. The importance of this mechanism for bidimensional stimuli is straightforward: It ensures continuity of sensation across the midline. However, for three-dimensional objects, it may have the additional function of allowing the comparison of the relative depth of stimuli straddling the midline.

The involvement of the corpus callosum in the processing of depth information is still a matter of debate. For example, Mitchell and Blakemore (1970), showed that a callosotomized subject failed to discriminate depth for disparate stimuli presented on either side of the midline but had no problem if both stimuli were presented eccentrically on one side. Using random dot stereograms, similar results were obtained with commissurotomized patients (Hamilton, Rodriguez, and Vermeire, 1987). On the other hand, Ledoux and colleagues (1977) found no deficit in a callosotomized subject whose anterior commissure was intact, suggesting that this commissure might suffice to mediate the function. However, this notion was challenged by Hamilton and colleagues (1987), who found that their patient L.B., with complete commissurotomy including the anterior commissure, was still able to discriminate stereopatterns in the midline. With regard to callosal agenesis, Jeeves (1991) compared acallosals and posterior callosotomized subjects to appropriate controls in their ability to stereoscopically evaluate the distance between line stimuli. The two experimental groups were found to have midline deficits for stimuli having uncrossed disparities. When crossed disparities were used or when the stimuli were presented eccentrically, no such problems were observed.

The experiments reported above assessed depth perception based essentially on binocular spatial disparity. However, there are a number of other cues to depth, some of which may operate even under monocular viewing conditions. One such cue is motion parallax. It is difficult to predict, for stimuli situated on either side of midline, how this cue may be integrated interhemispherically in subjects with callosal pathology, since perfect performance would require that they compare relative motion between the hemispheres. The first experiment attempting to assess the importance of the callosum for interhemispheric motion processing was carried out by Ramachandran, Cronin-Colomb, and Myers (1986), who showed that the direction of apparent motion produced by alternately flashing spots of light (similar to the phi phenomenon) presented on either side of the midline could be discriminated by callosotomized subjects. This finding was subsequently contested by Gazzaniga (1987) but partially supported by Naikar and Corballis (1996). The latter showed that the ability of split-brain patients to perceive apparent motion across the midline depends on spatiotemporal parameters. There was a marked decrease in performance when these parameters were below a critical level, which suggests that the compensatory (subcortical) structures are limited in spatial and temporal resolution.

In a study carried out in our laboratory, we tested whether callosal agenesis subjects could use motion parallax to judge the depth of two plates situated on each side of the midline (Rivest, Cavanagh, and Lassonde, 1994). Acallosal subjects and IQ-matched controls viewed the plates monocularly or binocularly while either holding the head in a fixed position or moving it side to side or up and down. When binocular spatial disparity was available, acallosal subjects showed no deficit in estimating the relative depth of two stimuli, each presented on one side of the midline. In the fixed-head condition, the two groups performed poorly, indicating that the task could not be resolved in the absence of both binocular and monocular depth cues. When horizontal and vertical movements were permitted, performance improved dramatically for the control subjects but not for the agenesis subjects. It therefore appears that motion parallax, as a cue for depth perception, cannot be integrated across the hemispheres in the absence of the corpus callosum.

As is the case with the visual modality, electrophysiological studies have shown that the somatosensory callosal system is closely associated with midline function. This privileged relationship between the corpus callosum and the body midline should result, in cases of callosal pathology, in functional deficits specific to the midline. In another experiment we aimed at exploring callosal involvement in somatosensory midline function. Two-point discrimination thresholds were measured in subjects with callosal section or congenital absence of the corpus callosum (Schiavetto, Lepore, and Lassonde, 1993). In concordance with the hypothesis, thresholds in these subjects were found to be higher than normal only for the trunk areas.

In the latter experiment, as in most studies carried out in the somatosensory system, a tactile discrimination task was used. The anatomical structures mediating this type of discrimination probably involve the dorsal-column medial lemniscal system, which is highly lateralized. This is why subjects manifest a clear disconnection syndrome following callosal transection for tactile tasks, such as stereognosis and texture discrimination. The somatosensory system, however, is also composed of a parallel system involving the anterolateral spinothalamic tract which is less lateralized. Thermal information is transmitted to central structures through this tract. Assessing thresholds with thermal stimulation therefore constitutes an ideal method for examining the efficiency of this parallel somatosensory pathway. This is precisely what we have done in an experiment in which thermal stimuli were presented to essentially the same regions of the body for which we tested two-point discrimination (Lepore et al., 1997). The results indicated that although the absolute value of the differential thresholds varied from region to region, the acallosals and their controls had comparable thresholds for any given region, including the axial areas. These results suggest that the corpus callosum is not required for transfer of sensation in a system that has a relatively large bilateral representation.

Few experiments have been carried out in humans with the objective of assessing the importance of the corpus callosum for midline fusion in the auditory modality. We conducted one such experiment on four acallosal subjects and matched controls (Poirier et al., 1993). Subjects had to point to a fixed auditory target presented on a sound perimeter. It was expected that acallosals would show a comparatively poorer performance at pericentral positions than control subjects. Contrary to our hypothesis, the data clearly showed that, in both groups, sound localization was significantly more precise for targets located in pericentral fields than in lateral fields, suggesting once more that the participation of the corpus callosum is not required in a system that has a more extensive bihemispheric representation.

Taken together, the results obtained in the various sensory modalities indicate that callosal involvement in midline function is important in the visual and lemniscal somatosensory systems but may be redundant in the auditory and spinothalamic somatosensory systems. In the latter systems there is considerable crossover of information at various levels, especially in the auditory system. Continuity of sensation across hemifields is thus not a problem, and the corpus callosum may contribute little to this function in those modalities. By contrast, the visual and somesthetic systems are essentially lateralized. In this context a mechanism that ensures continuity of sensation across sensory space is probably crucial.

Motor functions in callosal agenesis

Studies in split-brain patients suggest that the corpus callosum plays an important role in bilateral motor coordination and tactuomotor learning. Typically, these patients are impaired with respect to speed of bimanual coordination, and they have difficulties in maintaining a continued sequence of rapid asynchronous pronation-supination motions with the forearms (Zaidel and Sperry, 1977). In addition, they are unable to learn new

bimanual motor skills that require continuous mutual monitoring of both hands and bilateral interdependent motor control (Preilowski, 1972; Zaidel and Sperry, 1977). With regard to interhemispheric transfer of learning, poor intermanual performance has been reported on the rotary pursuit task (Zaidel and Sperry, 1977). Transection of the corpus callosum also abolishes transfer of tactuomotor formboard learning from the dominant to the nondominant hand (Goldstein and Joynt, 1975).

Similar deficits have been observed in individuals born without the corpus callosum. For example, acallosal patients are usually reported to be clumsy and slow on bimanual tasks (Jeeves, 1965; Chiarello, 1980; Sauerwein et al., 1981). Deficits in intermanual transfer of formboard learning and pencil maze learning have also been observed (Ferris and Dorsen, 1975; Gott and Saul, 1978; Jeeves, 1979), although results obtained on those tests are controversial: Some authors report good transfer of tactuomotor performance between the hands (Sauerwein et al., 1981, with a simpler formboard) and preserved transfer of stylus maze learning (Reynolds and Jeeves, 1977). A more recent study conducted by our group (Lassonde, Sauerwein, and Lepore, 1995) indicates that acallosal subjects fail to transfer a unilateral motor learning task from one hand to the other. Finally, acallosal subjects have been found to be as impaired as anterior commissurotomy patients on a bimanual tracking task requiring asymmetrical input from the two hands (Jeeves and Silver, 1988).

Subjects with callosal agenesis also display other types of motor deficits that, at first glance, might not appear to be related to the lack of interhemispheric communication. These include defects in grip formation as well as in reaching toward a visual stimulus (Jakobson et al., 1994; Lassonde, 1994; Silver and Jeeves, 1994). The failure to perform normally in these tests has generally been linked to the increased use of uncrossed, ipsilateral, motor projections in acallosals. It has been postulated that the reinforcement of ipsilateral connections in callosal agenesis results from the absence, during development, of the inhibitory action that the corpus callosum normally exerts on these projections (Dennis, 1976) for the crossed connections to prevail. Consequently, the uncrossed pathways would compete with the crossed ones and maintain control of the motor output, thereby reducing the overall level of performance (Dennis, 1976; Jeeves, 1986; Jeeves and Silver, 1988).

Sensorimotor integration in callosal agenesis

Poffenberger's paradigm (1912), developed more than 80 years ago, has provided a means of assessing how interhemispheric and intrahemispheric integration of sensory and motor functions takes place in the normal brain. As is described elsewhere in this volume, this paradigm makes use of the anatomical connections between a lateralized stimulus and the (lateralized) hand responding to it in a simple reaction time (RT) task. For instance, when a flash of light is presented in the left visual field, simple RTs made with the left hand (uncrossed condition) are faster than those made with the right hand (crossed condition). Conversely, the right hand is faster than the left when the stimulus is projected in the right hemifield. The difference in speed is assumed to reflect differences in length of the visuomotor pathways (direct versus indirect) that are utilized in the two conditions. In the uncrossed stimulus-response condition, the response is integrated intrahemispherically, since the hemiretinae receiving the stimulus project to the same hemisphere that controls the responding hand, whereas in the crossed stimulus-response condition, an interhemispheric integration is necessary to coordinate visual input and motor output. The difference between crossed and uncrossed RTs (crossed-uncrossed difference, or CUD) may then be regarded as an indirect measure of interhemispheric transmission time (ITT).

Interhemispheric transmission times have mostly been studied in the visual modality. A meta-analysis conducted by Marzi, Bisiacchi, and Nicoletti (1991) found a mean value across 16 studies of 3.8 ms in normal adults. By contrast, abnormally long ITTs have been found in patients who underwent a surgical section of the corpus callosum (Sergent and Myers, 1985; Di Stefano, Sauerwein, and Lassonde, 1992). This finding reinforces the notion that interhemispheric integration of simple visuomotor responses is mediated by the callosal pathway in the normal brain. Whether a specific part of the corpus callosum may be involved in this intermodal integration is still under discussion. An abnormal ITT has been reported in one callosotomized patient with sparing of the splenium (Di Stefano et al., 1992). However, normal ITTs have been found in eight patients with similar lesions (Tassinari et al., 1994; Iacoboni and Zaidel, 1995).

Many investigators have used Poffenberger's paradigm to study interhemispheric transfer in callosal agenesis subjects (see reviews by Marzi et al., 1991, and Milner, 1994). In general, the CUDs are larger than those found in normals (see Table 15.1), the uncrossed responses being systematically much shorter than the crossed responses. Furthermore, acallosals differ from normal subjects with regard to the laterality effects observed under the standard crossed-uncrossed conditions. While normal subjects show a left-visual-field and a right-hand advantage in this paradigm, acallosal sub-

TABLE 15.1

Mean crossed-uncrossed differences (CUDs) in studies involving callosal agenesis subjects

Study	Number of Subjects	CUD (ms)
Jeeves (1969)	3	32
Kinsbourne and Fisher (1971)	1	12.8
Milner (1982)	1	24.3
Milner et al. (1985)	1	22.3
Clarke and Zaidel (1989)	1	20
Di Stefano et al. (1992)	2	51.3
Tassinari et al. (1994)	1	24
Brodvedani et al. (1996)	1	18

jects fail to show any consistent laterality effect (see Marzi et al., 1991).

Acallosal subjects also have CUDs that are considerably larger than those of normals when they respond to lateralized flashes with both hands (Jeeves, 1969). This finding suggests that the pathway used in the absence of the corpus callosum is longer, probably involving additional synapses. Interestingly, both acallosal and normal subjects show a similar decrease of the CUD in the bimanual as compared to the unimanual condition, suggesting that both groups tend to synchronize their bilateral motor outputs in the bimanual condition.

Although ITTs in acallosals are abnormally long, they tend to be shorter than those observed in split-brain patients. While the CUD values in totally callosotomized patients may vary between 20 and 96 ms (see Tassinari et al., 1994; Marzi et al., 1991), those of patients with a complete absence of the corpus callosum vary between 12.8 and 52 ms with a greater proportion of cases showing CUDs in the 20-ms range. When unilateral and bilateral responses to lateralized flashes are performed by different effectors (distal, proximal, and axial muscles of the upper limbs), both acallosal and split-brain patients obtain CUD values that are greater for unilateral than for bilateral responses, and both show a decrease in CUDs along a distal-proximal-axial gradient (Aglioti et al., 1993). These results suggest that transfer is unnecessary when responses are effected by parts of the motor system that have a greater bilateral distribution (Berlucchi et al., 1995).

It has been argued that longer ITT in callosal agenesis subjects may be attributable to spatial compatibility between stimulus and response (Kinsbourne and Fisher, 1971). Spatial compatibility effects are routinely observed in choice RT experiments. Unlike in simple RT studies, in choice RT experiments, one factor determining the speed of visuomotor responses is the spatial correspondence between stimulus and response location. Choice RTs are shortest when stimulus and response are on the same side in space, regardless of the hand making the response. However, simple RTs have consistently been found to be faster for acallosal subjects when sensory input and motor output are coordinated in the same hemisphere, and this holds true whether the hand responds in the ipsilateral or contralateral hemispace (Milner, 1982; Milner et al., 1985; Di Stefano et al., 1992). Therefore, the CUDs observed in acallosals depend on anatomical connections rather than the spatial relationship between stimulus and response.

Further proof for the notion that the longer CUDs in callosal agenesis are directly attributable to the absence of the corpus callosum comes from the study of event-related potentials (ERPs) on symmetrical points on either side of the scalp. Recording visual ERPs while using Poffenberger's paradigm in normal subjects, Lines, Rugg, and Milner (1984) have shown a difference in latency between the early deflections obtained over the visual areas of the two occipital lobes. The response over the directly stimulated hemisphere (contralateral to the visual stimulus) and the indirectly stimulated (ipsilateral) hemisphere is thought to reflect the interhemispheric transmission time. The usual ITT measured under these conditions averages between 10 and 15 ms, and this value varies as a function of stimulus luminance. When acallosal subjects are tested under the same condition, normal visual ERPs are found over the directly stimulated hemisphere, but no corresponding deflections are found over the other hemisphere, thereby supporting the assumption that the response to the ipsilateral stimulation is normally mediated through the corpus callosum (Rugg, Milner, and Lines, 1985).

The finding of faster interhemispheric transmission times in individuals with congenital absence of the corpus callosum compared with patients who underwent callosal transection in adulthood may be considered as additional proof of cerebral plasticity. Just as for other types of interhemispheric integration, several compensatory mechanisms have been proposed to account for such plasticity. However, the fact that the transmission times of acallosals are also consistently longer than those of normal subjects points once more to the limits of plasticity in the acallosal brain.

Among the mechanisms that could account for the differences in the CUDs between acallosal and callosotomized subjects cross-cuing can be safely ruled out. Such behavioral strategies are routinely screened in all studies involving callosal agenesis subjects. More important, as Aglioti and colleagues (1993) pointed out,

although the interhemispheric transmission times observed in acallosals are longer than those in normal subjects, they are not long enough to suggest the use of a peripheral cross-cuing mechanism. Therefore, the large CUDs that are observed in callosal agenesis subjects are more likely to reflect the use of extracallosal pathways. In the absence of the corpus callosum, either ipsilateral motor pathways and/or secondary interhemispheric routes at the subcortical level could convey the appropriate motor response in the crossed S-R condition.

An enhancement of ipsilateral motor pathways, as discussed above, has often been postulated in cases of callosal agenesis (see Jeeves, 1986, 1994). If such a mechanism were used in the context of the Poffenberger's paradigm, the longer ITTs seen in acallosals would reflect a difference in proficiency between the contralateral and ipsilateral motor pathways. This would also imply that CUDs generally reflect an interhemispheric transfer over the motor areas. There is some evidence in favor of this latter assumption (see Berlucchi et al., 1995). For instance, abnormally large CUDs have been found in patients with frontal but not occipital lesions. More important, a normal CUD has been reported in a patient with an obstructive callosal dysgenesis affecting the posterior, and hence the visual part, of the corpus callosum (Berlucchi et al., 1995). The latter finding would indicate that the interhemispheric connections running in the anterior (motor) portion of the corpus callosum would suffice to achieve fast crossed reactions (Tassinari et al., 1994). As Berlucchi and colleagues (1995) have pointed out, however, data from this patient have yet to be replicated in other subjects. It is possible that in this particular patient the remaining corpus callosum contains visual fibers that have been rerouted through the anterior portion.

By contrast, most of the evidence suggests that the CUDs measured in acallosal subjects reflect a visual, rather than a motor, latency. Manipulation of stimulus luminances from near-threshold to high intensities have yielded variations in the CUDs obtained from two acallosal patients: The lower the intensity, the longer the CUD (Milner, 1994). A similar, albeit nonsignificant, trend was observed in an acallosal patient tested by Clarke and Zaidel (1989). Milner (1994) argues that the increments in luminance might not have been large enough in the latter study, as the mean response times only marginally increased with the change in luminance. Furthermore, unlike in neurologically intact subjects, the manipulation of stimulus eccentricities in acallosal subjects also modifies the CUD, at least in the acallosal patient tested by Lines and colleagues (1984). A similar trend was found in the acallosal patient studied by Clarke and Zaidel (1989). It would seem reasonable, therefore, to presume that the CUD of patients with complete callosal agenesis reflects a visually coded relay.

Again, the most likely pathways to convey such information from one hemisphere to the other are the anterior commissure or subcortical commissures such as the intertectal commissure (connecting the colliculi, an important relay in visual transmission) or the posterior commissure (connecting the posterior pretectal nuclei). As was mentioned earlier, it would appear that the anterior commissure is an important pathway that may be used by acallosals to transfer pattern information between the hemispheres (see Fischer et al., 1992). However, patients who underwent section of the corpus callosum with sparing the anterior commissure have CUDs in the same range as patients in whom both the callosum and the anterior commissure are divided. The extracallosal transfer observed in these split-brain patients would therefore appear to be mediated by subcortical commissures.

There is evidence that the same may apply to cases of callosal agenesis. We have recently obtained similar CUDs from a patient (S.P.) with agenesis of both the anterior and callosal commissures (Caillé et al., 1999). This subject is a 29-year-old, right-handed male with a verbal IQ of 138, which probably makes him the most intelligent acallosal subject reported to date in the literature. The crossed and uncrossed reaction times of S.P. were in the same range as those of the control subjects (Table 15.2). Consequently, the large CUD seen in this acallosal subject cannot simply be attributed to a global slowness in sensorimotor reaction time. However, while our estimate of interhemispheric transmission time in the controls (3.5 ms) was comparable to that reported by other authors (see Marzi et al., 1991), the CUD obtained from S.P. (23.5 ms) greatly exceeded that of the control group. Although the CUD of this patient is similar to that of other callosal agenesis subjects (see Table 15.1), it is smaller than that found in our acallosal patients with an intact anterior commissure who were tested in another study under the same conditions (see Table 15.1; Di Stefano et al., 1992). These results strongly suggest that in individuals with callosal agenesis the anterior commissure is not involved in the transfer of elementary

visual information such as used in the classical Poffenberger's paradigm. The intertectal or posterior commissure, the latter being visible on the MRI images of S.P., may be more likely candidates for subserving interhemispheric transfer of simple visual information in the acallosal brain. Furthermore, the finding of increased interhemispheric transmission times in this highly intelligent individual lends credibility to the notion that the agenesis of the commissures, rather than nonspecific attentional or intellectual impairments, is responsible for this phenomenon.

Conclusion

The neuropsychological investigation of callosal agenesis began almost concurrently with the analysis of the split-brain patients operated on by Bogen and Vogel in the early 1960s (Jeeves, 1965). The early work focused primarily on the contrast between these two types of "callosally deprived" patients. Thus, acallosal subjects were found to be devoid of many of the disconnection symptoms found in adult callosotomized patients, and cerebral plasticity was invoked to explain the lack of such symptoms. Acallosal patients were also reported to have cognitive deficits.

During the last two decades these views have sometimes been disputed as an increasing number of asymptomatic acallosal subjects has been described. It is now acknowledged that acallosal subjects can have normal and even superior intellectual abilities. The notion that the acallosal brain compensates for the lack of the principal interhemispheric commissure is also increasingly challenged. Most of the recent work emphasizes the limitations of the putative compensatory pathways used for interhemispheric transfer in callosal agenesis. One of the limitations concerns speed of transfer: Longer reaction times have been found in callosal agenesis both in simple RT experiments and in tasks involving interhemispheric transfer of more complex material. Notwithstanding these limitations, acallosal patients are in general capable of transferring elementary visual information and pattern or color information, and they are usually able to cross-match tactile information.

Limits to cerebral plasticity must also be invoked to account for the fact that callosal agenesis subjects do show disconnection symptoms that are similar in nature, albeit not in magnitude, to those observed in split-brain patients, at least in certain tasks. For instance, impairments in midline functions can be observed in the visual and tactile modalities in both acallosal and callosotomized patients. Furthermore, like split-brain patients, callosal agenesis subjects show deficits in many tasks involving a motor component. Thus, acallosals are com-

TABLE 15.2

Mean reaction times (ms) to a lateralized light stimulus obtained from the acallosal patient S.P. and his controls

Subjects	Crossed RTs	Uncrossed RTs	Mean CUD
S.P.	406.75	383.25	23.5
Controls (n = 10)	363.48	360.48	3.5
Range	(301–495)	(293–405 ms)	(−3.75–14.25)

monly reported to be clumsy and slow in bimanual operations. In fact, many of the deficits reported in acallosals appear to be related to activities mediated by the frontal regions (bimanual activities, transfer of motor learning, grasping, etc.) or the parietal areas (visual neglect, spatial analysis, visuomotor coordination, etc.). This can be expected, since the callosal fibers, apart from connecting the primary sensory areas involved in midline analysis, predominantly connect associative cortex. Therefore, just as in callosotomized patients, the pattern of disconnection deficits observed in callosal agenesis appears to reflect the disruption of anatomical connections between the two hemispheres.

Nevertheless, acallosal individuals appear to have access to a series of compensatory pathways or mechanisms, and some of these mechanisms may be privileged over others in certain individuals, thus producing different manifestations of the disconnection syndrome. In fact, it seems that there are many individual variants of cerebral organization in acallosal patients. The question arises as to whether there exist certain types of interhemispheric transfer that are consistently failed, or accomplished, in all acallosal subjects. In this context Berlucchi and colleagues (1995) have proposed an interesting avenue of investigation. They suggest that callosal agenesis subjects frequently show deficits in procedural tasks that do not require access to conscious knowledge but that they may perform normally on certain tests of interhemispheric integration that are based on declarative, or conscious, knowledge. According to this view, the adaptation seen in the acallosal brain would essentially represent an attempt at maintaining unity of consciousness in the absence of the most important commissural pathway. This unity may be achieved through bilateral wiring of sensory systems and crossover of information at lower levels of the brain.

ACKNOWLEDGMENTS   This work was support by grants from the Québec Formation de Chercheurs et Aide à la Recherche (FCAR) and the Natural Science and Engineering Research Council of Canada (NSERC) awarded to Maryse Lassonde.

REFERENCES

AGLIOTI, S., G. BERLUCCHI, R. PALLINI, G. F. ROSSI, and G. TASSINARI, 1993. Hemispheric control of unilateral and bilateral responses to lateralized light stimuli after callosotomy and in callosal agenesis. *Exp. Brain Res.* 93:51–165.

ANDERMANN, E., F. ANDERMANN, M. JOUBERT, G. KARPATI, S. CARPENTER, and D. MELANSON, 1972. Familial agenesis of the corpus callosum with anterior horn cell disease: A syndrome of mental retardation areflexia and paraparesis. *Trans. Am. Neurol. Assoc.* 97:232–244.

ATLAS, S. W., R. A. ZIMMERMAN, D. BRUCE, L. SCHUT, L. T. BILANIUK, D. B. HACKNEY, H. I. GOLDBERG, and R. I.

GROSSMAN, 1988. Neurofibromatosis and agenesis of the corpus callosum in identical twins: MR diagnosis. *Am. J. Neuroradiol.* 9:598–601.

BARANZINI, S. E., G. DEL REY, N. NIGRO, I. SZIJAN, N. CHAMOLES, and J. C. CRESTO, 1997. Patient with Xp21 contiguous gene deletion syndrome in association with agenesis of the corpus callosum. *Am. J. Med. Genet.* 70 (3):216–221.

BARR, M. L. 1972. *The Human Nervous System: An Anatomical Viewpoint.* New York: Harper and Row.

BERLUCCHI, G., S. AGLIOTTI, C. A. MARZI, and G. TASSINARI, 1995. Corpus callosum and simple visuomotor integration. *Neuropsychologia* 33:923–936.

BOGEN, J. E., and P. J. VOGEL, 1962. Cerebral commissurotomy in man. *Bull. Los Angeles Neurol. Soc.* 27:169–172.

BOGEN, J. E., and P. J. VOGEL, 1975. Neurologic status in the long term following cerebral commissurotomy. In *Les Syndromes de Disconnexion Calleuse Chez l'Homme*, F. Michel and E. Schott, eds. Lyon, France: Hôpital Neurologique, pp. 227–251.

BREMER, F., 1966. Le corps calleux dans la dynamique cérébrale. *Experientia* 22:201–208.

BREMER, F., 1967. La physiologie du corps calleux à la lumière de travaux récents. *Laval Medical* 38:835–843.

BROVEDANI, P., D. BRIZZOLARA, G. CIONI, and G. FERETTI, 1996. *Interhemispheric integration in partial callosotomy and callosal agenesis: Two developmental cases.* Poster presented at the NATO ASI meeting on the role of the human corpus callosum in sensory/motor integration: Individual differences and clinial applications. Castelvecchio Pascoli Lucca, Italy, Sept. 1–10, 1996.

CAILLÉ, S., A. SCHIAVETTO, F. ANDERMANN, A. BASTOS, E. DE GUISE, and M. LASSONDE, 1999. Interhemispheric transfer without forebrain commissures. *NeuroCase* 5:109–118.

CHIARELLO, C. 1980. A house divided? Cognitive functioning with callosal agenesis. *Brain Lang.* 11:128–158.

CIONI, G., E. BARTALENA, and A. BOLDRINI, 1994. Callosal agenesis: Postnatal sonographic findings. In *Callosal Agenesis: A Natural Split Brain?*, M. Lassonde and M. A. Jeeves, eds. New York: Plenum Press, pp. 69–77.

CLARKE, J. M., and E. ZAIDEL, 1989. Simple reaction times to lateralized light flashes. *Brain* 112:849–870.

COOK, N. D., 1986. *The Brain Code: Mechanisms of Information Transfer and the Role of the Corpus Callosum.* London: Methuen.

CORBALLIS, M. C., and M. J. MORGAN, 1978. On the biological basis of human laterality. I: Evidence for a maturational left-right gradient. *Behav. Brain Sci.* 1:261–269.

DAVIDOFF, L. M., and C. G. DYKE, 1934. Agenesis of the corpus callosum its diagnosis by pneumoencephalography. *Am. J. Neuroradiol.* 32:1–10.

DENNIS, M., 1976. Impaired sensory and motor differentiation with corpus callosum agenesis: A lack of inhibition during ontogeny? *Neuropsychologia* 14:455–469.

DENNIS, M., 1977. Cerebral dominance in three forms of early brain disorder. In *Topics in Child Neurology*, M. E. Blaw, I. Rapin, and M. Kinsbourne, eds. New York: Spectrum, pp. 189–212.

DENNIS, M., 1981. Language in an congenitally acallosal brain. *Brain Lang.* 12:33–53.

DI STEFANO, M. R., H. C. SAUERWEIN, and M. LASSONDE, 1992. Influence of anatomical factors and spatial compatibility on the stimulus-response relationship in the absence of the corpus callosum. *Neuropsychologia* 30 (2):177–185.

DONNENFELD, A. E., R. J. PACKER, E. H. ZACHAI, C. M. CHEE,

B. SELLINGER, and B. S. EMANUEL, 1989. Clinical cytogenic and pedigree findings in 18 cases of Aicardi syndrome. *Am. J. Med. Genet.* 32:461–467.

DONOSO, A. D., and M. SANTANDER, 1982. Sindrome de desconexion en agenesia del cuerpo calloso. *Nervol. Colombia* 6:177–180.

DOTY, R. W., N. NEGRAO, and K. YAMAGA, 1973. The unilateral engram. *Acta Neurobiol. Exp. (Warsz.)* 33:711–728.

ETTLINGER, G., C. B. BLAKEMORE, A. MILNER, and J. WILSON, 1972. Agenesis of the corpus callosum: A behavioural investigation. *Brain* 95:327–346.

FERRIS, G. S., and M. M. DORSEN, 1975. Agenesis of the corpus callosum: Neuropsychological studies. *Cortex* 11:95–122.

FISCHER, M., S. B. RYAN, and W. B. DOBYNS, 1992. Mechanisms of interhemispheric transfer and patterns of cognitive function in acallosal patients of normal intelligence. *Arch. Neurol.* 49:271–277.

GAZZANIGA, M. S., 1987. Perceptual and attentional processes following callosal section in humans. *Neuropsychologia* 25:119–133.

GEFFEN, G. M., G. M. FORRESTER, D. L. JONES, and D. A. SIMPSON, 1994a. Auditory verbal learning and memory in cases of callosal agenesis. In *Callosal Agenesis: A Natural Split Brain?*, M. Lassonde and M. A. Jeeves, eds. New York: Plenum Press, pp. 247–260.

GEFFEN, G. M., J. NILSSON, D. A. SIMPSON, and M. A. JEEVES, 1994b. The development of interhemispheric transfer of tactile information in cases of callosal agenesis. In *Callosal Agenesis: A Natural Split Brain?*, M. Lassonde and M. A. Jeeves, eds. New York: Plenum Press, pp. 185–198.

GEOFFROY, G., 1994. Other syndromes frequently associated with callosal agenesis. In *Callosal Agenesis: A Natural Split Brain?*, M. Lassonde and M. A. Jeeves, eds. New York: Plenum Press, pp. 55–62.

GOLDSTEIN, M. N., and R. J. JOYNT, 1975. The long-term effects of callosal sectioning: Report of a second case. *Arch. Neurol.* 32:52–53.

GOTT, P. S., and R. E. SAUL, 1978. Agenesis of the corpus callosum: Limits of functional compensation. *Neurology* 28:1272–1279.

HAMILTON, C. R., K. M. RODRIGUEZ, and B. A. VERMEIRE, 1987. The cerebral commissures and midline stereopsis. *Invest. Ophthalmol. Vis. Sci.* 28:294.

HOLTZMAN, J. D., 1984. Interaction between cortical and subcortical areas: Evidence from human commissurotomy patients. *Vision Res.* 24:801–813.

IACOBONI, M., and E. ZAIDEL, 1995. Channels of the corpus callosum: Evidence from simple reaction times to lateralized flashes in the normal and the split brain. *Brain* 118:779–788.

INBAR, D., G. J. HALPERN, R. WEITZ, M. SADEH, and M. SHOHAT, 1997. Agenesis of the corpus callosum in a mother and son. *Am. J. Med. Genet.* 69 (2):152–154.

JAKOBSON, L., P. SERVOS, M. A. GOODALE, and M. LASSONDE, 1994. Control of proximal and distal components of prehension. *Brain* 117:1107–1113.

JEEVES, M. A., 1965. Psychological studies of three cases of congenital agenesis of the corpus callosum. In *Function of the Corpus Callosum*, E. G. Ettlinger, ed., London: Macmillan, pp. 73–94.

JEEVES, M. A., 1969. A comparison of interhemispheric transmission times in acallosals and normals. *Psychon. Sci.* 16:245–246.

JEEVES, M. A., 1979. Some limits of interhemispheric integra-

tion in cases of callosal agenesis. In *Structure and Function of Cerebral Commissures*, I. S. Russel, M. W. Van Hof, and G. Berlucchi, eds. London: Macmillan, pp. 449–474.

JEEVES, M. A., 1986. Callosal agenesis: Neuronal and developmental adaptations. In *Two Hemispheres—One Brain: Functions of the Corpus Callosum*, F. Lepore, M. Ptito, and H. H. Jaspers, eds. New York: Alan Liss, pp. 403–421.

JEEVES, M. A., 1991. Stereopsis in callosal agenesis and partial callosotomy. *Neuropsychologia* 29:19–34.

JEEVES, M. A., 1994. Callosal agenesis—A natural split-brain: Overview. In *Callosal Agenesis: A Natural Split Brain?*, M. Lassonde and M. A. Jeeves, eds. New York: Plenum Press, pp. 285–300.

JEEVES, M. A., and P. H. SILVER, 1988. The formation of finger grip during prehension in an acallosal patient. *Neuropsychologia* 26:153–159.

JEEVES, M. A., P. H. SILVER, and I. JACOBSON, 1988. Bimanual coordination in callosal agenesis and partial commissurotomy. *Neuropsychologia* 26:833–850.

KARNATH, H. O., M. SCHUMACHER, and C. W. WALLESCH, 1991. Limitations of interhemispheric extracallosal transfer of visual information in callosal agenesis. *Cortex* 27:345–350.

KINSBOURNE, M., and M. FISHER, 1971. Latency of crossed and uncrossed reaction in callosal agenesis. *Neuropsychologia* 9:472–473.

LASSONDE, M., 1986. The facilitatory influence of the corpus callosum on intrahemispheric processing. In *Two Hemispheres—One Brain: Functions of the Corpus Callosum*, F. Lepore, M. Ptito, and H. H. Jaspers, eds. New York: Alan Liss, pp. 335–350.

LASSONDE, M., 1994. Disconnection syndrome in callosal agenesis. In *Callosal Agenesis: A Natural Split Brain?*, M. Lassonde and M. A. Jeeves, eds. New York: Plenum Press, pp. 275–284.

LASSONDE, M., M. P. BRYDEN, and P. DEMERS, 1990. The corpus callosum and cerebral speech lateralization. *Brain Lang.* 38:195–206.

LASSONDE, M., H. C. SAUERWEIN, A. J. CHICOINE, and G. GEOFFROY, 1991. Absence of disconnection syndrome in callosal agenesis and early callosotomy: Brain reorganization or lack of structural specificity during ontogeny? *Neuropsychologia* 29:481–495.

LASSONDE, M., H. C. SAUERWEIN, and F. LEPORE, 1995. Extent and limits of callosal plasticity: Presence of disconnection signs in callosal agenesis. *Neuropsychologia* 33:989–1007.

LASSONDE, M., H. C. SAUERWEIN, N. MCCABE, L. LAURENCELLE, and G. GEOFFROY, 1988. Extent and limits of cerebral adjustment to early section or congenital absence of the corpus callosum. *Behav. Brain Res.* 30:165–181.

LEDOUX, J. E., G. DENTSOH, D. H. WILSON, and M. S. GAZZANIGA, 1977. Binocular depth perception and the anterior commissure in man. *Psychologist* 20:55.

LEPORE, F., M. LASSONDE, N. VEILLETTE, and J. P. GUILLEMOT, 1997. Interhemispheric differential thresholds for temperature discrimination in acallosal and split-brain subjects. *Neurospychologia* 35:1225–1231.

LINES, C. R., M. D. RUGG, and A. D. MILNER, 1984. The effect of stimulus intensity on visually evoked potential estimates of interhemispheric transmission time. *Exp. Brain Res.* 22:215–225.

LOESER, J. D., and E. C. ALVORD, 1968. Agenesis of the corpus callosum. *Brain* 91:553–570.

LYNN, R., D. C. BUCHANAN, G. M. FERNICHEL, and F. R.

FREEMON, 1980. Agenesis of the corpus callosum. *Arch. Neurol.* 37:444–445.

MARTIN, A. A., 1985. A qualitative limitation on visual transfer via the anterior commissure. *Brain* 108:43–63.

MARZI, C. A., P. BISIACCHI, and R. NICOLETTI, 1991. Is interhemispheric transfer of visuomotor information asymmetric? Evidence from a meta-analysis. *Neuropsychologia* 29:1163–1177.

MEERWALDT, J. D., 1983. Disturbance of spatial perception in a patient with agenesis of the corpus callosum. *Neuropsychologia* 21:161–165.

MILNER, A. D., 1982. Simple reaction times to lateralized visual stimuli in a case of callosal agenesis. *Neuropsychologia* 20:411–419.

MILNER, A. D., 1994. Visual integration in callosal agenesis. In *Callosal Agenesis: A Natural Split Brain?*, M. Lassonde and M. A. Jeeves, eds. New York: Plenum Press, pp. 171–185.

MILNER, A. D., and M. A. JEEVES, 1979. A review of behavioural studies of agenesis of the corpus callosum. In *Structure and Function of Cerebral Commissures*, I. S. Russel, M. W. Van Hof, and G. Berlucchi, eds. London: Macmillan, pp. 428–448.

MILNER, A. D., M. A. JEEVES, P. H. SILVER, C. R. LINES, and J. G. WILSON, 1985. Reaction times to lateralized visual stimuli in callosal agenesis: Stimulus and response factors. *Neuropsychologia* 23:323–331.

MITCHELL, D. E., and C. BLAKEMORE, 1970. Binocular depth perception and the corpus callosum. *Vision Res.* 10:49–54.

MOSCOVITCH, M., 1977. Development of lateralization of language functions and its relations to cognitive and linguistic development: A review and some theoretical speculations. In *Language Development and Neurological Theory*, S. J. Segalowitz and F. A. Gruber, eds. New York: Academic Press, pp. 193–211.

NAIKAR, M., and M. C. CORBALLIS, 1996. Perception of apparent motion across the retinal midline following commissurotomy. *Neuropsychologia* 34:297–309.

PANDYA, D. N., E. A. KAROL, and P. P. LELE, 1973. The distribution of the anterior commissure in the squirrel monkey. *Brain Res.* 49:177–180.

POFFENBERGER, A. T., 1912. Reaction time to retinal stimulation with special reference to time lost in conduction through nerve centers. *Arch. Psychol. (NY)* 23:1–73.

POIRRIER, P., S. MILJOURS, M. LASSONDE, and F. LEPORE, 1993. Sound localization in acallosal human listeners. *Brain* 116:53–69.

PREILOWSKI, B. F. B., 1972. Possible contribution of the anterior forebrain commissures to bilateral motor coordination. *Neuropsychologia* 10:267–277.

RAMACHADRAN, V. S., A. CRONIN-COLOMB, and J. J. MYERS, 1986. Perception of apparent motion in commissurotomy patients. *Nature* 320:328–359.

RAUCH, R. A., and J. R. JINKINS, 1994. Magnetic resonance imaging of corpus callosum dysgenesis. In *Callosal Agenesis: A Natural Split Brain?*, M. Lassonde and M. A. Jeeves, eds. New York: Plenum Press, pp. 83–96.

REIL, J. C., 1812. Mangel des mittleren und freyen Theils des Balkens im Menschengehirn. *Arch. Physiol.* 11:314–344.

REYNOLDS, M. D., and M. A. JEEVES, 1977. Further studies of tactile perception and motor coordination in agenesis of the corpus callosum. *Cortex* 13:257–272.

RIVEST, J., P. CAVANAGH, and M. LASSONDE, 1994. Interhemispheric depth judgment. *Neuropsychologia* 32:69–76.

RUGG, M. D., A. D. MILNER, and C. R. LINES, 1985. Visual evoked potentials to lateralised stimuli in two cases of callosal agenesis. *J. Neurol. Neurosurg. Psychiatry* 48:367–373.

SAUERWEIN, H., and M. LASSONDE, 1983. Intra- and interhemispheric processing of visual information in callosal agenesis. *Neuropsychologia* 21:167–171.

SAUERWEIN, H., and M. M. LASSONDE, 1994. Cognitive and sensori-motor functioning in the absence of the corpus callosum: Neuropsychological studies in callosal agenesis and callosotomized patients. *Behav. Brain Res.* 64:229–240.

SAUERWEIN, H., M. LASSONDE, B. CARDU, and G. GEOFFROY, 1981. Interhemispheric integration of sensory and motor functions in agenesis of the corpus callosum. *Neuropsychologia* 19:445–454.

SCHIAVETTO, A., F. LEPORE, and M. LASSONDE, 1993. Somesthetic discrimination thresholds in the absence of the corpus callosum. *Neuropsychologia* 31:695–707.

SERGENT, J., and J. MYERS, 1985. Manual blowing and verbal simple reactions to lateralized flashes of light in commissurotomized patients. *Percept. Psychophys.* 37:571–578.

SERUR, D., J. S. JERET, and K. WISNIEWSKI, 1988. Agenesis of the corpus callosum: Clinical neuroradiological and cytogenic studies. *Neuropediatrics* 19:87–91.

SILVER, P. H., and M. A. JEEVES, 1994. Motor coordination in callosal agenesis. In *Callosal Agenesis: A Natural Split Brain?*, M. Lassonde and M. A. Jeeves, eds. New York: Plenum Press, pp. 207–219.

SPERRY, R. W., 1961. Cerebral organization and behavior. *Science* 133:1749–1757.

SPERRY, R. W., 1968. Plasticity of neural maturation. *Dev. Biol. Suppl.* 2:306–327.

SPERRY, R. W., 1970. Perception in the absence of the neocortical commissures. In *Perception and Its Disorders*, Research Publication of the Association for Research in Nervous and Mental Diseases, Vol. 48. Baltimore: Williams and Wilkins, pp. 123–138.

SPERRY, R. W., M. S. GAZZANIGA, and J. E. BOGEN, 1969. Interhemispheric relationships: The neocortical commissures: Syndromes of hemisphere disconnection. In *Handbook of Clinical Neurology*, Vol. 4: *Disorders of Speech Perception and Symbolic Behaviour*, P. J. Vinken and J. W. Bruyn, eds. Amsterdam: Elsevier, pp. 273–290.

TASSINARI, G., S. AGLIOTI, R. PALLINI, G. BERLUCCHI, and G. ROSSI, 1994. Interhemispheric integration of simple visuomotor responses in patients with partial callosal defects. *Behav. Brain Res.* 64:141–149.

TEMPLE, C. M., and I. ILSLEY, 1994. Sound and shapes: Language and spatial cognition in callosal agenesis. In *Callosal Agenesis: A Natural Split Brain?*, M. Lassonde and M. A. Jeeves, eds. New York: Plenum Press, pp. 261–273.

VANASSE, M., L. FOREST, and M. LASSONDE, 1994. Short- and middle-latency somatosensory evoked potentials in callosal agenesis. In *Callosal Agenesis: A Natural Split Brain?*, M. Lassonde and M. A. Jeeves, eds. New York: Plenum Press, pp. 199–206.

WISNIEWSKI, K., and J. S. JERET, 1994. Callosal agenesis: Review of clinical pathological and cytogenetic features. In *Callosal Agenesis: A Natural Split Brain?*, M. Lassonde and M. A. Jeeves, eds. New York: Plenum Press, pp. 7–19.

ZAIDEL, D., and R. W. SPERRY, 1977. Some long-term motor effects of cerebral commissurotomy in man. *Neuropsychologia* 10:103–110.

COMMENTARY 15.1

Sensorimotor Integration in Agenesis of the Corpus Callosum

MARCO IACOBONI, MAYIM H. BIALIK, AND ERAN ZAIDEL

ABSTRACT The interhemispheric transfer time measured by the Poffenberger paradigm typically differs between split-brain patients and acallosals. Is this due to the use of different interhemispheric routes or to a different efficiency of the same interhemispheric route in the two types of callosal patients? The data presented here are in support of the latter hypothesis.

In their article on agenesis of the corpus callosum, Lassonde and colleagues review experimental evidence on interhemispheric sensorimotor integration mechanisms in patients born without a corpus callosum. They suggest that this evidence is relevant to the understanding of general mechanisms of interhemispheric sensorimotor integration in the normal brain.

The interhemispheric transmission time (IHTT), as measured by the crossed-uncrossed difference (CUD) in simple reaction times to lateralized flashes, is typically faster in normal subjects than in patients with agenesis of the corpus callosum, who in turn have a faster IHTT than complete commissurotomy patients. The faster IHTT in acallosals can be accounted for by a faster transfer time through the anterior commissure in acallosals and a slower transfer time through subcortical routes in commissurotomy patients. However, this hypothesis, seems to be ruled out by case S.P., reported by Lassonde and colleagues. This patient shows agenesis of both corpus callosum and anterior commissure and a CUD that is quite similar to, or even smaller than, the CUD of acallosal patients with presence of anterior commissure. Lassonde and colleagues interpret the faster

IHTT in acallosals than in commissurotomized patients as evidence of compensatory mechanisms that are present in patients born without the corpus callosum but not present in the surgical split brain. However, the CUD in both acallosals and commissurotomized patients seems to be sensitive to the manipulation of visual parameters (Clarke and Zaidel, 1989; Milner, 1994). This may be compatible with the notion that similar interhemispheric routes are used in both types of patients.

The CUD in split-brain patients seems not to be sensitive to motor manipulation (Iacoboni and Zaidel, 1995). To test whether this is true in acallosals also, we recently tested a patient with agenesis of the corpus callosum (M.M.) in three different versions of the Poffenberger paradigm that were previously administered to 75 normal subjects, two complete commissurotomy patients, and a patient with partial callosotomy (Iacoboni and Zaidel, 1995). The versions of the task that are relevant here are a canonical version (basic task) and a version in which the complexity of the motor response was increased (motor task). (For a detailed description, see Iacoboni and Zaidel (1995) and Chapter 12 in this volume.) M.M. had a CUD of 10.95 ms in the basic task and of 11.97 ms in the motor task, thus confirming that acallosals tend to have IHTTs that are longer than those of normals but shorter than those of commissurotomized patients. Further, M.M. did not show any task by CUD interactions, similar to commissurotomized patients, and in contrast to normal subjects (Iacoboni and Zaidel, 1995).

Taken together, these findings and the findings summarized by Milner (1994) show that the manipulation of visual parameters affects the CUD in acallosals and commissurotomized patients but not in normal subjects, whereas the manipulation of motor parameters affects the CUD in normal subjects but not in acallosals and commissurotomized patients. These findings further

MARCO IACOBONI Ahmanson Lovelace Brain Mapping Center, Neuropsychiatric Institute, Brain Research Institute, David Geffen School of Medicine, University of California at Los Angeles, Los Angeles, California.

MAYIM H. BIALIK AND ERAN ZAIDEL Interdepartmental program in Neuroscience, University of California, Los Angeles, California.

370

support the notion that patients born without the corpus callosum and commissurotomized patients use similar interhemispheric routes in the Poffenberger paradigm, in spite of their differences in IHTT. It is possible that because acallosals were forced to use these routes since birth, whereas commissurotomy patients were able to use the callosal route at least until the surgical section of the cerebral commissures was made, the very same interhemispheric routes are more efficient in acallosals than in commissurotomized patients. However, we also have to keep in mind that the usually concomitant epilepsy and especially the associated pharmacological treatment in commissurotomy patients might contribute

to differences in IHTT between acallosals and surgical split-brain patients.

REFERENCES

CLARKE, J. M., and E. ZAIDEL, 1989. Simple reaction times to lateralized flashes: Varieties of interhemispheric communication routes. *Brain* 112:849–870.

IACOBONI, M., and E. ZAIDEL, 1995. Channels of the corpus callosum: Evidence from simple reaction times to lateralized flashes in the normal and the split brain. *Brain* 118:779–788.

MILNER, A. D., 1994. Visual integration in callosal agenesis. In *Callosal Agenesis*, M. Lassone, and M. A. Jeeves, eds. New York, Plenum Press.

COMMENTARY 15.2

Cerebral Plasticity in Callosal Agenesis Versus Callosotomy

JEFFREY M. CLARKE

ABSTRACT Individuals who are born without a corpus callosum (callosal agenesis) undergo considerably more brain reorganization than do split-brain patients whose cerebral commissures are transected in adolescence or adulthood for treatment of intractable epilepsy. Findings from two split-brain patients (L.B. and N.G.) indicate that certain subordinate anatomical pathways can sometimes play a more prominent role in these patients than is the case for normal, callosum-intact, individuals. The anatomical loci associated with interhemispheric transfer times in the Poffenberger (1912) task for acallosals, split-brain patients, and normals are speculated on and discussed.

Lassonde, Sauerwein, and Lepore's informative review of callosal agenesis discusses how certain sensory and motor interhemispheric functions are preserved in individuals born without a corpus callosum, while other functions follow an interhemispheric disconnection pattern. One of the important questions that emerges from this research is to what extent the interhemispheric, intrahemispheric, and subcortical pathways have been reorganized in acallosals to compensate for the lack of a corpus callosum. As Lassonde and colleagues discuss, one way of addressing this question is to compare findings from acallosals and commissurotomized (i.e., split-brain) patients. Whereas callosal agenesis is a neurogenesis disorder in which there is presumably considerable cerebral reorganization by birth, commissurotomy involves surgical section of the corpus callosum, and possibly other forebrain commissures, at an age when there is much less opportunity for significant neuronal reorganization. For example, acallosals typically can name items placed out of view in their left hand, while split-brain patients

JEFFREY M. CLARKE University of North Texas, Denton, Texas.

cannot. Apparently, early neuronal reorganization in acallosals includes the development of effective ipsilateral somatosensory connections (at least for touch) between their left hand and their left hemisphere, which, as in normals, is typically specialized for speech. Left-hand anomia persists in split-brain patients, even some 30 years after their surgeries, suggesting that a comparable cerebral plasticity within this sensory system is not possible in split-brain patients. In other sensory or motor domains, certain split-brain patients have exhibited signs of cerebral plasticity. I will now discuss two such cases.

Split-brain patients L.B. and N.G. are undoubtedly the most tested split-brain patients in history. All of the forebrain commissures, including the corpus callosum and the anterior and hippocampal commisures, were transected in these patients. Both L.B. and N.G. demonstrate the classic disconnection syndromes (Sperry, Gazzaniga, and Bogen, 1969), yet each exhibits unique evidence for cerebral plasticity. Unlike most split-brain patients, L.B. demonstrates unusually effective ipsilateral motor control of both hands (e.g., Zaidel and Sperry, 1977). This factor appears to play a role in L.B.'s performance on the Poffenberger (1912) task. L.B. was the only one of four split-brain patients whose crossed-uncrossed differences (CUDs) in reaction times were unaffected by changes in visual stimulus parameters (Clarke and Zaidel, 1989; see also Commentary 13.1 in this volume). Whereas subcortical visual interhemispheric pathways are presumably responsible for the CUDs in the other three split-brain patients, L.B.'s CUDs probably reflect an intrahemispheric effect that represents the difference in the efficiency of ipsilateral and contralateral motor pathways. This may also be the case for an acallosal patient whom we tested (Clarke and Zaidel, 1989; however, see Milner, 1994). As Lassonde and colleagues note, other acallosals have CUDs that do vary with visual stimulus parameters, which implicates interhemispheric transfer across visual pathways in these patients (i.e., anterior commissure or subcortical visual pathways). Acallosals also have enhanced ipsilateral motor control of their hands and yet their CUDs typically reflect visual transfer, suggesting that interhemispheric transfer along noncallosal visual routes is generally more efficient than ipsilateral motor pathways. This is consistent with Lassonde and colleagues' observation that the absence of a corpus callosum may produce disinhibition of ipsilateral motor pathways, which may, in turn, conflict with the contralateral motor system, resulting in poorer overall motor control.

Patient N.G. is unique among split-brain patients for being able to cross-compare left and right visual field stimuli (see Zaidel, 1995, for a review). As Zaidel and colleagues have recently shown, she can cross-compare nonverbalizeable geometric figures, as well as letters presented in the same case (e.g., AA) but not in different cases (e.g., Aa). She is less able to cross-compare colors. Importantly, N.G. can do these comparisons while being unable to name the stimulus in her left visual field. Presumably, visual information is being transferred between her hemispheres via subcortical visual pathways and is processed at a level that allows for perceptual comparisons but not verbal naming. The transfer may even be unidirectional, from the left hemisphere to the nonspeaking right hemisphere, which also would explain why she cannot name left-visual-field (right-hemisphere) stimuli (Zaidel, 1995). The subcortical visual system is sensitive to such rudimentary visual characteristics as movement, stimulus position, line orientation, and contrast. N.G. may have a particularly effective subcortical visual system that allows for cross-comparisons of stimuli based on such features as the orientation and thickness of the lines or edges that make up a stimulus. Acallosal patients may, like N.G., also have developed a highly effective visual subcortical system. As Lassonde and colleagues note, the subcortical visual system may be able to transfer certain types of visuospatial information, while more complex visual pattern information that, in turn, can be named is probably transferred across the anterior commissures in acallosal patients who have this structure. This latter function may be unique to acallosals, since interhemispheric transfer of visual pattern information is not possible in split-brain patients with intact anterior commissures (McKeever et al., 1981; Holtzman, 1984).

In both acallosals and split-brain patients, one should not rule out the possibility of interhemispheric cross-cuing or intrahemispheric guessing strategies that otherwise may be interpreted as noncallosal interhemispheric transfer. Reports that split-brain patients can transfer nonsensory abstract codes (e.g., Sergent, 1987) may actually be due to such strategies (e.g., Corballis and Trudel, 1993). Zaidel (1995) points out that such strategies are particularly effective for binary-choice tasks, in which a small set of easily learned, verbalizable stimuli are used.

Lassonde and colleagues note that most acallosals and split-brain patients tested to date on the Poffenberger sensorimotor integration task exhibit CUDs that are typically an order of magnitude larger than those in normals. Furthermore, unlike normals, the CUDs of many of these patients vary with visual stimulus parameters, such as stimulus eccentricity and/or intensity. As has already been discussed, this implicates a visual-sensory interhemispheric route in these patients. In split-brain patients who lack all of the forebrain commissures, the only possible visual interhemispheric route that remains is the subcortical intertectal (i.e., collicular) commissure. In acallosal patients, visual transfer may be possible via the intertectal commissure, the posterior commissure (which appears to have tectal targets; see Milner, 1994), and/or the anterior commissure. Lassonde and colleagues rule out the anterior commissure as contributing to the CUDs in acallosals who have this structure. If the intertectal commissure is responsible for the CUDs in acallosals, as appears to be the case in most split-brain patients, then one would expect the CUDs of acallosals and of split-brain patients to behave in a similar way. Yet differences are apparent across these two populations. As Lassonde and colleagues note, the CUDs of acallosals are typically smaller (~ 20 ms) than that of split-brain patients (20–96 ms). Furthermore, while stimulus eccentricity manipulations have similar effects on the CUDs of acallosals and split-brain patients, changes in stimulus intensity have greater effects on the CUDs in acallosals than in split-brain patients (Clarke and Zaidel, 1989). These differences between acallosals and split-brain patients could be due to either differences in organization of the subcortical pathways or a commissure other than the intertectal commissure being responsible for the CUDs in acallosals. The posterior commissure is one possibility, as suggested by Lassonde and colleagues' findings in acallosal patient S.P., whose posterior, but not anterior, commissure is intact. The anterior commissure is the other possible route in acallosal patients who have this structure. It would be somewhat surprising to find that the anterior commissure can transfer pattern information in acallosals but cannot transfer information pertaining to the presence of a light flash. The similarity in CUD measures between patient S.P., who lacks an anterior commissure, and other acallosals who have an anterior commissure suggests that interhemispheric transfer time is similar across anterior and posterior commissure pathways. Recall that the anterior commissure is apparently reorganized in acallosals to include visual pathways from the temporal lobe. Since this reorganization does not take place in split-brain patients whose anterior commissure is intact, this would explain why CUDs are equivalent for split-brain patients who either have or lack an anterior commissure.

The abnormally long CUDs in acallosals and in split-brain patients demonstrate that the corpus callosum is responsible for the CUD measures in neurologically normal individuals. Which callosum channel is responsible for this measure in normals? Several investigators have speculated that anterior, presumably motor, interhemispheric pathways are responsible. Since changes in visual stimulus parameters affect reaction times but not the CUDs of normals, this has been considered evidence that the transfer is nonvisual. While visual stimulus parameters do affect overall reaction times, it may be unreasonable to also expect measurable changes in a 3- to 6-ms CUD if it did actually represent interhemispheric visual transfer involving a monosynaptic connection. However, further arguments for motor transfer come from event-related potential (ERP) studies involving scalp recordings from normal individuals. On the basis of the latencies of the N160 component, Lines, Rugg, and Milner (1984) found electrophysiological measures of interhemispheric transfer time (ITT) to be 3 ms over central (motor) areas, and 13–16 ms over occipital (visual) areas. Interhemispheric motor pathways are implicated for the behavioral CUD, since the central ERP measures are most similar to the 3- to 6-ms behavioral CUD measures and since the occipital ITT measures are influenced by visual parameters while the central measures are not. We obtained somewhat different findings from ERP measures recorded directly from within the depths of the occipital lobes of three epileptic patients with intact corpora callosa who were neurosurgical candidates for treatment of their epilepsy (Clarke, Halgren, and Chauvel, 1999). ERPs were recorded while the patients participated in a lateralized go/no-go simple visual discrimination task. On the basis of their intracerebral N150 latencies, the average ITT from these patients was 5 ms. Although the sample size is small, it is interesting to note that the 5-ms mean ITT falls within the 3- to 6-ms behavioral CUD range of normals. This suggests that a visual callosum channel, within the splenium of the corpus callosum, may, under certain conditions (see below), account for the behavioral CUD values in callosum-intact individuals. This interpretation is supported by the finding that eight out of nine partial

callosotomy patients with intact spleniums demonstrated normal CUDs (see Lassonde et al., this volume). Apparently, both visual and motor interhemispheric routes can account for the CUDs in normals. In a Poffenberger task all cortical and subcortical interhemispheric channels are presumably activated in parallel, with processing terminating in a horse race fashion by the one that completes processing first (cf. Clarke and Zaidel, 1989). Following this model, particular channels may take precedence depending on particular stimulus and/or procedural factors. For example, Iacoboni, Fried, and Zaidel (1994) present evidence suggesting that motor, but not visual, transfer is responsible for normal CUDs when stimuli are presented at large eccentricities, whereas either motor or visual transfer can account for normal CUDs when stimuli are presented at smaller eccentricities.

In conclusion, comparisons between acallosals and split-brain patients can reveal the extent of cerebral plasticity in interhemispheric functions that is possible from noncallosal commissures. Following Lassonde and colleagues' example, future studies with acallosals will want to use MRI to determine which forebrain commissures are intact in their patients to further clarify the functional role of the different interhemispheric pathways.

REFERENCES

CLARKE, J. M., E. HALGREN, and P. CHAUVEL, 1999. Intracranial ERPs in humans during a lateralized visual oddball task: I. Occipital and peri-Rolandic recordings. *Clin. Neurophysiol.* 110:1210–1225.

CLARKE, J. M., and E. ZAIDEL, 1989. Simple reaction times to lateralized light flashes: Varieties of interhemispheric communication routes. *Brain* 112:849–870.

CORBALLIS, M. C., and C. I. TRUDEL, 1993. Role of the forebrain commissures in interhemispheric integration. *Neuropsychology* 7:306–324.

HOLTZMAN, J. D., 1984. Interactions between cortical and subcortical visual areas: Evidence from human commissurotomy patients. *Vision Res.* 24:801–813.

IACOBONI, M., I. FRIED, and E. ZAIDEL, 1994. Callosal transmission time before and after partial commissurotomy. *Neuroreport* 5:2521–2524.

LINES, C. R., M. D. RUGG, and A. D. MILNER, 1984. The effect of stimulus intensity on visual evoked potential estimates of interhemispheric transfer time. *Experimental Brain Res.* 57:89–98.

McKEEVER, W. F., K. F. SULLIVAN, S. M. FERGUSON, and M. RAYPORT, 1981. Typical cerebral hemisphere disconnection deficits following corpus callosum section despite sparing of the anterior commissure. *Neuropsychologia*, 18, 745–755.

MILNER, A. D., 1994. Visual integration in callosal agenesis. In *Callosal Agenesis*, M. Lassonde and M. A. Jeeves, eds. New York: Plenum Press, pp. 171–183.

POFFENBERGER, A. T., 1912. Reaction time to retinal stimulation, with special reference to the time lost in conduction through nerve centers. *Arch. Psychol.* 23:1–73.

SERGENT, J., 1987. A new look at the human split-brain. *Brain* 110:1375–1392.

SPERRY, R. W., M. S. GAZZANIGA, and J. E. BOGEN, 1969. Interhemispheric relationships: The neocortical commissures; syndromes of hemisphere disconnection. In *Handbook of Clinical Neurology*, P. J. Vinken and G. W. Bruyn, eds. Amsterdam: North-Holland, pp. 273–289.

ZAIDEL, D., and R. W. SPERRY, 1977. Some long-term motor effects of cerebral commissurotomy in man. *Neuropsychologia* 15:193–204.

ZAIDEL, E., 1995. Interhemispheric transfer in the split brain: Long-term status following complete cerebral commissurotomy. In *Brain Asymmetry*, R. J. Davidson and K. Hugdahl, eds. Cambridge, Mass.: MIT Press, pp. 491–532.

Commentary 15.3

Interhemispheric and Intrahemispheric Mechanisms of Visuomotor Integration in Callosal Agenesis

MARIROSA DI STEFANO AND CARLA SALVADORI

ABSTRACT We have measured in a "healthy" acallosal subject crossed and uncrossed reaction times with both distal and proximal movements. It is found that the crossed-uncrossed differences measured in the two hemifields are highly asymmetric in that, for both types of movements, the time lag between crossed and uncrossed reactions is very large for responses in the left hemifield and null or negative for responses in the right hemifield. This indicates that visuomotor integration between an input to the right hemisphere and an output from the left hemisphere (i.e., right hand responding to left stimuli) is abnormally long, whereas visuomotor integration is extremely fast when the right stimuli (which are detected by the left hemisphere) are responded to by the left hand. The striking laterality effect suggests a functional asymmetry in the hemispheric control of both distal and proximal motility of the ipsilateral hand. The fast visuomotor processing reflects involvement of the ipsilateral motor routes from the left hemisphere that make interhemispheric transmission unnecessary for the execution of the crossed responses by the left hand. On the contrary, the lengthened interhemispheric transfer, due to the callosum lack, is responsible for the long visuomotor integration shown on responses of the right hand to the left stimuli.

Functional superiority of the left hemisphere in controlling distal and proximal motility is not peculiar of the acallosal brains, as suggested by the recent magnetic resonance imaging results on normal subjects. In acallosal subjects, however, the direct access of the left hemisphere to the motility of the left hand becomes an especially efficient mechanism for mastering fast visuomotor integration.

Lassonde and colleagues discuss various issues related to interhemispheric integration in callosal agenesis. In this commentary, as was done in Commentary 15.2, we will focus on sensorimotor integration in particular, using the Poffenberger paradigm.

MARIROSA DI STEFANO AND CARLA SALVADORI Dipartimento di Fisiologia e Biochimica, Pisa, Italy.

The time needed for intrahemispheric and interhemispheric integration of simple visuomotor responses is classically estimated by the Poffenberger paradigm. The task compares the manual reaction times (RT) for stimuli briefly presented in the same (ipsilateral) or in the opposite (contralateral) visual field as the responding hand. Owing to the organization of visual and motor pathways, the uncrossed reactions performed on ipsilateral trials are faster than the crossed reactions of contralateral trials because the latter require an additional time for information transfer across the two sides of the brain. Ever since the pioneering study (Poffenberger, 1912) the crossed-uncrossed difference (CUD) is considered an estimate of the time needed for interhemispheric communication, and indeed, the CUD is found to be extremely long in patients with acquired or congenital absence of the corpus callosum (Hoptman and Davidson, 1994).

The crucial question raised by the Poffenberger paradigm concerns the nature—motor or visual—of the information that is interhemispherically transmitted in the crossed condition of response.

There is now converging evidence indicating that interhemispheric integration of visuomotor responses is subserved by both motor and visual callosal routes (Iacoboni and Zaidel, 1995). In normals the motor channel dominates, as indicated by the fact that manipulations of the brightness and the eccentricity of visual stimuli affect overall RT but do not modify the interhemispheric transmission time (Berlucchi et al., 1977; Clarke and Zaidel, 1989; Iacoboni and Zaidel, 1995).

One can argue, however, that interhemispheric transfer of the motor command might not occur when the responses to contralateral stimuli are performed by proximal movements. In fact, according to clinical and ex-

CONTROLS

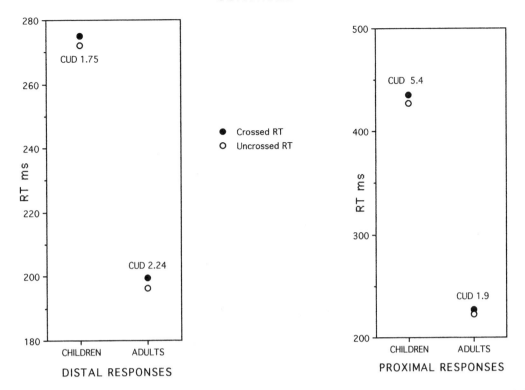

FIGURE 15.2. Crossed and uncrossed RT measured in normal controls with distal (keypress) and proximal (lever pull) movements. Data for adults are from Di Stefano et al. (1980). Data for children are from Di Stefano and Salvadori (1998).

perimental evidence, the proximal motility is likely to be subserved by bilateral motor pathways (Laget et al., 1977; Kuypers, 1989; Benecke, Meyer, and Freund, 1991), and then it is theoretically possible that a visual input channeled into a single hemisphere might directly initiate proximal movements on both sides of the body. If this were the case, the crossed proximal responses, being controlled by the same hemisphere that is receiving the visual stimulus, would not require interhemispheric integration, and the CUD would be absent.

In Figure 15.2 are reported the crossed and uncrossed RT measured in normal subjects—adults and children— on distal responses (consisting in a keypress by flexion of the thumb) and proximal responses (consisting in a lever pull by flexion of the forearm). The results point out that both types of movements are associated with small but significant CUDs due to the systematic prevalence in speed of the uncrossed reactions over the crossed ones. The finding is taken as an evidence that in normal subjects, the motor output does not interfere with visuomotor integration, since the crossed reactions, both distal and proximal, require additional time for interhemispheric information transfer (Di Stefano et al., 1980).

It has been suggested that the brains with congenital lack of the corpus callosum might rely on ipsilateral motor pathways more than normal brains do, as a compensatory mechanism for the absence of direct interhemispheric connections (Dennis, 1976; Laget et al., 1977). Accordingly, one might expect in acallosal subjects the annulment of CUD for proximal responses.

We have recently studied with the Poffenberger paradigm an acallosal boy, F.B., who has no other neurological deficits or lesions but the lack of a corpus callosum (Di Stefano and Salvadori, 1998). This "healthy" agenic subject performed visuomotor responses by distal and proximal movements under the same experimental conditions as the normals in Figure 15.2. F.B. was tested several times between 8 and 11 years of age and provided, overall, 480 distal RTs and 320 proximal RTs, that is, 120 distal and 80 proximal responses for each of the four hand/field combinations. The results are reported in Figures 15.3 and 15.4.

Figure 15.3 shows that with both types of movements, the crossed reactions of F.B. are much slower than the uncrossed ones, yielding crossed-uncrossed differences that are about 10 times longer than corresponding CUDs of the normal controls. From these results, one might infer that in callosal agenesis the ipsilateral motor routes are not involved in the crossed visuomotor integration. The reactions to contralateral stimuli are abnormally

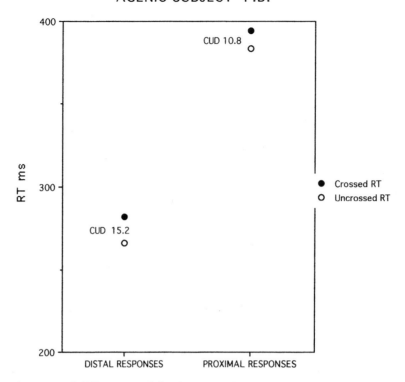

AGENIC SUBJECT F.B.

FIGURE 15.3. Crossed and uncrossed RT measured in the agenic subject F.B. under the same experimental conditions as the controls in Figure 15.3. Each value is the mean of the medians scored in each session in the two crossed and the two uncrossed hand-field combinations.

delayed, regardless of the type of movement performed for responding, and this suggests that in acallosal subjects the manual responses, both distal and proximal, are entirely controlled by the opposite hemisphere (Aglioti et al., 1993).

However, when the data of F.B. are analyzed according to the side of stimulus presentation, the rate of crossed visuomotor integration is found to be strikingly asymmetric between the two hemispheres.

Inspection of Figure 15.4 reveals that the extent of the CUDs measured in the two hemifields is quite different. In the left hemifield (LVF), for both types of movements the CUD is extremely long because of the extreme lengthening of the crossed reactions. In the right hemifield (RVF) for distal responses the CUD is virtually null, owing to the tendency of the crossed reactions to be as fast as the corresponding uncrossed RT; on proximal responses the right CUD is negative as a result of the significant prevalence in speed of the crossed RT. Statistical analyses rule out that the left/right asymmetry of distal and proximal CUDs might depend on unequal detection of the visual stimuli in the two hemifields and indicate that the laterality effect is related to the very different times that the left and the right hand require for reacting to contralateral stimuli.

It is found that the crossed visuomotor integration between stimuli in the LVF (detected by the right hemisphere, RH) and responses of the right hand is extremely slow. The finding is quite compatible with the view that this hand is under the full control of the opposite hemisphere and then an interhemispheric transfer is needed to execute the crossed reactions. The defective interhemispheric communication due to the callosal lack does account for the very long CUDs assessed in the LVF. Indeed, the almost identical distal and proximal CUDs (distal: 31.1 ms, proximal: 31.8 ms) strongly suggest that the crossed responses of the right hand, both distal and proximal, are dependent on a common mechanism of interhemispheric transmission with constant temporal characteristics.

On the assumption that the motor outcome of each hand is entirely controlled by the opposite hemisphere, the very fast integration between stimuli in the RVF (reaching the left hemisphere, LH) and responses by the left hand seems rather paradoxical. The contralateral processing (which would require the time-consuming interhemispheric transmission) is carried out with virtually no delay when the left hand responds with distal movements, as indicated by the near null CUD in the RVF. When the responses are performed by proximal

378   INTERHEMISPHERIC SENSORIMOTOR INTEGRATION: BEHAVIORAL STUDIES

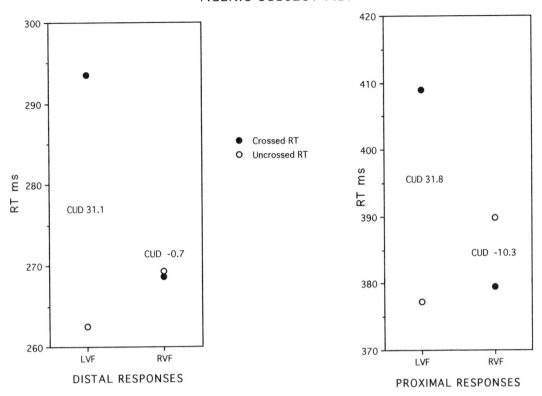

FIGURE 15.4. Crossed and uncrossed RT of F.B. as function of the side of stimulus presentation (left hemifield: LVF, right hemifield: RVF). Each value is the mean of the medians scored in each session in the four hand-field combinations.

movements, the crossed reactions of the left hand are even faster than the uncrossed responses of the right hand (advantaged by the processing in the same hemisphere of both stimulus and response), leading to a large and negative CUD in the RVF.

It is unlikely that the striking asymmetry in the velocity of visuomotor integration between the two hemispheres might result from a differential transmission rate through the indirect pathways subserving interhemispheric communication in the acallosal brains (Milner et al., 1985; Aglioti et al., 1993). It is most conceivable that the crossed integration between stimuli detected by the LH and responses by the left hand is not dependent on information transfer from the LH to the RH and is instead performed intrahemispherically within the LH.

All together, the results of the agenic subject suggest an additional motor control of the left hand through ipsilateral descending routes that make the interhemispheric transfer unnecessary for the execution of crossed responses. In this case the efficacy of the ipsilateral motor command determines the speed of the contralateral integration. If we consider that the crossed reactions of the left hand are subserved by this ipsilateral system, then its effectiveness in controlling the manual responses

might be hinted by the extent of distal and proximal CUDs in the RVF. As expected, the ipsilateral motor control seems to be mostly effective on the proximal movements. A large and negative CUD parallels in fact the consistent advantage of the proximal crossed responses of the left hand over the uncrossed responses of the right hand. Although on the distal responses there is no systematic prevalence of the crossed reactions, the null CUD shows that effectiveness of the ipsilateral pathway is good enough to command finger responses of the left hand that are as fast as the corresponding reactions of the right hand, controlled by the contralateral hemisphere.

In conclusion the different extent of the CUDs measured in the two hemifields of the agenic subject reveals that with both distal and proximal movements the visuomotor integration on the contralateral hand-field combinations is highly asymmetric in speed. The very fast processing of contralateral stimuli by the left hand can be ascribed to the functional superiority of the left hemisphere in controlling the ipsilateral motor output. In agreement with earlier neurological reports (De Renzi, 1989) recent magnetic resonance imaging studies have provided evidence that in normal subjects the left hemisphere is substantially activated during ipsilateral hand movements, unlike the right hemisphere (Kim et al., 1993; Roth et al., 1996). It may be argued that in the congenital lack of the corpus callosum, the direct access of the left hemisphere to the motility of the left hand becomes an especially efficient mechanism for mastering fast visuomotor integration, sparing a long interhemispheric transfer that, nevertheless, is needed when the crossed responses are performed by the right hand.

Finally, it is worth noting that the asymmetric pattern of visuomotor integration found in the acallosal boy F.B. with both distal and proximal responses is shared by three agenic subjects, comparable to F.B. for the lack of neural pathologies, whose results on distal responses are available from the literature (Kinsbourne and Fisher, 1971; Clarke and Zaidel, 1989; Tassinari et al., 1994). The reported data reveal that all these "healthy" acallosals present a very large CUD in the LVF and a very small or negative CUD in the RVF.

REFERENCES

AGLIOTI, S., G. BERLUCCHI, R. PALLINI, ET AL., 1993. Hemispheric control of unilateral and bilateral responses to lateralized light stimuli after callosotomy and in callosal agenesis. *Exp. Brain Res.* 95:151–165.

BENECKE, R., B. U. MEYER, and H. J. FREUND, 1991. Reorganization of descending motor pathways in patients after hemispherectomy and severe hemispheric lesions demonstrated by magnetic brain stimulation. *Exp. Brain Res.* 83:419–426.

BERLUCCHI, G., F. CREA, M. DI STEFANO, and G. TASSINARI, 1977. Influence of spatial stimulus-response compatibility on reaction time of ipsilateral and contralateral hand to lateralized light stimuli. *J. Exp. Psychol. Hum. Percept. Perform.* 3:505–517.

CLARKE, J. M., and E. ZAIDEL, 1989. Simple reaction times to lateralized light flashes: Varieties of interhemispheric communication routes. *Brain* 112:871–894.

DENNIS, M., 1976. Impaired sensory and motor differentiation with corpus callosum agenesis: A lack of callosal inhibition during ontogeny? *Neuropsychologia* 14:455–469.

DE RENZI, E., 1989. Apraxia. In *Handbook of Neuropsychology*, Vol. 2, F. Boller and J. Grafman, eds. Amsterdam: Elsevier, pp. 245–263.

DI STEFANO, M., M. MORELLI, C. A. MARZI, and G. BERLUCCHI, 1980. Hemispheric control of unilateral and bilateral movements of proximal and distal parts of the arms as inferred from simple RT to lateralized light stimuli in man. *Exp. Brain Res.* 38:197–204.

DI STEFANO, M., and C. SALVADORI, 1998. Asymmetry of the interhemispheric visuomotor integration in callosal agenesis. *NeuroReport* 9:1331–1335.

HOPTMAN, M. J., and R. J. DAVIDSON, 1994. How and why do the two cerebral hemispheres interact? *Psychol. Bull.* 116:195–219.

IACOBONI, M., and E. ZAIDEL, 1995. Channels of the corpus callosum: Evidence from simple RT to lateralized flashes in the normal and the split brain. *Brain* 118:779–788.

KIM, S. J., J. ASHE, K. HENDRICH, ET AL., 1993. Functional magnetic resonance imaging of motor cortex: Hemispheric asymmetry and handedness. *Science* 261:615–617.

KINSBOURNE, M., and M. FISHER, 1971. Latency of uncrossed and of crossed reaction in callosal agenesis. *Neuropsychologia* 9:471–473.

KUYPERS, H. G. J. M., 1989. Motor system organization. In *Encyclopedia of Neuroscience*, Suppl. 1, G. Adelman, ed. Boston: Birkhauser, pp. 107–110.

LAGET, P., A. M. D'ALLEST, R. FIHEY, and O. LORTHOLARY, 1977. L'interet des potentials evoques somesthesiques homolateraux dans les agenesies du corps calleux. *Rev. Electro-encephalogr. Neurophysiol. Clin.* 7:498–502.

MILNER, A. D., M. A. JEEVES, P. H. SILVER, ET AL., 1985. Reaction times to lateralized visual stimuli in callosal agenesis: Stimulus and response factors. *Neuropsychologia* 23:323–331.

POFFENBERGER, A. T., 1912. Reaction time to retinal stimulation with special reference to the time lost in conduction through nervous centers. *Arch. Psychol.* 23:1–73.

ROTH, M., J. DECETY, M. RAYBAUDI, ET AL., 1996. Possible involvement of primary motor cortex in mentally simulated movement: A functional magnetic resonance imaging study. *NeuroReport* 7:1280–1284.

TASSINARI, G., S. AGLIOTI, R. PALLINI, G. BERLUCCHI, and G. ROSSI, 1994. Interhemispheric integration of simple visuomotor responses in patients with partial callosal defects. *Behav. Brain Res.* 64:141–149.

Editorial Commentary 3

Current Directions in Behavioral Studies of Callosal Functions

Eran Zaidel and Marco Iacoboni

The section on partial and complete split-brain patients includes a chapter by Iacoboni and Zaidel on partial callosotomy. They argue that although callosal anatomy is more complex than was previously thought and a precise topographical arrangement of fibers connecting various cortical areas is probably restricted to limited regions of the corpus callosum (CC), it is nonetheless possible with a careful series of behavioral studies to define the functional status of callosal channels in patients with partial callosal section or partial callosal lesions.

Marzi and colleagues use ERP to investigate fast and slow callosal channels responsible for visuomotor transfer, compatible with the delays observed in chronometric studies in normals and partial split-brain patients. They observe some consistency but also some inconsistency between electrophysiological measures and behavioral measures in partial split-brain patients.

Hughdahl, in his commentary to Iacoboni and Zaidel's chapter, emphasizes the role of attentional channels that would be supramodal, not linked to any specific sensory modality. The presence of these channels may actually explain the inconsistency between the electrophysiological and behavioral measures.

In their commentary on Marzi and colleagues' chapter, Proverbio and Zani clarify the nature of interhemispheric sensorimotor interaction in the split brain by juxtaposing behavioral and ERP evidence in callosotomy patient J.W. While Marzi and colleagues show a discrepancy between behavioral and ERP measures of the CUD in SRT in two partial callosotomy patients,

Proverbio and Zani's commentary documents a parallel between behavioral and ERP evidence for interhemispheric transfer of sensorimotor signals in complete callosotomy patient J.W. Proverbio and Zani chose to focus on choice RT with stimuli consisting of horizontal and vertical gratings to engage the ventral visual stream and make the measurements more sensitive to visual parameters. They argue that targets consisting of small patches of light engage the dorsal stream conveyed by the collicular-parietal pathway and sensitive only to motion and location.

J.W. had much reduced early components (P1, N1) of the ERP over the hemisphere ipsilateral to the stimulus, consistent with visual disconnection. By contrast, late ERP components, specifically a P300 selective to target stimuli, did appear over the ipsilateral hemisphere at about normal latency and amplitude. This means that robust decision/response codes were immediately available to the nonviewing hemisphere. That is consistent with Reuter-Lorenz's thesis that early attentional processes show disconnection, whereas response initiation processes are shared between the disconnected hemispheres (see chapter, this volume).

However, Proverbio and Zani also describe a left neglect gradient in J.W., which they attribute to disconnection. We have not observed a similar gradient in any of four complete commissurotomy patients, including those who, like J.W., exhibited a CUD which is sensitive to eccentricity (Clarke and Zaidel, 1989).

Proverbio and Zani's discussion drives home the increased inferential power provided by the confluence of behavioral and physiological data in the same experiment, by analyzing separately the effects of crossed and uncrossed responses. First they show both behaviorally and physiologically that uncrossed (i.e., hemispherically pure) responses in the LH (RVF/right hand) exhibit a bias to the right (faster RT at 7° than at 4°) and a neglect of LVF targets. They proceed to contrast this pattern

ERAN ZAIDEL   Department of Psychology, University of California at Los Angeles, Los Angeles, California.

MARCO IACOBONI   Ahmanson Lovelace Brain Mapping Center, Neuropsychiatric Institute, Brain Research Institute, David Geffen School of Medicine, University of California at Los Angeles, Los Angeles, California.

with crossed responses (RVF/left hand, LVF/right hand). The behavioral data do not allow one to determine which hemisphere controls the responses in a crossed condition, but the physiological data can monitor responses in each hemisphere during these responses. Apparently, during crossed responses, there were substantial P300 amplitudes over the LH to LVF stimuli (comparable to P300 amplitudes over the right hemisphere (RH) to RVF stimuli) and the P300 to RVF stimuli was no longer larger for 7° than 4° eccentricities. In the behavioral data, too, crossed responses showed comparable RTs to LVF and RVF stimuli and similar RTs to 7° and 4° RVF stimuli. It thus appears that crossed responses are "processed" in the hemisphere ipsilateral to the stimulus VF and that the crossed conditions equilibrate or counteract the attentional bias across space in the two hemispheres of J.W.

The role of sensory, motor, and attentional manipulations in the Poffenberger paradigm and their effect in chronometric findings in complete split-brain patients is the main theme of Zaidel and Iacoboni's chapter. The data reviewed suggest a variety of parallel interhemispheric extracallosal routes in these patients. These routes are subject to individual differences that determine different responses to manipulations, across patients.

Corballis and Forster review data on the effects of visual parameters on interhemispheric transfer in commissurotomized patients. Taken all together, the data are in line with the findings of Zaidel and Iacoboni, suggesting that it is response information, not stimulus information, that is transferred in tasks requiring interhemispheric visuomotor integration.

Reuter-Lorenz addresses the question of whether the separated hemispheres can function as independent parallel processors, using various paradigms. She reports the paradoxical observation that a complete callosotomy patient had a greater redundancy gain than normal subjects and a partial split-brain patient. Reuter-Lorenz proposes that this paradoxical observation might be explained by a subcortically mediated gating mechanism.

Iacoboni and Zaidel, however, provide an alternative explanation for Reuter-Lorenz's findings. They propose that the amount of facilitation observed during parallel visuomotor tasks may be mediated by cortical modulation of subcortical structures. In support of this view, they report chronometric data from nine patients and fMRI data from two callosal agenesis patients.

The study of callosal agenesis is the central topic of Lassonde and colleagues' chapter. They review clinical, radiological, and behavioral findings in patients born without the corpus callosum. One of the question that emerges with regard to interhemispheric transfer in cal-

losal agenesis and split-brain patients is whether this transfer is qualitatively similar or not to the transfer of information observed in complete split-brain patients. Lassonde's data cannot directly address this question. In their commentary to Lassonde's article, Iacoboni and colleagues discuss some data obtained in callosal agenesis patients in various versions of the Poffenberger paradigm. They compare these findings with the findings obtained in complete split-brain patients and conclude that the quicker transfer observed in callosal agenesis patients is not due to a qualitatively different extracallosal channel used by acallosals. Probably, compensatory mechanisms due to the lack of the corpus callosum at birth can explain the different efficiencies of transfer between the two population of patients. A similar conclusion is reached by Clarke in his commentary.

In contrast, Di Stefano and Salvadori emphasize the hemispheric contribution to interhemispheric visuomotor integration that seems to play a prominent role in some patients born without the corpus callosum.

Banich's and Hugdahl's commentaries are distinguished by introducing new behavioral paradigms that go beyond SRT and study interhemispheric transfer in relation to hemispheric specialization. Their techniques will therefore be discussed in some detail.

The bilateral distribution advantage (BDA)

When two visual stimuli have to be compared and the task is simple enough, there is an advantage to comparisons within the same VF compared to comparisons between the two VFs. But when the task is complex enough, there is an advantage to comparisons between the two VFs relative to within either VF. This is termed the bilateral distribution advantage (BDA). The BDA seems to be independent of stimulus alignment (Jeeves and Lamb, 1988), and it is therefore not due to scanning habits. It disappears with sequential presentations (Hellige, 1987), and it can be reversed with practice (Liederman et al., 1985), presumably by making the task easier. The standard account of the BDA is that it allows parallel processing of an abstract code in each hemisphere, which more than compensates for the cost of callosal relay of the code for final comparison. This means that the BDA should occur only for tasks that show independent hemispheric processing, that is, direct access, and not for tasks that are strongly lateralized (cf. Berger and Perret, 1990).

Banich and her associates developed a paradigm designed to minimize confounds due to attentional scanning direction, stimulus eccentricity, scanning distance, and task information load (cf. Banich and Belger, 1990). Subjects have to decide whether a letter on the bottom of one VF matches either of two top letters, one in each VF. In this way, the stimulus display is the same for "within" and "between" comparisons. Unfortunately, subjects may need to compute both comparisons to get the answer. Indeed, there is evidence in Banich's data that subjects scan the top items in the display from left to right. Banich considers that both comparisons may be undertaken in parallel, horse race fashion, but this need not be the case.

In an attempt to test the BDA when perceptual load is equated in both types of comparisons and in both hemispheres, we ran experiments in which each display had four items: two in each hemisphere, one on the bottom and one on the top of the display.

Copeland (1995) has systematically compared the BDA in a task requiring letter matching by shape (A, A = same, A, a = different) or by name (a, A = same) within or between the VFs using two-, three- and four-item stimulus displays. Three-item tasks were more difficult than corresponding two-item tasks and showed a greater BDA in name matching, consistent with the hypothesis that the BDA reflects a resource limitation. Three-item experiments using the Banich paradigm showed evidence for left-to-right scanning (a distribution (within, between) × VF (left, right) interaction). One three-item version with attentional blocking required matching of the bottom item with the top item in the same VF (within condition) during one block or in the opposite VF (between condition) during another block. This version eliminated the undesirable left-to-right scanning, but it was slower than the corresponding two-item task, showing some automatic processing of, and resource expending by, the unattended stimuli. The four-item version of the task with attentional blocking (using a peripheral cue of the bottom item and instruction to match within the same or in the opposite visual field) was next compared with corresponding three-item tasks. The four-item version also eliminated left-to-right scanning. The introduction of an equal perceptual load on both hemispheres in the four-item tasks reduced but did not eliminate the BDA. This shows that the BDA in the Banich paradigm is partly due to a hemispheric perceptual imbalance. By contrast, the BDA in the four-item task reflects the cognitive imbalance in the within and between comparisons, that is, parallel processing in the between condition (Copeland and Zaidel, 1996). A final version of the experiment uses four-item displays with two peripheral cues to identify the items to be compared. This version was designed to avoid the possible strategic effects of attentional blocking while still eliminating the mental scanning introduced by the three-item task of Banich. Copeland found a latency BDA for the name task but not for the shape task. She also

found that, as expected, this task eliminated the scanning pattern.

Within each paradigm there was no relationship between task difficulty and the BDA, but across paradigms there was a significant negative correlation, likely due to the different information-processing characteristics of the different paradigms. This means that as the complexity of the letter-matching task changes, so do the cortical modules and the callosal channels that are engaged. Complexity here refers to the number of serial processing stages of the task rather than to the difficulty of each of them (cf. Merola and Liederman, 1990). Further, we posit that the BDA exists only for tasks (1) that require comparison of an abstract code common to both hemispheres (the common hemispheric code hypothesis) and (2) in which the codes are computed in hemispheric modules that have direct callosal connections (the privileged callosal channel hypothesis). Letter names have such a code.

Some support for this hypothesis comes from a recent trial-based fMRI experiment (Pollmann and Zaidel, submitted). We found that during the name (but not the shape) task, unilateral presentations yielded bilateral activation in letter-specific visual areas. Further, in the name task there was greater activation (hence, more processing resources) in the input hemisphere during unilateral presentation than during bilateral presentation. Finally, bilateral shape (but not name) matches showed increased activation in anterior and posterior cingulate cortex, consistent with increased interhemispheric coordination demands. Thus, the name task appears to exert fewer interhemispheric coordination costs than the shape task.

Copeland (1995) also showed that the signal detection measure of bias depends on the perceptual load imbalance in the two VFs and on the scanning pattern induced by multiple comparisons, in which a preliminary mismatch will induce a "different" bias. By contrast, the signal detection measure of d' may be sensitive to the cognitive load differences in the within and between comparisons but not to the perceptual load of the display. Here perceptual load refers to automatic processing of all stimuli, relevant or irrelevant, whereas cognitive load refers to attentional task-relevant processing.

The locus of attentional selection in these tasks appears to be intermediate rather than either early or late. Early selection, which should eliminate all processing of irrelevant items, would have resulted in equal performance in the three- and four-item cued tasks and the equivalent two-item tasks. On the other hand, selection at the level of decision making, after the completion of perceptual processing and elaboration of the items, would be unlikely to result in a large BDA, since only a "match" decision would remain to be made in either bilateral or unilateral trials. Neither possibility fits the data.

Banich shares our model of callosal structure and function as a set of channels for sensorimotor, cognitive, and control information. Her account of the BDA in terms of allocation of attentional resources is also consistent with our views. However, the role she assigns to the CC in selective attention remains vague.

The corpus callosum as an attentional modulator

Reaction times (RT) to lateralized flashes are typically faster when subjects respond with the hand ipsilateral to the stimulus (uncrossed condition) than when they respond with the contralateral hand (crossed condition). This difference, as the reader must know quite well by now, is called the crossed-uncrossed difference (CUD). The CUD may represent the conduction delay in the transfer of information required by the crossed condition but not by the uncrossed condition. Kinsbourne challenges this anatomical interpretation of the CUD. He suggests, instead, that the CUD may reflect different states of hemispheric activation. Kinsbourne argues that in the uncrossed condition, the hemisphere that controls the motor response has also received the visual stimulus and is relatively more activated than the hemisphere controlling the motor response in the crossed condition. The CC would rapidly equilibrate this imbalance in hemispheric activation—hence the longer CUDs in split-brain patients. We tested the anatomical and equilibrium hypotheses in a series of experiments.

In an initial series of experiments we tested whether simple detection of light flashes is influenced by context. Typically, RT to two light flashes is faster than RT to a single light flash. This is called the redundancy gain or the redundant target effect (Miller, 1982). In the first experiment, we observed that RT to two light flashes presented simultaneously (239 ms) was faster ($p = 0.03$) than RT to two light flashes presented with a stimulus onset asynchrony (SOA) of 30 ms (245 ms). In the second experiment, we mixed, in the same block, trials with a single light flash and trials with two light flashes, presented either simultaneously or with the SOA. As expected, RT to simultaneous redundant targets (248 ms) was faster ($p = 0.0001$) than RT to asynchronous light flashes (254 ms). Critical to our investigation, RTs to single flashes (251 ms) mixed with simultaneously presented light flashes were faster ($p = 0.003$) than RTs to single flashes (255 ms) mixed with asynchronous redundant targets, suggesting that contextual facilitation may be an important mechanism in sensorimotor integration.

Critical to our interest in the CUD and the role of the CC in generating it, these results suggested to us that context effects could be used to investigate the anatomical versus the equilibrium models of the CUD.

We consequently performed a meta-analysis of a series of experiments of simple RT to single or double simultaneous flashes that we had previously performed to study the redundant target effect. Altogether, we analyzed 138 normal subjects performing simple RT to lateralized flashes. In one task, only single flashes were presented (basic task). In another task, trials with single flashes were mixed with trials in which two flashes were presented in the two visual fields or two flashes were presented within a visual field (embedded task). If the CUD represents pure conduction delay, there should be no CUD difference between the two tasks (unless a shift in the callosal channel subserving the interhemispheric transfer is invoked). If the CUD represents an imbalance of hemispheric activation, trials with two flashes should balance hemispheric activation more, and the CUD should therefore be shorter in the embedded task. What we found was that the CUD in the embedded task (0.3 ms) was indeed shorter ($p < 0.02$) than the CUD in the basic task (3.0 ms). These findings are compatible with the notion that the CUD is a parameter that is sensitive to context effects and that it may reflect an imbalance of hemispheric activation rather than a conduction delay through callosal fibers. However, on the basis of normal data only, we cannot rule out the hypothesis that the shortening of the CUD is actually due to a shift in callosal channel involved in the interhemispheric transfer. Thus, we needed data from acallosal, partial, and complete split-brain patients to further explore this issue.

Most of the patients tested in our lab had actually performed both tasks, and we were in a position to carry out this analysis. What we observed was that there was no difference in the CUD in all but one patient (N.G.) between the basic and the embedded task. Thus, the combined data from the split brain seem to suggest that the difference in CUD observed in normals in the two tasks may be due to a shift in callosal channels subserving the transfer. An alternative explanation could be that most split-brain patients actually lack contextual modulation. Contextual modulation may be preserved only in N.G., the only patient showing a pattern similar to normals, with a shorter CUD in the embedded task.

It should be noted that our meta-analysis did not actually use the ideal paradigm to test the anatomical model against the equilibrium model of the CUD. In fact, in the embedded task we had trials with two flashes between the two visual fields (supposedly producing more equilibrium between the two hemispheres) but also trials with two flashes within one or the other visual field (supposedly producing more imbalance in hemispheric activation). Thus, we decided to design and perform an experiment to test more directly the anatomical model versus the equilibrium model. In this experiment, we tested 52 normal right-handers, and each subject was tested in the basic task and in two versions of the embedded task. In one version, trials with single flashes were mixed with trials in which two flashes were presented in the two visual fields (embedded between). In the other version, trials with single flashes were mixed with trials in which two flashes were presented within a visual field (embedded within). The predictions are straightforward: If the anatomical model of the CUD is valid, then there should be no difference in the CUD obtained in the basic task, in the embedded between task, and in the embedded within task. If the equilibrium model is correct, then the CUD in the basic task should be longer than the CUD in the embedded between task and should be shorter than the CUD in the embedded within task. The results were in line with the anatomical model of the CUD. No difference ($F = 0.32$, $p = 0.87$) was observed in the CUD obtained in the basic task (2.2 ms), in the embedded between task (3.8 ms), and in the embedded within task (2.7 ms). Note that even the direction of the changes in the magnitude of the CUD was not compatible with the equilibrium model.

Dichotic listening

Hugdahl's paper contrasts the role of the CC in relaying sensory auditory information and its role in modulating attention in the dichotic listening paradigm, using the syllables /ba/, /da/, /ga/, /pa/, /ta/, and /ka/. Hugdahl anchors this contrast in Aboitiz and colleagues' (1992 and Chapter 2 in this volume) distinction between sensorimotor channels that consist of large-diameter myelinated fibers and interconnect primary and secondary sensorimotor cortex, on the one hand, and higher cognitive channels that consist of small-diameter unmyelinated fibers and interconnect association cortex. This is consistent with the callosal channel doctrine (e.g., Zaidel, Clarke, and Suyenobu, 1990).

THE ANATOMICAL MODEL Hugdahl's discussion of dichotic listening to nonsense stop consonant-vowel (CV) syllables follows the anatomical model (cf. Zaidel, 1976, 1983). Specifically, he assumes (1) exclusive LH specialization for the phonetic identification of the syllables, (2) complete ipsilateral suppression, and (3) callosal relay of the left ear (LE) signal from the RH to the LH prior to

processing. Until recently, we believed these assumptions to be unchallenged, but some puzzling recent data give us pause. Here is a brief rundown.

First, regarding the assumption of *exclusive specialization*, we originally verified it in the split brain by showing that the disconnected RH cannot identify the syllables. The approach that we took was to probe each visual field with a letter probe (B, D, G, P, T, or K) while the patient heard a dichotic pair of syllables. The patient was required to indicate unimanually whether the probe matched the sound in either ear. When we probed the right visual field (RVF) (i.e., the LH), we found the same massive right-ear advantage (REA) observed with verbal responses. This confirms suppression of the ipsilateral LE signal in the LH. But probes in the LVF (RH) yielded chance performance for either ear. We concluded that the RH could not process the task at all. In fact, it could not even identify monaural stimuli to the LE when dichotic competition was removed. But there are a couple of problems. The result suggests RH incompetence, but consequently, it fails to demonstrate suppression of the RE in the RH. More important, perhaps the RH failed to match the sound syllable with a letter rather than to identify the sound itself.

We addressed this possibility by using an equivalent dichotic tape consisting of the syllables /bee/, /dee/, /gee/, /pee/, /tee/, and /kee/ and using letters (B, D, G, P, T, and K) as well as pictures (a bee, a girl (Dee Dee), a boy (French Guy), a pea pod, a tea cup, and a key) as probes. Letter probes showed the same massive REA in the LH and chance performance in the RH. Picture probes yielded the same massive REA in the LH but above-chance performance in the RH (commissurotomy patients L.B. and N.G.). In particular, patient L.B. showed a significant left-ear advantage (LEA), with chance performance in the RE, when picture probes were presented in the RH (Zaidel, 1983). Thus, the meaningfulness of the probe affected RH ability to identify the syllables.

ATTENTION Hugdahl shows that using his dichotic CVs in normal adults, attention to the right ear decreases the left-ear score and attention to the left ear increases the left-ear score, even reversing the REA to an LEA. Further, he notes a positive correlation between posterior callosum size and the LE score, but only in the LE focused attention condition. He attributes this correlation to a callosal channel that modulates attention via small-diameter unmyelinated fibers. This is consistent with the results of Aboitiz and colleagues (1992 and Chapter 2 in this volume), who predict morphometric correlates for cognitive but not for sensor in motor channels. It is noteworthy that the attentional channel is posterior rather than anterior, perhaps associated with parietal control of spatial orienting of attention. Apparently, the attentional channel associated with a particular sensorimotor channel is located near it in the callosum.

However, we have two mutually inconsistent lines of evidence regarding the conclusion that modulation of attention in the dichotic CV paradigm is mediated by the CC. The first is the difference in the effect of focused attention on the REA in the normal brain and the split brain. Using a dichotic CV tape (/dee/, /bee/, /gee/, /pee/, /tee/, /kee/), we found a much larger drop in the REA with LE attention in the split brain than in the normal brain (see Figures 4.11 and 4.12 in Zaidel, 1983). This suggests that the effect of attention on ipsilateral suppression is partly mitigated by the commissures.

In that case, what is the mechanism that mediates the effect of attention on the REA in the normal brain, found by Hugdahl? He argues that LE attention increases callosal connectivity from the RH to the LH. How? And how does RE attention reduce the LE signal? By decreasing callosal connectivity? And why is there a discrepancy between the sensitivity of the LE signal to focused attention in Hugdahl's normal subjects and that in ours?

The second line of evidence comes from preoperative and postoperative follow-ups of dichotic listening performance in a 30-year-old right-handed male patient with anterior callosotomy up to but sparing the splenium (Zaidel, Zaidel, and Bogen, 1996). Presurgically, the patient exhibited a normal REA in the divided attention condition of the dichotic CV syllables task with verbal responses. This changed to a massive REA right after surgery. Over the next two years the patient gradually started reporting more and more of the LE in the divided but not in the focused attention condition. This suggests that callosal relay of the LE signal in the divided and focused attention conditions occurs through different interhemispheric channels. The divided attention channel may have shifted from the isthmus to the anterior splenium or to subcallosal channels, whereas the focused attention channel remained disconnected. Thus, focused attention appears to be callosally mediated.

IPSILATERAL SUPPRESSION Hugdahl's arguments presuppose a complete and stable ipsilateral suppression that is not affected by attention. That assumption may not be valid. For example, 20 years ago we showed that patient L.B. had a higher sensitivity (d') for identifying RE syllables in the RH when the visual probes followed the dichotic CV syllables (0.5–1 s) ($d' = 1.2$) than when

they were simultaneous ($d' = 0$) (Zaidel, 1983). Attending to one ear in split-brain patient L.B. tended to increase its strength and decrease the strength of the other ear in the ipsilateral hemisphere, consistent with a reduction in ipsilateral suppression in both hemispheres (Zaidel, 1983). Furthermore, we recently administered a similar dichotic test with the CVC words /bale/, /dale/, /pail/, and /tail/ to split-brain patient L.B. and found different degrees of ipsilateral suppression in the LH, depending on whether the task required verbal responses or matching to lateralized (RVF) letter or picture probes. Thus, ipsilateral suppression can be modulated by top-down influences. It is therefore important to assess ipsilateral suppression in the split brain on a paradigm-by-paradigm basis. Of course, it is possible that ipsilateral suppression is normally modulated by the CC and might not be comparable in the split and in the normal brains. Some even believe that it is subject to individual differences (Sidtis, 1988).

CORRELATING THE LE SCORE WITH RE SCORE Hugdahl reasons that with limited resources there should be a negative correlation between the LE and RE scores, that is, the better the callosal channel connectivity the higher the LE score and the lower RE score. So far, so good. However, this does not mean, as Hugdahl argued, "that the better the left ear score is transferred during the FL (focused left) condition, the more negative should the correlation between the left and right ear become." Rather, the size and strength of the LE-RE correlation is associated with the degree of variability of callosal connectivity in the auditory channel versus variability of hemispheric specialization for the task. Under the callosal relay interpretation of the REA, a negative correlation between the two ears means that individual differences in callosal connectivity are greater than differences in left hemisphere (LH) competence. Conversely, a positive correlation means that individual differences in LH competence are greater than differences in callosal connectivity.

Earlier studies of this task rarely report the correlation between the two ear scores. When they do (Speaks, 1988; Zaidel et al., 1990), they generally find no significant correlation. Hugdahl reports a life-span developmental study in which the negative correlation under focused attention increases up to age 50 and decreases afterward. As was argued above, this does not mean that callosal connectivity increases up to age 50 and decreases again at higher ages. Rather, it means that individual variability in callosal connectivity is increasingly greater than variability in LH competence up to age 50. It is noteworthy that Hugdahl observed this trend only for focused attention (either ear) but not for divided attention. Why? Perhaps because, as was argued earlier, divided attention and focused attention are mediated by different interhemispheric/callosal routes. Then the developmental reversal observed by Hugdahl relates to callosal pathways for focused but not for divided attention. Thus, the different pathways show different developmental patterns across the life span; callosal mediation of focused attention is subject to greater and more changing individual variability than callosal mediation of divided attention.

We have correlated the LE and RE scores with divided attention in 30 subjects partitioned into high-masculine women, low-masculine women, high-masculine men, and low-masculine men, assessed with the Bem Sex Role Inventory. All groups, except the low-masculine men ($p > 0.05$) demonstrated significant negative correlations between the two ears at the 0.01 level: $r = -0.81$, -0.79, -0.82, and -0.47, respectively (Weekes et al., 1995). Thus, in all but the low-masculine men there was a greater individual difference in callosal connectivity than in hemispheric competence.

VALIDATING THE RIGHT-EAR ADVANTAGE (REA) Hugdahl used two methods for validating the REA as an index of LH specialization for language. First, he used Kimura's original procedure by comparing the REA with the results from temporary hemispheric anesthesia using the Wada test. The dichotic test showed 92% correct classification of side of language dominance. But it should be remembered that dichotic listening measures phonetic perception, whereas the Wada test usually measures speech dominance. The two functions might not lateralize identically. Second, Hugdahl used O^{15}-PET imaging during the dichotic test relative to a baseline tone discrimination test. The dichotic test activated the superior temporal gyrus bilaterally but more on the left. However, was there a correlation between the degree of behavioral REA and the degree of physiological asymmetry in temporal lobe activation?

We had used an alternative approach by tapping directly LH and RH competence for the dichotic task in split-brain patients. This has the advantage of being able to separate hemispheric competence from callosal connectivity and to assess degree of ipsilateral suppression in each hemisphere. But the approach presupposes that the data from the split brain generalize to the normal brain. Instead, it may be that the CC modulates ipsilateral suppression so that the pattern observed in the split brain will be different from what actually happens in the normal brain.

Thus, each approach has its advantages and disadvantages, and currently the best strategy is to use a convergent methodology.

REFERENCES

ABOITIZ, F., A. B. SCHEIBEL, R. S. FISHER, and E. ZAIDEL, 1992. Fiber composition of the human corpus callosum. *Brain Res.* 598:143–153.

BANICH, M. T., and A. BELGER, 1990. Interhemispheric interaction: How do the hemispheres divide and conquer a task. *Cortex* 26:77–94.

BERGER, J.-M., and E. PERRET, 1990. Interhemispheric integration of information in a surface estimation task. *Neuropsychologia* 24:743–746.

CLARKE, J. M., and E. ZAIDEL, 1989. Simple reaction times to lateralized light flashes: Varieties of interhemispheric communication routes. *Brain* 112:845–870.

COPELAND, S. A., 1995. *Interhemispheric interaction in the normal brain: Comparisons within and between the hemispheres.* Ph.D. Dissertation, Department of Psychology, University of California at Los Angeles.

COPELAND, S. A., and E. ZAIDEL, 1996. Contributions to the bilateral distribution advantage. *J. Int. Neuropsychol. Soc.* 2:29.

HELLIGE, J. B., 1987. Interhemispheric interaction: Models, paradigms and recent findings. In *Duality and Unity of the Brain*, D. Ottoson, ed. London: Macmillan, pp. 454–466.

JEEVES, M. A., and A. LAMB, 1988. Cerebral asymmetries and interhemispheric processes. *Behav. Brain Res.* 29:211–223.

LIEDERMAN, J., J. MEROLOA, and S. MARTINEZ, 1985. Interhemispheric collaboration in response to simultaneous bilateral input. *Neuropsychologia* 23:673–683.

MEROLA, J. L., and J. LIEDERMAN, 1990. The effect of task difficulty upon the extent to which performance benefits from between-hemisphere division of inputs. *Int. J. Neurosci.* 51:35–44.

MILLER, J., 1982. Divided attention: Evidence for coactivation with redundant signals. *Cogn. Psychol.* 14:247–279.

POLLMANN, S., and E. ZAIDEL, submitted. Interhemispheric resource in complex tasks: An efMRI study of the bilateral distribution advantage.

SIDTIS, J. J., 1988. Dichotic listening after commissurotomy. In *Handbook of Dichotic Listening: Theory, Methods and Research*, K. Hugdahl, ed. New York: John Wiley and Sons, pp. 161–184.

SPEAKS, C. E., 1988. Statistical properties of dichotic listening scores. In *Handbook of Dichotic Listening: Theory, Methods and Research*, K. Hugdahl, ed. New York: John Wiley and Sons, pp. 185–213.

WEEKES, N., D. W. ZAIDEL, and E. ZAIDEL, 1995. The effects of sex and sex role attributions on the ear advantage in dichotic listening. *Neuropsychology* 9:62–67.

ZAIDEL, E. 1976. Language, dichotic listening and the disconnected hemispheres. In *Conference on Human Brain Function*, D. O. Walter, L. Rogers, and J. M. Finzi-Fried, eds. Los Angeles: Brain Information Service/BRI Publications Office, UCLA, pp. 103–110.

ZAIDEL, E., 1983. Disconnection syndrome as a model for laterality effects in the normal brain. In *Cerebral Hemisphere Asymmetry: Method, Theory, and Application*, J. Hellige, ed. New York: Praeger, pp. 95–151.

ZAIDEL, E., J. CLARKE, and B. SUYENOBU, 1990. Hemispheric independence: A paradigm case for cognitive neuroscience. In *Neurobiology of Higher Cognitive Function*, A. B. Scheibel and A. F. Wechsler, eds. New York: Guilford Press, pp. 297–352.

ZAIDEL, E., D. W. ZAIDEL, and J. E. BOGEN, 1996. Disconnection syndrome. In *The Blackwell Dictionary of Neuropsychology*, G. Beaumont, P. M. Kenealy, and J. C. Rogers, eds. Oxford: Blackwell, pp. 279–285.

IV THE CORPUS CALLOSUM AND CLINICAL INVESTIGA- TIONS

16 Clinical Neuropsychological Assessment of Callosal Dysfunction: Multiple Sclerosis and Dyslexia

WARREN S. BROWN

ABSTRACT The contribution of the corpus callosum to human intelligence is not well understood. Clinical neuropsychological assessment and investigation of cognitive deficits related to callosal dysfunction will require appropriately sensitive measures. Multiple sclerosis (MS) involves degeneration of white matter, including the corpus callosum, and deficits in complex recent memory, concept formation, abstraction, and mental fluency. Callosal dysfunction has been reported in learning disabilities and dyslexia. This paper describes studies of callosal function in MS with a particular focus on the sensitivity of various measures of interhemispheric interaction. Data from adult dyslexics are presented regarding the detectability of callosal dysfunction in a syndrome with less clear callosal damage. Performance of these two clinical groups is compared to the performance of commissurotomy patients, individuals with agenesis of the corpus callosum, and normal adults and children. Several conclusions are suggested: (1) Not every test of callosal function will be adequately sensitive in a particular clinical population; (2) deficits are more apparent when tests demand interhemispheric transfer of more complex information; (3) a bimanual coordination task, the Tactile Performance Test, and the Finger Localization Test all proved to be particularly sensitive; and (4) evoked potentials to lateralized visual stimuli provide a direct measure of posterior callosal function.

The contribution of callosal function to neurocognitive abilities is not yet known. For example, commissurotomy (i.e., surgical cutting of all of the cerebral commissures, including the corpus callosum) does not dramatically alter measured I.Q. Similarly, individuals born without a corpus callosum (i.e., agenesis of the corpus callosum) can have normal scores on I.Q. tests. However, in both cases the individuals manifest subtle deficits in cognitive function that are likely due to callosal absence.

WARREN S. BROWN Travis Research Institute and The Graduate School of Psychology, Fuller Theological Seminary, Pasadena, California.

There are a number of neurological and neuropsychological syndromes that include cognitive deficits that may be attributable, at least in part, to dysfunction of the corpus callosum. However, in most cases the exact contribution of callosal dysfunction to the cognitive deficits is uncertain. Multiple sclerosis (MS) involves degeneration of white matter, including the corpus callosum, and neuropsychological deficits in complex recent memory, concept formation and abstraction, and mental fluency. However, little attention has been paid to the degree and nature of callosal dysfunction in MS patients and to the contribution of callosal dysfunction to cognitive deficits.

Callosal dysfunction has also been suggested to contribute to learning disabilities, developmental dyslexia, attention deficits, autism, and schizophrenia. In these cases there is at best only suggestive evidence of callosal neuropathology. Thus, callosal dysfunction may be a by-product of other neuropathology but contribute to the pattern of neuropsychological deficits.

Research questions

The study of interhemispheric interactions in clinical populations allows the researcher to ask two important kinds of questions:

• What can be learned about the relationship between callosal function and human cognitive ability from patients with known callosal pathology? What role does callosal pathology play in the cognitive symptoms of the particular group of patients? Dysfunction of which parts of the corpus callosum (i.e., callosal channels) disturb what specific sorts of interhemispheric transfer and cognitive function?

• What role does callosal pathology play in neurocognitive disorders that are not thought to be associated with dysfunction of the corpus callosum? Can one account for cognitive deficits by demonstrating callosal dysfunction in the patient group?

Studies of callosal function in MS patients will be described with reference to the first kind of question, that is, what we can learn about the role of the corpus callosum in human cognition by studying those with known callosal pathology. Data from adult dyslexics will be presented in which the second set of questions were the focus, that is, what role, if any, callosal dysfunction plays in dyslexia. Performance from these two clinical groups on tasks demanding interhemispheric interactions will be compared to the results from commissurotomy patients, individuals with agenesis of the corpus callosum, and normal adults and children to assess the contributions of callosal function to cognitive processing deficits.

Callosal function measures

Assessment of the contributions of callosal dysfunction to the neuropsychological profile of a particular clinical population can proceed only on the basis of measures of interhemispheric interactions that are well understood in terms of their sensitivity to various levels of callosal disturbance. Thus, for each proposed measure of callosal function, it is important to know the following:

• Whether the measure that is presumed to be dependent on the corpus callosum shows clear deficits in commissurotomy patients or individuals with agenesis of the corpus callosum
• Whether the measure is sufficiently sensitive to reflect more subtle changes in callosal function associated with normal child development
• Whether the kind or degree of callosal pathology in clinical populations affects the measure in a consistent manner

Studies of callosal function in clinical populations will be described that use measures presumably reflecting interhemispheric interactions. The measures used in our research include the following:

• Evoked potential indices of the time and efficiency of interhemispheric transmission (EP-IHTT)
• The bilateral visual field advantage, a measure of the ability to compare two complex visual stimuli (letters and patterns) when they are simultaneously flashed one to each visual field
• The ability to coordinate the speed of movement of the hands to accomplish a bimanual coordination task
• Transfer of complex tactile spatial learning between hands (hemispheres) in the Tactile Performance Test
• Intermanual transfer of the sequence of finger touches in the Finger Localization Test

• Intermanual transfer of learning of a complex tactile maze

These tests were selected because they have been frequently used in testing acallosal and commissurotomy patients. However, they do not represent a complete battery for assessment of callosal function.

Summary of subjects studied

Performance on this same battery of tests of callosal function will be summarized for six different groups with progressively decreasing degrees of callosal dysfunction.

COMMISSUROTOMY Patient L.B. from the California series of split-brain patients originally studied by Sperry and his colleagues (research summarized by Sperry, 1974; Bogen, 1993; Zaidel, Zaidel, and Bogen, 1999; patients described by Bogen, 1969) was tested in our laboratory on some of these measures, and data from other measures has been reported in the literature. This patient anchors the most extreme end of the hemispheric disconnection continuum in that not only is the corpus callosum severed, but all of the interhemispheric commissures are cut as well. Thus, L.B. provides performance levels indicative of the complete absence of interactions between the hemispheres via the forebrain commissures.

AGENESIS OF THE CORPUS CALLOSUM We have studied two individuals (M.M. and J.D.) who are both normally intelligent late adolescents who have succeeded in graduating from high school and are functioning relatively normally within the community (Brown et al., 1999). Because both individuals have an anterior commissure that is clearly visible in magnetic resonance imaging (MRI), they represent a lesser degree of commissural disturbance than that seen in L.B. Here, it can be argued that dysfunction in interhemispheric interaction is due specifically to callosal absence, while preservation of interhemispheric interactions may reflect contributions of the anterior commissure.

MULTIPLE SCLEROSIS MS is a progressive demyelinating neural disease that attacks the periventricular areas of the brain most vigorously. On the basis of MRI scans, callosal lesions are seen in 55% to as high as 93% of MS patients (Simon et al., 1986), and callosal atrophy in 40–60% of patients (Simon et al., 1986; Dietemann et al., 1988; Rao et al., 1989). Thus, MS subjects represent a group with varying degrees of callosal involvement. Some studies have directly compared MRI indices of lesion sizes and locations or degree of atrophy to deficits in interhemispheric transfer (e.g., Rao et al., 1989; Pelletier et al., 1993). We studied a group of 34 patients between 33 and 72 years of age with mild MS (Kurtzke Disability Scale from 3 to 7), compared to 30 matched normals (Burnison, Larson, and Brown, 1995; Larson, Brown, and Burnison, 1997). Because MRIs were not available on our patients, electrophysiological criteria were used to determine the degree of callosal involvement in our MS patients.

DYSLEXIC ADULTS   There is an accumulating literature suggesting callosal dysfunction among individuals with dyslexia (e.g., Gladstone and Best, 1985; Davidson, Leslie, and Saron, 1990; Davidson and Saron, 1992), but the exact relationship between callosal dysfunction and dyslexia has not been firmly established. The data that we report provide additional information regarding the existence and nature of callosal dysfunction in dyslexia. Also, since the functional and neuroanatomical data that exist do not suggest the severity of callosal dysfunction seen in many MS patients, dyslexics can be considered a group with minimal callosal dysfunction. We studied a group of 21 dyslexic adults (18–40 years old) who were sufficiently intelligent to be enrolled in a community college, compared to a group of 21 age-matched community college controls (Moore et al., 1995, 1996; Markee et al., 1996). Dyslexic individuals were included in our research on the basis of evidence of specific deficits in reading not associated with similar deficits in more general aspects of intelligence, language processing, or mathematics. Thus, our adult dyslexic group is not likely to include individuals with more general neuropsychological deficits or learning disabilities, a diagnostic difficulty in studying groups of dyslexic children.

NORMAL CHILDREN   Neuroanatomical research on human development suggests that the corpus callosum does not reach its adult levels of myelinization until early in the second decade (Yakovlev and Lecours, 1967; Rakic and Yakovlev, 1968). Thus, performance differences on callosal transfer tasks between younger (e.g., 6–9 years old) and older (e.g., 13–17 years old) children and adolescents allow one to observe the effects of even more subtle forms of callosal "dysfunction," that is, incomplete myelinization. For example, developmental differences in measures of callosal function have been observed in bimanually coordinated motor activity (Jeeves, Silver, and Jacobson, 1988), tactile evoked potentials (Salamy, 1978), and cross-hand versus uncrossed RTs (Brizzollara, et al., 1994).

NORMAL ADULTS   Data from all of the above groups are referenced to the results of various control groups of normal adults. With the application of good ex-

clusionary criteria for eliminating possible sources of subclinical brain dysfunction, normal adult controls represent individuals with presumably optimal callosal function.

Evoked potential interhemispheric transfer time

The unilateral projection of visual information from one visual field to the opposite (contralateral) hemisphere, and only subsequent transmission to the ipsilateral hemisphere via callosal fibers, is detectable using visual evoked potentials (EPs) (see Figure 16.1). The primary sensory components of the visual EP (i.e., P1 and N1)

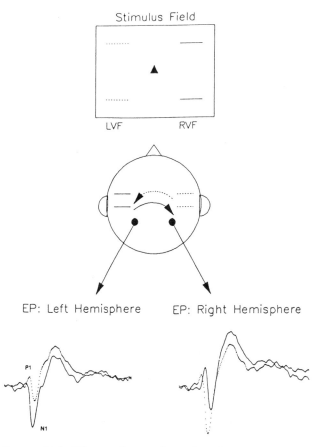

FIGURE 16.1. EP recording configuration. Stimulus presentation and EP recording configuration for the left visual field (dashed lines) and right visual field (solid lines) presentations used to elicit the EPs to calculate IHTT. Solid versus dashed lines suggest stimulus positions (upper rectangle), direct hemispheric visual projections (parallel lines within the head), callosal transfer (arrows crossing the midline of the head), and resultant EPs recorded over each hemisphere (at bottom) for each field of stimulation. (Figure reprinted from *Neuropsychologia*, volume 31, Brown and Jeeves, "Bilateral field advantage and evoked potential interhemispheric transmission time," pp. 267–1281, Copyright (1993), with kind permission from Elsevier Science Ltd., The Boulevard, Langford, Kidlington 0X5 1GB, UK.)

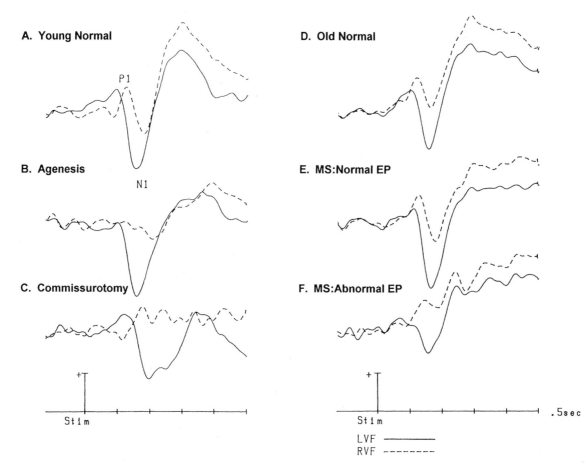

A. Young Normal

P1

N1

B. Agenesis

C. Commissurotomy

D. Old Normal

E. MS:Normal EP

F. MS:Abnormal EP

+

Stim

+

Stim   .5sec

LVF ————
RVF --------

FIGURE 16.2. Examples of EPs from various subjects and groups. All recordings are from a right parietal electrode to a left visual field stimulus (solid lines) compared to a right visual field stimulus (dashed lines). Responses are labeled as follows: (A) group mean EPs for 20 young normal adults, (B) EPs recorded from callosal agenesis patient J.D., (C) EPs recorded from commissurotomy patient L.B., (D) group mean EPs from a group of older normal adults matched in age to the MS pa-tients, (E) group mean EPs from the subgroup of MS patients with normal cross-callosal EPs, and (F) group mean EPs recorded from the subgroup of MS patients judged to have missing or severely diminished amplitude cross-callosal EPs. The vertical marker on the time scale at bottom indicates stimulus onset, the amplitude of which represents 7.5, 5.0, 2.5, 7.5, 7.5, and 7.5 μV of amplitude for the six sets of waves.

occur earlier in recordings made over the contralateral hemisphere than over the ipsilateral (cross-callosal) hemisphere. The difference in latency between these components when recorded over the contralateral and ipsilateral hemispheres has been used as an index of interhemispheric transmission time (IHTT) (see, for example Rugg, Lines, and Milner, 1984; Saron and Davidson, 1989). In normal adults the EP-IHTT varies from 15 to 25 ms for P1 and from 10 to 20 ms for N1 (Figures 16.2A and 16.2D). Interestingly, and as yet un-explainably, the EP-IHTT has been consistently found to be faster for right-to-left transmission than for left-to-right transmission (see data and meta-analysis by Brown, Larson, and Jeeves, 1994). A similar asymmetry in IHTT has been suggested for the crossed-uncrossed difference in simple reaction time (Marzi, Bisiacchi, and Nicoletti, 1991).

NORMAL CHILDREN As one might expect, evoked potential estimates of IHTT decrease progressively as a child's corpus callosum myelinates (Figure 16.3A). We have been able to show that N1 EP-IHTT decreases between a group of 7- to 9-year-olds (28 ms) and a group of 10- to 12-year-olds (12 ms) but does not continue to decrease in a group of 13- to 17-year-olds (14 ms) (Hagelthorn et al., 2000). That is, decreasing callosal transfer time reaches an asymptote early in the second decade of life. This result is consistent with the decreasing tactile EP-IHTT during late childhood reported by Salamy (1978). Thus, increasing myelinization

A. Development of EP-IHTT

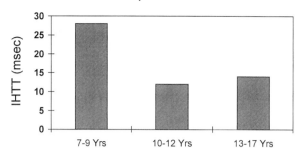

B. Development of BFA

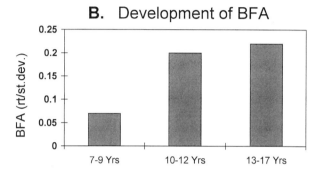

FIGURE 16.3. Results of developmental study of evoked potential interhemispheric transfer time (EP-IHTT) and bilateral field advantage (BFA). (A) Age-group mean EP-IHTT for the three age cohorts of normal children. (B) Age-group mean BFA for the same normal children. BFA is calculated as the difference between RTs for unilateral presentation minus bilateral presentation RT divided by the subjects' RT standard deviation over all trials. (Data from Hagelthorn et al., 2000.)

of the corpus callosum results in increasing speed of interhemispheric transfer of the visual EP; this speed reaches near-adult levels by around 10–12 years of age.

COMMISSUROTOMY AND AGENESIS PATIENTS   EPs recorded in commissurotomy and agenesis patients using this paradigm are particularly revealing. What is clear from the responses of both commissurotomy patients (Mangun et al., 1991; Brown et al., 1999) and those with agenesis of the corpus callosum (Rugg, Milner, and Lines, 1985; Brown et al., 1999) is that neither the P1 nor N1 components are detectable over the ipsilateral cortex (Figures 16.2B and 16.2C versus Figure 16.2A). That is, without a corpus callosum, interhemispheric transmission of the electrical activity evoked by visual stimulation does not cross between the hemispheres, and therefore, no P1 or N1 is recordable over the ipsilateral cortex.

From the point of view of electrophysiology, it is theoretically conceivable that the delayed-latency ipsilateral (cross-callosal) EP components recorded in normal adults or children are not evidence of electrical activity regen-

erated in the ipsilateral cortex but are instead a distant recording of the activity occurring in the hemisphere of direct projection (contralateral to the visual field of stimulation). If this were true, it would preclude both the interpretation of ipsilateral EPs as reflecting interhemispheric transfer and the use of EPs as an index of IHTT. However, the absence of an ipsilateral EP to unilateral visual stimulation in commissurotomy and callosal agenesis patients is critical proof of the dependence of ipsilateral visual EP components on callosal transfer and electrophysiological regeneration of the EP within the ipsilateral cortex. Consequently, the interpretation is supported that an interhemispheric latency difference in visual EP components is an index of IHTT.

MULTIPLE SCLEROSIS   The EP data from the commissurotomy and agenesis patients have been critical to the interpretation of our data from MS patients. Although the MS patients we tested (Burnison, Larson, and Brown, 1995) appeared as a group to have longer latency and lower amplitude cross-callosal EPs (compared to an age-matched group of normals), the highly variegated nature of lesions and demyelinization apparent on MRI scans within and between MS patients suggests the need for closer attention to the responses of individual patients. What this attention revealed was a subgroup of individuals with significantly diminished or absent P1 and N1 components in their ipsilateral, cross-callosal EPs (Figure 16.2E versus Figure 16.2F). That is, this subgroup of patients had a pattern of EPs that resembled that of the commissurotomy and agenesis patients (Figure 16.2F versus Figures 16.2B and 16.2C).

We interpreted these data as suggesting that these MS patients had significant damage to the posterior portion of the corpus callosum such that little early visual sensory information could be transmitted between the hemispheres. Consequently, these data suggest the possibility of some aspects of the disconnection syndrome (similar to that seen in split-brain individuals) within the subgroup of MS patients with diminished or absent cross-callosal EPs. Among the subgroup that had more normal-appearing cross-callosal EPs, no significant increase in IHTT could be demonstrated, suggesting either normal posterior callosal function or insufficient dysfunction to be detectable within the sensitivity of EP measures. The EP methodology thus has proven to be of value in detecting the presence or absence of significant posterior callosal dysfunction in MS patients.

ADULT DYSLEXICS   EP data from the group of adult dyslexics supports the hypothesis that dyslexia is related in some way to a deficiency in interhemispheric interaction (Markee et al., 1996). While the dyslexics differed from MS patients in that they all appeared to have clearly detectable cross-callosal EPs, the mean IHTT for this group was significantly longer than that of normal controls (14 ms versus 10 ms, respectively, for the N1 component). This result was not consistent with a similar study of EP-IHTT in dyslexic children reported by Davidson and Saron (1992). These investigators found *faster* EP-IHTT for dyslexics, particularly in the right-to-left direction. The source of this discrepancy is uncertain. Perhaps adult dyslexia is sufficiently different from dyslexia in children that they are associated with different forms of abnormality in interhemispheric interactions.

The bilateral visual field advantage

A commonly used interhemispheric transfer task is the comparison of two stimuli (e.g., letters) that are rapidly and simultaneously flashed one stimulus to each visual field. Subjects are asked to respond as rapidly as possible, indicating whether the stimuli match. A typical finding in these studies is that when the task is complex enough, responses are faster and more accurate for such bilateral field presentations than are responses to trials when both stimuli occur in the same visual field (e.g., Dimond and Beaumont, 1972; Liederman, Merola, and Martinez, 1985; Commentary 9.2 in this volume). This robust phenomenon is called a bilateral field advantage (BFA).

NORMAL ADULTS An example of the results from this test in 20 normal adults can be found in a paper from our laboratory (Brown and Jeeves, 1993). Subjects were asked to determine whether pairs of uppercase or lowercase As or Bs were a match in letter name (disregarding case) when presented for a 60-ms exposure in two of the four possible letter locations surrounding a constantly visible fixation point (Figure 16.4). Error rates were significantly smaller for bilateral presentations than for unilateral presentations (11.9% versus 16.6%, respectively; $p < 0.001$). Similarly, reaction times were significantly faster for bilateral trials than for unilateral trials (809 ms versus 897 ms, respectively; $p < 0.001$).

The reason for the occurrence of a BFA in these tests is not known. Because unilateral trials do not require callosal transfer, one might expect the opposite result, that is, faster and more accurate responses when stimuli are presented within the same visual field. Many suspect that the BFA occurs because bilateral presentations require each hemisphere to initially process only one stimulus (Dimond, 1970; Sereno and Kosslyn, 1991). This hypothesis is supported by the data, which show that as the complexity of the comparison to be made increases,

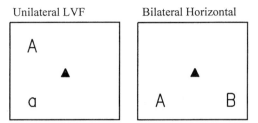

FIGURE 16.4. Examples of stimuli. The two rectangular fields represent examples of the stimuli of the letter-matching task. Labels above the rectangles indicate the type of trials. The solid triangle in the center was the constantly visible fixation point. The letters flashed for 56 ms for studies of younger normal adults, dyslexic adults, and callosal agenesis and commissurotomy patients. Stimulus duration was 200 ms for children, older adults, and MS patients.

the degree of advantage for bilateral presentations over unilateral presentations increases, as long as both hemispheres are capable of extracting the necessary information from the stimulus (Banich and Belger, 1990; Merola and Liederman, 1990; Norman et al., 1992). Regardless of the reasons for the bilateral advantage, the information in the stimuli must eventually be compared across visual fields (hemispheres). The point in the information-processing sequence at which information is integrated and compared is also not known. Nevertheless, the degree of BFA may reflect differences between clinical groups in callosal function.

NORMAL CHILDREN BFA in children was found to increase with increasing age (see Figure 16.3B) (Hagelthorn et al., 2000). That is, the RT advantage for bilateral presentations over unilateral ones (expressed as a proportion of the subject's standard deviation of RTs) was greater for older children (mean BFA = 0.20 for 10- to 12-year-olds) than for younger children (mean BFA = 0.07 for 7- to 9-year-olds) but did not change further in teenagers (mean BFA = 0.22 for 13- to 17-year-olds). BFA for response accuracy (i.e., percent error) showed the same developmental trend (mean BFA = 2%, 3%, and 4% for younger to older), but the effect was not statistically significant. These data parallel the developmental process reported for myelinization of the corpus callosum, as well as changes in EP-IHTT in the same subjects. Although the theory of independent hemispheric processing (Dimond, 1970; Sereno and Kosslyn, 1991) would suggest that increasing callosal function enhances hemispheric independence, some contribution to the BFA of more efficient interhemispheric transfer is also likely.

COMMISSUROTOMY AND AGENESIS PATIENTS As with the EP-IHTT measure, much can be learned about the BFA from the performance of individuals who lack a corpus callosum. However, in the case of BFA the results are quite different for these two types of acallosal patients (Brown et al., 1999). As one would expect from the many reports in the literature regarding the failure of interhemispheric transfer in split-brain patients, L.B. was unable to respond to bilateral letter-matching trials above the level of chance but compared letters within a single visual field well above chance level. Thus, L.B. had a substantial bilateral field disadvantage.

Agenesis patients, however, were clearly able to do bilateral letter comparisons above the level of chance. However, neither M.M. nor J.D. had a significant bilateral advantage in accuracy; that is, bilateral and unilateral trials were equally accurate. Although M.M. had a higher than normal overall error rate and slower overall RTs, J.D. was remarkably accurate (10% errors for both unilateral and bilateral) and fast (bilateral: 591 ms, unilateral: 606 ms). As was mentioned above, the MRIs of both of these agenesis patients clearly indicated the presence of the anterior commissure. This would suggest the hypothesis that bilateral visual field comparisons were able to be made in these patients via the anterior commissure but that this pathway was not sufficient to sustain a robust bilateral advantage. The hypothesis of bilateral visual comparisons via the anterior commissure is supported by a report from Fischer, Ryan, and Dobyns (1992), who compared an acallosal patient who had an anterior commissure to an acallosal patient who did not have an anterior commissure on tests of visual and tactile interhemispheric transfer. Results indicated that while the acallosal patient with the anterior commissure had normal interhemispheric transfer on these tests, the patient without the anterior commissure demonstrated impairment in both visual and tactile interhemispheric transfer.

The limits of interhemispheric transmission of visual information via the anterior commissure has been suggested by a second BFA experiment in the acallosals. This task required matching of patterns of dots rather than letters. Although this pattern-matching task is somewhat more difficult, normal adults still show a bilateral advantage (Larson and Brown, 1997). However, on this pattern comparison task agenesis patients had a significant bilateral disadvantage, that is, worse performance on bilateral trials compared to unilateral ones (Brown et al., 1999). Thus, on this more difficult comparison task individuals with callosal agenesis performed much more like a split-brain patient. These data suggest that there are limits to the visual information that can be adequately transferred over the anterior commissures— limits in either complexity or encodability of the items for comparison.

MULTIPLE SCLEROSIS PATIENTS While MS patients had a higher overall error rate and a slower overall reaction time than normals, they showed a very significant bilateral advantage in both RT and accuracy that was not different from that found in normals. The BFA for the two subgroups of MS patients (divided on the basis of the presence or absence of cross-callosal EPs) was also not found to differ significantly. Thus, while the MS subgroup lacking cross-callosal EPs had marked deficiencies in callosal transfer evident in visual EPs, they performed normally in making bilateral (interhemispheric) comparisons of the same letter stimuli from which the abnormal EPs were recorded. It may be that, as in the patients with agenesis of the corpus callosum, the anterior commissure of MS subjects is aiding the diseased corpus callosum in the interhemispheric transfer of visual letter information. Alternatively, it may be that BFA is a reflection of callosal channels other than the posterior channel carrying visual sensory-evoked potentials.

DYSLEXIC ADULTS The results from our study of adult individuals with dyslexia (Markee et al., 1996) are consistent with the findings from MS and callosal agenesis patients. That is, while dyslexics had significantly slower EP-IHTT, there was no evidence of this callosal deficit in the BFA data from this group. Although dyslexics made significantly more errors overall than controls and were somewhat (nonsignificantly) slower in overall RT, they had a large and robust BFA for both errors and reaction time that did not differ from that of normals. Here again, deficiencies in callosal transfer that were evident in EP-IHTT had no detectable effect on the speed or accuracy of making bilateral visual field letter comparisons.

The bimanual coordination task

In some of the early work on patients with commissurotomies, Preilowski (1972, 1975) demonstrated the usefulness of tests of bimanually coordinated motor activity in assessing callosal function. Preilowski's test involved an X-Y plotter modified so that the vertical axis was controlled by a handle that could be rotated by one arm and hand, while the horizontal axis was controlled by the other arm and hand. The task was to accurately and quickly draw an angled line, coordinating the speed of rotation of the two hands. Preilowski demonstrated deficits in this task among individuals who had the anterior portion of the corpus callosum surgically severed. He also found an asymmetry in performance such that performance was worse when the left hand had to contribute more to pen movement than the right hand.

Finally, Preilowski demonstrated particularly marked deficits when performance was attempted without visual feedback.

Preilowski's task can also be implemented by using an Etch-a-Sketch toy (Brown, 1991). This implementation of the bimanual coordination task (BCT) has the advantage of requiring hand and finger movements that have exclusively contralateral innervation for knob and cursor control, rather than arm movements, which have more bilateral representation. Our implementation of the BCT involves right- and left-hand unimanual trails, followed by three right-to-left angled target paths (22.5°, 45°, and 67.5°) and three left-to-right paths (112.5°, 135°, and 157.5°) (see Figure 16.5). Each of these angled paths is tested both with and without visual feedback for the last half of the target path while both time to complete the path and accuracy (either the number of times one leaves the demarcated path or the length of the line the subject draws in attempting to follow the path) is measured.

COMMISSUROTOMY AND AGENESIS PATIENTS L.B. performed well within the normal range in both speed and accuracy on the only portion of the BCT that we administered (i.e., right- and left-hand unimanual trials, and 22.5°, 45°, and 67.5°, all under visual control). Although our testing of L.B. was limited, our results are somewhat discrepant with the results of a BCT test of complete commissurotomy patients reported by Zaidel and Sperry (1977). Only three of eight commissurotomy patients reported by Zaidel and Sperry were able to do the test at all, and the three who could perform the task were reported to be unusually slow and inaccurate. Given our limited testing of L.B. and the absence of data from the more informative tests of BCT drawing without visual feedback, we can only conclude that split-brain patients working with the help of visual feedback do not always perform abnormally on the BCT, especially after many years since commissurotomy.

The BCT tests of our two patients with agenesis of the corpus callosum are more consistent with results for acallosals tested using the Preilowski version of this task (Jeeves, 1986; Jeeves et al., 1988). Both M.M. and J.D. were unremarkable in their performance when allowed visual feedback with respect to 15 age-matched normal adolescent boys, as well as in comparison to the data for normal children reported by Steese-Seda, Brown, and Caetano (1995) and adult normal controls reported by Moore and colleagues (1995). However, when visual feedback was removed, both agenesis patients were markedly deficient in their ability to continue bimanually coordinated activity. Jeeves (1986) and Jeeves and colleagues (1988) found that adults with agenesis of the

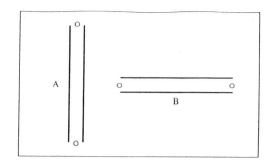

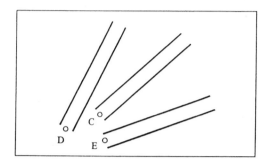

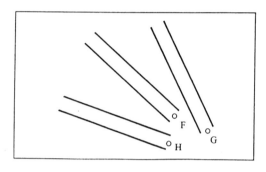

FIGURE 16.5. Target paths for the bimanual coordination task as they appeared on three Etch-a-Sketch overlays. Top: Two unimanual paths for right-hand (A = 90°) and left-hand (B = 0°) performance. Middle: Three right-angled paths for bimanual performance (C = 45°, D = 67.5°, E = 22.5°). Bottom: Three left-angle target paths for bimanual performance (F = 135°, G = 112.5°, H = 157.5°). Ratio of target path width to length is not to scale. (Figure reprinted from *Neuropsychologia*, volume 33, Moore, Brown, Markee, Theberge and Zvi, "Motor performance and interhemispheric collaboration in dyslexia," pp. 781–793, Copyright (1995), with kind permission from Elsevier Science Ltd., The Boulevard, Langford, Kidlington OX5 1GB, UK.)

corpus callosum performed slowly and inaccurately even after extensive practice but showed particularly marked abnormality when visual feedback was withdrawn.

In summary, these data suggest that absence of callosal connections does not necessarily disrupt the ability to coordinate the two hands in a task demanding continuous smooth modulations of the response speed of each hand, as long as visual feedback is available. However, testing in the absence of visual feedback reveals deficits in interhand coordination. Perhaps continuous visual scanning keeps hemispheric motor responses in harmony when callosal channels are absent.

NORMAL CHILDREN We have reported a study of BCT performance in 50 normal children between 6 and 13 years of age (Steese-Seda et al., 1995). The test involved only the subset of paths used with commissurotomy patient L.B. and therefore did not include performance without visual feedback. Speed and accuracy increased with age in a manner consistent with developmental progressions of motor ability; that is, bimanual time and errors were significantly correlated with age. Left-hand unimanual performance was most strongly age-related. Correlations between BCT measures and performance on the Tactile Performance Test (described below) suggested that facilitation of the nondominant hand may be an important callosal contribution to BCT performance. A replication of this research using a computerized version of the BCT in a new population of 68 normal school-aged children showed similar results. Most striking was the fact that the correlation with age for asymmetric hand performance (i.e., one hand must turn a response knob faster than the other hand) was significant ($r = -0.333$) even when covarying performance on symmetric angles (i.e., hands must turn knobs at the same speed) (Marion et al., 2000).

Jeeves and colleagues (1988) compared bimanual performance on the Preilowski version of the BCT in young adults (age 18–24) with that of younger and older children (ages 5–6 versus 9–11 years). Age differences were largest in early attempts on the bimanual task and converged with extensive practice. Performance of the younger group was more like adult acallosals when tested under conditions in which visual feedback was withdrawn halfway through a trial. Hence, younger children whose corpus callosum was not yet fully myelinated performed like individuals with callosal agenesis, while the older children who presumably had fully myelinated cerebral commissures performed more like normal adults. Fagard, Morioka, and Wolff (1985) also found that BCT performance of children was qualitatively different than that of adults in that children had directional asymmetries in errors that were not seen in

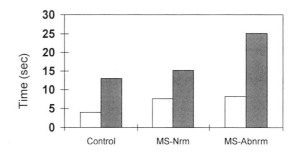

FIGURE 16.6. Performance on the BCT: MS patients. Mean times to complete target paths for unimanual (open bars) and bimanual (shaded bars) performance on the bimanual coordination test for age-matched older normal adults (Control), MS patients with normal cross-callosal EPs (MS-Nrm), and MS patients with abnormal cross-callosal EPs (MS-Abnrm).

adults, suggesting asymmetrical difficulties in the modulation of speed between the hands.

MULTIPLE SCLEROSIS MS patients were examined by using the Etch-a-Sketch version of the BCT (Larson et al., in press) and were found to be slower than non-patients on both unimanual trials (simple motor speed) and bimanual trials (intermanual coordination), consistent with their general neuromotor deficits associated with the demyelinization process. The subgroup of MS subjects with diminished-amplitude cross-callosal EPs was significantly slower than other MS patients on bimanual trials, even when statistically controlling for differences in unimanual speed (Figure 16.6). Thus, these data support the conclusion that significant deficits in interhemispheric coordination of motor activity occur in MS patients who show EP evidence of callosal dysfunction and interhemispheric transmission insufficiency.

ADULT DYSLEXICS The importance of deficits in bimanual coordination in dyslexia was suggested in the work of Gladstone and colleagues (1989). These authors demonstrated impairments in dyslexic boys on the Preilowski version of the BCT, particularly when individuals were required to make mirror-image responses with the two hands or when they were responding without the benefit of visual feedback. Similar results were found in a study of bimanual coordination in learning-disabled children (Rousselle and Wolff, 1991).

We recently reported evidence for BCT deficits in adult dyslexics (Moore et al., 1995). When compared to controls subjects, dyslexics showed deficits in BCT performance (both speed and accuracy) on all paths both with and without visual feedback. Consistent with the work of Gladstone and colleagues (1989), dyslexics had particular difficulty relative to normals when the left hand had to move faster than the right and when the hands had to make mirror-image movements. While our data seem to indicate most strongly a generalized motor deficit in adult dyslexics (e.g., significant differences found in both unimanual and bimanual speed), larger deficits for left-hand and mirror-image movements suggest additional problems with interhemispheric modulation of visuomotor control.

The Tactile Performance Test

The Tactile Performance Test (TPT) requires that the subject place differently shaped blocks into their proper locations on the test formboard while blindfolded (Halstead, 1947). First the test is done with the dominant hand; then the same blocks and formboard are tested with the nondominant hand. Normal adults show consistent savings in time to complete the puzzle for the nondominant hand relative to the previous dominant-hand performance. While the TPT measures tactile form perception, spatial learning, and spatial recall, successful performance of the nondominant hand relative to that of the dominant hand is believed to reflect sharing of spatial information between the hemispheres. Three versions of the TPT are available: six, eight, and ten blocks (Halstead, 1947; Russell, 1985).

NORMAL CHILDREN Sufficient normative data exist in the literature, and our testing of normal children on the TPT are consistent with these norms (Steese-Seda et al., 1995). Although the absolute savings in time for non-dominant-hand performance does not change much between 5 and 13 years of age, the percent savings increases progressively from around 15% to over 30% (Spreen and Gaddes, 1969). While increased learning efficiency may play a role in this developmental trend, these norms also suggest that progressive callosal myelinization during this developmental span is reflected in improved interhemispheric transfer of formboard information in the TPT.

COMMISSUROTOMY AND AGENESIS PATIENTS L.B. did relatively poorly but within the normal range on the first attempt with his dominant hand (z-score $= 1.65$ using the norms of Spreen and Strauss (1991)). However, as might be expected from the descriptions of the disconnection syndrome in split-brain patients (Sperry, 1974), L.B. showed no savings in his attempt with the nondominant hand; that is, time to finish the ten-block version of the puzzle with the left hand was longer than (showed no benefit from) the previous attempt with the dominant hand ($z = 9.95$). The same results were found with both agenesis patients, M.M. and J.D. While their performance was relatively poor with the dominant hand ($z = 5.35$ and 2.00, respectively), they were

markedly worse on the subsequent attempt with the nondominant hand ($z = 8.08$ and 9.75, respectively), indicating no interhemispheric (interhand) sharing of the spatial information regarding the layout of the formboard.

Deficits in TPT performance in individuals with agenesis of the corpus callosum has been reported by others (Fischer et al., 1992; Sauerwein and Lassonde, 1994). Although the degree of deficit in nondominant-hand performance differs between various reports, much of the differences can be accounted for by the difficulty of the TPT used. Sauerwein and colleagues (1981) reported unimpaired performance in two acallosals using a six-block TPT. Fischer and colleagues (1992) found only mild impairment using the intermediate (eight-block) version. Finally, Sauerwein and Lassonde (1994) have reported in their more recent work impaired performance on the ten-block TPT in two asymptomatic individuals with agenesis of the corpus callosum. Our results closely mirror these more recent data of Sauerwein and Lassonde. It can be concluded from these results that difficulty is an important variable in the sensitivity of the TPT to callosal absence. That is, while information relative to a simplified version of the TPT may cross via intact noncallosal channels (e.g., the anterior commissure), information regarding the more complex ten-block TPT cannot cross sufficiently to sustain normal performance, and results approach those of the split-brain individual. Thus, the level-of-difficulty versus transferability results in acallosals are consistent between the TPT test and the BFA experiment.

MULTIPLE SCLEROSIS Because of the general sensorimotor and memory deficits of MS patients, they were tested on the six-block TPT. Nevertheless, MS patients were somewhat deficient in dominant-hand performance when compared to the oldest available six-block norms, that is, 13-year-old children ($z = 2.43$). Subsequent nondominant-hand performance was relatively worse than dominant-hand performance ($z = 5.88$). Particularly interesting was the fact that individuals with abnormal cross-callosal EPs showed no savings on non-dominant-hand performance (i.e., took longer on non-dominant hand than on dominant hand) and were 3 standard deviations worse with the nondominant hand than individuals with normal cross-callosal EPs ($z = 7.87$ versus $z = 4.58$). These data indicate that even the simple version of the TPT is relatively difficult for individuals with mild MS and that deficits are markedly increased when interhemispheric transfer is demanded.

ADULT DYSLEXICS Our tests of TPT performance in adult dyslexics were entirely unremarkable. These individuals did not differ in either dominant- or nondominant-hand performance from matched controls, nor were they discrepant from available norms. However, we tested these adult individuals on the six-block version (primarily as a concession to the testing time required for our entire test battery). The data reviewed above relative to test complexity and deficits in agenesis patients is relevant to testing for callosal transfer deficits in dyslexics; that is, deficits are likely to appear only on more complex versions of this task. Thus, conclusions regarding TPT interhemispheric transfer in adult dyslexics must await further research.

The Finger Localization Test

The Finger Localization Test (FLT) assesses the ability of individuals to localize tactile stimulation of the fingertips and to transfer the information intermanually to indicate the fingers touched on the opposite hand while blindfolded (Geffen et al., 1985; Quinn and Geffen, 1986). On a particular block of trials, sequences of one, three, or four fingers are touched, and the subject is asked to replicate the sequence by touching the thumb to the appropriate fingers of the same or opposite hand. Comparisons of same-hand versus between-hand responding provides a measure of the interhemispheric transfer of the sequential-tactile information.

NORMAL CHILDREN   Transfer of finger localization information has been found to improve as a function of maturation in normal children (Quinn and Geffen, 1986; Geffen et al., 1985). Similarly, Galin and colleagues (1979) reported an increase in the accuracy of transfer of texture information as children develop. We have no additional data on FLT performance and callosal development in normal children.

COMMISSUROTOMY AND AGENESIS PATIENTS   Geffen and colleagues (1985) have reported data on FLT performance in L.B. For localization of a single stimulated finger, L.B. was unable to respond much above chance level on between-hand trials. Geffen and colleagues (1985) studied a total of 10 complete and partial commissurotomy patients. They found that opposite-hand responding for single-finger stimulation was 82% worse than same-hand responding in complete commissurotomy, 28% worse with only the trunk of the callosum severed, and only 7% worse in controls.

Our test of three- and four-finger stimulation in agenesis subjects showed mixed results. M.M. clearly had difficulty with this task generally (i.e., twice as many errors as controls on same-hand trials) but had particular difficulty with intermanual transfer (i.e., three times as many errors as controls on between hand trials). J.D., however, was clearly within the range of normal controls on both within- and between-hand trials. Several studies in the literature suggest that agenesis patients have difficulties with between-hand FLT responding (summarized by Geffen et al., 1994), although some studies have not found deficits in FLT in agenesis patients (e.g., Lassonde et al., 1988). Geffen and colleagues (1994) suggest that more difficult, multifinger stimulation tasks are necessary to reveal deficits in callosal agenesis patients. However, data from J.D. would suggest that deficits in a more difficult, multifinger FLT task are not necessarily the rule in agenesis patients. The reason for the lack of a transfer deficit in J.D. needs further study. It may be related to the fact that J.D. is left-handed and therefore may have a different cortical organization of the sensorimotor function of the hands. In addition, J.D. has a Probst bundle clearly evident in his MRI, and this structure is not visible in the MRI of M.M. (although the quality of the older MRI for M.M. makes it difficult to reach a firm conclusion).

MULTIPLE SCLEROSIS   It is difficult to come to firm conclusions from our data on FLT in MS patients, since we have not as yet collected age-appropriate normative data. However, comparison of the FLT data from MS patients with the somewhat younger normals of our dyslexia study is suggestive. MS patients who reported any paresthesia of the hands or fingers were not tested so as not to confound sensorimotor deficits with deficits in callosal transfer. The ratio of between-hand to same-hand correct responses (an index of callosal transfer adjusted for same-hand accuracy) was significantly smaller in MS patients than the dyslexic-study controls ($p < 0.04$). MS patients were 23% worse responding between hands than with the same hand, whereas the controls were only 14% worse. Thus, MS patients appear to have a deficit in callosal transfer that is not attributable to more general sensorimotor problems that would be associated with same-hand responding. However, this apparent deficit in callosal transfer of finger localization information did not differ between the two subgroups of MS patients (no cross-callosal EP: 24% worse, clear cross-callosal EP: 22% worse). Thus, deficits in transfer of tactile information in the FLT are not related to the kind of deficits in callosal transfer that are manifest in the visual EPs of MS patients.

ADULT DYSLEXICS   Results of our study of FLT in adult dyslexics have been reported by Moore and colleagues (1996). Comparing the FLT ratio of correct responses (between-hand/same-hand) of dyslexics and controls yielded a nonsignificant trend suggesting less efficient intermanual transfer in dyslexics ($p = 0.13$). Dyslexics were 24% worse responding with the opposite hand than with the same hand, while the controls were 14% worse. However, on the basis of the work of Temple, Jeeves, and Villaroya (1989, 1990) suggesting difficulties in rhyming in patients with callosal agenesis, we combined the dyslexic and normal groups and redivided the subjects on the basis of a ratio comparing their rhyming fluency with their general verbal fluency (the FAS task). Split this way, there were very significant differences between groups in the FLT ratio ($p < 0.006$). Good rhymers did on the average 10% worse between hands, while poor rhymers did 27% worse. It seems, then, that reading ability as indexed by the diagnostic schema for dyslexia is not as related to callosal dysfunction as the more specific ability in phonological processing that is required to do rhyming tasks. This result in individuals who (presumably) all have a corpus callosum is entirely consistent with the results of Temple, Jeeves, and Villaroya for tests of individuals with agenesis of the corpus callosum in demonstrating a relationship between callosal function and phonological-processing ability.

Tactile maze

This test requires the blindfolded completion of a tactile maze involving a 10×10 grid of metal buttons with a single correct path from the lower left to upper right corners (patterned after Milner, 1965). Ten learning trials are given with the dominant hand, then alternate blocks of two trials are given with the nondominant, dominant, and nondominant hands, respectively. Of particular interest is the interhand (interhemispheric) transfer of maze learning (Jeeves, 1979). Normal individuals are as fast and accurate when switched to their nondominant hand as they were on previous trials with the dominant hand; that is, intermanual transfer of the maze learning occurs without loss.

COMMISSUROTOMY AND AGENESIS PATIENTS   Although we have no data on this task from L.B., it is clear that individuals with agenesis of the corpus callosum show deficiencies in intermanual transfer of tactile maze performance. After 10 consecutive learning trials with the dominant hand, both agenesis adolescents were taking approximately 1 minute to complete the maze. Their response times did not differ from the comparison group of age-matched normals (M.M.: $z = -0.61$, J.D.: $z = -0.51$). However, when they were switched to the nondominant hand, time increased markedly for both individuals as compared to the normal controls, whose time did not change (M.M.: $z = 3.40$, J.D.: $z = 1.40$). A similar pattern was evident in errors. Thus, there is a deficit in intermanual transfer of maze learning in these two individuals with agenesis of the corpus callosum.

MULTIPLE SCLEROSIS   MS patients are the only other clinical group for whom we have results from tests of tactile maze performance. MS patients performed normally on this task in that their time and error scores for both dominant and nondominant hands were generally within the range of those of our adolescent boys who were used as controls for the agenesis patients. What is more, each switch between dominant and nondominant hand was accompanied by slightly better performance in time and error rate. Thus, not only did tactile learning transfer, but also performance continued to improve, suggesting that the continued benefits of practice were accessible to both hands in these MS patients.

Summaries of callosal function in MS and dyslexia

The data reported above are summarized in Table 16.1. All of the tests used to assess callosal function in our clinical studies of MS and adult dyslexia showed abnormalities in both the commissurotomy patient (when data were available) and the callosal agenesis patients (with the exception of inconsistent outcomes for FLT). In addition, in the three tests in which the effect of child development were studied (EP-IHTT, BFA, and BCT), as well as one test in which developmental trends in intermanual transfer were suggested by published norms (TPT), children show increasing efficiency of callosal function up to around 10–12 years of age, with little evidence of further change thereafter. This progression is consistent with what is known of callosal myelinization during this developmental span. Thus, the test battery that we have used in these clinical studies appears to be valid and sensitive to callosal dysfunction.

MULTIPLE SCLEROSIS   There is no argument over the fact that MS affects the corpus callosum in a large percentage of patients (Simon et al., 1986; Dietemann et al., 1988; Rao et al., 1989). However, the effects of callosal lesions and/or atrophy on interhemispheric interactions in MS patients has only recently been appreciated (e.g., Rao et al., 1989; Pelletier et al., 1993). The results reported herein strongly support the conclusion that MS patients can suffer from deficits reminiscent of the disconnection syndrome shown by split-brain or, to a lesser degree, callosal agenesis patients. Deficits in interhemispheric interactions were evident in MS patients on four of the six measures in our battery.

More important, these data highlight the value of evoked potential methods in the clinical diagnosis of callosal dysfunction in MS. While finger localization was

Table 16.1

Summary of results[1]

Test \ Group	Commissurotomy	Agenesis of the Corpus Callosum	Normal Children	Multiple Sclerosis	Adult Dyslexia
EP Interhemisph. Transfer Time (EP-IHTT)	Abnormal Absent Cross-Callosal EPs	Abnormal Absent Cross-Callosal EPs	Age-related IHTT decreases	Abnormal Absent Cross-Callosal EPs	Abnormal Slowed IHTT
Bilateral Field Advantage (BFA)	Abnormal Failure of bilateral matching	Abnormal Bilateral matching OK, but no BFA	Age-related BFA increases	Normal	Normal
Bimanual Coordination Test (BCT)	No Data[2] [Difficulty when without visual feedback]	Abnormal Difficulty when no visual feedback	Age-related Improved performance [greatest age effect for no-feedback]	Abnormal Relatively greater deficit on bimanual paths for abnormal EP subgroup	Abnormal Slower on all bimanual paths
Tactile Performance Test (TPT)	Abnormal No intermanual transfer	Abnormal Deficit in intermanual transfer of learning	No Data [Increasing % savings on published norms]	Abnormal Largest deficit for abnormal EP subgroup	Normal Only 6-block version tested
Finger Localization Test (FLT)	No Data [Lack of transfer would be expected]	Inconsistent MM is abnormal JD appears normal	No Data [age-related changes reported for tactile comparisons]	Abnormal Inflated error rate for between hand	Abnormal Inflated error rate for between hand
Tactile Maze (Maze)	No Data [Lack of transfer would be expected]	Abnormal Deficit in intermanual transfer of learning	No Data	Normal	No Data

[1] Statements in brackets [ ] indicate reasonable conclusions that can be made from the published literature.

[2] Some data are available on LB, but the critical data without visual feedback are missing.

abnormal in both MS subgroups, it was only the subgroup of MS patients with abnormal cross-callosal EPs for which abnormalities of bimanual coordination (BCT) and interhand transfer of tactile-spatial information (TPT) could be detected. Thus, visual EPs can provide an important index of the degree of dysfunction of the posterior callosum, which, in these data, was predictive of deficits in visuomotor and tactile-spatial intermanual performance.

The contribution of callosal dysfunction to the neuropsychological profile of MS (e.g., deficits in memory, abstraction, and mental fluency) needs further study. However, aided by EP and MRI methods of revealing degree and location of callosal dysfunction, further study of MS patients should contribute considerably to understanding the importance of interhemispheric interactions via the corpus callosum for various higher mental abilities in humans.

DYSLEXIA While callosal dysfunction has been demonstrated in several previous studies (Gladstone et al., 1989; Davidson et al., 1990; Davidson and Saron, 1992), the existence of callosal deficits in dyslexia is not well established, nor is the nature of such deficits well understood. Our study of adult dyslexics (Moore et al., 1995, 1996; Markee et al., 1996) yielded evidence of callosal dysfunction in EP-IHTT, bimanual coordination, and finger localization. The only test of callosal function for which adequate data were available that did not show evidence of callosal dysfunction was the BFA, which was also normal in both subgroups of MS patients.

Callosal dysfunction as revealed in these measures might not be a direct cause of the reading disability. Several other possibilities must be considered. First, callosal dysfunction may be a separate dysfunction related to dyslexia only in that the two conditions tend to co-occur. Second, it may be that callosal problems relate to an intervening, more general neuropsychological variable such as attention that in turn affects reading. Or third, deficits in tests of callosal transfer may be secondary to abnormalities of processing and neuropathology in cortical areas of origin or destination of callosal fibers. Galaburda and colleagues (1985), for example, have evidence for neuronal ectopias and architectonic dysplasias in the perisylvian region of the left hemisphere in dyslexic individuals. Finally, it may be that normal callosal activity is critical for a subfunction of reading but not the entire process. That callosal function is related to, but not critical for, reading is supported by the work of Temple and colleagues (1989, 1990), who did not find evidence of dyslexia in a group of individuals with agenesis of the corpus callosum, although a consistent disorder of phonological processing was noted in these patients.

Our data from bimanual coordination and finger localization (Moore et al., 1995, 1996) illustrate the interaction between types and definitions of reading disability and specific tests of callosal function. On the BCT, deficits were seen in the dyslexic group on all aspects tested, suggestive of more general neurological impairments in this group. Involvement of callosal function more specifically was evident in the larger differences between normals and dyslexics when left-hand or mirror image responding was demanded. However, BCT performance was not associated with performance on our test of phonological-processing ability (rhyming). In direct contrast, deficits in intermanual transfer of finger localization information could not be significantly demonstrated for the group of individuals who were diagnosed as dyslexic (although a trend was apparent). However, phonological-processing ability was found to be very significantly related to the ratio of between- to same-hand performance on the FLT. While it seems clear that callosal function deficits play some role in dyslexia, further work needs to be done with increased attention to the linguistic subcomponents of reading ability, the age and gender of the dyslexic individuals, and the kind of interhemispheric interactions being tested.

Neuropsychological assessment of callosal dysfunction

The data presented in this chapter illustrate a number of important points regarding the clinical neuropsychological assessment of callosal function:

• Not every test that appears to tap callosal function will be adequately sensitive. The letter-matching version of the BFA task was not sensitive to callosal dysfunction in dyslexia or in either subgroup of MS patients.
• Complexity of information to be transferred is an issue that needs attention. Deficits are more likely to be apparent when transfer of more complex information is demanded.
• EPs to lateralized visual stimuli provide an important direct measure of posterior callosal function.
• Ability of the BCT and TPT to differentiate between MS patients grouped on the basis of EP evidence of callosal malfunction suggests the sensitivity of these measures to callosal dysfunction in the individual MS patient.
• FLT was able to reveal callosal dysfunction even in MS patients who did not show abnormal EPs.

Neuropsychological test batteries seldom include tests of callosal function. The studies described in this chapter demonstrate that callosal function can be adequately and sensitively assessed, that improving callosal function is an important aspect of child neuropsychological development, and that callosal dysfunction contributes to at least two neuropsychological syndromes (i.e., MS and dyslexia). Perhaps more attention needs to be paid to the routine assessment of adequacy of callosal function.

ACKNOWLEDGMENTS The research on multiple sclerosis reported herein was supported by a grant from the National Multiple Sclerosis Society ("Disconnection Syndromes in Multiple Sclerosis," W. S. Brown, P.I., PP0244). The author gratefully acknowledges the following of his current and former students who contributed so significantly to this research: Eric Larson, Debra Burnison, Taryn Markee, Larry Moore, David Theberge, Deborah Steese-Seda, Carla Caetano, Vicki McWain, Lynn Paul, Kathleen (Thompson) Hagelthorn, and Stacy Amano. Larry Moore gave helpful comments on earlier versions of this text. The author also recognizes the collaboration on some of this research, and influence on the entire research project, of Professor Malcolm Jeeves of the University of St. Andrews, Scotland.

REFERENCES

BANICH, M. T., and A. BELGER, 1990. Interhemispheric interaction: How do the hemispheres divide and conquer a task? *Cortex* 26:77–94.

BOGEN, J. E., 1969. The other side of the brain. I: Dysgraphia and dyscopia following cerebral commissurotomy. *Bull. Los Angeles Neurol. Soc.* 34:73–105.

BOGEN, J. E., 1993. The callosal syndromes. In *Clinical Neuropsychology*, 3rd ed., J. M. Heilman and E. Valenstein, eds. New York: Oxford University Press, pp. 337–407.

BRIZZOLARA, D., G. FERRETTI, P. BROVEDANI, C. CASALINI, and L. COWAN, 1994. Is interhemispheric transfer time related to age? A developmental study. *Behav. Brain Res.* 64:179–184.

BROWN, W. S., 1991. *The Bimanual Coordination Test: Version 1.* Pasadena, CA: The Travis Institute Papers.

BROWN, W. S., and M. JEEVES, 1993. Bilateral field advantage and evoked potential interhemispheric transmission time. *Neuropsychologia* 31:1267–1281.

BROWN, W. S., M. A. JEEVES, R. DIETRICH, and D. S. BURNISON, 1999. Bilateral field advantage and evoked potential interhemispheric transmission in commissurotomy and callosal agenesis. *Neuropsychologia*, 37:1154–1180.

BROWN, W. S., E. B. LARSON, and M. JEEVES, 1994. Directional asymmetries in interhemispheric transmission time: Evidence from visual evoked potentials. *Neuropsychologia* 32:439–448.

BURNISON, D. S., E. B. LARSON, and W. S. BROWN, 1995. Evoked potential interhemispheric transmission and the bilateral field advantage in multiple sclerosis [Abstract]. *J. Int. Neuropsychol. Soc.* 1:182.

DAVIDSON, R. J., S. C. LESLIE, and C. D. SARON, 1990. Reaction time measures of interhemispheric transfer time in reading disabled and normal children. *Neuropsychologia* 28:471–485.

DAVIDSON, R. J., and C. D. SARON, 1992. Evoked potential measures of interhemispheric transfer time in reading disabled and normal boys. *Dev. Neuropsychol.* 8:261–277.

DIETEMANN, J. L., C. BEIGELMAN, L. RUMBACH, M. VOUGE, T. TAJAHMADY, C. FAUBERT, M. Y. JEUNG, and A. WACKENHEIM, 1988. Multiple sclerosis and corpus callosum atrophy: Relationship of MRI findings to clinical data. *Neuroradiology* 30:478–480.

DIMOND, S. J., 1970. Hemispheric refractoriness and control of reaction time. *Q. J. Exp. Psychol.* 22:610–617.

DIMOND, S. J., and G. BEAUMONT, 1972. Processing in perceptual integration between and within the cerebral hemispheres. *Br. J. Psychol.* 63:509–514.

FAGARD, J., M. MORIOKA, and P. H. WOLFF, 1985. Early stages in the acquisition of bimanual motor skill. *Neuropsychologia* 23:535–543.

FISCHER, M., S. B. RYAN, and W. B. DOBYNS, 1992. Mechanisms of interhemispheric transfer and patterns of cognitive function in acallosal patients of normal intelligence. *Arch. Neurol.* 49:271–277.

GALABURDA, A. M., G. F. SHERMAN, G. D. ROSEN, F. ABOITIZ, and N. GESCHWIND, 1985. Developmental dyslexia: Four consecutive patients with cortical anomalies. *Ann. Neurol.* 18:222–233.

GALIN, D., J. JOHNSTONE, L. NAKELL, and J. HERRON, 1979. Development of the capacity for tactile information transfer between hemispheres in normal children. *Science* 204:1330–1332.

GEFFEN, G., J. NILSSON, K. QUINN, and E. L. TENG, 1985. The effects of lesions of the corpus callosum on finger localization. *Neuropsychologia* 23:497–514.

GEFFEN, G., J. NILSSON, D. A. SIMPSON, and M. A. JEEVES, 1994. The development of interhemispheric transfer of tactile information in cases of callosal agenesis. In *Callosal Agenesis*, M. Lassonde and M. A. Jeeves, eds. New York: Plenum.

GLADSTONE, M., and C. T. BEST, 1985. Developmental dyslexia: The potential role of interhemispheric collaboration in reading acquisition. In *Hemispheric Function and Collaboration in the Child*, C. T. Best, ed. San Francisco: Academic Press, pp. 87–118.

GLADSTONE, M., C. T. BEST, and R. J. DAVIDSON, 1989. Anomalous bimanual coordination among dyslexic boys. *Dev. Psychol.* 25 (2):236–246.

HAGELTHORN, K. M., W. S. BROWN, S. AMANO, and R. ASARNOW, 2000. Normal development of bilateral field advantage and evoked potential interhemispheric transmission time. *Dev. Neuropsychol.*, in press.

HALSTEAD, W. C., 1947. *Brain and Intelligence*. Chicago: University of Chicago Press.

JEEVES, M. A., 1979. Some limits to interhemispheric integration in cases of callosal agenesis and partial commissurotomy. In *Structure and Function of the Cerebral Commissures*, I. S. Russell, M. W. van Hof, and G. Berlucchi, eds., London: Macmillan.

JEEVES, M. A., 1986. Callosal agenesis: Neuronal and developmental adaptations. In *Two Hemispheres—One Brain*, F. Lepore, M. Ptito, and H. H. Jasper, eds. New York: Alan R. Liss, pp. 403–421.

JEEVES, M. A., P. H. SILVER, and I. JACOBSON, 1988. Bimanual coordination in callosal agenesis and partial commissurotomy. *Neuropsychologia* 26:833–850.

LARSON, E. B., and W. S. BROWN, 1997. Bilateral field interactions, hemispheric specialization and evoked potential interhemispheric transmission time. *Neuropsychologia* 35:573–581.

LARSON, E. B., D. S. BURNISON, and W. S. BROWN. Callosal function in multiple sclerosis: Bimanual motor coordination. *Cortex*, in press.

LASSONDE M., H. SAUERWEIN, N. McCABE, L. LAURENCELLE, and G. GEOFFROY, 1988. Extent and limits of cerebral adjustment to early section or congenital absence of the corpus callosum. *Behav. Brain Res.* 30:165–181.

LIEDERMAN, J., J. MEROLA, and S. MARTINEZ, 1985. Interhemispheric collaboration in response to simultaneous bilateral input. *Neuropsychologia* 23:673–683.

MANGUN, G. R., S. J. LUCK, M. S. GAZZANIGA, and S. A. HILLYARD, 1991. Electrophysiological measures of interhemispheric transfer of visual information: Studies of split-brain patients. *Soc. Neurosci.* 17:340–344.

MARION, S., S. KILLIAN, T. NARAMOR, and W. BROWN, 2000. Normal development of callosal and visuomotor aspects of bimanual coordination [Abstract]. *J. Int. Neuropsychol. Soc.* 6:116.

MARKEE, T. E., W. S. BROWN, L. H. MOORE, D. C. THEBERGE, and J. C. ZVI, 1996. Callosal function in dyslexia: Evoked potential interhemispheric transfer time and bilateral field advantage. *Dev. Neuropsychol.* 12:409–428.

MARZI, C. A., P. BISIACCHI, and R. NICOLETTI, 1991. Is interhemispheric transfer of visuomotor information asymmetric? Evidence from a meta-analysis. *Neuropsychologia* 29:1163–1177.

MEROLA, J., and J. LIEDERMAN, 1990. The extent to which between-hemisphere division of inputs improves performance depends upon task difficulty. *J. Clin. Exp. Neuropsychol.* 10:69.

MILNER, B., 1965. Visually-guided maze learning in man: Effects of bilateral hippocampal, bilateral frontal and unilateral cerebral lesions. *Neuropsychologia* 3:317–338.

MOORE, L. H., W. S. BROWN, T. E. MARKEE, D. C. THEBERGE, E. and J. ZVI, 1995. Motor performance and interhemispheric collaboration in dyslexia. *Neuropsychologia* 33:781–793.

MOORE, L. H., W. S. BROWN, T. E. MARKEE, D. C. THEBERGE, and J. C. ZVI, 1996. Callosal transfer of finger localization information in phonologically dyslexic adults. *Cortex* 32:311–322.

NORMAN, W. D., M. A. JEEVES, A. MILNE, and T. LUDWIG, 1992. Hemispheric interactions: The bilateral advantage and task difficulty. *Cortex* 28:623–642.

PELLETIER, J., M. HABIB, O. LYON-CAEN, G. SALAMON, M. PONCET, and R. KHALIL, 1993. Functional and magnetic resonance imaging correlates of callosal involvement in multiple sclerosis. *Arch. Neurol.* 50:1077–1082.

Preilowski, B., 1972. Possible contributions of the anterior forebrain commissures to bilateral motor coordination. *Neuropsychologia* 10:267–277.

Preilowski, B., 1975. Bilateral motor interaction: Perceptual and motor performance of partial and complete "split-brain" patients. In *Cerebral Localization*, K. J. Zulch, O. Creutzfeldt, and G. C. Galbraith, eds. Berlin: Springer, pp. 115–132.

Quinn, K., and G. Geffen, 1986. The development of tactile transfer of information. *Neuropsychologia* 24:793–804.

Rakic, P., and P. I. Yakovlev, 1968. Development of the corpus callosum and cavum septi in man. *J. Comp. Neurol.* 132:45–72.

Rao, S. M., L. Bernardin, G. J. Leo, L. Ellington, S. B. Ryan, and L. S. Burg, 1989. Cerebral disconnection in multiple sclerosis: Relationship to atrophy of the corpus callosum. *Arch. Neurol.* 46:918–920.

Rousselle, C., and P. H. Wolff, 1991. The dynamics of bimanual coordination in developmental dyslexia. *Neuropsychologia* 29:907–924.

Rugg, M. D., C. R. Lines, and A. D. Milner, 1984. Visual evoked potentials elicited by lateralized stimuli and the measurement of interhemispheric transmission time. *Neuropsychologia* 22:215–225.

Rugg, M. D., A. D. Milner, and C. R. Lines, 1985. Visual evoked potentials to lateralized stimuli in two cases of callosal agenesis. *J. Neurol. Neurosurg. Psychiatry* 48:367–373.

Russell, E. W., 1985. Comparison of the TPT 10 and 6 hole form board. *J. Clin. Psychol.* 41:68–81.

Salamy, A., 1978. Commissural transmission: Maturational changes in humans. *Science* 200:1409–1411.

Saron, C. D., and R. J. Davidson, 1989. Visual evoked potential measures of interhemispheric transfer time in humans. *Behav. Neurosci.* 103:1115–1138.

Sauerwein, H. C., and M. Lassonde, 1994. Cognitive and sensori-motor functioning in the absence of the corpus callosum: Neuropsychological studies in callosal agenesis and callosotomized patients. *Behav. Brain Res.* 64:229–240.

Sauerwein, H. C., M. Lassonde, B. Cardu, and G. Geoffroy, 1981. Interhemispheric integration of sensory and motor functions in callosal agenesis. *Neuropsychologia* 19:445–454.

Sereno, A. B., and S. M. Kosslyn, 1991. Discrimination within and between hemifields: A new constraint on theories of attention. *Neuropsychologia* 29:659–675.

Simon, J. H., S. L. Holtas, R. B. Schiffer, R. A. Rudick, R. M. Herndon, D. K. Kido, and R. Utz, 1986. Corpus callosum and subcallosal-periventricular lesions in multiple sclerosis: Detection with MR. *Radiology* 160:363–367.

Sperry, R. W., 1974. Lateral specialization in the surgically separated hemispheres. In *The Neurosciences Third Study Program*, F. O. Schmitt and F. G. Worden, eds. Cambridge, Mass.: MIT Press, pp. 5–19.

Spreen, O., and W. H. Gaddes, 1969. Developmental norms for 15 neuropsychological tests of age 6 to 15. *Cortex* 5:171–191.

Spreen, O., and E. Strauss, 1991. *A Compendium of Neuropsychological Tests: Administration, Norms and Commentary.* New York: Oxford University Press.

Steese-Seda, D., W. S. Brown, and C. Caetano, 1995. Development of bimanual visuomotor coordination in school aged children: The bimanual coordination task. *Dev. Neuropsychol.* 11:181–199.

Temple, C. M., M. A. Jeeves, and O. Vilarroya, 1989. Ten pen men: rhyming skills in two children with callosal agenesis. *Brain Lang.* 37:548–564.

Temple, C. M., M. A. Jeeves, and O. O. Vilarroya, 1990. Reading in callosal agenesis. *Brain Lang.* 39:235–253.

Yakovlev, P. I., and A. R. Lecours, 1967. The myelogenetic cycles of regional maturation in the brain. In *Regional Development of the Brain in Early Life*, A. Minowski, ed. Oxford, Engl.: Blackwell, pp. 98–114.

Zaidel, D. W., and R. W. Sperry, 1977. Some long-term motor effects of cerebral commissurotomy in man. *Neuropsychologia* 97:263–272.

Zaidel, E., D. W. Zaidel, and J. E. Bogen, 1999. The split brain. In *Encyclopedia of Neuroscience*, 2nd ed., G. Adelman and B. Smith, eds. Amsterdam: Elsevier, pp. 1930–1936. (Also on CD-ROM)

COMMENTARY 16.1

Interhemispheric Conduction Delay in Multiple Sclerosis

FRANCESCO TOMAIUOLO, MARCO IACOBONI, M. ALTIERI, VITTORIO DI PIERO, CARLO POZZILLI, GIAN L. LENZI, AND CARLO A. MARZI

ABSTRACT The serial information-processing model (see Chapter 12 in this volume) and the equilibrium model (see Chapter 10 in this volume) of callosal functions were contrasted in this study. The timing of interhemispheric visuomotor integration was investigated in a group of multiple sclerosis (MS) patients with mild disability and various degrees of callosal atrophy. Interhemispheric transfer time in MS patients was similar to that of normal controls. In contrast, a patient with complete callosotomy had an interhemispheric transfer time much longer than those of normals and MS patients. These findings reinforce the notion that interhemispheric visuomotor integration is subserved by specific callosal channels that may be selectively impaired by specific lesion locations but that are generally spared by a nonspecific process of atrophy of the corpus callosum. These data are more naturally explained by the serial information-processing model of callosal functions during visuomotor interhemispheric integration.

As Brown demonstrates in his chapter, a number of behavioral and electrophysiological studies have shown interhemispheric disconnection symptoms in patients with multiple sclerosis (MS). This is not surprising, given the available magnetic resonance imaging (MRI) evidence of callosal lesions and callosal atrophy in a high percentage of MS patients (Huber et al., 1987; Pozzilli et al., 1991). Here, we used a classic paradigm to investigate interhemispheric mechanisms of basic sensorimotor integration in a series of MS patients with relapsing-remitting form.

Since the beginning of the century, simple reaction times to lateralized flashes have been used to estimate interhemispheric conduction delay (Poffenberger, 1912). In this task, simple visual stimuli are presented to the left or right visual hemifield. On detection of the stimulus, subjects are required to respond with the left or the right hand. When stimuli and response are contralateral (crossed condition), it is necessary to transfer information from the hemisphere that receives the visual stimulus to the hemisphere that controls the motor response. When stimuli and responses are ipsilateral (uncrossed condition), in contrast, there is no need for interhemispheric transfer. When one subtracts reaction times (RT) of the two uncrossed conditions (left hand/left visual hemifield and right hand/right visual hemifield) from those of the two crossed conditions (left hand/right visual hemifield and right hand/left visual hemifield) and divides by 2, one obtains an estimate of the interhemispheric conduction delay called crossed-uncrossed difference (CUD).

A variety of interhemispheric routes may, in principle, subserve the integration of visual stimuli and motor responses between the two hemispheres (Clarke and Zaidel, 1989). However, empirical evidence suggests that the shortest interhemispheric transfer occurs through the corpus callosum. Indeed, normal subjects have an interhemispheric conduction delay of about 4 ms (Marzi, Bisiacchi, and Nicoletti, 1991), whereas patients with complete surgical section of the corpus callosum carried out to obtain relief from intractable epilepsy have a much longer interhemispheric conduction delay, ranging from 25 ms to 75 ms (Iacoboni and Zaidel, 1995; Marzi et al., 1991). Furthermore, patients born without a corpus callosum tend to have an intermediate inter-

FRANCESCO TOMAIUOLO IRCCS Fondazione Santa Lucia, Rome, Italy.

MARCO IACOBONI Ahmanson Lovelace Brain Mapping Center, Neuropsychiatric Institute, Brain Research Institute, David Geffen School of Medicine, University of California at Los Angeles, Los Angeles, California.

M. ALTIERI, VITTORIO DI PIERO, AND GIAN L. LENZI Clinica Neurologica, Department of Neurological Sciences, University La Sapienza, Rome, Italy.

CARLO POZZILLI Clinica Neurologica, Department of Neurological Sciences, University La Sapienza, Rome, Italy.

CARLO A. MARZI Department of Neurological and Visual Sciences, University of Verona, Verona, Italy.

hemispheric conduction delay, usually ranging from 15 to 20 ms (Marzi et al., 1991).

Recent anatomical studies on the fiber composition of the human corpus callosum have demonstrated that callosal fibers have wide differences in diameter size. Myelinated callosal fibers tend to have larger diameter than the unmyelinated ones (Aboitiz et al., 1992). Among myelinated fibers, assuming that the conduction velocity of callosal fibers varies with diameter size as in the peripheral nervous system and that the values of conduction velocity observed in the peripheral nervous system can be generalized to callosal fibers, only the largest fibers, with a diameter size ranging from 3 μm to 5 μm, would subserve the fast interhemispheric transfer time seen in normal subjects (Marzi et al., 1991; Aboitiz et al., 1992; Iacoboni and Zaidel, 1995). This population of fibers is represented in two relatively small contingents of callosal axons, one located in the midbody of the corpus callosum and the other located in the posterior tip of the splenium of the corpus callosum (Aboitiz et al., 1992). Studies in neurological patients seem to suggest that the fastest callosal transfer occurs at the level of the contingent of large-diameter callosal fibers located in the midbody (Iacoboni, Fried, and Zaidel, 1994; Geschwind et al., 1995; Tomaivolo et al., 2001). Thus, from a probabilistic standpoint, given the smallness of this contingent of fibers and the nature of the disease process in MS, in which lesion location is generally randomly distributed, demyelinating lesions located in this small contingent of fibers subserving fast transfer are unlikely. Hence, it is unlikely that MS patients show an abnormally prolonged interhemispheric conduction delay.

The serial information-processing model that assumes a fast transfer of a simple bit of information through a small number of large-diameter fibers, however, has been recently challenged by other models that assume that the role of the corpus callosum in sensorimotor integration is of dynamically equilibrating the opposite activation of large neuronal ensembles of the two hemispheres (see Chapters 10 and 13 in this volume). These models explain the difference in RT between crossed and uncrossed responses to lateralized light flashes as being due to the equilibrating role of the corpus callosum in hemispheric activation. When a given hemisphere receives a visual stimulus, it becomes more activated than the contralateral one. The presence of the corpus callosum equilibrates this imbalance of activation very rapidly, and therefore only a small difference in RT between crossed and uncrossed responses is observed. In split-brain patients, the lack of the callosum makes the imbalance of hemispheric activation much larger, such

that during crossed responses the initiation of motor command in the less activated hemisphere is much slower than the initiation of a motor command in the activated hemisphere (directly receiving the visual input) during uncrossed responses.

All these equilibrium models assume the cooperativity of several neuronal pools, and therefore several callosal axons, in interhemispheric integration. Given this assumption, a natural prediction of these models would be that MS patients should show abnormal interhemispheric integration, because randomly located demyelinating lesions are likely to "hit" these axonal ensembles and interfere with their functioning. In contrast, the serial information model of interhemispheric transfer would not predict impairment of MS patients unless there is specific massive damage to the callosal sites of fast transfer. Our study is aimed at testing the opposite predictions of these contrasting models of callosal functions.

Six male and six female right-handed MS patients with normal or corrected vision participated in the study. Their mean age was 28.9 years (range 20–44 years). All of them had a relapsing-remitting form of MS. Informed consent according to the ethical guidelines of the University La Sapienza of Rome was obtained from each patient. Selected patients had no gross motor or sensory defects, and their score on the Kurtzke Expanded Disability Status scale (EDSS) (Kurtzke, 1987) was not greater than 1.5. The EDSS is a scale with a score range up to 5 (the higher the score, the higher patients' impairment) and is heavily biased toward motor functions. A score not greater than 1.5 on the EDSS ensures that no gross motor deficits that might influence reaction times performance were present in the group of MS patients.

We also tested a complete callosotomy patient to compare his interhemispheric conduction delay with those of MS patients. This patient (M.E.) is a right-handed 25-year-old male who suffers from drug-resistant epilepsy resulting from a head trauma that occurred in a traffic accident when he was 8 years old. About 9 years before testing, M.E. underwent complete surgical callosotomy in two stages for the relief of his severe epilepsy. This resulted in a favorable change in both severity and frequency of the seizures. Pharmacological treatment with phenobarbital has been continued throughout the postoperative period. The completeness of the callosal section and the integrity of the anterior commissure have been confirmed by MRI, which also revealed a lesion in the right frontal pole. In addition, MRI analysis demonstrated a smaller lesion on the orbital aspect of the left frontal lobe. Both lesions occurred as a result of the traffic accident and of the surgical removal of a subdural hematoma. Since the last operation, standard clinical testing has revealed ideo-motor dyspraxia and anomia in the left hand as well as alexia in the left hemifield. Further details on this patient are available elsewhere (Aglioti et al., 1993; Tassinari et al., 1994; Berlucchi, Aglioti, and Tassinari, 1997).

Seven males and five females, all right-handed, with normal or corrected-to-normal vision and no evidence or history of neurological disorder, participated in this study as normal controls. Their mean age was 29.6 years (range 24–38 years).

MRI scanning was performed on the same day as be-havioral testing in six of the MS patients. In the re-maining six patients, MRI scanning was performed no later than 10 days after the behavioral testing session. Each patient underwent conventional sagittal and trans-verse spin-echo for T1-WI (TR/TE 650/25), T2-WI (TR/TE 2500/90), and proton-density-weighted images (PD-WI) of 6-mm thickness using a 1.5T supraconduct-ing magnet. The matrix size was 256×256 pixels, and the field of view was 230 mm. Contrast-enhanced T1-WI transverse MR images were obtained by using gadolinium-penta-acetic acid. The MRI scans were evaluated by a neuroradiologist who was unaware of the behavioral data. Callosal damage was ranked on a five-point scale (absent = 0, very mild = 1, mild = 2, moderate = 3, severe = 4).

Subjects sat on a stool in a quiet, diffusely illuminated room with the head positioned on a head and chin rest 57 cm from a computer screen. The stimulus, a lumi-nous square of $1°$ of visual angle, was presented for 50 ms on the computer screen, to either the left or the right visual field, at $8°$ of eccentricity from a continu-ously present fixation point represented by a cross. A 100-ms acoustic tone was used as a warning signal; the interval between warning signal and visual stimulus was randomized within a time window of 1–3 s. The subject was instructed to fixate the cross in the center of the screen and to press a button with the index finger as quickly as possible after stimulus appearance. Eye move-ments were controlled by directly watching the subject's eyes. Each subject was tested in four sessions composed of four blocks of 40 trials each. The callosotomized patient was tested in only one session. On half of the blocks, subjects were asked to use the left hand; on the other half they were requested to use the right hand. The stimuli were presented in the right visual hemifield in half of the trials and in the left visual hemifield in the other half of the trials. The sequence of hemifield stim-ulations within each block was randomized. RTs faster than 150 ms (anticipations) and those slower than 900 ms (retards) were rejected without replacement.

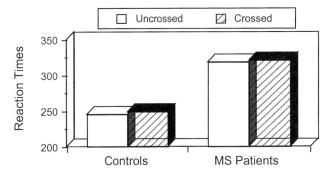

FIGURE 16.7. Mean reaction times for MS patients and nor-mal controls in the crossed and uncrossed hemifield/hand conditions.

As to speed of response, the main effect of group was significant, with MS patients showing overall RTs longer than controls (MS patients = 319.26 ms, controls = 246.97 ms; $F(1, 20) = 21.49$, $p < 0.001$) (Figure 16.7). No effect of gender was found ($F(1, 11) = 0.08$), while the experimental condition factor was significant with an overall CUD of 3.47 ms (crossed condition = 285.63 ms, uncrossed condition = 282.16 ms; $F(1, 11) = 13.93$, $p = 0.001$). The crucial interaction group by experimental condition was not significant ($F(1, 20) = 0.03$), thus indicating that the CUD was similar in MS patients (CUD = 3.8 ms) and control subjects (CUD = 3.1 ms).

MRI disclosed a different degree of callosal damage in the 12 patients who were imaged during the study. Cal-losal damage ranged from very mild, as in patient T.R., who had a small lesion in the lower portion of the callosal isthmus, to a severe atrophy as in patient P.E. Spearman correlation analyses between the EDSS score and the CUD of MS patients ($r = 0.209$, $p = 0.521$) and between callosal damage score and the CUD of MS pa-tients ($r = 0.163$, $p = 0.589$) were far from showing even a trend to significance.

Figure 16.8 shows the CUDs for individual controls and MS subjects; clearly, there was a large overlap be-tween the two groups, even though the two tails of the distribution in the MS group are wider than those in the control group. Given that the longest CUDs were all in the MS groups (Patients I.P., L.S., and P.E.), we for-mally tested the difference between the distribution of CUDs in the two groups with a Kolgomorov-Smirnov analysis. The result, however, was again far from signif-icant ($p = 0.527$).

To have a more detailed description of the behavioral performance in normal subjects and neurological pa-tients, we also plotted the CUD of the commissurotom-ized patient M.E. (Figure 16.8). It is clear from Figure 16.8 that M.E.'s CUD is a stray point, whereas the cu-

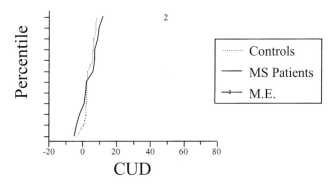

FIGURE 16.8. Cumulative distribution functions of CUDs in MS patients and normal controls. When formally tested with a Kolgomorov-Smirnov analysis, the two distributions do not differ ($p = 0.527$). The CUD of callosotomized patient M.E. (50 ms) is also plotted here. M.E.'s CUD is clearly a stray point, reaffirming that normal controls and MS patients have very similar CUDs. Note also that CUDs similar to M.E.'s have been observed repeatedly in split-brain patients.

mulative distributions of CUDs in normal controls and MS patients are largely overlapping. This finding supports the notion that the MS patients tested here are much more similar to a normal subject than to a callosum-sectioned subject in basic interhemispheric visuomotor behavior. Note that the CUD in M.E. is very similar to the CUD observed in split-brain patients in previous studies (Marzi et al., 1991; Iacoboni and Zaidel, 1995).

When compared to a group of normal subjects, MS patients with mild disability do not show any slowing down in mean interhemispheric transfer time. Also, when the distribution of interhemispheric conduction delays in each group is considered, no differences emerge. Imaging the callosum of MS patients shows various degrees of callosal atrophy but no callosal lesions critically located in the midbody and potentially interfering with large-diameter fibers with fast conduction velocity. Correlation analyses do not show any relationship between overall callosal damage and CUD or between disability score and CUD. Taken together, these findings are more compatible with the view that the callosum selectively transfers information through specific channels (Iacoboni and Zaidel, 1995) than with the view that the callosum equilibrates hemispheric activation (see Chapter 10 in this volume).

One might argue, however, that our failure to show a correlation between overall callosal damage and CUD is due to a rather coarse assessment of callosal damage as evidenced by MRI, owing to absence of a quantitative analysis of callosal morphometry in our study. For this reason, then, the empirical evidence presented here

might not be considered conclusive. It must be noticed, however, that the distribution of the CUD in the group of patients largely overlap the distribution of the CUD in normal subjects (Figure 16.8). This makes it rather unlikely that a more precise assessment of callosal damage would disclose a correlation between the morphometry of the callosum in MS patients and their CUD. In fact, if such a correlation were to be found, its interpretation would be rather puzzling, in that a similar correlation between callosal morphometry and CUD should be expected in normals, too, given that the two groups have CUD distributions that, when formally tested, show a probability level in favor of the null hypothesis greater than 50%.

Our findings seem to be in line with the serial information-processing model of callosal functions in basic sensorimotor integration. According to this model, a selective lesion affecting fast transfer channels should produce a significant slowing down of conduction delay. In keeping with this, in a patient with alien hand syndrome following a very selective vascular callosal lesion located in the midbody of the callosum, a conspicuous slowing down of conduction delay was observed when the patient responded with the hand not affected by the alien hand symptomatology (Geschwind et al., 1995). Still in keeping with this model, in a patient with anterior section of the corpus callosum sparing only the splenium where visual callosal fibers are grouped, interhemispheric transfer time was found to be sensitive to retinal eccentricity variations of the light stimulus only after callosotomy (Iacoboni et al., 1994). This can be explained by the topographical arrangement of callosal fibers connecting the visual cortices of the two hemispheres. Indeed, callosal fibers connect occipital visual areas only up to about 5° of retinal eccentricity from the vertical meridian (Marzi, 1986). Thus, any unilateral input that is more peripheral than 5° from the vertical meridian must synapse one more time before getting transferred to the contralateral hemisphere. Before callosotomy, when the large-diameter fibers in the midbody of the corpus callosum are available, changes in retinal eccentricity do not affect interhemispheric transfer time because a fast callosal transfer could take place at the level of central callosal channels. After callosotomy only visual callosal channels are available, and changes in retinal eccentricity of the light stimulus did affect interhemispheric conduction delay (Iacoboni et al., 1994).

Recently, it has been shown that transcranial magnetic stimulation (TMS) of extrastriate visual areas produces an inhibitory effect on RT only during crossed responses, when an interhemispheric transfer is needed (Marzi et al., 1998). This suggests that extrastriate visual areas are a relevant pathway in interhemispheric integration of visuomotor information. Since extrastriate areas are known to send major visual inputs to frontal lobe areas relevant to voluntary action (Passingham, 1993), it is conceivable that at least some of the large-diameter fibers located in the midbody of the callosum connect heterologous cortical areas, that is, higher-order visual and premotor areas, and that this pathway may be the most efficient in basic interhemispheric sensorimotor integration processes. This hypothesis would be in line with an emerging concept of callosal anatomy, according to which axons connecting heterologous areas are an important component of callosal fibers (Cavada and Goldman-Rakic, 1989a, 1989b; Commentary 2.1 in this volume). This would also explain complex integrative interhemispheric phenomena that are observed behaviorally in normal subjects when motor and visual components of basic visuomotor integration are manipulated (Iacoboni and Zaidel, 1995). In keeping with this, TMS of frontal eye fields carried out in one cerebral hemisphere in normal subjects while blood flow was measured in a PET scanner did produce blood flow changes in heterologous areas in the opposite hemisphere, notably posterior parietal regions (Paus et al., 1997).

However, we cannot exclude alternative interpretations of our data that might still be compatible with equilibrium models of callosal functions. First of all, our subjects did not suffer from a severe form of disease. To avoid confounding factors in the interpretation of RT to lateralized flashes, we selected only patients without gross motor or sensory defects. Given that callosal atrophy progresses in parallel with the progression of the disease, we cannot exclude the possibility that our sample of patients did not reach a critical threshold of callosal atrophy necessary to determine callosal dysfunction. Second, it is possible that the role of callosal fibers in selectively transferring information through specific channels and in equilibrating hemispheric activation are not mutually exclusive. In principle, it is conceivable that basic integrative behavior is subserved by serial processing (transfer models) while complex integrative behavior is subserved by both serial and parallel processing (transfer and equilibrium models coexisting).

To conclude, our data suggest that basic visuomotor integration mechanisms are not disrupted in the early stages of MS, in spite of the presence of callosal atrophy in some patients. What remains to be tested is whether selective demyelinizing lesions in strategic location of the corpus callosum can produce disconnection in basic visuomotor behavior as seen after stroke lesions (Geschwind et al., 1995; Tomaiuolo et al., 2001).

REFERENCES

ABOITIZ, F., A. SCHEIBEL, R. FISHER, and E. ZAIDEL, 1992. Fiber composition of the human corpus callosum. *Brain Res.* 598:143–153.

AGLIOTI, S., G. BERLUCCHI, R. PALLINI, G. F. ROSSI, and G. TASSINARI, 1993. Hemispheric control of unilateral and bilateral responses to lateralized light stimuli after callosotomy and in callosal agenesis. *Exp. Brain Res.* 95:151–165.

BERLUCCHI, G., S. AGLIOTI, and G. TASSINARI, 1997. Rightward attentional bias and left hemisphere dominance in a cue-target light detection task. *Neuropsychologia* 35:941–952.

CAVADA, C., and P. S. GOLDMAN-RAKIC, 1989a. Posterior parietal cortex in rhesus monkey. I: Parcellation of areas based on distinctive limbic and sensory corticocortical connections. *J. Comp. Neurol.* 287:422–445.

CAVADA, C., and P. S. GOLDMAN-RAKIC, 1989b. Posterior parietal cortex in rhesus monkey. II: Evidence for segregated corticocortical networks linking sensory and limbic areas with the frontal lobe. *J. Comp. Neurol.* 287:422–445.

CLARKE, J., and E. ZAIDEL, 1989. Simple reaction times to lateralized flashes: Varieties of interhemispheric communication routes. *Brain* 112:849–870.

GESCHWIND, D. H., M. IACOBONI, M. S. MEGA, D. W. ZAIDEL, T. CLOUGHESY, and E. ZAIDEL, 1995. Alien hand syndrome: Interhemispheric motor disconnection due to a lesion in the midbody of the corpus callosum. *Neurology* 45:802–808.

HUBER, S. J., G. W. PAULSON, E. C. SHUTTLEWORTH, D. CHAKERES, L. E. CLAPP, A. PAKALNIS, K. WEISS, and K. RAMMOHAN, 1987. Magnetic resonance imaging correlates of dementia in multiple sclerosis. *Arch. Neurol.* 44:732–736.

IACOBONI, M., I. FRIED, and E. ZAIDEL, 1994. Callosal transmission time before and after partial commissurotomy. *NeuroReport* 5:2521–2524.

IACOBONI, M., and E. ZAIDEL, 1995. Channels of the corpus callosum: Evidence from simple reaction times to lateralized flashes in the normal and the split brain. *Brain* 118:779–788.

KURTZKE, J. F., 1987. Rating neurologic impairment in multiple sclerosis: An expanded disability status scale (EDDSS). *Neurology* 33:1444–1452.

MARZI, C. A., 1986. Transfer of visual information after unilateral input to the brain. *Brain Cogn.* 5:163–173.

MARZI, C. A., P. BISIACCHI, and R. NICOLETTI, 1991. Is interhemispheric transfer of visuomotor information asymmetric? Evidence from a meta-analysis. *Neuropsychologia* 29:1163–1177.

MARZI, C. A., C. MINIUSSI, A. MARAVITA, L. BERTOLASI, G. ZANETTE, J. C. ROTHWELL, and J. N. SANES, 1998. Transcranial magnetic stimulation selectively impairs interhemispheric transfer of visuo-motor information in humans. *Exp. Brain Res.* 118:435–438.

PASSINGHAM, R. E., 1993. *The Frontal Lobes and Voluntary Action.* New York: Oxford University Press.

PAUS, T., R. JECH, C. J. THOMPSON, R. COMEAU, T. PETERS, and A. C. EVANS, 1997. Transcranial magnetic stimulation during positron emission tomography: A new method for studying connectivity of the human cerebral cortex. *J. Neurosci.* 17:3178–3184.

POFFENBERGER, A., 1912. Reaction time to retinal stimulation with special reference to the time lost in conduction through nervous centers. *Arch. Psychol.* 23:1–73.

Pozzilli, C., S. Bastianello, A. Padovani, D. Passafiume, E. Millefiorini, L. Bozzao, and C. Fieschi, 1991. Anterior corpus callosum atrophy and verbal fluency in multiple sclerosis. *Cortex* 27:441–445.

Tassinari, G., S. Aglioti, R. Pallini, G. Berlucchi, and G. Rossi, 1994. Interhemispheric integration of simple visuo-motor responses in patients with partial callosal defects. *Behav. Brain Res.* 64:141–149.

Tomaiuolo, F., U. Nocentini, L. Grammaloo, C. Cattagirone, 2001. Interhemispheric transfer time in a patient with a portical lesion of the corpus collosum. *NeuroReport* 12:1469–1472.

COMMENTARY 16.2

Redundancy Gain as a Measure of Implicit Sensorimotor Integration

MARCO IACOBONI AND ERAN ZAIDEL

Brown and Tomaiuolo and colleagues suggest that the Poffenberger paradigm and its variation can be used in clinical populations to assess specific functions that we may expect to be disrupted or preserved by the disease. They tested normal subjects and patients with multiple sclerosis, reasoning that the callosal atrophy that is often observed in multiple sclerosis patients might have impaired transfer of sensorimotor information. It did not. In this commentary we briefly review some other evidence on the use of simple reaction times to lateralized flashes in patients with neurological disorders.

Marzi and colleagues (1996), for instance, used a variation of the task, the redundant target paradigm, to test patients with visual extinction. (For further information on this paradigm, see Chapter 14 and Commentary 14.1 in this volume.) Briefly, this paradigm compares the reaction times to multiple copies of the same target with the reaction times to a single target. Marzi and colleagues reasoned that if there is some level, however implicit, of processing of the extinguished target in these patients, then the reaction times to two targets should be different from the reaction times to a single target (Marzi et al., 1996). This should be valid even though both single-target trials and redundant-target trials would elicit in the patient awareness of a single stimulus in the right visual hemifield. Supporting the hypothesis of implicit processing for extinguished trials, the reaction times to two stimuli, even when the contralesional one was extinguished, were faster than the reaction times to single ipsilesional stimuli. Moreover, the redundancy gain that was obtained under these conditions was found to fit the neural summation model rather than the prob-

abilistic horse race model of redundancy gain (see also Chapter 14 in this volume).

Tomaiuolo and colleagues used the same redundant-target paradigm to investigate blindsight in hemispherectomy patients (Tomaiuolo et al., 1997). They reasoned that if the redundant target was presented in the blind field of a hemispherectomy patient, a speeding up of reaction times would signal some level of processing of the visual stimulus. In this series, some patients did show the effect, and some others did not. At this time, it is not clear what determines the differential effect between patients. Tomaiuolo and colleagues observed no evidence for anatomical differences between the patients who showed the redundant-target effect in the blind field and patients who did not show it. It is possible that the efficiency of subcortical pathways, and especially of the so-called second visual system, may be a factor in these interpatient differences.

We used the same approach to test residual vision in a patient with complete cortical blindness (Iacoboni, Saver, and Zaidel, 1996). The target stimuli that were used were auditory stimuli, and the redundant stimuli were visual stimuli. We also added a condition with redundant auditory stimuli to test whether the simple additivity of stimuli could account for the predicted facilitatory effect. The patient, a 65-year-old man, had coronary artery bypass surgery complicated by a hypertensive episode and a bilateral occipital stroke. Simple reaction times to bimodal (auditory and visual) stimuli were compared to simple RT to auditory stimuli only. The patient had four different response conditions: (1) single auditory stimuli, (2) double auditory stimuli presented simultaneously, (3) bimodal (single auditory and single visual) stimuli presented simultaneously, and (4) double bimodal (two auditory and two visual) stimuli presented simultaneously. Sixteen blocks (four per condition) of 40 trials each were administered, and the response hand (left or right) was counterbalanced across

MARCO IACOBONI Division of Brain Mapping, Department of Neurology, UCLA School of Medicine, Los Angeles, California.

ERAN ZAIDEL Department of Psychology, University of California at Los Angeles, Los Angeles, California.

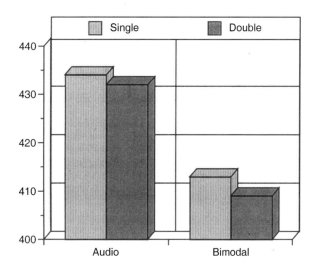

FIGURE 16.9. Reaction times for single and double auditory and bimodal stimuli.

to bimodal (single auditory and single visual) stimuli (413 ms) (see Figure 16.9).

Taken together, our results clearly suggest that the shortening in RT is due to intersensory facilitation of auditory and visual stimuli and not to the mere effect of two stimuli presented simultaneously. Since there is evidence for a robust intersensory facilitation of auditory and visual stimuli in the superior colliculus, we believe that our data support the role of visual processing in the superior colliculus in generating blindsight as opposed to being related to residual visual cortical processing in extrastriate areas.

To conclude, it seems to us that paradigms that are generally used in experimental psychology can be successfully employed to study brain-behavior relationships in clinical populations and may ultimately be used to assess or even predict recovery of function after brain damage.

blocks. RTs faster than 150 ms were considered anticipatory errors, and RTs slower than 700 ms were considered attentional errors. Both anticipatory and attentional errors (9% of total trials) were removed from the analysis. RTs to double auditory stimuli (432 ms) were not faster ($F = 0.091$, $p > 0.7$) than RTs to single auditory stimuli (434 ms). RTs to bimodal (auditory and visual) stimuli (413 ms) were faster ($F = 13.3$, $p < 0.001$) than RTs to single auditory stimuli (434 ms). RTs to double bimodal (two auditory and two visual) stimuli (409 ms) were not faster ($F = 0.165$, $p > 0.6$) than RTs

REFERENCES

IACOBONI, M., J. SAVER, and E. ZAIDEL, 1996. Second visual system and blindsight: Evidence from simple reaction times to bimodal (auditory and visual) stimuli. *Eur. J. Neurol.* 3:167–168.

MARZI, C. A., N. SMANIA, M. MARTINI, G. GAMBINA, G. TOMELLERI, A. PALAMARA, F. ALESSANDRINI, and M. PRIOR, 1996. Implicit redundant-targets effect in visual extinction. *Neuropsychologia* 34:9–22.

TOMAIUOLO, F., M. PTITO, C. A. MARZI, T. PAUS, and A. PTITO, 1997. Blindsight in hemispherectomized patients as revealed by spatial summation across the vertical meridian. *Brain* 120:795–803.

17 Alexithymia as a Consequence of Impaired Callosal Function: Evidence from Multiple Sclerosis Patients and Normal Individuals

MICHEL HABIB, GÉRALDINE DAQUIN, JEAN PELLETIER, MICHELE MONTREUIL, AND FABRICE ROBICHON

ABSTRACT The term *alexithymia* refers to special personality traits found in both normal and various pathological populations whereby people experience more or less difficulty in verbalizing their emotions and affects. An alexithymic profile has been found with high frequency in patients with multiple sclerosis (MS). In two separate studies of MS patients we tested the hypothesis that this high incidence of alexithymia might be related to impaired callosal transfer of emotional information between the emotional right hemisphere and the verbal left hemisphere. In the first study, we tried to correlate callosal measurement obtained on magnetic resonance imaging sagittal slices with indices of interhemispheric function and evaluation of alexithymia profile. In the second study, a dichotic paradigm allowed us to evaluate separately interhemispheric transfer of verbal and emotional information. Results show (1) a significant correlation between callosal size, in particular in its posterior (visual) part, and degree of alexithymia; (2) a significant impairment in MS patients compared to matched controls in degree of transfer of emotional information; and (3) a correlation between degree of alexithymia and transfer of verbal information from the right to the left rather than transfer of emotional information from the left to the right.

The term *alexithymia* was initially proposed by Nemiah and Sifneos (1970) as a concept characterizing, in psychosomatic medicine, the mode of mental functioning of certain patients who experience more or less conscious

MICHEL HABIB, GÉRALDINE DAQUIN, AND JEAN PELLETIER Neurology Clinic and Cognitive Neurology Laboratory, Faculty of Medicine, CHU Timone, Marseille, France.
MICHELE MONTREUIL Fédération de Neurologie, Hôpital de la Salpêtrière, Paris, France.
FABRICE ROBICHON L.E.A.D., Université de Bourgogne, Dijon, France.

difficulties in verbalizing emotions, affects, and bodily sensations. Subsequently, this concept has been used for normal populations, leading to alexithymia's being considered a personality trait that is distributed across the general population as a continuous variable (Taylor and Bagby, 1988).

Several neurological models have been put forward to account for alexithymia: disconnection between limbic system and neocortex (MacLean, 1949), dysfunction of the right hemisphere (Sifneos, 1988), and interhemispheric disconnection (namely, the language-dominant left hemisphere would be deprived of emotional information processed in the emotion-dominant right hemisphere). In support of the latter hypothesis, Hoppe and Bogen (1977) and TenHouten and colleagues (1985) have shown that patients who have undergone surgical callosotomy demonstrate significant alexithymic profile on standardized questionnaires, suggesting that alexithymia could, in certain cases, result from functional interhemispheric disconnection. More recently, Zeitlin, Richard, and Lane (1989) have found in a population of veterans with posttraumatic stress disorder a relationship between interhemispheric transfer of sensorimotor information and the degree of alexithymia. Finally, Montreuil and Lyon-Caen (1993) have shown that patients with multiple sclerosis (MS), a frequent, incapacitating disease of unknown etiology mainly affecting young women, are significantly more often alexithymic (over 50%) than controls (less than 10%).

In the latter condition, on the basis of evidence of anatomical and functional involvement of the corpus callosum (Lindeboom and Horst, 1988; Rao et al., 1989;

Pelletier et al., 1993), interhemispheric disconnection is often considered a prominent feature of the disease, and therefore MS is a valuable model to use in investigating interhemispheric relationships.

Our purpose here was then to test the interhemispheric disconnection hypothesis of alexithymia and further explore the mechanisms of alexithymia in MS. To investigate this issue, we carried out two different studies. In the first one we measured the corpus callosum (CC) on magnetic resonance imaging (MRI) images obtained in 21 unselected MS patients and found that the size of the CC, in particular its posterior part, was smaller in alexithymic patients. In a second, more controlled, study on 20 MS patients and 20 matched controls, we addressed specifically the issue of whether interhemispheric transfer of emotional information is deficient in alexithymic individuals.

Study 1

SUBJECTS AND METHODS Twenty-one consecutive MS patients (15 females, 6 males, 19 right-handers, 2 non-right-handers), with a mean age of 36.3 ± 9.7 years, a Kurtske disability score of 3.6 ± 1.53 (moderate), and evolution of illness of 6.4 ± 3 years, were assessed for alexithymia by means of two different methods. One was the Toronto Alexithymia Scale (TAS), a 26-item self-administered questionnaire that is commonly used in psychosomatic research.* The other was a newly devised clinical tool, the Parallel Visual Information Processing Test (PVIPT) (Montreuil et al., 1991), whose results have been found to be highly correlated with more "classical" questionnaires in various normal and pathological populations. This test explores subjects' ability to retrieve consciously the emotional content of photographs encoded implicitly during a simultaneous dual task (Figure 17.1).

All patients also received a brain MRI scan to measure the degree of global and regional callosal atrophy on the midsagittal section, according to a method previously reported by our group (Habib et al., 1991; Pelletier et al., 1993) using a computer program that automatically calculates total callosal area, anterior and posterior halves, and six subareas (Figure 17.2).

RESULTS First, our two measurements of alexithymia correlated with each other, indicating the validity of their application to this group (Figure 17.3). As can be seen

---

* Each of the 26 questions of the TAS—for example, "I find it hard to describe how I feel about people" or "When I cry I always know why"—is rated from 1 to 5, providing a general score from 26 to 130. People who score 74 and over are considered significantly alexithymic.

on this plot, the score of the majority of patients on the TAS was above the critical level of 73 defining alexithymia, confirming that this sample of MS patients is globally more alexithymic than the general population.

Moreover, both alexithymia scores correlated with callosal area measurements (Figure 17.4), especially the posterior part for TAS, in that more alexithymic patients had smaller posterior callosal areas. In other words, it appears that alexithymia may be related to the loss of callosal axons in MS, but this relationship holds only for the posterior part of the callosum, thus suggesting that the relevant mechanism must involve interhemispheric transfer or sharing of "posterior" (sensory) brain functions.

The effect was even clearer and more specific to the splenial area with PVIPT, which may logically be related to the visual nature of this task. One may hypothesize that patients' abilities to verbalize their emotions is related to their left hemisphere's capacity for drawing complex sensory information processed in the right hemisphere's association cortices, whose interhemispheric connections are known to cross the posterior part of the callosum. In particular, performing the PVIPT may strongly rely on subjects' ability to verbally retrieve the emotional content of visual scenes, a process that likely depends on the integrity of the splenial-presplenial callosal regions.

To summarize, Study 1 provides preliminary evidence for a relationship between callosal size and alexithymia. We then carried out a second study aimed at investigating the proper mechanisms underlying the link between callosal function and alexithymia. More specifically, using a contrasted verbal/emotional dichotic paradigm, we addressed the issue of whether alexithymia might be related to reduced availability to the left hemisphere of emotional information primarily processed by the right hemisphere.

In this study, we also tried to circumscribe more accurately the population, by selecting only milder MS cases, compared to carefully matched normal controls.

Study 2

SUBJECTS AND METHODS This study involved 20 MS patients and 20 matched controls, each group including half males and half females.

All 40 subjects were right-handed; that is, they scored above 75% on the Edinburgh Handedness Inventory. For the MS sample, the mean age was 34 ± 7 years, Kurtske disability score < 3 (mild), and disease evolution 4.5 ± 3 years.

Patients and controls completed the TAS and received the PVIPT.

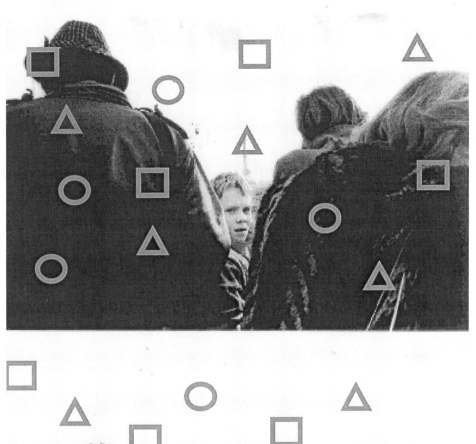

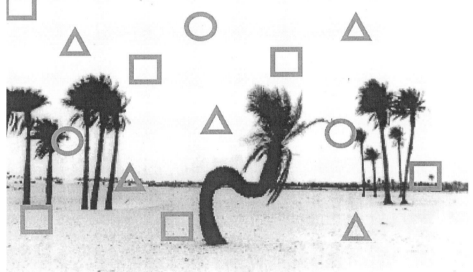

FIGURE 17.1. Parallel visual information-processing test. Subjects are presented with four different pictures representing emotionally loaded scenes. Superimposed on the pictures is a transparency with printed squares, circles, and triangles. Patients are required to trace a line joining the squares. Then all the material is removed, and the patient is asked to recall the maximum elements from the pictures. Alexithymic behavior is characterized by the poverty of explicit spontaneous recall of emotional elements.

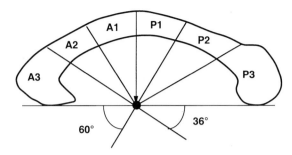

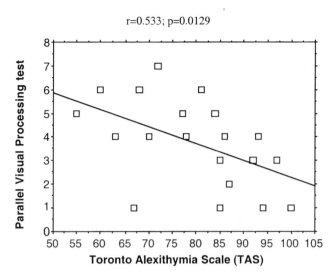

r=0.533; p=0.0129

FIGURE 17.2. Mode of segmentation of callosal areas obtained from the midsagittal MRI sections (Habib et al., 1991). A center of gravity of the total callosal area is calculated and projected on the horizontal line tangent to the inferior limit of the callosum. Then subareas are automatically calculated. This method, better than others using vertical parcellation, takes into account the variations in curvature of the callosum across individuals.

FIGURE 17.3. Study 1: Correlation between the two modes of assessment of alexithymia in 21 MS patients. For the TAS, scores over 73 are considered suggestive of alexithymia.

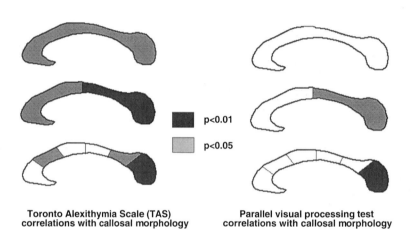

Toronto Alexithymia Scale (TAS) correlations with callosal morphology

Parallel visual processing test correlations with callosal morphology

FIGURE 17.4. Study 1: Correlations between MS patients' scores on alexithymia evaluation and callosal morphology. Results of Spearman correlation tests computed on measurements of total callosal area (top), anterior and posterior halves (middle), and six subregions (bottom).

Emotional transfer was assessed through a dichotic paradigm derived from P. Bryden's procedure (see Bryden and MacRae, 1989; Bryden et al., 1991), using four different nonwords recorded by a professional actor pronouncing each nonword with one of four different emotional tones (fear, disgust, sadness, anger). Auditory stimuli were carefully aligned using a computer program. We chose negative emotions because these have been shown to induce larger laterality effects than positive emotions.

The different combinations yielded 72 pairs, which, after ear reversal, gave 144 trials provided in two different experimental conditions, each in four blocks. In the verbal condition, subjects had to detect the occurrence of one given phoneme; in the emotional condition,

subjects had to detect the occurrence of one given emotional tone.

Our hypotheses for this experiment were (1) that we should find an overall right-ear advantage for the verbal condition and a left-ear advantage for the emotional condition, (2) that callosal disconnection in MS patients should manifest as a left-ear deficit for verbal and a right-ear deficit for emotional stimuli, and (3) that the degree of right-ear extinction for emotional stimuli should correlate with the degree of alexithymia.

RESULTS   Figure 17.5 shows the mean performance for each ear in the two groups for the verbal condition (left) and emotional condition (right). The first important result is that, as expected, there is an overall right-ear ad-

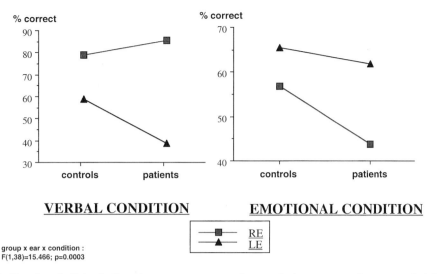

% correct

VERBAL CONDITION   EMOTIONAL CONDITION

RE
LE

group x ear x condition :
F(1,38)=15.466; p=0.0003

FIGURE 17.5. Study 2: Results of dichotic listening test performed in 20 MS patients and 20 controls in two contrasted conditions: Detect one given phoneme (verbal condition) or one given emotional tone (emotional condition). Both patients and controls demonstrate the expected right-ear advantage for the verbal condition and left-ear advantage for emotional condition (laterality effect).

vantage in the verbal condition and a left-ear advantage in the emotional condition. This meets our expectation, based on data with the dichotic listening procedure, that in both patients and controls, the left hemisphere would be more involved and/or more efficient in processing phonetic judgment on verbal materials and the right hemisphere would be more efficient in processing emotional components of the same stimuli (Bryden and MacRae, 1989; Bryden et al., 1991). However, there also was a clear group effect: Whereas MS patients are globally less efficient than controls, this difference is significant only for the left ear in the verbal condition and the right ear in the emotional condition. This means that MS patients, compared to controls, showed an impaired left-ear performance at detecting a given phoneme but an impaired right-ear performance at detecting a given emotion. In other words, the ear ipsilateral to the hemisphere that is presumably dominant for one given condition (crossed pathway) is specifically poorer in MS, whereas performance to the other ear (uncrossed pathway) does not differ from that of controls. This is completely consistent with the idea that, inasmuch as MS is associated with damage to callosal fibers, such callosal damage has impaired right-to-left transfer of verbal information and left-to-right transfer of emotional information.

In addition, and rather surprisingly, there was a group × ear interaction for the verbal condition only, due to a slightly better right ear in patients than controls in this condition (Figure 17.6). This is what we may ex-

pect if the cross-callosal LE signal is weaker and thus less effective in competing with the RE signal for processing resources. A similar effect has been observed in split-brain patients (Zaidel, 1983). This may also be interpreted as a consequence of impaired callosal function, due to a possible release, in MS patients, from transcallosal inhibition from the nondominant hemisphere on the dominant hemisphere. Transcallosal inhibition has been repeatedly demonstrated in experimental and neuropsychological settings and may be one crucial component of the corpus callosum function (Clarke et al., 1993).

Finally, since there is evidence from the literature that the degree of verbal lateralization may vary according to sex, we also looked for an effect of sex. We did not find any gender effect for the verbal condition, for either controls or patients. We did find such a gender effect, however, for the emotional condition, with females significantly outperforming males, especially for the left ear for controls and the right ear for patients. In other words, the laterality effect that is found in normals is present only in females, whereas the disconnection effect found in patients is present only in males.

We will not discuss these results in detail, although they obviously provide interesting insights into the issue of sex differences in brain lateralization. Schematically, they suggest that (1) the superiority of the right hemisphere for processing emotional intonations is more pronounced in the female brain and (2) brain processing of emotional material relies more heavily on callosal con-

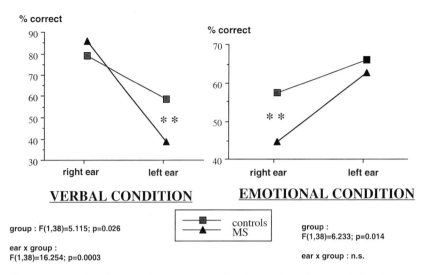

FIGURE 17.6. Study 2: Comparison of patients and controls. Only performance on the ear ipsilateral to the hemisphere dominant for either condition (crossed pathway) significantly differs between the two groups (disconnection effect).

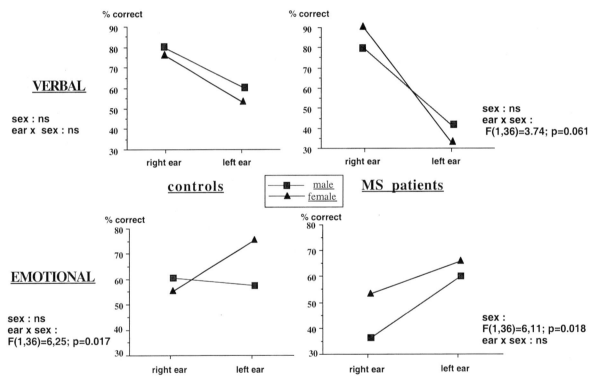

FIGURE 17.7. Gender effects. Significant sex differences appear only in the emotional condition, with females outperforming males overall, especially for the left ear in controls (more of a laterality effect) and the right ear in patients (less of a disconnection effect).

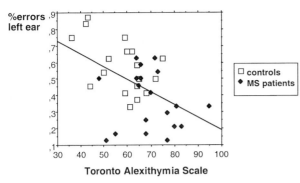

%errors left ear

Toronto Alexithymia Scale

□ controls
◆ MS patients

total : r=0.488; p=0.0019
controls : r=0.565; p=0.0287
MS patients : r=0.155; n.s.

FIGURE 17.8. Correlation between alexithymia scores (TAS) and left-ear performance on dichotic listening in the verbal condition.

nections in males than in females. (See also Galaburda, Rosen, and Sherman, 1990, for a discussion of the possible neuroanatomical substrate of gender differences in bihemispheric functioning.)

Turning now to the main point of this research, namely, alexithymia, we were somewhat disappointed, since there were, contrary to predictions, very few correlations between ear effects and alexithymia scores. In particular, there was no correlation with either right-ear or left-ear performance in the emotional condition. The only correlation was found between the TAS and left-ear errors in the verbal condition (Figure 17.8).

Thus, this experiment failed to confirm our hypothesis that alexithymia is related to impaired interhemispheric transfer of emotional information. However, one can notice that the emotional disconnection effect measured by the rate of errors on the right ear explores only transfer of emotional information from the left to the right hemisphere and not from the right to the left, as was initially proposed as a basis for alexithymia. In this regard, our results remain compatible with the initial hypothesis, inasmuch as one considers the direction of interhemispheric transfer to be more pertinent than the nature of information transferred. Moreover, as is illustrated on the plot in Figure 17.8, this correlation is significant both in the total (patients plus controls) and normal populations. The nonsignificant trend for the MS population only may be due to the fact that, in spite of careful selection, the MS sample remains more heterogeneous than the control population.

Discussion

Taken together, the results of our two studies provide convincing separate and complementary evidence in fa-

vor of the interhemispheric disconnection hypothesis of alexithymia. From both anatomical and functional viewpoints it seems that increased incidence of alexithymia in MS is related to impaired communication between the hemispheres, especially in their posterior regions. In addition, results from Study 2 show that this also holds true for a normal population: In spite of the fact that on the TAS most controls do not generally reach the cutoff point of 73 indicating "pathologic" alexithymia, the continuum observed within the normal range proved to be proportional to the capacity for the left hemisphere to process phonemic information primarily received by the right hemisphere. In any case our results are not compatible with the current theory ascribing alexithymia to impaired right-hemisphere function. In that case, one would have expected left-ear performance in the emotional condition to be inversely proportional to the degree of alexithymia, a prediction that is made plausible by the global superiority of the left ear, especially in females from the two groups. Instead, the only significant correlation of alexithymia was with the left ear but in the verbal condition.

Finally, some points concerning specifically MS deserve to be discussed. First, our study provides a striking confirmation that callosal involvement is a common feature of this disease. Even in mildly affected patients, like those selected for Study 2, with a disease duration of about 3 years, impaired callosal function can be consistently demonstrated. It must be noticed that alexithymia scores were not correlated with disease duration or severity, suggesting that even the mildest cases may be alexithymic. This observation raises the issue of the significance of alexithymia and its relation to callosal involvement in the course of the illness. In a previous study (Pelletier et al., 1993), we showed that callosal involvement was already significant in a subgroup of patients in early stages of the disease, in particular without significant white matter hemispheric lesions. Similarly, one may wonder whether alexithymia, being a personality trait that is found even in normal populations, would represent a preexisting characteristic of patients who are at risk for developing MS. Although it is not easy to disentangle these symptoms from those due to brain changes or even to psychological consequences of the disabling course of the illness, the authors' clinical experience with MS patients is that inappropriateness of mood and affective reactions to situations and life events is a common finding among these patients and often reveals profound emotional premorbid fragility. The notion of a pathological premorbid personality in MS patients has long been envisaged in early psychiatric accounts of the disease, which often stress the "hysterical" character structure of MS patients (Langworthy, 1948) as well as emotional and psychosexual immaturity (Philippopoulos, Wittkower, and Cousineau, 1958).

Thus, one fascinating hypothesis, which could serve as a basis for future studies, would be that such premorbid traits actually reflect special anatomofunctional brain organization, in particular in terms of interhemispheric connectivity, which would play a facilitating or even causal role in the development of this still mysterious disease.

In conclusion, this work offers interesting perspectives not only to understand the mechanisms of some behavioral characteristics and disorders in multiple sclerosis, which could eventually enhance our understanding of the pathophysiology of this disease, but also as an illustration of what can be expected from a neuropsychological approach to complex aspects of normal human behavior.

REFERENCES

BRYDEN, M. P., T. FREE, S. GAGNE, and P. GROFF, 1991. Handedness effects in the detection of dichotically-presented words and emotions. *Cortex* 27:229–235.

BRYDEN M. P., and L. MACRAE, 1989. Dichotic laterality effects obtained with emotional words. *Neuropsychiatry Neuropsychol. Behav. Neurol.* 1:171–176.

CLARKE, J. M., R. B. LUFKIN, and E. ZAIDEL, 1993. Corpus callosum morphometry and dichotic listening performance: Individual differences in functional interhemispheric inhibition? *Neuropsychologia* 31:547–557.

GALABURDA, A. M., G. D. ROSEN, and G. F. SHERMAN, 1990. Individual variability in cortical organization: Its relationship to brain laterality and implications to function. *Neuropsychologia* 28:529–546.

HABIB, M., D. GAYRAUD, A. OLIVA, J. REGIS, G. SALAMON, and R. KHALIL, 1991. Effects of handedness and sex on the morphology of the corpus callosum: A study with brain magnetic resonance imaging. *Brain. Cogn.* 16:41–61.

HOPPE, K. D., and J. E. BOGEN, 1977. Alexithymia in twelve commissurotomized patients. *Psychother. Psychosom.* 28:148–155.

LANGWORTHY, O. R., 1948. Relation of personality problems to onset and progression of multiple sclerosis. *Arch. Neurol. Psychiatr.* 59:13–20.

LINDEBOOM, J., and R. T. HORST, 1988. Interhemispheric disconnection effects in multiple sclerosis. *J. Neurol. Neurosurg. Psychiatry* 51:1445–1447.

MACLEAN, P. D., 1949. Psychosomatic disease and "the visceral brain": Recent developments bearing on the Papez theory of the emotions. *Psychosom. Med.* 11:338–353.

MONTREUIL, M., R. JOUVENT, S. CARON, C. BUNGENER, and D. WIDLÖCHER, 1991. Parallel visual information processing test. *Psychother. Psychosom.* 56:212–219.

MONTREUIL, M., and O. LYON-CAEN, 1993. Troubles thymiques et relations entre alexithymie et troubles du transfert dans la sclerose en plaques. *Rev. Neuropsychol.* 3:287–304.

NEMIAH, J. C., and P. E. SIFNEOS, 1970. Psychosomatic illness: A problem in communication. *Psychother. Psychosom.* 18:154–160.

PELLETIER, J., M. HABIB, O. LYON-CAEN, G. SALAMON, M. PONCET, and R. KHALIL, 1993. Functional and magnetic resonance imaging correlates of callosal involvement in multiple sclerosis. *Arch. Neurol.* 50:1077–1082.

PHILIPPOPOULOS, G. S., E. D. WITTKOWER, and A. COUSINEAU, 1958. The etiologic significance of emotional factors in onset and exacerbations of multiple sclerosis. *Psychosom. Med.* 20:458.

RAO, S. M., L. BERNARDIN, G. J. LEO, L. ELLINGTON, S. B. RYAN, and L. S. BURG, 1989. Cerebral disconnection in multiple sclerosis: Relationship to the atrophy of the corpus callosum. *Arch. Neurol.* 46:918–920.

SIFNEOS, P. E., 1988. Alexithymia and its relationship to hemispheric specialisation, affect, and creativity. *Psychiatr. Clin. North Am.* 3:287–292.

SIFNEOS, P. E., 1973. The prevalence of alexithymic characteristics in psychosomatic patients. *Psychother. Psychosom.* 22:255–262.

TAYLOR, G. J., and M. R. BAGBY, 1988. Measurement of alexithymia: Recommendations for clinical practice and future research. *Psychiatr. Clin. North Am.* 3:351–365.

TENHOUTEN, W. D., K. D. HOPPE, J. E. BOGEN, and D. WALTER, 1985. Alexithymia: An experimental study of commissurotomy patients and normal control subjects. *Am. J. Psychiatry* 143:312–316.

ZAIDEL, E., 1983. Disconnection syndrome as a model for laterality effects in the normal brain. In *Cerebral Hemisphere Asymmetry: Method, Theory and Application*, J. Hellige, ed. New York: Praeger.

ZEITLIN, S. B., M. S. RICHARD, and D. C. LANE, 1989. Interhemispheric transfer deficit and alexithymia. *Am. J. Psychiatry* 146:1434–1439.

18 Functional Consequences of Changes in Callosal Area in Tourette's Syndrome and Attention Deficit/ Hyperactivity Disorder

M. YANKI YAZGAN AND MARCEL KINSBOURNE

ABSTRACT In this chapter we discuss the functional and clinical significance of observed structural abnormalities and alterations and their presumed impact on interhemispheric integration in Gilles de la Tourette's syndrome (TS) and attention deficit/hyperactivity disorder (ADHD). TS is a chronic neuropsychiatric disorder of childhood-onset characterized by multiple motor and vocal tics and associated symptoms such as impulsivity, distractibility, and obsessive-compulsivity. Impulsivity, inattention, and hyperactivity are also cardinal features of ADHD. Theories implicating abnormal patterns of cortical and subcortical development in TS and ADHD, particularly in systems that are involved in the anterior and posterior regulatory and attentional processes, receive support from the findings of reduced size in genu, rostrum, and splenium regions of the CC.

Among functions that have been proposed for the CC is mediation of interaction between the extensive territories of the hemispheres that it links homotopically. The richness of callosal interhemispheric connections has a role in determining the degree of behavioral laterality.

We also discuss the results from the studies in which tests of behavioral laterality (line bisection, turning bias, dichotic listening test) and a covert orienting task, also known as Posner's task, were administered to a group of individuals whose callosal areas were measured on the MR images.

In these studies, TS patients showed slower RTs than their normal controls. Validity effects decreased as the callosal area became smaller, supporting the role of intact corpus callosum in integrating hemisphere's orienting responses. TS patients, who had smaller CC areas than did controls, manifested reduced validity effects, indicating inadequate utilization of cues. The degree of reduction in validity effects was significantly associated with increased tic severity. These findings suggest an association between inefficient callosal functioning and more severe expression of the illness in adult patients with TS. They also support the idea that the corpus callosum, although smaller in size, continues to play an integrative role in patients similar to its role in normals. An insult at the early phases of a patient's life may have caused a compensatory redistribution of channels. The likelihood of compensatory processes to take place is high. Whether the onset of symptoms of both TS and ADHD (as well as those of the other developmental neuropsychiatric disorders) is related to plasticity-related changes in the callosum will be an interesting question to answer in future studies.

The patient presents himself or herself to a physician with a variety of symptoms. The physician often, if not always, utilizes his or her "professional mind," which is organized to recognize the cluster of the patient's symptoms consistent with the accumulated experience in the field, and makes a diagnosis. Pathogenesis is the process underlying and leading to a particular constellation of symptoms (i.e., diagnosed as a disease). Curious clinicians have long speculated about the pathogenesis of what they have seen in their patients. The techniques available in their times have determined the degree to which they have been able to confirm their hypotheses and generate new ones for further testing. The pathogenesis of a particular disorder is expressed concurrently at different levels and systems of the organism in which the disorder embodies itself. Neuroanatomy is one of these levels for disorders in the clinical fields of psychiatry and neurology. Efforts to understand the neuroanatomical substrate of developmental neuropsychiatric disorders have increased in parallel to the availability of postmortem and in vivo imaging techniques. These

M. YANKI YAZGAN Department of Psychiatry and Child Psychiatry, Marmara University Faculty of Medicine, Istanbul, Turkey.

MARCEL KINSBOURNE Department of Psychology, New School University, New York, New York.

423

studies were mostly based on hypotheses driven by phenomenology of the disorders. For example, Gilles de la Tourette's syndrome (TS) a childhood-onset neuropsychiatric disorder, has been investigated for abnormalities in the basal ganglia because of the predominance of movement-related symptoms seen in TS patients. The logic is straightforward: Movement programs are executed by the basal ganglia, and lesions of the basal ganglia, as in Parkinson's disease or vascular infarctions, may result in abnormal movements. Tics, therefore, may be associated with changes in the basal ganglia.

Developments in neuroimaging technology bring answers to some of the long-standing questions applied to neuropsychiatric disorders in which there are no structural lesions. New questions arise as the old ones are answered. One of the new questions is: What is the functional and clinical significance of the observed structural abnormalities and alterations?

In this chapter we address that question with respect to abnormality of a particular structure, the corpus callosum (CC), reported for two closely related developmental neuropsychiatric disorders: TS and attention deficit/hyperactivity disorder (ADHD). In accord with the main theme of this book, we limit the content of this chapter to the presumed impact of CC alterations on interhemispheric integration in TS and ADHD. We begin with descriptions of the disorders and the line of reasoning that brings the CC into question for its possible role in the pathogenesis of these particular disorders. We follow with a summary of previous research related to our topic. We then present the data we collected on a group of TS patients whose midsagittal cross-sectional CC areas were reported to be smaller than those of normal controls. Finally, we discuss briefly the findings in the context of interhemispheric interaction and the pathogenesis and natural history of developmental (early-onset) neuropsychiatric disorders.

Phenomenology of the disorders

Gilles de la Tourette's syndrome Gilles de la Tourette's syndrome (TS) is a chronic neuropsychiatric disorder of childhood onset characterized by multiple motor and vocal tics and associated symptoms such as impulsivity, distractibility, and obsessive-compulsivity. More recently, sensorimotor phenomena and psychasthenia associated with the performance of tics have been described as significant clinical features. Diagnosis of TS is almost always unequivocal, and diagnostic criteria are well established. The prevalence is thought to be between one and six cases per 1000 boys, and milder variants of the syndrome may occur in 2–10% of the population (Leckman, Pauls, and Cohen, 1995).

Motor tics are involuntary, rapid, repetitive, and stereotyped movements of individual muscle groups. Vocal/phonic tics are involuntary sounds produced by moving air through the nose, ear, and throat. Tics can also occur as a response to an urge to perform the movement that temporarily relieves the sensation (involuntary). Sensory phenomena are described in three forms: premonitory urges associated with tics, heightened sensory awareness of particular anatomical locations, and disinhibition (feeling tempted to do whatever they are not supposed to do) (Leckman, Walker, and Cohen, 1993).

Age of onset, duration and severity of symptoms, and the type of tics (motor, phonic) are important for classification and clinical course of the disorder. The average age of onset is 6–7 years, with a range between 2 and 17 years of age. Males are severalfold more frequently affected than females.

Up to 50% of all TS patients may present with attention deficit/hyperactivity disorder (ADHD) symptoms of inattention, impulsivity, and hyperactivity, which usually precede the onset of tics.

Neurobiological Research in TS TS has been of interest to researchers as a model neuropsychiatric disorder that may provide clues to understanding the interaction of genetic, environmental, and neurobiological factors.

Genetic A single, major autosomal dominant gene is thought to play a role, as is suggested by family segregation analyses and twin studies. However, differences in tic severity, even between monozygotic (MZ) TS patients, cannot be accounted for by genetic influences alone.

Perinatal Birth weight differences between MZ twins have been associated with changes in tic severity. Prenatal stress has also been proposed as an epigenetic factor in mediating the TS phenotype and altering CNS lateralization (Cohen and Leckman, 1994).

Sex Differences The higher risk of TS among males does not fit the current transmission model, which dictates equal risk to both sexes. Males are exposed to androgenic steroids early in fetal life, and this exposure (via steroid receptors) exerts an influence on the formation of structural CNS dimorphisms, including the CC (Fitch et al., 1990). There are reports of positive response to antiandrogenic medications in severe TS, which have led Leckman and Peterson (1993) to hypothesize that androgenic steroids acting at key developmental periods (the prenatal period when the brain is being formed, adrenarche, and puberty) may be involved in determining the natural history of TS and related disorders.

These findings and ideas have led researchers to investigate the role of particular brain structures in the pathobiology of TS. The neurobiological research has focused on the basal ganglia and the neural circuitry that involves the basal ganglia. A major finding about the pathogenesis of TS was the absence of normal asymmetry of the basal ganglia in the MR images of child and adult TS brains (Peterson et al., 1993; Singer et al., 1993). The only report about the morphometrics of the CC in TS followed this finding of lack of asymmetry (Peterson et al., 1994).

Attention deficit/hyperactivity disorder Impulsivity, inattention, and hyperactivity are cardinal features of attention deficit/hyperactivity disorder (ADHD). This is a fairly common disorder of childhood (6%) that extends into adulthood. Although a significant amount of research on ADHD is ongoing, the heterogeneity of the disorder and the pervasive presence of its symptoms across several diagnoses pose an open problem for the neurobiological and neuropsychological studies of ADHD. The majority of TS patients have ADHD symptoms severe enough to warrant energetic treatment. ADHD and TS are associated with a greater-than-chance risk within families. Core neuropsychological problems in ADHD are formulated as defective response inhibition, difficulties in sustained attention, increased distractibility, and impulsivity, all of which may easily be considered typical of TS as well (Harris, 1995).

The magnetic resonance imaging (MRI) technique has been applied to ADHD in a somewhat similar fashion to its application in TS. The caudate nuclei and lenticular nuclei, both subregions of the basal ganglia that are reported to be abnormal in TS, were found to be smaller in size, leading to absence of normal asymmetry in two separate studies (Singer et al., 1993; Castellanos et al., 1994). The reports of structural changes in cortical and subcortical regions in both TS and ADHD were followed by the structural studies of the CC. Some of the rationales for choosing the CC for studying TS and ADHD are stated in the articles listed. These rationales have not included hypotheses about the functional implications of callosal changes in terms of hemispheric interaction in TS and ADHD. (See below for a discussion of the functional implications of callosal changes.)

The CC and "attention"

One of the main functions of the CC is the allocation of attention and relative arousal levels of the two hemispheres (Kinsbourne, 1974, and Chapter 10, this volume; Guiard, 1980; Levy, 1985). The structural changes

in the CC may reflect disturbances in interhemispheric connectivity in addition to abnormalities in the cortical sources of the fibers traversing it, thus providing at least two sources of an attentional disturbance (Giedd et al., 1994). Theories implicating abnormal patterns of cortical and subcortical development in TS and ADHD, particularly in systems involved in the anterior and posterior regulatory and attentional processes, receive support from the findings of smaller genus, rostra, and splenia of the CC, thus connecting diverse cortical regions in two hemispheres (Castellanos, unpublished lecture at the Tourette Syndrome Association Meeting, New York, October 1999). For example, a PET study in ADHD subjects (Zametkin et al., 1990) showed lowered glucose metabolism in the premotor area and superior prefrontal cortex (which is essential to the suppression of relatively automatic responses to certain sensory stimuli). The rostrum of the CC, which includes projections from the premotor and supplementary motor areas, also contains projections from the caudate/orbital prefrontal region that were implicated in SPECT and structural MRI studies of TS and ADHD (Lou et al., 1989; Singer et al., 1993). These cortical regions are all known to contribute to different aspects of attention and impulse regulation that are the basic functions believed to be impaired in TS and ADHD.

We must emphasize that these reports have limited discussions of the relation of their findings to hypothesized cortical changes. In particular, the interpretation of the results has not included comments about interhemispheric interaction. Neuropsychological correlates received little emphasis in these reports, even when neuropsychological measures were administered. For example, the CC area was not significantly correlated with the "attentional" battery used in Giedd and colleagues' (1994) study, and the groups did not differ on the neuropsychological battery. Despite the explanation that the battery included only attentional measures, there were also measures such as the go/no-go task that would reflect defective response inhibition presumed (by the authors) to be associated with the rostral callosal area. A significant CC-symptom correlation was in fact observed: The rostral area was smaller in subjects with higher impulsivity scores.

Rationales for investigating the role of the corpus callosum in TS and ADHD

MORPHOLOGICAL RATIONALES

Index of abnormal development CC abnormality may be considered an index of abnormal brain development such as disturbances in interhemispheric connectivity in addition to abnormalities in the cortical origins of the fibers traversing through it. Regional differences in the CC may be viewed as markers of the development of particular cortical areas connected through specific regions.

Neighboring regions The CC develops closely with the hippocampal formation and the cingulate cortex (which has been implicated in TS and related disorders), along with others (LaMantia and Rakic, 1990).

MR images The CC is anatomically distinct in its midsagittal cross section, and its cross-sectional area is proportional to its complement of axons, particularly the relatively small axons that interconnect association cortices (Aboitiz et al., 1992a, 1992b). Because the size of the CC reflects its neural complement more than is the case for most cerebral structures, the CC lends itself to a test of the manner in which gross structure relates to function in the human cerebrum. Its fibers course uniformly in the coronal plane, and therefore, a sagittal MRI slice through the CC indexes the number of small-diameter axons transmitted through it.

FUNCTIONAL RATIONALES Among functions that have been proposed for the CC is mediation of interaction between the extensive territories of the hemispheres that it links homotopically. The CC is said to transmit "excitatory and inhibitory channel-specific control codes the proportion of which may vary over different callosal regions. The participation of these channels and regions are dictated by the cortical localization of the functions required to perform a particular task" (Clarke and Zaidel, 1994).

The richness of callosal interhemispheric connections affects the degree of behavioral laterality. Behavioral laterality is related to hemispheric interaction between the homologous regions. When stimuli for the same task are presented separately to the two hemispheres, the hemispheres differ systematically in the level of performance they generate. This systematic discrepancy between hemispheres is expressed as a laterality index, and the asymmetry expressed by this index is referred to as a laterality effect. Three tests of behavioral laterality (line bisection, turning bias, dichotic listening test) were administered to a group of individuals whose callosal areas on the MR images were computed (Yazgan et al., 1995b). The results suggest that as one side of the brain has to take control of the behavior in these tasks, the smaller CC leaves the specialized hemisphere in control (yielding a larger laterality effect), whereas the larger CC distributes this role more equitably between the two sides.

In tasks for which specialization is not strict, cross-callosal excitation may serve to enlarge the amount of cortex that is available for computation (Kinsbourne

and Hicks, 1978). By excitation, we mean the facilitation of the processes in the other hemisphere by the activated hemisphere. A larger CC area may also yield a performance advantage for difficult and demanding tasks, on the assumption that the relevant computations benefit from the availability of wider areas of cortex (McFarland and Ashton, 1978).

PHENOMENOLOGICAL RATIONALES Phenomenological rationales for a possible involvement of the CC in mediating tics in TS have not been proposed in earlier studies. The only published study of the CC in TS was driven by a finding of lack of asymmetry in the basal ganglia (Peterson et al., 1994). Higher frequency of midline and proximal locations of tics may be considered suggestive of callosal involvement in the pathogenesis of tics.

A traditional method employed in brain-behavior studies is making inferences from observations on brain-lesioned patients. Lesions of the CC may be vascular (e.g., infarctions), neoplastic (e.g., tumors), or degenerative (MS plaques). These lesions may result in callosal syndromes (Bogen, 1993). There is no reason to think of either TS or ADHD as a callosal syndrome in the conventional neurological sense, nor is the callosum the pathological site responsible for symptom production. However, certain characteristics of callosal disconnection syndromes are worth discussing in relation to tics. For example, in the callosal dissociative phenomenon, bodily action is dissociated from what is said or what is being done by either hand. Signs of release from frontal control are also observed. These include stereotypic and repetitive behaviors in response to an external stimulus. TS patients also have limited control over their bodily actions (just like callosal patients) and describe their tics as being against their will.

FUNCTIONAL QUESTIONS REGARDING STRUCTURAL ALTERATIONS Following are functional questions about structural alterations in the CC in TS and ADHD:

1. Do the structural alterations in the CC influence functions served by the CC? That is, if groups differ on structural measures, do they also differ on related behavioral/functional measures?

2. Do the CC alterations change callosal structure-function correlations? That is, do the normal correlations persist in the clinical groups with the CC alterations?

3. Are these functional changes associated with the clinical characteristics?

We attempted to answer these questions in a group of individuals with TS and with significant alterations in their callosal area. The findings about the structural callosal changes in this group and the structure-function correlations have been previously reported by our group (Peterson et al., 1994; Yazgan et al., 1995b; Chapter 10 in this volume).

Task selection in TS and ADHD to reflect callosal changes We previously studied in a healthy group the relationships between individual variations in callosal area and behavioral measures that would require CC participation (Yazgan et al., 1995b). One of the measures we employed was a dual task of verbal-motor interference. The dual task is based on the observation that when subjects are required to perform two tasks at the same time, one involving each hemisphere, they do better than when both tasks rely on the same hemisphere (Kinsbourne and Cook, 1971; Kinsbourne and Hiscock, 1983). In our study, we measured the slowing influences of speech on unimanual motor activity. Two conditions occur: within hemisphere (right hand/speech) and between hemispheres (left hand/speech). The amount of dual task interference was strongly inversely correlated with the CC area in both within-hemisphere (right-hand) and between-hemispheres (left-hand) conditions. We explained our findings with a cross-excitation model in which a larger CC favors a larger and better-integrated system by facilitating recruitment of additional sectors of the network in the other hemisphere, thus resulting in less interference. We examined TS subjects' performance on this task and also correlated it with their callosal areas.

The second measure that we hypothesized to be related to callosal area is a covert orienting task, also known as Posner's task, in which response time is measured by reaction time to events that occur at a location to which attention is cued or miscued. Covert orienting is described as reflexive, early automatic orienting to salient visual stimuli in the peripheral visual field. A cue directs the subject's attention toward the most likely target location. The presence of the cue signals the start of a trial and acts as a general warning signal as well as telling the subjects where the target is most likely to occur. The cue is peripheral, is close to the target, and tends to summon the subjects' attention (Posner, 1980, 1991). At cue-target intervals of 100 ms, subjects respond more rapidly if the cue and target are at the same location than the cue (valid) and more slowly if the target is at a different location (invalid). We defined the *validity effect*, the parameter that we used in our work, as the time difference between two cue-target conditions, computed as (invalid RT − valid RT). This may represent the extra time necessary to shift attention from an invalid cue to a target. Posner and colleagues (1987) as well as others (e.g., Hughes and Zimba, 1987) postulated the presence

of interhemispheric cooperation for shifting attention across the vertical meridian. The hypothesis of callosal participation in shifting attention seemed to be weakened when costs associated with both horizontal and vertical shifts of attention were reported to be comparable (Rizzolatti et al., 1987). However, previous reports of the CC's participation in both interhemispheric and intrahemispheric processing provides an alternative explanation for the altered validity effects in both conditions in relation to the CC area (Lassonde, 1986; Yazgan et al., 1995b).

In the Posner task of covert orienting, we found shifting attention across the CC (and shifting control between hemispheres) to be associated with the CC area on the MR image, which in turn represents small-diameter fibers that would mediate these effects (Chapter 10 in this volume). The data that we will present from the TS group should be read in conjunction with the findings for the normals by Yazgan and colleagues (1995b).

Neuropsychological-clinical rationales for task selection

While selecting the tasks to reflect CC differences between the TS and normal adults, we based our assumptions on the following thoughts and clinical and neuropsychological findings about TS and ADHD:

• Patients pay more attention to irrelevant stimuli and less attention to relevant stimuli than do normal controls, as demonstrated in electrophysiological studies (van der Woerkom, Roos, and van Dijk, 1994; Yazgan et al., 1996).

• "Overefficient" attentional processing of the environment and the body in TS patients leads to increased somatic awareness and consequent tics (Kane, 1994).

• Problems are observed in shifting attention between relevant and irrelevant information while utilizing cues.

• A dual task was employed in a group of ADHD children. Their performance on the primary task improved with treatment, while performance on the secondary task remained the same. Medication made switching attention difficult (Carlson et al., 1991).

• Pervasive attention problems and visuomotor precision difficulties in children with ADHD were reported (Korkman and Pesonen, 1994).

• A reduced validity effect was observed in the ADHD children for the longer delay intervals (800 ms), suggesting a difficulty in sustaining, rather than a shift of, attention that would occur in shorter delays (100 ms) such as the ones we used (Swanson et al., 1991; Posner, 1991).

Distractibility is a cardinal feature in both TS and ADHD. This feature commonly manifests itself as rapid, unnecessary shifts between targets and difficulty with utilizing relevant environmental cues while attending to stimuli. TS patients attend to irrelevant stimuli more than normal controls do (van Woerkom et al., 1994). This may result in their paying less attention to relevant stimuli and in their responding to irrelevant stimuli by ticking. This condition may be described as a state of hyperarousal-vigilance in which resources for relevant cognitive tasks are used inefficiently. A somewhat over-efficient attentional processing of the environment and the body in TS patients has been reported by patient/authors such as Bliss (1980) and Kane (1994). Over-attention in the somatic modality is proposed as a basic mechanism in the pathogenesis of tics. Posner's task may provide a good measure of efficiency of shifting attention between relevant and irrelevant information.

Hypotheses for testing the functional consequences of callosal alterations

COVERT ORIENTING OF ATTENTION (POSNER'S TASK)   We predicted that the TS patients would shift their attention from a previously cued location to a target more easily than their normal controls, resulting in a reduced validity effect. An implication of this prediction was that, because of their smaller CCs, the TS patients would demonstrate this difference particularly while shifting attention horizontally.

VERBAL-MANUAL INTERFERENCE (DUAL TASK)   Previous research showed that a greater CC enhances the ability to time-share between tasks. CC size influenced both hemispheres. Therefore, we predicted that the TS patients would demonstrate increased interference in both hemispheres owing to their smaller CC size and reduced cerebral functional space available for computations (Kinsbourne and Hicks, 1978).

Methods in brief

For testing our hypotheses, we recruited adult subjects with TS who had previously been shown to have smaller callosa (as a group) than controls (see the appendix to this chapter). As in any study of clinical disorders, groups differed only in having TS and associated disorders. They were carefully screened for other factors (such as non-consistent right-handedness) that could confound findings associated with the CC. In particular the controls were screened for familial loading for TS and ADHD, which cosegregate in family studies, as well as for obsessive-compulsive disorder and bipolar disorder because of the strong genetic links between these disorders. Tic severity in each patient was rated by using

an interview schedule (Yale Global Tic Severity Scale) that was specifically designed for this purpose by James Leckman and colleagues at the Yale Child Study Center. Other symptoms that may be related to the comorbid disorders such as ADHD and OCD were also carefully assessed.

Findings

GROUP DIFFERENCES

Covert orienting task   The performance of normal subjects was consistent with the previous reports using the same paradigm. Shorter cue-target intervals shortened the reaction time when cue and target were in the same location and prolonged the reaction time when cue and target were in different locations regardless of the "same-sidedness." An increased validity effect when attention was shifted horizontally (i.e., extra time necessary for shifting attention from a precued location to another as in invalid trials) was associated with a greater CC area (Yazgan et al., 1995b).

TS patients were overall slower in responding to targets, and this was the major significant difference between patients and controls. However, patients did not show significantly reduced validity effects, despite their smaller CC sizes.

Verbal-manual interference   An asymmetry with better performance for the tasks lateralized to different hemispheres was observed in normals as predicted. The amount of dual-task interference in normals was strongly inversely correlated with the CC area in both within-hemisphere (right-hand) and between-hemispheres (left-hand) conditions. Left-hand slowing was significantly higher than previously reported, reflecting the increased demands and complexity of the task we used.

The amount of dual-task interference in the TS group was smaller than in normals, particularly in the right hand. This difference reduced the normal dual-task interference asymmetry in the patient group. TS patients who had smaller than normal CCs also had smaller than normal interference. However, the correlation between hand slowing and the CC area in the TS group was not significant.

CLINICAL CORRELATIONS   Task performances were correlated with the severity of the clinical presentation, controlling statistically for the possible influence of the CC area on symptom severity. TS subjects showed significantly greater tic severity with smaller validity effects. In other words, the patients who had greater validity effects for shifting attention, regardless of shifting direction, showed less symptom severity. Greater lifetime phonic tic severity was associated with increased hand slowing in the dual task.

In the control group, individuals who showed less validity effects while shifting their attention horizontally had more verbal interference on their manual activity. No such relationship was observed in the TS group.

SUMMARY OF THE IMPORTANT FINDINGS Normal subjects' performance was consistent with the previous reports using tasks based on the same paradigms.

Slower: TS patients showed overall slower reaction times than normals in the Posner's task.

Less interference: The amount of dual-task interference in the TS group was smaller, particularly in the right hand.

Callosal area: In the normal group only, with smaller callosal area, validity effects decreased. In addition, the amount of dual-task interference increased in both within-hemisphere (right-hand) and between-hemispheres (left-hand) conditions.

Symptoms: More severe tics were associated with reduced validity effects and increased hand slowing in the dual task.

Task-task: Reduced validity effects were associated with more verbal interference on their manual activity in the normal control group.

Discussion

NORMALS Increased validity effect, (i.e., extra time necessary for shifting attention from a precued location to another) was associated with greater CC area.

DIFFERENCES BETWEEN GROUPS TS patients were overall slower in responding to targets, and this was the major significant difference between patients and controls. Smaller callosal size may be associated with reduced speed of information processing (Jäncke and Steinmetz, 1994), as callosal section is associated with reduced overall performance (Kinsbourne, 1974). Overall slowing in the absence of a lateralized difference between patients and controls has also been reported for ADHD children, who are believed to have attentional difficulties similar to those of most TS patients (Swanson et al., 1991). The overall slowing reported above might be due to a dysregulation in arousal that was reported to be associated with callosal functioning (Levy, 1985). A dysregulated arousal system would interact with the efficiency of the covert orienting system, as suggested by reduced validity effects with the use of NE blocking agents such as clonidine, which alters the arousal state (Posner, 1991).

Patients did not show significantly reduced validity effects despite their smaller CC sizes. Reduced validity effects were reported in callosotomized subjects (Reuter-Lorenz and Friedrich, 1990), and the CC has been postulated to play a role in integrating attentional orienting between the two hemispheres in target detection tasks based on Posner's paradigm (Posner et al., 1987; Luck et al., 1994). Lack of a significant reduction in validity effects of the TS subjects may simply be due to absence of an association between covert shifting of attention (and validity effects) and the CC area in the patient group. This relationship, although not significant, was in the same direction. Absence of significantly reduced validity effects is likely due to small sample size; that is, some patients' CCs may not be small enough to have functional consequences.

TS patients who had smaller than normal CCs also had less than normal interference. This effect was manifest especially on their right hands, in contrast to what would be predicted by the normal data. TS subjects were perhaps able to use extracallosal pathways to distribute the load (better than they could with a normal CC). An alternative explanation is that since the arousal effects associated with novel tasks and with stress originate in the right hemisphere and spread to the left via the CC (Posner, 1991), a smaller CC will result in a smaller left-hemisphere share of the arousal. The overall slowing is also present in the dual-task performance of the TS subjects, and the obtained slowing indices do not correlate with the CC area. Reduced validity effects due to presumably high levels of arousal observed in the covert orienting task are consistent with the (assumed) arousal related changes in the dual task.

CORRELATIONS BETWEEN TIC SEVERITY AND NEUROPSYCHOLOGICAL MEASURES TS subjects showed greater tic severity with reduced validity effects and increased hand slowing with concurrent speech. The reduced tendency to use peripheral cues may be due to high levels of arousal (as discussed above) stimulated by detection of the warning signal and/or related stressful states. This difficulty in restricting attention to the target will appear in daily life as abnormal distractibility. Tic severity associated with an increase in distractibility is consistent with Kane's (1994) and Bliss's (1980) descriptions of tic experiences. Tics are induced, exacerbated, or exaggerated by mental or physical (e.g., thermal) stress (Leckman et al., 1995). Electrophysiological (van Woerkom et al., 1994) reports of central gating deficits, increased distractibility, and increased attention to irrelevant stimuli provide further support to this formulation.

LIMITATIONS Our findings in this small sample of TS patients are confounded by several factors, which limit our discussion to hypothesis generation rather than definitive explanations. The small sample size reduces the chances that a true difference between the groups is detected. It does not allow multivariate analyses that could be employed to assess the influence of multiple factors such as sex, age, age of onset, and comorbid diagnoses. Although some of our analyses were hypothesis driven, several post hoc exploratory analyses were performed, further reducing our power.

Our tasks might not be specific enough, reducing their sensitivity to detect differences. Since we used the overall callosal area in our analyses, regional differences in the CC and possible plastic changes in regional redistribution of neural channels cannot be considered. These would be important in a disorder associated with the developmental process.

Despite these limitations, the strong task-structure correlations in the normal group as well as the task-clinical severity correlations deserve further study. We must note that a follow-up study in a larger sample using the same neuropsychological battery revealed similar group differences and symptom-task performance relationships for TS and ADHD patients. A larger sample of patients including children needs to be imaged and tested for answering the questions raised by the findings in this report.

Conclusions

TS patients showed slower RTs than their normal controls. Validity effects decreased as the callosal area became smaller, supporting the role of intact corpus callosum in integrating the hemispheres' orienting responses. TS patients, who had smaller CC areas than their controls, manifested reduced validity effects, indicating inadequate utilization of cues. This difference did not reach significance. However, the degree of reduction in validity effects was significantly associated with increased tic severity. These findings are suggestive of an association between inefficient callosal functioning and more severe expression of the illness in adult patients with TS. They also suggest that the corpus callosum, although smaller in size, continues to play an integrative role in patients, similar to its role in normals. The limitations of our study described above notwithstanding, these findings, together with the earlier TS and ADHD reports, support the notion that the presumed early insult may have caused "a redistribution of channels, leading to compensatory shifts and even apparent paradoxical increases in connectivity" (Zaidel, Clarke, and Suyenobu, 1986). The likelihood that compensatory processes take place is high, since "cerebral plasticity is linked to the extent of the functional maturity of the le-

sioned structure" and "plasticity may be extended by hormonal influences" (Lassonde et al., 1991). Whether the onset of symptoms of both TS and ADHD (as well as of other developmental neuropsychiatric disorders) is related to plasticity-related changes in the callosum will be an interesting question to answer in future studies. Novel hypotheses about the role of interhemispheric integration in TS and ADHD should consider the role of plasticity. The natural history of the disorder suggests that TS, a chronic disorder with exacerbations and remissions, is difficult to explain without considering its plasticity as a syndrome. Thus, the corpus callosum appears to be an excellent candidate for structural MRI studies, thanks to its plastic nature, which may accommodate the life course of a plastic disorder.

ACKNOWLEDGMENTS The data reported in this paper were collected while the first author was at the Yale Child Study Center in collaboration with Drs. James F. Leckman, Bradley Peterson, and Bruce E. Wexler. The study described in the chapter was supported in part by NIH grants MH44843, MH49351, HD03008, RR00125 (General Clinical Research Center), and MH30929 (Mental Health Clinical Research Center) to the Yale Child Study Center.

REFERENCES

ABOITIZ, F., A. B. SCHEIBEL, R. S. FISHER, and E. ZAIDEL, 1992a. Fiber composition of the human corpus callosum. *Brain Res.* 598:143–153.

ABOITIZ, F., A. B. SCHEIBEL, R. S. FISHER, and E. ZAIDEL, 1992b. Individual differences in brain asymmetries and fiber composition in the human corpus callosum. *Brain Res.* 598:154–161.

BLISS, J., 1980. Sensory experiences of Gilles de la Tourette syndrome. *Arch. Gen. Psychiatry* 37:1343–1347.

BOGEN, J. E., 1993. The callosal syndromes. In *Clinical Neuropsychology*, 3rd ed., K. M. Heilman and E. Valenstein, eds. New York: Oxford University Press, pp. 337–408.

CARLSON, C. L., W. E. PELHAM, J. SWANSON, and J. L. WAGNER, 1991. A divided attention analysis of the effects of methylphenidate. *J. Child Psychol. Psychiatry* 32:463–471.

CASTELLANOS, F. X., J. N. GIEDD, P. ECKBURG, W. L. MARSH, D. KAYSEN, S. D. HAMBURGER, and J. L. RAPOPORT, 1994. Quantitative morphology of the caudate nucleus in attention deficit hyperactivity disorder. *Am. J. Psychiatry* 151:1791–1796.

CLARKE, J. M., and E. ZAIDEL, 1994. Anatomical-behavioral relationships: Corpus callosum morphometry and hemispheric specialization. *Behav. Brain Res.* 64:185–202.

COHEN, D. J., and J. F. LECKMAN, 1994. Developmental psychopathology and neurobiology of Tourette's syndrome. *J. Am. Acad. Child Adolesc. Psychiatry* 33:2–15.

FITCH, R. H., A. S. BERREBI, P. E. COWELL, L. M. SCHROTT, and V. H. DENENBERG, 1990. Corpus callosum: Effects of neonatal hormones on sexual dimorphism in the rat. *Brain Res.* 515:111–116.

GIEDD, J., F. CASTELLANOS, B. CASEY, ET AL., 1994. Quantitative morphology of the corpus callosum in attention deficit/hyperactivity disorder. *Am. J. Psychiatry* 151: 665–669.

GUIARD, Y., 1980. Cerebral hemispheres and selective attention. *Acta Psychol.* 46:41–61.

HARRIS, J. C., 1995. Attention deficit disorder-hyperactivity disorder. In *Developmental Neuropsychiatry*, J. C. Harris, ed. New York: Oxford University Press.

HUGHES, H. C., and L. D. ZIMBA, 1987. Natural boundaries for the spatial spread of directed visual attention. *Neuropsychologia* 25:5–18.

JÄNCKE, L., and H. STEINMETZ, 1994. Interhemispheric transfer time and corpus callosum size. *NeuroReport* 5:2385–2388.

KANE, M. J., 1994. Premonitory urges as "attentional" tics. *J. Am. Acad. Child Adolesc. Psychiatry* 33:803–808.

KINSBOURNE, M., 1974. Mechanisms of hemispheric interaction in the brain. In *Hemispheric Disconnection and Cerebral Function*, M. Kinsbourne and W. L. Smith, eds. Springfield, Ill.: Thomas, pp. 260–285.

KINSBOURNE, M., and J. COOK, 1971. Generalized and lateralized effects of concurrent verbalization on a unimanual skill. *Q. J. Exp. Psychol.* 23:341–345.

KINSBOURNE, M., and R. E. HICKS, 1978. Functional cerebral space: A model for overflow, transfer and interference effects in human performance. In *Attention and Performance VII*, M. Requin, ed. Hillsdale, N.J.: Lawrence Erlbaum.

KINSBOURNE, M., and HISCOCK, M., 1983. Asymmetries of dual-task performance. In *Cerebral Hemisphere Asymmetry: Method, Theory and Application*, J. B. Hellige, ed. New York: Praeger.

KORKMAN, M., and A. E. PESONEN, 1994. A comparison of neuropsychological profiles of children with ADD and/or LD. *J. Learn. Disabil.* 27:383–392.

LaMANTIA, A.-S., and P. G. RAKIC, 1990. Cytological and quantitative characteristics of four cerebral commissures in the rhesus monkey. *J. Comp. Neurol.* 291:520–537.

LASSONDE, M., 1986. The facilitatory influence of the corpus callosum on intrahemispheric processing. In *Two Hemispheres—One Brain: Functions of the Corpus Callosum*, F. Lepore, M. Ptito, and H. H. Jasper, eds. New York: Liss, pp. 385–401.

LASSONDE, M., H. SAUERWEIN, A.-J. CHICOINE, and G. GEOFFEOY, 1991. Absence of disconnexion syndrome in callosal agenesis and early callosotomy. *Neuropsychologia* 29:481–492.

LECKMAN, J. F., D. L. PAULS, and D. J. COHEN, 1995. Tic disorders. In *Psychopharmacology: The Fourth Generation of Progress*, F. Bloom and D. Kupfer, eds. New York: Raven Press.

LECKMAN, J. F., and B. PETERSON, 1993. The pathogenesis of Tourette's syndrome: Epigenetic factors active in early CNS development. *Biol. Psychiatry* 34:425–427.

LECKMAN, J. F., D. WALKER, and D. J. COHEN, 1993. Premonitory urges in Tourette syndrome. *Am. J. Psychiatry* 150:98–102.

LEVY, J., 1985. Interhemispheric collaboration. In *Hemisphere Function and Collaboration in the Child*, C. T. Best, ed. New York: Academic Press.

LOU, H. C., L. HENRIKSEN, P. BRUHN, and B. NIELSEN, 1989. Striatal dysfunction in attention deficit and hyperkinetic disorder. *Arch. Neurol.* 46:48–52.

LUCK, S. J., S. A. HILLYARD, G. R. MANGUN, and M. S. GAZZANIGA, 1994. Independent hemispheric attentional systems mediate visual search in split-brain patients. *J. Cogn. Neurosci.* 6:84–91.

McFARLAND, K. A., and R. ASHTON, 1978. The influence of concurrent task difficulty on manual performance. *Neuropsychologia* 16:735–741.

PETERSON, B. S., M. A. RIDDLE, D. J. COHEN, L. D. KATZ, J. C. SMITH, M. T. HARDIN, and J. F. LECKMAN, 1993. Reduced basal ganglia volumes in Tourette's syndrome using three-dimensional reconstruction techniques from magnetic resonance images. *Neurology* 43:941–949.

PETERSON, B. S., J. F. LECKMAN, R. WETZLES, J. DUNCAN, M. A. RIDDLE, M. T. HARDIN, and D. J. COHEN, 1994. Corpus callosum morphology from MR images in Tourette's syndrome. *Psychiatry Res. Neuroimaging* 55:85–99.

POSNER, M. I., 1980. Orienting of attention. *Q. J. Exp. Psychol.* 32:3–25.

POSNER, M. I., 1991. Interaction of arousal and selection in the posterior attention network. In *Attention: Selection, Awareness and Control. A tribute to Donald Broadbent*, A. Baddeley and L. Weiskrantz, eds. New York: Academic Press.

POSNER, M. I., J. A. WALKER, F. A. FRIEDRICH, and R. D. RAFAL, 1987. How do parietal lobes direct covert attention? *Neuropsychologia* 25:135–145.

REUTER-LORENZ, P., and R. FRIEDRICH, 1990. Orienting attention across the vertical meridian: Evidence from callosotomy patients. *J. Cog. Neurosci.* 2:232–238.

RIZZOLATTI, G., L. RIGGIO, I. DASCOLA, and C. UMILTA, 1987. Reorienting attention across the horizontal and vertical meridians: Evidence in favor of a premotor theory of attention. *Neuropsychologia* 25:31–40.

SINGER, H. S., A. L. REISS, J. E. BROWN, E. H. AYLWARD, B. SHIH, E. CHEE, E. L. HARRIS, M. J. READER, G. A. CHASE, R. N. BRYAN, and M. B. DENCKLA, 1993. Volumetric MRI changes in basal ganglia of children with Tourette's syndrome. *Neurology* 43:950–956.

SWANSON, J., M. POSNER, S. POTKIN, S. BONFORTE, D. CANTWELL, and F. CRINELLA, 1991. Activating tasks for the study of visual-spatial attention in ADHD children: A cognitive anatomic approach. *J. Child Neurol.* 6:S119–S127.

VAN WOERKOM, T. C. A. M., R. A. C. ROOS, and J. G. VAN DIJK, 1994. Altered attentional processing of background stimuli in Gilles de la Tourette syndrome. *Acta Neurol. Scand.* 90:116–125.

YAZGAN, M. Y., B. PETERSON, B. E. WEXLER, and J. F. LECKMAN, 1995a. Behavioral laterality in individuals with Gilles de la Tourette's syndrome and basal ganglia alterations. *Biol. Psychiatry* 38:386–390, 1995.

YAZGAN, M. Y., B. E. WEXLER, M. KINSBOURNE, B. PETERSON, and J. F. LECKMAN, 1995b. Functional significance of individual variations in callosal area. *Neuropsychologia* 33:769–781.

YAZGAN, M. Y., S. ZAIMOGLU, and S. KARAMURSEL, 1996. *Auditory ERPs evoked in an oddball paradigm in TS*. Paper presented at the American Psychiatric Association Meeting, New York.

ZAIDEL, E., J. M. CLARKE, and A. M. SUYENOBU, 1986. Hemispheric independence: A paradigm case for cognitive neuroscience. In *Neurobiology of Higher Cognitive Function*, A. B. Scheibel and A. F. Wechsler, eds. New York: Guilford.

ZAMETKIN, A., T. E. NORDAHL, M. GROSS, A. KING, J. RUMSEY, and R. COHEN, 1990. Cerebral glucose metabolism in adults with hyperactivity of childhood onset. *N. Engl. J. Med.* 323:1361–1366.

About the methods

Subject characteristics and clinical diagnostic procedures have been published by Yazgan and colleagues (1995a). Scanning procedures and image analysis are detailed by Peterson and colleagues (1994).

Neuropsychological tasks

COVERT ORIENTING OF ATTENTION (POSNER'S TASK)   Each subject ran in a single 35-minute session that started with an approximately 1-minute practice session of 10 trials. After this, subjects completed 352 trials in four blocks, with both hands. Subjects had 1- to 3-minute intervals between blocks.

Before each trial began, a 0.5° cross appeared on the center and remained there for 250 ms before being erased. This cross was a signal to the subjects that a trial was starting and provided a central fixation point. After the cross disappeared, five 1° boxes appeared, four of which formed the corners of a 10° wide box; the fifth was in the center of the box. After those boxes were presented for 1000 ms, a cue appeared. The cue was a larger box that appeared around one of the four peripheral boxes selected at random and equiprobably. The target (a 0.8° asterisk) occurred at the center of one of the boxes at 100, 200, 700, or 1200 ms after the onset of the cue. If the target was presented at the same location as the cue, it was called a true cue. If the target was presented at a noncued location, it was called a false cue. The center box was never cued. In catch trials, a cue but no target appeared.

The subjects' task was to press the response key as rapidly as possible when they detected the target. There was an intertrial interval of 1500 ms, and the computer waited 3000 ms for a response on each trial before terminating the trial and moving on to the next trial. Subjects were instructed to keep their eyes fixed on the center. Previous work has shown that they are unlikely to move their eyes when performing a task such as this that does not require visual acuity. This is particularly true for trials with shorter than 150-ms stimulus onset asynchrony (SOA).

There were 88 trials in each block; 20% of trials were valid trials. In 40% of invalid trials the target appeared in the same visual field, although it appeared in a different location ("same false"). Remaining invalid trials consisted of cue and targets appearing in opposite visual fields. Eight were catch trials. Cue-target intervals (SOA) were distributed between four intervals (100, 200, 700, and 1200 ms). Of particular interest to us were the 100-ms SOA trials.

Reaction times less than 100 ms were eliminated to reduce any anticipations. Reaction times longer than 3000 ms were also eliminated, since the computer program moved on to the next trial if no response had been made by then. For the remaining trials, median values for each subject for each condition were calculated, and mean values were calculated across subjects.

VERBAL-MANUAL INTERFERENCE TASK (VMI)   This procedure, based on the dual-task paradigm, measures the impact of lateralized concurrent language activity on a timed unimanual task. For a baseline condition, subjects were asked to complete a motor task for each hand (right and left). As an interference condition, they were asked to do the motor task concurrently with a language task. The order of first hand use was randomized to avoid transfer of learning effects. The motor task was the Trail Making Test, Part B. In this test, subjects connect circles with alternating contents of sequential numbers and letters. The language task instruction was to respond vocally by conjugating into past tense a heard list of commonly used irregular verbs. The time interval between verbs was 2–3 seconds. Subjects were instructed to do the best they could in performing both tasks at the same time rather than focusing on one of the tasks during the dual-task condition. The time for completion of tasks under each condition was determined in seconds. The number of errors in motor and language performance were also recorded. Interference is expressed as proportional decrements in right- and left-hand performances (23). The decrements are calculated as X% = 100 × (time for dual-task performance − time for single-task performance)/ time for single task performance for each hand (R% and L%).

19 Using the Corpus Callosum as an Effective Anatomical Probe in the Study of Schizophrenia

PATRICIA E. COWELL, VICTOR DENENBERG, GARY BOEHM, ANDREW KERTESZ, AND HENRY NASRALLAH

ABSTRACT In an area of research that lacks consensus about normative patterns of group variation, investigation of patient-control differences sets out with a clear disadvantage. Such is the state of affairs with respect to the study of corpus callosum (CC) anatomy in schizophrenia. In this chapter we explore several approaches for maximizing effectiveness of the CC as an anatomical probe for studying schizophrenia. One such approach advocates the use of correlational models for understanding patterns of neuromorphological variation in the CC. Another approach advocates examination of patient-control-differences in neurobehavioral relationships. Both techniques are put forward as methods that have shown more reliable outcomes in the study of normative CC variation than the more commonly used comparison of group means. The study of the CC has proven more complex than was originally conceived at the advent of its large-scale study in the early 1980s. The study of schizophrenia, in its various clinical, neuropsychological, and neurobiological manifestations, is also a process that often yields more new questions than answers. However, if appropriate techniques are used, regional callosal anatomy may be viewed as a highly sensitive and useful probe in the systematic study of neurocognitive variation in neuropsychiatric and normative populations.

The corpus callosum (CC) in its midline perspective is an attractive candidate for neuroanatomical study owing to

PATRICIA E. COWELL Department of Human Communication Sciences, University of Sheffield, Sheffield, United Kingdom.
VICTOR DENENBERG Biobehavioral Sciences and Psychology, University of Connecticut, Storrs, Connecticut.
GARY BOEHM Department of Psychology, Texas Christian University, Fort Worth, Texas.
ANDREW KERTESZ Department of Clinical Neurological Sciences, University of Western Ontario, London, Ontario, Canada.
HENRY NASRALLAH Professor of Psychiatry, Neurology, and Medicine, University of Mississippi School of Medicine, Jackson, Mississippi.

its relative ease of measurement (Figure 19.1). This ease of access is heightened when researchers are able to obtain neuroanatomical data from live human subjects via magnetic resonance imaging (MRI). Yet anyone who has ever worked with the CC or tried to digest the growing literature on CC research knows that while it is a convenient structure to measure, it is also a vexing one. Trying to pin down the sources of variation that affect this structure in normative human populations, as well as in patients with various behavioral and psychiatric disorders, has been a difficult task. The literature in this area is fraught with controversy, and as a result, the CC has gained a reputation with some scientists as being a structure that is too variable to measure and analyze with any degree of confidence.

In this chapter we propose that rather than being "too variable," the CC is instead highly sensitive to a range of factors that, once understood, can be formally incorporated into experimental design and analysis. Several clues to the types of factors that may influence the development and function of the CC in schizophrenia are already present in the literature on normative patterns of variation in CC anatomy. One aim of this chapter is to discuss how information from the study of the CC in healthy research subjects may be incorporated, both theoretically and methodologically, into the mainstream of neurobiological research on the CC in schizophrenia.

Research on the CC in schizophrenia is discussed from several perspectives. First, the context within which research on the CC fits into the broader study of schizophrenia from theoretical, clinical, neuropsychological, analytical, and interpretational perspectives is addressed. Next, the study of individual differences and how group comparisons of regional CC anatomy in normative human populations can inform the study of the CC in

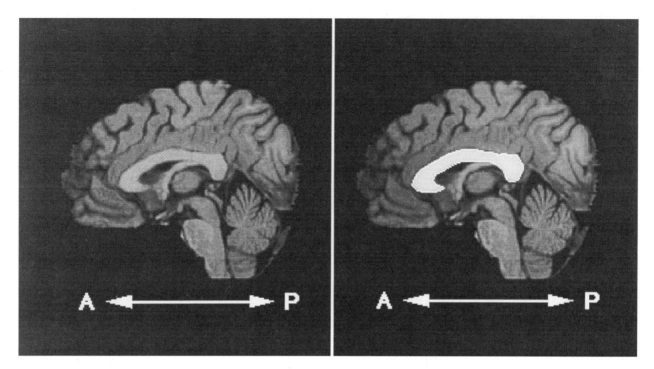

FIGURE 19.1. Midline view of the human brain from a magnetic resonance image (left). The corpus callosum (CC) has been outlined and filled (right) to demonstrate that the CC is anatomically distinct from other structures and therefore relatively easy to measure. (A = anterior; P = posterior).

schizophrenia are covered. In the final sections of this chapter, two approaches, taken from the study of the CC in normative samples, are applied to the investigation of callosal anatomy in a sample of patients with schizophrenia.

Context: Finding a place for the corpus callosum in schizophrenia research

How does investigation of the CC fit into the broader spectrum of biomedical research on schizophrenia? A colleague once referred to the literature on schizophrenia as "that great thicket of putative explanations for schizophrenia." This is an apt description of the field in light of the extraordinary scope and breadth of research efforts to understand the complexity of this debilitating neuropsychiatric disorder. A presentation of the entire neurobiological literature relating to schizophrenia is beyond the scope of this chapter. However, research on the CC, if used to its fullest advantage, may provide information that helps us navigate through the "great thicket." This chapter describes several ways in which this might be accomplished.

David (1994) makes specific reference to the fact that just about every brain region examined in schizophrenia has revealed some sort of anomaly. This concept may also be applied to the many behavioral and cognitive dimensions that have been found to differ between healthy comparison subjects and patients with schizophrenia. The number of individual reports concerning the CC in schizophrenia hovers somewhere between 200 and 300. This represents a very small fraction of the myriad scientific articles on schizophrenia that have been published in the past 30 years. Indeed, there is relatively limited evidentiary warrant to support a primary role for the CC in the etiology of the acute symptoms of schizophrenia such as hallucinations, delusions, bizarre behavior, and thought disorder.

In comparison, a much higher proportion of schizophrenia research has been dedicated to the study of neurophysiological phenomena that contribute directly to developments in patient care. For example, much scientific investigation has centered on trying to understand how disturbances in neurotransmitter systems contribute to the onset and expression of this disorder. This body of research has led to the discovery of drugs that allow psychiatrists to pharmaceutically treat the acute psychotic symptoms of schizophrenia. Another key area of scientific inquiry is neurodevelopmental, and it implicates early prenatal damage to structures in the temporal lobe such as the entorhinal cortex (Arnold et al., 1991) and the hippocampus, followed by the postpubertal emergence of dysfunction in prefrontal cortical systems (Lipska, Jaskiw, and Weinberger, 1993). Such research may lead to discoveries that can be applied to the development of early intervention techniques or preventive therapies. Some authors have emphasized the role of cerebral laterality in the emergence of schizophrenia (see Cowell, Fitch, and Denenberg, 1999, for a review). However, even if a particular emphasis is placed on the development of brain asymmetry and interhemispheric relationships, it seems likely that the CC plays a supporting role rather than a primary role in the intricate profile of neurobehavioral and neurocognitive processes underlying and accompanying schizophrenia.

Where exactly does investigation of the CC fit among the many other aspects of brain function and structure that have also been implicated in schizophrenia? Perhaps more importantly, we must ask whether research on the CC, and on interhemispheric relationships in general, contributes to the understanding, prevention, and effective treatment of this neuropsychiatric disorder. One aim of this chapter is to demonstrate that research on interhemispheric relationships, including the structure and function of the CC, will help to further our ability to understand schizophrenia and treat patients, but it will do so only as part of a much larger picture.

This larger picture goes beyond the acute clinical symptoms of schizophrenia and their immediate treatment to incorporate a broad array of underlying cognitive traits, some of which persist despite medication (Cannon et al., 1994). Such cognitive characteristics may be related in varying degrees to the CC and its role in interhemispheric function. A number of investigations have employed behavioral paradigms designed to tap directly into interhemispheric function and have yielded results that suggest differences in the effectiveness of callosal transfer in patients with schizophrenia (David, 1994; Green, Hugdahl, and Mitchell, 1994; Woodruff et al., 1997). The CC has also been indirectly implicated in studies showing that key neuropsychological features of schizophrenia have their basis in disturbances of functional asymmetry. In a sample of patients without histories of drug or alcohol abuse, cognitive functions that showed the most marked differences compared to controls were semantic memory, visual memory, and verbal learning (Saykin et al., 1991). There is evidence from the neuropsychology and neuroimaging literature that these disturbances in learning and memory may be related to disruptions in lateralized cortical function. In patients with schizophrenia, deficits in verbal recall were correlated with left-hemisphere abnormalities in glucose metabolism (Harper Mozley et al., 1996).

At first glance, research on the CC might appear to be relatively remote from the mainstream of schizophrenia research that is highlighted by advances in the understanding of neurotransmitter systems (possibly leading to new drug treatments) and neurodevelopmental mechanisms (possibly leading to earlier clinical interventions).

However, if the characterization of schizophrenia is expanded to include deficits in cognitive performance, and in particular measures related to lateralized or interhemispheric functions, the potential for using neuroanatomical measures of the CC to examine brain-behavior correlations becomes evident. Such a research program could be extended to incorporate the study of correlations between the CC and clinical manifestations of schizophrenia such as negative symptoms, thought disorder, and auditory hallucinations whose severity has been linked to degree of asymmetry in outlying regions of cortical anatomy (Barta et al., 1990; Shenton et al., 1992; Bilder et al., 1994; Petty et al., 1995; Turetsky et al., 1995). In this way, links could be made among the various cognitive, clinical, and callosal components of schizophrenia.

Having established theoretically that there is a potential niche for CC research in schizophrenia, how can we proceed methodologically to maximize the applicability and relevance of currently available data to future investigations? As described in the preceding paragraphs, the CC may be viewed as a potential mediator of disorders in interhemispheric relationships, lateralized cognitive function, and clinical symptomatology. One of the fundamental elements in coordinating the multidimensional research program necessary to investigate these various roles is a clear understanding of the CC's anatomy and its organization in schizophrenia. To effectively achieve such an understanding, it is essential to first look at the research in normative human populations. This will reveal factors that contribute significantly and reliably to individual differences in regional CC anatomy. It would be of particular interest to see whether variables such as sex and age, which affect CC anatomy in healthy humans subjects, have similar relationships to the CC in patients with schizophrenia and then to examine how these effects may be associated with outlying cortical structures.

The CC is a fiber tract interconnecting many regions of the right and left cerebral cortex. Therefore, by viewing it in its midsagittal perspective, one has access to a rough index of what is happening in the outlying cortex.[1] In this manner, regional anomalies in the CCs of patients with schizophrenia may be used to detect probable sites in outlying cortex for further neuroanatomic investigation.

---

[1] The anterior-to-posterior layout of the CC as mapped by various researchers can be viewed only as an approximate index of homotopically interconnected cortical regions, since there are also heterotopic connections and dorsoventral distinctions in the topography of the midsagittal CC.

Knowledge about the factors that affect CC structure and function in schizophrenia has been acquired using a variety of methods. The between-group comparison of area or regional size is the most commonly employed procedure in neuroanatomical investigations of the CC. In such studies, anatomical measures are taken for a group of patients and then compared to equivalent measures in a group of controls to explore differences in CC size between the samples. (The results from a review of these studies are discussed below.) In addition, mathematical models have been used to investigate group differences in callosal form (Bookstein, 1996/7; Casanova et al., 1990a, 1990b; Chapters 4 and 5 in this volume). One such method for examining differences in callosal form is based on factor analysis (Denenberg et al., 1991b) and is explored below.

There are also correlational techniques that may be used to study brain-behavior relationships between CC size and the various functional attributes of schizophrenia. Some studies have examined the nature of the relationship between CC size and severity of clinical symptomatology or performance on cognitive tasks involved in interhemispheric functions (Raine et al., 1990; Colombo et al., 1993; Woodruff et al., 1997; Tibbo et al., 1998).[2] An indirect correlational approach could also be used to investigate, in patients, the neurocognitive basis for behaviors that have been shown to vary systematically with CC function in normative samples. For example, recent research has found that in specific situations, brain-behavior relationships between CC size and measures of interhemispheric function may be placed along a similar functional continuum in patients and controls (Woodruff et al., 1997). However, if callosal systems are severely damaged or dysfunctional in schizophrenia, then different neural systems may be recruited to execute interhemispheric functions. In such a situation it is possible that brain-behavior correlations seen in normative samples might not be observed in all patients with schizophrenia. Such an approach provides the basis of one of our analyses later in this chapter.

Differences in CC structure may be used to provide insights at many levels of neuroanatomical analysis. At the most localized level, findings from regional callosal analyses may reflect only differences in the CC itself and the specific cortical cells that send fibers through the callosal regions in question. Alternatively, findings in the CC may reflect more global phenomena that extend to the outlying regional cortical white matter and perhaps even to the related gray matter. Finally, it is always possible that a proportion of the variation in CC anatomy reflects overall variation in whole brain, head, or even body size (Jäncke et al., 1997). Therefore, the task of studying the CC in schizophrenia is further complicated by the wide array of options available for interpreting the meaning of differences in callosal size, form, or relationships with behavioral measures.

In this review of the literature that examines group differences in CC area and regional CC size, few, if any, reliable effects were observed. Some studies have found the CC to be larger in patients, whereas others have shown the opposite pattern or no differences at all. The notion that decreased cortical gray matter should result in proportionately more white matter and larger CC size in schizophrenia is supported by studies showing that patients have larger CCs than controls. Indeed, it has been shown that patients have longer CCs than controls (Mathew et al., 1985), that only female patients have larger CCs (Nasrallah et al., 1986; Raine et al., 1990), and that the increase in CC size is carried by one clinical subgroup of early-onset patients (Coger and Serafetinides, 1990).

Other studies have found CC size to be smaller in patients than in controls. These results have been used to support the notion that decreased gray matter should result in fewer cortical cells, fewer CC fibers, and a smaller CC. A smaller CC was observed for whole patient samples (Rossi et al., 1989; Takeuchi, 1992; Woodruff et al., 1995), in male patients only (Raine et al., 1990; Woodruff et al., 1993; Tibbo et al., 1998), and in particular clinical subgroups classified by first-episode female patients in one study (Hoff et al., 1994) and late-onset patients with positive symptoms in another (Coger and Serafetinides, 1990). There are also reports of no significant size differences between patients' and controls' CCs (Hauser et al., 1989; Casanova et al., 1990b; Colombo et al., 1993; Woodruff et al., 1997).

This collection of contradictory reports is reminiscent of the perplexing array of findings published on the topic of sex differences in normative human samples (Bishop and Wahlsten, 1997). Another peculiar aspect of the schizophrenia literature is that a similar neuroanatomical underpinning (reductions in gray matter) has been used to account for reports of both increased and decreased CC size. Recent research has sought to clarify these issues through the study of axon density and number in men and women with schizophrenia compared to controls (Highley et al., 1999). In the following sections

---

[2] Right-ear advantage in dichotic listening of auditory verbal stimuli is believed to reflect the left-hemisphere advantage in normal language processing. Dichotic listening in patients with schizophrenia has been studied by multiple research groups with mixed results, suggesting heterogeneity in cerebral lateralization across patient samples, paralleled possibly by varying degrees of CC dysfunction.

we suggest two techniques to address issues of CC complexity and heterogeneity using methods applicable at the gross anatomical level.

Normative variation in the corpus callosum: Its relevance to the study of the callosum in schizophrenia

In light of the studies reviewed above, who is "correct" and where does one go from here? In response to the first part of this question, perhaps all the authors are correct, that is, correct about their particular samples of patients and controls. In response to the latter part, unless the approach to the study of CC anatomy in schizophrenia is significantly revised, we are destined only to add to the controversy. Therefore, it is critical to stop and take stock of the various factors that have been found to contribute to normative variation in CC size. Before we can understand all the variables that contribute to callosal heterogeneity in patients with a disorder as complex and varied in its clinical manifestations as schizophrenia, we must first come to grips with some of the factors that contribute to variability of this structure in the normative population. The remainder of this chapter is dedicated to the search for approaches derived from research in healthy human subjects that have the potential to shed light on the study of not only the CC, but also the outlying cerebral cortex, in patients with schizophrenia. Applications of these approaches to the analysis of the CC in a sample of patients with schizophrenia are then explored.

To appreciate the research findings described below, it is important to first have a general understanding of the assessment techniques that are used. The CC measurement procedure, summarized below, is described in detail by Denenberg and colleagues (1991a) and is an adaptation of a method that was originally used to quantify the CC in rodents. The scientific perspectives that we brought to bear on the study of the CC in schizophrenia were not clinically driven but based in the traditions of developmental psychobiology and the biobehavioral sciences. Thus, before we performed studies of group differences of any kind, we set out to design a method for measuring and subdividing the CC in a manner that would yield results as sensitive and reliable as those we obtained from our experiments on the CC in rodents (Fitch et al., 1990, 1991).

Our program to investigate the human CC was initially based in an animal research facility. Therefore, our raw data were MRIs obtained through collaborations with other scientists. Various researchers sent us their samples that were comprised of, or from which we could obtain, tracings of the CC at midline. These outlines of the midsagittal CC were digitized on a computer

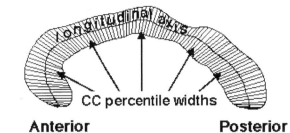

FIGURE 19.2. Sample outline of a human CC taken from a magnetic resonance image. After being digitized, each CC tracing is displayed as shown with the 99 CC percentile widths and the longitudinal axis. (This figure has been adapted from Cowell et al., 1993, with permission from Lippincott-Raven Publishers.)

tablet with an interactive software program (Denenberg et al., 1991a). Once a CC case was digitized, an output consisting of callosal area, perimeter, 99 percentile widths along the curved longitudinal axis, and axis length was displayed. The 99 widths were formed by dividing the dorsal (upper) and ventral (lower) perimeters into percentiles and connecting the correspondingly numbered points. Axis length was constructed by connecting the midpoints of the 99 widths. Our measurement procedure used the criterion that the sum of the 99 widths was to be a minimum, which was obtained by retracing the CC until a satisfactory solution was reached. The 99 CC widths and longitudinal axis are depicted in Figure 19.2.

Once the minimum 99 widths solution was obtained, five tracings were made for each case and averaged to control for measurement error. In our first study, this procedure was performed for a large sample of healthy men and women aged 18–49 years. Once we had digitized the CCs for this group, we applied a correlational model that would allow the data to reveal its own integral organization through objective mathematical analyses. The multiple anatomical measures (99 CC widths, CC area, CC perimeter, CC length, and midsagittal brain area) for 103 human subjects were entered into a factor analysis. The solution was expressed as a significantly reduced number of semi-independent callosal factors that accounted for almost 90% of variance from the original data. Each of the emergent seven width factors, depicted in Figure 19.3, represented a highly intercorrelated cluster of adjacent CC widths. CC length and perimeter were associated with the posteriormost CC width factor, CC area was not uniquely associated with any factor, and midsagittal brain area was represented by an eighth factor. This factor analysis solution was originally published by Denenberg and colleagues (1991b), to which readers are referred for more details on the procedures summarized above.

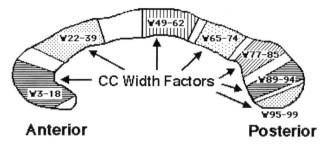

FIGURE 19.3. After a large sample of CCs have been digitized, the raw anatomical data are factor analyzed. The seven factor widths from the factor analytic solution published by Denenberg and colleagues (1991b) are overlaid onto a CC outline for graphical display. (This figure has been adapted from Cowell et al., 1993, with permission from Lippincott-Raven Publishers.)

Through extensive investigation, we found the CC factor structure to have a remarkably high degree of congruence, or similarity, across two large independent groups of human subjects (Cowell et al., 1994). In contrast to the controversial literature on both normative sex differences and patient-control differences in schizophrenia, our factor structure represented one of the few characteristics of CC anatomy that had been replicated. This high degree of consistency across normative samples, which differed along multiple demographic dimensions such as the age and hand preference composition, suggested that factor analysis might prove to be an effective probe in the search for neuroanatomical traits associated with clinical disorders such as schizophrenia.

Factor analysis proved to be a reliable method for quantifying CC form; but just as importantly, the groupings of CC widths along the seven factors provided us with a nonarbitrary basis for subdividing the CC into subregions for purposes of studying group differences in regional CC size (see Figure 19.3). The research of Fitch and colleagues (1990, 1991) had demonstrated the utility of regional subdivisions of the CC based on factor analyses in rodents, particularly in the area of sex differences and CC development. Application of this method to the study of sex differences in human CC across the life span was a logical next step. It involved the measurement of 146 human CCs from men and women ranging from 2 to 79 years of age (Cowell et al., 1992) and used a polynomial trend analysis to examine the differential effects of age on the CC in men and women.

Our findings demonstrated that normative sex differences in this structure were far more complex than originally thought (Cowell et al., 1992). First, they were localized to specific CC regions; second, they were expressed differently at various stages of the human life span. For example, the anteriormost CC width factor, W3–18 (Figure 19.4), which, on the basis of tract tracing

work in monkeys, is believed to interconnect the prefrontal cortex (Pandya and Seltzer, 1986), was at its maximum size for the age group representing the third decade of life in men (at which point it was larger than in women of the same age). In women the data suggested that this region of the CC may increase in size through the fifth decade of life (at which point it tended to be larger than in men of the same age) and only afterward show decreases in mean width indicative of decline in CC size with advancing age. This pattern was specific to the anterior (W3–18 and W22–49) and posterior of the CC (W95–99) and was not found in other CC regions. For example, in the midbody (W49–62), which is believed to interconnect sensorimotor cortex (Pandya and Seltzer, 1986), growth and decline of CC width was the same for men and women.

It is not difficult to deduce how this type of variability in normative samples may have multiple effects on the study of the CC in schizophrenia. If one were, for example, to examine the anterior CC in the typical fashion of comparing regional CC size in patients to controls, it is possible that the magnitude (and possibly even the direction) of the difference between the groups would be affected by variation related more to the particular sex and age range of the healthy comparison subjects than actual neuropsychiatric differences. It is also possible that CC measures in patients would be affected by the interactive effects of sex and age, though possibly, as suggested by longitudinal work (DeLisi et al., 1997), in ways that are unique to this disorder. Once one appreciates the complexity of these phenomena, it becomes clear that failure to control carefully for variability in the sex and age distributions of patient and control samples may have been a contributing factor to the heterogeneity of findings in the literature on patient-control differences in regional CC anatomy.

Sex and age are not the only sources of variation in normative human populations. We found that the interactions between sex, direction of hand preference (right versus left), and degree (consistent versus nonconsistent) of hand preference also contributed significantly to normative variability in regional CC anatomy (Denenberg et al., 1991b; Cowell et al., 1993).[3] Our findings replicated and expanded on the original findings of Witelson (1989), who discovered that in right-handed men but not

---

[3] Cowell and colleagues (1993) showed that there are distinct relationships between degree of right-hand versus degree of left-hand preference and the CC. Thus, both direction (right versus left) and degree (consistent versus nonconsistent) of hand preference appear to affect CC size. Studies that failed to find effects of hand preference in the CC isthmus often collapsed across one of these dimensions of hand preference.

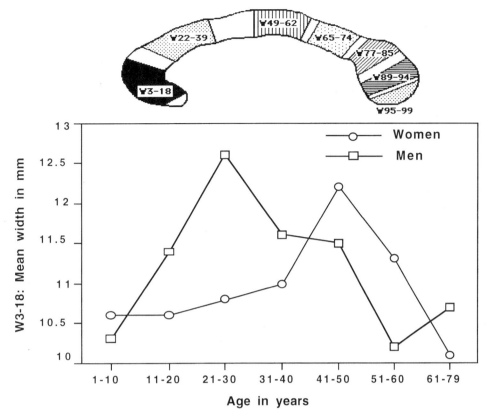

Figure 19.4. CC width (in millimeters) of regional factor W3-18 (filled with black, above) for men and women ($N = 146$) is plotted as a function of age group (divided into approximate 10-year age groups, below). Note that this anteriormost CC region is at its maximum width in men during the third decade of life, but in women this region is at maximum width during the fifth decade of life. (This figure has been adapted from Cowell et al., 1992, with permission from Elsevier Science Publishers.)

right-handed women, size of the isthmus region in the CC was related to degree of consistency (the isthmus is roughly equivalent to our W77–85). Thus, men who always performed manual activities with the right hand (consistent right-handers, CRH) had smaller CCs in this region than men who performed some manual activities with the left or both hands (nonconsistent right-handers, NCRH). This finding was replicated across several independent laboratories (Witelson, 1989; Denenberg et al., 1991b; Habib et al., 1991) and has been associated with parallel effects in outlying regions of the cerebral cortex (Witelson and Kigar, 1992).

Therefore, if not carefully controlled, variability associated with hand preference may also contribute to unreliable findings in the study of the CC in schizophrenia. The effects of hand preference may influence comparisons of patients and controls by affecting CC size in either, or possibly both, groups. However, these variables could be incorporated into a research design that subclassified patients and controls by sex and degree of right-hand consistency. Such a design would serve as the basis for investigating patterns of variability in the

CC anatomy of patients using an approach that has yielded stable and neurocognitively relevant results in controls.

Piloting methods for the effective investigation of corpus callosum anatomy in schizophrenia

In the preceding section, two stable characteristics of CC anatomy in normative samples were discussed. The first was the factor structure of the human CC, and the second was the relationship between degree of right-hand consistency and regional CC size found in men but not women. It is the aim of this section to investigate the feasibility of using these two stable characteristics as the basis for designing neuroanatomical probes for the study of the CC in schizophrenia.

We conducted some exploratory pilot analyses with a sample of right-handed patients with DSM-III diagnoses of schizophrenia (H. Nasrallah's data). This sample of patient data was large enough for a factor analysis and comprised subjects with sufficient variation in degree of right-hand preference. A sample of control subjects

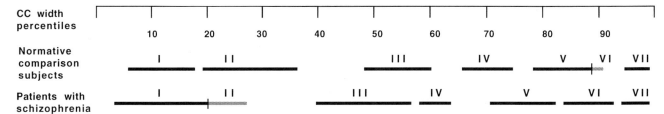

FIGURE 19.5. Comparison of the factor structures for a sample of normative comparison subjects and a sample of patients with schizophrenia. The first factor structure (top) was from a previous study (Cowell et al., 1994) and contained healthy right-handed men and women ($N = 51$). The second factor structure (bottom) contained right-handed men and women with schizophrenia ($N = 66$). (The gray-toned and vertical bars are used to visually separate two adjacent factors.) (This figure has been adapted from Cowell et al., 1994, with permission from Academic Press.)

was available with this particular patient sample. However, having originally been collected for research analyses other than the ones we wanted to perform, the sample was not large enough for a separate factor analysis, nor did it contain a sufficient number of nonconsistent right-handers. Therefore, we opted to demonstrate how factor structure and right-hand consistency comparisons might be used to study the CC in schizophrenia, by comparing the results from Nasrallah's patients to those from a well-characterized normative sample of right-handed men and women from another laboratory (A. Kertesz's data). These subjects were studied as part of several previous investigations of CC anatomy (Kertesz et al., 1987; Denenberg et al., 1991b; Cowell et al., 1993, 1994). Because the samples of subjects were from two different research sites, we emphasize to the reader that the methodological approach is being promoted in this chapter rather than the specific findings per se.

In the first stage of our pilot study, we performed a factor analysis with the CC measurements of 66 right-handed patients with schizophrenia using methods summarized above (Denenberg et al., 1991b). The factor analysis for the normative comparison group was originally part of a larger study of factor structure stability published by Cowell and colleagues (1994).[4] The results of these two analyses are depicted in graphic form in Figure 19.5.

The purpose of our comparative factor analysis is to reveal both similarities and differences in factor struc-

ture that may point to commonalities and disparities in the organization of CC structure across the various subject groups studied. In the current comparison the same number of width factors emerged in both patients and controls. Some differences were found in the extreme anterior and posterior CC, including an anterior shift in factors V and VI. However, the most prominent differences between the two factor structures appeared in the midbody of the CC. In patients there appeared to be a marked anterior shift of factors occurring in the callosal body. This shift was the result of two specific differences in the factor structure of patients compared to controls. The first difference was a shortening of factor II to approximately half the size of that seen in the normative comparison group. The second difference was an anterior shift of factors III and IV in patients to fill a space that was "factorless" in the normative sample.[5]

It is possible that a shift or displacement of CC factors such as that seen in our exploratory comparison of patients with schizophrenia may indicate actual anatomical shifts in patterns of interhemispheric connections. In a study of cerebral blood flow, Gur and colleagues (1994) showed that appropriately lateralized task-activated changes in patients with schizophrenia occurred in brain regions anterior and posterior to those seen in controls.

---

[4]Before factor analysis the CC data for the patient and comparison groups were standardized to z-scores as a function of sex and right-hand consistency classification and then pooled to control for mean differences that were shown to affect the factor structure (Cowell et al., 1994). Of the 66 right-handed patients, one man who had incomplete hand preference questionnaire data was included as a NCRH for the standardization procedure. This subject was later excluded for the portion of the pilot study that specifically examined mean differences in regional CC size.

---

[5]Another aspect of the factor structure that may be used to learn more about neuroanatomical organization in schizophrenia is the relationship between the regional widths and the more global parameters such as length, perimeter, and CC area. In the normative samples studied, perimeter and length were associated with the posteriormost regional width (W95–99), and CC area was not uniquely associated with any CC factor. This was probably because this areal measure of overall CC size was correlated with every region but not distinctly more so with one width factor over another. However, in the patient group, CC area loaded on a factor with W94–99, perimeter, and length. In this fashion, factor analysis may be used to elucidate relationships among regional and global CC parameters, particularly those that may be disrupted in patients with schizophrenia.

TABLE 19.1
Means for regional CC factor widths of patients with schizophrenia and normative comparison subjects subclassified by sex and right-hand consistency

Groups	Consistency	W65-74		W77-85	
		Women	Men	Women	Men
Normative comparison	CRH W: $N = 12$ M: $N = 11$	6.267 [0.372]	6.590 [0.388]	10.303 [0.451]	10.07 [0.471]
	NCRH W: $N = 15$ M: $N = 14$	6.505 [0.333]	7.838 [0.344]	10.341 [0.404]	12.106 [0.418]
Patients	CRH W: $N = 17$ M: $N = 33$	5.784 [0.312]	6.418 [0.224]	10.133 [0.379]	10.109 [0.272]
	NCRH W: $N = 5$ M: $N = 10$	5.935 [0.576]	6.395 [0.407]	10.284 [0.699]	9.315 [0.494]

W = women; M = men; CRH = consistent right-handers; NCRH = nonconsistent right-handers. Standard errors are in brackets.

Normative data are reprinted from Cowell et al. (1993) with permission from Lippincott-Raven Publishers.

Such shifts in cortical activity may be functional correlates of the anatomical shifts demonstrated in the CC factor structure of patients.

Principal components analysis of CC subareas and their cellular components has been used with a combined sample of patients and controls to delineate regional subgroupings for further anatomical analyses (Highley et al., 1999). However, the results of our analyses above suggest that the factor structure itself may be affected in schizophrenia. Thus, comparative factor analysis could be used, in conjunction with functional brain imaging studies, to investigate cortical reorganization related to neurodevelopmental precursors to this neuropsychiatric disorder.

Our second pilot analysis promotes the use of Witelson's (1989) classification of subjects into groups by sex and right-hand consistency as a way to investigate, in schizophrenia, a characteristic of CC anatomy that has been found to be relatively stable across independent normative samples. The data used in this portion of the pilot study were from the same samples of patients and normative subjects that were used in the above factor analyses.[6] Mean widths and standard errors of our W65–74 and W77–85 are listed in Table 19.1. These two CC width factors overlap most closely with Witelson's (1989) anatomically defined regions of the posterior body and isthmus and were also shown to be most sensitive to the interactive effects of sex and right-hand consistency in our previous study (Denenberg et al., 1991b).

When one examines the pattern of means within the normative sample, it is apparent that for both W65–74 and W77–85 the measurements are very similar for CRH women, NCRH women, and CRH men. However, there is a notable deviation in the mean size of these CC widths in NCRH men that accounted for the significant sex × right-hand consistency effects in our previous reports (Denenberg et al., 1991b; Cowell et al., 1993). Within the patient sample, however, there does not seem to be any evidence for a larger regional CC width in NCRH men. Taken together, the patterns of means in our normative and patient samples demonstrate how having an increased number of NCRH men in a given study's control group could potentially bias the results of that study toward a finding of smaller regional CC size in patients.

We recommend that readers interpret the preliminary findings of these exploratory comparisons with caution. However, should these findings hold up to the rigors of future replication, they could have implications for understanding cortical disorganization and the development of interhemispheric connections in schizophrenia. For example, Witelson and Kigar (1992) showed that the larger CC isthmus that is seen in NCRH men corresponded with a more symmetrical Sylvian fissure com-

[6] Note that there are 52 right-handed controls, compared to the 51 used in the factor analysis. Deletion of this subject from the factor analysis is described by Denenberg and colleagues (1991b). Also note that one male patient has been deleted from the handedness analysis owing to lack of complete hand preference data.

pared to CRH men. A similar effect was documented with respect to the planum temporale (Aboitiz et al., 1992). Given that some researchers have found reductions or absence of the normative left-greater-than-right asymmetry pattern in the Sylvian fissure and temporal lobe structures of patients (Falkai et al., 1992; Hoff et al., 1992; Rossi et al., 1992; Petty et al., 1995), one might expect a larger CC isthmus in schizophrenia. However, the basis for anatomical laterality in regions of temporal cortex that project fibers through the CC isthmus appears to differ between patients and controls. In studies using normative subjects, symmetry of the planum temporale was due to a larger right side (Galaburda et al., 1987; Habib, 1989), whereas in patients with schizophrenia, symmetry of the planum was due, at least in part, to decreased left temporal lobe size (Young et al., 1991; Breier et al., 1992; Falkai et al., 1992; Rossi et al., 1992; Shenton et al., 1992; Turetsky et al., 1995).[7] A recent meta-analysis showed that lack of planum asymmetry in patients was due to a combined effect of non-significant decreases in left planum size together with significant increases in right planum size compared to controls (Shapleske et al., 1999). This finding suggests a more complex and multidimensional neurodevelopmental etiology for disruptions in cortical laterality and interhemispheric connections in schizophrenia than was perhaps originally suspected.

Conclusions

The research described in this chapter suggests that the study of the CC in schizophrenia can be informed by the study of normative variation in this structure's size and shape. Our pilot investigations emphasize the importance of going beyond the study of simple patient–control group comparisons in anatomical size in trying to unravel the complexities of schizophrenia. Although independent, large-scale studies of the CC in patients with schizophrenia will be needed to provide support for the reliability and generalizability of our preliminary findings, we propose that by using neurobehavioral probes that have established stability in normative samples, researchers may increase the likelihood of cross-study consistency when investigating the CC in schizophrenia patients. Only by adopting methodological and analytical approaches that harness the CC's sensitivity can one use the study of this structure to shed light on the demographic, behavioral, and clinical factors that

shape the neurocognitive development and expression of schizophrenia.

REFERENCES

ABOITIZ, F., A. SCHEIBEL, and E. ZAIDEL, 1992. Morphometry of the sylvian fissure and the corpus callosum, with emphasis on sex differences. *Brain* 15:1521–1541.

ARNOLD, S. E., B. T. HYMAN, G. W. VAN HOESEN, and A. R. D'AMASIO, 1991. Some cytoarchitectural abnormalities of the entorhinal cortex in schizophrenia. *Arch. Gen. Psychiatry* 48:625–632.

BARTA, P. E., G. D. PEARLSON, R. E. POWERS, S. S. RICHARDS, and L. E. TUNE, 1990. Auditory hallucinations and smaller superior temporal gyral volume in schizophrenia. *Am. J. Psychiatry* 147:1457–1462.

BILDER, R. M., H. WU, B. BOGERTS, G. DEGREEF, M. ASHTARI, J. M. J. ALVIR, P. J. SNYDER, and J. A. LIEBERMAN, 1994. Absence of regional hemispheric volume asymmetries in first-episode schizophrenia. *Am. J. Psychiatry* 151:1437–1447.

BISHOP, K. M., and D. WAHLSTEN, 1997. Sex differences in the corpus callosum: Myth or reality? *Neurosci. Biobehav. Rev.* 21:581–601.

BOOKSTEIN, F. L., 1996/7. Landmark methods for forms without landmarks: Morphometrics of group differences in outline shape. *Med. Image Anal.* 1:225–243.

BREIER, A., R. W. BUCHANAN, A. ELKASHEF, R. C. MUNSON, B. KIRKPATRICK, and F. GELLAD, 1992. Brain morphology and schizophrenia: A magnetic resonance imaging study of limbic, prefrontal cortex, and caudate structures. *Arch. Gen. Psychiatry* 49:921–926.

CANNON, T. D., L. EYLER ZORILLA, D. L. SHTASEL, R. E. GUR, R. C. GUR, E. J. MARCO, P. MOBERG, and R. A. PRICE, 1994. Neuropsychological functioning in siblings discordant for schizophrenia and healthy volunteers. *Arch. Gen. Psychiatry* 51:651–661.

CASANOVA, M., R. SANDERS, T. GOLDBERG, L. BIGELOW, G. CHRISTISON, E. F. TORREY, and D. WEINBERGER, 1990b. Morphometry of the corpus callosum in monozygotic twins discordant for schizophrenia: A magnetic resonance imaging study. *J. Neurol. Neurosurg. Psychiatry* 53:416–421.

CASANOVA, M., M. ZITO, T. GOLDBERG, R. SUDDATH, E. F. TORREY, L. BIGELOW, R. SANDERS, and D. WEINBERGER, 1990a. Corpus callosum curvature in schizophrenic twins. *Biol. Psychiatry* 27:83–84.

COGER, R., and E. SERAFETINIDES, 1990. Schizophrenia, corpus callosum and inter-hemispheric communication: A review. *Psychiatry Res.* 34:163–184.

COLOMBO, C., A. BONFANTI, S. LIVIAN, M. ABBRUZZESE, and S. SCARONE, 1993. Size of the corpus callosum and auditory comprehension in schizophrenics and normal controls. *Schizophr. Res.* 11:63–70.

COWELL, P. E., L. S. ALLEN, A. KERTESZ, N. S. ZALATIMO, and V. H. DENENBERG, 1994. Human corpus callosum: A stable mathematical model of regional neuroanatomy. *Brain Cogn.* 25:52–66.

COWELL, P. E., L. S. ALLEN, N. S. ZALATIMO, and V. H. DENENBERG, 1992. A developmental study of sex and age interactions in the human corpus callosum. *Dev. Brain Res.* 66:187–192.

COWELL, P. E., R. H. FITCH, and V. H. DENENBERG, 1999.

---

[7] A similar explanation has been put forth by Galaburda (1993) to account for anomalous patterns of cerebral laterality observed in dyslexia, a language-related reading disorder with a neurodevelopmental basis.

Laterality in animals: Relevance to schizophrenia. *Schizophr. Bull.* 25:41–62.

COWELL, P. E., A. KERTESZ, and V. H. DENENBERG, 1993. Multiple dimensions of handedness and the human corpus callosum. *Neurology* 43:2353–2357.

DAVID, A. S., 1994. Schizophrenia and the corpus callosum: Developmental, structural and functional relationships. *Behav. Brain Res.* 64:203–211.

DELISI, L. E., M. SAKUMA, W. TEW, M. KUSHNER, A. L. HOFF, and R. GRIMSON, 1997. Schizophrenia as a chronic active brain process: A study of progressive brain structural change subsequent to the onset of schizophrenia. *Psychiatry Res. Neuroimaging Section* 74:129–140.

DENENBERG, V. H., P. E. COWELL, R. H. FITCH, A. KERTESZ, and G. H. KENNER, 1991a. Corpus callosum: Multiple parameter measurements in rodents and humans. *Physiol. Behav.* 49:433–437.

DENENBERG, V. H., A. KERTESZ, and P. E. COWELL, 1991b. A factor analysis of the human's corpus callosum. *Brain Res.* 548:126–132.

FALKAI, P., B. BOGERTS, B. GREVE, U. PFEIFFER, B. MACHUS, B. FOLSCH-REETZ, C. MAJTENYI, and I. OVARY, 1992. Loss of sylvian fissure asymmetry in schizophrenia. A quantitative post mortem study. *Schizophr. Res.* 7:23–32.

FITCH, R. H., A. S. BERREBI, P. E. COWELL, L. M. SCHROTT, and V. H. DENENBERG, 1990. Corpus callosum: Effects of neonatal hormones on sexual dimorphism in the rat. *Brain Res.* 515:111–116.

FITCH, R. H., P. E. COWELL, L. M. SCHROTT, and V. H. DENENBERG, 1991. Corpus callosum: Ovarian hormones and feminization. *Brain Res.* 542:313–317.

GALABURDA, A., 1993. Neurology of developmental dyslexia. *Curr. Opin. Neurobiol.* 3:237–242.

GALABURDA, A., J. CORSIGLIA, G. ROSEN, and G. SHERMAN, 1987. Planum temporale asymmetry: Reappraisal since Geschwind and Levitsky. *Neuropsychologia* 25:853–868.

GREEN, M. F., K. HUGDAHL, and S. MITCHELL, 1994. Dichotic listening during auditory hallucinations in patients with schizophrenia. *Am. J. Psychiatry* 151:357–362.

GUR, R. E., J. JAGGI, D. SHTASEL, J. D. RAGLAND, and R. C. GUR, 1994. Cerebral blood flow in schizophrenia: Effects of memory processing on regional activation. *Biol. Psychiatry* 35:3–15.

HABIB, M., 1989. Anatomical asymmetries of the human cerebral cortex. *Int. J. Neurosci.* 47:67–79.

HABIB, M., D. GAYRAUD, A. OLIVA, J. REGIS, G. SALAMON, and R. KHALIL, 1991. Effects of handedness and sex on the morphology of the corpus callosum: A study with brain magnetic resonance imaging. *Brain Cogn.* 16:41–61.

HARPER MOZLEY, L., R. C. GUR, R. E. GUR, P. D. MOZLEY, and A. ALAVI, 1996. Relationships between verbal memory performance and the cerebral distribution of fluorodeoxyglucose in patients with schizophrenia. *Biol. Psychiatry* 40: 443–451.

HAUSER, P., D. DAUPHINAIS, W. BERRETTINI, L. DELISI, J. GELERNTER, and R. POST, 1989. Corpus callosum dimensions measured by magnetic resonance imaging in bipolar affective disorder and schizophrenia. *Biol. Psychiatry* 26:659–668.

HIGHLEY, J. R., M. M. ESIRI, B. MCDONALD, M. CORTINA-BORJA, B. M. HERRON, and T. J. CROW, 1999. The size and fibre composition of the corpus callosum with respect to gender and schizophrenia: A post-mortem study. *Brain* 122:99–110.

HOFF, A. L., C. NEAL, M. KUSHNER, and L. E. DELISI, 1994. Gender differences in corpus callosum size in first-episode schizophrenics. *Biol. Psychiatry* 35:913–919.

HOFF, A. L., H. RIORDAN, D. O'DONNELL, P. STRITZKE, C. NEALE, A. BOCCIO, A. K. ANAND, and L. E. DELISI, 1992. Anomalous lateral sulcus asymmetry and cognitive function in first-episode schizophrenia. *Schizophr. Bull.* 18:257–270.

JÄNCKE, L., J. F. STAIGER, G. SCHLAUG, Y. HUANG, and H. STEINMETZ, 1997. The relationship between corpus callosum size and forebrain volume. *Cereb. Cortex* 7:48–56.

KERTESZ, A., M. POLK, J. HOWELL, and S. BLACK, 1987. Cerebral dominance, sex and callosal size in MRI. *Neurology* 37:1385–1388.

LIPSKA, B. K., G. E. JASKIW, and D. R. WEINBERGER, 1993. Postpubertal emergence of hyperresponsiveness to stress and to amphetamine after neonatal excitotoxic hippocampal damage: A potential animal model of schizophrenia. *Neuropsychopharmacology* 9:67–75.

MATHEW, R. J., C. L. PARTAIN, R. PRAKASH, M. V. KULKARNI, T. P. LOGAN, and W. H. WILSON, 1985. A study of the septum pellucidum and corpus callosum in schizophrenia with MR imaging. *Acta Psychiatr. Scand.* 72:414–421.

NASRALLAH, H., N. ANDREASEN, J. COFFMAN, S. OLSON, V. DUNN, J. EHRHARDT, and S. CHAPMAN, 1986. A controlled magnetic resonance imaging study of corpus callosum thickness in schizophrenia. *Biol. Psychiatry* 21:274–282.

PANDYA, D., and B. SELTZER, 1986. The topography of commissural fibers. In *Two Hemispheres—One Brain: Functions of the Corpus Callosum*, F. Lepore, M. Ptito, and H. Jasper, eds. New York: Alan Liss, pp. 47–73.

PETTY, R. G., P. E. BARTA, G. D. PEARLSON, I. K. MCGILCHRIST, R. W. LEWIS, A. Y. TIEN, A. PULVER, D. D. VAUGHN, M. F. CASANOVA, and R. E. POWERS, 1995. Reversal of asymmetry of the planum temporale in schizophrenia. *Am. J. Psychiatry* 152:715–721.

RAINE, A., G. HARRISON, G. REYNOLDS, C. SHEARD, J. COOPER, and I. MEDLEY, 1990. Structural and functional characteristics of the corpus callosum in schizophrenics, psychiatric controls, and normal controls. *Arch. Gen. Psychiatry* 47:1060–1064.

ROSSI, A., P. STRATTA, M. GALLUCCI, R. PASSARIELLO, and M. CASACCHIA, 1989. Quantification of corpus callosum and ventricles in schizophrenia with nuclear magnetic resonance imaging: A pilot study. *Am. J. Psychiatry* 146:99–101.

ROSSI, A., P. STRATTA, P. MATTEI, M. CUPILLARI, A. BOZZAO, M. GALLUCCI, and M. CASACCHIA, 1992. Planum temporale in schizophrenia: A magnetic resonance study. *Schizophr. Res.* 7:19–22.

SAYKIN, A. J., R. C. GUR, R. E. GUR, P. D. MOZLEY, L. H. MOZLEY, S. M. RESNICK, D. B. KESTER, and P. STAFINIAK, 1991. Neuropsychological function in schizophrenia: Selective impairment in memory and learning. *Arch. Gen. Psychiatry* 48:618–624.

SHAPLESKE, J., S. L. ROSSELL, P. W. R. WOODRUFF, and A. S. DAVID, 1999. The planum temporale: A systematic, quantitative review of its structural, functional and clinical significance. *Brain Res. Rev.* 29:26–49.

SHENTON, M. E., R. KIKINIS, F. A. JOLESZ, S. D. POLLAK, M. LEMAY, C. G. WIBLE, H. HOKAMA, J. MARTIN, D. METCALF, M. COLEMAN, R. W. MCCARLEY, 1992. Abnormalities of the left temporal lobe and thought disorder in schizophrenia. *N. Engl. J. Med.* 327:604–612.

Takeuchi, K., 1992. Studies of the correlations between morphological brain changes on MRI and computerized EEG changes in schizophrenics. *Seishin Shinkeigaku Zasshi Psychiatria et Neurologia Japonica* 94:584–604. [English abstract cited]

Tibbo, P., P. Nopoulos, S. Arndt, and N. C. Andreasen, 1998. Corpus callosum shape and size in male patients with schizophrenia. *Biol. Psychiatry* 44:405–412.

Turetsky, B. I., P. E. Cowell, R. C. Gur, R. I. Grossman, D. L. Shtasel, and R. E. Gur, 1995. Frontal and temporal lobe brain volume in schizophrenia: Relationship to symptoms and clinical subtype. *Arch. Gen. Psychiatry* 52: 1061–1070.

Witelson, S., 1989. Hand and sex differences in the isthmus and genu of the human corpus callosum. *Brain* 112:799–835.

Witelson, S. F., and D. L. Kigar, 1992. Sylvian fissure morphology and asymmetry in men and women: Bilateral differences in relation to handedness in men. *J. Comp. Neurol.* 323:326–340.

Woodruff, P. W. R., I. C. McManus, and A. S. David, 1995. Meta-analysis of corpus callosum size in schizophrenia. *J. Neurol. Neurosurg. Psychiatry* 58:457–461.

Woodruff, P., G. Pearlson, M. Geer, P. Barta, and H. Chilcoat, 1993. A computerized magnetic resonance imaging study of corpus callosum morphology in schizophrenia. *Psychol. Med.* 23:45–56.

Woodruff, P. W. R., M. L. Phillips, T. Rushe, I. C. Wright, R. M. Murray, and A. S. David, 1997. Corpus callosum size and inter-hemispheric function in schizophrenia. *Schizophr. Res.* 23:189–196.

Young, A. H., D. H. R. Blackwood, H. Roxborough, J. K. McQueen, M. J. Martin, and D. Kean, 1991. A magnetic resonance imaging study of schizophrenia: Brain structure and clinical symptoms. *Br. J. Psychiatry* 158:158–164.

20 Interhemispheric Abnormalities in Schizophrenia and Their Possible Etiology

ROBERT W. DOTY

ABSTRACT The extreme diversity of symptoms in this illness presents a severe challenge to identifying its etiology. Eleven characteristics are briefly listed that form the core of what must be explained. Data drawn from a variety of sources suggest that a viral or other agent, entering the CNS via the olfactory epithelium either in utero or in later life, would be transported retrogradely into the serotonergic raphe of the mesencephalon. If in utero, perturbation of the serotonergic system would account for many of the reported anatomical abnormalities associated with schizophrenia and, given the extraordinary bilaterality of the system, could also underlie the common disturbances in laterality of hemispheric functions that form such a prominent feature of schizophrenia. In addition, this concept is consonant with the newly discovered efficacy of therapeutic agents influencing serotonergic function that are now revising its pharmacological treatment.

Schizophrenia is a protean illness, devastating lives throughout the world with intractable and often bizarre delusions, continual assault from hallucinated voices, anhedonia, incoherent thought, and/or poverty of action ranging into catatonia. An excellent overview of the disease and its complexities is provided by Crow and Johnstone (1987). Further cogent details can be found in the work of Flack, Miller, and Wiener (1991), Straube and Oades (1992), and Andreasen (1997), for example, and in the prelude to this chapter, Doty (1989). In the interest of brevity, references in this chapter have been selected primarily to provide leads to the literature.

What needs to be explained

The following 11 characteristics of schizophrenia need to be explained:

ROBERT W. DOTY Department of Neurobiology and Anatomy, University of Rochester School of Medicine and Dentistry, Rochester, New York.

1. Through the use of neuroimaging, it has become apparent that almost any form of intellectual activity engages both cerebral hemispheres and forms complex patterns of interhemispheric activation. For schizophrenic subjects such bihemispheric patterns are decidedly abnormal (Andreasen, 1997; Woodruff et al., 1997b). Crow (1997) interprets this abnormality as being a diminution of the strong hemispheric dominance associated with human phylogeny and the acquisition of speech; and, indeed, a number of studies do show a lessened asymmetry in schizophrenic patients. There is evidence of reduced callosal size and fiber density (e.g., Hoff et al., 1994; Woodruff et al., 1997a; Highley et al., 1999) and a long and diverse list of other abnormal hemispheric asymmetries in cerebral size, function, or chemistry without any clear disturbance of handedness (e.g., Nasrallah, 1986; Bracha, 1987; Delisi et al., 1997; Zaidel, Esiri, and Harrison, 1997; Tiihonen et al., 1998; Wiser et al., 1998; Gruzelier, 1999; Petty, 1999).

2. Although varying considerably in incidence with time and locale, the disorders called schizophrenia afflict about 1% of the population worldwide at one or another time in their life (Crow, 1997).

3. The symptoms are extremely heterogeneous and idiosyncratic (Dollfus et al., 1996), to the point at which many now consider that schizophrenia merges without clear boundaries with depression and bipolar disorder (Crow, 1997; Maier et al., 1993).

4. There are definitive signs, such as ventriculomegaly (Marks and Luchins, 1990), temporal lobe abnormalities (e.g., Shenton, 1996), or cerebellar (Chua and McKenna, 1995; Jacobsen et al., 1997) abnormalities, that indicate a prenatal or perinatal insult in the majority, but by no means all, of the cases.

5. In light of the preceding characteristic, it is deeply puzzling as to what transpires in the interim between

damage that is present at birth and the initiation of florid postpubertal symptoms. True, there are many effects that are noticeable during childhood (Walker, Lewine, and Neumann, 1996) that adumbrate the definitive illness, but the correlation is primarily ex post facto, and there remains the added challenge of explaining a delay into later decades of life (Basso et al., 1997; Castle et al., 1997).

6. Also, given characteristics 4 and 5, it is equally mysterious as to why and how remission occurs in roughly 30% of the cases, admittedly to varying degrees but ranging into essentially full normality (Bleuler, 1978; Fenton and McGlashan, 1987; Ram et al., 1992). The recently discovered ability of the hippocampus to generate new neuronal and glial elements in adult primates (Eriksson et al., 1998; Kornack and Rakic, 1999) will certainly be examined in this regard.

7. There is clearly a factor of heredity, both in familial risk of the disorder and in detectable signs in near relatives. However, there are also a great many instances in which such connection is lacking, as in monozygotic twins who are entirely discrepant for the illness (Torrey et al., 1994).

8. Accompanying disorders of movement (preceding or unassociated with drug therapy) are common (Manschrek, 1986), such as high frequency of blinking (Karson, Dykman, and Paige, 1990) or, particularly noteworthy, disruption of ocular pursuit (Levy et al., 1993; Friedman et al., 1995; Crawford et al., 1998).

9. Some of the symptoms of schizophrenia are so closely imitated by psychotomimetic drugs (Rosse et al., 1994) or temporal lobe epilepsy (Trimble, 1991) as to be cursorily indistinguishable from the disease itself.

10. In many cases very significant symptomatic relief is obtained by agents that block dopamine D2 receptors, now recently augmented by additional blockade of serotonergic 5-HT2 receptors (e.g., Lieberman et al., 1998; Kapur, Zipursky, and Remington, 1999).

11. To the many intellectual and psychophysiological peculiarities of the disorder must be added the stubborn inability of many patients to recognize that they are actually abnormal, that is, an unawareness of illness (Young, Davila, and Scher, 1993; Amador et al., 1994; Cuesta and Peralta, 1994).

Explanation, level 1: Etiology

It is hypothesized herewith that the primary, initial insult that eventually leads to schizophrenic illness is the entry of a virus or another agent into the central nervous system via the olfactory nerves. Transported into the olfactory bulb, the agent is there available for uptake and retrograde transport into neuronal groups, particu-

larly the serotonergic raphe or cholinergic systems of the diagonal band that centrifugally innervate the bulb (see Shipley, 1985; Halász, 1990). These systems, in turn, are then compromised in their function and furthermore allow diffusion of the agent into adjacent neurons in these pools. Since both of these systems project widely and profusely, their perturbation can ramify accordingly into essentially any system of the brain.

Depending on the precise timing of this putative invasion in fetal life, one or another neuronal system may or may not be affected by this process, either by direct damage to invaded neurons or from indirect consequence of such perturbation. Thus, the great diversity and subtlety of anatomical effects, in ventriculomegaly or histological abnormalities in the medial temporal lobe or cerebellum, can be explained by the vagaries of the initial spread and subsequent disruption of functioning of the serotonergic or cholinergic systems. There is, of course, no a priori reason to exclude the possibility that the olfactory system might also be capable of transporting the responsible agent or agents in later life similarly to produce schizophrenic illness. If so, however, some distinguishing characteristic of this later origin should be expected, such as absence of gross morphological changes or a different pattern of symptoms, given the great changes in the neuronal milieu consequent to development.

Because of its bilaterality and its effect on neuronal development, the serotonergic system is of unique interest here. Neurons on either side of the raphe may project to either side of the brain. The contralateral projection ranges from 10–20% for hippocampus (Amaral and Cowan, 1980) to 10–30% for neocortex (Doty, 1983; Wilson and Molliver, 1991) in macaques; and the major input to the raphe comes from the habenulo-interpeduncular system, perhaps the most diverse system of the vertebrate brain in regard to laterality (e.g., Lenn and Whitmore, 1989). The perturbed cerebral asymmetry so commonly observed in schizophrenia (characteristic 1 above) could have its origin here. Equally relevant, it is apparent that serotonergic innervation has important trophic influence on neuronal survival and organization during development (e.g., Sikich, Hickok, and Todd, 1990; Chubakov, Tsyganova, and Sarkisova, 1993; Lauder, 1993; Lebrand et al., 1996; Lavdas et al., 1997; Levitt et al., 1997; Mansour-Robaey et al., 1998; Rhoades et al., 1998; Brezun and Daszuta, 1999). A remnant of this disturbance of the serotonergic system may be reflected in the abnormal survival of 5-HT_{1a} receptors in the cerebellum of schizophrenic subjects (Slater, Doyle, and Deakin, 1998) as well as in autism (Chugani et al., 1999).

It is worth emphasizing that a viral infection in utero, via the olfactory route proposed, would likely leave no immunological or histological (glial) trace, thus being consonant with findings in the great majority of searches along these lines on schizophrenic patients (but see Stevens (1982), who found such occasional traces, possibly reflecting adult acquisition, as noted above). Of course, the possibility exists of a lingering infection, as in the case of herpes simplex or shingles, but to date rather extensive explorations along these lines have been essentially negative (Taller et al., 1996). Although still controversial (Wyatt, Apud, and Potkin, 1996), there have been several analyses strongly suggesting an association of subsequent schizophrenia with influenza sustained by the mother in the second trimester (e.g., Menninger, 1926/1994; Mednick, Huttunen, and Machon, 1994; O'Callaghan et al., 1994).

Were the olfactory system to serve as a portal for entry of a schizophrenogenic virus, the perspective on underlying genetic factors in the disease would be grossly altered. The question would be not what genetic defect produced alterations in the brain, but what characteristics of the olfactory epithelium predisposed to viral entry. Since the olfactory system is governed by a huge number of genes, perhaps as many as 1000 (Buck, 1996), an enormous selectivity is possible (see Johnson, 1980; Stroop and Baringer, 1989; Barnett, Cassell, and Perlman, 1993).

The paradigmatic demonstration of the credibility of the foregoing thesis is given by Mohammed and colleagues (1992). After infusing a droplet of vesicular stomatitis virus, an RNA viral relative of rabies, into the nostrils of 12-day-old rat pups, they analyzed the behavior and brains of the adult (18-month-old) animals. The treated animals swam normally but were subnormal in solving the Morris water maze. It was found that two thirds of the neurons in the dorsal and median raphe had degenerated and that serotonin levels in neocortex and hippocampus were drastically reduced. No other histopathological changes were found, perhaps not unexpectedly, since the olfactory introduction of the virus occurred well after formation of most of the central nervous system, and the characteristics of this virus may provide only limited analogy to the putative schizophrenogenic agent.

Explanation, level 2: Symptoms

The vagaries of timing and penetration and the genetic variation in virus and host(s) (there being two for the in utero case plus medications of the mother) are, as was noted above, clearly capable of producing a vast range of effects throughout the nervous system. The predilection of cerebellum, hippocampal system, and prefrontal cortex to such disruption, probably reflected in ven-

triculomegaly, can all be loosely attributed to disruption of the developmental influence of the serotonergic raphe. A tentative suggestion of the olfactory entrance can perhaps be seen in the poor olfactory discrimination of schizophrenic subjects (Wu et al., 1993; Malaspina et al., 1994; Kopala et al., 1995; Brewer et al., 1996; Moberg et al., 1997; Stedman and Clair, 1998). One would like to see better control for the presence of the heavy smoking, which is common in schizophrenia, and testing of each nostril separately, since a remarkable separation of the airway allows probing of individual hemispheres; and there is normally a strong right-hemispheric superiority for olfactory discrimination (Yousem et al., 1997; Dade et al., 1998).

Most critical is the issue of disturbed interhemispheric relations, a pervasive feature of schizophrenia whenever examined, be it with neurochemistry (Arato et al., 1991), anatomy (Shenton, 1996; Delisi et al., 1997; Petty, 1999), electrophysiology (Tiihonen, et al., 1998; Gruzelier, 1999), neuroimaging (Catafau et al., 1994; Buckley, 1998), dichotic listening (Green, Hugdahl, and Mitchell, 1994), or psychometric testing (Gruzelier, 1999). Were the raphe indeed to be the underlying focus of the initial pathogenic effect, the unusual bilaterality of its projections provides ample means of influencing interhemispheric symmetry, both ab initio and in the subsequent psychotic state. The fact that the hemispheres work in conjunction with brain stem systems is often overlooked. Hemispheric interaction occurs not only via the forebrain commissures, but also via a multifarious loop (Doty, 1989, 1995) that intimately involves brain stem systems in reciprocal interchange with the cortex. In other words, while the corpus callosum achieves massive hemispheric coupling, it does so in a neuronal setting in which each hemisphere is receiving and returning input from and to the modulatory systems of raphe and nucleus basalis.

If the psychopathology of schizophrenia owes much to the disruption of hemispheric interchange, the question arises as to whether the experienced hallucinations and delusions arise because the left hemisphere fails to recognize their origin in the right hemisphere (Nasrallah, 1986) or because an overactive left hemisphere produces disorganized thought when unchecked by the right. Since neither hallucinations nor delusions occur in split-brain patients (e.g., Sperry, 1984), some peculiarity of commissural interchange, or better, the multifarious loop, must account for the ensuing pathology. As perceptively reviewed by Cutting (1990), lesions in the right hemisphere induce a range of effects that have an astonishing parallel to many aspects of schizophrenia, including unawareness of illness (also see Bisiach et al., 1986; Geschwind et al., 1995). Again, of course, since right-hemispherectomy patients are not schizophrenic, something else is at work in addition to absent right-hemisphere tissue.

Recent endeavors to explain auditory hallucinations illustrate this problem of hemispheric origin. Cleghorn and colleagues (1992) and Woodruff and colleagues (1997b), with PET imaging, found a decrease in left-hemisphere activation and an increase on the right in hallucinating patients; and using dichotic listening, Green, Hugdahl, and Mitchell (1994) found the left hemisphere to be abnormal. On the other hand, McGuire, Shah, and Murray (1993), also with PET, found an increase in the left prefrontal cortex (Broca's area), and Silbersweig and colleagues (1995) report a number of sites from which it is difficult to discern much in relation to asymmetry and hallucinations. The majority of the data would thus seem to favor a right-hemispheric origin for the hallucinated material, but only at a gross conceptual level.

The contrary evidence seems equally strong. Dierks and colleagues (1999) show an increased activation of Heschl's gyrus closely correlated with time when hallucinations are occurring. Furthermore, the left hemisphere alone can produce hallucinations if it is cut off from the right by callosal agenesis (Swayze et al., 1990). The permissive condition for hallucinations may thus be a left hemisphere freed of the constraint of right-hemispheric confirmation. An example of such an effect occurs in an entirely different context. Negrão and I (see Doty, 1970) were able to produce a convincing hallucination in macaques by electrical stimulation of peristriate cortex. In analogy to that reported by a similarly stimulated human patient, we called it a "hallucinated butterfly." The animal at first slowly tracked a non-existent object downward with its eyes, then made a sudden catching, grasping movement and, intently peering at its clenched fist, slowly opened it as if to see what it had caught. This phenomenon was produced in several animals, but only in those in which the corpus callosum had been cut. We inferred that in the intact animal the hallucination was countermanded by the absence of correlated activity in the other hemisphere, even though the hallucinating animal could use either ipsilateral or contralateral hand for the "capture." Never being successful at catching anything, the animals, unlike the schizophrenic patients lacking insight into their condition, soon tired of the game, precluding further study.

A consistent undercurrent in this discussion of schizophrenia is the still undefined nature and role of altered neurochemistry. The fact that chemical agents are capable of both imitating and alleviating the symptoms of schizophrenia is prima facie evidence that not every-thing is likely to be explained by structure alone. Here, too, the role of the serotonergic system seems paramount (Abi-Dargham et al., 1997). It is not just serotonin per se, however, but the type and distribution of serotonin receptors that are important. Burnet, Eastwood, and Harrison (1996), for instance, find a 23% increase in $5HT_{1a}$ receptors and a 27% decrease in $5HT_{2a}$ receptors in dorsolateral prefrontal cortex in brains of schizophrenics. Control studies in rats indicated that such changes are not attributable to the chronic administration of the haloperidol medication given to these individuals. There is now, in addition, abundant evidence for the therapeutic efficacy (Lieberman et al., 1998) of drugs affecting the serotonergic system and for its control or modulation of dopaminergic (e.g., Dewey et al., 1995; Moukhles et al., 1997; Kapur et al., 1999) and cholinergic (Morilak and Ciaranello, 1993) neurons.

Finally, it bears mention that the serotonergic raphe plays a strikingly permissive role in the rapid eye movement (REM), dreaming stage of sleep. The bizarre quality of dreams has often been likened, however crudely, to some of the mental confusions that characterize schizophrenia. It is unequivocally clear that the REM stage of sleep is under the control of ponto-mesencephalic cholinergic and serotonergic systems. A dramatic corollary of this is that neurons of the raphe fall silent during REM; local serotonin release likewise decreases drastically. Now, in cats, infusion of an agent producing such curtailment of serotonin output has been shown to precipitate the REM state (Portas et al., 1996). Is there, perhaps, some partial expression of this raphe modulation that produces the dreamlike distortion of reality that so many schizophrenic patients are unable to either recognize as such or to awaken from its compelling spell?

ACKNOWLEDGMENT   I am most grateful for the support of the Margo Cleveland Fund, which fostered my exploration of the thesis set forth herein and encouraged my continuing efforts.

REFERENCES

ABI-DARGHAM, A., M. LARUELLE, G. K. AGHAJANIAN, D. CHARNEY, and J. KRYSTAL, 1997. The role of serotonin in the pathophysiology and treatment of schizophrenia. *J. Neuropsychiatry Clin. Neurosci.* 9:1–17.

AMADOR, X. F., M. FLAUM, N. C. ANDREASEN, D. H. STRAUSS, S. A. YALE, S. C. CLARK, and J. M. GORMAN, 1994. Awareness of illness in schizophrenia and schizoaffective and mood disorders. *Arch. Gen. Psychiatry* 51:826–836.

AMARAL, D. G., and W. M. COWAN, 1980. Subcortical afferents to the hippocampal formation in the monkey. *J. Compar. Neurol.* 189:573–591.

ANDREASEN, N. C., 1997. Linking mind and brain in the study of mental illness: A project for a scientific psychopathology. *Science* 275:1587–1593.

ARATO, M., E. FRECSKA, D. J. MACCRIMMON, R. GUSCOTT, B. SAXENA, K. TEKES, and L. TOTHFALUSI, 1991. Serotonergic interhemispheric asymmetry: Neurochemical and pharmaco-EEG evidence. *Prog. Neuro-Psychopharmacol. Biol. Psychiatry* 15:759–764.

BARNETT, E. M., M. D. CASSELL, and S. PERLMAN, 1993. Two neurotropic viruses, herpes simplex virus type 1 and mouse hepatitis virus, spread along different neural pathways from the main olfactory bulb. *Neuroscience* 57:1007–1025.

BASSO, M. R., H. A. NASRALLAH, S. C. OLSON, and R. A. BORNSTEIN, 1997. Cognitive deficits distinguish patients with adolescent- and adult-onset schizophrenia. *Neuropsychiatry Neuropsychol. Behav. Neurol.* 10:107–112.

BISIACH, E., G. VALLAR, D. PERANI, C. PAPAGANO, and A. BERTI, 1986. Unawareness of disease following lesions of the right hemisphere: Anosognosia for hemiplegia and anosognosia for hemianopia. *Neuropsychologia* 24:471–482.

BLEULER, M., 1978. *The Schizophrenic Disorders: Long-Term Patient and Family Studies.* New Haven, Conn.: Yale University Press.

BRACHA, H. S., 1987. Asymmetric rotational (circling) behavior, a dopamine-related asymmetry: Preliminary findings in unmedicated and never-medicated schizophrenic patients. *Biol. Psychiatry* 22:995–1003.

BREWER, W. J., J. EDWARDS, V. ANDERSON, T. ROBINSON, and C. PANTELIS, 1996. Neuropsychological, olfactory, and hygiene deficits in men with negative symptom schizophrenia. *Biol. Psychiatry* 40:1021–1031.

BREZUN, J. M., and A. DASZUTA, 1999. Depletion in serotonin decreases neurogenesis in the dentate gyrus and the subventricular zone of adult rats. *Neuroscience* 89:999–1002.

BUCK, L. B., 1996. Information coding in the vertebrate olfactory system. *Ann. Rev. Neurosci.* 19:517–544.

BUCKLEY, P. F., 1998. Structural brain imaging in schizophrenia. *Psychiatr. Clin. North Am.* 21:77–92.

BURNET, P. W. J., S. L. EASTWOOD, and P. J. HARRISON, 1996. 5-HT1a and 5-HT2a receptor mRNAs and binding site densities are differentially altered in schizophrenia. *Neuropsychopharmacology* 15:442–455.

CASTLE, D. J., S. WESSELY, R. HOWARD, and R. M. MURRAY, 1997. Schizophrenia with onset at the extremes of adult life. *Int. J. Geriatr. Psychiatry* 12:712–717.

CATAFAU, A. M., E. PARELLADA, F. J. LOMENA, M. BERNARDO, J. PAVIA, D. ROS, J. SETOAIN, and E. GONZALEZ MONCLUS, 1994. Prefrontal and temporal blood flow in schizophrenia: Resting and activation technetium-99m-HMPAO SPECT patterns in young neuroleptic-naive patients with acute disease. *J. Nucl. Med.* 35:935–941.

CHUA, S. E., and P. J. MCKENNA, 1995. Schizophrenia—a brain disease: A critical review of structural and functional cerebral abnormality in the disorder. *Br. J. Psychiatry* 166:563–582.

CHUBAKOV, A. R., V. G. TSYGANOVA, and E. F. SARKISOVA, 1993. The stimulating influence of the raphe nuclei on the morphofunctional development of the hippocampus during their combined cultivation. *Neurosci. Behav. Physiol.* 23:271–276.

CHUGANI, D. C., O. MUZIK, M. BEHEN, R. ROTHERMEL, J. J. JANISSE, J. LEE, and H. T. CHUGANI, 1999. Developmental changes in brain serotonin synthesis capacity in autistic and nonautistic children. *Ann. Neurol.* 45:287–295.

CLEGHORN, J. M., S. FRANCO, B. SZECHTMAN, R. D. KAPLAN, H. SZECHTMAN, G. M. BROWN, C. NAHMIAS, and E. S. GARNETT, 1992. Toward a brain map of auditory hallucinations [see comments]. *Am. J. Psychiatry* 149:1062–1069.

CRAWFORD, T. J., T. SHARMA, B. K. PURI, R. M. MURRAY, D. M. BERRIDGE, and S. W. LEWIS, 1998. Saccadic eye movements in families multiply affected with schizophrenia: The Maudsley Family Study. *Am. J. Psychiatry* 155:1703–1710.

CROW, T. J., 1997. Is schizophrenia the price that Homo sapiens pays for language? *Schizophr. Res.* 28:127–141.

CROW, T. J., and E. C. JOHNSTONE, 1987. Schizophrenia: Nature of the disease process and its biological correlates. In *Handbook of Physiology, Section 1: The Nervous System*, Vol. 5: *Higher Functions of the Brain*, V. B. Mountcastle, F. Plum, and R. Geiger, eds. Bethesda, Md.: American Physiological Society, pp. 843–869.

CUESTA, M. J., and V. PERALTA, 1994. Lack of insight in schizophrenia. *Schizophr. Bull.* 20:359–366.

CUTTING, J., 1990. *The Right Cerebral Hemisphere and Psychiatric Disorders.* Oxford, Engl.: Oxford University Press.

DADE, L. A., M. JONES-GOTMAN, R. J. ZATORRE, and A. C. EVANS, 1998. Human brain function during odor encoding and recognition: A PET activation study. *Ann. N.Y. Acad. Sci.* 855:572–574.

DELISI, L. E., M. SAKUMA, M. KUSHNER, D. L. FINER, A. L. HOFF, and T. J. CROW, 1997. Anomalous cerebral asymmetry and language processing in schizophrenia. *Schizophr. Bull.* 23:255–271.

DEWEY, S. L., G. S. SMITH, J. LOGAN, D. ALEXOFF, Y. S. DING, P. KING, N. PAPPAS, J. D. BRODIE, and C. R. ASHBY, 1995. Serotonergic modulation of striatal dopamine measured with positron emission tomography (PET) and in vivo microdialysis. *J. Neurosci.* 15 (1, Pt. 2):821–829.

DIERKS, T., D. E. J. LINDEN, M. JANDL, E. FORMISANO, R. GOEBEL, H. LANFERMANN, and W. SINGER, 1999. Activation of Heschl's gyrus during auditory hallucinations. *Neuron* 22:615–621.

DOLLFUS, S., B. EVERITT, J. M. RIBEYRE, F. ASSOULY-BESSE, C. SHARP, and M. PETIT, 1996. Identifying subtypes of schizophrenia by cluster analyses. *Schizophr. Bull.* 22:545–555.

DOTY, R. W., 1970. On butterflies in the brain. In *Electrophysiology of the Central Nervous System*, V. S. Rusinov, B. Haigh, and R. W. Doty, eds. New York: Plenum Press, pp. 97–106.

DOTY, R. W., 1983. Nongeniculate afferents to striate cortex in macaques. *J. Comp. Neurol.* 218:159–173.

DOTY, R. W., 1989. Schizophrenia: A disease of interhemispheric processes at forebrain and brainstem levels? *Behav. Brain Res.* 34:1–33.

DOTY, R. W., 1995. Brainstem influences on forebrain processes, including memory. In *Neurobehavioral Plasticity: Learning, Development, and Response to Brain Insults*, N. E. Spear, L. P. Spear, and M. L. Woodruff, eds. Hillsdale, N.J.: Erlbaum, pp. 349–370.

ERIKSSON, P. S., E. PERFILIEVA, T. BJORK-ERIKSSON, A. M. ALBORN, C. NORDBORG, D. A. PETERSON, and F. H. GAGE, 1998. Neurogenesis in the adult human hippocampus. *Nature Med.* 4:1313–1317.

FENTON, W. S., and T. H. McGLASHAN, 1987. Sustained remission in drug-free schizophrenic patients. *Am. J. Psychiatry* 144:1306–1309.

FLACK, W. F. J., D. R. MILLER, and M. WIENER, eds. 1991. *What Is Schizophrenia.* New York: Springer-Verlag.

FRIEDMAN, L., J. A. JESBERGER, L. J. SIEVER, P. THOMPSON, R. MOHS, and H. Y. MELTZER, 1995. Smooth pursuit performance in patients with affective disorders or schizophrenia and normal controls: Analysis with specific oculomotor measures, rms error and qualitative ratings. *Psychol. Med.* 25:387–403.

GESCHWIND, D. H., M. IACOBONI, M. S. MEGA, D. W. ZAIDEL, T. CLOUGHESY, and E. ZAIDEL, 1995. Alien hand syndrome: Interhemispheric motor disconnection due to a lesion in the midbody of the corpus callosum. *Neurology* 45:802–808.

GREEN, M. F., K. HUGDAHL, and S. MITCHELL, 1994. Dichotic listening during auditory hallucinations in patients with schizophrenia. *Am. J. Psychiatry* 151:357–362.

GRUZELIER, J. H., 1999. Functional neuropsychophysiological asymmetry in schizophrenia: A review and reorientation. *Schizophr. Bull.* 25:91–120.

HALÁSZ, N., 1990. *The Vertebrate Olfactory System: Chemical Neuroanatomy, Function and Development.* Budapest, Hungary: Akadémiai Kiadó.

HIGHLEY, J. R., M. M. ESIRI, B. McDONALD, M. CORTINA-BORJA, B. M. HERRON, and T. J. CROW, 1999. The size and fibre composition of the corpus callosum with respect to gender and schizophrenia: A post-mortem study. *Brain* 122 (1):99–110.

HOFF, A. L., C. NEAL, M. KUSHNER, and L. E. DELISI, 1994. Gender differences in corpus callosum size in first-episode schizophrenics. *Biol. Psychiatry* 35:913–919.

JACOBSEN, L. K., J. N. GIEDD, P. C. BERQUIN, A. L. KRAIN, S. D. HAMBURGER, S. KUMRA, and J. L. RAPOPORT, 1997. Quantitative morphology of the cerebellum and fourth ventricle in childhood-onset schizophrenia. *Am. J. Psychiatry* 154:1663–1669.

JOHNSON, R. T., 1980. Selective vulnerability of neural cells to viral infections. *Brain* 103:447–472.

KAPUR, S., R. B. ZIPURSKY, and G. REMINGTON, 1999. Clinical and theoretical implications of 5-HT2 and D2 receptor occupancy of clozapine, risperidone, and olanzapine in schizophrenia. *Am. J. Psychiatry* 156:286–293.

KARSON, C. N., R. A. DYKMAN, and S. R. PAIGE, 1990. Blink rates in schizophrenia. *Schizophr. Bull.* 16:345–354.

KOPALA, L., K. GOOD, J. MARTZKE, and T. HURWITZ, 1995. Olfactory deficits in schizophrenia are not a function of task complexity. *Schizophr. Res.* 17:195–199.

KORNACK, D. R., and P. RAKIC, 1999. Continuation of neurogenesis in the hippocampus of the adult macaque monkey. *Proc. Natl. Acad. Sci. U.S.A.* 96:5768–5773.

LAUDER, J. M., 1993. Neurotransmitters as growth regulatory signals: Role of receptors and second messengers. *Trends Neurosci.* 16:233–240.

LAVDAS, A. A., M. E. BLUE, J. LINCOLN, and J. G. PARNAVELAS, 1997. Serotonin promotes the differentiation of glutamate neurons in organotypic slice cultures of the developing cerebral cortex. *J. Neurosci.* 17:7872–7880.

LEBRAND, C., O. CASES, C. ADELBRECHT, A. DOYE, C. ALVAREZ, S. ELMESTIKAWY, I. SEIF, and P. GASPAR, 1996. Transient uptake and storage of serotonin in developing thalamic neurons. *Neuron* 17:823–835.

LENN, N. J., and L. WHITMORE, 1989. Modification of left-right pairing during the development of individual crest synapses in the rat interpeduncular nucleus. *J. Comp. Neurol.* 281:136–142.

LEVITT, P., J. A. HARVEY, E. FRIEDMAN, K. SIMANSKY, and E. H. MURPHY, 1997. New evidence for neurotransmitter influences on brain development. *Trends Neurosci.* 20:269–274.

LEVY, D. L., P. S. HOLZMAN, S. MATTHYSSE, and N. R. MENDELL, 1993. Eye tracking dysfunction and schizophrenia: A critical perspective. *Schizophr. Bull.* 19:461–536.

LIEBERMAN, J. A., R. B. MAILMAN, G. DUNCAN, L. SIKICH, M. CHAKOS, D. E. NICHOLS, and J. E. KRAUS, 1998. Serotonergic basis of antipsychotic drug effects in schizophrenia [Review]. *Biol. Psychiatry* 44:1099–1117.

MAIER, W., D. LICHTERMANN, J. MINGES, J. HALLMAYER, R. HEUN, O. BENKERT, and D. F. LEVINSON, 1993. Continuity and discontinuity of affective disorders and schizophrenia: Results of a controlled family study. *Arch. Gen. Psychiatry* 50:871–883.

MALASPINA, D., A. D. WRAY, J. H. FRIEDMAN, X. AMADOR, S. YALE, A. HASAN, J. M. GORMAN, and C. A. KAUFMANN, 1994. Odor discrimination deficits in schizophrenia: Association with eye movement dysfunction. *J. Neuropsychiatry Clin. Neurosci.* 6:273–278.

MANSCHRECK, T. C., 1986. Motor abnormalities in schizophrenia. In *Handbook of Schizophrenia*, Vol. 1: *The Neurology of Schizophrenia*, H. A. Nasrallah and D. R. Weinberger, eds. Amsterdam: Elsevier, pp. 65–96.

MANSOUR-ROBAEY, S., N. MECHAWAR, F. RADJA, C. BEAULIEU, and L. DESCARRIES, 1998. Quantified distribution of serotonin transporter and receptors during the postnatal development of the rat barrel field cortex. *Brain Res. Dev Brain Res.* 107:159–163.

MARKS, R. C., and D. J. LUCHINS, 1990. Relationship between brain imaging findings in schizophrenia and psychopathology. In *Modern Problems in Pharmacopsychiatry. Schizophrenia: Positive and Negative Symptoms and Syndromes*, Vol. 24, N. C. Andreasen, ed. Basel, Switzerland: Karger, pp. 89–123.

McGUIRE, P. K., G. M. S. SHAH, and R. M. MURRAY, 1993. Increased blood flow in Broca's area during auditory hallucinations in schizophrenia. *The Lancet* 342:703–706.

MEDNICK, S. A., M. O. HUTTUNEN, and R. A. MACHON, 1994. Prenatal influenza infections and adult schizophrenia. *Schizophr. Bull.* 20:263–267.

MENNINGER, K. A., 1994. Influenza and schizophrenia—An analysis of post-influenzal dementia precox, as of 1918: And five years later further studies of the psychiatric aspects of influenza [reprinted]. *Am. J. Psychiatry* 151 (6, Suppl.):183–187.

MOBERG, P. J., R. L. DOTY, B. I. TURETSKY, S. E. ARNOLD, R. N. MAHR, R. C. GUR, W. BILKER, and R. E. GUR, 1997. Olfactory identification deficits in schizophrenia: Correlation with duration of illness. *Am. J. Psychiatry* 154:1016–1018.

MOHAMMED, A. K., J. MAEHLEN, O. MAGNUSSON, F. FONNUM, and K. KRISTENSSON, 1992. Persistent changes in behaviour and brain serotonin during ageing in rats subjected to infant nasal virus infection. *Neurobiol. Aging* 13:83–87.

MORILAK, D. A., and R. D. CIARANELLO, 1993. 5-HT2 receptor immunoreactivity on cholinergic neurons of the pontomesencephalic tegmentum shown by double immunofluorescence. *Brain Res.* 627:49–54.

Moukhles, H., O. Bosler, J. P. Bolam, A. Vallee, D., Umbriaco, M. Geffard, and G. Doucet, 1997. Quantitative and morphometric data indicate precise cellular interactions between serotonin terminals and postsynaptic targets in rat substantia nigra. *Neuroscience* 76:1159–1171.

Nasrallah, H. A., 1986. Cerebral hemisphere asymmetries and interhemispheric integration in schizophrenia. In *Handbook of Schizophrenia*, Vol. 1: *The Neurology of Schizophrenia*, H. A. Nasrallah and D. R. Weinberger, eds. Amsterdam: Elsevier, pp. 157–174.

O'Callaghan, E., P. C. Sham, N. Takei, G. Murray, G. Glover, E. H. Hare, and R. M. Murray, 1994. The relationship of schizophrenic births to 16 infectious diseases. *Br. J. Psychiatry* 165:353–356.

Petty, R. G., 1999. Structural asymmetries of the human brain and their disturbance in schizophrenia. *Schizophr. Bull.* 25:121–139.

Portas, C. M., M. Thakkar, D. Rainnie, and R. W. McCarley, 1996. Microdialysis perfusion of 8-hydroxy-2-(di-n-propylamino)tetralin (8-OH-DPAT) in the dorsal raphe nucleus decreases serotonin release and increases rapid eye movement sleep in the freely moving cat. *J. Neurosci.* 16:2820–2828.

Ram, R., E. J. Bromet, W. W. Eaton, C. Pato, and J. E. Schwartz, 1992. The natural course of schizophrenia: A review of first-admission studies. *Schizophr. Bull.* 18:185–207.

Rhoades, R. W., N. L. Chiaia, R. D. Lane, and C. A. Bennett-Clarke, 1998. Effect of activity blockade on changes in vibrissae-related patterns in the rat's primary somatosensory cortex induced by serotonin depletion. *J. Comp. Neurol.* 402:276–283.

Rosse, R. B., J. P. Collins, M. Fay McCarthy, T. N. Alim, R. J. Wyatt, and S. I. Deutsch, 1994. Phenomenologic comparison of the idiopathic psychosis of schizophrenia and drug-induced cocaine and phencycliding psychoses: A retrospective study. *Clin. Neuropharmacol.* 17:359–369.

Shenton, M. E., 1996. Temporal lobe structural abnormalities in schizophrenia: A selective review and presentation of new magnetic resonance findings. In *Psychopathology*, S. Matthysse, D. L. Levy, J. Kagan, and F. M. Benes, eds. Cambridge, Engl.: Cambridge University Press, pp. 51–99.

Shipley, M. T., 1985. Transport of molecules from nose to brain: Transneuronal anterograde and retrograde labeling in the rat olfactory system by wheat germ agglutinin-horseradish peroxidase applied to nasal epithelium. *Brain Res. Bull.* 15:129–142.

Sikich, L., J. M. Hickok, and R. D. Todd, 1990. 5-HT1A receptors control neurite branching during development. *Brain Res. Dev. Brain Res.* 56:269–274.

Silbersweig, D. A., E. Stern, C. Frith, C. Cahill, A. Holmes, S. Grootnook, J. Seaward, P. McKenna, S. E. Chua, L. Schorr, T. Jones, and R. S. J. Frackowiak, 1995. A functional neuroanatomy of hallucinations in schizophrenia. *Nature* 378:176–179.

Slater, P., C. A. Doyle, and J. F. Deakin, 1998. Abnormal persistence of cerebellar serotonin-1A receptors in schizophrenia suggests failure to regress in neonates. *J. Neural Transm.* 105:305–315.

Sperry, R. W., 1984. Consciousness, personal identity and the divided brain. *Neuropsychologia* 22:661–673.

Stedman, T. J., and A. L. Clair, 1998. Neuropsychological, neurological and symptom correlates of impaired olfactory identification in schizophrenia. *Schizophr. Res.* 32:23–30.

Stevens, J. R., 1982. Neuropathology of schizophrenia, *Arch. Gen. Psychiatry* 39:1131–1139.

Straube, E. R., and R. D. Oades, 1992. *Schizophrenia: Empirical Research and Findings.* San Diego: Academic Press.

Stroop, W. G., and J. R. Baringer, 1989. Neurotropic viruses: Classification and fundamental aspects. In *Handbook of Clinical Neurology: Viral Disease*, Vol. 12, R. R. McKendall, ed. Amsterdam: Elsevier, pp. 1–23.

Swayze, V. W., N. C. Andreasen, J. C. Ehrhardt, W. T. C. Yuh, R. J. Alliger, and G. A. Cohen, 1990. Developmental abnormalities of the corpus callosum in schizophrenia. *Arch. Neurol.* 47:805–808.

Taller, A. M., D. M. Asher, K. L. Pomeroy, B. A. Eldadah, M. S. Godec, P. G. Falkai, B. Bogert, J. E. Kleinman, J. R. Stevens, and E. F. Torrey, 1996. Search for viral nucleic acid sequences in brain tissues of patients with schizophrenia using nested polymerase chain reaction. *Arch. Gen. Psychiatry* 53:32–40.

Tiihonen, J., H. Katila, E. Pekkonen, I. P. Jaaskelainen, M. Huotilainen, H. J. Aronen, R. J. Ilmoniemi, P. Rasanen, J. Virtanen, E. Salli, and J. Karhu, 1998. Reversal of cerebral asymmetry in schizophrenia measured with magnetoencephalography. *Schizophr. Res.* 30:209–219.

Torrey, E. F., A. E. Bowler, E. H. Taylor, and I. I. Gottesman, 1994. *Schizophrenia and Manic-Depressive Disorder: The Biological Roots of Mental Illness as Revealed by the Landmark Study of Identical Twins.* New York: Basic Books.

Trimble, M. R., 1991. *The Psychoses of Epilepsy.* New York: Raven.

Walker, E. F., R. R. Lewine, and C. Neumann, 1996. Childhood behavioral characteristics and adult brain morphology in schizophrenia. *Schizophr. Res.* 22:93–101.

Wilson, M. A., and M. E. Molliver, 1991. The organization of serotonergic projections to cerebral cortex in primates: Retrograde transport studies. *Neuroscience*, 44:555–570.

Wiser, A. K., N. C. Andreasen, D. S. O'Leary, G. L. Watkins, L. L. Boles Ponto, and R. D. Hichwa, 1998. Dysfunctional cortico-cerebellar circuits cause "cognitive dysmetria" in schizophrenia. *NeuroReport* 9:1895–1899.

Woodruff, P. W., M. L. Phillips, T. Rushe, I. C. Wright, R. M. Murray, and A. S. David, 1997a. Corpus callosum size and interhemispheric function in schizophrenia. *Schizophr. Res.* 23:189–196.

Woodruff, P. W., I. C. Wright, E. T. Bullmore, M. Brammer, R. J. Howard, S. C. Williams, J. Shapleske, S. Rossell, A. S. David, P. K. McGuire, and R. M. Murray, 1997b. Auditory hallucinations and the temporal cortical response to speech in schizophrenia: A functional magnetic resonance imaging study. *Am. J. Psychiatry* 154:1676–1682.

Wu, J., M. S. Buchsbaum, K. Moy, N. Denlea, P. Kesslak, H. Tseng, D. Plosnaj, M. Hetu, S. Potkin, S. Bracha, et al., 1993. Olfactory memory in unmedicated schizophrenics. *Schizophr. Res.* 9:41–47.

Wyatt, R. J., J. A. Apud, and S. Potkin, 1996. New directions in the prevention and treatment of schizophrenia: A biological perspective. *Psychiatry* 59:357–370.

YOUNG, D. A., R. DAVILA, and H. SCHER, 1993. Unawareness of illness and neuropsychological performance in chronic schizophrenia. *Schizophr. Res.* 10:117–124.

YOUSEM, D. M., S. C. R. WILLIAMS, R. O. HOWARD, C. ANDREW, A. SIMMONS, M. ALLIN, R. J. GECKLE, D. SUSKIND, E. T. BULLMORE, M. J. BRAMMER, and R. L. DOTY, 1997. Functional MR imaging during odor stimulation: Preliminary data. *Radiology* 204:833–838.

ZAIDEL, D. W., M. M. ESIRI, and P. J. HARRISON, 1997. The hippocampus in schizophrenia: Lateralized increase in neuronal density and altered cytoarchitectural asymmetry. *Psychol. Med.* 27:703–713.

EDITORIAL COMMENTARY 4

Current Directions in Clinical Studies of Callosal Functions

ERAN ZAIDEL AND MARCO IACOBONI

This part of the book discusses behavioral, physiological, and anatomical evidence for abnormal callosal function in selective clinical syndromes, including multiple sclerosis (MS) (Brown, Habib et al., Tomaiuolo et al.), schizophrenia (Cowell et al., Doty), alexithymia in multiple sclerosis (Habib et al.), dyslexia (Brown), and Tourette's syndrome and attention deficit/hyperactivity disorder (Yazgan and Kinsbourne).

Multiple sclerosis

Brown measured interhemispheric transfer time (IHTT) using event-related potential (ERP) to unilateral letter stimuli and found a subgroup of patients with significantly diminished or absent P1 or N1 components in their ipsilateral, that is, cross-callosal, evoked potentials. By contrast, Tomaiuolo and colleagues did not observe any slowing down of IHTT in their patients of the relapsing-remitting variety using the crossed-uncrossed difference (CUD) in simple reaction time (SRT). These results are not necessarily discrepant with each other. IHTT obtained from N1 or P1 with visual ERP routinely yields cross-callosal transfer times between 20 and 25. This suggests that the ERP measures transfer through different callosal channels than the one that mediates crossed responses in SRT, which typically yields transfer times of about 3 ms.

An important feature of Brown's paper is the presentation of converging evidence and the cross-validation of measures. For example, Brown does not assume that the ipsilateral P1 and N1 components of lateralized vi-

ERAN ZAIDEL   Department of Psychology, University of California at Los Angeles, Los Angeles, California.
MARCO IACOBONI   Ahmanson Lovelace Brain Mapping Center, Neuropsychiatric Institute, Brain Research Institute, David Geffen School of Medicine, University of California at Los Angeles, Los Angeles, California.

sual ERP reflect callosal relay. He verifies this directly with split-brain patients. Furthermore, he compares callosal pathology to developmental immaturity by administering his measures to normal children. Brown also compares frank disconnection following commissurotomy with the more subtle transfer deficits of agenesis of the corpus callosum (CC). His MS population, in turn, offers an attractive opportunity to relate (1) anatomical measures of callosal atrophy to (2) physiological (ERP) measures of callosal transfer and (3) behavioral measures of transfer. Unfortunately, no MRIs of the MS patients were available. Further, no behavioral measure of interhemispheric transfer time was collected and reported.

Tomaiuolo and colleagues use their MS data to decide between two competing models of callosal function. They posit an anatomical model that incorporates a discrete fast motor channel through the callosal midbody, in contrast with an attentional model that is more diffusely represented throughout the CC. They reason that, probabilistically, their patients are unlikely to have selective damage to the fast motor channel but likely to have damage to the diffuse attentional "channel." Thus, the anatomical model predicts no significant change in the CUD in MS, whereas the attentional model predicts a significant increase in the CUD. The data show no difference and are thus consistent with the anatomical model. However, the assumption of a diffuse attentional "channel" might not be valid. For example, we have evidence for distinct auditory callosal channels that are attention-specific and nonspecific (Zaidel et al., 1996).

The paper by Habib and colleagues (henceforth HEA) is a beautiful example of the application of sophisticated methodology from laterality research to a psychiatric condition in a neurological disorder. The psychiatric condition is alexithymia, the inability to verbalize emotions. Among other goals, HEA set out to test the hypothesis that alexithymia is due to (1) right-hemisphere dysfunction, leading to impoverishment of affect, and (2) functional callosal disconnection, leading to inaccessibility of right-hemisphere (RH) emotions to left-hemisphere (LH) verbalization. Since the neurological disorder MS is associated with white matter degeneration in general and CC atrophy in particular, it is a valuable model system for testing the disconnection hypothesis of alexithymia.

HEA selected Bryden's words/emotions dichotic tape for testing their predictions. In this test, the stimuli consist of four words (*bower*, *dower*, *power*, and *tower*) expressed in four different emotional intonations (angry, sad, neutral, and happy). The verbal task requires detecting a target word, say, "bower," and the emotional task requires detecting, say, the emotion "sad," while dividing attention between the two ears. The task yields a right-ear advantage (REA) in the verbal task and a left-ear advantage (LEA) in the emotion task. This is explained by the fact that the dichotic condition results in suppression of the ipsilateral left ear (LE) → RH and right ear (RE) → RH projections. (The auditory nerves cross both in the brain stem (superior olive) and in the inferior colliculus.)

Now, if the verbal stimuli are processed exclusively in the LH, then the RE has privileged access to its processing resources, whereas the LE must first traverse the CC from the RH to the LH before being processed in the LH (Zaidel, 1976, 1983; Zaidel, Zaidel, and Bogen, 1990; Zaidel, Clarke, and Suyenobu, 1990). Furthermore, there are data suggesting that auditory interhemispheric transfer occurs largely through the isthmus of the CC (e.g., Alexander et al., 1989). Thus, posterior callosal dysfunction should result in a failure of LE transfer and a reduced LE score in the verbal task. This is exactly what HEA observed for MS patients relative to normal controls. We might even expect an increased RE score due to release from competition for resources by the LE signal, but this wasn't quite significant. A similar, symmetric, argument applies to emotion processing in the RH. In this case, MS patients have a lower RE score, presumably because the RE signal must traverse the CC from left to right before being processed. In this task, the left ear of MS patients does not tend to surpass that of controls, perhaps because emotional processing in the RH of MS patients is also impaired, as predicted by HEA.

But the argument advanced above is valid only if (1) the stimuli indeed yield ipsilateral suppression on both sides and (2) the tasks are exclusively specialized in the opposite hemispheres. Are these assumptions true? They can be tested critically in the split brain. The assumptions are best tested in a patient with complete cerebral commissurotomy, L.B., who appears to have compe-

tence for at least one task in each hemisphere. When L.B. was asked to respond by verbally identifying the word or emotion heard in either ear, he showed a massive REA for word identification and a massive LEA for emotion identification. The simplest account of this pattern of results is that (1) there is good ipsilateral suppression for both tasks in both hemispheres; (2) the LH specializes for and dominates the identification of the words, exhibiting an expected massive REA; (3) the RH specializes for and dominates the identification of the emotions, yielding a massive LEA; and (4) verbal identification of the emotions reflects either RH speech or LH verbalization of the emotion, or a code identifying it, which is transferred subcallosally from the RH to the LH. On this account, HEA's argument is valid.

But the plot thickens. Bryden and HEA used a slightly different paradigm. Instead of using verbal identification, they used target detection, in which subjects were asked to detect one nominated target word (say, "tower") and one nominated target emotion (say, "sad") in either ear. This paradigm also yields the expected REA for words and LEA for emotions. But does it satisfy the assumptions of ipsilateral suppression and exclusive specialization? The data for this paradigm in L.B. do not quite satisfy all the assumptions. For words the RE score was 100%, the LE score was 42% (chance = 50%), and the false alarm rate ("yes" responses to pairs that did not contain the target in either ear) was 28%. For emotions the RE score was 72%, the LE score was 64%, and the false alarm rate was 1%. Thus the word task did yield a massive REA with chance performance in the LE, consistent with ipsilateral suppression and LH competence. It is noteworthy, however, that the LE score was at, rather than below, chance, suggesting that L.B. does not hear only a single word and that he can identify the source of the LE signal but not its content. The emotions task yields unexpected results: There was an REA, with above-chance performance in the RE but not in the LE, suggesting LH processing, which shows only partial competence. The target detection task confirms the conclusion from verbal identification, namely, that there is LE suppression in the LH for the word task. But is LH specialization exclusive? We addressed this question with a third paradigm, requiring matching of the sound to lateralized letter probes (B, D, P, and T). Unfortunately, this task yielded high biases and low sensitivities, so the data are inconclusive.

We conclude that as far as our data go, they are consistent with HEA's interpretation, but further experimentation is necessary to establish exclusive LH specialization for word identification in the words/emotions dichotic listening task. Until that is done, HEA's results must be considered as only tentative.

Schizophrenia

Surprisingly, we could find no satisfactory comparisons of the CUD in lateralized SRT with unimanual responses between schizophrenics and controls. Shelton and Knight (1984) did report no difference in the CUD between 12 active schizophrenics on neuroleptics and 12 controls with personality disorders or alcohol abuse. However, (1) their task was unusual in including an equal number of trials with targets and catch trials, (2) there were only 15 targets per hand × VF combination, (3) RTs were exceptionally long for this task (∼590 ms for controls, ∼780 ms for schizophrenics), and (4) the task yielded no significant response hand (Rh) (left, right) × VF (left, right) or group (schizophrenia, controls) × Rh × VF interaction. Therefore, the task is ill-behaved. The pattern of results was different in the two groups, and the CUD in the patients (15 ms) was actually somewhat shorter than that in the controls (20 ms).

Cowell and colleagues argue that the CC is likely to play a supporting rather than a primary role in the complex neurocognitive profile of schizophrenia. Because specific channels of the CC interconnect specific cortical modules in the two hemispheres, a regional anomaly in the CC of schizophrenics may provide a clue about the location of associated cortical anomalies. It is also possible that normal callosal functions are so disrupted in schizophrenia that abnormal or compensatory brain-behavior relationships are established. Our understanding of such compensatory mechanisms is still poor. For example, do alleged decreases in cortical gray matter in schizophrenia yield proportionally more white matter and larger CC size, or, on the contrary, do they yield fewer cortical cells, fewer CC fibers, and a smaller CC?

A critical question in analyzing regional CC structure is how to partition it into functionally significant regions. Witelson proposed a scheme in terms of half, one third, and one fifth of the longest line connecting the anterior and posterior poles of the CC. This scheme has a gross functional motivation, but it is quantitatively somewhat arbitrary. Cowell and colleagues propose a more coherent scheme based on a factor analysis of regional callosal size. Seven factors emerged. Furthermore, the factor-based regional callosal size turns out to depend on an interaction of age, sex, and handedness. For example, CC size is normally larger in non-right-handed males than in right-handed males but shows no handedness effect in females (cf. Commentary 15.2 in this volume). This relationship did not hold in schizophrenia.

When these individual difference variables were carefully controlled, Cowell and colleagues found that the CC factors of the schizophrenics and controls differed especially in the midbody of the CC, with a marked anterior shift in the patients. Does this finding explain observed behavioral differences in hemispheric specialization and interaction in schizophrenia?

Doty proposes a provocative explanation for abnormal laterality in schizophrenia by a perturbation of the serotonergic raphe system. But actual data on disturbances of hemispheric function or of interhemispheric transfer in schizophrenia are contradictory. Doty cites evidence for reduced asymmetry in schizophrenia on the one hand and for reduced callosal function on the other. First, one would expect behavioral/anatomical asymmetry to be negatively correlated with callosal transfer (Zaidel, Aboitiz, and Clarke, 1995). Second, our own data conflict with both claims. These data are described next.

Narr and colleagues (submitted) mounted a sophisticated attack on this problem. They used a simple behavioral laterality paradigm that measures separately hemispheric asymmetry in word recognition and interhemispheric transfer of lexical status. The paradigm involved lateralized presentation of an orthographically legal (word or nonword) target character string for lexical decision indicated by a unimanual two-choice button press. The underlined target is accompanied by a word or nonword distractor in the opposite visual hemifield. This lexical decision task can be processed independently in each hemisphere and normally yields a consistent right visual field advantage (RVFA), indicating left hemisphere superiority for lexical decision—stronger for words than for nonwords. Furthermore, there was a lexicality priming effect between distractors and targets: Word targets were decided faster with word distractors than with nonword distractors, especially in the LVF. This priming effect is interhemispheric: It does not occur with target and distractor in the same visual field (Zaidel et al., 1998).

Narr tested 34 chronic schizophrenics and 20 normal controls matched for sex, handedness, and education. She found decreased accuracy in the patients but similar hemispheric asymmetries (RVF advantage) in the two groups. The patients also used standard psycholinguistic strategies in both hemispheres. However, the patients showed greater lexicality priming than did the controls. Narr concluded that the asymmetry of the modules activated by lexical decision is less affected by schizophrenia than are the callosal channels that interconnect these modules. Are these channels implicated by Cowell and colleagues? Indeed, the isthmus (widths 65–76, region IV; see Chapter 19 in this volume) is the one most anteriorly displaced in schizophrenics relative to the normative comparison subjects.

Narr and colleagues also correlated the presence of positive or negative symptoms in the schizophrenic sample with the lateralized behavioral measures. Positive symptoms refer to hallucinations, delusions, and formal thought disorders; negative symptoms refer to blunted affects, withdrawal, and reduction in speech or movement. Positive symptoms correlated positively with degree of functional asymmetry in latency (LVF − RVF), i.e., (LVF − RVF)/(LVF + RVF), $r = 0.39$, $p = 0.0246$), whereas negative symptoms correlated negatively with LVF (RH) latency ($r = -0.409$, $p = 0.014$). Neither positive nor negative symptoms correlated with the lexicality priming measure of interhemispheric transfer. Thus, our data only partly support the view that schizophrenia is associated with decreased asymmetry.

Narr also administered a divided attention dichotic listening test to the same schizophrenic patients. The test consisted of stop consonant-vowel nonsense syllables (/ba/, /da/, /ga/, /pa/, /ta/, and /ka/) accompanied by lateralized visual probes of letters (B, D, G, P, T, and K) flashed to one visual field. Subjects responded unimanually by pressing one button if the probe matched the sound in either ear and another button otherwise. There was an equal REA in accuracy in patients and controls. On the assumption that this task is "callosal relay," that is, exclusively specialized to the LH (Zaidel, 1983), the LE signal partly reflects auditory callosal relay, and group differences in the efficiency of auditory callosal channels should have been reflected in group differences in the LE score and consequently in the REA. (A higher LE score leads to a lower RE score and to a lower REA.) Significantly, the callosal channel that mediates auditory transfer is again the isthmus (Alexander and Warren 1988).

We are thus faced with an apparent discrepancy. Schizophrenics show greater lexicality priming, associated with increased efficacy of the isthmus of the CC, but the same patients fail to show an increased LE score in dichotic listening, associated with unchanged connectivity through the isthmus. The solution may be that there are distinct lexical and auditory/phonetic channels around the isthmus and that the former is hyperactive in our schizophrenic sample, whereas the latter is not.

To complicate the story further, Narr's dichotic listening data seem to contrast with a previous study with a similar dichotic listening test in hallucinating and non-hallucinating psychotic patients (Green, Hugdahl, and Mitchell, 1994). The nonhallucinating patients showed a normal REA, whereas the hallucinating patients showed an increased LE score, a reduced RE score, and a reduced REA. This suggests that hallucinations are associated with increased callosal function in the auditory channel. By contrast, in Narr's data the only significant

negative correlation was between the RE score and positive symptoms (including hallucinations) ($r = -0.3857$, $p = 0.0388$). This suggests an association between positive symptoms and LH dysfunction in schizophrenia. Thus, different aspects of the disease appear to be associated with modulation of different asymmetric cortical modules and different callosal channels.

Yazgan and Kinsbourne's chapter emphasizes the role of the CC in regulating attentional processes in the two hemispheres. This is a counterpoint to the usual view of the CC as a set of channels for the transfer of information between the two hemispheres. It goes beyond Banich, who addresses both perceptual and attentional aspects of callosal functions during interhemispheric perceptual matching tasks. Some, but not all, of Yazgan and Kinsbourne's data support their view of the role of the CC in interhemispheric attentional regulation. Thus, they found that Tourette patients showed smaller validity effects in the Posner paradigm (covert orienting of spatial attention), the smaller the sizes of their CCs. This is consistent with the finding that interhemispheric cross-cuing is reduced in callosotomy (Arguin et al., 2000; Chapter 14 in this volume), but it is also inconsistent with the finding of some increased interhemispheric cross-cuing effects in commissurotomy patients (Zaidel, 1995), implicating subcallosal channels in interhemispheric attentional priming and the CC in modulating them (Zaidel et al., in press).

Yazgan and Kinsbourne point out that structural changes in the CC might reflect disturbances in interhemispheric connectivity, as well as abnormalities in the cortical sources of the fibers transversing the callosum, thus providing at least two sources of attentional disturbances. As they point out, the richness of callosal interhemispheric connections affects the degree of behavioral laterality. Indeed, Geschwind and Galaburda (1985) suggested that hemispheric specialization is negatively correlated with associated callosal connectivity, and we found some anatomical (Aboitiz et al., 1992) and behavioral (Clarke and Zaidel, 1994) support for this view (see also Zaidel, Aboitiz, and Clarke, 1995).

Yazgan and Kinsbourne report using a verbal-motor dual task with normal subjects and finding, surprisingly, that the amount of dual-task interference was inversely correlated with the CC area in both within-hemisphere (right-hand) and between-hemisphere (left-hand) conditions. They explained their findings with a cross-excitation model, in which a larger CC favors a larger and better-integrated system by facilitating recruitment of resources from the other hemisphere. This model better explains the results for within-hemisphere interference than for between-hemisphere interference. Perhaps a larger CC includes better anterior control channels for inhibiting cross-hemisphere interference. In any case, the important message from Yazgan and Kinsbourne is that the CC participates in both interhemispheric and intrahemispheric processing.

REFERENCES

ABOITIZ, F., A. B. SCHEIBEL, and E. ZAIDEL, 1992. Morphometry of the Sylvian fissure and the corpus callosum, with emphasis on sex differences. *Brain* 115:1521–1541.

ALEXANDER, M. P., and R. L. WARREN, 1988. Localization of callosal auditory pathways: A CT case study. *Neurology* 38:802–804.

CLARKE, J. M., and E. ZAIDEL, 1994. Anatomical-behavioral relationships: Corpus callosum morphometry and hemispheric specialization. *Behav. Brain Res.* 64:185–202.

GESCHWIND, N., and A. M. GALABURDA, 1985. Cerebral lateralization: Biological mechanisms, associations and pathology. *Arch. Neurol.* 42:428–459.

GREEN, M. F., K. HUGDAHL, and S. MITCHELL, 1994. Dichotic listening during auditory hallucinations in patients with schizophrenia. *Am. J. Psychiatry* 151:357–362.

NARR, K., M. F. GREEN, L. CAPETILLO-CUNLIFFE, A. W. TOGA, and E. ZAIDEL, submitted. Lateralized lexical decision in schizophrenia: Hemispheric specialization and interhemispheric lexicality priming.

NARR, K., E. ZAIDEL, L. CAPETILLO-CUNLIFFE, A. W. TOGA, and M. F. GREEN, 2000. Hemispheric specialization and interhemispheric interaction in schizophrenia. *J. Int. Neuropsychol. Soc.* 6:242.

SHELTON, E. J., and R. G. KNIGHT, 1984. Inter-hemispheric transmission times in schizophrenics. *Br. J. Clin. Psychol.* 23:227–228.

ZAIDEL, E. 1976. Language, dichotic listening and the disconnected hemispheres. In *Conference on Human Brain Function*, D. O. Walter, L. Rogers, and J. M. Finzi-Fried, eds. Los Angeles: BRI Publications Office, UCLA, pp. 103–110.

ZAIDEL, E., 1983. Disconnection syndrome as a model for laterality effects in the normal brain. In *Cerebral Hemisphere Asymmetry: Method, Theory and Application*, J. Hellige, ed. New York: Alan R. Liss, pp. 95–151.

ZAIDEL, E., 1995. Interhemispheric transfer in the split brain: Long-term status following complete cerebral commissurotomy. In *Brain Asymmetry*, R. J. Davidson and K. Hugdahl, eds. London: MIT Press, pp. 491–532.

ZAIDEL, E., A. ABOITIZ, and J. CLARKE, 1995. Sexual dimorphism in interhemispheric relations: Anatomical-behavioral convergence. *Biol. Res.* 28:27–43.

ZAIDEL, E., J. M. CLARKE, and B. SUYENOBU, 1990. Hemispheric independence: A paradigm case for cognitive neuroscience. In *Neurobiology of Higher Cognitive Function*, A. B. Scheibel and A. F. Wechsler, eds. New York: Guilford Press, pp. 297–355.

ZAIDEL, E., M. IACOBONI, D. W. ZAIDEL, and J. BOGEN, in press. The callosal syndromes. In *Clinical Neuropsychology*, 4th ed., K. M. Heilman and E. Valenstein, eds. New York: Oxford University Press.

ZAIDEL, E., D. W. ZAIDEL, and J. E. BOGEN, 1990. Testing the commissurotomy patient. In *Neuromethods: Methods in Human Neuropsychology*, Vol. 15, A. A. Boulton, G. B. Baker, and M. Hiscock, eds. Clifton, NJ: Humana Press, pp. 147–201.

V FROM ANATOMY TO BEHAVIOR: THE CASE OF PURE ALEXIA

21 The Role of Homotopic and Heterotopic Callosal Connections in Humans

STEPHANIE CLARKE

ABSTRACT There are two complementary views of the human callosal connections. One is that human callosal connections are organized in a very similar way to those of other primates or, indeed, of other mammals. The second view is based on the fact that in humans several functions are lateralized and that callosal afferents reflect this human specialization. Both of these views are supported by recent hodological studies of human visual callosal connections. As in nonhuman primates, human visual callosal afferents link representations of the vertical meridian and are thus landmarks for several retinotopically organized visual areas. Many influential models of human cognitive functions have presumed that human callosal connections link predominantly symmetrical parts of cortex; these same assumptions are still present in recent models. Our recent results challenge this view by revealing a large array of heterotopic callosal connections in humans.

Hierarchical organization of visual areas

The work of the past 25 years has demonstrated that macaque extrastriate cortex is not a homogeneously organized association cortex but an array of functional units that obey clearly defined organizational principles (for a review, see Felleman and Van Essen, 1991). First, it contains a large number of visual areas that are defined by their topographical representation, functional specialization, architecture, and connectivity; recent estimates exceed 30 areas. V1 (the primary visual area) and other early-stage visual areas have a rather precise retinotopic representation of the contralateral hemifield. Several extrastriate areas are highly specialized for some aspects of visual perception; the most striking examples are V4 (the fourth visual area), with a high proportion of neurons selective for color (Zeki, 1973), and V5/MT

STEPHANIE CLARKE Division de Neuropsychologie, Centre Hospitalier Universitaire Vaudois, Lausanne, Switzerland.

(the fifth visual area, also called MT by analogy), with a high proportion of neurons selective for motion (Zeki, 1974; Van Essen, Maunsell, and Bixby, 1981). Second, different aspects of visual information, such as color, shape, and motion, appear to be processed at the cortical level in parallel; separate compartments for these attributes were described in V1 and V2 (the secondary visual area) as well as specific connections of these compartments to specialized extrastriate areas (Livingstone and Hubel, 1984, 1987a; Shipp and Zeki, 1985). Third, macaque visual areas seem to constitute a hierarchical system. The level within the hierarchy is determined by the coding properties of the neurons and by the pattern of intrahemispheric corticocortical connections originating and terminating within a given area. The bottom of the hierarchy is formed by V1, and the top levels by parietal and temporal visual areas that are involved in complex cognitive functions (Felleman and Van Essen, 1991).

Human visual cortex appears to be organized in a very similar way. First, anatomical evidence indicates that human extrastriate cortex contains several visual areas (see below). Recent evidence from fMRI studies shows that at least four areas are retinotopically organized: V1, V2, V3 (the third visual area), VP (the ventroposterior visual area, defined as such in New World monkeys; the term has recently been used to denote ventral V3 in macaque and humans), V3A (the visual area anterior to the third visual area) (Sereno et al., 1995; DeYoe et al., 1996). Human extrastriate cortex contains regions that deal specifically with some aspects of visual information. Distinct regions were selectively activated by color (Lueck et al., 1989; Corbetta et al., 1990; Gulyas and Roland, 1991; Zeki et al., 1991) or motion stimuli (Corbetta et al., 1990; Zeki et al., 1991; Watson et al., 1993). Second, color, shape, and motion are processed separately by the human visual system, as indicated by psychophysical (Livingstone and Hubel, 1987b) and hodological evidence (Burkhalter and Bernardo, 1989). Third, human visual areas are most likely hierarchically organized. This point has never been directly demonstrated in humans, but there is rather convincing circumstantial evidence based on the strong similarities to macaque visual cortex and on the increasing specialization of the more anterior visual areas.

Human visual callosal connections

There are two complementary views of the human callosal connections. One is that human callosal connections are organized in a very similar way to those of other primates or, indeed, of other mammals. The second view is based on the fact that in humans several functions are lateralized and that callosal afferents reflect this human specialization. Both these views are supported by recent hodological studies of human visual callosal connections.

REGIONS OF ORIGIN   Several parts of the human visual cortex have been shown to form callosal connections: the inferomedial and superolateral parts of the occipital cortex and the posteroinferior part of the temporal cortex (Van Valkenburg, 1908; Clarke and Miklossy, 1990; Di Virgilio and Clarke, 1997). The evidence comes from cases with small lesions in which degenerating axon segments were demonstrated in the corpus callosum or in the contralateral target territories. The posterior parietal cortex most likely gives rise to callosal connections as well, but no unequivocal evidence has been yet presented.

The radial distribution of callosal neurons in humans is largely unknown. It has been proposed that the large pyramidal neurons in lower layer III within the subarea OBgamma of Von Economo and Koskinas (1925) send axons through the corpus callosum. Circumstantial evidence comes from acallosal patients, who were reported to lack these neurons, as do rhesus monkeys after callosotomy (Shoumura, Ando, and Kato, 1975; Glickstein and Whitteridge, 1976).

REGIONS OF TERMINATION   Recent anatomical studies demonstrated that the intracortical distribution of visual callosal afferents in the human cortex forms a complex pattern of callosal-rich and -poor regions. The tracing method used was a modification of the Nauta method for anterogradely degenerating axons (Clarke and Miklossy, 1990; Clarke et al., 1995). Human brains with unilateral occipital or occipitotemporal lesions were silver-impregnated for degenerating axons, thus reveal-ing callosal afferents from the infarction to the intact, contralateral hemisphere. Charts of individual sections from the hemisphere contralateral to the lesion revealed a patchy distribution of degenerating axon segments, that is, callosal afferents (Figure 21.1). A band of callosal afferents was found along the 17/18 boundary, reaching more into area 18 than 17. Area 17 outside this thin band was devoid of callosal afferents. A 15- to 45-mm-wide stripe of area 18 adjacent to the callosal band along the 17/18 boundary was callosal-poor. Patches of callosal afferents of different width alternated with callosal-free regions more laterally in areas 18 and 19. In a first study, the medial part of the occipital lobe of three cases was unfolded (Clarke and Miklossy, 1990). It showed an alternating pattern of anteroposteriorly oriented bands of callosal-rich and -poor regions (Figure 21.2a). This resembled the situation in macaque monkeys, in which similar bands of callosal afferents are concentrated along the representation of the vertical meridian, providing useful landmarks for some boundaries between visual areas.

More recently, we extended the analysis of callosal afferents (Clarke et al., 1995). The whole posterior third of the hemisphere was flattened using an algorithm developed by Heather Drury and David Van Essen (Clarke et al., 1995; Van Essen et al., 1995). Two important results emerged. First, callosal connections originating in the medio-occipital and the inferior temporo-occipital cortex spread widely over the whole occipital and the posterior temporal and parietal cortices. Second, as shown in the flattened reconstructions, patches of callosal-poor regions exist also on the lateral aspect of the hemisphere, probably in areas V3A and dorsal V4.

Visual callosal afferents are landmarks for several visual areas

Although cytoarchitecture and myeloarchitecture vary considerably within the human extrastriate visual cortex, they do not on their own provide precise landmarks for a functional subdivision (for a review, see Zilles and Clarke, 1997). In this respect, the pattern of callosal afferents constitutes a unique set of landmarks.

The tangential distribution of callosal afferents in the occipital cortex is discontinuous in all mammalian species so far studied (for a review, see Innocenti, 1986). In the macaque the first coherent scheme was proposed by Zeki (1970), consisting of six bands of callosal afferents through areas 18 and 19. Later, maps of callosal afferents were related to the electrophysiologically defined areas of the occipital cortex (Zeki, 1977, 1978; Van Essen and Zeki, 1978; Van Essen, Newsome, and Bixby, 1982). Callosal afferents were shown to characterize vi-

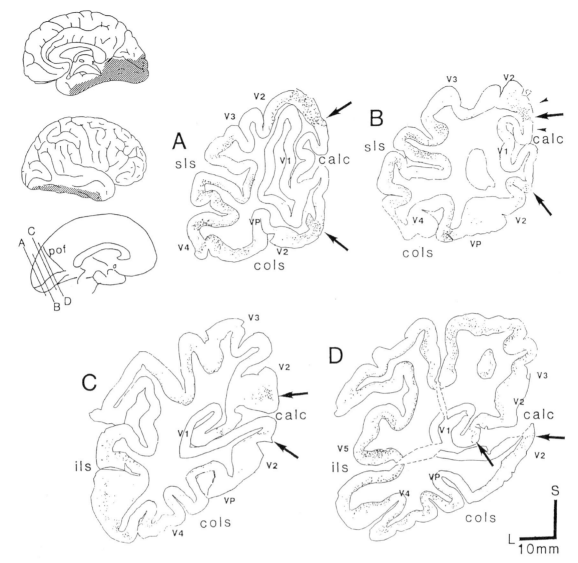

FIGURE 21.1. Distribution of visual callosal connections within individual sections of the occipital lobe. The approximate positions of these sections (left hemisphere) as well as the location and extent of the lesion (right hemisphere) from which the connections were traced are shown in the brain inset. The contours of the section and the limit between layer VI and the white matter are indicated by continuous lines. Each dot represents one degenerating axon segment. The boundary between areas V1 and V2 are indicated with arrows. Note the discontinuous distribution of callosal afferents. (Adapted from Clarke and Miklossy, 1990.)

sual area boundaries that contain the representation of the vertical meridian: V1/V2, V3/V3A, V3/V4 and VP/V4 boundaries. The remaining parts of V1, V2, VP, V3, V3A, and V4, including the V2/V3 and V2/VP boundaries, are devoid of, or very poor in, callosal afferents. The pattern of callosal afferents becomes more blurred in the more anterior visual areas. The same organizational principle is likely to apply to the human visual cortex, and the pattern of human callosal afferents is likely to constitute landmarks for some visual area boundaries. We have thus identified the location of human visual areas V1, V2, V3, and VP as well as the medial boundary of V4 (Figures 21.2a and 21.2b).

FURTHER EVIDENCE FOR EXTRASTRIATE VISUAL AREAS IN HUMANS   Although the proposed subdivision of the human occipital cortex relies largely on the pattern of callosal afferents, some human visual areas appear to have distinct architectonic features as well as connectivity pattern.

Cortical architecture   We have found rather well defined myeloarchitectonic landmarks for three extrastriate visual areas: V2, VP, and V5/MT (Figures 21.2b and 21.2c; see Clarke and Miklossy, 1990). The latter area may correspond to the macaque motion area that is found in the superior temporal sulcus (Zeki, 1974; Van

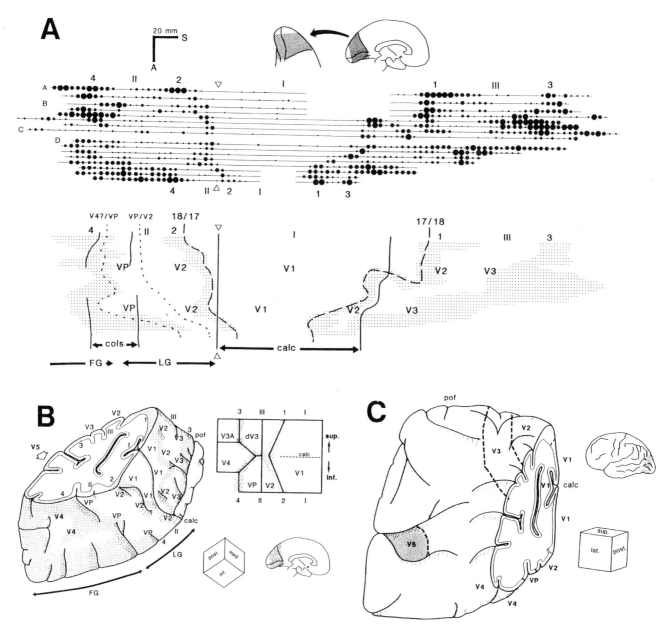

FIGURE 21.2. (A) Flat reconstruction of the medial part of the left occipital lobe showing the distribution of callosal afferents (same case as shown in Figure 21.1; from Clarke and Miklossy, 1990). The reconstructed region corresponds to the shaded portion of the brain insets but comprises also the cortex within the sulci. The spacing of charted sections is represented here by the distance between the horizontal lines. In each section, segments of callosal axons were projected onto a line running halfway between the pial surface and the bottom of the cortex. Different sizes of solid circles represent the number of callosal axons within a 2.3-mm-wide bin along this line. Open arrowheads show the position of the inferior lip of the calcarine fissure along which the sections were aligned. Roman numerals denote callosal-poor regions; I contains most of area V1, II contains area V2 medially and VP laterally, and III contains V2 medially and V3 laterally. Arabic numerals denote callosal-rich bands. In the lower half of the figure, bands of callosal afferents are represented in stippling and the position of visual areas is related to them. (B) The distribution of callosal afferents (stippled) and the locations of visual areas in a three-dimensional view of the left hemisphere of the case shown in Figures 21.1 and 21.2A (from Clarke and Miklossy, 1990). The reconstructed region corresponds to the shaded portion of the brain insets in Figures 21.1; its orientation is as shown on the cube (side = 10 mm). (C) The location of human area V5/MT (stippled), identified as a heavily myelinated region on the occipital convexity (from Clarke and Miklossy, 1990). The region reconstructed corresponds to the shaded portion of the brain inset in Figures 21.1; its orientation is as shown on the cube (side = 10 mm).

Essen et al., 1981) and can be anatomically delineated by its heavy myelination. Cytoarchitectonic correlates of human extrastriate visual areas are less clear. On the inferior part of the occipital lobe, areas V2, VP, and V4 each have a distinct architecture and show strong resemblance with areas OB, OA₁, and OA₂ (= OAₘ) of Von Economo and Koskinas (1929), respectively (Clarke and Miklossy, 1990).

Pattern of cytochrome oxidase activity The pattern of cytochrome oxidase activity was shown to vary between some of the human extrastriate visual areas (Clarke, 1994a). Cytochrome oxidase is a mitochondrial enzyme that is particularly active in regions with high metabolic activity (Wong-Riley, 1979). Histochemical revelation of cytochrome oxidase activity has proved to be useful for studying the organization of the primate visual system (for a review on macaque V1, see Wong-Riley, 1993). In the human extrastriate cortex, comparison of the cytochrome oxidase staining with cytoarchitecture and myeloarchitecture in adjacent sections led to the identification of characteristic patterns of several human extrastriate areas (Clarke, 1994a). The overall intensity of staining varied between areas: VP was very light; V2, V3, and V4 were darker; and V5/MT was very dark. Tangential sectioning of the flattened cortex confirmed differences between some of the visual areas and showed compartments of darker and lighter staining within some of the visual areas (Tootell and Taylor, 1995).

Intrahemispheric and intrinsic connectivity Very little is known about the intrahemispheric connectivity of human extrastriate visual areas, but available evidence supports a model of parallel and serial processing such as that derived from work in nonhuman primates.

By applying the carbocyanine dye DiI to human areas V1 and V2, Burkhalter and Bernardo (1989) demonstrated reciprocal connections between V1 and V2. These formed a patchy pattern, linking preferentially specific compartments in these areas and thus resembling the connectivity pattern described in macaque monkeys. The laminar origin and termination of connections between V1 and V2 suggest that these areas are organized hierarchically, V2 representing a processing stage above V1. Backprojections from V2 to V1 were partially compatible with selective connections within the magnocellular stream. Within V1, intrinsic connections were shown to connect preferentially blob or interblob regions.

The connectivity of a higher order visual area, located in the superolateral part of area 19, was studied with the Nauta method for anterogradely degenerating axons (Clarke, 1994b). Circumstantial evidence suggested that

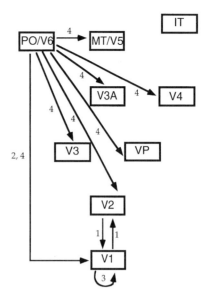

FIGURE 21.3. Intrahemispheric connectivity and putative hierarchical order of human visual areas. Macaque visual areas have been shown to be heavily interconnected in a hierarchical and parallel network (Felleman and Van Essen, 1991). Much less is known about the human intrahemispheric connections. A study using the carbocyanin dye DiI (Burkhalter and Bernardo, 1989) and another using the Nauta method (Clarke, 1994b) described efferent connections from V1 and V2 and from putative area V6/PO, respectively. The overall pattern of connections resembles that of macaque monkeys, but more studies are needed to understand fully the processing pattern within human visual cortex. (1 = Burkhalter and Bernardo, 1989; 2 = Clarke and Miklossy, 1990; 3 = Burkhalter et al., 1993; 4 = Clarke, 1994b.)

the lesion lay anterolateral to visual areas V3 and V3A (Figure 21.3), probably in the human equivalent of V6 (Zeki, 1986) or PO (Colby et al., 1988). The damaged part of cortex formed dense intrahemispheric connections to V1, V2, V3, and probably the lateral part of V4, as well as weaker connections to VP and V5/MT. The backprojections to V1 and to V2 were mainly directed to the representation of the lower paramedian part of the visual field. The pattern of long intrinsic connections within or around area V6/PO (the sixth visual area, possibly an analog of area PO) was patchy. This study revealed several principles concerning the organization of intrahemispheric connections. First, intrahemispheric connections are numerous within the occipital lobe. Second, there is a preferential connectivity between particular parts of the visual cortex. Third, there are rather strong intrahemispheric connections between areas belonging to the magnocellular stream (here putative area V6/PO) and those belonging to the parvocellular stream (here V4). Fourth, backprojections from higher-order to early-stage visual areas can be retinotopically organized. Five, the patchy pattern of intrinsic connections in V6/PO suggests that this area is segregated into functionally distinct subunits.

Thalamic connectivity of the human extrastriate cortex also suggests the existence of functionally distinct areas. Retrograde degeneration studies showed that human extrastriate visual cortex receives projections from the pulvinar (Van Buren and Borke, 1972). Anterograde tracing, using the Nauta method in a case of right fusiform gyrus infarction, demonstrated that human fusiform gyrus has a high-density projection to a subpart of the inferior pulvinar nucleus and a low-density projection to the medial pulvinar nucleus as well as in the posteroinferior part of the reticular nucleus (Clarke et al., 1999c). The lesion in this case included regions that are known to be involved in face and color recognition (for comparison with neuropsychological studies and a review of the literature, see Clarke et al., 1997, 1998b; Schoppig et al., 1999). Thus, there is a precise topographic relationship between parts of the extrastriate cortex and the pulvinar, suggesting segregated thalamocortical pathways for different parts of the extrastriate cortex.

HETEROTOPIC VISUAL CALLOSAL AFFERENTS ARE WIDELY SPREAD AND LINK HIERARCHICALLY DIFFERENT REGIONS Many influential models of human cognitive functions have presumed that human callosal connections link predominantly symmetrical parts of cortex (e.g., Geschwind, 1965, 1975). These same assumptions are still present in recent models (McIntosh et al., 1996).

PUTATIVE ROLE OF HOMOTOPIC CALLOSAL CONNECTIONS According to the locations they link, homotopic callosal connections may play different roles. In areas with precise retinotopic representation, callosal connections are found along representations of the vertical meridian (for a review, see Innocenti, 1986). Their main role is believed to be midline fusion, that is, the unification of the two hemifield representations. They have been proposed to link groups of neurons at either side of the vertical meridian in the same way as intracortical fibers link nearby neuronal representations within the same hemifield (Hubel and Wiesel, 1967). Neurons with receptive fields stretching over the midline were shown to depend for the ipsilateral part of their receptive field on callosal connections (Berlucchi and Rizzolatti, 1968; Gross, Bender, and Mishkin, 1977).

A very different role can be expected for homotopic callosal connections between functionally lateralized areas. Hemispheric specialization has often been described as the capacity of one hemisphere to process a certain type of information and to transmit it to the opposite hemisphere (see, e.g., Geschwind, 1965). Convincing demonstrations of the lack of interhemispheric transmission are left-hand apraxia and anomia following callosal section (see the specialized chapters in this volume). In the first case a motor program is elaborated in the left hemisphere but fails to be transmitted to the right hemisphere, which ensures the guidance of the left hand. In the second case, tactile information from the left hand is analyzed by the right hemisphere but fails to reach speech areas in the left hemisphere.

EXAMPLES OF HETEROTOPIC VISUAL CALLOSAL CONNECTIONS THAT MAY PLAY A PARTICULAR ROLE IN HUMAN COGNITION The distinct role that heterotopic callosal connections may play can be appreciated through a simplified model of the human striate and extrastriate visual cortex (Figure 21.4). This can be roughly subdivided into three levels. Level 1 comprises retinotopi-

Heterotopic callosal connections

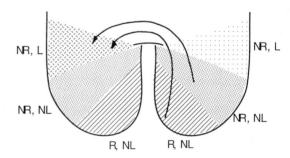

FIGURE 21.4. Heterotopic callosal connections. Schematic representation of the posterior parts of the cerebral hemispheres. Human visual areas have been subdivided into areas that are retinotopically (R) or nonretinotopically (NR) organized. Furthermore, a distinction has been made between cortical parts that support lateralized (L; e.g., speech, reading) or nonlateralized (NL; e.g., color or motion perception within early-stage visual areas) functions. Retinotopically organized, nonlateralized areas are V1, V2, V3, and VP; nonretinotopically or only loosely retinotopically organized, nonlateralized areas are V4, V5/MT, V3A, and perhaps parts of the inferior temporal cortex; nonretinotopically organized lateralized regions are the angular gyrus and Wernicke's areas, as far as the latter can be considered related to vision. The differently shaded regions may represent different levels of visual information processing. Widely spread heterotopic callosal connections may link different levels of processing and have been shown to do so in two instances: The right medio-occipital region (= R, NL) projects to the left angular gyrus (= NR, L; Clarke et al., 1995), and the right inferior temporal cortex (= NR, NL) projects to Wernicke's area (NR, L; Di Virgilio and Clarke, 1997).

cally organized visual areas V1, V2, V3, and VP. These treat visual information that falls within the contralateral visual hemifield and do not show hemispheric specialization. Level 2 comprises visual areas with a loose retinotopic organization supporting nonlateralized functions such as color or motion perception. Examples of such areas are V4, V5/MT, V3A, and possibly parts of the inferior temporal cortex. Level 3 comprises non-retinotopically organized cortex that supports lateralized functions, such as speech or reading. Examples of such cortical regions are the angular gyrus and Wernicke's area.

Heterotopic callosal connections may provide a direct link between these three levels:

1. Connections from level 1 (V1, V2, V3, VP) to level 3 (supporting lateralized functions). These connections may play a very similar role to that of the intrahemispheric connections from early-stage visual areas to lateralized regions. However, because of their region of origin, the callosal connections cover only information from parts of the visual field near the vertical meridian.

2. Connections from level 2 (e.g., V4, V5/MT, V3A, and possibly parts of the inferior temporal cortex) to level 3 (supporting lateralized functions). Nonretinotopically or only loosely retinotopically organized areas of level 2 receive information from both visual hemifields, and the whole of such an area has access mostly to the corpus callosum.

3. Backprojections from level 3 (regions supporting lateralized functions) to levels 1 or 2. These connections may play a very similar role to that of the intrahemispheric connections from lateralized regions to early-stage visual areas. However, because of their region of termination, the callosal connections will be able to influence only information processing that is pertinent to the visual field near the vertical meridian.

The role of heterotopic callosal connections between two levels may be very different from other possible routes between the two levels. Thus, direct, heterotopic callosal connections from level 1 to contralateral level 3 bypass processing in either contralateral level 1 or ipsilateral level 3.

Callosal pathways putatively involved in reading In a recent study, interhemispheric connections originating in the medial part of the right occipital lobe were traced by using the Nauta method (Clarke et al., 1995). Serial coronal sections from the posterior third of the hemisphere contralateral to the lesion were stained and analyzed for anterogradely degenerating axons, that is, interhemispheric afferents from the damaged site. The pattern of callosal afferents within early-stage visual areas was as described in a previous paper (Figures 21.1 and 21.2; Clarke and Miklossy, 1990). However, the newly analyzed cortex included also the posterior parietal and temporal cortex. Both these regions received medium to high density of callosal afferents originating in the contralateral medio-occipital cortex. Among the callosal-recipient regions was the (left) angular gyrus.

Dejerine (1882) reported a case of pure alexia following lesion in the left calcarine region and the splenium of the corpus callosum (Dejerine and Vialet, 1883). The alexia was attributed to disconnection of the right, non-injured calcarine region from the left angular gyrus, which was proposed to be involved in reading. There are at least three possible routes by which visual information from the right calcarine region might reach the left angular gyrus. The first route is a combination of homotopic callosal connections from the right calcarine region to the left one and then association connections from the left calcarine region to the left angular gyrus. The second route is a heterotopic callosal connection from the right calcarine region directly to the left angular gyrus. The third route is a combination of association connections from the right calcarine region to the right angular gyrus and then a homotopic callosal connection from the right angular gyrus to its homologue on the left side. Neuropsychological evidence shows that the ability to read does not rely critically on the first route. Lesions that were limited to the medial and inferior occipital lobe alone were not found to be associated with reading deficits; a lesion of the callosal pathway was needed for alexia to occur (Binder and Mohr, 1992). The second route, that is, a monosynaptic pathway from the right calcarine region to the left angular gyrus has been described in humans (see above), but it is unknown whether this route alone can sustain reading.

The more general question that arises is whether different callosal pathways can support different reading strategies. It might be argued that heterotopic callosal connections from the right calcarine region to the left angular gyrus transmit low-level visual information, which is then treated by the left-hemisphere paradigms. The alternative route from the right calcarine region via the right angular gyrus to the left angular gyrus might participate in right-hemisphere paradigms of reading (Zaidel and Peters, 1981). One hypothesis that I would like to propose and that would be amenable to experimental studies is that the heterotopic route (i.e., the second in the above scheme) is essential for normal reading strategies and that the homotopic route via the right angular gyrus plays a role in alternative reading strategies, such as are observed in deep dyslexia. Although precise anatomical correlates are unknown, reading capacities that are spared in deep dyslexia are believed to depend on right-hemisphere processing (Coltheart, 1980).

For reasons of simplification the above account of possible reading pathways concentrates on three possible routes. It is obvious, however, that a multitude of other pathways could be involved, including homotopic and heterotopic callosal connections of other parts of the extrastriate cortex.

Visual callosal input to speech areas: Where vision and speech meet Recently, we analyzed interhemispheric connections from the right inferior temporal lobe to Broca's and Wernicke's areas (Di Virgilio and Clarke, 1997). The lesion from which connections were traced was in the middle portion of the fusiform and parahippocampal gyri and the hippocampal formation. Serial sections through Broca's and Wernicke's areas were stained and analyzed for anterogradely degenerating axons. Degen-erating axon segments were found in the posterior part of the superior temporal gyrus, the planum temporale, and the supramarginal gyrus—that is, in all parts that are believed to belong to Wernicke's area. They were also found, but in lesser densities, in the triangular and opercular parts of the inferior frontal gyrus, that is, in Broca's area.

The right inferior temporal cortex is known to be involved in high-level visual functions. The lesion from which the interhemispheric connections were traced was within a region that is known to be activated selectively in tasks of recognition of known faces (comparison of lesion site and activation foci reported by Sergent, Ohta, and MacDonald, 1992) and the lesion of which is accompanied by prosopagnosia (Clarke et al., 1997). The interhemispheric pathways described here are part of what is most likely a large network linking higher-order visual and speech areas, including widely spread intra-hemispheric and homotopic and heterotopic interhemi-spheric connections (Figure 21.5). When parts of this

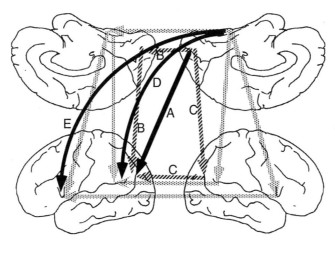

Direct heterotopic interhemispheric connections:
A: from right calcarine region to left angular gyrus
D: from right inferior temporal cortex to Wernicke's area
E: from right inferior temporal cortex to Broca's area

Multistage pathways with homotopic interhemispheric connections (as proposed by classical models):
✏ from right calcarine region to left angular gyrus (presumed role in reading)
▦ from right inferior temporal cortex to Wernicke's and Broca's areas (putative role in naming)

FIGURE 21.5. Heterotopic interhemispheric connections that have been demonstrated anatomically in humans (black arrows) and the pathways that were proposed in classical models (shaded arrows). (A) Direct, monosynaptic connections were found to link the right calcarine region to the left angular gyrus (Clarke et al., 1995); this may be one of several pathways (B, C) involved in reading (see text). (D, E): Direct, monosynaptic connections were demonstrated from the inferior temporal cortex to Wernicke's and Broca's areas (Di Virgilio and Clarke, 1997); this is part of a most likely large network linking higher-order visual and speech areas and sustaining visuoverbal functions. (From Clarke, 1998.)

network are damaged, processing within the remaining parts determines spared capacities. It is conceivable that connections from the right inferior temporal cortex to the speech areas may play a role in successful phonemic cuing observed in otherwise anomic patients (see, e.g., a case reported by Semanza and Sgaramella, 1993). Simultaneous auditory (i.e., the first phoneme of the target name) and visual input (i.e., the presented object or face) in both Wernicke's and Broca's areas may be strong enough to initiate correct naming.

EXTRASPLENIAL VISUAL INTERHEMISPHERIC PATHWAYS Human primary, secondary, third, and fourth visual areas have been shown to have a strict retinotopic representation of the contralateral visual hemifield, whereas the motion area V5/MT has a bilateral representation (Tootell et al., 1995). In analogy to nonhuman primates it has been proposed that activation by stimuli presented in the visual hemifield ipsilateral to the analyzed area V5/MT is mediated via the corpus callosum. We have tested this hypothesis by examining the interhemispheric transfer of visual information in a patient who sustained damage to the posterior half of the corpus callosum (Clarke et al., 2000b). On tachistoscopical left-hemifield presentation the patient was severely impaired in reading letters, words, and geographical names and moderately impaired in naming pictures and colors. In contrast, interhemispheric transfer of visual motion information was preserved. Pattern of cerebral activation elicited by apparent motion stimuli was studied with fMRI and compared to that of normal subjects. In normal subjects, apparent motion stimuli, as compared to darkness, activated strongly striate and extrastriate cortex. When stimuli were presented to one hemifield only, the contralateral calcarine region was activated, while regions on the occipital convexity, including putative area V5, were activated bilaterally. A similar activation pattern was found in the patient with the posterior callosal lesion; unilateral left- or right-hemifield stimulation was accompanied by activation on contralateral and ipsilateral occipital convexity. This observation suggests that interhemispheric transfer of visual motion information does not rely uniquely on the posterior two thirds of the corpus callosum and that other probably subcortical parallel pathways may be involved (Tordif and Clarke, 2002).

Parallel processing and parallel pathways outside the visual cortex

There is increasing evidence that different aspects of auditory information are processed in parallel. Studies of brain-damaged patients demonstrated that different types of sound analysis can be disrupted independently: discrimination of the acoustic trace belonging to one sound source from a background (segregation of sound objects); semantic identification; and asemantic recognition, defined as the capacity to judge whether two different sound samples belong to the same object (Clarke et al., 1996). In a recent study of auditory short-term memory in normal subjects, we further demonstrated the independence of processing concerned with sound content and that concerned with sound localization (Clarke et al., 1998a). This dichotomy between recognition and localization was confirmed by our subsequent observations of selective deficits in patients with circumscribed hemispheric lesions. On the basis of anatomoclinical correlations of our cases and comparison with our previous anatomical studies, we have proposed the existence of two anatomically distinct auditory-processing pathways (Clarke et al., 2000a).

Anatomical studies have revealed several organizational characteristics that are compatible with parallel processing of auditory information. Histochemical studies of normal human brains visualized several distinct areas around the primary auditory cortex (Rivier and Clarke, 1987). Using cytochrome oxidase staining, we visualized distinct compartments (stripes) in the human primary auditory cortex (Clarke and Rivier, 1998). Thus, the human auditory cortex displays two characteristics that have been shown to be closely linked to parallel processing within the visual system: a compartmentalization within the primary cortex and the presence of multiple early-stage areas.

Parallel interhemispheric pathways are found beyond the human visual cortex. In a recent study we investigated the connectivity of the human anterior commissure in six adult cases that had circumscribed hemispheric lesions in temporal, frontal, parietal, or occipital cortices or in infrapallidal white matter; the method used was the Nauta method for anterogradely degenerating axons (Di Virgilio et al., 1999). We confirmed that a large number of anterior commissure axons originate in the inferior temporal cortex, but we also showed that in humans other regions, such as the inferior part of the occipital lobe, the occipital convexity, and possibly the central fissure and the prefrontal convexity, contribute also to the anterior commissure (Figure 21.6). Axons originating in the inferior temporal cortex terminated not only in homotopic but also in heterotopic targets in the opposite hemisphere. Among the latter were the amygdala and possibly the orbitofrontal cortex. These data suggest that the human anterior commissure conveys axons from much larger territories than expected from work on nonhuman primates.

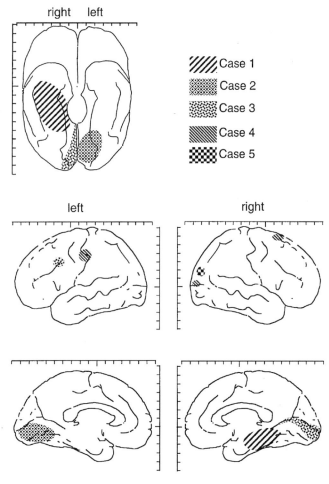

FIGURE 21.6. The locations of lesions that yielded anterograde degeneration in the anterior commissure (from Di Virgilio et al., 1999). The lesions were assessed in Talairach coordinates to allow interindividual comparisons.

REFERENCES

BERLUCCHI, G., and G. RIZZOLATTI, 1968. Binocularly driven neurons in visual cortex of split-chiasm cats. *Science* 159: 308–310.

BINDER, J. R., and J. P. MOHR, 1992. The topography of callosal reading pathways: A case-control analysis. *Brain* 115:1807–1826.

BURKHALTER, A., and K. L. BERNARDO, 1989. Organization of corticocortical connections in human visual cortex. *Proc. Natl. Acad. Sci. U.S.A.* 86:1071–1075.

CLARKE, S., 1994a. Modular organisation of human extrastriate visual cortex: Evidence from cytochrome oxidase pattern in normal and macular degeneration cases. *Eur. J. Neurosci.* 6:725–736.

CLARKE, S., 1994b. Association and intrinsic connections of human extrastriate visual cortex. *Proc. R. Soc. Lond. B* 257: 87–89.

CLARKE, S., 1998. Neural basis for neuropsychological rehabilitation. *Swiss Arch. Neurol. Psychiatry* 149:73–79.

CLARKE, S., M. ADRIANI, and A. BELLMANN, 1998a. Distinct short-term memory systems for sound content and sound localization. *NeuroReport* 9:3433–3437.

CLARKE, S., A. BELLMANN, F. DE RIBAUPIERRE, and G. ASSAL, 1996. Non-verbal auditory recognition in normal subjects and brain-damaged patients: Evidence for parallel processing. *Neuropsychologia* 34:587–603.

CLARKE, S., A. BELLMANN, R. A. MEULI, G. ASSAL, and A. J. STECK, 2000a. Auditory agnosia and auditory spatial deficits following left hemispheric lesions: Evidence for distinct processing pathways. *Neuropsychologia* 38:797–807.

CLARKE, S., A. LINDEMANN, P. MAEDER, F. X. BORRUAT, and G. ASSAL, 1997. Face recognition and postero-inferior hemispheric lesions. *Neuropsychologia* 35:1555–1563.

CLARKE, S., P. MAEDER, R. MEULI, F. STÁUB, A. BELLMANN, L. REGLI, N. DE TRIBOLET, and G. ASSAL, 2000b. Interhemispheric transfer of visual motion information after posterior callosal lesion: Neuropsychological and fMRI study. *Exp. Brain Res.* 132:127–133.

CLARKE, S., and J. MIKLOSSY, 1990. Occipital cortex in man: Organization of callosal connections, related myelo- and cytoarchitecture, and putative boundaries of functional visual areas. *J. Comp. Neurol.* 298:188–214.

CLARKE, S., S. RIAHI-ARYA, E. TARDIF, A. C. COTTIER ESKENASY, and A. PROBST, 1999. Thalamic projections of the fusiform gyrus in man. *Eur. J. Neurosci.* 11:1835–1838.

CLARKE, S., and F. RIVIER, 1998. Compartments within human primary auditory cortex: Evidence from cytochrome oxidase and acetylcholinesterase staining. *Eur. J. Neurosci.* 10:741–745.

CLARKE, S., D. C. VAN ESSEN, N. HADJIKHANI, H. DRURY, and T. A. COOGAN, 1995. Understanding human area 19 and 37: Contribution of two-dimensional maps of visual callosal afferents. *Hum. Brain Mapp. Suppl.* 1:33.

CLARKE, S., V. WALSH, A. SCHOPIG, G. ASSAL, and A. COWEY, 1998b. Colour constancy impairments in patients with lesions of the prestriate cortex. *Exp. Brain Res.* 123:154–158.

COLBY, C. L., R. GATTASS, C. R. OLSON, and C. G. GROSS, 1988. Topographical organization of cortical afferents to extrastriate visual area PO in the macaque: A dual tracer study. *J. Comp. Neurol.* 269:392–413.

COLTHEART, M., 1980. Deep dyslexia: A right-hemisphere hypothesis. In *Deep Dyslexia*, K. E. Patterson and J. C. Marshall, eds. London: Routledge and Kegan Paul, pp. 326–380.

CORBETTA, M., F. M. MIEZIN, S. DOBMEYER, G. L. SHULMAN, and S. E. PETERSEN, 1990. Attentional modulation of neuronal processing of shape, color, and velocity in humans. *Science* 248:1556–1559.

DEJERINE, J., 1892. Contribution à l'étude anatomo-pathologique et clinique des différentes variétés de cécité verbale. *C. R. Hebdomadaires Scéances Mémoires Soc. Biol.* 4:61–90.

DEJERINE, J., and J. N. VIALET, 1893. Contribution à l'étude de la localisation de la cécité verbale pure. *C. R. Hebdomadaires Scéances Mémoires Soc. Biol.* 5:790–793.

DEYOE, E. A., G. CARMAN, P. BANDETTINI, S. GLICKMAN, J. WIESER, R. COX, D. MILLER, and J. NEITZ, 1996. Mapping striate and extrastriate visual areas in human cerebral cortex. *Proc. Natl. Acad. Sci. U.S.A.* 93:2382–2386.

DI VIRGILIO, G., and S. CLARKE, 1997. Direct interhemispheric visual input to human speech areas. *Hum. Brain Mapp.* 5:347–354.

Di Virgilio, G., S. Clarke, G. Pizzolato, and T. Schaffner, 1999. Cortical regions contributing to the anterior commissure in man. *Exp. Brain Res.* 124:1–7.

Felleman, D. J., and D. C. Van Essen, 1991. Distributed hierarchical processing in the primate cerebral cortex. *Cereb. Cortex* 1:1–47.

Geschwind, N., 1965. Disconnexion syndromes in animals and man. *Brain* 88:237–294, 585–644.

Geschwind, N., 1975. The apraxias: Neural mechanisms of disorders of learned movement. *Am. Scientist* 63:188–195.

Glickstein, M., and D. Whitteridge, 1976. Degeneration of layer III pyramidal cells in area 18 following destruction of callosal input. *Brain Res.* 104:148–151.

Gross, C. G., D. B. Bender, and M. Mishkin, 1977. Contributions of the corpus callosum and the anterior commissure to visual activation of inferior temporal neurons. *Brain Res.* 131:227–239.

Gulyas, B., and P. E. Roland, 1991. Cortical fields participating in form and colour discrimination in the human brain. *NeuroReport* 2:585–588.

Hubel, D. H., and T. N. Wiesel, 1967. Cortical and callosal connections concerned with the vertical meridian of visual fields in the cat. *J. Neurophysiol.* 30:1561–1573.

Innocenti, G. M., 1986. General organization of callosal connections in the cerebral cortex. In *Cerebral Cortex*, Vol. 5, E. G. Jones and A. Peters, eds. New York: Plenum Press, pp. 291–353.

Livingstone, M. S., and D. H. Hubel, 1984. Anatomy and physiology of a color system in the primate visual cortex. *J. Neurosci.* 4:309–356.

Livingstone, M. S., and D. H. Hubel, 1987a. Connections between layer 4B of area 17 and the thick cytochrome oxidase stripes of area 18 in the squirrel monkey. *J. Neurosci.* 7:3371–3377.

Livingstone, M. S., and D. H. Hubel, 1987b. Psychophysical evidence for separate channels for the perception of form, color, movement, and depth. *J. Neurosci.* 7:3416–3468.

Lueck, C. J., S. Zeki, K. J. Friston, M. P. Deiber, P. Cope, V. J. Cunningham, A. A. Lummertsma, C. Kennard, and R. S. J. Frackowiak, 1989. The colour centre in the cerebral cortex of man. *Nature* 430:386–389.

McIntosh, A. R., C. L. Grady, J. V. Haxby, L. G. Ungerleider, and B. Horwitz, 1996. Changes in limbic and prefrontal functional interactions in a working memory task for faces. *Cereb. Cortex* 6:571–584.

Rivier, F., and S. Clarke, 1997. Cytochrome oxidase, acetylcholinesterase and NADPH-diaphorase staining in human supratemporal and insular cortex: Evidence for multiple auditory areas. *NeuroImage* 6:288–304.

Schoppig, A., S. Clarke, V. Walsh, G. Assal, and A. Cowey, 1999. Short-term memory for colour following posterior hemispheric lesions in man. *NeuroReport* 10:1379–1384.

Semanza, C., and T. M. Sgaramella, 1993. Production of proper names: A clinical case study of the effects of phenemic cueing. *Memory* 1:249–263.

Sereno, M. I., A. M. Dale, J. B. Reppas, K. K. Kwong, J. W. Belliveau, T. J. Brady, B. R. Rosen, and R. B. H. Tootell, 1995. Borders of multiple visual areas in humans revealed by functional magnetic resonance imaging. *Science* 268:889–893.

Sergent, J., S. Ohta, and B. MacDonald, 1992. Functional neuroanatomy of face and object processing: A positron emission tomography study. *Brain* 115:15–36.

Shipp, S., and S. Zeki, 1985. Segregation of pathways leading from area V2 to areas V4 and V5 of macaque monkey visual cortex. *Nature* 315:322–325.

Shoumura, K., T. Ando, and K. Kato, 1975. Structural organization of "callosal" OBg in human corpus callosum agenesis. *Brain Res.* 93:241–252.

Tordif, E., and S. Clarke, 2002. Commissural connections of human superior colliculus. *Neuroscience* 111:363–372.

Tootell, R. B. H., J. B. Reppas, K. K. Kwong, R. Malach, R. T. Born, T. J. Brady, B. R. Rosen, and J. W. Belliveau, 1995. Functional analysis of human MT and related visual cortical areas using magnetic resonance imaging. *J. Neurosci.* 15:3215–3230.

Tootell, R. B. H., and J. B. Taylor, 1995. Anatomical evidence for MT and additional cortical visual areas in humans. *Cereb. Cortex* 5:39–55.

Van Buren, J. M., and C. Borke, 1972. *Variations and Connections of the Human Thalamus.* New York: Springer-Verlag.

Van Essen, D. C., S. Clarke, N. Hadjikhani, H. Drury, T. A. Coogan, G. Carman, and R. Kraftsik, 1995. Two-dimensional maps of visual callosal projections in human extrastriate cortex. *Soc. Neurosci. Abstr.* 20:428.

Van Essen, D. C., J. H. R. Maunsell, and J. L. Bixby, 1981. The middle temporal visual area in the macaque: Myeloarchitecture, connections, functional properties and topographic organization. *J. Comp. Neurol.* 199:293–326.

Van Essen, D. C., W. T. Newsome, and J. L. Bixby, 1982. The pattern of interhemispheric connections and its relationship to extrastriate visual areas in the macaque monkey. *J. Neurosci.* 2:265–283.

Van Essen, D. C., and S. M. Zeki, 1978. The topographic organization of rhesus monkey prestriate cortex. *J. Physiol.* 277:193–226.

Van Valkenburg, C. T., 1908. Zur anatomie der projektions- und balkenstrahlung des hinterhauptlappens sowie des cingulum. *Monatsschr. Psychiatr. Neurol.* 24:320–339.

Von Economo, C., and G. N. Koskinas, 1925. *Die Cytoarchitectonik der Hirnrinde des Erwachsenen Menschen.* Berlin: Julius Springer.

Watson, J. D., R. Myers, R. S. Frackowiak, J. V. Hajnal, R. P. Woods, J. C. Mazziotta, S. Shipp, and S. Zeki, 1993. Area V5 of the human brain: Evidence from a combined study using positron emission tomography and magnetic resonance imaging. *Cereb. Cortex* 3:79–94.

Wong-Riley, M. T. T., 1979. Changes in the visual system of monocularly sutured or enucleated cats demonstrable with cytochrome oxidase histochemistry. *Brain Res.* 171:11–28.

Wong-Riley, M. T. T., 1993. Primate visual cortex: Dynamic metabolic organization and plasticity revealed by cytochrome oxidase. In *Cerebral Cortex*, Vol. 10, A. Peters and K. S. Rockland, eds. New York: Plenum Press, pp. 291–353.

Zaidel, E., and A. M. Peters, 1981. Phonological encoding and ideographic reading by the disconnected right hemisphere: Two case studies. *Brain Lang.* 14:205–234.

Zeki, S. M., 1970. Interhemispheric connections of prestriate cortex in monkey. *Brain Res.* 19:63–75.

Zeki, S. M., 1973. Colour coding in rhesus monkey prestriate cortex. *Brain Res.* 53:422–427.

Zeki, S. M., 1974. Functional organization of a visual area in the posterior bank of the superior temporal sulcus of the rhesus monkey. *J. Physiol. (Lond.)* 236:549–573.

ZEKI, S. M., 1977. Simultaneous anatomical demonstration of the vertical and horizontal meridians in areas V2 and V3 of rhesus monkey visual cortex. *Proc. R. Soc. Lond. B* 195:517–523.

ZEKI, S. M., 1978. Functional specialization in the visual cortex of the rhesus monkey. *Nature* 274:423–428.

ZEKI, S., 1986. The anatomy and physiology of area V6 of macaque monkey visual cortex. *J. Physiol. (Lond.)* 381:62P.

ZEKI, S., J. D. WATSON, C. J. LUECK, K. J. FRISTON, C. KENNARD, and R. FRACKOWIAK, 1991. A direct demonstration of functional specialization in human visual cortex. *J. Neurosci.* 11:641–649.

ZILLES, K., and S. CLARKE, 1997. Architecture, connectivity and transmitter receptors of human extrastriate cortex: Comparison with non-human primates. In *Cerebral Cortex*, Vol. 12: *Extrastriate Cortex in Primates*, K. S. Rockland, J. H. Kaas, and A. Peters, eds. New York: Plenum Press, pp. 673–742.

Commentary 21.1

Learning to Read and Write Shapes the Anatomy and Function of the Corpus Callosum

ALEXANDRE CASTRO-CALDAS, ALEXANDRA REIS, PEDRO CAVALEIRO MIRANDA, AND
EDUARDO DUCLA-SOARES

ABSTRACT The function and shape of the corpus callosum may be influenced by literacy. Two pieces of evidence are reported. The first one addressed the study of hand movements controlling a target in a screen. There were differences in performance between literate and illiterate subjects. In the second study the morphology of the corpus callosum was compared in two groups, literate and illiterate women. The region where interparietal fibres are thought to cross is thinner in illiterates.

The study of callosal function embodies almost all chapters of cognitive neuroscience. This book deals with anatomic and functional aspects of the corpus callosum, in particular the effects of stimulus and task manipulations on the normal interhemispheric crossing of information. The book also addresses the clinical manifestations of pathologic states such as agenesis, callosotomy, and multiple sclerosis.

Among these aspects, the relationship between reading abilities and callosal function remains to be understood. Clarke addresses homotopy and heterotopy in posterior callosal connections. Here, we focus on the relationship between the morphometry of callosal channels and their functions. Although the exact nature of the connection between callosal structure and function is unknown, differences in the shape of the corpus callosum have been reported between normal readers and dyslexics (Duara et al., 1991; Hynd et al., 1995). The reports vary concerning the region of the corpus cal-

ALEXANDRE CASTRO-CALDAS Language Research Laboratory, Centro de Estudos Egas Moniz, Hospital de Santa Maria, Lisbon, Portugal.
ALEXANDRA REIS Area Departamental de Psicologia, F.C.H.S., Campus de Gambelas, Universidade do Algarve, Faro, Portugal.
PEDRO CAVALEIRO MIRANDA AND EDUARDO DUCLA-SOARES Institute of Biophysics and Biomedical Engineering, Centro de Neurociências de Lisboa, Hospital de Santa Maria, Lisbon, Portugal.

losum involved in this difference and whether it corresponds to a small or large contingent of crossing fibers. Within the dyslexic population, variations have been shown in the anatomy as well as the function of the corpus callosum. The findings reported by Brown (1996) in adult dyslexics have shown that interhemispheric transfer time (IHTT) was greater when compared to normal readers. This is particularly interesting in comparison to results reported in children (Davidson and Saron, 1992), as dyslexic children have faster IHTT than do controls.

It has been established that the corpus callosum changes in structure, shape, and function with age (Cowell et al., 1992; Pujol et al., 1993). Genetics play an important role in this maturational process, as was shown in the study by Oppenheim and colleagues (1989) with identical twins. However, in that same study, small differences were apparent between brothers, suggesting a certain degree of external influence in the development of the biological process. A study of musicians further supports the hypothesis that the training of a certain task may influence biological development (Elbert et al., 1995).

It is precisely the matter of the influence of external factors on the morphology of the brain that motivated our present research on illiteracy. First, a definition of the experimental population must be presented. All studies are performed comparing two populations that differ, as exclusively as possible, in the ability for matching graphemes to phonemes. They are matched for intelligence, cultural background, gender, and age. A significant part of the population is illiterate in certain regions of Portugal as the result of social factors. Fifty years ago, schools were scarce, and children were frequently required to walk long distances to attend classes. Most of the older girls did not acquire a formal education because they were needed at home to care for younger siblings. It is very common nowadays to find sisters living close by and leading similar lives, the older being illiterate and the younger literate.

Comparing the performances of these two groups revealed differences in oral language processing. These differences became apparent in testing both normal and brain-damaged subjects (Castro-Caldas, Reis, and Parreira, 1994; Reis and Castro-Caldas, 1997). Those who never learned how to match a phoneme to a grapheme in childhood have difficulties in repeating plausible pseudo-words, being untrained in using language phonology. The illiterate subjects prefer to use a semantic reference system. When these subjects became aphasic, their repetition of words and phrases deteriorated when oral comprehension was poor; that is, there were only rare cases of transcortical sensory aphasia in illiterates (Castro-Caldas et al., 1994). At the same time, the pattern of activation observed with PET scans also revealed differences, suggesting that if illiterate subjects are poor performers in a task, this is because they are not using the same neural substrate as do literate subjects (Castro-Caldas et al., 1998b).

What may be concluded so far is that the absence of the formal learning of a specific task of matching a phoneme to a grapheme at the proper age affects or determines the future functional organization of the brain.

Bearing in mind this information and considering the results reported in dyslexia, we decided to study the corpus callosum of illiterate subjects from both the functional (Reis and Castro-Caldas, 1997) and morphological points of view (Castro-Caldas et al., 1999).

Functional study

The processing of written language is a lateralized function that interacts constantly with processes of both sides of the brain. Reading activity brings together the visual scanning of space, which is dependent on the right hemisphere, and graphemic-phonemic matching, which is dependent on the left hemisphere. Writing activity also stimulates parallel processing in both hemispheres, which certainly stimulates transcallosal crossing of information. Therefore, the acquisition of reading and writing habits may promote an increase in transfer of information between the right and left hemispheres. The purpose of the present study was to design a functional task simulating the visuomotor components of writing and compare the performance of literate and illiterate non-brain-damaged subjects on the task.

MATERIAL AND METHODS

Subjects Twenty-two women from the same sociocultural background were selected. Eleven were illiterate

(mean age $= 64.2 \pm 3.1$), and eleven were literate (mean age $= 61.1 \pm 4.7$; mean years of schooling $= 5.6 \pm 2.3$). All the subjects were strongly right-handed (assessed by a 10-item questionnaire). Subjects were matched for intelligence on the basis of a questionnaire adapted for low cultural levels, and brain lesions were carefully ruled out by clinical methods. None of the subjects in either group had had any previous experience in handling the mouse of a computer.

Procedures The experiments were run on an IBM-compatible personal computer, with stimuli being displayed on a color screen (22×16 cm). One hundred and sixty target stimuli (yellow squares; 80 left visual field, 80 right visual field), appeared randomly on the screen. The subjects were required to signal lateralized target stimuli (a yellow square turns red) by handling the mouse of the computer. Subjects fixated on a point located at the center of the screen between the appearances of the stimuli. Execution time between target appearance and target detection was measured. Half of the subjects started with their right hand, the other half with their left, alternating hands every 20 stimuli. There was a training session with both hands.

RESULTS

To analyze the effect of being literate or illiterate on the variables involved (right/left hand and right/left side of the screen) a three-way ANOVA was done (repeated measures), using the sum of execution time (in milliseconds) for each subject as the dependent variable. This analysis included three factors: (1) subject's literacy (G, illiterate versus literate); (2) hand used in the task (H, right versus left); (3) side of the screen where the stimulus was presented (SS, right versus left).

As can be seen in Table 21.1, there was a group effect ($p = 0.002$), no hand effect ($p = 0.076$), and no interaction between group and hand ($p = 0.74$), suggesting that the two groups behave similarly regarding individual hand performance (Figure 21.7a). Figure 21.7a also shows that literate subjects were faster than illiterate

TABLE 21.1

Analysis of variance, G (group) $\times$ H (hand) $\times$ SS (side of screen)

Source of Variance	$F(1, 20)$	p
Group (G)	13.1	0.002
Hand (H)	3.5	0.076
Side of screen (SS)	14.2	0.001
G $\times$ H	0.11	0.74
G $\times$ SS	11.6	0.003
H $\times$ SS	0.0003	0.99
G $\times$ H $\times$ SS	0.14	0.72

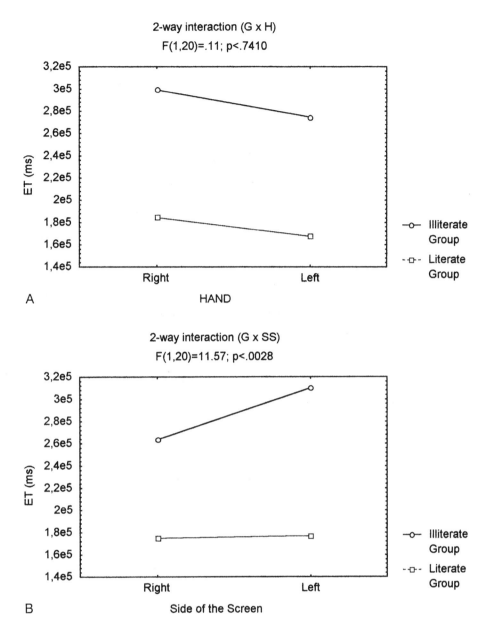

2-way interaction (G x H)

F(1,20)=.11; p<.7410

A

HAND

2-way interaction (G x SS)

F(1,20)=11.57; p<.0028

B

Side of the Screen

FIGURE 21.7. (A) Literate subjects are faster than illiterate ones with both hands, but there is no evidence of different hand preference between the groups. (B) Illiterate subjects are slow when the stimulus appeared in the left side of the screen.

ones, with both the right hand (Mann-Whitney Test, $U = 22$; $p = 0.012$) and the left hand (Mann-Whitney Test, $U = 16$; $p = 0.0035$), but no significant differences between right and left hands were found for either group (Wilcoxon matched pairs test; for illiterate, $T = 23$, $p = 0.37$, and for literate, $T = 14$, $p = 0.09$). This explains the absence of an interaction between group and hand.

As can be seen in Table 21.1, the side of the screen where the stimuli were presented was also a source of significant difference ($p = 0.001$), and there was also a significant interaction of this variable with group ($p = 0.003$). Figure 21.7b shows that the illiterate group

was slower when the stimulus appeared on the left side of the screen than when it was on the right side (Wilcoxon matched pairs test, $T = 5$, $p = 0.012$). This was not the case for the literate group (Wilcoxon matched pairs test, $T = 27$, $p = 0.59$).

COMMENTS The results of this experiment for the illiterate subjects showed that the overall execution time was slower on the left side of the screen. It is possible that these differences indicate that the absence of learning to read and write at the proper time of life influences the development of bihemispheric processing of information related to visuomotor activities. Reading and writing are highly trained visuospatial processes, involving space scanning and motor planning. There is right-hemisphere superiority in tasks involving left-side scanning and a left-hemisphere preference for propositional motor planning. In this view, the practice in reading and writing increases the cross-talk between the hemispheres, and it is in the crossed condition that illiterate subjects are slower.

The observation of this functional difference between literate and illiterate subjects prompted us to look for morphological differences in their callosa.

Morphological study

MATERIALS AND METHODS Owing to potential variations in callosal shape and size with gender, handedness, and age, only true right-handed women, 50–70 years of age, were included in the study. The sample population thus consisted of 41 right-handed women, of whom 18 were illiterate (with an average age of 62.6 ± 5.6) and 23 were literate (with an average age of 59.9 ± 6.1 and a range of 3–16 years of literacy instruction, mean = 8.5 ± 5.1). Hand preference was assessed by a standard questionnaire about common hand use for nine tasks. Selection of cases was based on the same criteria as defined for the first study.

MRI examinations of the midsagittal section were performed with a GE (Signa) 1.5 T scanner, typically using a T1-weighted image, matrix size of 256×192 and a slice thickness of 5 mm.

The outline of each CC was digitized by manually tracing over the film using a digitizing stylus (3Space from Polhemus). The procedure was carried out blindly by two independent examiners after having mutually agreed on the limits of the CC. The precision of the digitizer was approximately 0.3 mm.

The contours were analyzed according to the method described by Denenberg and colleagues (1991), in which the CCs are divided into 100 parts. Two points are chosen, one in the genu and one in the splenium, and the ventral and dorsal perimeters are divided into 100 segments of equal length. Corresponding pairs of points in the two perimeters are joined, forming 99 widths. The criterion for choosing the two terminal points is that the sum of the widths, Σw, should be minimum.

For each set of tracings, the mean size of each width was calculated separately for the two populations. The differences in widths between the literate and illiterate populations were tested for statistical significance by using the (two-tailed) Mann-Whitney test.

RESULTS The first stage of the data analysis produced two estimates of the 99 widths for 41 CCs. For each

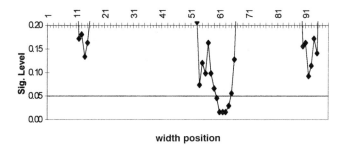

FIGURE 21.8. The p-value for the difference between the widths. In region 60–64 the mean widths for the illiterate population are significantly smaller ($p < 0.05$). The average width over the five slices 60–64 is 5.0 ± 0.2 mm for the literate subjects and 4.2 ± 0.2 mm for the illiterate ones ($p < 0.05$). The right side of the figure corresponds to posterior region of the CC, and the left corresponds to the anterior region. The section in which the difference is significant corresponds to the crossing of parietal fibers.

width the probability plots indicate departures from the normal distribution. The two population means were therefore compared by using the Mann-Whitney test.

The two sets of traces were comparable and were therefore averaged together. The results for the latter case are shown in Figure 21.8. The region around width 62 is consistently and significantly smaller in illiterate subjects in each of the two sets of traces as well as in their average. This region corresponds to fibers connecting parietal associative areas (Pandya and Kuypers, 1969).

Further statistical analysis based on factor analysis revealed six factors. There was a significant interaction between some factors and literacy. Literates had larger regions around the posterior midbody (widths 46–64), whereas illiterates had larger regions at the rostral and caudal tips of the callosum (widths 1–4 and 94–99) (Castro-Caldas et al., 1999).

COMMENTS Connection between the two parietal cortices occurs in the most anterior part of the posterior third of the CC (Pandya and Kuypers, 1969). In our study, some differences were found, suggesting a smaller contingent of fibers crossing the CC coming from association parietal cortices in illiterate subjects.

We suggest that the absence of a frequent practice of reading and writing, which stimulates the bihemispherical parallel neural network, leads to a poor development of transcallosal connections in that specific region, resulting in developmental arrest of this portion relative to normally schooled individuals. This result may support the findings reported in the functional study.

Furthermore, recent evidence suggests that the knowledge of orthography contributes to an increased cross-talk between parietal areas of both hemispheres.

Taking in consideration several regions of interest, activity measured in PET during word and pseudo-word repetition was compared between hemispheres. The differences between groups showed a dissociation between the superior and inferior parts of the angular/supramarginal regions. The superior part was more active on the left than on the right in illiterate subjects compared to literate subjects, while the inferior part and the precuneous were more active on the right than on the left in illiterate subjects compared to literate subjects (Castro-Caldas et al., 1998a).

ACKNOWLEDGMENTS Supported in part by JNICT: project Praxis XXI (A.R.) and project STRIDE (352/92).

REFERENCES

BROWN, W. S., 1996. *Clinical Syndromes of Callosal Malfunction and Cognitive Dysfunction*. Paper presented at the NATO Advanced Studies Institute, Italy, September.

CASTRO-CALDAS, A., P. CAVALEIRO MIRANDA, I. CARMO, A. REIS, F. LEOTE, C. RIBEIRO, and E. DUCLA-SOARES, 1999. Influence of learning to read and write on the morphology of the corpus callosum. *Eu. J. Neurol.* 6:23–28.

CASTRO-CALDAS, A., K. M. PETERSON, A. REIS, S. ASKELOF, and M. INGVAR, 1998a. Differences in inter-hemispheric interactions related to literacy, assessed by PET. *Neurology* 50:A43.

CASTRO-CALDAS, A., K. M. PETERSON, A. REIS, S. STONE-ELANDER, and M. INGVAR, 1998b. The illiterate brain: Learning to read and write during childhood influences the functional organization of the adult brain. *Brain* 121:1053–1063.

CASTRO-CALDAS, A., A. REIS, and E. PARREIRA, 1994. *Word Repetition by Illiterate Aphasics: The Importance of the Phonological Awareness*. Paper presented at Research Group Aphasia and Cognitive Disorders, W.F.N., Budapest, Hungary, June 17–18.

COWELL, P. E., L. S. ALLEN, N. S. ZALATIMO, and V. H. DENENBERG, 1992. A developmental study of sex and age interactions in the human corpus callosum. *Dev. Brain Res.* 66:187–192.

DAVIDSON, R. J., and C. D. SARON, 1992. Evoked potential measures of interhemispheric transfer time in reading disabled and normal children. *Dev. Neuropsychol.* 8:261–277.

DENENBERG, V. H., P. E. COWELL, R. H. FITCH, A. KERTESZ, and G. H. KENNERS, 1991. Corpus callosum: Multiple parameter measurements in rodents and humans. *Physiol. Behav.* 49:433–437.

DUARA, R., A. KUSHCH, K. GROSS-GLENN, W. BARKER, B. JALLAD, S. PASCAL, D. A. LOEWENSTEIN, J. SHELDON, M. RABIN, B. LEVIN, and H. LUBS, 1991. Neuroanatomic differences between dyslexic and normal readers on magnetic imaging scans. *Arch. Neurol.* 48:410–416.

ELBERT, T., C. PANTEV, C. WIENBRUCH, B. ROCKSTROH, and E. TAUB, 1995. Increased cortical representation of the fingers of the left hand in string players. *Science* 270:305–307.

HYND, G. W., J. HALL, E. S. NOVEY, D. ELIOPULOS, K. BLACK, J. GONZALEZ, J. E. EDMONDS, C. RICCIO, and M. COHEN, 1995. Dyslexia and corpus callosum morphology. *Arch. Neurol.* 52:32–38.

OPPENHEIM, J. S., J. E. SKERRY, M. J. TRAMO, and M. S. GAZZANIGA, 1989. Magnetic resonance imaging morphology of the corpus callosum in monozygotic twins. *Ann. Neurol.* 26:100–104.

PANDYA, D. N., and H. G. J. M. KUYPERS, 1969. Cortico-cortical connections in the rhesus monkey. *Brain Res.* 13:13–36.

PUJOL, J., P. VENDRELL, C. JUNQUÉ, J. L. MARTI-VILALTA, and A. CAPDEVILLA, 1993. When does human brain development end? Evidence of corpus callosum growth up to adulthood. *Ann. Neurol.* 34:71–75.

REIS, A., and A. CASTRO-CALDAS, 1997. Illiteracy: A cause of biased cognitive development. *J. Int. Neuropsychol. Soc.* 3:444–450.

REIS, A., and A. CASTRO-CALDAS, 1997. Learning to read and write increases the efficacy of reaching a target in two dimensional space. *J. Int. Neuropsychol. Soc.* 3:222.

22 Optic Aphasia and Pure Alexia: Contribution of Callosal Disconnection Syndromes to the Study of Lexical and Semantic Representation in the Right Hemisphere

CLAUDIO G. LUZZATTI

ABSTRACT The relevance of the corpus callosum as the major pathway connecting the right and left hemispheres was identified as long ago as the latter decades of the nineteenth century. The importance of this connection became particularly clear after the identification of lateralized functions in the hemispheres, especially of the language and praxic left lateralization. For decades, observations on focal brain injury patients have supplied important data that have supported descriptions of the nature of interhemispheric connections and interactions. This chapter opens with a review of the classic neuropsychological disorders that have been explained by a callosal disconnection between hemispheres. The deficits arising from a splenial interruption of the corpus callosum are described in greater detail. Special attention is given to the cognitive models of object naming and of reading aloud and their implications for the interpretation of optic aphasia and pure alexia. A final purpose of the chapter is to discuss the relevance of focal injuries of the callosal pathways to describe the right hemisphere lexical and semantic linguistic capacity. It is suggested that the variable pattern of optic aphasia, associative visual agnosia, and pure alexia may be explained by a different amount of verbal and/or semantic knowledge in the right hemisphere.

Early neuropsychological observations

In 1889 Carl Samuel Freund described a patient with right homonymous hemianopia who could not name objects from sight but retained the ability to identify

them. Freund labeled this impairment *optic aphasia* (OA) and explained the deficit on the basis of a left parieto-occipital lesion producing right-side hemianopia and a splenial disconnection of the intact right occipital visual areas from the left-hemisphere (LH) speech areas (see Figure 22.1).

A few years later, Joseph-Jules Déjerine (1892) described the case of a patient with a pure reading disorder that he called *verbal blindness*. The reading disorder was due to a lesion of the left occipital lobe and of the callosal fibers connecting the visual areas of the right hemisphere (RH) to those of the LH and to the language areas (see Figure 22.2).

The relationship between *ideomotor apraxia* and the corpus callosum was first identified by Hugo Liepmann (1900, 1905), who described and modeled the LH lateralization of higher-level motor functions. A LH lesion along Liepmann's pathway causes *ideomotor apraxia*, a disorder of the complex voluntary motor behavior that manifests not only on the right hand, but also on the left. It implies that the RH control of the left-hand movements is subordinated to a motor program controlled by the LH.

Dependence of the left-hand eupraxic movement on the LH through the anterior part of the corpus callosum was first suggested and then demonstrated by Liepmann in a series of papers published from 1900 to 1920. According to his model, a lesion of the anterior callosal pathways determines an apraxic deficit for the left hand only (see Figure 22.3). Liepmann and Maas (1907) made a similar observation in a right-handed patient who also

CLAUDIO G. LUZZATTI Dipartimento di Psicologia, Università di Milano-Bicocca, Milano, Italy.

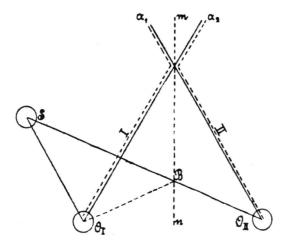

FIGURE 22.1. Freund's (1889) model of optic aphasia. S = language centers; O' and O'' = left and right occipital visual cortex; m–n = sagittal axis between the hemispheres; B = posterior part of the corpus callosum; a_1, a_2 = retinal input from the left and right eye, respectively.

suffered from *left-hand agraphia*. The deficit could not be explained as being due to constructive apraxia because the patient did not show any impairment in copying complex drawings or printed words with his left hand. Furthermore, it could not be explained as a classic dysgraphic disorder because spontaneous writing with the right hand was preserved, and he had no deficit in oral spelling of words.

A further typical symptom of callosal disconnection is *left-hand tactile anomia*. It usually follows a lesion of the medial area of the corpus callosum. Geschwind and Kaplan (1962) described in detail a patient suffering from this deficit who could not name simple objects by tactile manipulation and produced rough semantic substitutions and circumlocutions. However, the patient could identify the objects he could not name after tactile manipulation, since the left hand spontaneously performed the actions appropriate to the objects. Left-hand tactile anomia should therefore be distinguished from astereognosic tactile agnosia.

Information-processing accounts to optic aphasia

A visuoverbal disconnection (Freund, 1889) has not always been accepted as an explanation of OA. Freud (1891), Wolff (1904), Goldstein (1906), and Kleist (1934) maintained, for instance, that the disorder underlying OA was not distinguishable from visual agnosia (Lissauer, 1890) or anomia. Many decades later, Norman Geschwind (1965) interpreted visual agnosia itself in terms of visuoverbal disconnection, claiming that most cases of visual agnosia had to be reinterpreted as a

"confabulatory visual anomia interfering with otherwise intact gnostic capacities" (Geschwind and Fusillo, 1966).

More recently, other authors described patients with behavioral characteristics similar to those first described by Freund but in an information-processing frame. Figure 22.4 shows a contemporary model for object identification and naming. According to Marr's (1982) theory, after a low-level processing stage, the image of an object undergoes a further level of analysis to transform the actually perceived pattern into an abstract representation that is independent of the viewer's perspective. This episodic object-centered structural description of the perceived object is then matched with the stored object-centered structural representation of the objects an individual has experienced in his or her past. This matching permits recognition of the object, after which all visual and associative semantic information are activated, and the appropriate lexical representation is retrieved henceforth from the phonological output lexicon.

Following presentation of this schematic processing model, the different explanations of the cognitive mechanisms underlying OA will be briefly discussed. (For a more extensive analysis of these different explanations, see Luzzatti, Rumiati, and Ghirardi, 1998.)

OA AS A DISCONNECTION BETWEEN VISUAL AND VERBAL SEMANTIC SYSTEMS Lhermitte and Beauvois (1973), Beauvois (1982), and Shallice (1988) explained OA in the frame of the multiple semantic systems theory, suggesting that symptoms are the outcome of damage to the interaction between a modality-specific visual and a verbal semantic system.

OA AS ACCESS VISUAL AGNOSIA In Riddoch and Humphreys's (1987) theory the patients' deficits are interpreted as an impairment in accessing complete semantic representations of objects from vision. More recently, Hillis and Caramazza (1995) proposed a similar explanation.

OA AS A DISRUPTION OF A NONSEMANTIC ROUTE FOR NAMING Ratcliff and Newcombe (1982) suggested that OA is caused by damage to a route for naming that bypasses the semantic system and leads directly from the pictogen (i.e., the structural description of an object) to the phonological output lexicon. There is an obvious analogy with the explanation given for deep dyslexia by Schwartz and colleagues (1980), that is, damage to a direct lexical nonsemantic route for reading. However, if the connection from the pictogen to the semantic system and from the semantic system to the phonological output lexicon is spared, OA patients could use this indirect

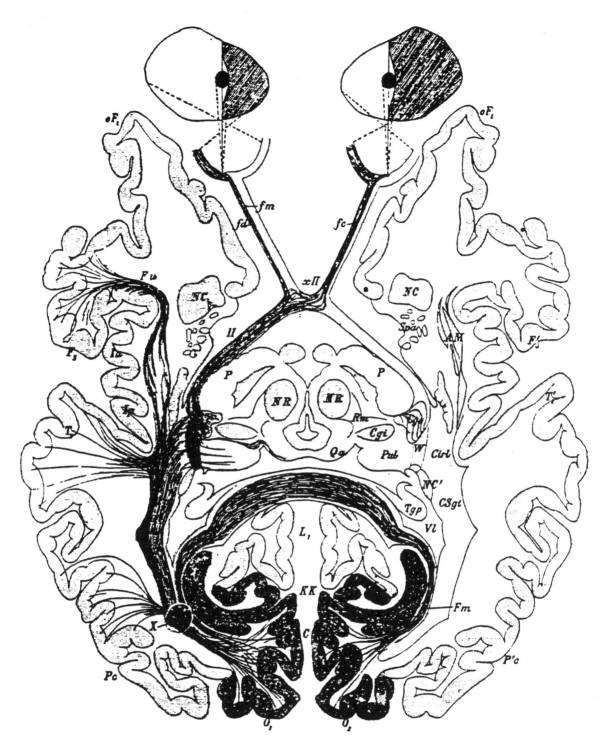

FIGURE 22.2. Déjerine's (1892) model of verbal blindness (pure alexia).

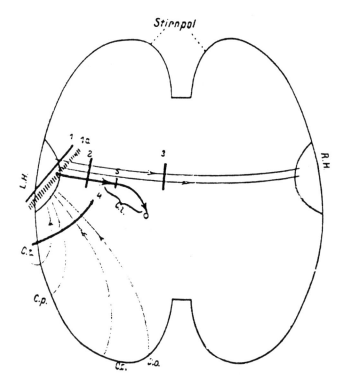

FIGURE 22.3. Liepmann's (1900, 1905) model of callosal (left-hand) ideomotor apraxia.

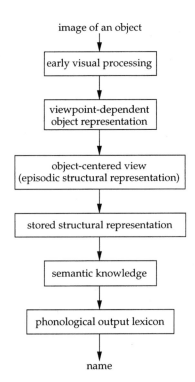

image of an object

↓

early visual processing

↓

viewpoint-dependent object representation

↓

object-centered view (episodic structural representation)

↓

stored structural representation

↓

semantic knowledge

↓

phonological output lexicon

↓

name

FIGURE 22.4. Information-processing model for object identification and naming.

pathway when naming pictures. To account for the anomic behavior and to explain the large number of semantic errors, Ratcliff and Newcombe (1982) had to assume a further functional lesion that causes a fuzziness in mapping semantic onto phonological representations.

OA AS A DISCONNECTION BETWEEN RIGHT- AND LEFT-HEMISPHERE SEMANTICS Coslett and Saffran's (1989b, 1992) account updates Freund's original theory of OA as a visuoverbal disconnection within an information-processing frame. Owing to the left occipital lesion and the splenial disconnection, all visual and identification processing is accomplished in the RH, and the resulting flow of information cannot reach the LH semantic and LH lexical representations. The merit of Coslett and Saffran's theory is that they mapped a model of object recognition and naming and their account of OA to neuroanatomy. However, the explanation they offer lacks detail regarding the concept of RH and LH semantics.

To support the claim that OA can be explained only by a theory that takes into account both a detailed cognitive model and its anatomical constraints, especially the effect of a callosal disconnection, Luzzatti and colleagues (1998) studied a patient who showed the typical OA deficit pattern in confrontation naming. The study

also aimed to demonstrate that the best cognitive model to match the concept of RH and LH semantics is the multiple semantic systems theory (Shallice, 1988). This model offers the best explanation for a left/right semantic difference, when one considers that visual semantics as well as the other sensory semantic systems are represented symmetrically in the two hemispheres, whereas verbal semantics is located predominantly in the LH.

The patient, A.B., was a 74-year-old Italian housewife with five years of education. In August 1993 she suffered a CVA in the territory of the left posterior cerebral artery, determining a malacic lesion of the left occipital inferior and mesial cortex and of the underlying white matter (see Figure 22.5). Her major impairments were a complete right hemianopia, a severe naming deficit on visual presentation, and full alexia.

To better understand the nature of her naming deficit, A.B. was tested by means of a set of tasks tapping the retrieval of object names and the different processing levels represented in Figure 22.4. The results are summarized in Table 22.1.

Naming Her ability to name objects from tactile exploration (23/30, 77%) was significantly better than her ability to name them from visual presentation (7/30,

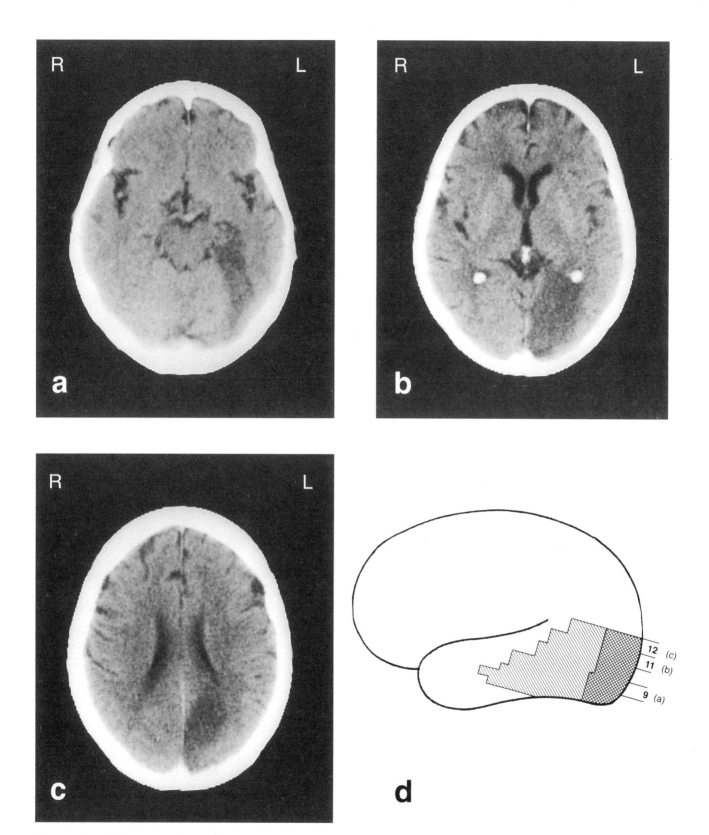

FIGURE 22.5. CT scan showing A.B.'s vascular lesion in the territory of the left posterior cerebral artery, involving the left occipital inferior and mesial cortex and the underlying white matter.

TABLE 22.1

A.B.'s performance on the naming, visual processing, semantic, and gesturing tasks

Tasks	Normal	Mild Deficit	Severe Deficit
Naming			
Naming real objects			
Visual			−
Tactile	+		
Naming to definition	+		
Naming line drawings			−
Early Visual Processing			
Poppelreuter-Ghent	+		
Copying of geometrical drawings	+		
Access to Structural Description			
Object decision	+		
Drawing from memory		+/−	
Spoken Word-to-Picture Matching	+		
Access to Semantics			
Picture-to-picture matching			−
Word-to-word matching	+		
Selecting pictures belonging to the same category	+		
Sorting pictures into categories			
Without name of categories			−
With name of categories	+		
Word and Letter Naming			
Word naming			−
Letter naming			−
Letter-name-to-letter matching		+/−	
Apraxia			
Reproduction of gestures			−
Use of objects		+/−	

23%) ($\chi^2(1) = 17.1$; $p < 0.0001$). Naming to definition was at ceiling for concrete objects and actions (30/30, 100%) and still within the normal range for abstract concepts (25/30, 83%). A.B. was asked to name drawings of 44 natural objects and 59 artificial objects from Snodgrass and Vanderwart's norms (1980); she was able to name only 21% of the drawings, without significant difference between natural (16%) and artificial (25%) items. Overall, A.B. showed a naming deficit of visually presented objects, suggesting that her impairment was not due to a lexical access deficit or to a loss of knowledge within a unitary semantic system. If A.B.'s naming deficits had been located on either of these processing levels, her naming performance should have been affected equally for all input modalities. The majority of errors were circumlocutions (42%) and perseverations (22%), and she made only one visual and a few (7%) semantic errors. This pattern of disruption is hardly compatible with the explanation of OA as an access visual agnosia (Riddoch and Humphreys, 1987), which would require a prevalence of visual and visual-semantic errors.

Early visual processing A.B.'s ability to produce an on-line representation of visual stimuli was in the normal range, both on a figure-ground discrimination task (Poppelreuter-Ghent) and on the copying of geometric line drawings.

Access to the structural description system The integrity of the structural description system was demonstrated by a normal performance (34/34) on an object decision task (i.e., the patient had to decide whether an object depicted by a line drawing is real) and by an almost normal ability to draw from memory.

Spoken word-to-picture matching   A.B. was asked to point to the picture corresponding to the item spoken aloud by the examiner within a matrix of six to eight line drawings taken from the same category as the target picture. She performed this task without any error or hesitation (109/109), showing a normal access to structural representations of objects from their names.

Access to semantics   A.B.'s performance on an associative matching task with pictures (Pyramids and Palm Tree Test) was severely impaired (17/30, 57%), and the score she achieved was below that obtained by a sample of global aphasic patients (22.9 ± 5.4), while her performance on a spoken version of the task was unimpaired (27/30, 90%). Finally, A.B.'s ability to sort pictures of objects into categories derived a significant benefit from lexical cueing; when given the names of the categories to which the objects belonged, she was able to sort pictures (96/106, 91%), whereas she hesitated and made significantly more mistakes (78/106, 74%) when the names of the categories were not given and had to be gained from inspection of the pictures themselves. Overall, these results could support an explanation of OA as an access deficit of semantic knowledge from visual input. However, this explanation (Riddoch and Humphreys, 1987; Hillis and Caramazza, 1995) does not account for the isolated involvement of categorical/associative knowledge and for the results on the sorting task, which differ according to the presence or absence of lexical cueing. This difference can be explained only by assuming that A.B.'s performance deteriorates when a task requires the retrieval of associative and categorical knowledge that is basically lexical in nature.

Word and letter naming   A.B. was not able to read either words or nonwords aloud (0/86 and 0/28, respectively), nor was she able to match written words to pictures. Naming of isolated letters was also severely impaired, and she could read only 17/48 letters (35.5%). Her performance on a letter-name-to-letter matching task was relatively less impaired (33/48 letters, 69%) than her letter naming.

Apraxia   It is said that OA patients tend to compensate for their confrontation naming deficit by demonstrating the use of objects they are not able to name. This dissociation does not seem to be the rule, however; A.B. showed a severe deficit in imitating gestures (37/72; De Renzi, Motti, and Nichelli, 1980) and a mild impair-

ment in demonstrating the use of objects and tools (11/14; De Renzi, Pieczuro, and Vignolo, 1968). Thus, the lesion that disconnected the RH visual centers from the LH language areas must also have disconnected the same visual centers from the LH parietal ideatory and ideomotor representations.

In conclusion, A.B., presented typical OA features, that is, a modality-specific visual naming deficit with fair tactile naming and spared naming from definitions. Her visual naming deficit was not due to an early recognition problem, since A.B. was able to discriminate shapes adequately. She was also able to gain an episodic structural description of objects and to access stored structural knowledge of objects from both visual and verbal stimuli. Her good performance on the word-to-picture matching task is not consistent with those of other OA patients (e.g., Beauvois, 1982; Riddoch and Humphreys, 1987), who presented bidirectional damage from visual-to-verbal and from verbal-to-visual representations. The best explanation of A.B.'s deficit on the picture-to-picture matching task and when sorting pictures into categories without lexical cueing may be found in the framework of the multiple semantic systems theory (Shallice, 1988). A.B. was able to access her visual semantic knowledge without difficulty, but this did not hold true for the verbal categorical and associative knowledge that is also required in a "purely" visual task such as the Pyramid and Palm Tree Test. However, the multiple semantic theory does not explain in detail the pathogenesis of the OA symptomatology. A more explicit anatomofunctional interpretation is offered by the account of OA as a disconnection between RH and LH semantics (Coslett and Saffran, 1989b). This theory, however, in turn lacks detail regarding the functional and cognitive difference between RH and LH semantics. Thus, it is only after integration of this concept into the more detailed cognitive model of a disconnection between visual and verbal semantics that the theory assumes its full heuristic capacity, providing the best theoretical framework for the explanation of A.B.'s performance.

The diagram in Figure 22.6 summarizes the processing units that are available in each hemisphere and shows which units are damaged in A.B. The major difference between the right and left hemispheres concerns the orthographic and phonological output lexicons and the sub-word-level conversion routines that are usually represented in the LH only. The organization of the phonological and orthographic input lexicons and of the semantic knowledge is also asymmetrical; compared to the full lexical and associative/categorical semantic representation of the LH, the RH has a coarser

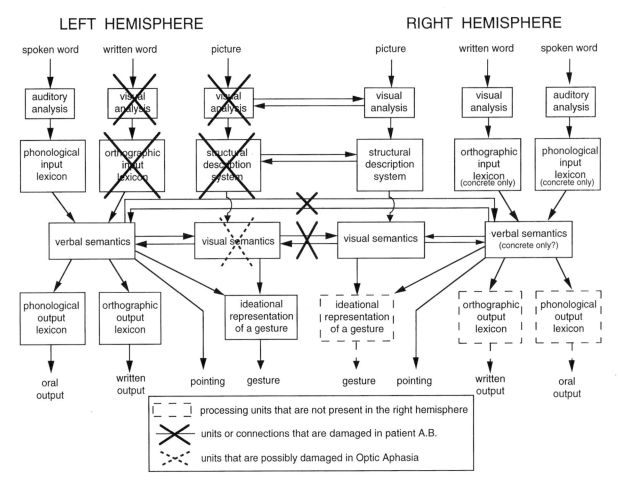

FIGURE 22.6. Diagram summarizing the processing units that are available in each hemisphere and showing which of these units are damaged in the OA patient described by Luzzatti and colleagues (1998).

representation for concrete, morphologically simple words only. Owing to the left occipital and callosal damage, visual analysis and access to visual semantic knowledge can be achieved only by the RH. However, the RH representations cannot access full verbal semantic, categorical associative and lexical representation. This also explains A.B.'s ideomotor and ideatory apraxia from visual stimuli.

FUNCTIONAL AND NEUROANATOMICAL INTERACTION OF OPTIC APHASIA AND ASSOCIATIVE VISUAL AGNOSIA Classic neuropsychology made a clear distinction between the concept of OA and that of associative visual agnosia (VA), stating that OA is a lexical deficit, whereas VA is a disorder of object identification. However, this distinction has not been universally accepted (Freud, 1891; Wolff, 1904; Goldstein, 1906; Geschwind, 1965; Riddoch and Humphreys, 1987; Hillis and Caramazza,

1995), and even if it were accepted in principle, it is not always easy to make a clear-cut distinction between the disorders because (1) it is often difficult to prove or exclude the identification of objects, (2) some cases show intermediate patterns or shift from one condition to the other, and (3) except for a few cases in which VA was caused by a bilateral lesion of both visual integrative areas, OA and VA cases usually share a very similar underlying brain lesion, that is, a left occipital lesion associated with a disconnection of the occipital callosal pathways.

An interpretation of this interaction has been given by Schnider, Benson, and Scharre (1994). They discussed the case of a 71-year-old right-handed man suffering from a relatively pure visual recognition and/or naming disorder caused by a left occipital and posterior temporal lobe infarct. No impairment emerged in naming either from verbal description or when the use of a tool was demonstrated by the examiner, but the patient was not able to name a visually presented object or make the appropriate pantomime. Errors were predominantly confabulations and perseverations. It was possible to suppress confabulations by providing the patient with a name for the object, which could be correct or false. The patient only had to answer yes or no, which he always did correctly. "Under this condition the patient pantomimed each tool's use. Thus, this simple maneuver temporarily changed the disorder from visual agnosia to optic aphasia." In fact, after each correct pantomime the patient was also able to name the target object, apparently on the basis of the kinesthetic feedback from performing the pantomime. It is therefore not clear whether the maneuver actually did "change the disorder temporarily to OA" or whether it revealed the real disorder of the patient, that is, a visuoverbal disconnection due to the left mesial occipital lesion. To answer the question of which anatomical substrate would allow the transition of VA to OA, the authors compared the CT and MRI scans of the principal cases suffering from VA and OA, concluding that "Both groups show inferior temporo-occipital lesions. The splenium, however, is involved only in patients who could... demonstrate the use of visually presented objects and who had no difficulty using objects, i.e., optic aphasics."

However, from an inspection of the lesion templates collected by the authors, this contraposition is not fully convincing, as the lesions shown by the two groups of patients are almost identical. Furthermore, the data presented by Schnider and colleagues (1994) are more likely to support the hypothesis that their patient was actually able to identify the visually presented objects. However, as is often the case, the disconnection syndrome prevented him from clearly demonstrating his ability to identify the visual stimuli. Thus, the performance obtained after suppression of the confabulations is open to another interpretation: Instead of showing a "temporary change of the deficit," it is evidence of the true underlying cognitive capacity, which has been altered by the visuoverbal disconnection.

In conclusion, it is true that the distinction between associative VA and OA may in some cases be vague and in others almost impossible to discern; however, the difference between these symptomatologies should not be interpreted on the basis of the more or less extensive damage of the callosal pathways, but rather on the basis of a variability in the RH verbal semantic representation that subjects had before the onset of cerebral damage (De Renzi and Saetti, 1997; Luzzatti et al., 1998; De Renzi, 1999). Hence, a left occipital lesion that is associated with a posterior callosal disconnection will deter-

mine different patterns of symptoms, interspersed as a continuum ranging through VA to OA, color anomia, or alexia, in relation to the more or less extensive verbal and visual semantic representation in the RH.

Acquired dyslexia following left-hemisphere lesions

Pure Alexia and Déjerine's Classical Model of Written Language   In 1891 and 1892 Joseph-Jules Déjerine described two patients with reading disorders in the absence of any other major verbal deficits. The reading disorders of the first case were associated with a writing deficit (*cécité verbale avec agraphie*, i.e., verbal blindness with agraphia) following a left angular gyrus infarction. The reading deficit of the second patient was pure and followed an infarction of the mesial and inferior surface of the left occipital lobe extending to the retroventricular white matter and a portion of the callosal splenium. On the basis of his observations Déjerine suggested that the left angular gyrus is the site of the verbal optic images that are critical for normal recognition of letters and words and for normal spelling ability. According to Déjerine the RH is word-blind; therefore, the visual images of letters and words have to reach the LH angular gyrus to be identified. The flowchart in Figure 22.7 is an adaptation of Déjerine's model (Figure 22.2) into a contemporary cognitive flowchart.

Visual recognition of letters and words requires the interaction of the occipital visual centers with the center of visual memory of letters and words, which is located in the left angular gyrus. Comprehension of written words requires the connection of the center of visual

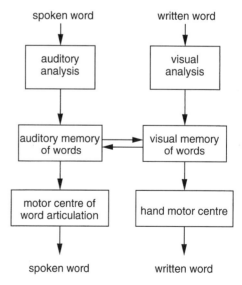

Figure 22.7. Dejerine's model transformed into an information-processing flowchart.

memory of letters and words to the center of auditory memory of words (Wernicke's area), whereas reading aloud requires the association of the center of visual memory of letters and words to the motor center of word articulation (Broca's area). Writing to dictation requires the activation of the auditory center of words and its association to the center of visual memory of letters and words and thus the activation of the corresponding graphic patterns from the hand motor center.

According to Déjerine, alexia with agraphia follows damage of the left angular gyrus, which is the image store of written words. Pure alexia, on the other hand, is due to damage of the LH visual areas and a disconnection of the RH visual areas from the preserved word images stored in the left angular gyrus.

COGNITIVE MODELS OF WRITTEN LANGUAGE   The interpretation of reading disorders given by classic aphasiology could not explain some qualitative aspects of dyslexic behavior, such as semantic substitutions, visual errors, or morphological errors. Furthermore, reading tasks did not take into account certain relevant orthographic and psycholinguistic aspects, such as orthographic regularity, length of stimuli, word frequency, imageability, part of speech effect, and the performance with nonlexical stimuli.

On the basis of these observations Marshall and Newcombe (1966, 1973) suggested and demonstrated the need for two distinct reading pathways. During the following years their model was progressively developed to account more accurately for the processing of written language. Figure 22.8 shows an updated version of the model proposed by Morton and Patterson in 1980.

Contemporary reading models have two main differences compared with Déjerine's model. First, the visual representation of letters and words, identified by Déjerine in the left angular gyrus, has been substituted with two separate and independent orthographic representations for reading and writing (orthographic input and output lexicons). Second, written material may be processed along two distinct pathways: On one side, there is a lexical routine for regular or irregular words, the orthography of which has been learned previously; on the other side, there are sub-word-level conversion routines that are used both for regular words, of which the orthography is unknown to the subject, and for regular nonlexical orthographic strings (nonwords): the Grapheme-to-Phoneme Conversion (GPC) routine and the Phoneme-to-Grapheme Conversion (PGC) routine, respectively.

Regular words may be read along both the lexical and the sub-word-level routine, whereas irregular words may

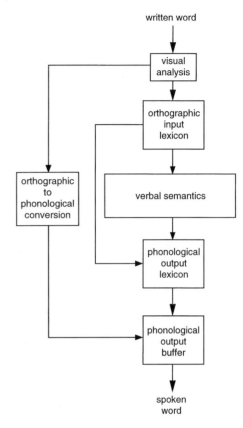

FIGURE 22.8. Morton and Patterson's (1980) model (modified).

be read along the lexical routine only. Irregular words usually contain letter strings that may correspond to different phonological realizations. For instance, the orthographic string EA may be read [i:] in the word VEAL, [e] in the word HEAD, [ε:] in the word BEAR, [a:] in the word HEART, or [ei] in the word STEAK. Other words have a full irregular transcription, as in YACHT [jɔt] and PINT [paint].

Multiple-routine reading and writing models have been confirmed by observations of neuropsychological patients with specific written language deficits. On the one hand, there are patients who, after a lesion of the lexical route, are still able to read regular words and nonwords along the GPC routine but are unable to read irregular words. They make regularization errors; for example, the word PINT may be read as [pint] instead of [paint]. This reading disorder is called *surface dyslexia*. On the other hand, there are patients who, after a functional lesion of the GPC routine, are still able to read overlearned words but are unable to read simple legal meaningless orthographic strings (nonwords) such as TOOF [tu:f] or BLICK [blik]. This reading deficit is called *phonological dyslexia*.

Schwartz and colleagues (1980) described a further type of reading disorder in a patient who was able to read irregular words aloud, the meaning of which she did not understand. This pattern of deficits was called *direct dyslexia* and suggested the division of the lexical route into two distinct subroutines: a direct lexical and a lexical-semantic one. The authors explained the patient's reading behavior as a breakdown of semantic knowledge in which the direct lexical routine is spared.

Finally, there is a peculiar reading disorder called *letter-by-letter (LBL) dyslexia* (Alajouanine, Lhermitte, and Deribaucourt-Ducarne, 1960; Kinsbourne and Warrington, 1962; Benson and Geschwind, 1969; Hecaen and Kremin, 1976; Patterson and Kay, 1982). LBL dyslexia is, in its pure form, a peripheral reading disorder in which a written word cannot be processed either by the lexical route or by the sub-word-level routine. However, the patient is still able to name the single letters of the string. If letter naming is spared, the patient may be able to retrieve the phonological representation of written words using an inverse spelling procedure based on his or her preserved orthographic ability. However, this procedure is very slow and laborious, with a clear length effect and no frequency, imageability, or part-of-speech effects.

Different explanations of LBL reading have been given over the last decades. They range from a perceptual account such as simultanagnosia (Kinsbourne and Warrington, 1962) to an early orthographic-processing deficit (Warrington and Shallice, 1980; Patterson and Kay, 1982).

THE CASE OF DEEP DYSLEXIA AND THE ROLE OF THE RIGHT HEMISPHERE   There is a peculiar variation of phonological dyslexia in which semantically but non-phonologically related responses may occur (semantic paralexia). A patient sees the word HOUND and reads [dɔg] or misreads WOOD as [tri:]. This abnormal reading behavior is called *deep dyslexia* (Coltheart, Patterson, and Marshall, 1980). Semantic errors in reading aloud suggest that deep dyslexic patients attempt to read via the semantic system, which, however, is damaged. Patients are often able to identify words in a lexical decision task, and this suggests that the orthographic input lexicon is still unimpaired but is disconnected from the phonological output lexicon. The inability to read nonwords also suggests an impairment of the orthographic-to-phonological conversion. Indeed, damage to both the sub-word-level and direct lexical routes appears to be a necessary condition for semantic errors to occur. Furthermore, letter naming is severely impaired, thus ruling out a LBL reading strategy. The patients also show an

imageability effect (concrete nouns are better read than abstract) and a part-of-speech effect (nouns are better read than verbs and function words).

In an alternative to an information-processing explanation of deep dyslexia, Coltheart (1980, 1983) suggested that this pattern of symptoms may be the consequence of severe damage to the LH reading processes and that the residual reading abilities are the expression of the patient's RH. This explanation is obviously in contrast with the claim of a full verbal blindness of the RH and of its complete lack of lexical-semantic capacity.

Evidence in support of a RH representation of written language arises from Schweiger, Zaidel, Field, and Dobkin's (1989) study of a deep dyslexic patient. R.W. was a 38-year-old right-handed woman who suffered a large LH infarct extending anteriorly into the posterior-inferior frontal lobe and posteriorly to the superior part of the temporal lobe and the parietal lobe. At the time of the first testing session (a few months after disease onset), the patient presented a moderate Broca's aphasia with mild agrammatism, a right hemiplegia, but no visual field defect. Her reading disorder corresponded to the pattern of a deep dyslexia, with no PGC ability (nonwords = 0%), many semantic errors in reading words, and dramatic part-of-speech and imageability effect (concrete nouns = 47%, adjectives = 36%, verbs = 35%, abstract nouns = 26%, function words = 16%). This profile is similar to that of the disconnected RH of split-brain patients (Zaidel, 1990). The only difference is that because the RH of commissurotomized patients has no control over speech and has no access to the speech mechanisms in the LH, these patients do not produce semantic errors in reading aloud; however, semantic errors arise in reading comprehension tasks (Zaidel, 1982).

R.W.'s reading abilities were first tested by means of a lexical decision task (*go* if stimulus is a word). A set of words and nonwords were flashed for 150 ms in either the right or the left visual field. R.W. showed almost equal accuracy for the left and right visual fields (> 80%). However, the reaction time for presentation in the left visual field (1000 ms) was significantly shorter than that for the right visual field presentation (1400 ms). The difference could not be accounted for by a shorter anatomical route (the RH-to-left-hand path as compared to the LH-to-RH-to-left-hand path) because a similar difference could not be found in a letter-counting task (*go* if stimulus contains more than four letters). An interhemispheric difference also emerged from word naming. A set of real, high-frequency English nouns were flashed for 90 ms to either the right or left visual field. R.W. made almost three times as many semantic errors in the left visual field, whereas in the right visual field she could name a few more items but made more visual and derivational errors.

These data support the claim that the RH has a rather diffuse or undifferentiated semantic representation, at least for imageable high-frequency nouns. The results also provide evidence regarding the asymmetrical functional architecture of the dual-route model for reading: The LH has full representation for the nonlexical as well as the lexical-semantic routes, whereas the RH has only lexical orthographic input and semantic representation (at least for concrete high-frequency nouns). In deep dyslexic patients, both the LH nonlexical and lexical route are impaired, owing to the left-side lesion. The alternative RH lexical route to semantics is spared, as well as the LH ability to retrieve the phonological address of a word. When lexical access fails in the LH, the RH provides semantic access, which is then transmitted through the intact callosum to the LH for phonological encoding and production. But as the semantic address provided by the RH is diffuse and less constrained by phonology, the output often consists of semantic substitutions.

Further evidence in support of the RH hypothesis of deep dyslexia comes from a study on regional cerebral blood flow (rCBF) in a deep dyslexic patient during visual word recognition and spoken word production (Weekes, Coltheart, and Gordon, 1997). For the deep dyslexic patient, rCBF was greater in the RH than in the LH. No such difference was found on the same task in either a surface dyslexic patient or two control subjects with no cerebral damage. Furthermore, the RH major activation could not simply be explained by the effect of the LH cerebral lesion, since the spoken word production task generated much greater activation in the LH than in the RH.

Anomalous Patterns in Pure Alexia and Letter-by-Letter Reading Over the years, many investigators replicated Déjerine's original observations, thus confirming the principle of a full RH linguistic blindness (e.g., Warrington and Shallice, 1980; Patterson and Kay, 1982). More recently, however, observations have been made on the cases of a number of patients who had full damage to the left occipital visual areas but still showed capacities that appear to be inconsistent with the traditional account of pure alexia as a disconnection of the "word-blind" left visual field (RH) from the LH language areas. However, it is also true that their residual reading capacities do not fit easily with the cognitive accounts of dyslexia. Many pure alexic patients are in fact able to read, although slowly and sometimes laboriously, by means of a LBL reading strategy. The critical

features of LBL reading are, on the one hand, the linear increment in the time the patients need to read increasingly longer words, and, on the other, the deleterious effects of tachistoscopic presentation. In this condition, reading becomes impossible once the time of exposure becomes shorter than the time required for an effective LBL strategy. As we have already seen, LBL reading is a compensatory behavior for different types of visual-processing disorders, in particular for simultanagnosia (Kinsbourne and Warrington, 1962). Owing to a primary perceptual deficit or to damage of the standard orthographic procedures, subjects process each single letter as a separate image, identify it, retrieve the letter name, and eventually retrieve the phonological representation of the target word by means of an inverse spelling strategy. However, this account of LBL reading is in contrast with the implicit reading capacity these patients often show while reading words, in spite of their dramatic deficit in identifying and reading aloud the same words.

A first account of this dissociation was given by Landis, Regard, and Serrat (1980). They described the case of a 39-year-old patient presenting dense hemianopia and pure alexia after resection of a left occipital brain tumor. Under tachistoscopic presentation the patient was not able to read any of the stimulus words but was actually able to point to the corresponding objects among 10 alternatives displayed on a table in front of him. Shallice and Saffran (1986) described a similar patient whose letter naming was almost normal, whereas word naming was slow and laborious, with a clear length effect. Lexical decision under tachistoscopic presentation was significantly better than chance, and the patient showed some comprehension of words he denied having either read or understood. For instance, on a map of Britain he could point to the correct location of geographic names he could not read. The authors compared this phenomenon to that observed in normal subjects after subliminal tachistoscopic presentation (Marcel, 1983) and to the blindsight phenomenon, that is, a disorder observed in patients with dense hemianopia who are unable to identify any object in the hemianopic field but who are nevertheless able to point to the location of an "unseen" object (e.g., Weiskrantz, 1983). Another proof of the RH lexical processing of written words is to be found in a study of a pure alexic patient (J.V.) and his capacity to identify letters in real words and nonwords (Bub, Black, and Howell, 1989). The patient, just like the normal subjects, still showed a word superiority effect (Reicher, 1969; Wheeler, 1970); that is, he performed better on identifying letters in real words than on random letter strings. This result suggested that the patient's RH visual areas were not verbal blind and were still able to activate stored lexical information.

A more extensive study on the RH reading ability was performed by Coslett and Saffran (1989a, 1994). They studied five patients with pure alexia and two patients in whom alexia was associated with optic aphasia. The reading disorder of the five pure alexic patients showed the typical features of a LBL dyslexia: Letter naming was spared, and reading speed was a function of the word length. (The patient J.G., for instance, read three-letter words in about 9″, four-letter words in 13″, five-letter words in 17″, and six-letter words in 27″.) The reading performance of the two optic aphasic patients was, as usual, nil. In spite of the fact that their word naming was nil or slow and laborious, all patients showed a clear implicit reading capacity with the features already described for the RH lexical and semantic processing. Implicit reading could be demonstrated by means of a lexical decision and a semantic judgment task. In the lexical decision task, irrespective of their reading disorders, all seven patients were able to discriminate between simple words and plausible nonwords after tachistoscopic presentation (i.e., at an exposure time that was largely shorter than that required for an effective use of the LBL reading strategy). A similar pattern of performance resulted from the semantic judgment task: Irrespective of their reading deficit, all patients were able to decide whether stimuli were names of animals and, in a second condition, names of edible items.

Another peculiar aspect of the LBL reading disorder that emerged in Coslett and Saffran's (1994) patients was a diminished ability to judge low-frequency and/or low-imageability words and morphologically complex items. Their performance on these items was in decided contrast to their good capacity for making lexical decisions on simple high-frequency and highly imageable words. A poor performance pattern with free and bound grammatical morphemes and with less frequent and less imageable items is very similar to the pattern described for the RH processing in patients with (posterior) callosal disconnection (e.g., Michel, Henaff, and Intrilligator, 1996).

In many patients pure alexia is a symptom that may remain unchanged for many years or may modify into a less severe reading disorder. One of the cases described by Coslett and Saffran (1994) evolved over an eight-year follow-up period from LBL into a deep/phonological dyslexia, with imageability and part-of-speech effects (Buxbaum and Coslett, 1996), a pattern of impairment that has already been discussed as typical of the RH processing capacity of written language. This interpretation is patently supported by the fact that whereas LH

transcranial magnetic stimulation did not modify the patient's reading ability, after RH stimulation the original LBL reading strategy reappeared, and the patient's reading performance declined from 71% to 21% (Coslett and Monsul, 1994).

Overall, the characteristics of implicit reading may be summarized as follows: (1) the patients do not access either the phonological output lexicon or the GPC routine; (2) although their LBL reading is null or slow and laborious, patients access implicitly written word representations and meaning; (3) this dissociation emerges when LBL reading is suppressed, as is the case with tachistoscopic presentations. Implicit reading is sensitive to imageability and word frequency, in that there is a poor processing of free and bound grammatical morphemes (function words and affixes), whereas performance is not susceptible to word length.

However, these results are not consistent with the results obtained from some other dyslexic cases. Warrington and Shallice (1980) described a patient (R.A.V.) who could not make any lexical decisions or semantic judgments on words he could not read. Patterson and Kay (1982) examined four patients with pure alexia and LBL reading and did not find any compelling evidence that the patients were able to comprehend words that they could not explicitly identify. Patterson and Besner (1984) cited the absence of reading ability in a patient with pure alexia as compelling evidence against the right-hemisphere reading hypothesis. Finally, Behrmann, Black, and Bub (1990) described the case of a patient with almost pure LBL dyslexia (D.S.) who could name letters with normal accuracy and speed. Word naming, however, was very slow and laborious; the patient had to name letters sequentially and could name words of four letters or more only by means of the inverse spelling strategy. The same laborious solution was used on a lexical decision and a semantic judgment task (sad words, animals, etc.), on which the patient showed a progressive increase in the reaction time for words of increasing length (from 5 seconds for three-letter words to 9 and 14 seconds for five- and seven-letter words, respectively, that is, approximately 2 seconds per letter). Lexical decision and semantic judgments were at chance level when stimuli were presented tachistoscopically (3-second exposure). Finally, using the methodology devised by Bub and colleagues (1989), the authors did not find any word superiority effect. Coslett and Saffran (1994) suggested that the inconsistency of these findings with their own results (i.e., presence of implicit RH reading) is the consequence of the different experimental paradigms used: Authors who could not find implicit reading effects have presented the items with an overly long exposure time and did not hinder patients from LBL reading, a

TABLE 22.2
Dyslexia +/− implicit processing (patient P.V.)

Visual and Auditory Lexical Decision: % of Correct Responses

	$n =$	Free Visual Presentation	Tachistoscopic Presentation	Oral Presentation
Function words	18	44	78	100
Abstract nouns	18	44	100	100
Concrete nouns (natural objects)	18	78	94	100
Concrete nouns (artifacts)	18	56	89	100
Illegal nonwords	18	83	67	100
Legal nonwords	18	83	22	100
Improperly suffixed words	18	67	33	100
Suffixed nonwords	18	67	17	100
Total hits	144	65	63	100

Semantic Judgments ("Is it a coarse word or not"?)

	$n =$	Response	Written (% hits)	Oral (% hits)
Coarse words	14	yes	100	100
Neutral words	12	no	14	100

procedure that is a prerequisite for direct access to the RH lexical and lexical-semantic representations.

The inconsistent pattern of symptoms following left occipital damage has also been justified by the difference in size of the underlying callosal lesions (Binder and Mohr, 1992). However, an anatomical correlative study on Coslett and Saffran's series did not agree with this account, since the sites of the lesions causing LBL reading disorders varied considerably, with different degrees of impairment of the callosal pathway (Saffran and Coslett, 1998).

Alternatively, it should be considered that if covert processing depends on the RH and there are individual differences in the RH linguistic capacities, then this kind of variability across subjects was clearly to be expected (see Coltheart, 1998, for a more extensive discussion). A similar variability of performance emerged also from the written lexical decision and semantic judgments of commissurotomized patients (see Baynes and Eliassen, 1998, for a review).

Different performances under unlimited and tachistoscopic exposure were also found in two Italian dyslexic patients whom we had the opportunity to test for their covert reading abilities. Both patients presented severe impairment in reading words and nonwords and performed lexical decision at chance level but showed contrasting behavior on semantic judgment tasks.

The first patient was a 48-year-old bank employee (P.V.) suffering from right hemianopia, mild fluent aphasia, and alexia owing to a left temporoparieto-occipital infarct. Word naming was slow and laborious, with length effect and the remaining features of LBL reading. Writing was unimpaired. P.V.'s performance on an auditory and a visual lexical decision task is summarized in Table 22.2. Under the visual modality and with unlimited time exposure he accepted most of the concrete natural words, rejected most of the nonwords, but performed at chance with concrete artifacts, abstract words, and function words. In the tachistoscopic condition he rejected most of the illegal nonwords but accepted most of the phonologically legal and pseudo-suffixed nonwords and of the improperly suffixed words. Overall, the patient varied the response pattern according to whether the presentation was free or tachistoscopic: He overgeneralized the no decision with the unlimited exposure and the yes decision in the tachistoscopic condition. Table 22.2 also shows P.V.'s performance on a semantic decision task in which he had to judge whether a stimulus was or was not a coarse word. Under written tachistoscopic presentation the patient considered most of the neutral words as coarse words. Here too he seemed to follow a yes solution, deciding in almost all cases for a coarse word. In conclusion, P.V. had little RH visual lexical processing and little, if any, implicit semantic processing.

The second case was an 18-year-old patient (D.M.) suffering from right hemianopia and severe language disorder with the features of a mixed transcortical apha-

TABLE 22.3

Dyslexia +/− implicit processing (patient D.M.)

Repetition and Naming of Words and Nonwords

	$n =$	Repetition (%)	Word Naming (%)
Function words	16	88	0
Natural concrete objects	15	93	0
Artifacts	15	93	0
Abstract nouns	15	80	0
Simple nonwords	15	73	0
Pseudo-derived nonwords	15	93	0

Visual and Auditory Lexical Decision (% of Correct Responses)

	$n =$	Tachistoscopic Presentation	Oral Presentation
Function words	18	44	72
Abstract nouns	18	61	83
Concrete nouns (natural objects)	18	78	100
Concrete nouns (artifacts)	18	67	100
Illegal nonwords	18	94	100
Legal nonwords	18	61	78
Improperly suffixed words	18	44	94
Suffixed nonwords	18	56	83
Total hits	144	63	89

Semantic Judgments (% of Hits): Coarse Word Identification ("Is it a coarse word or not"?),
    Edible Item Discrimination ("Is it edible or not"?)

	$n =$	Coarse Words (% hits)	Edible Items (% hits)
Yes	14	92	77
No	12	93	77

sia. A CT scan showed a left occipital infarct extending to the temporoparietal regions. Letter naming was severely impaired (21/48). Table 22.3 shows her repetition and reading performance with words and nonwords, and her performance on an auditory and visual lexical decision task. In the visual condition she was at chance level with function words, abstract nouns, legal nonwords, improperly suffixed words, and suffixed nonwords, whereas she performed significantly better than chance with concrete nouns and illegal nonwords. Table 22.3 also shows her performance on two semantic judgment tasks under written tachistoscopic presentation; the patient was able to discriminate coarse from neutral words and to distinguish edible from inedible items. Overall, in the lexical decision task D.M. showed a clear part of speech and imageability effect with words but performed almost randomly with nonwords. Her se-

mantic judgments, by contrast, were close to normal or only moderately impaired. D.M.'s performance pattern thus conforms with the hypothesis of an implicit RH lexical and semantic processing. As expected, however, her implicit processing is limited to high-frequency and morphologically simple concrete nouns. The dissociation between D.M.'s almost normal performance on both semantic judgments and her poor performance on the lexical decision task is not easy to explain within the framework of the usual information-processing models, as these results are a cue for a spared access to semantics, with impaired access, however, to the orthographic input lexicon. A possible explanation is that reading with the RH lexical pathway is not only implicit but also automatic. D.M. is able to access semantic information without consciously accessing the orthographic input level. Lexical decision is thus possible only as a top-down process and only for concrete words that activate some semantic information.

Reading in the RH: Data from left hemispherectomy Further support for RH contribution to language processing comes from the study of a patient who underwent left hemispherectomy due to Rasmussen encephalitis (Patterson, Vargha-Khadem, and Polkey, 1989). A 17-year-old girl (N.I.) came for neurological observation due to a progressive degeneration of the left cerebral hemisphere with recurrent epileptic seizures and, subsequently, epilepsia partialis continua. The patient therefore underwent left hemispherectomy. After surgery the seizures ceased completely. Spontaneous speech was very limited with severe anomia and mild agrammatism. Her residual lexical and semantic abilities showed strong similarities to those of deep dyslexic patients and to the semantic abilities of split-brain patients who were given reading tasks lateralized to the left visual field.

N.I.'s reading performance was impaired, showing the pattern of phonological dyslexia: (1) identification of letters was perfect, but their naming was poor and possible only through enumeration from A to the target letter; (2) lexical decision was impaired particularly for lower-frequency elements; (3) naming of words and word-to-picture-matching were moderately impaired with frequency, imageability, and part-of-speech effect; and (4) reading of nonwords was null.

These results showed that the isolated RH of a right-handed subject may have enough lexical orthographic input and semantic abilities, at least for concrete nouns, as well as phonological output abilities. The classic explanation given to justify RH language skills in patients after commissurotomy is that they have suffered from epilepsy since childhood, and this may have determined an incomplete lateralization of cognitive functions. However, this explanation can hardly be applied to N.I., whose anatomical and functional development was completely normal until the age of 13.

Conclusions

Since Freund's (1889) description, optic aphasia has been at the center of the controversy on the functional interaction between hemispheres. In more recent years the study of this selective naming impairment has also thrown light on the issue of RH lexical-semantic competence. A functional model based on a multiple semantic system representation and on a bilateral but diversified organization of lexical-semantic abilities supplies the best theoretical account of OA symptomatology. The reading performance of deep dyslexic patients and of LBL readers also shows that the RH has

at least partial linguistic competence, though usually limited to the basic representation of highly imageable and morphologically simple content words. Studies of commissurotomized patients and patients who sustained left hemispherectomy have supplied converging evidence of RH lexical and semantic processing.

Most of the studies that analyzed RH linguistic competence also documented a high level of interindividual variability either for type or for degree of impairment. This can be seen in the variable pattern of impairment that emerges after a left occipital lesion with functional damage to the splenial pathways (ranging from pure alexia to associative VA) or in the irregular emergence of implicit reading in pure alexia. Different hypotheses were suggested to explain this variability. While Schnider and colleagues (1994) tried to explain the OA/VA dichotomy with a different extent of callosal damage, De Renzi (1999) hinted at a premorbid variability of RH lexical-semantic competence: "It is this premorbid individual feature that determines the degree to which the RH can compensate for the left side's lack of contribution to visual semantic processing and whether the clinical profile of the patient is more skewed towards optic aphasia or visual agnosia" (p. 384). This explanation also accounts for the inconsistent emergence of implicit reading in pure alexia and for lateralized left visual field (RH) stimulation in commissurotomized patients.

REFERENCES

ALAJOUANINE, T., F. LHERMITTE, and B. DE RIBAUCOURT-DUCARNE, 1960. Les alexies agnosiques et aphasiques. In *Les Grandes Activités du Lobe Occipital*, T. Alajouanine, ed. Paris: Masson.

BAYNES, K., and J. C. ELIASSEN, 1998. The visual lexicon. In *Right Hemisphere Language Comprehension: Perspectives from Cognitive Neuroscience*. Mahwah, NJ: Lawrence Erlbaum Associates, pp. 79–104.

BEAUVOIS, M. F., 1982. Optic aphasia: A process of interaction between vision and language. *Philos. Trans. R. Soc. Lond. B* 289:35–47.

BEHRMANN, M., S. E. BLACK, and D. N. BUB, 1990. The evolution of pure alexia: A longitudinal study of recovery. *Brain Lang.* 39:405–427.

BENSON, D. F., and N. GESCHWIND, 1969. The alexias. In *Handbook of Clinical Neurology*, Vol. 4, P. J. Vinken and G. W. Bruyn, eds. Amsterdam: North-Holland, pp. 112–140.

BINDER, J. R., and J. P. MOHR, 1992. The topography of callosal reading pathways: A case control analysis. *Brain* 115:1807–1826.

BUB, D. N., S. BLACK, and J. HOWELL, 1989. Word recognition and orthographic context effects in a letter-by-letter reader. *Brain Lang.* 36:357–376.

BUXBAUM, L., and H. B. COSLETT, 1996. Deep dyslexic phenomena in a pure alexic. *Brain Lang.* 54:136–167.

COLTHEART, M., 1980. Deep dyslexia: A right hemisphere hypothesis. In *Deep Dyslexia*, M. Coltheart, K. E. Patterson, and

J. C. Marshall, eds. London: Routledge and Kegan Paul, pp. 326–380.

COLTHEART, M., 1983. The right hemisphere and disorders of reading. In *Functions of the Right Cerebral Hemisphere*, A. W. Young, ed. London: Academic Press, pp. 171–201.

COLTHEART, M., 1998. Seven questions about pure alexia (letter-by-letter reading). *Cogn. Neuropsychol.* 15:1–6.

COLTHEART, M., K. E. PATTERSON, and J. C. MARSHALL, EDS., 1980. *Deep Dyslexia*. London: Routledge and Kegan Paul.

COSLETT, H. B., and N. MONSUL, 1994. Reading and the right hemisphere: Evidence from transcranial magnetic stimulation. *Brain Lang.* 46:198–211.

COSLETT, H. B., and E. M. SAFFRAN, 1989a. Evidence for preserved reading in 'pure alexia.' *Brain* 112:327–359.

COSLETT, H. B., and E. M. SAFFRAN, 1989b. Preserved object recognition and reading comprehension in optic aphasia. *Brain* 112:1091–1110.

COSLETT, H. B., and E. M. SAFFRAN, 1992. Optic aphasia and the right hemisphere: A replication and extensions. *Brain Lang.* 43:148–161.

COSLETT, H. B., and E. M. SAFFRAN, 1994. Mechanics of implicit reading in alexia. In *The Neuropsychology of High-level Vision*, M. J. Farah and G. Ratcliff, eds. Hillsdale, NJ: Lawrence Earlbaum Associates, pp. 299–330.

DÉJERINE, J., 1891. Sur un cas de cécité verbale avec agraphie, suivi d'autopsie. *C. R. Séances Mém. Soc. Biol.* 3:197–201.

DÉJERINE, J., 1892. Contributions à l'étude anatomo-pathologique et clinique de différentes variétés de cécité verbale. *C. R. Séances Mém. Soc. Biol.* 4:61–90.

DE RENZI, E., 1999. Agnosia. In *Handbook of Experimental Neuropsychology*. Hove, UK: Psychology Press, pp. 371–407.

DE RENZI, E., F. MOTTI, and P. NICHELLI, 1980. Imitating gestures: A quantitative approach to ideomotor apraxia. *Arch. Neurol.* 37:6–10.

DE RENZI, E., A. PIECZURO, and L. A. VIGNOLO, 1968. Ideational apraxia: A quantitative study. *Neuropsychologia* 6:41–52.

DE RENZI, E., and M. C. SAETTI, 1997. Associative agnosia and optic aphasia: Qualitative or quantitative difference. *Cortex* 33:115–130.

FREUD, S., 1891. *Zur Auffassung der Aphasien.* Leipzig and Vienna, Deuticke.

FREUND, C. S., 1889. Ueber optische aphasie und seelenblindheit. *Arch. Psychiatrie Nervenkrankheiten* 20:276–297, 371–416. Engl. translation and commentary by A. Beaton, J. Davidoff, and U. Erstfeld, 1991. On optic aphasia and visual agnosia. *Cogn. Neuropsychol.* 8:21–38.

GESCHWIND, N., 1965. Disconnection syndromes in animals and man. *Brain* 88:585–644.

GESCHWIND, N., and M. FUSILLO, 1966. Color-naming defects in association with alexia. *Arch. Neurol.* 15:137–146.

GESCHWIND, N., and E. KAPLAN, 1962. A human cerebral deconnection syndrome. *Neurology* 12:675–685.

GOLDSTEIN, K., 1906. Zur frage der amnestischen aphasie und ihrer abgrenzung gegenüber der transcorticalen und glossopsychischen aphasie. *Arch. Psychiatrie Nervenkrankheiten* 41:911–950.

HECAEN, H., and H. KREMIN, 1976. Neurolinguistic research on reading disorders resulting from left hemisphere lesions: Aphasic and "pure" alexia. In *Studies in Neurolinguistics*, Vol. 2, H. Whitaker and H. A. Whitaker, eds. New York: Academic Press.

HILLIS, A., and A. CARAMAZZA, 1995. Cognitive and neural mechanisms underlying visual and semantic processing: Implication from "Optic Aphasia." *J. Cogn. Neurosci.* 7:457–478.

KINSBOURNE, M., and E. K. WARRINGTON, 1962. A disorder of simultaneous form perception. *Brain* 85:461–485.

KLEIST, K., 1934. Kriegsverletzungen des Gehirns in ihrer Bedeutung für die Hirnlokalisation und Hirnpathologie. In *Handbuch der ärztlichen Erfahrungen im Weltkrieg*, vol. 4, B. von Schjerning and K. Bonhoeffer, eds. Leipzig: Barth, pp. 343–1416.

LANDIS, T., M. REGARD, and A. SERRAT, 1980. Iconic reading in a case of alexia wihout agraphia caused by a brain tumor: A tachistoscopic study. *Brain Lang.* 11:45–53.

LHERMITTE, F., and F. BEAUVOIS, 1973. A visual-speech disconnection syndrome: Report of a case with Optic Aphasia, agnosic alexia and colour agnosia. *Brain* 96:695–714.

LIEPMANN, H., 1900. Das Krankheitsbild der Apraxie ("motorischen Asymbolie"). *Monatsschr. Psychiatr. Neurol.* 8, 15–44, 102–132, 182–197.

LIEPMANN, H., 1905. Die linke Hemisphäre und das Handeln. *Münch. Med. Wochenschr.* 49:2322–2326, 2375–2378.

LIEPMANN, H., 1920. Apraxie. *Ergebnisse Gesamten Med.* 1:516–543.

LIEPMANN, H., and O. MAAS, 1907. Ein fall von linksseitiger agraphie und apraxie bei rechtsseitiger lähmung. *J. Psychol. Neurol.* 10:214–227.

LISSAUER, H., 1890. Ein fall von seelenblindheit nebst einem beitrage zur theorie derselben. *Arch. Psychiatr. Nervenkrankheiten* 21:222–270.

LUZZATTI, C., R. RUMIATI, and G. GHIRARDI, 1998. A functional model of visuo-verbal disconnection and the neuroanatomical constraints of optic aphasia. *Neurocase* 4:71–87.

MARCEL, A. J., 1983. Conscious and unconscious perception. Experiments on visual masking and word recognition. *Cogn. Psychol.* 15:197–237.

MARR, D. 1982. *Vision.* San Francisco: W. H. Freeman.

MARSHALL, J., and F. NEWCOMBE, 1966. Syntactic and semantic errors in paralexia. *Neuropsychologia* 4:169–176.

MARSHALL, J., and F. NEWCOMBE, 1973. Patterns of paralexia: A psycholinguistic approach. *J. Psycholinguist. Res.* 2:175–199.

MICHEL, F., M. A. HENAFF, and J. INTRILLIGATOR, 1996. Two different readers in the same brain after a posterior callosal lesion. *NeuroReport* 7:786–788.

MORTON, J., and K. PATTERSON, 1980. A new attempt at an interpretation, or an attempt at a new interpretation. In *Deep Dyslexia*, M. Coltheart, K. E. Patterson, and J. C. Marshall, eds. London: Routledge and Kegan Paul, pp. 91–118.

PATTERSON, K., and D. BESNER, 1984. Is the right hemisphere literate? *Cogn. Neuropsychol.* 1:315–341.

PATTERSON, K., and J. KAY, 1982. Letter-by-letter reading: Psychological descriptions of a neurological syndrome. *Q. J. Exp. Psychol. Hum. Exp. Psychol.* 34A:411–441.

PATTERSON, K., F. VARGHA-KHADEM, and C. E. POLKEY, 1989. Reading with one hemisphere. *Brain* 112:39–63.

RATCLIFF, G., and F. NEWCOMBE, 1982. Object recognition: Some deductions from the clinical evidence. In *Normality and Pathology in Cognitive Functions*, A. W. Ellis, ed. New York: Academic Press, pp. 147–171.

REICHER, G. M., 1969. Perceptual recognition as a function of meaningfulness of stimulus material. *J. Exp. Psychol.* 81:275–328.

RIDDOCH, M. J., and G. W. HUMPHREYS, 1987. Visual object processing in a case of optic aphasia: A case of semantic access agnosia. *Cogn. Neuropsychol.* 4:131–185.

SAFFRAN, E. M., L. C. BOGYO, M. F. SCHWARTZ, and O. S. M. MARIN, 1980. Does deep dyslexia reflect right hemisphere reading? In *Deep Dyslexia*, M. Coltheart, K. E. Patterson, and J. C. Marshall, eds. London: Routledge and Kegan Paul.

SAFFRAN, E. M., and H. B. COSLETT, 1998. Implicit vs. letter-by-letter reading in pure alexia: A tale of two systems. *Cogn. Neuropsychol.* 15:141–165.

SCHNIDER, A., D. F. BENSON, and D. W. SCHARRE, 1994. Visual agnosia and optic aphasia: Are they anatomically distinct? *Cortex* 30:445–457.

SCHWARTZ, M. F., E. M. SAFFRAN, and O. S. M. MARIN, 1980. Fractionating the reading process in dementia: Evidence for word-specific print-to-sound associations. In *Deep Dyslexia*, M. Coltheart, K. E. Patterson, and J. C. Marshall, eds. London: Routledge and Kegan Paul, pp. 259–269.

SCHWEIGER, A., E. ZAIDEL, T. FIELD, and B. DOBKIN, 1989. Right hemisphere contribution to lexical access in an aphasic with deep dyslexia. *Brain Lang.* 37:73–89.

SHALLICE, T., 1988. *From Neuropsychology to Menal Structure.* Cambridge, Engl.: Cambridge University Press.

SHALLICE, T., and E. SAFFRAN, 1986. Lexical processing in the absence of explicit word identification: Evidence from a letter-by-letter reader. *Cogn. Neuropsychol.* 3:429–458.

SNODGRASS, J. G., and M. VANDERWART, 1980. A standardized set of 260 pictures: Norms for name agreement, image agreement, familiarity, and visual complexity. *J. Exp. Psychol. Hum. Percept. Perform.* 6:174–215.

WARRINGTON, E. K., and T. SHALLICE, 1980. Word form dyslexia, *Brain* 103:99–112.

WEEKES, B., M. COLTHEART, and E. GORDON, 1997. Deep dyslexia and right hemisphere reading: A regional cerebral blood flow study. *Aphasiology* 11:1139–1158.

WEISKRANTZ, L., 1983. Evidence and scotomata. *Behav. Brain Sci.* 6:464–467.

WHEELER, D. D., 1970. Processes in word recognition. *Cogn. Psychol.* 1:59–85.

WOLFF, G., 1904. *Klinische und kritische Beiträge zur Lehre von den Sprachstörungen.* Leipzig: Veit.

ZAIDEL, E., 1982. Reading in the disconnected right hemisphere: An aphasiological perspective. In *Dyslexia: Neuronal, Cognitive and Linguistic Aspects*, Y. Zotterman, ed. Oxford: Pergamon Press, pp. 67–91.

ZAIDEL, E., 1990. Language functions in the two hemispheres following complete cerebral commissurotomy and hemispherectomy. In *Handbook of Neuropsychology*, Vol. 4, F. Boller and J. Graffman, eds. Amsterdam: Elsevier, pp. 115–150.

COMMENTARY 22.1

Right Hemisphere Contributions to Word Recognition in Pure Alexia

ELISABETTA LÀDAVAS

ABSTRACT In this commentary the assumption that the right hemisphere mediates the reading performance of letter-by-letter readers is considered in the light of results obtained in split-brain patients in tasks that are more closely matched to ones used by investigators for pure alexic patients. The conclusion is that the hypothesis appears more suggestive than conclusive. In contrast, an attempt has been made to interpret the performance of pure alexic patients as an impairment of visual processing associated with LH damage.

In this commentary on the chapter by Luzzatti, I consider the literature pertaining to the representation of language in the right hemisphere of callosotomy patients to determine whether it provides an empirical basis for the assertion that the right hemisphere mediates the reading errors of pure alexic patients. These patients do not appear to be able to read in the sense of fast, automatic word recognition, although they are able to use a compensatory strategy that involves naming letters in a serial fashion. They read, in effect, letter by letter. Recently, however, several investigators have demonstrated that alexic patients are able to perform tasks such as lexical decision and semantic categorization on letter strings that are presented too rapidly to permit effective use of the letter-by-letter procedure (Shallice and Saffran, 1986; Landis, Regard, and Serrat, 1987; Coslett and Saffran, 1989). Though lexical decision and categorization are performed at above-chance levels, the patients are able to explicitly identify only a small percentage of these words at rapid presentations. It has been suggested that the implicit lexical and semantic performance may be mediated by the right hemisphere (Coslett and Saffran, 1989), which has an orthographic input lexicon and some semantic knowledge about words. When the left-hemisphere (LH) nonlexical route

fails because the exposure time is too short, and when the alternative lexical route to semantics in the right hemisphere (RH) is spared, the RH provides a semantic access, which is then transmitted through the intact callosum to the LH for phonological encoding and production.

The RH reading hypothesis has been put forward many times, from diverse sources and for diverse reasons (see references in Luzzatti's chapter) but has met with numerous objections (Coltheart, 1983; Patterson and Besner, 1984; Baynes, 1990). One potential way to clarify this point is to specify the visual mechanisms that are disrupted in pure alexic patients (see point 1 below) and to compare the results obtained in split-brain patients in those tasks that are more closely matched to ones used by other investigators in pure alexic patients (see points 2 and 3).

1. As was stated earlier, the hypothesis that the RH mediates the reading errors of pure alexic patients is motivated by the good performance these patients show on lexical and semantic tasks.

An argument that has been put forward against this position is the failure to demonstrate the effect of lexical and semantic categorization with brief exposure in all patients. However, Coslett and colleagues (1993) demonstrated the fragility of lexical and semantic effects by noting that it can be disrupted if naming is required first. Although it is possible that this effect may be manifested without requiring patients to explicitly read the letter string, it has been shown recently that this might not be the only reason to account for the absence of lexical and semantic effects. Làdavas and colleagues (in preparation) have documented the existence of two types of letter-by-letter readers, each of them showing a specific visual-processing deficit. The deficit may be related to an impairment in simultaneous processing of two visual targets located in two different spatial locations (spatial simultagnosia) or to a deficit in letter iden-

ELISABETTA LÀDAVAS Dipartimento di Psicologia, University of Bologna, Bologna, Italy; Centro di Neuroscience Cognitive, Cesena, Italy.

tification. These two different types of visual impairment interact differently with the ability to access visually lexical and semantic information.

In the first case, when the single letters forming a word or a nonword were presented tachistoscopically and sequentially on the same spatial position, the patient was able to read aloud the letter string, as normal subjects do. In contrast, when the single letters forming a letter string were presented simultaneously in different spatial locations along the horizontal dimension, the patient was not able to read the letter strings. This pattern of results was manifested with both letters and visual objects, demonstrating that it was not specific to linguistic processing. In addition, this patient performed at chance level on lexical and semantic tasks, showing that the letter string did not activate the corresponding representation in the lexicon and the semantic system.

In contrast, the other letter-by-letter reader performed at a level above chance both lexical and semantic tasks. However, his performance in reading aloud the letter string did not improve as much when the letters were presented in the same position. In contrast, his performance did improve when the interval between the presentation of each letter was increased, showing that the deficit was more at the level of letter identification (see Howard, 1990, for a similar explanation). The letter identification problem probably forced the patient to use a slow and serial letter processing in the reading-aloud task. In contrast, when the patient was instructed to give a quick glance at the stimulus, the normal, or close-to-normal, parallel-processing mode led to a representation of the whole string that, though degraded by the letter identification deficit, was able to activate the corresponding representation in the lexicon.

It is worthwhile to remember that although this second patient, as well as all other patients described in the literature, could carry out lexical and semantic decisions, he could not read aloud or identify the letter string after the categorization tasks. This probably occurs because the lexical and categorical discriminations can be carried out with a weaker or noisier output of the orthographic system than that required for reading aloud. The degraded output of the orthographic system is sufficient to support the correct category discrimination without being sufficient for the identification of the specific item itself. This is essentially analogous to the explanation given for related phenomena in neglect patients by Farah (1994) and in semantic access dyslexia by Hinton and Shallice (1991).

The results of Làdavas and colleagues (in preparation) clearly show that the deficit underlying the letter-by-letter reading is, in one patient, due to the presence of simultagnosia, which impedes parallel access of letter information to a visual word form, and as a consequence the patient cannot make lexical and semantic judgments on a string of letters that are briefly presented or read aloud the letter string by using the lexical route. This forced the patient to use the phonological route, which is serial and slow. In contrast, in the other patient, parallel visual processing was possible, but the locus of the deficit was more at the level of letter identification, which forced the patient to use slow and serial letter processing when the letter string was presented for a long exposure time. In contrast, the brief presentation of the letter string impeded the reading-aloud task but not the lexical and semantic tasks, which could be carried out with a weaker output from the orthographic system.

This way of interpreting the pattern of performance shown in pure alexic patients is entirely compatible with the notion that the performance might be carried out by the LH and, as a consequence, there is no need to invoke the orthographic input lexicon and the semantic knowledge in the RH. In fact, as we will see below, the linguistic competence of this hemisphere is far from clear.

2. Another way to clarify the role of the RH in mediating the performance of letter-by-letter readers is to compare the results obtained in split-brain patients in tasks that are more closely matched to tasks used by investigators for pure alexic patients. Both lexical and semantic tasks will be considered.

Some letter-by-letter readers seem to be able to perform lexical decision tasks at a level above chance. If we maintain the hypothesis that the RH mediates letter-by-letter readers' performance, we have to show that the RH of split-brain patients has an orthographic input lexicon.

The first report of visual lexical decision in the split-brain was made by Zaidel (1983), describing the work of Radant (1981). Using concrete imageable frequent words of unspecified length with a 100-ms exposure duration, all patients (L.B., R.Y., and N.F.) except N.G. were reported to be "bilaterally competent" at making lexical decisions. However, when Eviatar and Zaidel (1991) used four-, five-, and six-letter words as stimuli for a lexical decision task, L.B., R.Y., and N.G. were not able to respond at above-chance level to LVF/RH trials.

A similar conclusion can be drawn from Gazzaniga's patients (Baynes and Eliassen, 1997). When J.W., V.P., and D.R. were tested for LVF accuracy in lexical judgment for words and pseudo-words across a variety of experiments, it was clear that they had difficulty in performing the task at above chance level; moreover, there was a variability within subjects under differing experimental conditions.

In conclusion, if the RH of a split brain cannot perform lexical tasks, how can it mediate the lexical decision tasks of letter-by-letter readers, who perform this task at above chance level?

3. Despite the difference between the RH of split-brain patients and letter-by-letter readers in the lexical decision tasks, there are some similarities as far as the semantic tasks are concerned. As was stated earlier, letter-by-letter readers can make judgments about which of two broad superordinate categories a word is in (the easiest semantic decision). However, when the decision between alternatives requires the patient to identify the target word, because the semantic connection requires an inference (inferential judgment), performance is especially poor.

The same pattern of results has been demonstrated by the RH of split-brain patients. The RH of commisurotomy patients has neither control of speech mechanisms nor access to the speech mechanisms in the LH; as a consequence it cannot be tested for semantic errors in reading-aloud tasks, but only in reading comprehension tasks. Reading comprehension as measured by the ability to match written words with pictures appears to be accurate in both the East Coast (Gazzaniga's patients) and West Coast (Zaidel's patients) split-brain patients, although there are exceptions. D.R.'s RH is unable to read tachistoscopically presented stimuli to match words with pictures, although she could make lexical decisions in this time frame (Baynes, Tramo, and Gazzaniga, 1992).

However, as Zaidel (1990, p. 125) pointed out, "when the picture decoys in the multiple-choice arrays were all semantically associated with the target, the RH made many errors." In other words, when the semantic task requires more than a simple decision about which of two broad superordinate categories a word is in, as would be required in the case in which the semantic connection requires an inference about common semantic features, then performance is poor. These results are very similar to those found in pure alexic patients when they perform semantic tasks.

On the other hand, the conclusion that the RH has a full semantic representation of a written word appears more suggestive than conclusive when evaluated with studies in which semantic priming was used. The presence of semantic priming in a lexical decision task has been used to demonstrate semantic knowledge. Five complete commisurotomy patients were tested on their ability to respond to targets in a lexical decision task and then to targets with visual and auditory primes (Zaidel, 1983). Only one patient (L.B.) showed a priming effect with visual primes and only in the LH.

In conclusion, it seems from this short review that evidence for the hypothesis that the RH mediates the reading performance of letter-by-letter readers is more suggestive than conclusive. In contrast, it seems that a careful analysis of the impairment of visual processing in letter-by-letter readers may account for the dissociation between the performance in the reading task and lexical/semantic tasks in the LH.

REFERENCES

BAYNES, K., 1990. Language and reading in the right hemisphere: Highways or byways of the brain? *J. Cogn. Neurosci.* 2:159–179.

BAYNES, K., and J. C. ELIASSEN, 1997. The visual lexicon: Its access and organization in commisurotomy patients. In *Right Hemisphere Language Comprehension: Perspectives from Cognitive Neuroscience*, M. Beeman and C. Chiarello, eds. Mahwah, N.J.: Lawrence Erlbaum Associates, pp. 79–104.

BAYNES, K., M. J. TRAMO, and M. GAZZANIGA, 1992. Reading with a limited lexicon in the right hemisphere of a callosotomy patient. *Neuropsychologia* 30:187–200.

COLTHEART, M., 1983. The right hemisphere and disorders of reading. In *Functions of the Right Cerebral Hemisphere*, A. Young, ed. London: Academic Press.

COSLETT, H. B., and E. M. SAFFRAN, 1989. Evidence for preserved reading in pure alexia. *Brain* 112:327–329.

COSLETT, H. B., E. M. SAFFRAN, S. GREENBAUM, and H. SCHWARTZ, 1993. Reading in pure alexia. *Brain* 116, 21–37.

EVIATAR, Z., and E. ZAIDEL, 1991. The effects of word length and emotionality on hemispheric contribution to lexical decision. *Neuropsychologia* 29:415–428.

FARAH, M. J., 1994. Visual perception and visual awareness after brain damage: A tutorial overview. In *Attention and Performance XV*, C. Umiltà and M. Moscovitch, eds. Cambridge, Mass.: MIT Press, pp. 37–75.

HINTON, G. E., and T. SHALLICE, 1991. Lesioning an attractor network: Investigations of acquired dyslexia. *Psychol. Rev.* 98:74–95.

HOWARD, D., 1990. Letter-by-letter readers: Evidence for parallel processing. In *Basic Processes in Reading*, D. Besner and G. Humphreys, eds. Hillsdale, N.J.: Lawrence Erlbaum Associates, pp. 34–76.

LADAVAS, E., and G. DI PELLEGRINO, in preparation, Impairment of visual processing in letter-by-letter readers.

LANDIS, T., M. REGARD, and A. SERRAT, 1987. Iconic reading in case of alexia without agraphia caused by a brain tumor: A tachistoscopic study. *Brain Lang.* 11:45–53.

PATTERSON, K., and D. BESNER, 1984. Is the right hemisphere literate? *Cogn. Neuropsychol.* 1:315–341.

RADANT, A., 1981. *Facilitation in a lexical decision task: Effects of visual field, sex, handedness and anxiety*. Unpublished Honor Undergraduate Thesis, Department of Psychology, University of California at Los Angeles.

SHALLICE, T., and E. M. SAFFRAN, 1986. Lexical processing in the absence of explicit word identification: Evidence from a letter-by-letter reader. *Cogn. Neuropsychol.* 3:429–458.

ZAIDEL, E., 1983. Disconnection syndrome as a model for laterality effects in the normal brain. In *Cerebral Hemisphere Asymmetry: Method, Theory and Application*, J. E. Hellige, ed. New York: Praeger, pp. 95–151.

ZAIDEL, E., 1990. Language functions in the two hemispheres following complete cerebral commisurotomy and hemispherectomy. In *Handbook of Neuropsychology*, Vol. 4, F. Boller and G. Grafman, eds. New York: Elsevier Science Publishers, pp. 115–150.

COMMENTARY 22.2

Right Hemisphere Contributions to Residual Reading in Pure Alexia: Evidence from a Patient with Consecutive Bilateral Strokes

PAOLO BARTOLOMEO, ANNE-CATHERINE BACHOUD-LÉVI, JEAN-DENIS DEGOS, AND FRANÇOIS BOLLER

ABSTRACT This commentary focuses on the proposal that the disconnection approach may fruitfully interact with cognitive neuropsychology. In particular, we concentrate on pure alexia by providing a review of some explanatory accounts and a longitudinal case study. This patient became a letter-by-letter reader after a left occipitotemporal hematoma. Seven months later, she suffered a second, mirror-image hematoma in the right hemisphere, after which her residual reading capacity deteriorated dramatically, in terms of both accuracy and reading latencies for words and isolated letters. Our findings thereby support the hypothesis that the right hemisphere contributes to residual reading in pure alexic patients.

One of the main tenets of Luzzatti's chapter is that the classical disconnection approach may be updated with the models and methods of cognitive neuropsychology. Luzzatti provides convincing examples of the advantages that can be obtained by combining these two approaches. In particular, as Luzzatti notes, the renewed interest in disconnection syndromes has emphasized the need to anchor cognitive models to their neuroanatomical foundations. It may be noted that this approach is by no means universally accepted and that other investigators think that neuroanatomical constraints play at best an ancillary role in drawing inferences on normal cognition (Caramazza, 1992). However, Luzzatti's approach proves fruitful for the two main foci of his paper: optic aphasia and pure alexia. In this commentary we concentrate on pure alexia, presenting a brief review of the proposed explanatory accounts and some experimental data from our laboratory.

Pure alexia, or letter-by-letter reading, is an acquired reading disorder caused by lesions in the posterior regions of the left hemisphere (LH). Patients typically read slowly, letter by letter, and consequently show a length effect in word reading, that is, a monotonic increase of reading time with word length. Writing is characteristically spared, but patients are unable to read their own written production. Déjerine (1892) articulated his famous "Contribution to the Pathological and Clinical Investigation of Different Varieties of Verbal Blindness" by elaborating on Wernicke's theoretical predictions. He contrasted two case studies: patient Séj . . . , who showed alexia with agraphia and whose brain lesion was localized in the inferior part of the left angular gyrus (Déjerine, 1891), and M.C., who was alexic but not agraphic. M.C.'s reading deficit was particularly severe: "Even the letters presented in isolation are unrecognizable; he can only recognize them after a long hesitation and by tracing their contour" (Déjerine, 1892, p. 66). Writing was preserved until 10 days before his death, when M.C. suddenly became aphasic and agraphic. Autopsy disclosed two LH lesions: a recent one centered on the angular gyrus and the inferior parietal lobule and an old one restricted to the cuneus, the posterior part of the fusiform and lingual gyri, and the mesial temporo-occipital sulcus. The right hemisphere (RH) was intact. The pattern of impairments and the lesion location in these two cases, together with the evolution of M.C.'s deficits after his first and second strokes, convinced Déjerine that "in pure verbal blind-

PAOLO BARTOLOMEO INSERM Unit 324, Paris, France; Neuroscience Department, Hôpital Henri-Mondor, Créteil, France.
ANNE-CATHERINE BACHOUD-LÉVI LSCP, EHESS, CNRS, Paris, France; Neuroscience Department, Hôpital Henri-Mondor, Créteil, France.
JEAN-DENIS DEGOS Deceased.
FRANÇOIS BOLLER INSERM Unit 324, Paris, France.

ness with integrity of writing ... the center of the optic images of letters—the angular gyrus—is intact, but the lesion separates, isolates it from the common visual center" (p. 90). In other words, pure alexia would be due to an impaired access of visual information to intact visual representations of letters in the left angular gyrus. Geschwind (1965; Geschwind and Fusillo, 1966) assumed this explanation without modifications, as it nicely accommodated his own theoretical framework. More recently, the neurological account was challenged by cognitively based hypotheses. Pure alexia was then attributed to impaired activation of the visual word form (Warrington and Shallice, 1980) or to impaired access to lexical entries (Patterson and Kay, 1982). The notion of a reading-specific deficit was challenged in another set of studies. Pure alexia was thus considered to part of a more general problem with automatic identification of visual input (Friedman and Alexander, 1984) or an impairment in rapidly processing complex visual stimuli, both verbal and nonverbal (Kinsbourne and Warrington, 1962; Levine and Calvanio, 1978; Farah and Wallace, 1991). As Farah and Wallace (1991) note, these accounts present the advantage of not postulating dedicated neural hardware for a phylogenetically recent ability such as reading. However, these purely perceptual hypotheses fail to account for the specificity of LH, as opposed to RH, lesions in determining pure alexia. Rapp and Caramazza (1991) argued for a spatially determined deficit characterized by a left-to-right gradient of processing efficiency but found it difficult to specify more precisely the nature of this spatially based deficit as opposed to neglect dyslexia resulting from RH injury.

In a somewhat intermediate position between language-related hypotheses and more general perceptual-spatial accounts, a deficit occurring at the letter identification level is increasingly being recognized as a possible basis for pure alexia. Thus, Bub, Black, and Howell (1989) suggested that their patient J.V. might suffer from a subtle letter identification deficit, since the mere presence of a letter before the onset of another letter pair made their analysis difficult. However, Bub and colleagues considered it unlikely that this deficit was the cause of dyslexia. Reuter-Lorenz and Brunn (1990) demonstrated for their patient W.L. a deficit in processing the constituent letters in words. Howard (1991) argued for a problem in the identification of items, such as letters or letter features, whose number increases with word length. However, Howard noted that his data did not point specifically to a deficit of letter identification, that this deficit could be but a residual sign of an object agnosia, and that the relation of letter reading to word reading is not a transparent one. Arguin and Bub (1993) hypothesized for their patient D.M. a deficit in extract-

ing the perceptual identity of alphanumeric stimuli. Similarly, Behrmann and Shallice (1995, patient D.S.) argued for a visual disorder in the activation of individual letters that disrupts their rapid identification and proposed to consider this impairment as the default explanation of pure alexia. Perri, Bartolomeo, and Silveri (1996) explicitly addressed the issue of a causal relationship between letter and word reading deficits. They described a pure alexic patient, S.P., who produced misreading errors on both letters in isolation and words. Perri and colleagues found that errors in word reading were predictable from those in letter reading. In both cases, most errors were perceptual: S.P., like Patterson and Kay's (1982) patients, exhibited a tendency to confuse structurally similar letters. Perri and colleagues proposed an account of pure alexia based on an access deficit to the abstract visual representations of letters. This deficit would prevent an efficient (i.e., parallel) letter identification, forcing the patient to read letter by letter in order to afford one perceptual problem at a time. Furthermore, in agreement with Arguin and Bub (1993), Perri and colleagues (1996) argued that some differences that are observed among pure alexic patients might be quantitative, rather than qualitative. In particular, the letter identification problem might vary from mild to severe forms, producing, respectively, a simple letter-by-letter behavior (as in D.M. and D.S.) or some letter misidentifications even on reading letters in isolation, as in S.P.

A further issue in the discussion of pure alexia concerns the role of the intact RH in the reading behavior of pure alexic patients. An indispensable corollary of classical disconnectionistic accounts of pure alexia is the complete illiteracy of the RH; should the RH have some reading capacity, a disconnection of its visual areas from the LH would produce more complex patterns of behavior than the absolute inability to process visual verbal material postulated by Déjerine and Geschwind. Following a pure disconnection account, even reading letter by letter should not be possible, as was indeed the case with Déjerine's (1892) patient, who could not identify any single letter. However, most patients with pure alexia can read letter by letter, and some of them can even show some access to the identity of words that are presented too rapidly to permit overt reading. For example, pure alexic patients have been shown to perform tasks of lexical decision and semantic categorization on words that they do not name (Shallice and Saffran, 1986; Coslett and Saffran, 1989; see Luzzatti's chapter for a review of these implicit reading phenomena). Lexical decision may even be more efficient with short exposure times than with long ones, thus suggesting that alternative, competing strategies are employed for this task and for reading letter by letter. On the basis of this and other arguments, the observed implicit reading abilities have been attributed to a RH contribution (Landis et al., 1980; Coslett and Saffran, 1989, 1994). Coslett and Saffran (1994) proposed an information-processing account of single-word reading, with several levels of processing being implemented in the two hemispheres, thus providing a good example of mutual influence between cognitive neuropsychology and the disconnection anatomic approach (see Luzzatti's chapter). In this model, visual information proceeds in parallel in both hemispheres from early visual-processing levels through an object recognition system to a conceptual system; each of these levels is connected to its contralateral homologue by interhemispheric links. The LH and RH conceptual systems receive input from two further levels: a letter identification level and a visual word form system, which are specific to reading and bilaterally represented but not connected by callosal fibers. A phonological output system is represented uniquely in the LH and receives input from the LH conceptual system. In pure alexia, letter information would reach the LH via the object recognition system (in either hemisphere?); this mechanism would not permit parallel identification of letters in words, thus leading to letter-by-letter reading. Letter information would in turn activate the appropriate visual word forms in the LH through a reverse spelling procedure. On the other hand, implicit reading would be mediated by RH-based processing from early visual levels to the RH conceptual system, which has no direct connection with the phonological output lexicon (see Luzzatti's chapter). Some independent evidence supporting this model was provided by Coslett and Monsul (1994) using transcranial magnetic stimulation, which is assumed to transiently block the neural function of the underlying brain regions. They stimulated the posterior regions of the RH or the LH of a partially recovered pure alexic and found that stimulation of the RH but not of the LH disrupted oral reading.

Longitudinal studies of patients with consecutive brain lesions provide a different approach to test hypotheses about the hemispheric contributions to reading. For example, Heilman and colleagues (1979, case 1) described the case of a left-brain-damaged aphasic patient who was able to read but lost this ability after a second RH stroke. The authors speculated that the LH may use a grapheme-to-phoneme transcoding strategy in reading, while the RH may be able to read ideographically, without phonological processing (see Zaidel, 1990, for a related proposal based on evidence from commisurotomized patients). In another study on the effect of subsequent lesions on dyslexia, Roeltgen (1987) described a

deep dyslexic patient who lost his residual reading ability after a second LH stroke. According to Roeltgen, this sequence of events challenged the RH reading hypothesis advanced by Coltheart (1980) for deep dyslexia. However, it may be noted that Roeltgen's patient had sustained a previous right frontal lesion, whose role in the subsequent sequence of events remains unclear.

The follow-up study of LH-damaged pure alexic patients who suffered a second RH stroke would provide a unique opportunity to test directly the RH reading account in pure alexia. We were able to study one such patient, who became alexic after a LH temporal-occipital lesion and whose residual reading capacities markedly worsened following a second, mirror-image RH lesion.

Case report

Madame D. is a 74-year-old right-handed housewife who had worked as a secretary. She had enjoyed reading and painting as hobbies until May 1995, when she complained of suddenly occurring blurred vision in the right visual field. A computerized tomography scan showed a hematoma located across the left temporo-occipital sulcus, involving the middle occipital gyrus and the inferior temporal gyrus (Brodmann areas 18, 19, and 37). She presented with a right homonymous hemianopia and showed a mild anomia for visually presented items, without any comprehension or repetition deficit, that subsided after some weeks. She showed no signs of recognizing the items she could not name; naming by definition was spared, suggesting that she suffered from a mild form of object agnosia. The only other linguistic deficit, and the patient's major complaint, was difficulty in reading. At clinical onset she read slowly and letter by letter, with occasional confusion among letters. Writing was preserved. Some weeks afterward, when experimental testing began, her visual field defect on confrontation testing had resolved. Goldmann perimetry showed a residual right paracentral scotoma, which disappeared with IV/4 test. On a simple motor reaction time (RT) task to lateralized visual stimuli (Bartolomeo, 1997), she was moderately slow on right-sided targets, possibly on account of some subtle form of spatial neglect, but performed in the range of age-matched controls when responding to left-sided (ipsilesional) stimuli.

In December 1995 Madame D. suffered a second, right-sided hematoma, almost symmetrical to the first. The lesion was centered on the middle occipital gyrus, just posterior to the temporo-occipital sulcus, involving areas 19 and 18 and the underlying white matter (Figure 22.9).

To her dismay, Madame D., who was beginning to recover to some extent and to enjoy reading again,

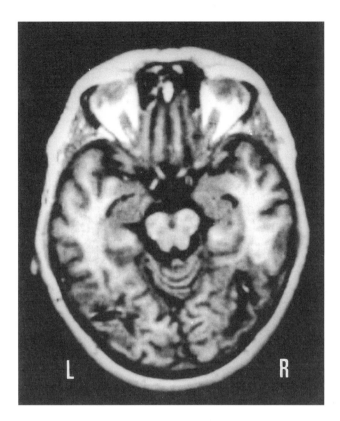

FIGURE 22.9. T1-weighted magnetic resonance image showing the first left hemispheric lesion (on the right side of the figure) and the second right hemispheric lesion (left side of the figure).

found herself once again alexic, to a much greater extent than before. Moreover, she had become severely prosopagnosic, object agnosic, and achromatopsic. The unfortunate occurrence of the second brain lesion brought our experimental testing to an abrupt stop, preventing us from studying covert reading in this patient. She had full visual field on confrontation testing. Goldmann perimetry showed a small central scotoma with II/4 test. Visual evoked responses with black-and-white pattern were normal for latency and amplitude. She was unable to name any black-and-white realistic drawings. When asked to name real objects presented by the examiner, she was 13/35 correct on visual presentation, claiming that she was unable to recognize the other items. She named the same objects without any hesitation or error when they produced a characteristic noise (e.g., jiggling keys) or on tactile presentation. After some weeks, she had regained some minimal ability to identify alphanumeric characters. When presented with words or letters, she appeared at a loss, examining the stimulus for a long time before producing a doubtful response. She was asked to point to individual letters and single-digit numbers named by the examiner. The characters were printed in Times 72 font on paper strips scattered on the

table in front of her. She was 4/26 correct for letters and 1/10 correct for digits. At that time, the patient obtained a verbal IQ of 109 on the WAIS-R. When presented with items from two oral confrontation picture-naming tests (Snodgrass and Vanderwart, 1980; Deloche et al., 1996), she was 39/90 (43%) and 94/167 (56%) correct, respectively. She showed no sign of recognizing the items she could not name. She performed correctly the screening test and the space perception test of the Visual Object and Space Perception Battery (VOSP) (Warrington and James, 1991) but failed on all the object perception tests. On a test of line orientation judgment (Benton et al., 1983), she obtained a corrected score of 25, well within the normal limits. She produced a plausible copy of the drawing of a landscape (Gainotti et al., 1986). Her RTs to left-sided targets in the simple motor RT task did not differ from response latencies recorded before the occurrence of the second lesion.

Material

WORD READING Two hundred words of four, five, six, seven, and eight letters in length were presented free field, printed in lowercase on a paper strip, without a time limit. Half of the stimuli were high-frequency words (>3000 from Content, Mousty, and Radeau's (1990) word count), and half were low-frequency words (<1300). Accuracy and reading time were recorded manually by the examiner, who started a stopwatch on stimulus presentation and stopped it when the response was complete. The word list was presented twice on separate occasions: after the first stroke and after the second stroke.

LETTER READING The 26 letters of the French alphabet were randomly presented in lowercase on paper strips for unlimited time. Accuracy was recorded. Reading latencies for letters were measured for Madame D. and her 74-year-old, right-handed husband, who was free from neurological deficit. Again, all the letters of the French alphabet were used. Letters were presented in lowercase Trip font size 8 (subtending a visual angle of about 1°30′) at the center of the plasma screen of a Toshiba T-5200 computer. A microphone was connected to an OROS AU-22 digital board programmed to function as a voice key, which measured naming time to the nearest millisecond and digitized the naming response. Subjects were instructed to name the letter as soon as it appeared on the screen and to respond as fast as possible. The target letter remained visible until a vocal response was made or 5 seconds had elapsed. Responses were followed for 2 seconds by a blank screen before the next trial began. Naming latencies were mea-

TABLE 22.4

Mean correct reading latencies for words (in seconds), following the first and the second stroke

	Word Length (letters)		
	4–5	6	7–8
LH lesion	2.6	3.5	4.8
LH + RH lesions	9.4	15.9	14.3

sured from the appearance of the letter on the display to the onset of a response. The set of 26 letters was presented four times for each session in a random order. The experiment was divided into two blocks. Each block contained twice the complete alphabet and was preceded by 13 practice trials. Madame D. and her husband performed three sessions; after her second stroke, Madame D. performed two additional sessions.

READING TESTS: INITIAL ASSESSMENT   Some weeks after her LH lesion, Madame D. read aloud correctly 398/400 (99%) words. She had the impression of reading faster than she was able to do soon after the stroke, even though she was still distressed by her reading difficulties. She showed a linear relationship between word length and reading time ($r = 0.77$), with a slope of 0.50 s per additional letter ($t = 24.02$, $p < 0.0001$; the intercept was removed, forcing the model through the origin, as it makes no sense to measure the reading time for a 0-letter word) (see Table 22.4). The observed length effect was in the range of previous reports on letter-by-letter readers (see Shallice, 1988, Table 4.1, p. 74). High-frequency words were read faster than low-frequency words ($t(2) = -3.20$, $p < 0.05$).

When reading lowercase letters presented for unlimited time, Madame D. was 156/156 (100%) correct. On the time-limited computer presentation she was 295/312 (94%) correct. Her husband scored 307/312 (98%) correct, thus performing in the same range ($\chi^2(1) = 0.41$, $p > 0.5$). However, as concerns reading latency, Madame D. was about 230 ms slower than her husband (Madame D.: mean RT = 697 ms (S.D.: 98); control: mean RT = 464 ms (S.D.: 31); $t(50) = 11.54$, $p < 0.0001$). This finding suggests that Madame D. suffered from a subtle deficit of letter identification. The longest RTs were observed for the same subset of letters on which patient S.P. (Perri et al., 1996) made most of his reading errors; this finding provides some support for a possible generalizability of our account.

READING TESTS: SECOND ASSESSMENT   After the RH lesion, Madame D. was presented with the same stimulus material used in the preceding test sessions. In contrast with her near perfect accuracy in reading words and isolated letters after the first stroke, she was now only 156/400 (39%) correct when reading words and 22/52 (42%) correct when reading lowercase letters. Word reading latencies were significantly increased with respect to latencies before the second lesion ($t(504) = -14.50$, $p < 0.0001$). The patient now needed about 13 s on average to read a single word. She continued to use a letter-by-letter strategy but now made several letter identification errors. For example, when trying to read the word *rescapé* [survivor], the patient took 59 s to say: "n...o...s...c...u...p... Moscou? [Moscow]." A word length effect was still present ($r = 0.75$) but with the steeper slope of 2.01 s per additional letter ($t = 14.07$, $p < 0.0001$). Mean correct RTs for words of different lengths are displayed in Table 22.4. Madame D. showed a trend toward reading high-frequency words faster ($t(122) = -1.43$, $p = 0.077$, one-tailed) than low-frequency words, but reading accuracy was comparable across the two sets of stimuli (86/200 correct for high-frequency words, 70/200 for low-frequency words; Fisher's $p = 0.12$). Her mean vocal RT to isolated letters was now 1197 ms (S.D.: 166).

Discussion

We have described a patient who showed a typical pure alexia after a left occipitotemporal lesion. Her reading difficulties markedly increased following a second, mirror-image lesion in the right hemisphere. The deterioration of word and letter reading performance involved both accuracy and response time.

Our patient's increased reading latency cannot be ascribed to a nonspecific slowing due to the brain lesions, as she performed in the normal range when responding to left-sided visual stimuli on a simple motor RT task. Her impaired reading accuracy after the second stroke cannot be explained by a low-level visual deficit, given her good performance on copying drawings, on line orientation judgments, and on the spatial subtests of the VOSP. Moreover, both magnetic resonance imaging and visual evoked potentials suggest that early visual processing was substantially spared in Madame D. Thus, the deterioration of reading accuracy after the second stroke seems to indicate that some mechanisms that Madame D. used to compensate for her alexia were impaired by the RH lesion. These putative compensatory mechanisms were apparently involved in both word and letter identification.

After her first lesion Madame D. showed a length effect on word reading latencies, arguably because she used a strategy of serial letter identification. The fact that a length effect was still present after the second stroke suggests that Madame D. continued to employ such a strategy. However, after the second lesion the serial letter identification was much less efficient, being both slower and less accurate. The finding that our patient continued to read letter by letter after the RH lesion supports the claim that this strategy represents a residual LH reading mechanism in pure alexia (Zaidel, 1998), but the fact that letter-by-letter reading was slower and less accurate after the RH lesion seems to suggest that the RH can also contribute to it.

Lexical frequency inversely affected word reading latencies after the LH lesion; this effect became less reliable after the RH lesion. A word frequency effect in pure alexia can be easily explained as a top-down effect in the framework of a hierarchical model of reading (McClelland and Rumelhart, 1981), which postulates that word nodes for high-frequency words have resting levels higher than nodes for low-frequency words. A weak or ambiguous input from the letter level can then activate the nodes for high-frequency words faster and more reliably than the nodes for low-frequency words. This account implies, of course, that the word level was entirely spared in our patient, an assumption that challenges the proposed breakdown of the visual word form system in pure alexia (Warrington and Shallice, 1980). As the RH lexicon seems to contain representations of concrete high-frequency nouns, it is tempting to relate the observed decrease of frequency effect after the RH lesion to an impaired RH contribution to reading. Alternatively, practice could have reduced the effect of lexical frequency by rendering low-frequency items as easy to read as high-frequency items; however, this is unlikely because months elapsed between testing sessions, and Madame D. never gave signs of remembering words she had previously encountered.

Taken together, our data provide converging evidence for the claim that the right hemisphere plays a role in the residual reading of pure alexic patients (Coslett and Saffran, 1989). Because of the posterior location of our patient's lesions, the sequence of events that we observed might in fact be considered a lesional equivalent to Coslett and Monsul's (1994) transcranial magnetic stimulation experiment. In particular, our pattern of results suggests that after the LH lesion our patient used RH-based mechanisms to increase accuracy and speed of letter and word identification, even in the absence of right-sided hemianopia. However, it is unlikely that her residual reading capacities were entirely attributable to the RH, as some patients with isolated LH lesions show a higher degree of impairment than Madame D. (see, e.g., Perri et al., 1996). Rather, the RH seemed to cooperate with some LH residual mechanisms

in our patient. If we are correct in interpreting the underlying mechanism of Madame D.'s alexia after the LH lesion as a letter identification problem, then a RH-based shape recognition mechanism might have contributed to letter identification at this stage. This process, not being specific to reading, would presumably be less efficient than its LH counterpart; it would not thereby allow parallel identification of letters in words, thus leading to letter-by-letter reading. On the other hand, the mutually constraining activities of a partially functioning LH letter identification process and of an intact RH shape recognition mechanism would account for the accurate, if slow, reading performance that is observed at this stage. As was mentioned earlier in this commentary, Coslett and Saffran (1994) argue for a similar explanation of pure alexia, though in their view, the LH has no access whatsoever to visual information (which is actually the case only in hemianopic patients). Coslett and Saffran's model fits with our results, in that they postulate that the RH object recognition mechanism is callosally connected with its LH homologue, thus providing the LH with information about individual letters that are processed as familiar visual forms. This information would in turn activate the appropriate visual word forms in the LH through a reverse spelling procedure. Madame D.'s second lesion might have resulted in an impairment of the RH object recognition system, thus leading to further disruption of letter identification, which became error-prone and much slower than before. In turn, this more severe letter identification deficit might have caused the deterioration of word reading. Support for this interpretation comes from the appearance, after the RH lesion, of a stable object agnosia.

ACKNOWLEDGMENTS We acknowledge with thanks the help of Beatrice de Gelder and Victor Rosenthal in testing the patient. Some results from the present case report appeared in a previously published article (Bartolomeo et al., 1998).

REFERENCES

ARGUIN, M., and D. N. BUB, 1993. Single-character processing in a case of pure alexia. *Neuropsychologia* 31:435–458.

BARTOLOMEO, P., 1997. The novelty effect in recovered hemineglect. *Cortex* 33:323–332.

BARTOLOMEO, P., A. C. BACHOUD-LÉVI, J. D. DEGOS, and F. BOLLER, 1998. Disruption of residual reading capacity in a pure alexic patient after a mirror-image right hemispheric lesion. *Neurology* 50:286–288.

BEHRMANN, M., and T. SHALLICE, 1995. Pure alexia: A nonspatial visual disorder affecting letter activation. *Cogn. Neuropsychol.* 12:409–454.

BENTON, A. L., K. HAMSHER, N. R. VARNEY, and O. SPREEN, 1983. *Contributions to Neuropsychological Assessment.* Oxford, Engl.: Oxford University Press.

Bub, D. N., S. Black, and J. Howell, 1989. Word recognition and orthographic context effects in a letter-by-letter reader. *Brain Lang.* 36:357–376.

Caramazza, A., 1992. Is cognitive neuropsychology possible? *J. Cogn. Neurosci.* 4:80–95.

Coltheart, M., 1980. Deep dyslexia: A right hemisphere hypothesis. In *Deep Dyslexia*, M. Coltheart, K. E. Patterson, and J. Marshall, eds. London: Routledge and Kegan Paul, pp. 22–47.

Content, A., P. Mousty, and M. Radeau, 1990. Brulex, une base de données lexicales informatisée pour le français écrit et parlé. *L'Année Psychol.* 90:551–566.

Coslett, H. B., and N. Monsul, 1994. Reading with the right hemisphere: Evidence from transcranial magnetic stimulation. *Brain Lang.* 46:198–211.

Coslett, H. B., and E. M. Saffran, 1989. Evidence for preserved reading in 'pure alexia.' *Brain* 89:327–359.

Coslett, H. B., and E. M. Saffran, 1994. Mechanisms of implicit reading in alexia. In *The Neuropsychology of High-Level Vision: Collected Tutorial Essays*, M. J. Farah and G. Ratcliff, eds. Hillsdale, N.J.: Lawrence Erlbaum Associates, pp. 299–330.

Déjerine, M. J., 1891. Sur un cas de cécité verbale avec agraphie, suivi d'autopsie [On a case of word blindness with agraphia, followed by autopsy]. *Mém. Soc. Biol.* 3:197–201.

Déjerine, M. J., 1892. Contribution à l'étude anatomo-pathologique et clinique des différentes variétés de cécité verbale [Contribution to the pathological and clinical investigation of different varieties of word blindness]. *Mém. Soc. Biol.* 4:61–90.

Deloche, G., D. Hannequin, M. Dordain, D. Perrier, B. Pichard, S. Quint, M. C. Metz-Lutz, H. Kremin, and D. Cardebat, 1996. Picture confrontation oral naming: Performance differences between aphasics and normals. *Brain Lang.* 53:105–120.

Farah, M. J., and M. A. Wallace, 1991. Pure alexia as a visual impairment: A reconsideration. *Cogn. Neuropsychol.* 8:313–334.

Friedman, R. B., and M. P. Alexander, 1984. Pictures, images, and pure alexia: A case study. *Cogn. Neuropsychol.* 1:9–23.

Gainotti, G., P. D'Erme, D. Monteleone, and M. C. Silveri, 1986. Mechanisms of unilateral spatial neglect in relation to laterality of cerebral lesions. *Brain* 109:599–612.

Geschwind, N., 1965. Dysconnexion syndromes in animals and man. *Brain* 88:237–294.

Geschwind, N., and M. Fusillo, 1966. Color naming defects in association with alexia. *Arch. Neurol.* 15:137–146.

Heilman, K. M., L. Rothi, D. Campanella, and S. Wolfson, 1979. Wernicke's and global aphasia without alexia. *Arch. Neurol.* 36:129–133.

Howard, D., 1991. Letter-by-letter readers: Evidence for parallel processing. In *Basic Processes in Reading: Visual Word Recognition*, D. Besner and G. W. Humphreys, eds. Hillsdale, N.J.: Lawrence Erlbaum Associates, pp. 34–76.

Kinsbourne, M., and E. K. Warrington, 1962. A disorder of simultaneous form perception. *Brain* 85:461–486.

Landis, T., M. Regard, and A. Serrat, 1980. Iconic reading in a case of alexia without agraphia caused by a brain tumor: A tachistoscopic study. *Brain Lang.* 11:45–53.

Levine, D. N., and R. Calvanio, 1978. A study of the visual defect in verbal alexia-simultanagnosia. *Brain* 101:65–81.

McClelland, J. L., and D. E. Rumelhart, 1981. An interactive activation model of context effects in letter perception: 1. An account of basic findings. *Psychol. Rev.* 88:375–407.

Patterson, K., and J. Kay, 1982. Letter-by-letter reading: Psychological description of a neurological syndrome. *Q. J. Exp. Psychol.* 34A:411–441.

Perri, R., P. Bartolomeo, and M. C. Silveri, 1996. Letter dyslexia in a letter-by-letter reader. *Brain Lang.* 53:390–407.

Rapp, B. C., and A. Caramazza, 1991. Spatially determined deficits in letter and word processing. *Cogn. Neuropsychol.* 8:275–311.

Reuter-Lorenz, P. A., and J. L. Brunn, 1990. A prelexical basis for letter-by-letter reading: A case study. *Cogn. Neuropsychol.* 7:1–20.

Roeltgen, D. P., 1987. Loss of deep dyslexic reading ability from a second left-hemispheric lesion. *Arch. Neurol.* 44:346–348.

Shallice, T., 1988. *From Neuropsychology to Mental Structure.* New York: Cambridge University Press.

Shallice, T., and E. M. Saffran, 1986. Lexical processing in the absence of explicit word identification. *Cogn. Neuropsychol.* 3:429–458.

Snodgrass, J. G., and M. Vanderwart, 1980. A standardized set of 260 pictures: Norms for name agreement, image agreement, familiarity and visual complexity. *J. Exp. Psychol. Hum. Learn. Mem.* 6:174–215.

Warrington, E. K., and M. James, 1991. *The Visual Object and Space Perception Battery.* Bury St. Edmunds, Engl.: Thames Valley Test Company.

Warrington, E. K., and T. Shallice, 1980. Word-form dyslexia. *Brain* 103:99–112.

Zaidel, E., 1990. Language functions in the two hemispheres following complete cerebral commisurotomy and hemispherectomy. In: *Handbook of Neuropsychology*, F. Boller and J. Grafman, eds. Amsterdam: Elsevier, pp. 115–150.

Zaidel, E., 1998. Language in the right hemisphere following callosal disconnection. In *Handbook of Neurolinguistics*, B. Stemmer and H. Whitaker, eds. New York: Academic Press, pp. 369–383.

COMMENTARY 22.3

Letter-by-Letter Reading: Regional Cerebral Blood Flow Correlates

MARCO IACOBONI, PATRIZIA PANTANO, AND VITTORIO DI PIERO

ABSTRACT A 28-year-old right-handed female developed a letter-by-letter reading strategy following a large demyelinating lesion in temporo-occipital white matter of the left hemisphere. Regional cerebral blood flow (rCBF) was measured with single photon emission computerized tomography (SPECT) and Tc-99m HM-PAO at rest and during a reading task. During reading, a significant rCBF increase in the right temporoparietal and occipital areas was observed, in comparison with the rest condition. Findings may argue for the existence of a right-hemisphere visual word form system that operates by sequential access.

Luzzatti suggests that letter-by-letter reading in pure alexia is subserved by the damaged left hemisphere. Here we present evidence from brain activation during reading in pure alexia, suggesting that letter-by-letter reading is subserved by the undamaged right hemisphere.

Recall that letter-by-letter reading is a form of acquired dyslexia in which patients read single words by identifying one letter at a time. Reading is very fatiguing, and latencies increase linearly with the number of letters in a word. In the last decade, different studies, using detailed information-processing analyses, have proposed sophisticated cognitive models to explain the disorder (Warrington and Shallice, 1980; Patterson and Kay, 1982; Friedman and Alexander, 1984; Shallice and Saffran, 1986; Doctor, Sartori, and Saling, 1990; Hanley and Kay, 1992), whereas cascade-processing models have been alternatively offered to explain mechanisms of reading (McClelland and Rumelhart, 1981; Rumelhart and McClelland, 1982).

Evidence from single-case studies has suggested that letter-by-letter readers could have a deficit of the visual

MARCO IACOBONI Ahmanson Lovelace Brain Mapping Center, Neuropsychiatric Institute, Brain Research Institute, David Geffen School of Medicine, University of California at Los Angeles, Los Angeles, California.

PATRIZIA PANTANO AND VITTORIO DI PIERO Department of Neurological Sciences, University La Sapienza, Rome, Italy.

word-form system (Warrington and Shallice, 1980) or, alternatively, that they have lost the ability to transmit letter information in parallel to it (Patterson and Kay, 1982). The visual word form is a representation of the orthography of the letter string in which the individual letters are combined into ordered, familiar chunks (Compton et al., 1991; Warrington and Shallice, 1980). Other single-case studies have argued for a prelexical basis of this disorder, with damage to an early visual processing component (Friedman and Alexander, 1984; Reuter-Lorenz and Brunn, 1990). The lack of consistency in previous studies might be explained by different strategies employed by letter-by-letter readers to carry out the task of reading (Doctor et al., 1990; Hanley and Kay, 1992).

Recent studies employing positron emission tomography (PET) have investigated the functional anatomy of word reading in normals (Petersen et al., 1989, 1990), showing a network of specific areas involved in reading visual words that include a left ventral occipital area, a right temporal area, and a left inferior prefrontal area. The left ventral occipital area is activated by both words and orthographically regular nonwords (Peterson et al., 1989, 1990), and it has been proposed as the anatomical correlate of the visual word-form system (Peterson et al., 1990). The right temporal area is activated by all strings used and appears to be activated when subjects are required to detect a feature. It is thought to constitute a visual prelexical representation (Corbetta et al., 1990; Compton et al., 1991). The left frontal area is activated by words but not by nonwords when the subjects deal with the meaning of the word.

To our knowledge, only a few studies have applied functional neuroimaging techniques to letter-by-letter readers. In the first study an activation reading paradigm was performed, but the investigation was severely limited by the low resolution of the bidimensional nontomographic technique employed (Halsey et al., 1980), whereas in the second, a PET study, activation reading tasks were not carried out (Silver et al., 1988).

Here we report evidence from SPECT to measure activity-related changes in regional cerebral blood flow to identify brain regions that are active during a reading task in a letter-by-letter reader.

F.C., a 28-year-old right-handed female high-school graduate, presented with fever and abdominal pain. Four days after the onset of symptoms she developed hypostenia in the left limbs. After a week she experienced lower limb paresthesiae, reduced vision, and awareness that she could not read. She was admitted to the Department of Neurological Sciences of the University La Sapienza of Rome for evaluation and treatment.

On admission, examination disclosed blood pressure of 150/100 mm Hg; her pulse was 70 beats per minute and regular. Except for abdominal pain, results of a general examination were unremarkable. The patient could speak fluently and comprehend spoken but not written language. She had right homonymous hemianopia, a slightly decreased right corneal reflex, paraparesis and left upper limb weakness, tactile hypoesthesia of the lower limbs, and ataxia in all limbs. Deep tendon reflexes were diminished in the left upper limb and increased in the lower limbs. She had a bilateral plantar extensor response. She also presented with disturbances of micturition. CSF study showed mononuclear pleocytosis and a slight increase of total protein content and IgG. The IgG index also showed an increased value. However, oligoclonal bands were not seen. Viral antigens were not demonstrated in CSF. Visual and tactile evoked responses and blink reflexes were altered, while brain stem auditory evoked responses were not. A magnetic resonance imaging study disclosed a high-intensity lesion, in both T1- and T2-weighted images, involving pes medullae and cervical spinal cord. In another set of high-intensity T1- and T2-weighted images, a large lesion was demonstrated in the white matter of the left temporal and occipital lobe, involving the forceps major and the paraventricular region of the occipital horn. Another set of high-intensity T1- and T2-weighted images demonstrated a small lesion in the paraventricular white matter of the left frontal lobe. All lesions showed enhancement after administration of gadolinium-DTPA. The patient was treated with Methil-Prednisolone, 1000 mg i.v. per day, for 10 days. After this treatment she showed a good motor recovery, but reading disorders and visual field defects did not improve. The patient was discharged with the diagnosis of postinfectious leukoencephalomyelitis.

On neuropsychological evaluation her spontaneous speech was fluent, articulate, and prosodic without any kind of errors. She had no difficulty in auditory comprehension. Repetition of words, nonwords, and sentences was intact. She was able to fluently repeat words and nonwords spelled aloud by the examiner (spelling identification). She was also able to spell words or nonwords (oral spelling). She had no difficulty in naming colors and objects. On the Boston Naming Test she scored 46/60 correct responses without cues. She was able to decipher ideograms, such as $, %, and =. Her writing capabilities were unimpaired, except for her motor difficulties. She showed a profound impairment in word reading, but her ability to read individual letters was less impaired. Therefore, she developed a letter-by-letter reading strategy, which made the task laborious. To read a three-letter word by this means would take F.C., on average, 13 seconds. Reading errors were visually similar to the target ("b" for "d," "n" for "u"; i.e., visual paralexias). She did not show semantic paralexias. Number reading was slightly impaired, and calculation was poor.

She was able to match briefly presented written words to line drawings of objects. The patient was presented with 12 words printed in uppercase lettering, each for 2 seconds, timed with a stopwatch. The patient's task was to choose among five line-drawn objects, the names of which all began with the same letter and had approximately the same length (e.g., penna, pane, pino, pera, and pesca). F.C. responded correctly on nine of the 12 trials (75%). Her performance was significantly above chance (20%) on a binomial test ($p < 0.0001$).

Finger agnosia was intact, and right-left discrimination was normal. Facial recognition and limb and facial praxis were also intact. On the Wechsler Adult Intelligence Scale (WAIS) the patient scored 90 on verbal I.Q., which was affected by her poor calculation ability; 85 on performance I.Q., the latter being affected mainly by slowness in time-dependent tasks; and 87 on full-scale I.Q. Her verbal memory was faulty. On the Wechsler Memory Scale (WMS) she scored 73. She correctly remembered only six words on immediate recall and three words on delayed recall of the Auditory Verbal Learning Test. She did not remember, in three trials, any of the hard associates of the subtest Paired Associate Learning of the WMS. On the Logical Memory Subtest, she correctly rehearsed only five items on Immediate Recall and three on the Delayed Recall.

Reading tasks

EXPERIMENT 1: WORD-LENGTH EFFECT In letter-by-letter readers the pronunciation of a printed or written word is accomplished through the activation of a reversed spelling strategy (Warrington and Shallice, 1980).

The prediction here is that reading time should increase with the number of letters in the stimulus. In addition, if the patient has no perceptual and/or attentional disorders, topographic transformation (vertical form) of stimuli should affect neither latencies nor accuracy of the reading processes. The prediction here is that vertical reading shows the same pattern of errors and the same reading latencies as horizontal reading.

F.C. was presented with a set of 50 horizontally oriented abstract and concrete words, ranging from three to seven letters. There were 10 words of each length. Each word was written in uppercase letters on a separate index card. A second list of 50 abstract and concrete words, written in uppercase letters with the same distribution of word length, oriented in a vertical column, was presented, one word per index card. The words in the two lists were randomized and presented to F.C. one at a time for oral reading. There were five trials of 20 words per trial. Time and accuracy were recorded for each word. F.C.'s speed of reading was timed with a stopwatch. For scoring purposes, only the first response and the time needed to reach the first response were recorded, although, if F.C. asked, she was told whether or not her response was correct and was allowed to try again.

F.C. made reading errors in response to 13/50 (26%) horizontally oriented words and 12/50 (24%) vertically oriented words. The only stimulus parameter that was found to significantly affect her reading speed and accuracy was word length. Concreteness and word frequency (Bortolini, Tagliavini, and Zampolli, 1968) did not affect either accuracy or latencies. Reading errors and reading latencies revealed a strong positive linear relationship with the length of the words, either horizontally or vertically oriented, on linear regression analysis (Table 22.5). Reading time increased by approximately 6–8 seconds per letter in each orientation. A qualitative analysis of reading errors showed a strong visual simi-

larity effect (b, d, p). Error position analysis did not reveal a prevalence of errors on the first or the second half of the words, in either horizontal or vertical orientation. The results of this experiment confirmed that letter-by-letter reading was affected mainly by stimulus length and that visual similarities were the major cause of reading errors. The absence of different results between horizontal and vertical reading and of a specific spatial distribution error pattern suggests the absence of perceptual and/or attentional disorders in F.C.

EXPERIMENT 2: ORAL READING OF WORDS AND NON-WORDS In the dual-route model of reading processes (Andreewsky, 1974; Coltheart, 1985), reading is assumed to involve two routes that can be used to reach naming. The first reading process is analytical at the visual level and phonological at the linguistic one. It is called the indirect route or phonological reading process, involving grapheme-to-phoneme correspondence rules. It is the route that is normally used to read nonwords aloud. The second reading process is global at the visual level and lexical or semantic at the linguistic one. Only lexical and meaningful stimuli can be read by means of this reading process, which is called direct, lexical, or nonphonological reading.

Assuming that words and nonwords are processed by the same mechanisms in letter-by-letter readers and not via separate routes as in normals, the letter identification and reversed spelling strategy (spell out the letters, then recognize the word auditorily) should be applied with the same degree of success for words and nonwords. The prediction here is that reading accuracy and reading latencies for words are comparable to those of nonwords in F.C.

We presented a list of 50 words and a list of 50 pronounceable nonwords. Nonwords were derived from real words by changing one or two letters. The letter strings were three to seven letters long, 10 letter strings per length. Each letter string was printed on an index card. Presentation was randomized. This task was performed in five blocks of 20 letter strings per block. In this experiment we again used a stopwatch to measure reading latencies.

Data are summarized in Table 22.6. Reading latencies and accuracy were scored separately for words and nonwords as a function of stimulus length. F.C. made reading errors in 12/50 (24%) words and 11/50 (22%) nonwords. F.C.'s reading errors were usually related to the written target word by visual similarities (so-called visual paralexias) rather than by similar meaning (semantic paralexias). Erroneous responses in either condition were both real words and nonwords. Mann-Whitney U test was used for latencies, and Fisher's exact test was

TABLE 22.5

Oral reading error scores (percentage) and latencies (seconds) given separately for horizontally and vertically oriented words

| | Number of Letters | | | | | |
	3	4	5	6	7	p
Accuracy						
Horizontal	10	20	30	30	40	<0.01
Vertical	10	10	30	30	40	<0.02
Latencies						
Horizontal	13.85	22.56	26.61	31.69	42.73	<0.01
Vertical	14.12	20.79	26.79	32.47	42.88	<0.01

TABLE 22.6
Oral reading error scores (percentage) and latencies (seconds) given separately for words and nonwords

	Number of Letters				
	3	4	5	6	7
Accuracy					
Words	10	10	20	40	40
Nonwords	10	10	30	30	30
p	ns	ns	ns	ns	ns
Latencies					
Words	15.33	22.94	25.95	32.65	43.47
Nonwords	15.27	22.12	26.14	32.48	43.40
p	ns	ns	ns	ns	ns

TABLE 22.7
Lexical decision task accuracy for words, nonwords, and total

			p
Words	17/20	85%	
Nonwords	16/20	80%	
Total	33/40	83%	<0.001

p = binomial probability distribution.

used for accuracy. On both measures, there were no differences between the two conditions at each stimulus length. The patient again showed a linear increase in reading latencies and error rate as the stimuli increased in length. The results of this experiment suggest that the reversed spelling process is intact in F.C., and by means of it the patient could read nonwords as well as words.

EXPERIMENT 3: LEXICAL DECISION Some "pure alexics" patients can perform significantly better than chance on lexical decision and forced-choice semantic categorization tasks with briefly presented letter strings that they could not explicitly identify (Caplan and Hedley-White, 1974; Coslett and Saffran, 1989; Shallice and Saffran, 1986). On the assumption that in these patients' comprehension of printed words necessarily involves a reversed spelling strategy, evidence of word recognition on brief presentation would suggest that reversed spelling strategy is not the only processing strategy available to letter-by-letter readers.

We visually presented 20 words and 20 nonwords to F.C., one at a time. All stimuli were four letters in length. Nonwords were derived from real words by changing one or two letters in the third and fourth positions. We assumed that F.C., having a mean reading latency of approximately 4 seconds per letter, could not reach the third position of a letter string in 2 seconds by using a left-to-right scanning strategy. All the stimuli were written on index cards, and they were visible for only approximately 2 seconds (calculated with the stopwatch). Their presentation was randomized. F.C. had to decide whether the stimulus was a word. Despite her complaints that she was unable to do so, we had her choose one way or another, following her instinct. In addition, after the lexical decision was made, we asked the patient whether she had recognized the word or the nonword.

Table 22.7 shows F.C.'s performance on the lexical decision task. F.C. identified exactly 17 words out of 20 and 16 nonwords out of 20. On the other hand, our patient exactly recognized only one word after the brief exposure of the stimulus. A binomial probability distribution test revealed that the values were significantly greater than would be expected by chance ($p < 0.001$). Our patient performed surprisingly well on the lexical decision task, although she was unable to explicitly identify most of the stimuli.

EXPERIMENT 4: MIRROR-REVERSED READING F.C. clearly used a letter-by-letter reading strategy characterized by naming aloud the individual letters of a word, as indicated by a clear increase in reading latencies when the length of the letter string increases and by the capability to read nonwords. In addition, this patient showed a clear difficulty in the discrimination of similar letters; the majority of her letter confusions occurred within visually similar clusters (b, d, etc.). These findings suggest a deficit in the early visual processing of individual letters features (Reuter-Lorenz and Brunn, 1990; Reuter-Lorenz and Gazzaniga, 1991). Word recognition is a process not dissimilar in its general form to that involved in visual object recognition (Caramazza and Hillis, 1990). The process involves the computation of several different levels of representation (Marr and Nishihara, 1978; Marr, 1982). We assumed that if the early stages of reading are disrupted, F.C. should have major difficulty in processing letters presented in an unusual way. To verify the assumption, we presented mirror-reversed letters and words (Patterson and Wilson, 1990). The prediction here was that if the reading disorder in F.C. was due to an early visual-processing deficit, the anomalous presentation of the stimuli might break down the reading performance.

F.C. was presented with 10 mirror-reversed letters and the same letters normally oriented. The order of presentation was randomized. Then two lists of 50 words were presented, in both normal and mirror-reversed orientation. Words ranged from three to seven letters in length, 10 words of each length. All letter strings were presented individually. Presentation was randomized.

TABLE 22.8

*Oral reading error scores (percentage) and latencies (seconds) given
separately for normally oriented and mirror-reversed words*

	Number of Letters				
	3	4	5	6	7
Accuracy					
Normally oriented words	10	10	30	30	40
Mirror-reversed words	10	20	30	40	40
p	ns	ns	ns	ns	ns
Latencies					
Normally oriented words	14.60	21.98	26.69	31.82	42.95
Mirror-reversed words	15.22	20.38	27.91	32.80	43.51
p	ns	ns	ns	ns	ns

This task was performed in five blocks of 20 letter strings per block. Stimuli for mirror-reversed reading were made by photocopying the words printed in block letters onto transparencies and flipping the transparencies with a white paper background. Latencies were calculated with a stopwatch.

The number of words that were read correctly and the time it took to read them are shown in Table 22.8. Again, the patient showed a linear increase in reading latency and errors as words increased in length. Data analysis relied on the Mann-Whitney U test for latencies. A Fisher's exact test was carried out for accuracy.

There were no differences in reading time and accuracy between normally oriented and reversed letters or words. The patient did not show the expected breakdown in mirror-reversed reading.

SPECT study

A regional cerebral blood flow (rCBF) study was obtained by using a Tomomatic 564 (Medimatic, Denmark) SPECT device and Tc-99m HM-PAO. The patient was studied at rest and during a reading task. The split-dose method was employed to perform repeated rCBF measurements in the same study session (Pantano et al., 1992). After intravenous injection, Tc-99m HM-PAO brain uptake is almost complete within a few minutes and is stable for up to 5 hours. Its distribution is proportional to rCBF. One of the advantages of this tracer is the possibility of injecting the patient during an activation task and scanning him or her later without significant changes in tracer's brain distribution. Thus, a subsequent rCBF assessment reflects the brain activity during the activation task.

The first scan was performed in a dimly lit room with the patient lying on a couch, at rest. The patient's head was positioned by using a laser reference system and was aligned to the orbitomeatal line. A continuous infusion of isotonic saline solution was administered intravenously to allow atraumatic serial tracer injections. The rest scan was obtained by injecting 6 mCi of labeled HM-PAO and collecting about 800,000 counts per slice in 15 minutes of acquisition time. The second study was performed during a reading task. The task consisted of reading aloud different concrete words, with a word length ranging from three to six letters. Each word was written in uppercase letters on a separate index card. Three minutes after the start of this task, 18 mCi of Tc-99m HM-PAO were injected while the patient was still performing the task. The patient continued to read for the following 5 minutes, during the entire period of tracer's brain uptake. At the end of the activation the patient was repositioned in the camera as in the previous scan by means of a laser reference system. About 1,500,000 counts per slice were collected in 5 minutes.

For each scan, 3 slices were obtained at +0.5 cm, +4.5 cm, and +8.5 cm above the orbitomeatal line. Spatial resolution was 9 mm, and slice thickness was 10 mm, full-width at half-maximum. Data analysis of the scans was performed by using a semiquantitative method by calculating a ratio between the counts of each single region of interest (ROI) and the counts of the whole slice. Irregular ROIs were manually drawn over the first scan images according to an anatomical reference atlas (Talairach and Tournoux, 1988) and then automatically transferred on the second scan images.

We measured the regional CBF values and their variability for repeated SPECT scans in five healthy controls, studied twice at rest. rCBF changes were calculated by evaluating the percentage differences between the same ROI ratios (single ROI/whole slice) in the two rest scans. The test-retest rCBF changes in the control group were $-0.2\% \pm 5.0\%$, on average. An rCBF change was considered significant when the difference of regional values between the reading activation scan and the basal one was higher than the mean plus 2 S.D. of the rCBF changes measured in the test-retest study in the control group. Thus, we consider significant a rCBF change higher than 9.8% (mean plus 2 S.D.).

At rest, there were no relevant rCBF reductions in the left cortical areas and in the left thalamus compared to the contralateral homologous regions as well as to the control group ones. During reading activation a significant rCBF increase in the right temporoparietal (+10%) and medial occipital (+12%) areas was observed, compared to the rest condition (Table 22.9).

TABLE 22.9

Ratio between counts in each ROI and the total counts of the corresponding slice

	Rest		Reading		Diff %	
	LH	RH	LH	RH	LH	RH
Frontal	1.23	1.28	1.28	1.29	0.05	0.01
Frontotemporal	1.29	1.27	1.3	1.23	0.01	−0.04
Temporal	1.32	1.25	1.34	1.32	0.02	0.07
Temporoparietal	1.14	1.14	1.16	1.24	0.02	**0.1**
Medial occipital	1.2	1.26	1.23	1.38	0.03	**0.12**
Thalamus	1.13	1.18	1.15	1.24	0.02	0.06

Numbers in bold are values higher than the mean plus 2 S.D. of the CBF changes in the test-retest study (two rest conditions) in controls (Tc99m-HMPAO split-dose method).

Discussion

Here we report for the first time data from an activation reading task using single photon emission tomography technique in a letter-by-letter reader. The patient's reading ability shared many features with those of letter-by-letter readers previously described in literature. In fact, she read one letter at a time, showed a significant word-length effect in both accuracy and latency of word reading, and could read nonwords as well as words. In addition, she evidenced implicit processing skills on a lexical decision task, a phenomenon that is commonly present in some of these patients (Shallice and Saffran, 1986; Coslett and Saffran, 1989), though absent in others (Warrington and Shallice, 1980; Patterson and Kay, 1982).

We observed that at rest there was only a slight, non-significant hypoperfusion, in the left occipital lobe. During the reading task activation two regions of the right hemisphere showed a significant increase in rCBF: the medial occipital area and the temporoparietal one. This finding is at variance with a bilateral occipital rCBF increase that was previously reported in a patient with alexia during a reading activation task using a low-resolution bidimensional nontomographic technique (Halsey et al., 1980).

However, the right temporoparietal activation observed in our study is in accordance with recent PET studies showing a similar activated area in normals when they are required to detect a feature and is presumed to be due to a visual prelexical representation (Corbetta et al., 1990). PET activation studies in normals showed also that visually presented words and pseudowords (nonwords that follow orthographic rules) produce re-

sponses in the left medial extrastriate cortex that are not seen with false fonts or random letter strings (Peterson et al., 1990). This activation is thought to be the functional anatomical correlate of the visual word form system (Petersen et al., 1989), a left-hemisphere-based mechanism that serves to process visual verbal information and provides for word identification (Warrington and Shallice, 1980). In our case we observed only a small, non-significant increase (+3%) of rCBF in the left medial occipital area during reading. These data may account for the presumed failure of the left-hemisphere visual word form system in letter-by-letter readers (Warrington and Shallice, 1980).

An evident increase of the rCBF in the contralateral right medial occipital area (12%) was observed during the reading task activation. This response may be explained with the simple processing at the level of complex visual features. However, in recent years a growing body of evidence from studies on normals, split-brain patients, and brain-damaged patients has supported the hypothesis that the two cerebral hemispheres may represent two complete cognitive systems, each capable of processing most environmental information and controlling the behavior of the organism as a whole (Zaidel, 1989). The thesis of hemispheric independence, assuming that the two hemispheres work independently and in parallel, suggests also that the strategies employed to compute solutions might be different; for example, one hemisphere might solve a particular problem bottom-up and the other top-down, or one hemisphere in parallel and the other serially, allowing effective monitoring and error detection (Zaidel, Clarke, and Suyenobu, 1990).

With these suggestions in mind, we may hypothesize that a right-hemisphere-based system, usually not activated during reading in normal subjects, becomes active in letter-by-letter readers because of the functional impairment of the left visual word form system. It has been previously proposed that the disturbance in letter-by-letter readers arises from a restriction on information transmission from a letter-analysis stage to a stage of orthographic processing at which multiletter segments are identified for subsequent analysis. In normals this stage is thought to operate on letter information in a parallel fashion; it has been postulated that it can also accept letter information sequentially and that it operates in this sequential mode in letter-by-letter readers (Patterson and Kay, 1982). Our findings suggest that the serial transmission of information from the letter-analysis stage to the word-form system in these patients may depend on sequential access to the right visual word-form system. This model may also be supported by the case of a patient who recovered from alexia due to a large vascular lesion in the left hemisphere but subsequently became profoundly and permanently alexic after a second right hemisphere vascular lesion (Heilman et al., 1979).

In conclusion, we believe that although our data have some methodological limitations with respect to PET studies (limited spatial resolution, quantification, number of repeated scans, etc.) (Frith et al., 1991; Haxby et al., 1991; Tikofsky and Hellman, 1991; Wise et al., 1991), they suggest the existence of a right visual word-form system. Further experimental designs combining the use of functional neuroimaging techniques with activation paradigms coming from cognitive neuropsychology or lateralization tasks might be fruitful for investigating cognitive processes, both in normals and in brain-damaged patients.

REFERENCES

ANDREEWSKY, E., 1974. Un modèle sèmantique. Application a la pathologie du language: Alexia aphasique. *Informations* 2:3–27.

BORTOLINI, U., C. TAGLIAVINI, and A. ZAMPOLLI, 1968. *Lessico di Frequenza della Lingua Italiana Contemporanea*. Bari: Laterza.

CAPLAN, L. R., and T. HEDLEY-WHITE, 1974. Cueing and memory dysfunction in alexia without agraphia: A case report. *Brain* 97:251–262.

CARAMAZZA, A., and A. E. HILLIS, 1990. Levels of representation, co-ordinate frames, and unilateral neglect. *Cogn. Neuropsychol.* 7:391–445.

COLTHEART, M., 1985. Cognitive neuropsychology and reading. In *Attention and Performance*, Vol. 11, M. Posner and O. S. M. Marin, eds. Hillsdale, N.J.: Lawrence Erlbaum Associates.

COMPTON, P. E., P. GROSSENBACHER, M. I. POSNER, and D. M. TUCKER, 1991. A cognitive-anatomical approach to attention in lexical access. *J. Cogn. Neurosci.* 3:304–312.

CORBETTA, M., F. M. MIEZIN, P. T. FOX, S. M. DOBMEYER, and S. E. PETERSEN, 1990. Right infero-temporal cortex PET activation during object recognition tasks in human. *Soc. Neurosci. Abstr.* 260:10.

COSLETT, H. B., and E. M. SAFFRAN, 1989. Evidence for preserved reading in "pure alexia." *Brain* 112:327–359.

DOCTOR, E. A., G. SARTORI, and M. M. SALING, 1990. A letter-by-letter reader who could not read nonwords. *Cortex* 26:247–262.

FRIEDMAN, R. B., and M. P. ALEXANDER, 1984. Pictures, images, and pure alexia: A case study. *Cogn. Neuropsychol.* 1:9–23.

FRITH, C. D., K. J. FRISTON, P. F. LIDDLE and R. S. J. FRACKOWIACK, 1991. A PET study of word finding. *Neuropsychologia* 29:1137–1148.

HALSEY, J. H., U. W. BLAUENSTEIN, E. M. WILSON and E. L. WILLS, 1980. rCBF activation in a patient with right homonymous hemianopia and alexia without agraphia. *Brain Lang.* 9:137–140.

HANLEY, J. R., and J. KAY, 1992. Does letter-by-letter reading involve the spelling system? *Neuropsychologia* 30:237–256.

HAXBY, J. V., C. L. GRADY, L. G. UNGERLEIDER, and B. HORWITZ, 1991. Mapping the functional neuroanatomy of the intact human brain with brain work imaging. *Neuropsychologia* 29:539–555.

HEILMAN, K. M., L. ROTHI, D. CAMPANELLA, and S. WOLFSON, 1979. Wernicke's and global aphasia without alexia. *Arch. Neurol.* 36:129–133.

MARR, D., 1982. *Vision*. New York: W.H. Freeman.

MARR, D., and H. K. NISHIHARA, 1978. Representation and recognition of the spatial organisation of three-dimensional shapes. *Proc. R. Soc. Lond. B* 200:269–294.

MCCLELLAND, J. L., and D. E. RUMELHART, 1981. An interactive activation model of context effects in letter perception: 1. An account of basic findings. *Psychol. Rev.* 88:375–407.

PANTANO, P., V. DI PIERO, M. RICCI, C. FIESCHI, L. BOZZAO, and G. L. LENZI, 1992. Motor stimulation response by technetium-99m hexamethilpropilene amine oxime split-dose method and single photon emission tomography. *Eur. J. Nucl. Med.* 19:939–945.

PATTERSON, K. E., and J. KAY, 1982. Letter-by-letter reading: Psychological descriptions of a neurological syndrome. *Quart. J. Exp. Psychol.* 34A:411–441.

PATTERSON, K., and B. WILSON, 1990. A ROSE is a ROSE or a NOSE: A deficit in initial letter identification. *Cogn. Neuropsychol.* 7:447–477.

PETERSEN, S. E., P. T. FOX, M. I. POSNER, M. MINTUN, and M. E. RAICHLE, 1989. Positron emission tomographic studies of the processing of single words. *J. Cogn. Neurosci.* 1:153–170.

PETERSEN, S. E., P. T. FOX, A. Z. SNYDER, and M. E. RAICHLE, 1990. Activation of extrastriate and frontal cortical areas by visual words and word-like stimuli. *Science* 249:1041–1044.

REUTER-LORENZ, P. A., and J. L. BRUNN, 1990. A pre-lexical basis for letter-by-letter reading: A case study. *Cogn. Neuropsychol.* 7:1–20.

REUTER-LORENZ, P. A., and M. S. GAZZANIGA, 1991. Localization of function: A perspective from cognitive neuropsychology. In *Neurobehavioral Aspects of Cerebrovascular Disease*, R. A. Bornstein and G. Brown, eds. New York: Oxford University Press.

RUMELHART, D. E., and J. L. MCCLELLAND, 1982. An interactive activation model of context effects in letter perception: 2. The contextual enhancement effect and some tests and extension of the model. *Psychol. Rev.* 89:60–94.

SHALLICE, T., and E. SAFFRAN, 1986. Lexical processing in the absence of explicit word identification: Evidence from a letter-by-letter reader. *Cogn. Neuropsychol.* 3:429–458.

SILVER, F. L., J. B. CHAWLUK, T. M. BOSLEY, M. ROSEN, R. DANN, R. C. SERGOTT, A. ALAVI, and M. REIVICH, 1988. Resolving metabolic abnormalities in a case of pure alexia. *Neurology* 38:730–735.

TALAIRACH, J., and P. TOURNOUX, 1988. *Co-planar Stereotaxic Atlas of the Human Brain. 3-Dimensional Proportional System: An Approach to Cerebral Imaging*. New York: Thieme Medical Publishers.

TIKOFSKY, R. S., and R. S. HELLMAN, 1991. Brain single photon emission computed tomography: Newer activation and intervention studies. *Sem. Nucl. Med.* 21:40–57.

WARRINGTON, E. K., and T. SHALLICE, 1980. Word-form dyslexia. *Brain* 103:99–112.

WISE, R., F. CHOLLET, U. HADAR, K. FRISTON, E. HOFFNERN, and R. J. S. FRACKOWIACK, 1991. Distribution of cortical neural networks involved in word comprehension and word retrieval. *Brain* 114:1803–1817.

ZAIDEL, E., 1989. Hemispheric independence and interaction in word recognition. In *Brain and Reading*, C. von Euler, I. Lundberg, and G. Lennerstrand, eds. Hampshire, Engl.: Macmillan, pp. 77–97.

ZAIDEL, E., J. M. CLARKE, and A. M. SUYENOBU, 1990. Hemispheric independence: A paradigm case for cognitive neuroscience. In *Neurobiology of Higher Cognitive Functioning*, A. B. Scheibel and M. D. Wechsler, eds. New York: Guilford Press, pp. 297–355.

EDITORIAL COMMENTARY 5

The Case Study of Pure Alexia: Sensorimotor Integration in the Split Brain

ERAN ZAIDEL AND MARCO IACOBONI

Luzzatti reviews comprehensively four prominent syndromes that are often associated with callosal lesions and occasionally with right hemisphere (RH) lexical processing: left-hand apraxia to verbal command, optic aphasia, pure alexia, and deep dyslexia. How do split-brain data bear on these issues? Consider first left-hand apraxia to verbal command. Some patients with natural anterior callosal lesions cannot follow verbal commands with the left hand as well as being unable to imitate actions or show appropriate object use with the left hand (Heilman and Rothi, 1993). The acute split brain usually includes severe apraxia to verbal command, and the chronic split brain usually includes a mild form of the syndrome. Yet even when split-brain patients cannot follow a spoken or written command with the left hand, they can nonetheless often match the command with a pictorial representation of the action and they can imitate the action (Zaidel, 2001). One explanation for the discrepancy between the natural partial callosal lesion data and the surgical complete callosotomy data is that there is an individual difference in degree of language comprehension and of praxis control in the normal RH (Heilman and Rothi, 1993). A possible explanation for the inability to follow the command while demonstrating comprehension and imitation in the disconnected RH is a combined mild dual lesion: one in comprehension, the other in execution. Neither lesion is symptomatic by itself, but together they yield a deficit.

Consider optic aphasia next. The patients cannot name visual stimuli and read words aloud, but they can name to definition or to tactile or auditory presentation, and they can (often?) mime to visual presentations. Luz-

zatti offers a disconnection account that elaborates Coslett and Saffran's model (1992), itself a modern version of Freund's (1889) visual-verbal disconnection theory. This account posits two separate semantic systems in the two hemispheres, but it also distinguishes separate visual and verbal semantic systems in each hemisphere and argues for individual differences in the strength of these systems in the RH. Luzzatti further suggests that optic aphasia and associative visual agnosia fall on a continuum that is determined by individual variability in verbal and visual semantic representation in the RH (cf. De Renzi and Saetti, 1997). Thus, what distinguishes visual agnosia from optic aphasia and in turn from color anomia or alexia is not the extent of callosal damage (e.g., Schnider et al., 1994). This account has the virtue that it can be tested in the normal brain using chronometric hemifield tachistoscopy. For example, it predicts that normal subjects will vary more in their left visual field (LVF) than right visual field (RVF) associative matching (Pyramid and Palm Tree Test, a measure of visual semantics) or in their LVF ability to sort objects into categories (a measure of verbal semantics).

The classic disconnection account is, of course, the anatomic model of pure alexia attributed to Déjerine (1892). (But as Damasio and Damasio (1983) point out, Déjerine himself did not emphasize the role of the splenial damage in the etiology of the syndrome.) Pure alexics cannot read words overtly except by a laborious letter-by-letter (LBL) sounding process. They occasionally exhibit covert reading in response to tachistoscopic presentations in which they can point to multiple-choice pictures. Luzzatti cogently argues that overt LBL reading is a residual left-hemisphere (LH) strategy, whereas covert reading is a RH strategy. The data are supportive but inconclusive. One difficulty is that some LBL readers do and some do not exhibit covert reading. Luzzatti appeals again to individual differences in RH linguistic capacities.

ERAN ZAIDEL Department of Psychology, University of California at Los Angeles, Los Angeles, California.
MARCO IACOBONI Ahmanson Lovelace Brain Mapping Center, Neuropsychiatric Institute, Brain Research Institute, David Geffen School of Medicine, University of California at Los Angeles, Los Angeles, California.

Ladavas's commentary on Luzzatti offers an alternative explanation. She distinguishes two types of LBL readers. The first type reflects an impairment in simultaneous processing of two visual targets located in two different locations (spatial simultagnosia) and does not show covert reading. The second type reflects a deficit in letter identification but intact covert reading. Ladavas explains intact lexical decision and semantic judgment without naming by a degraded output of the orthographic system, which is sufficient for category discrimination without being sufficient for identification. This enables her to favor a LH interpretation of covert reading without the need to appeal to a RH system that has lexical semantics but not output phonology.

What are the arguments for RH support of covert reading in LBL reading? Two types of arguments have been proposed, both with mixed evidence. The first argument is by analogy with reading in the disconnected RH. Luzzatti reads the evidence as demonstrating RH capacity for lexical decision and semantic judgment; Ladavas reads it as not demonstrating such a capacity. In fact, the data from both the California series (Zaidel, 2001) and the Dartmouth-Toledo series (Baynes and Eliassen, 1998) show some lexical decision in the disconnected RHs, though it is subject to individual differences and underestimates the reading ability of the same RH. Complete commissurotomy patients N.G., R.Y., and A.A. from the California series and callosotomy patients V.P., J.W., and D.R. from the Dartmouth series have all shown limited competence for lexical decision in the disconnected RH, and L.B. from the California series has shown substantial such ability (see Table 1 in Zaidel, 2001).

We used a series of lateralized lexical decision tasks and interpreted the findings in terms of the hemispheric dual-route model of word recognition. The model distinguishes a lexical ("sight vocabulary") route, characterized by lexical semantic effects, and a nonlexical route ("phonic" reading), characterized by an orthographic regularity effect. Length effects characterize an early, common stage of input normalization into a sequence of abstract letter identities. In English the lexical route is said to be more efficient than the nonlexical route. Does the lexical route, in either hemisphere, incorporate a pattern recognition process? In that case, format distortion (e.g., vertical or zigzag presentations) should interact with lexical semantic variables and affect decisions in one or the other visual field. The model also posits (1) that each hemisphere can store abstract letter identities, (2) that each hemisphere has access to "its own" lexical route, but (3) that only the LH has access to a nonlexical route.

We used targets that varied in length, orthographically regular nonwords, and sometimes words that varied in concreteness, emotionality, frequency, and regularity of grapheme-phoneme translation. We found that the disconnected RHs of five commissurotomy patients (four complete, L.B., N.G., R.Y., N.W., and one partial, N.F.) could perform lexical decision above chance (Zaidel, 1989). The LHs were superior in accuracy but not in latency. Using signal detection measures, the LHs had greater sensitivity, but the bias in the RH (which tended to be less than 1, that is, the RH tends to respond "yes") varied independently of LH bias (which was both less than and greater than 1). A model that posits that the lexical decision process in the RH is similar to that in the LH, but with a smaller vocabulary, predicts a consistently smaller sensitivity but larger bias in the RH. The data did not support this model. Rather, the results suggest independent and different lexical decision processes in the two hemispheres.

A series of five lexical decision experiments disclosed (1) similar length effects in both disconnected hemispheres, stronger for nonwords than for words; (2) a lexicality effect (advantage of words over nonwords) in both hemispheres; (3) similar frequency, emotionality, and concreteness effects in both hemispheres; (4) no regularity effect in either hemisphere; (5) equal format distortion effects in both hemispheres, affecting words more than nonwords; and (6) similar format distortion effects in both hemispheres, showing an increased length effect, especially for nonwords. The latter result is in contrast to experiments with normal subjects that showed a greater format distortion for words in the RVF (Zaidel et al., 1999). Thus, the split-brain data are generally consistent with the hemispheric dual-route model, although they show a rather similar lexical organization in the two disconnected hemispheres. Less support for the hemispheric dual-route model comes from hemifield tachistoscopic experiments with normal subjects (cf. Zaidel, 1998).

Our data suggest that the lexicons in the two disconnected hemispheres share some organizational principles (by frequency, concreteness, etc.) but that they use different strategies for lexical access. Results with normal subjects suggest that all effects (length, wordness, frequency, and regularity) are possible but none is necessary in either VF. In this view, an effect occurs in a particular condition only when resources are limited (cf. Eviatar and Zaidel, 1991). Consequently, the serial position effects in a word superiority task observed by Reuter-Lorenz and Baynes (1992) do not imply that the RH always uses a serial processing strategy in word recognition.

Thus, like covert LBL readers, the disconnected RH shows a frequency effect in lexical decision, but unlike them it also shows a length effect. But we have argued that these effects reflect task-dependent resource limitations rather than characteristic processing strategies.

Arguin (personal communication, April 14, 1996) also argues for a dual-process theory of LBL reading but opts for an opposite hemispheric interpretation. He distinguishes two pathways for reading: (1) the normal efficient abstract orthographic pathway and (2) a compensatory "token" or shape-specific pathway that is essential for overt word recognition. LBL readers use the token pathway but also preserve rapid access to an abstract orthographic pathway, which controls covert reading tasks. Further, Arguin believes that the token pathway is supported by normal RH reading, whereas implicit reading in pure alexics is supported by the residual LH system. This is based on the assumption that the RH has no abstract letter identities. The evidence is from (1) Reuter-Lorenz and Baynes (1992), who showed a length effect in a variant of the word superiority effect in the LVF of J.W., and (2) Marsolek and colleagues (1992), who show selective same-case stem completion priming in the LVF of normal subjects. However, the relevance of these tasks to reading is questionable, and there is ample evidence that the normal and disconnected RHs can form abstract letter identities (Zaidel, 1982; Eviatar and Zaidel, 1994).

The second type of argument for RH support of covert reading in LBL readers is more direct. It consists of imaging hemispheric activation during LBL reading or disrupting it with natural or artificial lesions. But here again the data are scanty and inconsistent. On the one hand, Coslett and Monsul (1994) showed that right but not left temporoparietal transcortical magnetic stimulation disrupted implicit/covert reading in pure alexia. On the other hand, Iacoboni and colleagues (Commentary 22.3 in this volume) showed greater right posterior than left Broca's area SPECT activation during LBL reading of a patient. (However, the choice of control task in this study was not optimal.) Conversely, Bone and colleagues (2000) used fMRI to image a patient with pure alexia and with slow serial explicit reading but fast and parallel implicit reading. They showed RH mediation of implicit but not explicit reading.

Coslett and Saffran (1994) view reading in pure alexia and in optic aphasia as falling on a continuum of callosal disconnection. They posit that only phylogenetically old functions with bilateral representation are subserved by homotopic areas of the two cerebral hemispheres and have direct callosal connections. Such connections exist, therefore, between the object recognition systems (through more posterior callosal channels) and the higher conceptual systems (through more anterior channels) in the two hemispheres but not between the recent visual word form systems in the two hemispheres. Thus, LBL reading reflects disconnection of early visual information but not of the object recognition pathways. This allows letters to be transmitted and recognized serially, as objects, from the RH to the LH. In optic aphasia, on the other hand, the interhemispheric object recognition pathways are disconnected as well, so LBL reading (or object naming) is no longer possible. On this account, both pure alexics and optic aphasics show intact implicit reading in the RH.

Clarke uses anatomical studies of the patterns of intrahemispheric and interhemispheric connectivity in visual areas of the human cortex to infer the organizational principles of striate and extrastriate cortex. Since in areas with precise retinotopic representation, callosal connections are found along representations of the vertical meridian (serving midline fusion), the distribution of visual callosal afferents can be used as landmarks for demarcating several visual areas. The disconnection syndromes illustrated in this section of the book presuppose that callosal connections predominantly connect homotopic cortical modules, but Clarke challenges this view. She reasons that hemispheric specialization calls for callosal connections from lower to higher levels in a cognitive hierarchy and thus for heterotopic connectivity.

Indeed, Clarke and colleagues (1995) found heterotopic connections from the medial part of the right occipital lobe not only to early visual areas in the other hemisphere but also to left posterior parietal and temporal cortex and to left angular gyrus. Clarke proposes the radical hypothesis that heterotopic callosal connections from the right calcarine region to the left angular gyrus are used by normal LH reading strategies, whereas the alternative route from the right calcarine region to the right angular gyrus to the left angular gyrus may be used by alternative RH reading strategies, such as in deep dyslexia.

Critically needed are organizational principles that segregate homotopic and heterotopic callosal connections by their function on the one hand and by their localization in the callosum on the other.

Bartolomeo and colleagues' commentary describes a patient with a left occipitotemporal lesion who became a pure alexic and whose residual reading worsened following a subsequent mirror-image lesion in the RH. The patient's reading aloud after the first lesion was accurate but showed a length effect as well as a frequency effect.

She could also read letters correctly, if somewhat slowly. After the second lesion, her ability to read words and letters worsened, the length effect was stronger, and the frequency effect was reduced. This suggests to the authors that the RH was involved in residual reading after the first lesion and that it contributed to the length effect, that is, to LBL reading. The authors suggest that the letters were recognized as objects in the RH, then transferred to the LH for "reverse reading." Unfortunately, no testing of covert reading was undertaken. This account is therefore consistent with RH covert reading in pure alexia but also posits some RH contribution to LH LBL reading. In light of our own data from both normal subjects and split-brain patients (Zaidel, 1998, 2001), we would not identify a length effect with LBL reading, especially given Bartolomeo and colleagues' patient's accurate reading after the first lesion. In fact, we would expect length effects to occur whenever resources are taxed and hence to appear in the RH before they occur in the LH. Thus, Bartolomeo and colleagues' data do not challenge either the RH hypothesis of covert reading or the LH hypothesis of LBL reading in pure alexia.

The standard approach to analyzing structure-function relationships is to observe changes in behavior, in our case reading, following changes to the anatomy, in our case disconnection of the splenium. This is the approach taken in the papers by Luzzatti, Bartolomeo and colleagues, and Iacoboni and colleagues. In dramatic contrast, Castro-Caldas and colleagues analyze the possible anatomic changes, in this case to callosal morphometry, following changes in linguistic experience, in this case literacy training. Castro-Caldas and colleagues explore the provocative hypothesis that reading acquisition requires interhemispheric interaction and results in increasing functional and anatomical connectivity in the anterior isthmus, which interconnects associative parietal areas. They show that (1) illiterates are deficient in a task that requires motor orienting to lateral targets; and (2) illiterates have smaller anterior isthmuses than matched literates. These results are suggestive but circumstantial. First, does the motor orienting task actually depend on interhemispheric interaction? Does it in fact successfully simulate the visuomotor interhemispheric requirements of writing (spatial scanning in the RH, motor planning in the LH)? Second, does extent of deficit in the task correlate with degree of literacy/writing ability? Third, does either correlate with the size of the anterior isthmus? These questions suggest a fascinating line of research on a direct coupling between language experience/competence and callosal anatomy. For example, do languages that are read from right to left stimulate selective anatomical and functional callosal development?

Luzzatti's chapter focuses on the role of the splenium in the etiology of acquired reading disorders, but these are just a few examples of the consequences of partial disconnection.

Anatomical, physiological, and behavioral/clinical data converge on the view that the corpus callosum contains modality- and function-specific channels whose anteroposterior organization follows the anteroposterior arrangement of the corresponding cortical modules. However, effects of partial disconnection are still incompletely understood. Some conflicting data exist between surgical disconnection on the one hand and disconnection due to traumatic/cerebrovascular accidents on the other. Sorely needed is a standardized battery for measuring levels of callosal efficiency in different callosal channels.

1. *Callosotomy sparing the anterior commissure.* Patients with complete callosotomy sparing the anterior commissure exhibit the generalized but not the specific disconnection syndrome (Sidtis et al., 1981). They exhibit somatosensory disconnection, auditory disconnection, and usually, but not always, visual disconnection. Left hemialexia/hemianomia may (Risse et al., 1978) or may not (McKeever et al., 1981) be present. They do not exhibit olfactory disconnection (Risse et al., 1989). Di Virgilio and colleagues (1999) show interhemispheric inferotemporal and occipital projections through the anterior commissure in humans and suggest that it may mediate visuosemantic information. Lauro-Grotto and colleagues (in preparation) describe a callosotomy patient M.E. with a right frontal polectomy (prefrontal cortex). The patient was unable to read LVF words but could name some LVF pictures and make semantic decisions on pictures. The authors attributed these to LH control following visuosemantic transfer via the anterior commissure.

2. *Splenial section.* Splenial section results in visual disconnection but variable hemianomia and hemialexia. Complete section of the splenium, including the tip, is necessary and sufficient for visual disconnection (Maspes, 1948). The ventral splenium may transfer nonverbal visual information, whereas the dorsal splenium may transfer verbal visual information (Gersh and Damasio, 1981). The posterior splenium (and genu) was severed in a Japanese who attempted suicide with an ice pick (Abe et al., 1986). There was a more severe left hemialexia for kana (phonological script) than for kanji (logographic script). Perhaps kanji was controlled by the RH. Cohen and Dehaene (1996) described a patient with an infarct in the posterior half of the corpus callosum. There was

disconnection for Arabic digits and numerosity but transfer for approximate magnitude.

3. *Lesions of the body of the corpus callosum.* These lesions often result in more or less severe tactile (or motor) disconnection (Jeeves, 1979; Bentin, Sahar, and Moscovitch, 1984; Mayer, Koenig, and Panchaud, 1988). Section of the posterior body of the corpus callosum results in tactile disconnection, that is, failure of interhemispheric tactile transfer and left hand tactile anomia. Section of the anterior body may result in left-hand apraxia to verbal commands. Section of the posterior body may result in left-hand agraphia.

4. *Section of the isthmus.* Section of the isthmus usually (Alexander and Warren, 1988) but not always (Sugishita et al., 1995) results in auditory disconnection. The involvement of the anterior splenium in auditory interhemispheric transfer may be subject to individual differences.

5. *Commissurotomy/callosotomy sparing the splenium.* Surgical section of the anterior two thirds of the corpus callosum can result in few or no disconnection symptoms. Auditory disconnection may be present, depending on the posterior extent of the lesion. There may be mild deficits in bimanual coordination and in tactile or motor transfer. Memory for new events is also impaired (Gordon, 1990). This contrasts with natural lesions to the parts of the corpus callosum that may prevent crossmodal associations and splenial transfer.

6. *Left-hand agraphia.* Callosal lesions often result in left-hand agraphia. Some believe that three separate components are required for writing and that they are mediated by different callosal channels (Roeltgen, 1993): verbal motor programs through the genu, important for oral spelling; visual-kinesthetic engrams through the body, important for the motor execution of writing in space and time, lesions which result in "apraxic agraphia"; and linguistic information through the splenium, which is important, say, for anagram writing or typing, lesions which result in "aphasic agraphia." Furthermore, splenial lesions sometimes result in agraphia in kana but not in kanji (Sugishita et al., 1980; Yamadori et al., 1980).

Two partial disconnection syndromes deserve special mention. The first is left-hand apraxia to verbal command. The second syndrome is intermanual conflict (diagnostic dyspraxia, Akelaitis, 1944–45), autocriticism, and alien hand (Brion and Jedynak, 1972). These refer to opposing well-organized intentional actions by the two hands, often accompanied by denial of conscious control of one of them (usually the left), sometimes with an associated inability to recognize that hand as the patient's own (alien hand).

1. *Intermanual conflict (anarchic hand).* An example of this occurs in buttoning and unbuttoning a shirt. This symptom was observed with all series of split-brain patients (Akelaitis, California, Dartmouth, Toledo, and Yale), but it is usually only temporary, restricted to the acute disconnection. The symptom is also associated with partial vascular or tumoral lesions of the corpus callosum. Then it may be more severe and persisting. There are two variants with natural lesions (Goldberg et al., 1981): mesial frontal lesions and callosal lesions (Tanaka, 1996). Both lesions may be necessary for intermanual contact.

There is a form of agonistic apraxia (Lavados et al., submitted) in a patient with a vascular lesion to the body of the corpus callosum. The patient had temporary left-hand apraxia to verbal command, intermanual conflict, sensation of a "third" hand, and persisting automatic execution of actions with one hand when verbally instructed to use the other.

2. *Alien hand.* This form may be associated with anterior callosal lesions and mesial loss of inhibition due to frontal cortical damage (Dela Sala, Marchetti, and Spinnler, 1991).

3. *Autocriticism.* Split-brain patients are aware of the apparent independence of left-hand actions or of processing of LVF stimuli. But they express persistent surprise, even anger, at it and sometimes rationalize or even confabulate about it.

REFERENCES

ABE, T., N. NAKAMURA, M. SUGISHITA, Y. KATO, and M. IWATA, 1986. Partial disconnection syndrome following penetrating stab wound of the brain. *Eur. Neurol.* 25:233–239.

AKELAITIS, A. J., 1944–45. Studies on the corpus callosum: IV. Diagnostic dyspraxia in epileptics following partial and complete section of the corpus callosum. *Am. J. Psychiatry* 101:594–599.

ALEXANDER, M. P., and R. L. WARREN, 1988. Localization of callosal auditory pathways: A CT case study. *Neurology* 38:802–804.

BAYNES, K., and J. C. ELIASSEN, 1998. The visual lexicon: Its access and organization in commissurotomy patients. In *Right Hemisphere Language Comprehension: Perspectives from Cognitive Neuroscience*, M. Beeman, C. Chiarello, eds. Mahwah, NJ. Erlbaum, pp. 79–104.

BAYNES, K., J. C. ELIASSEN, H. L. LUTSEP, and M. S. GAZZANIGA, 1998. Modular organization of cognitive systems masked by interhemispheric integration. *Science* 280:902–905.

BENTIN, S., A. SAHAR, and M. MOSCOVITCH, 1984. Interhemispheric information transfer in patients with lesions in the trunk of the corpus callosum. *Neuropsychologia* 22:601–611.

BONE, R. B., L. MAHER, W. MAO, and F. HAIST, 2000. Functional neuroimaging of implicit and explicit reading in patients with pure alexia. *J. Int. Neuropsychol. Soc.* 6:157.

BRION, S., and C. P. JEDYNAK, 1972. Troubles du transfert interhémisphérique [callosal disconnection] à propos de trois observations de tumeurs du corps calleux. Le signe de la main etrangère. *Rev. Neurol.* 126:257–266.

CLARKE, S., F. DE RIBAUPIERRE, V. M. BAJO, E. M. ROUILLER, and R. KRAFTSIK, 1995. The auditory pathway in cat corpus callosum. *Exp. Brain Res.* 104:534–540.

COHEN, L., and S. DEHAENE, 1996. Cerebral networks for number processing: Evidence from a case of posterior callosal lesion. *Neurocase* 2:155–174.

COSLETT, H. B., and N. MONSUL, 1994. Reading with the right hemisphere: Evidence from transcranial magnetic stimulation. *Brain Lang.* 46:198–211.

COSLETT, H. B., and E. M. SAFFRAN, 1992. Optic aphasia and the right hemisphere: A replication and extension. *Brain Lang.* 43:148–161.

COSLETT, H. B., and E. M. SAFFRAN, 1994. Mechanisms of implicit reading in alexia. In *The Neuropsychology of High-Level Vision*, M. J. Farah and G. Ratcliff, eds. Hillsdale, N.J.: Lawrence Erlbaum Associates, pp. 299–330.

DAMASIO, A. R., and H. DAMASIO, 1983. The anatomic basis of pure alexia. *Neurology (Cleveland)* 33:1573–1583.

DÉJERINE, J., 1892. Contributions a l'étude anatomopathologique et clinique des différentes variétés de cécité verbale. *C. R. Séances Mém. Soc. Biol.* 44 (vol. 4 of Series 9):61–90.

DELA SALA, S., C. MARCHETTI, and H. SPINNLER, 1991. Right-sided anarchic (alien) hand: A longitudinal study. *Neuropsychologia* 29:113–117.

DE RENZI, E., and M. C. SAETTI, 1997. Associative agnosia and optic aphasia: Qualitative or quantitative difference? *Cortex* 33:115–130.

DI VIRGILIO, G., S. CLARKE, G. PIZZOLATO, and T. SCHAFFNER, 1999. Cortical regions contributing to the anterior commissure in man. *Exp. Brain. Res.* 124:1–7.

EVIATAR, Z., and E. ZAIDEL, 1991. The effects of word length and emotionality on hemispheric contribution to lexical decision. *Neuropsychologia* 29:415–428.

EVIATAR, Z., and E. ZAIDEL, 1994. Letter matching within and between the disconnected hemispheres. *Brain Cogn.* 25:128–137.

FREUND, C. S., 1889. Ueber optische aphasie und seelenblindheit. *Arch. Psychiatrie Nervenkrankheiten* 20:276–297, 371–416.

GERSH, F., and A. R. DAMASIO, 1981. Praxis and writing of the left hand may be served by different callosal pathways. *Arch. Neurol.* 38:634–636.

GORDON, H. W., 1990. Neuropsychological sequelae of partial of partial commissurotomy. In *Handbook of Neuropsychology*, Vol. 4, F. Boller and J. Grafman, eds. Amsterdam: Elsevier.

GOLDBERG, G., N. H. MAYER, and J. U. TOGLIA, 1981. Medial frontal cortex infarction and the alien hand sign. *Arch. Neurol.* 38:683–686.

HEILMAN, K. M., and L. J. G. ROTHI, 1993. Apraxia. In *Clinical Neuropsychology*, 3rd ed., K. M. Heilman and E. Valenstein, eds. New York: Oxford University Press, pp. 141–163.

JEEVES, M. A., 1979. Some limits to interhemispheric integration in cases of callosal agenesis and partial commissurotomy. In *Structure and Function of the Cerebral Commissures*, I. S.

Russel, M. V. Van Hof, and G. Berlucchi, eds. London: Macmillan, pp. 449–474.

LAURO-GROTTO, R., G. TASSINARI, and T. SHALLICE, submitted. Interhemispheric transfer of visual-semantic information in the callosotomized brain.

LAVADOS, M., X. CARRASCO, M. PENA, D. W. ZAIDEL, E. ZAIDEL, and F. ABOITIZ, submitted. A new sign of callosal disconnection syndrome: Agnostic dyspraxia. A case study. *Neurocase.*

MARSOLEK, C. J., S. M. KOSSLYN, and L. R. SQUIRE, 1992. Form-specific visual priming in the right cerebral hemisphere. *J. Exp. Psychol. Learn. Mem. Cogn.* 18:492–508.

MASPES, P. E., 1948. Le syndrome experimental chez l'homme de la section de splenium du corps calleux: alexia visuelle pure hemianopsique. *Rev. Neurol. (Paris)* 80:100–113.

MAYER, E., O. KOENIG, and A. PANCHAUD, 1988. Tactual extinction without anomia: Evidence of attentional factors in a patient with a partial callosal disconnection. *Neuropsychologia* 26:851–868.

McKEEVER, W. F., K. F. SULLIVAN, S. N. FERGUSON, and M. RAYPORT, 1981. Typical cerebral hemisphere disconnection deficits following corpus callosum section despite sparing of the anterior commissure. *Neuropsychologia* 19:745–755.

REUTER-LORENZ, P. A., and K. BAYNES, 1992. Modes of lexical access in the callosotomized brain. *J. Cogn. Neurosci.* 4:155–164.

RISSE, G., J. GATES, G. LUND, R. MAXWELL, and A. RUBENS, 1989. Interhemispheric transfer in patients with incomplete section of the corpus callosum. *Arch. Neurol.* 46:437–443.

RISSE, G. L., J. LEDOUX, S. P. SPRINGER, D. H. WILSON, and M. S. GAZZANIGA, 1978. The anterior commissure in man: Functional variation in a multisensory system. *Neuropsychologia* 16:23–31.

ROELTGEN, D. P., 1993. Agraphia. In *Clinical Neuropsychology*, K. M. Heilman, and E. Valenstein, eds. New York: Oxford Press, pp. 63–89.

SCHNIDER, A., D. F. BENSON, and D. W. SCHARRE, 1994. Visual agnosia and optic aphasia: Are they anatomically distinct? *Cortex* 30:445–457.

SIDTIS, J. J., B. T. VOLPE, D. H. WILSON, M. RAYPORT, and M. S. GAZZANIGA, 1981. Variability in right hemisphere language function after callosal section: Evidence for a continuum of generative capacity. *J. Neurosci.* 1:323–331.

SUGISHITA, M., K. OTOMO, K. YAMAZAKI, H. SHIMIZU, M. YOSHIOKA, and A. SHINOHARA, 1995. Dichotic listening in patients with partial section of the corpus callosum. *Brain* 118:417–427.

SUGISHITA, M., Y. TOYOKURA, M. YOSHIOKA, and R. YAMADA, 1980. Unilateral agraphia after section of the posterior half of the truncus of the corpus callosum. *Brain Lang.* 9:215–225.

TANAKA, Y., A. YOSHIDA, N. KAWAHATA, and T. OBAYASHI, 1996. Diagnostic dyspraxia. Clinical characteristics, responsible lesion and possible underlying mechanism. *Brain* 119:859–873.

YAMADORI, A., Y. OSUMI, H. IKEDA, and Y. KANAZAWA, 1980. Left unilateral agraphia and tactile anomia: Disturbances seen after occlusion of the anterior cerebral artery. *Arch. Neurol.* 37:88–91.

ZAIDEL, E., 1982. Reading in the disconnected right hemisphere: An aphasiological perspective. In *Dyslexia: Neuronal, Cognitive and Linguistic Aspects*, Y. Zotterman, ed. Oxford: Pergamon Press.

ZAIDEL, E., 1989. Lexical decision and semantic facilitation in the split brain. Unpublished manuscript, Department of Psychology, UCLA.

ZAIDEL, E., 1998. Language in the right hemisphere following callosal disconnection. In *Handbook of Neurolinguistics*, B. Stemmer and H. Whitaker, eds. San Diego: Academic Press.

ZAIDEL, E. 2001. Hemispheric specialization for language in the split brain. In *Handbook of Neuropsychology*, 2nd ed., Vol. 2, *Language and Aphasia*, R. Berndt, vol. ed., F. Boller and J. Grafman, series eds. Amsterdam: Elsevier, pp. 393–418.

ZAIDEL, E., M. BLOCH, and M. ARGUIN, 1999. Pattern perception in hemispheric word recognition. *Brain Lang.* 69:379–382.

ABOUT THE AUTHORS

Note: Biographical sketches of the lead author of each article and commentary follow. Affiliations for all contributors appear on the chapter-opening pages and in the contributor listing that follows this section.

Francisco Aboitiz received his M.Sc. degree in biology at the University of Chile in 1983 and then traveled to Boston to work at Beth Israel Hospital for two years. There he studied the anatomical bases of cerebral asymmetries in humans and collaborated in postmortem analyses of dyslexic brains. In 1985 he joined the Ph.D. program in neuroscience at UCLA.
His dissertation was on the fiber composition of the human corpus callosum and its relation to brain lateralization. After obtaining his Ph.D. in 1991, Aboitiz worked as a postdoctoral fellow performing anatomical studies in the corpus striatum. In 1992 he was appointed assistant professor in neuroanatomy at the Faculty of Medicine of the University of Chile. In 1997 he was promoted to associate professor, and in 1998 he was appointed chairman of the morphology program of the Institute for Biomedical Sciences at the Faculty of Medicine. Most recently, Aboitiz was appointed professor in the department of psychiatry of the Catholic University of Chile in Santiago. Aboitiz's research interests concern the anatomical bases of brain laterality and interhemispheric communication, its genetic control, and more generally the evolution of the human brain.

Marie T. Banich's interest in cognitive neuroscience can probably be traced to growing up right-handed in a family of left-handers, who, she was told, had special brains. They had egalitarian and equal hemispheres, whereas each of her hemispheres was lopsided and distinct, something of a mismatch. It occurred to her, however, that the two hemispheres
of her brain seemed to interact pretty seamlessly, like those special couples who know each other intimately and intuitively. She figured that by studying interhemispheric interaction, she might learn a thing or two about effective communication.

Paolo Bartolomeo was born in Avezzano, Italy, in 1962. He graduated in Medicine in 1987 and completed his residency in Neurology in 1991 at the Catholic University of Rome, where he worked in the laboratory of Guido Gainotti. After receiving his Ph.D. in Neuroscience, he moved to Paris, France, where in 1998 he was appointed senior researcher in
the laboratory of Frannois Boller. His research interests are centered on neuropsychology (clinical, experimental, and cognitive), particularly in reference to unilateral neglect, visual attention, mental imagery, pure alexia, and patterns of cognitive impairment in dementia.

Born in 1935 and committed to brain research for over 40 years, **Giovanni Berlucchi** clearly belongs to the old guard of neuroscience, though, he adds, hopefully not to the rearguard. After graduating in Medicine from the University of Pavia, Berlucchi had the privilege of being trained in research by Giuseppe Moruzzi in Pisa, Roger Sperry in Pasadena, and James Sprague in Philadelphia. Hence, he says, his former
students can quite justifiably argue that the main difference between them and him is that he had some really great teachers. One of Berlucchi's credos is that there is no psychology without neurophysiology, but also no neurophysiology without psychology.

After Peace Corps service as a science teacher in Africa, **Steve Berman** received a Ph.D. in Experimental Cognition from The City University of New York in 1986. He completed a postdoctoral fellowship at Columbia University's Psychiatric Institute, studying the development of electrophysiological signs of attention and memory during childhood. Dr.
Berman came to UCLA in 1990 to characterize adolescent electrophysiological, neuropsychological, personality, and genetic markers for alcoholism vulnerability with Ernest Noble. Although this productive work continues, Dr. Berman is also currently collaborating with UCLA neuroscientists Eran Zaidel (psychophysiology of hemispheric specialization/communication), Emeran Mayer (psychophysiology of functional disorders), Edythe London (studying drug addiction with brain imaging), and California State University, Northridge's Maura Mitrushina (electrophysiological correlates of aging and dementia).

Fred L. Bookstein works on the rhetoric of quantitative reasoning across the sciences. He is the central figure in the small band of biologists and mathematicians who, beginning about 1980, established morphometrics (the statistics of biological shape) as a respectable statistical specialty. He takes particular delight in the unfundable aspects of this
quest, which range from its historic origins in the graphic arts through public presentations of dancing grids. Bookstein is a Distinguished Senior Research Scientist at the University of Michigan, Ann Arbor, Michigan, where he teaches rhetoric of science.

Born in Ottawa in 1953, **Claude Braun** was baptized Catholic and given the religious middle name Marie-Joseph. He opted for the scientific world outlook, trying to specialize in behavioral neurology, neuropsychiatry, epistemology, magnetic resonance imaging spectroscopy, experimental neuropsychology, neuropsychoendocrinology, and neuropsychoimmunology. Obviously, he has not specialized very much at all. He has lived in the United States, several European countries, and several Canadian provinces, and is now settled in Montreal, Quebec. He is a full professor of Psychology at the Université du Québec à Montréal and has been affiliated with neurology and psychiatry and psychology departments around the Montreal area.

Warren S. Brown is a professor at the Graduate School of Psychology, Fuller Theological Seminary, and Director of the Travis Research Institute. He is involved in research on cognitive and psychosocial disabilities in callosal agenesis. Previous research includes: (1) callosal function in dyslexia, ADHD, and multiple sclerosis; (2) evoked potential (EP) changes in aging and dementia; (3) EP indices of language comprehension; (4) brain wave changes in kidney disease; and (5) attentional deficits in schizophrenia. Brown has also written on science and religion, and is the editor of *Whatever Happened to the Soul? Scientific and Theological Portraits of Human Nature* (1998).

Alexandre Castro-Caldas was born 1948 in Lisbon. He is a Professor of Neurology at the Lisbon Faculty of Medicine and Head of the Neurological Department at the Hospital de Santa Maria. He was President of the International Neuropsychological Society (2000–2001).

Jeffrey M. Clarke began his studies of the corpus callosum as a graduate student at UCLA under the direction of Eran Zaidel. UCLA had just obtained its first MRI machine, and Jeff was able to get scans of his participants by literally running them from the graduate dorm to the medical center whenever there was an unexpected cancellation for a clinical session. As an Assistant Professor of Psychology (University of North Texas; Brooklyn College, CUNY), Jeff has examined inter-relationships between corpus callosum morphometry, behavioral measures of interhemispheric functions, and neurophysiological indices of interhemispheric interactions (scalp and intracranial ERPs). Jeff is now at Mattel Corporation in Los Angeles.

Stephanie Clarke holds a Swiss National Science Foundation fellowship for a joint appointment in the Division of Neuropsychology and in the Institute of Physiology at the University of Lausanne, and she is "professeur assistant" at the Medical Faculty. Her group is currently carrying out research projects that combine investigations of cognitive functions and of the functional organization of the human cerebral cortex. They are particularly interested in the functional subdivision and connectivity of the visual and auditory cortices. Their work with normal subjects and brain-damaged patients concerns mainly visual and auditory recognition.

Michael C. Corballis was born and partly educated in New Zealand. He came of age in Montreal, Canada, where he completed his Ph.D. at McGill University and taught from 1968 until 1978, when he returned to the University of Auckland as Professor of Psychology. He has written articles and books on telling left from right, cerebral asymmetry, visual imagery, and human evolution, including one book called *The Lopsided Ape* that might be thought of as autobiographical but isn't. He currently works mainly on the split brain and has recently published a book on the gestural origins of language, called *From Hand to Mouth*.

Patricia E. Cowell's interest in interhemispheric relations was inspired by her undergraduate psychology professor Jackie Liederman at Boston University. It was she who advised Patty to apply to the University of Connecticut for graduate study. She was invited to interview with Vic Denenberg, and that summer started working on her Ph.D. in developmental psychobiology. At the University of Connecticut, Cowell worked with Holly Fitch, investigating how sex hormones and early environment affect corpus callosum development in rodents. Her own dissertation looked at similar factors but in humans. She did her postdoctoral work with Raquel and Ruben Gur at the University of Pennsylvania, where her previous callosum work gave her insight into the study of cortical sex differences and their application to research on normal ageing and schizophrenia. In 1996 she established a cognitive neuroscience research laboratory at the University of Sheffield, England. Her current interests are in the area of individual differences in human brain and behavior across the life span. This includes sensorimotor mechanisms in speech and language, hormones and cortical plasticity, laterality, and, of course, the corpus callosum.

Marirosa Di Stefano is Researcher of the Department of Physiology and Biochemistry at the University of Pisa, Italy. She was born in Naples, where she graduated in medicine and received a specialization in neurology. She has been a visiting professor at Montreal and Perth Universities. Her major research interests are the mechanisms of functional recovery following cortical lesions and the role of interhemispheric interactions in development of the hemispheric asymmetries. For some years she has studied the dependence of binocular functions on the integrity of the corpus callosum in strabismic cats.

Robert William Doty, born 10 Jan 1920. Noticed by Elizabeth Natalie Jusewich, evening college biology class, 6 March 1941; married 30 Aug 1941 until death in 1999. U.S. Army, 11 Sep 1942–9 Aug 1946 Pvt to Captain, Transport Commander; Afrikakorps Kriegsgefangenen; ship sunk 1943 prior to Anzio; 7 voyages, last with "war brides"; discharged 27 Apr 1964, Major, Medical Service Corps. University of Chicago, BS 1948, MS 1949, PhD 1950, in Physiology: Physics from Fermi, Physical Chemistry from Libby, Neuroscience from Sperry, Klüver, Kleitman, Riesen, Halstead, Hess; Gerard thesis advisor. Postdoc with McCulloch, Founding Council Society for Neuroscience; President, 1976, Chief Editor Neuroscience Translations (Russian) 1963–1970; Visiting Professor University of Mexico, Osaka University. Organization of deglutition, including split brainstem, afferent code for triggering; vision in cats after cortical lesions at birth; luxotonic units in primate striate cortex (with John Bartlett); interhemispheric processing and memory in primates. Lord of 90 acres of farm, forest and swamp; gardener, beekeeper, deerslayer—devout atheist who believes, with Sperry, that, being conscious, he has free will, and that machines will not—the quintessential problem of science.

Michel Habib is a neurologist, trained in clinical neuropsychology, and deeply involved in clinical research. He is currently the director of a newly created laboratory of cognitive neurology at the Faculty of Medicine of Marseille. He is also working in an increasingly close collaboration with the laboratory of Côte des Neiges Hospital at Montreal, which is affiliated with the University of Montreal, Canada. Habib's interests cover a wide array of neuropsychologic domains, from developmental dyslexia to dementia, from phonemic representation to emotional disorders. His publications, including several books, cover these different domains. He is convinced that neuropsychology is conceivable only in terms of a close relationship between clinical and basic research and that the best way to do this is to be both a clinician and a researcher, which obviously takes time and energy. Undoubtedly, his model is the late Norman Geschwind, probably the most amazingly eclectic neurologist of the last century.

Kenneth Hugdahl is professor of biological and medical psychology at the University of Bergen, Norway. His research interests involve experimental and clinical studies of brain asymmetry, including cognitive and emotional stimuli. He has been particularly interested in auditory laterality and the application of dichotic listening techniques to problems of brain asymmetry. Hugdahl is the editor of *Handbook of Dichotic Listening*, published in 1988, co-editor of the recent volume *Brain Asymmetry*, published in 1995, and co-editor of *The Asymmetrical Brain*, published in 2002. He is currently on the editorial board of the journal *Laterality*.

Marco Iacoboni is a member of the UCLA Brain Mapping Center, where he heads the Transcranial Magnetic Stimulation Laboratory. Trained as a neurologist and neuroscientist in Italy, he has collaborated with Eran Zaidel since 1993. His main interest is sensorimotor integration and its lateralization. He is currently studying imitation, combining  different imaging techniques, such as functional MRI and positron emission tomography, as well as transcranial magnetic stimulation. Iacoboni's failures are more noteworthy than his accomplishments. He used to play the trumpet but quit when he realized he could never come close to his models, Chet Baker and Miles Davis. He has also written and directed a couple of short independent movies. One of them was favorably reviewed in an independent film festival in Italy. It is not clear why he did not pursue this interest further. Perhaps because as a neurologist he witnessed the effects of a stroke on famed director Federico Fellini. He even attempted to write fiction but soon realized that the task was beyond his skills. When he finally decided, by default, to become a scientist, he settled for the comfortable canonical writing form, Introduction-Methods-Results-Discussion, of scientific papers. Iacoboni really likes his corpus callosum and he displays it around wherever possible.

Giorgio M. Innocenti was born in Italy and obtained his medical degree and a specialization in Neurology and Psychiatry from the University of Turin. He has worked at the universities of Turin, Rome, Catania, Ferrara, Lausanne, and at the Max Planck in Göttingen. He is now Professor at the Karolinska Institutet in Stockholm. He has applied electrophysiological, anatomical, and computational techniques to the study of cortical organization, of interhemispheric interactions and their development. His work has shown that massive overproduction of transient axons occurs in cortical development and may provide the substrate for developmental plasticity and evolution of cerebral cortex.

Lutz Jäncke was the head of the Department of General Psychology at the Otto-von-Guericke-University Magdeburg until his recent move to the Department of Psychology, Division of Neuropsychology, of the University of Zurich. His research interests are functional neuroanatomy and cognitive neurosciences, with a special focus on sensorimotor integration, auditory perception, laterality, and higher cognitive func-

tions. After studying biology and psychology at the universities of Bochum, Braunschweig, and Düsseldorf, he received his diploma in psychology in 1984 from the Heinrich-Heine-University of Düsseldorf. In 1989 he received his Ph.D (Dr. rer. nat.), also from the Heinrich-Heine-University Düsseldorf, with a dissertation entitled "Auditory Feedback Control of Phonation." Since 1989 he has collaborated with Dr. Helmuth Steinmetz in studying the relationship between human brain anatomy and psychological functions. In 1995 he worked as a visiting scientist at the Harvard Medical School (Beth Israel Hospital) and also that year received his habilitation from the Heinrich-Heine-University Düsseldorf, which also was awarded by the faculty of natural sciences of this university.

Marcel Kinsbourne is Professor of Psychology at the New School University and Research Professor of Cognitive Studies at Tufts University. Kinsbourne trained in medicine at Oxford University, England, and subsequently subspecialized in pediatric neurology. Concurrently, he began investigations in experimental neuropsychology and developmental dis- abilities. Following a University Lectureship in Psychology at Oxford, he moved to the United States, where he was Associate Professor of Pediatrics and Neurology at Duke University, Durham, North Carolina (1967–1974) and Chief of the Division of Pediatric Neurology. He was then Professor of Pediatrics (Neurology) at the University of Toronto and Director of the Learning Clinic at the Hospital for Sick Children in Toronto. In 1980 Kinsbourne assumed the position of Director of the Department of Behavioral Neurology at the Eunice Kennedy Shriver Center and in 1995 he joined the New School faculty. He has served as president of the International Neuropsychological Society and president of the Society for Philosophy and Psychology and is the author of nearly 400 scientific papers and the author or editor of eight books, mostly on the topics of cognitive processes and their brain basis, in normal and developmentally delayed children, normal and focally damaged adults, and elderly people. Kinsbourne's current research projects center on issues of ADHD, neuropsychology, and the brain basis of consciousness.

Elisabetta Làdavas is Professor of Neuropsychology. Over the past 20 years she has conducted research in the Department of Psychology, University of Bologna, and authored numerous articles on cognitive neuropsychology. She is interested mainly in human selective attention in vision, hearing and touch, cross-modal integration, the mental represen- tation of space in relation to perception and action, word recognition, cerebral hemisphere asymmetry, and neuropsychological deficits in all these processes, their relation to normal function, and their possible rehabilitation.

Maryse C. Lassonde was born and happily raised in Quebec. After completing her undergraduate studies at the Université de Montréal, she studied at Stanford University with Karl H. Pribram, who taught her, among other things, how basic cellular mechanisms may ultimately lead to the understand- ing of the human brain. Lassonde spent an agreeable time in several laboratories around the world, including those of Aaron Smith in Michigan and Giovanni Berlucchi in Verona. She has worked a great deal on callosal agenesis and is striving to pursue other research interests (multimodal plasticity, cognitive effects of mild concussions and childhood epilepsy), but her many invitations to participate in conferences always seem to bring her back to the corpus callosum. Her career in science as well as her involvement in scientific policies has led her to receive several awards, among them a fellowship of the Royal Society of Canada and a knighthood from the Government of Quebec.

Jacqueline Liederman obtained her doctoral degree from the University of Rochester via qualifying exams in physiological psychology, neurophysiology, and developmental psychology. She is now Director of the Brain, Behavior and Cognition Program at Boston University. Her early work centered on the development of cerebral laterality and the effects of

its disruption on cognition and manual preference. She is still quite interested in the effects of early brain damage on the genesis of neurodevelopmental disorders, such as dyslexia, and how this brain damage may differ between the sexes. Her other major interest is on the role of cortico-cortical fibers in cognition. She has written extensively on the role of *inter*hemispheric cortico-cortical fibers during information processing. Her most recent work explores the role of *intra*hemispheric cortio-cortical fibers. In particular, she is interested in the role of feedback projections from higher-order to lower-order areas, in terms of attention, "binding," and improvements in perceptual learning. She is investigating these questions with the aid of functional magnetic resonance imaging.

Claudio G. Luzzatti started his career at the University of Milan in clinical neurology and neuropsychology. His early research focused on unilateral neglect and later shifted to neurolinguistics. In this latter context he worked on language disorders and rehabilitation, with particular emphasis on morphosyntactic disorders in agrammatism and on acquired

deficits of written language. He has taught clinical neuropsychology and neurorehabilitation at the Medical School of the University of Milan and physiological psychology at the University of Padova. Following an appointment as a Professor of Psychology at the University La Sapienza in Rome, he is now a professor in the Department of Psychology at the University of Milano-Bicocca.

Carlo A. Marzi is a professor of psychology at the Faculty of Medicine of the University of Verona, Italy. He has been President of the European Brain and Behavior Society and is President Elect of the International Neuropsychology Symposium. He is Section Editor (Behavioral Sciences and Neuropsychology) of the journal *Experimental Brain Research*.

His research interests include interhemispheric transmission in normal and brain-damaged human subjects; visual spatial attention in normals and in hemineglect and extinction patients; and the redundant signal effect and the stop-signal paradigm as tools for studying implicit perception in normal and brain-damaged subjects.

Carlo Miniussi was educated in experimental psychology in Padua and in Verona, where he studied with Professor Carlo A. Marzi and received a Ph.D. in neuroscience. He was a postdoctoral fellow in the Department of Experimental Psychology at Oxford University. His research interests include interhemispheric transfer in normal and pathological

subjects and inhibitory and facilitatory mechanisms of attention and temporal attention. Currently, Miniussi is at the IRCCS S. Giovanni di Dio in Brescia, Italy.

Alice Mado Proverbio received a degree in experimental psychology from the University of Rome "La Sapienza" and a doctoral degree in psychology from the University of Padua. From 1993 to 1994 she was a postdoctoral scholar at the Center for Neuroscience of the University of California at Davis, where she was supervised by Professor George Ron Mangun. Following an assistant professorship of Psycho-

physiology and Cognitive Electrophysiology at the University of Trieste, Italy (Department of Psychology), Proverbia is now at the Department of Psychology at the University of Milano-Bicocca.

Dr. Proverbio is the author of many papers on ERPs and mechanisms for visual attention and language comprehension. She recently edited a book on cognitive psychophysiology (Proverbio and Zani, Eds., Carocci Editore, Rome, 2000).

Maurice Ptito, a Canadian citizen, received his Ph.D. from the Université de Montréal in 1974. Under a fellowship from the Medical Research Council of Canada, he spent two years at the Stanford University Medical School Department of Psychiatry. In 1976 he joined the Department of Psychology at the Université du Québec à Trois-Rivières, where he

founded and directed the Groupe de Recherche en Neuropsychologie Expérimentale. In 1988 he moved to the Department of Psychology at the Université de Montréal as full professor and director of the newly formed Groupe de Recherche en Neuropsychologie Expérimentale. Since 1993 he has been adjunct professor of Neurology and Neurosurgery at the Montreal Neurological Institute and an active member of the Centre de Recherche en Sciences Neurologiques (Université de Montréal). In 1986 he co-edited (with F. Lepore and H. H. Jasper) a volume on the functions of the corpus callosum. His research interests include the behavioral and anatomical aspects of cerebral plasticity in brain-damaged animals and humans, and he has collaborated with colleagues in the United States, Europe, Australia, and the Caribbean. His leisure-time pursuits include sports (especially tennis and skiing with his four daughters), fine wines, and South American art.

Patricia A. Reuter-Lorenz's roots in cognitive neuroscience go back to the study of laterality and emotion as an undergraduate at SUNY, Purchase. Heading north to the University of Toronto, her attention was captured by the neurological phenomenon of unilateral neglect and its implications for hemispheric asymmetries of attention, which pro-

ceeded to guide her scientific pursuits throughout her graduate career and beyond. As a postdoctoral fellow, she had the opportunity to study the fascinating individuals who have undergone brain bisection and who provide the inspiration for her contribution to this volume. Now an associate professor at the University of Michigan, she continues to be grateful to her mentors along the way, Richard Davidson, Morris Moscovitch, Marcel Kinsbourne, Michael Posner, and Michael Gazzaniga.

Glenn D. Rosen received an A.B. in biology and psychology from Swarthmore College and a Ph.D. in developmental psychobiology from the University of Connecticut. His research interests have included circadian rhythms, learning and memory, lateralization of structure and function, and developmental dyslexia. He is currently involved in the development

of animal models for three of the differences that have been noted between the brains of dyslexics and those of normal readers. These differences are (1) symmetry of normally asymmetric brain regions, (2) cerebrocortical malformations, and (3) defects in fast processing of sensory information.

Clifford D. Saron received a B.A. in biology from Harvard College in 1976 and his Ph.D. in neuroscience from the Albert Einstein College of Medicine in 1999. He has had 27 years of research experience in human psychophysiology, working in the areas of cerebral lateralization, hemispheric interaction, and sensorimotor integration with Dr. Richard Davidson at the University of Wisconsin and Dr. Herbert Vaughan and colleagues at Einstein. Currently, he is an Associate Research Neuroscientist, working with Dr. G. Ron Mangun in the new Center for Mind and Brain at the University of California at Davis.

Paul M. Thompson is an Assistant Professor in the Department of Neurology at UCLA. His research focuses on the neuroscience, mathematics, computer science, software engineering, and clinical aspects of neuroimaging and brain mapping. Thompson obtained his M.A. in mathematics and classical languages from Oxford University, England, and his Ph.D. in neuroscience from UCLA. Recent awards include the Fulbright and Hughes Fellowships (1993–1998), the SPIE Medical Imaging Award (1997), the Di Chiro Outstanding Scientific Paper Award (1998), and the 1998 Eiduson Neuroscience Award. In collaboration with scientists at UCLA and around the world, Thompson's articles and chapters describe novel mathematical and computational strategies for analyzing brain image databases, for detecting pathology in individual patients and groups, and for creating disease-specific atlases of the human brain. His recent work has focused on mapping dynamic (4D) processes during brain development and degeneration, brain mapping in Alzheimer's disease, schizophrenia and neuro-oncology, and creating population-based digital brain atlases.

Francesco Tomaiuolo obtained his "Laurea in Psicologia" at the University of Padua and completed his Thesis in Experimental Psychology under the supervision of C. A. Marzi. Subsequently, he earned a Ph.D. in neuroscience in the Department of Neurological and Visual Sciences of the University of Verona, again under the supervision of Marzi. As part of his Ph.D. program he carried out research at McGill University, both in the Neuropsychology Unit and at the Brain Imaging Center of the Montreal Neurological Institute and Hospital under the supervision of T. Paus, M. Petrides, and L. B. Taylor. He has also collaborated with M. Ptito and A. Ptito on topics in cognitive neuroscience. Currently, Tomaiuolo is a researcher at the IRCCS Fondazione Santa Lucia in Rome, where he is working on the morphology and morphometry of the human brain in relation to cognitive functions.

M. Yanki Yazgan, currently an associate professor of Psychiatry at the Marmara University Faculty of Medicine, completed his medical education (1983) and general psychiatry residency training (1991) in Turkey. After a research fellowship in childhood-onset neuropsychiatric disorders at the Yale University Child Study Center (1992), he completed a clinical fellowship in child and adolescent psychiatry at the Child Study Center/Yale-New Haven Hospital program (1995). His research interest is in the neurobiology and phenomenology of developmental neuropsychiatric disorders across the life span.

Eran Zaidel was born in Kibbutz Yagur in Israel in 1944. The Kibbutz is undoubtedly the source of some of his social skills, on the one hand, and of some of his emotional hang-ups, on the other. After military service in Israel (1961–1963), Zaidel attended Columbia College in the city of New York (1963–1967), where he started majoring in physics but ended up majoring in mathematics (no experiments to botch up), and where he befriended some leading hippies and agitators of the time. In 1967 Zaidel joined the new Information Science (Computer Science) department at Caltech in Pasadena, California. There he worked with Fred Thompson on natural language interface for the computer until he realized that he might learn more about the human mind by studying how natural language is implemented in the brain than on a computer. He then joined Roger Sperry's lab in the Biology Division, completing his dissertation on natural language in the right hemisphere of split brain and hemispherectomy patients (1973). Thus, Zaidel was a latent cognitive psychologist, masquerading as a computer scientist, studying linguistics, doing neuroscience, but thinking philosophy. Although he has never taken a formal psychology class throughout his educational career, Zaidel joined the psychology department at UCLA in 1979. He is now a professor of Behavioral Neuroscience and of Cognition there and a member of UCLA's Brain Research Institute. He says that he enjoys teaching and appreciates being an employee of the state: serving as a representative of the people in the quest for knowledge. His research interests are cognitive neuroscience and hemispheric specialization, a field that allows him to study any and all aspects of the human experience, including consciousness.

CONTRIBUTORS

ABOITIZ, FRANCISCO   Departamento de Psiquiatría, Pontificia Universidad Católica de Chile, Santiago, Chile

ACHIM, ANDRÉ   Centre de Neurosciences Cognitive, Université du Québec a Montréal, Montreal, Quebec, Canada

ALTIERI, M.   Clinica Neurologica, Department of Neurological Sciences, University La Sapienza, Rome, Italy

BACHOUD-LÉVI, ANNE-CATHERINE   LSCP, EHESS, CNRS, Paris, France; Neuroscience Department, Hôpital Henri-Mondor, Créteil, France

BANICH, MARIE T.   Departments of Psychology and Psychiatry, University of Colorado, Boulder, Colorado

BARTOLOMEO, PAOLO   INSERM Unit 324, Paris, France; Neuroscience Department, Hôpital Henri-Mondor, Créteil, France

BERLUCCHI, GIOVANNI   Dipartimento di Scienze Neurologiche e della Visione, Seziòne di Fisiologia Umana, Università di Verona, Verona, Italy

BERMAN, STEVEN   Neuropsychiatric Institute, Universisty of California at Los Angeles, Los Angeles, California

BIALIK, MAYIM H.   Interdepartmental Program in Neuroscience, University of California, Los Angeles, California

BLANTON, REBECCA E.   Laboratory of Neuro Imaging, Department of Neurology, Division of Brain Mapping, UCLA School of Medicine, Los Angeles, California

BOEHM, GARY   Department of Psychology, Texas Christian University, Fort Worth, Texas

BOIRE, DENIS   École d'Optometrie, Université de Montréal, Montreal, Quebec, Canada

BOLLER, FRANÇOIS   INSERM Unit 324, Paris, France

BONGIOVANNI, L. G.   Department of Neurological and Visual Sciences, University of Verona, Verona, Italy

BOOKSTEIN, FRED L.   Institute of Anthropology, University of Vienna, Vienna, Austria; Institute of Gerontology, University of Michigan, Ann Arbor, Michigan

BRAUN, CLAUDE M. J.   Centre de Neurosciences Cognitives, Université du Québec a Montréal, Montreal, Quebec, Canada

BRESSOUD, RAYMOND   Institut de Biologie Cellulaire et Morphologie, Lausanne, Switzerland

BROWN, WARREN S.   Travis Research Institute and The Graduate School of Psychology, Fuller Theological Seminary, Pasadena, California

CASTRO-CALDAS, ALEXANDRE   Language Research Laboratory, Centro de Estudos Egas Moniz, Hospital de Santa Maria, Lisbon, Portugal

CLARKE, JEFFREY M.   University of North Texas, Denton, Texas; currently at Worldwide Sales Research, Mattel, Inc., El Segundo, California

CLARKE, STEPHANIE   Division de Neuropsychologie, Centre Hospitalier Universitaire Vaudois, Lausanne, Switzerland

CORBALLIS, MICHAEL C.   Department of Psychology, University of Auckland, Auckland, New Zealand

COWELL, PATRICIA E.   Department of Human Communication Sciences, University of Sheffield, Sheffield, United Kingdom

DAQUIN, GÉRALDINE   Neurology Clinic and Cognitive Neurology Laboratory, Faculty of Medicine, CHU Timone, Marseille, France

DENENBERG, VICTOR   Biobehavioral Sciences and Psychology, University of Connecticut, Storrs, Connecticut

DI PIERO, VITTORIO   Clinica Neurologica, Department of Neurological Sciences, University La Sapienza, Rome, Italy

DI STEFANO, MARIROSA   Dipartimento di Fisiologia e Biochimica, Pisa, Italy

DOTY, ROBERT W.   Department of Neurobiology and Anatomy, University of Rochester School of Medicine and Dentistry, Rochester, New York

DUCLA-SOARES, EDUARDO   Institute of Biophysics and Biomedical Engineering, Centro de Neurosciências de Lisboa, Hospital de Santa Maria, Lisbon, Portugal

FORSTER, BETTINA   School of Psychology, Birkbeck College, London, United Kingdom

FOXE, JOHN J.   Cognitive Neurophysiology Laboratory, Program in Cognitive Neuroscience and Schizophrenia, The Nathan S. Kline Institute for Psychiatric Research, Orangeburg, New York; Departments of Neuroscience and Psychiatry, Albert Einstein College of Medicine, Bronx, New York

HABIB, MICHEL   Neurology Clinic and Cognitive Neurology Laboratory, Faculty of Medicine, CHU Timone, Marseille, France

HUGDAHL, KENNETH   Department of Biological and Medical Psychology, University of Bergen, Bergen, Norway

IACOBONI, MARCO   Ahmanson Lovelace Brain Mapping Center, Neuropsychiatric Institute, Brain Research Institute, David Geffen School of Medicine, University of California at Los Angeles, Los Angeles, California

IDE, ANDRÉS   Departamento de Morfología Experimental, Facultad de Medicina, Universidad de Chile, Santiago, Chile

INNOCENTI, GIORGIO M.   Division of Neuroanatomy and Brain Development, Department of Neuroscience, Karolinska Institutet, Stockholm, Sweden

JÄNCKE, LUTZ   Department of Psychology, Division of Neuropsychology, University of Zurich, Zurich, Switzerland

KERTESZ, ANDREW   Department of Clinical Neurological Sciences, university of Western Ontario, London, Ontario, Canada

KINSBOURNE, MARCEL   Department of Psychology, New School University, New York, New York

LÀDAVAS, ELISABETTA   Dipartimento di Psicologia, University of Bologna, Bologna, Italy; Centro di Neuroscience Cognitive, Cesena, Italy

LAROCQUE, CAROLINE   Centre de Neurosciences Cognitives, Montreal, Quebec, Canada

LASSONDE, MARYSE C.   Groupe de Recherche en Neuropsychologie Expérimentale, Département de Psychologie, Université de Montréal, Montreal, Quebec, Canada

LENZI, GIAN L.   Clinica Neurologica, Department of Neurological Sciences, University La Sapienza, Rome, Italy

LEPORE, FRANCO   Groupe de Recherche en Neuropsychologie Expérimentale, Département de Psychologie, Université de Montréal, Montreal, Quebec, Canada

LIEDERMAN, JACQUELINE   Brain, Behavior and Cognition Program, Boston University, Boston, Massachusetts

LUZZATTI, CLAUDIO G.   Dipartimento di Psicologia, Università di Milano-Biccoca, Milano, Italy

MARAVITA, ANGELO   Institute of Cognitive Neuroscience, University College London, London, United Kingdom

MARZI, CARLO A.   Department of Neurological and Visual Sciences, University of Verona, Verona, Italy

MINIUSSI, CARLO   IRCSS S. Giovanni di Dio, Brescia, Italy

MIRANDA, PEDRO CAVALEIRO   Institute of Biophysics and Biomedical Engineering, Centro de Neurosciências de Lisboa, Hospital de Santa Maria, Lisbon, Portugal

MONTREUIL, MICHELE   Fédération de Neurologie, Hôpital de la Salpêtrière, Paris, France

NARR, KATHERINE L.   Laboratory of Neuro Imaging, Department of Neurology, Division of Brain Mapping, UCLA School of Medicine, Los Angeles, California

NASRALLAH, HENRY   Professor of Psychiatry, Neurology, and Medicine, University of Mississippi School of Medicine, Jackson, Mississippi

OLIVARES, RICARDO   Facultad de Ciencias, Veterinarias, Universidad de Chile, Santiago, Chile

PANTANO, PATRIZIA   Department of Neurological Sciences, University La Sapienza, Rome, Italy

PELLETIER, JEAN   Neurology Clinic and Cognitive Neurology Laboratory, Faculty of Medicine, CHU Timone, Marseille, France

POZZILLI, CARLO   Clinica Neurologica, Department of Neurological Sciences, University La Sapienza, Rome, Italy

PROVERBIO, ALICE MADO   Department of Psychology, University of Milano-Bicocca, Milano, Italy

PTITO, MAURICE   Ecole D'Optometrie, Université de Montréal, Montreal, Quebec, Canada

REIS, ALEXANDRA   Area Departamental de Psicologia, F.C.H.S., Campus de Gambelas, Universidade do Algarve, Faro, Portugal

REUTER-LORENZ, PATRICIA A.   Department of Psychology, University of Michigan, Ann Arbor, Michigan

ROBICHON, FABRICE   L.E.A.D., Université de Bourgogne, Dijon, France

ROSEN, GLENN D.   Dyslexia Research Laboratory and Charles A. Dana Research Institute, Beth Israel Deaconess Medical Center; Division of Behavioral Neurology, Beth Israel Deaconess Medical Center Hospital, Boston, Massachusetts; Harvard Medical School, Boston, Massachuesetts

SALVADORI, CARLA   Dipartimento di Fisiologia e Biochimica, Pisa, Italy

SARON, CLIFFORD D.   Center for Mind and Brain, University of California at Davis, Davis, California

SAUERWEIN, HANNELORE C.   Groupe de Recherche en Neuropsychologie Expérimentale, Département de Psychologie, Université de Montréal, Montreal, Quebec, Canada

SIMPSON, GREGORY V.   Department of Radiology, University of California at San Francisco, San Francisco, California

SMANIA, NICOLA   Rehabilitation Unit, Ospedale Civile Borgo Roma, Verona, Italy

STEINMETZ, HELMUTH   Department of Neurology, Johann Wolfgang Goethe University, Frankfurt, Germany

THOMPSON, PAUL M.   Laboratory of Neuro Imaging, Department of Neurology, Division of Brain Mapping, UCLA School of Medicine, Los Angeles, California

TOGA, ARTHUR W.   Laboratory of Neuro Imaging, Department of Neurology, Division of Brain Mapping, UCLA School of Medicine, Los Angeles, California

TOMAIUOLO, FRANCESCO   IRCCS Fondazione Santa Lucia, Rome, Italy

VAUGHN, HERBERT G.   Departments of Neurology and Neuroscience, Albert Einstein College of Medicine, Bronx, New York

YAZGAN, M. YANKI   Department of Psychiatry and Child Psychiatry, Marmara University Faculty of Medicine, Istanbul, Turkey

ZAIDEL, ERAN   Department of Psychology, University of California at Los Angeles, Los Angeles, California

ZANI, ALBERTO   Department of Psychology, Consiglio Nazionale delle Ricerche, Rome, Italy

NAME INDEX

A

Abe, T., 518
Abel, P. L., 12
Abi-Dargham, A., 448
Aboitiz, Francisco, 33–44, 51, 53, 59, 60, 70–72, 93, 95, 107, 113, 116, 131–136, 159, 175, 208, 210, 222, 242, 262, 266, 277, 302, 305, 314, 386, 408, 426, 442, 455
Abukmeil, S. S., 116
Achim, André, 175, 237–254, 259–261, 263–265
Adelson, E. H., 337
Adesanya, T., 53
Aggoun-Zouaoui, D., 19–23, 27, 208
Aglioti, S., 6, 172, 237, 238, 242, 243, 250, 264, 296, 299, 326, 332, 360, 364, 365, 378, 379, 409
Ahlfors, Seppo, 212
Aine, C. J., 178, 183
Akelaitis, A. J., 519
Alajouanine, T., 489
Alazraki, N., 108
Albert, M. L., 113
Alexander, M. P., 55, 454, 456, 490, 507, 519
Allard, F., 310
Allen, L. S., 54, 60, 95, 96, 102, 120
Allendoerfer, K. L., 21
Al-Senawi, D., 250
Altieri, M., 407–411
Alvord, E. C., 357
Amadeo, M., 238
Amador, X. F., 446
Amano, Stacy, 404
Amaral, D. G., 446
Amit, Y., 121
Andermann, E., 358
Anderson, J. A., 272
Andersson, L., 58, 307, 310
Ando, T., 159, 462
Andreasen, N. C., 116, 253, 445
Andreassi, J. L., 174, 178
Andreewsky, E., 509
Anllo-Vento, L., 297
Annett, M., 56
Antonini, A., 151, 334
Anzola, G. P., 206, 207, 238, 246, 247
Appel, E. M., 52
Appel, F. W., 52
Appenteng, K., 207
Apud, J. A., 447
Arato, M., 447
Arguin, M., 351, 456, 501, 517
Arieli, A., 202
Armstrong, E., 108
Arnold, S. E., 108, 434
Arnsten, A. F. T., 103

B

Babiloni, F., 179, 181, 183, 199
Bachoud-Lévi, Anne-Catherine, 500–505
Badian, N. A., 172
Bagby, M. R., 415
Bajcsy, R., 98
Bakke, S., 314
Baleydier, C., 144, 334
Banich, Marie T., 211, 266–269, 352, 382–384, 396
Baranzini, S. E., 358
Barbaresi, 152, 278
Barbas, H., 272
Baringer, J. R., 447
Barkovich, A. J., 101, 102
Barnett, E. M., 447
Barr, M. L., 361
Barrett, G., 174
Barrett, S. E., 160
Barta, P. E., 435
Bartley, A. J., 117, 118
Bartolomeo, Paolo, 500–505, 517–518
Bashore, T. R., 172, 237, 238
Basso, A., 224, 292, 303, 331, 446
Bauer, H., 230
Baughman, R. W., 166
Baumgardner, T. L., 51, 93, 103, 104, 118
Baynes, K., 321, 492, 497–499, 516, 517
Bean, R. B., 53, 54
Beaton, Alan A., 39, 95, 96, 211, 315–317
Beaumont, G., 396
Beauvois, F., 480, 485
Beck, E., 47
Beck, S. G., 252
Beech, A. R., 34
Behrmann, M., 491, 501
Beigon, A., 107
Belger, A., 267, 382, 396
Bell, A. D., 102
Bender, D. B., 466
Benecke, R., 167, 210, 377
Bennett, M. V. L., 17, 207, 208

Asanuma, H., 158, 167
Asbjørnsen, A. E., 59, 307, 308, 310
Ashburner, J., 101
Ashby, F. G., 342
Ashton, R., 426
Astur, R. S., 160
Atkinson, D. S., 51
Atlas, S. W., 358
Atluri, P. P., 158
Austin, G., 157
Avella, C., 297
Aziz-Zadeh, L., 263, 319, 325, 330

Benson, D. F., 486, 489
Bentin, S., 519
Benton, A. L., 503
Berardi, N., 244, 251
Berbel, P., 11, 19, 22, 23, 27, 28
Berger, J.-M., 382
Berlucchi, Giovanni, 6, 17, 30, 35, 140, 144, 154–156, 166–168, 172, 175, 182, 207, 220, 224, 232, 233, 238, 242, 243, 246, 247, 250, 253, 264, 274, 292, 301–304, 306, 323, 330, 332, 360, 361, 364, 365, 367, 376, 409, 466
Berman, Steven, 133, 230–231, 252
Bernardi, Eric, 24
Bernardo, K. L., 462, 465
Berrebi, A. S., 60
Bertoloni, G., 242
Besner, D., 491, 497
Best, C. T., 393
Bialik, Mayim H., 370–371
Bianki, V. L., 244, 252, 253
Biegon, A., 111, 113
Bieser, D. G., 352
Bigelow, L. B., 117, 118
Bilder, R. M., 435
Binder, J. R., 467, 492
Bisazza, A., 33
Bishop, G. H., 167
Bishop, K. M., 37, 54, 64, 66, 69, 96, 98, 116, 118, 242, 436
Bisiach, E., 447
Bisiacchi, P., 5, 172, 175, 176, 242, 243, 260–262, 301, 339, 364, 394, 407
Bisti, S., 244
Bixby, J. L., 461, 462
Bjerke, M. D., 175
Black, S. E., 111, 113, 490, 491, 501
Blacker, D., 108
Blakemore, C., 149, 362
Blanton, Rebecca E., 93–123
Bleier, R., 54, 95, 96
Blessed, G., 108
Bleuler, M., 446
Blinkov, S. M., 52, 53, 277
Bliss, J., 428
Blumhardt, L. D., 174
Bobrow, D. G., 262
Boecker, H., 198
Boehm, Gary, 433–442
Bogen, J. E., 93, 133, 139, 319, 320, 325, 341, 357, 360, 366, 372, 386, 392, 415, 426, 454
Bogerts, B., 116
Boire, Denis, 22, 30–32
Boller, François, 500–505
Bone, R. B., 517
Bongiovanni, L. G., 287–294
Bookstein, F. L., 75–90, 95, 97–99, 101, 109, 113, 132, 436

Lehmann, D., 181
Lehmann, P., 18, 19, 27, 208
Lele, P. P., 361
Lemon, R., 197
Lenn, N. J., 446
Lenzi, G. L., 407–411
Leonard, C. M., 38
Leporé, Franco, 23, 140, 144–146,
  150–152, 211, 212, 242, 357–367, 372
Leslie, S. C., 172
Levander, M. B., 253
Levine, D. N., 501
Levitsky, W., 37, 111
Levitt, P., 19, 446
Levy, D. L., 446
Levy, J., 24, 161, 163, 164, 237, 238, 247,
  321, 347, 351, 352, 425, 429
Lewine, J. D., 160, 162, 167, 168, 209
Lewine, R. R., 446
Lhermitte, F., 480, 489
Lieberman, J. A., 446, 448
Liederman, Jacqueline, 211, 268, 275,
  282–286, 382, 383, 396
Liepert, J., 167, 210
Liepmann, Hugo, 2, 479
Lim, K. O., 120
Lindeboom, J., 415
Lindsley, D. B., 179
Lines, C. R., 6, 174, 175, 240, 242, 243,
  246, 264, 266, 276–277, 287, 297, 323,
  365, 374, 394, 395
Lipska, B. K., 434
Lissauer, H., 480
Littman, T., 22
Liu, Y., 267
Livingstone, M. S., 17, 337, 461, 462
Llinas, R., 17
Loeser, J. D., 357
Loewenstein, D. A., 111
Loftus, W. C., 39
Lomber, S. G., 140, 158, 209, 274, 302
Lou, H. C., 425
Lowel, S., 22
Luchins, D. J., 445
Luck, S. J., 297, 348, 351, 429
Lueck, C. J., 461
Lufkin, R. B., 72, 310
Luh, K., 163
Lund, R. D., 23
Luppino, G., 192, 197
Luxenberg, J., 108
Luybymov, N. N., 144
Luzzatti, Claudio, G., 479–494, 497, 500,
  501, 507, 515, 518
Lynn, R., 358
Lyon-Caen, O., 415
Lyoo, I. K., 103, 111, 113

M

Maas, O., 479
Maccabe, J. J., 334
MacDonald, B., 468
MacDonald, David, 123
MacDonald, K. A., 132

Machon, R. A., 447
Mack, C. M., 67, 68
MacLean, P. D., 415
MacRae, L., 418, 419
Maffei, L., 244
Maier, W., 445
Mailhoux, C., 240
Mailloux, C., 206
Makarova, I. A., 244
Malaspina, D., 447
Malin, J.-P., 167, 210
Mall, F. P., 52, 53, 54
Mandelkern, M., 133
Mangun, G. R., 164, 221, 287, 299, 350,
  351, 395
Manschreck, T. C., 446
Mansour-Robaey, S., 446
Manzoni, T., 11, 12, 151, 152, 155, 208,
  212, 278
Maravita, A., 220–223
Marchetti, C., 519
Mardia, K. V., 75, 77
Markee, Taryn E., 175, 393, 395, 397,
  398, 403
Marks, R. C., 445
Marr, D., 480, 510
Marsh, L., 116
Marsh, N. W. A., 238
Marshall, J. C., 163, 488, 489
Marsolek, C. J., 517
Martin, A. A., 360, 361
Martinez, S., 396
Martinez-Garcia, F., 208
Martinez-Millan, L., 208
Marzi, C. A., 5, 172, 176, 207, 220–223,
  221, 225, 243, 260, 277, 287–294, 296,
  301, 302, 329, 339, 342, 360, 364, 366,
  381, 394, 407–411, 413
Mascetti, G. G., 167, 168
Maspes, P. E., 518
Masterton, R. B., 42, 158
Masuda, T., 276
Mathew, R. J., 436
Matsubara, J., 17
Matsunami, K., 166
Maunsell, J. H., 178, 461
Maxfield, L., 161, 211
Mayer, E., 519
Mazziotta, John C., 94, 98, 102, 105, 120,
  121, 123, 133
McClelland, J. L., 505, 507
McCourt, M. E., 18
McCulloch, W. S., 174
McFarland, K. A., 426
McGlashan, T. H., 446
McGlone, J., 54
McGuire, P. K., 448
McIntosh, A. R., 466
McKeever, W. F., 119, 160, 161, 238,
  242, 247, 373, 518
McKenna, P. J., 445
McKhann, G., 108
McManus, I. C., 51, 93
McWain, Vicki, 404
Mecacci, L., 251
Mednick, S. A., 447

Meerwaldt, J. D., 361
Mega, Michael S., 122, 123
Meissirel, C., 11, 172, 302
Mek, J., 1
Melzer, P., 23
Menninger, K. A., 447
Menon, R. R., 116, 225
Meredith, M. A., 41
Merola, J. L., 383, 396
Messenger, T. B., 273
Messirel, C., 272
Mesulam, M. M., 31
Meyer, A., 47
Meyer, B. U., 167, 210, 243, 377
Meyer, David E., 342, 345, 346, 353
Michalland, S., 42
Michel, F., 491
Miklossy, J., 35, 47, 48, 158, 176,
  462–465, 467
Miller, A. C., 267
Miller, B., 22, 23, 27, 28
Miller, D. R., 445
Miller, J., 195, 288, 328, 342, 355, 384
Miller, M. I., 94, 98, 101, 121
Miller, S. M., 253
Milleret, C., 12, 27, 176, 277–278
Milner, A. D., 6, 172, 174, 175, 240, 242,
  243, 246, 264, 266, 276–277, 287, 297,
  305, 306, 323, 332, 360, 364, 365, 370,
  372–374, 379, 394, 395, 402
Miniussi, C., 220–223, 288, 342
Miranda, Pedro Cavaleiro, 473–477
Mirra, S. S., 108
Mishkin, M., 209, 211, 466
Mitchell, D. E., 149, 362
Mitchell, S., 435, 447, 448, 456
Moberg, P. J., 447
Mochizuki, Y., 51
Moffat, S. D., 41, 55
Mogenson, G. J., 155
Mohammed, A. K., 447
Mohr, B., 155
Mohr, J. P., 467, 492
Molliver, M. E., 446
Monsul, N., 491, 502, 505, 517
Morton, J., 488
Montreuil, Michele, 415–422
Moody, D. M., 54
Moore, D., 22
Moore, J. A., 207
Moore, Larry H., 393, 399, 401, 403,
  404
Mooshagian, E., 332
Mora, F., 151
Mordkoff, J. T., 262
Moreau, T., 253
Morgan, M. J., 359
Moriarty, J., 51, 253
Morilak, D. A., 448
Morioka, M., 399
Morrell, F., 179
Morrell, L. K., 179
Moruzzi, Giuseppe, 168
Moscovitch, M., 247, 301, 359, 519
Motti, F., 495
Moukhles, H., 448

Sly, S. E., 238
Small, G. W., 111
Smania, N., 287–294
Smith, A., 157
Smith, L. C., 247, 301
Smith, R. C., 118
Snodgrass, J. G., 484, 593
Sobire, G., 94
Sobotka, S., 160
Softky, W., 18
Sohn, Y. S., 268
Somogyi, P., 208
Sonesson, B. G., 253
Sonneville, L., 51
Soong, A. C., 179
Southard, D. L., 250
Sparks, R., 310
Speaks, C. E., 386
Spekreijse, H., 178
Speransky, A. D., 271
Sperling, G., 163
Sperry, R. W., 24, 139, 151, 154, 156,
    157, 168, 272, 275, 320, 321, 325, 341,
    346, 347, 352, 357, 359, 360, 363, 372,
    392, 398, 400, 447
Spiers, P. A., 163
Spinelli, D., 251
Spinnler, H., 111, 519
Sprague, James, 156, 168, 325
Spreen, O., 307, 400
Staib, L. H., 101
Stancák, A., Jr., 198
Stanczak, L., 267
Stanford, L. R., 17
Stanton, P. K., 155
Stedman, T. J., 447
Steere, J. C., 103
Steese-Seda, Deborah, 398–400
Stein, B. E., 41
Stein, J. F., 117
Steinmetz, Helmuth, 51–60, 64–72, 120,
    131, 133, 210, 308, 429
Stensaas, S. S., 177
Stern, M., 174
Sterzi, R., 224, 292, 303, 331
Stevens, J. R., 113, 115, 120, 447
Stievenart, J. L., 95, 97
St. John, R., 6, 7, 172, 240, 242, 263, 304
Stomonyakov, V., 251
Stone, J., 181
Straube, E. R., 445
Strauss, E., 55, 59, 94, 111, 307, 400
Streissgurth, Ann, 90
Strick, P. L., 193, 197
Strik, W. K., 121
Stroop, W. G., 447
Subsol, S., 98
Sugihara, I., 17
Sugishita, M., 519
Sugita, Y., 154
Sugiura, S., 113
Sullivan, E. V., 120
Sullivan, K. F., 161
Sundet, K., 314
Supek, S., 183
Sutton, J. P., 272

Suyenobu, B., 59, 68, 271, 284, 307, 385,
    430, 454, 512
Swadlow, H. A., 158, 208
Swanson, J. M., 174, 206, 207, 212, 224,
    245, 276, 427, 429
Swayze, V. W., 103–104, 116, 117, 253,
    448

T

Tagliavini, C., 509
Takeda, T., 276
Takeuchi, K., 436
Talairach, J., 98, 109, 113, 120, 511
Taller, A. M., 447
Tamaiuolo, F., 292
Tamas, G., 208
Tanaka, Y., 519
Tanji, J., 193, 197
Tassinari, G., 151, 172, 237, 243, 246,
    250, 253, 303–304, 332, 360, 364, 365,
    380, 409
Taylor, G. J., 415
Taylor, J. B., 465
Tegenthoff, M., 167, 210
Temple, C. M., 103, 361, 402, 404
Teng, E. L., 275, 321, 347
TenHouten, W. D., 415
Terry, R. D., 108
Tettoni, L., 18
Thalluri, J., 18
Theberge, David C., 398
Theoret, H., 274
Thirion, J.-P., 98, 101, 104, 106, 121
Thomas, D. G., 178, 242, 246
Thompson, Paul M., 93–123, 132
Thut, G., 224
Tibbo, P., 436
Tieman, S. B., 144
Tiihonen, J., 445, 447
Tikofsky, R. S., 513
Timney, B., 149
Timo-Iaria, C., 252
Todd, R. D., 102, 446
Toga, Arthur W., 93–123
Tokuno, H., 193, 197
Tolchenova, G. A., 252
Tomaiuolo, F., 342, 407–411, 413, 453
Tomasch, J., 159
Tomlinson, B. E., 108
Tootell, R. B. H., 175, 211, 465, 469
Torrey, E. F., 446
Tournoux, P., 98, 109, 120, 511
Townsend, J. T., 342
Toyama, K., 208
Toyoshima, K., 197
Tramo, M. J., 175, 211, 287, 499
Treisman, A., 348
Tremblay, F., 140, 141
Trevarthen, C., 24, 140, 161–163, 272,
    274–275, 278, 320, 347, 351, 352
Trimble, M. R., 446
Trope, I., 6
Trudel, C. I., 320, 373
Truwit, C. L., 102, 116

Tsyganova, V. G., 446
Tucker, D. M., 274
Turetsky, B. L., 435, 442

U

Uematsu, M., 117, 118
Ugawa, Y., 167
Ulinski, P. S., 41
Updyke, B. V., 325
Urbano, A., 183, 197, 198
Uusitalo, M. A., 179

V

Vaal, J., 103, 253
Vallar, G., 224, 292, 303, 304, 331
Vallortigara, G., 33
Vanasse, M., 361
van Buren, J. M., 47, 466
van den Abel, T., 285
van der Heijden, A. H. C., 347
van der Twell, L. H., 178
Vanderwart, M., 484, 593
van der Woerkom, T. C. A. M., 427–429
VanDeventer, A. D., 238
van Dijk, J. G., 427
van Essen, David C., 176, 178, 461, 462,
    465
van Hoesen, G. W., 48
van Orden, K. J., 251
van Valkenberg, C. T., 47, 462
Vargha-Khadem, F., 157, 494
Variend, S., 102
Vassilev, A., 251
Vaughan, Herbert G., Jr., 171–212, 276
Vermeire, B. A., 160, 362
Vermersch, P., 93, 113
Vialet, J. N., 467
Vignolo, L. A., 247, 485
Vilapakkam, S., 238
Villaroya, O. O., 402
Villenueve, L., 243, 246, 253
Vogel, P. G., 139, 357, 360, 366
Voigt, H., 96
Volkmann, J., 57, 72
Volpe, B. T., 349
Von Cramon, D., 183
Von Economo, C., 462, 465
Von Hofsten, C., 102

W

Wada, J., 59, 94, 111, 308, 387
Waddington, J. L., 115, 116
Wagner, N., 163, 247
Wahba, G., 181
Wahlsten, D., 37, 54, 64, 66, 95, 96, 98,
    116, 118, 436
Wahlund, L. O., 111
Waldemar, G., 108
Walker, E. F., 446
Wallace, M. J., 501

SUBJECT INDEX

binocular stimulation (continued)
  input elimination and callosal
    connectivity, 30–32
  memory, hemispheric associations with,
    162
  reaction time to, 2
  split-chiasm interhemispheric transfer,
    145–149
  See also visual system
blindsight, 324
  boutons, callosal axons
  contributions from, 17
  development of, 21
  selection in differentiation, 22
brain electrical source analysis (BESA),
  183–184
brain-imaging techniques. *See* structure of
  corpus callosum
brain lateralization
  anatomical asymmetry vs. behavioral
    asymmetry, 38
  behavioral, interhemispheric transfer
    and, 134–136
  bilateral redundancy, 319
  callosal structure, 37
  corpus callosum, size of, 55–59, 68
  dichotic listening tests. *See* dichotic
    listening and brain lateralization
  dyslexia and. *See* dyslexia, inter-
    hemispheric visuomotor integration
  evolution of, 42–44
  hemispheric selection, controlled by
    corpus callosum, 271–286
    coactivation, 276–277
    cross-sectional callosal fiber area and
      performance, 277–278
    Poffenberger's paradigm and,
      275–277
    reciprocal inhibition, 272–275
    switchboard model, 272
    switching dominance, 162–164
  language in acallosal subjects, 359, 360.
    See also callosal agenesis
  memory, hemispheric associations with,
    161–162
  motor activation in intrahemispheric
    conditions, 197–200. *See also*
    sensorimotor (visuomotor)
    integration, callosal
  See also function correlations with
    structure; handedness
brain size and callosal variability, 51–60,
  64–72
  brain lateralization, 55–59, 68,
    71–72
  forebrain volume (FBV), 52–54,
    64–69, 96
  IHTT and, 158–159
  normalizing for brain size, 70–72
  regional size measurement, 66–67
  schizophrenia, 436
  sex differences, 54–55, 67–68, 96
  See also structure of corpus callosum,
    mapping
brain stem visual system, 324

brightness and reaction time, split-brain
  subjects, 322–326, 337

C

CA (callosal cross-sectional area) and
  performance, 277–278
callosal agenesis, 357–367
  cognitive abilities, 358–359
  interhemispheric communication,
    359–361
  midline sensory integration, 361–363
  motor functions, 363
  plasticity. *See* plasticity of callosal
    axons
  sensorimotor and visuomotor
    integration, 363–366, 370–371
    inter- and intrahemispheric
      mechanisms, 376–380
  See also split-brain subjects
callosal axons, 11–24, 140
  binocular input elimination, 30–32
  callosally mediated inhibition, 166–168,
    208–211
    corpus callosum as attentional
      equilibrator, 383–385
    reciprocal inhibition, 272–275
    redundancy gain, 343–345
  connection complexity, 47–49
  cortical plate injury, 27–29
  differentiation, stages in, 19–22
  hemispheric asymmetry and
    connectivity, 40
  interhemispheric transmission velocity.
    See IHTT
  myelination. *See* myelination of callosal
    axons
  operations implemented by, 13–17
  plasticity. *See* plasticity of callosal axons
  regression events, 22
  regulation and development, 22–23. *See
    also* development of callosal
    connections
  rules for connections, 11–12
  temporal transformations, 17–19
  topography of, 47. *See also* mapping the
    corpus callosum
callosal connectivity. *See* interhemispheric
  connectivity
callosal dysfunction. *See* dysfunction,
  callosal
callosal fiber area, performance and,
  277–278
callosal relay time. *See* IHTT
  (interhemispheric transfer time)
callosal sensorimotor integration. *See*
  sensorimotor (visuomotor)
  integration, callosal
callosal transfer model, 59
callosotomy. *See* partial callosal
  disconnection; split-brain subjects
cats, split-chiasm studies on, 139–152
  callosal plasticity, 144–145
  new perspectives from, 151–152

visual information, interhemispheric
  transfer of, 140–144
    midline fusion hypothesis, 149–151,
      154–156
    stereoperception, 145–149
CC. *See* corpus callosum
cerebral asymmetry. *See* hemispheric
  asymmetry
cerebral commissurotomy. *See* split-brain
  subjects
chemicals associated with interhemispheric
  transfer, 151–152
childhood disorders and callosal
  development, 102–104
  reciprocal inhibition, 273
chromosomal aberrations and callosal
  development, 253
chronic callosal disconnection, 320–321
coactivation of callosal function, 276–277
  corpus callosum as attentional
    equilibrator, 383–385
  Poffenberger's paradigm, 275–277
  testing model for, 282–286
cognitive function. *See* neurocognitive
  function
cognitive relay, interhemispheric, 5–6. *See
  also* IHTT
color-contingent response time, split-brain
  subjects, 338
color naming and matching, schizophrenia
  and, 119
commissurotomy. *See* agenesis of corpus
  callosum; forebrain commissures;
  split-brain subjects
conduction aphasia, 273
conduction velocity of callosal axons,
  17–19
confrontation naming studies, 482–484
connectional maps, callosal axons,
  13–17
  cortical plate injury, 27–29
  formation, 19
connectivity, callosal. *See* callosal axons;
  interhemispheric connectivity
conscious experience via interhemispheric
  transfer, 157–164
  alexithymia, 415–422
  hemispheric specialization, 159–161
  heterotopic visual callosal connections,
    466–469
  memory, 161–162
  nature of neuronal signals, 158–159
  switching hemispheric dominance,
    162–164
  See also neurocognitive function
consecutive bilateral strokes and pure
  alexia, 500–505. *See also* pure alexia
continuous mapping, interpolating discrete
  data for, 181
convergence of callosal axons, 15–17
corpus callosum (CC)
  absence of. *See* plasticity of callosal axons
  anterior commissure, fibers between, 48
  atlas-based pathology detection,
    121–122

as attentional equilibrator, 383–385
brain size and morphological variability,
    51–60, 64–72
    brain lateralization, 55–59, 68,
        71–72
    forebrain volume (FBV), 52–54
    normalizing for brain size, 70–72
    regional size measurement, 66–67
    sex differences, 54–55, 67–68, 96
callosal agenesis, 357–367
    cognitive abilities, 358–359
    interhemispheric communication,
        359–361
    midline sensory integration, 361–363
    motor functions, 363
    plasticity. *See* plasticity of callosal axons
    sensorimotor and visuomotor
        integration, 363–366, 370–371,
        376–380
    See also split-brain subjects
callosal axons. *See* callosal axons
forebrain commissures. *See* forebrain
    commissures
handedness/dominance differences. *See*
    handedness (dominance)
hemispheric asymmetry
    anatomy and variability, 34
    complexity of connectivity, 47–49
    developmental aspects and
        evolutionary speculations, 40–44
    interhemispheric communication,
        39–40
    interindividual differences, 37
    perisylvian region, 37–39, 109, 111
    regional and age differences, 35–37
    sex differences, 38
hemispheric selection, controlling,
    271–286
    coactivation, 276–277
    cross-sectional callosal fiber area and
        performance, 277–278
    Poffenberger's paradigm and,
        275–277
    reciprocal inhibition, 272–275
    switchboard model, 272
    switching dominance, 162–164
interhemispheric transfer time. *See*
    IHTT
lesions. *See* split-brain subjects
neurocognitive disorders. *See*
    neurocognitive function
relationship with conscious mind,
    157–168
    attentive processes, 163–164, 168
    hemispheric specialization, 159–161
    memory, 161–162
    switching hemispheric dominance,
        162–164
sensorimotor integration. *See*
    sensorimotor (visuomotor)
    integration, callosal
sex differences. *See* sex differences
shape. *See* shape of corpus callosum
split-brain subjects. *See* split-brain
    subjects

structure. *See* structure of corpus
    callosum
topography within, 47
visual system. *See* visual system
cortical ingrowth, 21
cortical plate injury, callosal axons and,
    27–29
corticotopic mapping, callosal axons,
    15–17
cross-sectional callosal fiber area,
    277–278
crossed hand positions, 207
crossed retinothalamocortical pathway,
    stereopsis via, 145–149
CSD (current source density) analysis,
    181–182
CUD (crossed-uncrossed difference) in
    measuring IHTT, 2–7, 172, 206,
    207, 224–229, 238–239
    amplitudes, 247, 262–263
    bilateral activation, 275–277
    bimanual response conditions, 249–250,
        331–332
    corpus callosum as attentional
        equilibrator, 383–385
    effects from measurement technique, 246
    historical account
        empirical claims, 263–265
        methodological claims, 262–263
        theoretical claims, 259–262
    interindividual variability, 245–246, 263
    lateralized flashing experiments. *See*
        retinal eccentricity manipulations
        on interhemispheric transfer
    multiple sclerosis (MS) patients,
        409–410, 453–454
    sex differences, 240–242
    short-term memory, 242
    split-brain subjects, 288, 292–293, 296,
        319
        acallosal subjects, 364, 370–371,
            376–380
        motor vs. visual fibers. *See* motor
            relay effect to visual evoked
            potential
        redundancy gain, 341–353, 356
        SRT, lateralized flashing, 322–332
        visuomotor integration, callosal,
            337–339
        See also split-brain subjects
    See also Poffenberger's paradigm for
        interhemispheric reaction time
current source density (CSD) analysis,
    181–182
cytochrome oxidase activity in visual
    areas, 465

D

data interpolation of discrete spatial
    sampling, 181
decomposition. *See* partitioning the corpus
    callosum
deformable brain atlases, 98

Déjerine's classical model of written
    language, 487–494
dementia and callosal structure, 107–113
    aging vs., 111
    schizophrenia and, 113
density of spatial sampling (electrodes),
    179–181
deep dyslexia, 489, 491
depth perception, split-brain experiments
    on, 145–149, 361–362
development of callosal connections, 19
    binocular input elimination, 30–32
    cortical plate injury and, 27–29
    disease and pathology effects, 102–104,
        253–254
    mapping structural alternations during,
        101–107
        childhood and adolescence, 102
        childhood disorders, 102–104
        embryonic period, 101
        reciprocal inhibition, 273
dichotic listening and brain lateralization,
    55–59, 72, 135, 385–386
    acallosal subjects, 359, 360, 363. *See also*
        callosal agenesis
    attentional modulation of auditory
        IHTT, 307–317
        left-ear performance and callosal
            efficiency, 311, 314–317, 385
        right-ear advantage (REA), 310,
            385–387
        two-channel model for callosal
            transfer, 312–314
    coactivation/equilibration model,
        283–284
differentiation of callosal axons, 19–22
direct access model, 59
direct dyslexia, 489
directional asymmetry in interhemispheric
    transfer time, 176, 243–244, 251,
    260–263
    acallosal subjects, 378–380
    ERP evidence for, 263
disconnection syndrome, 139, 319–321
    acallosal subjects, 361
    See also split-brain subjects
discrimination, visual. *See* visual system
disinhibition. *See* inhibition by
    intrahemispheric processing
distributed callosal activation. *See*
    hemispheric selection, corpus
    callosum as control for
divergence of callosal axons, 15–17
divided attention effects, 329–330
DL. *See* dichotic listening and brain
    lateralization
dominance effects. *See* handedness
double simultaneous completion, 275
Down syndrome, callosal development
    and, 103
dual-task studies, split-brain subjects,
    345–347
dynamic mapping of callosal growth
    patterns, 104–107
dynamogenic effect, 2

dysfunction, callosal
alexithymia, 415–422
atlas-based detection, 121–122
hemispheric disconnection. *See* partial
callosal (split-brain) disconnection;
split-brain subjects
multiple sclerosis (MS) and callosal
dysfunction, 391–404
bilateral visual field advantage (BFA),
397
bimanual coordination, 399
evoked potential IHTT, 395,
453–454
finger localization, 401
interhemispheric transfer time
(IHTT), 407–411
tactile maze, 402
tactile performance, 400
neurocognitive disorders. *See*
neurocognitive function
schizophrenia, 433–442
etiology of interhemispheric
abnormalities, 445–448
Tourette's syndrome (TS) and ADHD,
423–430
callosal development, 103
dyslexia
acquired following left-hemisphere
lesions, 487–494
callosal development, 103
callosal dysfunction and, 391–404
bilateral visual field advantage (BFA),
397
bimanual coordination, 399
callosal pathways involved in, 467
evoked potential IHTT, 395–396
finger localization, 401
tactile performance, 400
interhemispheric visuomotor
integration, 171–212
bilateral motor activation, 197–200
callosal pathways involved in, 467
effects of task demand, 176–177
ERPs and reaction times, 205
experiment design, 177–184
experimental findings, 184–205
measuring interhemispheric transfer
time, 172–177
motor activation as reaction time
predictor, 200–204
visual responses in motor regions,
193–197
visual vs. motor transfer times,
190–193

E

eccentricity. *See* retinal eccentricity
manipulations on interhemispheric
transfer
ECCs (extrinsic cortical connections),
272–273
fiber size and, 277–278
intrahemispheric, 273
Edgewarp software family, 90

electrode density, spatial and temporal,
179–181
electromyographic activity (EMG), 179
elongation of callosal axons, 19–21
embryonic corpus callosal development,
mapping, 101
reciprocal inhibition, 273
schizophrenia and, 116
EMG (electromyographic activity), 179
emotional transfer difficulties
(alexithymia), 415–422
encoding brain variation data, 121
engram unilaterality, 161–162
equilibration of callosal function. *See*
coactivation of callosal function
ERPs (event-related potentials) and IHTT,
174–175, 212, 230–231, 262
acallosal subjects, 365
callosal dysfunction and, 393–396,
·453–457
directional asymmetry of IHTT, 263
effects of callosal lesions, 289–293,
297–298
measuring reaction times, 205
retinal eccentricity. *See* retinal
eccentricity manipulations on
interhemispheric transfer
evoked potential. *See* ERPs and IHTT
evolutionary speculations on corpus
callosum morphology, 41
exclusive specialization, 385. *See also*
hemispheric specialization
exogenous cuing, 348–349
extinction effects, parallel processing and,
351–352
extracallosal pathways. *See* forebrain
commissures; split-brain subjects;
subcallosal channels in split-brain
subjects
extrasplenial visual interhemispheric
pathways, 469
extrastriate visual areas, 461–470
extrinsic cortical connections (ECCs),
272–273
fiber size and, 277–278
intrahemispheric, 273

F

face recognition and hemispheric
specialization, 160
facilitation/inhibition by intrahemispheric
processing, 166–168, 208–211
reciprocal inhibition, 272–275
redundancy gain, 343–345
factor analysis of regional callosal
differences, 132–133
FBV. *See* forebrain volume
female differences. *See* sex differences
fetal alcohol syndrome, callosal
development and, 103–104
fiber area (callosal), performance and,
277–278
finger alternation manipulation conditions,
248–249, 331–332

Finger Localization Test (FLT), 401
flashing, lateralized. *See* retinal eccentricity
manipulations on interhemispheric
transfer
FLT (Finger Localization Test), 401
focus attention effects, 328–329
forebrain commissures (split-chiasm
studies), 139–152
callosal dysfunction, assessing, 392
bilateral visual field advantage (BFA),
396–397, 408–410
bimanual coordination, 397–400
evoked potential IHTT, 395
finger localization, 401
tactile maze, 402
tactile performance, 400
callosal plasticity, 144–145
conscious experience via
interhemispheric transfer, 157–164
hemispheric specialization, 159–161
memory, 161–162
nature of neuronal signals, 158–159
switching hemispheric dominance,
162–164
new perspectives from, 151–152
visual information, interhemispheric
transfer of, 140–156
See also split-brain subjects
forebrain volume (FBV), 52–54, 64–69,
96
form discrimination, axon conduction
velocity and, 17
formation of callosal connections, 19
binocular input elimination, 30–32
cortical plate injury and, 27–29
disease and pathology effects, 102–104,
253–254
mapping structural alternations during,
101–107
childhood and adolescence, 102
childhood disorders, 102–104
embryonic period, 101
reciprocal inhibition, 273
four-dimensional maps of callosal
development, 104–105
Fourier series approach to expressing
brain shape, 101
foveal stimulation, reaction time to, 2
function correlations with structure,
132–133
learning to read/write, 473–477
schizophrenia, 118. *See also*
schizophrenia
switching hemispheric dominance,
162–164
See also brain lateralization; structure of
corpus callosum

G

gender differences. *See* sex differences
Gilles de la Tourette's syndrome. *See*
Tourette's syndrome
GPC (grapheme-to-phoneme conversion)
routine, 488–489

H

hand alternation conditions, 248–249, 331–332
hand images as visual targets, 330
handedness (dominance)
  corpus callosal size, 55–59, 68, 307
  dyslexia and. *See* dyslexia, interhemispheric visuomotor integration
  hemispheric asymmetry and communication, 39–40
  hemispheric dominance switching, 162–164
  IHTT measurements, 2–7, 243, 251
    CUD differences, 246–247
  memory, hemispheric associations with, 161–162
  response gating, 352
  schizophrenia, 438–439
  sex differences and isthmus size, 71
  Tactile Performance Test (TCT), 400
  See also brain lateralization
haptic recognition and dyslexia, 172
hemispheric asymmetry, 311
  acallosal subjects and visuomotor integration, 378–380
  Alzheimer's disease progression, 111
  callosal connectivity, 23, 40
    complexity of, 47–49
    interhemispheric communication, 39–40
  corpus callosum morphology and, 33–44
    anatomy and variability, 34
    developmental aspects and evolutionary speculations, 40–44
    interindividual differences, 37
    perisylvian region, 37–39, 109, 111
    regional and age differences, 35–37
    sex differences, 38
  directional asymmetry in interhemispheric transfer time, 176, 243–244, 251, 260–263
    ERP evidence for, 263
  ear-related, 58–59
  exclusive specialization, 385
  functional laterality vs., 38
  hemispheric connectivity. *See* interhemispheric connectivity
  hemispheric selection, controlled by corpus callosum, 271–286
    coactivation, 276–277
    cross-sectional callosal fiber area and performance, 277–278
    Poffenberger's paradigm and, 275–277
    reciprocal inhibition, 272–275
    switchboard model, 272
    switching dominance, 162–164
  See also interhemispheric connectivity; interhemispheric transfer
hemispheric specialization, 159–161, 243
  attention as right-hemisphere specialty, 168. *See also* attentional modulation, hemispheric

callosal connectivity and, 134–136
connectivity and, 134–136
effects on IHTT, 177, 251
hemispheric selection, controlled by corpus callosum, 271–286
  coactivation, 276–277
  cross-sectional callosal fiber area and performance, 277–278
  Poffenberger's paradigm and, 275–277
  reciprocal inhibition, 272–275
  switchboard model, 272
  switching dominance, 162–164
memory, 161–162
switching hemispheric dominance, 162–164
See also handedness
heterotopic/homotopic callosal connectivity, 48
  behavioral laterality, 252
  callosal axons, 13–15
  cortical plate injury and, 28
  crossed responses, 1
  partial callosotomy and, 302–303
  role of, in humans, 461–470
    cognition and, 466–469
horse race model of IHTT, 243, 262
  redundancy gain, 342, 355

I

ideomotor apraxia, 479, 485
IHRS (interhemispheric relay strength), 247, 262–263
IHRT (interhemispheric relay time). *See* IHTT
IHTT (interhemispheric transfer time), 1–7, 172–177
  age differences, 36–37
  asymmetric (directionally), 176, 243–244, 251, 260–263
    ERP evidence for, 263
  attentional effects. *See* attentional modulation, hemispheric
  brain lateralization, 43–44
  callosal dysfunction and, 393–396
    multiple sclerosis (MS), 395, 407–411, 453–454
  conduction delay of callosal axons, 17–19
  CUD measurements and, 224–229
    empirical claims, 263–265
    methodological claims, 262–263
    motor vs. visual fibers. *See* motor relay effect to visual evoked potential
    theoretical claims, 259–262
  distributed callosal activation. *See* selecting hemispheres, corpus callosum as control for
  evolution of concept of, 237–254
    balance-of-cost metaphor, 245–250, 267
    complex behavioral paradigms, 237–239
    future research directions, 250–254

horse race model, 243, 262, 342, 355
  network-gradient metaphor, 244, 262, 266
  single- and two-cable metaphors, 240–244
lateralized flashing experiments. *See* retinal eccentricity manipulations on interhemispheric transfer
measuring with ERPs. *See* ERPs and IHTT
motor relay effect on visual evoked potential, 190–193, 243, 253, 263. *See also* sensorimotor (visuomotor) integration, callosal
regional differences, 35–36
redundancy gain. *See* redundant signal paradigm
retinal eccentricity. *See* retinal eccentricity manipulations on interhemispheric transfer
schizophrenia, 119
sex and handedness differences, 39–40
size and, 158–159
split-brain subjects. *See* split-brain subjects
task demand effects, 176–177
illiteracy. *See* reading and writing disabilities
individual differences. *See* interindividual variability
information flow model, coactivation/equilibration model vs., 282–286
inhibition by intrahemispheric processing, 166–168, 208–211
  corpus callosum as attentional equilibrator, 383–385
  reciprocal inhibition, 272–275
  redundancy gain, 343–345
intelligence. *See* neurocognitive function
intercollicular commissure, 144
interhemispheric asymmetry. *See* hemispheric asymmetry
interhemispheric commissure formation, 19
interhemispheric connectivity. *See also* interhemispheric transfer
  alternative (noncallosal) pathways, 319–334
  acallosal subjects, 360
  bilateral redundancy, 319
  interfield visual comparisons vs. left field naming, 321–322
  interindividual variability, 323
  redundant signal paradigm and, 355–356, 413–414
  simple reaction time (SRT), lateralized flashing, 322–332
  attentional effects. *See* attentional modulation, hemispheric
  balance-of-cost metaphor, 245–250
  bimanual response conditions, 249–250
  physiological mechanisms, possible, 250
brain asymmetry and, 39–40
callosal agenesis, 359–361
connectional maps, 13–17

cortical plate injury and, 27–29
hemispheric selection, controlled by
    corpus callosum, 271–286
    coactivation, 276–277
    cross-sectional callosal fiber area and
        performance, 277–278
    Poffenberger's paradigm and,
        275–277
    reciprocal inhibition, 272–275
    switchboard model, 272
    switching dominance, 162–164
heterotopic/homotopic. See heterotopic/
    homotopic callosal connectivity
illiteracy effects, 476
network-gradient metaphor, 244, 262,
    266
neurocognitive disorders, role in,
    391–404
    alexithymia, 415–422
    bilateral visual field advantage (BFA),
        396–397, 408–410
    bimanual coordination, 397–400
    evoked potential IHTT, 393–396
    finger localization, 401
    optic aphasia (verbal blindness),
        479–494
    schizophrenia, 433–442
    tactile maze, 402
    tactile performance, 400
    Tourette's syndrome (TS) and
        ADHD, 423–430
    visual agnosia (VA), 486–487
neuroimaging patterns of, 224–229
schizophrenia and, 117
single-cable metaphor, 240–242
specialization and, 134–136
transfer time. See IHTT
two-channel model, 242–244, 312–317
interhemispheric distance, brain
    lateralization and, 43–44
interhemispheric transfer. See also
    interhemispheric connectivity
    alternative (noncallosal) pathways,
        319–334
    acallosal subjects, 360
    bilateral redundancy, 319
    interfield visual comparisons vs. left
        field naming, 321–322
    interindividual variability, 323
    redundant signal paradigm and,
        355–356, 413–414
    simple reaction time (SRT),
        lateralized flashing, 322–332
    See also plasticity of callosal axons
anterior commissure and visual
    information, 397
attention modulation. See attentional
    modulation, hemispheric
chemicals associated with, 151–152
conscious experience via, 157–164
    hemispheric specialization, 159–161
    memory, 161–162
    nature of neuronal signals, 158–159
    switching hemispheric dominance,
        162–164

facilitation/inhibition by
    intrahemispheric processing,
    166–168, 208–211
corpus callosum as attentional
    equilibrator, 383–385
reciprocal inhibition, 272–275
redundancy gain, 343–345
interhemispheric integration. See
    sensorimotor (visuomotor)
    integration, callosal
split-chiasm studies. See forebrain
    commissures; split-brain subjects
transfer time. See IHTT
interindividual variability
    callosum cross-sectional area, 277–278
    corpus callosum asymmetry, 37
    CUD measurements, 245–246, 263
    SCD (scalp current density) analysis,
        184
intermanual conflict and autocriticism,
    320, 341
interpolation of discrete spatial sampling,
    181
interstimulus intervals (ISIs), 178
intertectal commissure, 144–145
inverse problem, 183–184
ipsilateral motor pathways in acallosal
    subjects, 365
ISIs (interstimulus intervals), 178
isthmus regions
    childhood development, 102
    size and sex/handedness differences,
        71
IT. See IHTT; interhemispheric transfer

J

juvenile callosal axons, 22–23

L

Laplacian waveforms, 182–183, 205
latency vs. strength, CUD, 247, 262–263
laterality, behavioral. See behavioral
    laterality
lateralization, anatomical. See brain
    lateralization
lateralized flashing. See retinal eccentricity
    manipulations on interhemispheric
    transfer
LBL (letter-by-letter) dyslexia, 489–494,
    497–499, 515–518. See also pure
    alexia
    regional cerebral blood flow (rCBF),
        490, 507–513
learning disabilities and callosal
    dysfunction, 391–404
    bilateral visual field advantage (BFA),
        397
    bimanual coordination, 399
    evoked potential IHTT, 395–396
    finger localization, 401
    tactile performance, 400

left-ear performance and callosal
    efficiency, 311, 314–317, 385
left-hand agraphia, 480, 487–494
left-hand tactile anomia, 480
lesions and split-brain subjects. See partial
    callosal (split-brain) disconnection;
    split-brain subjects
letter-by-letter (LBL) reading. See LBL
    dyslexia
letter matching and shape discrimination
    BDA (bilateral distribution advantage),
        382–383
    behavioral laterality, 134–136
    interfield visual comparisons vs. left field
        naming, 321–322
    mediated reciprocal inhibition, 275
    shape-contingent response time, split-
        brain subjects, 338
    See also dyslexia; optic aphasia
lexical decision tasks, 135, 510, 516
lexical representation. See optic aphasia;
    reading and writing disabilities
literacy. See reading and writing
    disabilities
local callosal structure, detecting, 101
localized callosum atrophy from
    Alzheimer's disease, 109
long-term depression (LTD) of synaptic
    transmission, 155
long-term potentiation (LTP) of synaptic
    transmission, 155
luminance and reaction time, split-brain
    subjects, 322–326, 337

M

magnocellular processing and handedness,
    251
male differences. See sex differences
manual dominance. See handedness
mapping the corpus callosum. See structure
    of corpus callosum
maze, tactile, 402
meaningfulness of stimulus and reaction
    time, 325
medial intraparietal cortex (MIP), 195
memory
    hemispheric specialization, 161–162,
        167–168
    short-term memory and CUD, 242
menstrual cycle and interhemispheric
    relay, 252
microgyria, callosal connectivity and,
    27–29
midline fusion hypothesis, 149–151
    acallosal subjects, 361–363
    limitations of, 154–156
mind. See conscious experience via
    interhemispheric transfer
mirror-reversed reading, 510
MIP (medial intraparietal cortex), 195
mnemonic processing. See memory
modularity of interhemispheric transfer,
    6–7

corpus callosal shape, 75–84
  group shape differences, 78–81
  Procrustes method, 76–78
  thin-plate splines, 81–84
corpus callosum structure, 107–113
  etiology of interhemispheric
    abnormalities, 445–448
  interhemispheric transfer, 119
  patient homogeneity, 120
  sex, age, and hand preference
    differences, 118, 438–439
selecting hemispheres, corpus callosum as
    control for, 271–286
  coactivation, 276–277
  cross-sectional callosal fiber area and
    performance, 277–278
  Poffenberger's paradigm and, 275–277
  reciprocal inhibition, 272–275
  switchboard model, 272
  switching dominance, 162–164
selection in callosal axon differentiation,
    22
selective attention. *See* attentional
    modulation, hemispheric
semantic representation in right
    hemisphere. *See* optic aphasia
sensorimotor (visuomotor) integration,
    callosal, 131–136
  acallosal subjects, 363–366, 370–371,
    373, 376–380. *See also* callosal
    agenesis
  limitations of midline fusion hypothesis,
    154–156
  motor relay effect. *See* motor relay effect
    to visual evoked potential
  neuroimaging techniques, 224–229
  pure alexia, 515–519. *See also* pure
    alexia
  retinal eccentricity. *See* retinal
    eccentricity manipulations on
    interhemispheric transfer
  spatiotemporal data on
    interhemispheric visuomotor
    integration, 171–212
    effects of task demand, 176–177
    experiment design, 177–184
    experimental findings, 184–205
    measuring interhemispheric transfer
      time, 172–177
  split-brain subjects and interhemispheric
    transfer, 139–156, 296–299,
    319–334, 337–339
    acallosal subjects, 363–366
    bilateral redundancy, 319
    callosal plasticity, 144–145
    color- and shape-contingent response,
      338
    conscious experience via
      interhemispheric transfer,
      157–164
    eccentricity-contingent response, 337
    interfield visual comparisons vs. left
      field naming, 321–322
    luminance-contingent response, 337
    new perspectives from, 151–152
    partial callosotomy, 301–306

simple reaction time (SRT),
    lateralized flashing, 322–332
  subcortical transfer, 297–299
  visual information, interhemispheric
    transfer of, 140–144
serial information-processing model, 408
serotonin and interhemispheric relay, 252
  schizophrenia, 446
sex differences and corpus callosum,
    95–98
  age and, 84–87
  callosal transfer in dichotic listening
    experiments, 315–316
  cross-section callosal size vs. brain size,
    54–55, 67–68, 307
  CUD measurements, 240–242
  handedness and isthmus size, 71
  hemispheric asymmetry and
    communication, 39–40
  schizophrenia, 118, 438
  Tourette's syndrome, 424
shape-contingent response time, split-
    brain subjects, 338
shape discrimination and letter matching
  BDA (bilateral distribution advantage),
    382–383
  behavioral laterality, 134–136
  hand images as visual targets, 330
  interfield visual comparisons vs. left field
    naming, 321–322
  mediated reciprocal inhibition, 275
  shape-contingent response time, split-
    brain subjects, 338
  See also dyslexia; optic aphasia
shape of corpus callosum, 75–90
  approaches to mapping, 98–101. *See also*
    structure of corpus callosum
  function, covariance between, 87–88
  group shape differences, 78–81
  Procrustes method for measuring,
    76–81, 98–99
    age and sexual dimorphism, 85–86
  schizophrenia and, 75–84
    group shape differences, 78–81
  shape-theoretic approaches to callosal
    mapping, 98–101
  thin-plate splines, 81–84
short-term memory and CUD, 242
simple reaction time. *See* reaction time
simultaneous bimanual response
    conditions, 250
single-cable metaphor for hemispheric
    connectivity, 240–242
size, brain. *See* brain size and callosal
    variability
SMA (supplementary motor area),
    192–193
  activation measurements and reaction
    time, 200–202
  bilateral motor activation, 197
somatosensory callosal system, 361–362
spatial compatibility effects on reaction
    time, 206–207, 237–332
spatial discrimination, dual-task split-brain
    experiments, 346
spatial electrode density, 179–181

spatial-precuing paradigm, 348–352
spatial uncertainty and reaction time,
    326–327
spatiotemporal data on interhemispheric
    visuomotor integration, 171–212
  effects of task demand, 176–177
  experiment design, 177–184
    data analysis and modeling, 181–184
    data collection, 179–181
    design elements, 178
  experimental findings, 184–205
    bilateral motor activation, 197–200
    ERPs and reaction times, 205
    motor activation as reaction time
      predictor, 200–204
    visual responses in motor regions,
      193–197
    visual vs. motor transfer times,
      190–193
  measuring interhemispheric transfer
    time, 172–177
  See also sensorimotor (visuomotor)
    integration, callosal
specialization, hemispheric. *See*
    hemispheric specialization
speech
  alexithymia, 415–422
  inability to repeat, 273
  optic aphasia (verbal blindness),
    479–494
    visual agnosia (VA) and, 486–487
  pure alexia, 467, 515–519
    regional cerebral blood flow (rCBF),
      409, 507–513
    right-hemisphere contribution,
      487–494, 497–499
    stroke patients studies, 500–505
    visual callosal input and, 468
  See also auditory stimulation
spherical spline interpolation, 181
spline interpolation, 181
split-brain subjects
  acallosal subjects. *See* callosal agenesis
  callosal dysfunction, assessing, 392
    bilateral visual field advantage (BFA),
      396–397, 408–410
    bimanual coordination, 397–400
    evoked potential IHTT, 395
    finger localization, 401
    tactile maze, 402
    tactile performance, 400
  disconnection syndrome, 139, 319–321
    acallosal subjects, 361
  effects on IHTT, 287–294
    ERPs (event-related potentials),
      289–293, 297–298
    partial callosal lesions, 288–292,
      296–297
    possible transfer pathways, 292
    unilateral cortical lesions, 292–294
  intermanual conflict and autocriticism,
    320, 341
  motor relay effect to visual evoked
    potential, 319–334
    alternating finger and bimanual
      responses, 331–332

split-brain subjects (continued)
  motor relay effect to visual evoked
      potential (continued)
    bilateral redundancy, 319
    interfield visual comparisons vs. left
        field naming, 321–322
    Poffenberger's paradigm and CUD
        measurements, 301–306
    simple reaction time (SRT),
        lateralized flashing, 322–332
  optic aphasia and pure alexia, 499. See
      also optic aphasia
  parallel processing model, 333,
      341–353
    dual-task studies, 345–347
    extinction effects, 351
    visual attention and spatial-precuing
        paradigm, 347–352
  plasticity. See plasticity of callosal
      axons
  split-chiasm studies of interhemispheric
      transfer, 139–152
    callosal plasticity, 144–145
    conscious experience via
        interhemispheric transfer,
        157–164, 158–159, 159–161,
        161–162, 162–164
    new perspectives from, 151–152
    visual information, interhemispheric
        transfer of, 140–156
  visuomotor integration, 296–299
    subcortical transfer, 297–299
SRT (simple reaction time). See reaction
    time
stereoperception, 145–149
stimulus-driven laterality effect, 311
stimulus meaningfulness and reaction
    time, 325
stimulus-response compatibility effects on
    RT, 238
structure of corpus callosum, 93–123
  aging and Alzheimer's disease, 107–113
  atlas-based pathology detection,
      121–122
  challenges of, 93
  during development, 101–107
  learning to read and write, 473–477
  schizophrenia, 113–121, 433–442
    structure vs. function, 118
  sex differences, 95–98
  shape-theoretic approaches, 98–101
subcallosal channels in split-brain subjects,
    319–334
  acallosal subjects, 360
  bilateral redundancy, 319
  interfield visual comparisons vs. left field
      naming, 321–322
  interindividual variability, 323
  redundant signal paradigm and,
      355–356
  simple reaction time (SRT), lateralized
      flashing, 322–332
  See also plasticity of callosal axons
subcortical branching of callosal axons,
    21

subcortical transfer in split-brain subjects,
    297–299
superiority, hemispheric, 160–164
supplementary motor area (SMA),
    192–193
  activation measurements and reaction
      time, 200–202
  bilateral motor activation, 197
surface dyslexia, 488
switchboard model for hemispheric
    selection, 272
switching hemispheric dominance,
    162–164
Sylvian fissure asymmetry and callosal
    structure, 37–39, 109, 111
synaptic overproduction, 22
synaptic refinement, 102
synaptogenesis, 21
synchronicity of callosal axons, 17–19, 155

T

tactile response. See also handedness
  finger alternation manipulation
      conditions, 248–249, 331–332
  Finger Localization Test (FLT), 401
  left-hand tactile anomia, 480
  tactile discrimination, acallosal subjects,
      362–363
  tactile maze, 402
  Tactile Performance Test (TCT), 400
TAS (Toronto Alexithymia Scale), 416
temporal electrode density, 179–181
temporal maps of callosal development,
    104
temporal parameters of callosal axons,
    17–19
tensor maps of callosal growth,
    105–106
terminal columns (callosal), 17
texture discrimination, acallosal subjects,
    362–363
thin-plate splines for relating callosum
    shape, 81–84
TMS (transcranial magnetic stimulation),
    210, 410–411
Toronto Alexithymia Scale (TAS), 416
Tourette's syndrome (TS) and ADHD,
    423–430
  callosal development and, 104
TPT (Tactile Performance Test), 400
transcranial magnetic stimulation (TMS),
    210, 410–411
transient projections, callosal axons, 19
transmission velocity, callosal. See IHTT
two-channel model for callosal transfer,
    242–244, 312–317

U

unilateral cortical lesions, IHTT and,
    292–294
unilateral engrams, 161–162

unmyelinated phylogenetically primitive
    fibers, 253. See also myelination of
    callosal axons

V

VA (visual agnosia), 486–487
variability. See interindividual variability
vascular dementia. See dementia and
    callosal structure
velocity of interhemispheric transfer. See
    IHTT
verbal blindness (optic aphasia), 479–494
  pure alexia, 467, 515–519
    regional cerebral blood flow (rCBF),
        409, 507–513
    right-hemisphere contribution,
        487–494, 497–499
    stroke patients studies, 500–505
  visual agnosia (VA) and, 486–487
verbal-manual interference (VMI)
    paradigm, 284, 428, 432
verbalization of emotions (alexithymia),
    415–422
vertical partitioning of the corpus
    callosum, 95, 97
virtual electrodes (virtrodes), 183
visual agnosia (VA), 486–487
visual system
  anatomy of interhemispheric transfer,
      140–144
  attentional effects. See attentional
      modulation, hemispheric
  bilateral visual field advantage (BFA),
      396–397, 408–410
  blindsight and brain stem visual system,
      324
  callosal connectivity
    binocular input elimination and,
        30–32
    development based on visual activity,
        22
  color naming and matching,
      schizophrenia and, 119
  depth perception, split-brain
      experiments on, 145–149
    acallosal subjects, 361–362
  dyslexia. See dyslexia
  eccentricity. See retinal eccentricity
      manipulations on interhemispheric
      transfer
  emotional transfer (alexithymia) tests,
      416–417, 421
  ERPs and IHTT. See ERPs and IHTT
  hemispheric specialization, 159–161
  heterotopic connections between visual
      areas, 48, 461–470
  interfield visual comparisons, split-brain
      subjects, 321–322
  lateralized flashing. See retinal
      eccentricity manipulations on
      interhemispheric transfer
  memory, hemispheric associations with,
      161–162